Women's Bodies, Women's Wisdom

Women's Bodies, Women's Wisdom

Creating Physical and Emotional
Health and Healing

REVISED AND UPDATED

Christiane Northrup, M.D.

BANTAM BOOKS
NEW YORK

Published in the United States by Bantam Books, an imprint of Random House, a division of Penguin Random House LLC, New York.

BANTAM BOOKS and the HOUSE colophon are registered trademarks of Penguin Random House LLC.

ISBN 978-0-525-48611-4

This book is for all who believe that it is possible to flourish, regardless of our present or past circumstances.

It is for all who acknowledge the daily presence in our lives of mystery, uncertainty, and hope.

It is for those who yearn to be well and know that there is something more to healing than simply external substances or techniques.

This book is for every physician, nurse, healthcare practitioner, healer, or patient who keeps an open heart and an open mind and acknowledges the fact that scientific truth is constantly changing.

It is for those who know that we heal and flourish to the degree that we consciously invite the sacred into our lives.

This book is dedicated with appreciation to the scientists and healers of the past, present, and future who have had and will have the courage to speak their truth and go forward in faith, hope, and joy, despite the deadening effects of conventional thinking.

Contents

List of Figures   xv

List of Tables   xvii

Acknowledgments   xix

Introduction to the Fifth Edition: The Medicine of Empowerment   xxi

Part One:
From External Control to Inner Guidance

1 The Patriarchal Myth: The Origin of the
   Mind/Body/Emotion Split   3
   Our Cultural Inheritance
   Patriarchy Results in Addiction
   Fundamental Beliefs of the Dominator System
   Reclaiming the Authority of Our Own Feelings

2 Feminine Intelligence and a New Mode of Healing   29
   Energy Fields and Energy Systems
   Understanding the Bodymind
   Feminine Intelligence: How Thoughts Become Embodied
   Beliefs Are Physical
   Healing Versus Curing

3 Inner Guidance   56
   Listening to Your Body and Its Needs
   Emotional Cleansing: Healing from the Past
   Dreams: A Doorway to the Unconscious
   Intuition and Intuitive Guidance
   How Inner Guidance Works

4 The Female Energy System   77
     The Matter-Energy Continuum
     Earth's Energy
     The Chakras
     The Lower Female Centers: Chakras One to Three
     Other Chakra Issues

Part Two:

The Anatomy of Women's Wisdom

5 The Menstrual Cycle   117
     Our Cyclical Nature
     Our Cultural Inheritance
     Menstrual Cramps (Dysmenorrhea)
     Premenstrual Syndrome (PMS)
     Irregular Periods
     Excessive Buildup of the Uterine Lining (Endometrial
         Hyperplasia, Cystic and Adenomatous Hyperplasia)
     Dysfunctional Uterine Bleeding (DUB)
     Heavy Periods (Menorrhagia)
     Healing Our Menstrual History: Preparing Our Daughters

6 The Uterus   191
     Our Cultural Inheritance
     Energy Anatomy
     Chronic Pelvic Pain
     Endometriosis
     Uterine Prolapse
     Fibroid Tumors

7 The Ovaries   237
     Anatomy
     Ovarian Cysts
     Polycystic Ovary Syndrome (PCOS)
     Ovarian Cancer

8 Reclaiming the Erotic   268
     We Are Sexual Beings
     Our Cultural Inheritance
     Reclaiming Our Erotic Selves

9 Vulva, Vagina, Cervix, and Lower Urinary Tract   315
     Our Cultural Inheritance
     Anatomy

Human Papilloma Virus (HPV)
Herpes
Cervicitis
Cervical Dysplasia (Abnormal Pap Tests)
Vaginal Health: What Is Normal?
Vaginitis
A Note on Sexually Transmitted Diseases
Chronic Vulvar Pain (Vulvodynia)
Lichen Sclerosus
Vaginal Cosmetic Surgery
Interstitial Cystitis (Painful Bladder Syndrome)
Recurrent Urinary Tract Infections
Stress Urinary Incontinence

10 Breasts 387
Our Cultural Inheritance
Anatomy
Breast Self-Exams
Benign Breast Symptoms: Breast Pain, Lumps,
    Cysts, and Nipple Discharge
Treatment for Benign Breast Symptoms
Mammography
Breast Cancer
Program to Promote Healthy Breast Tissue
Cosmetic Breast Surgery

11 Our Fertility 464
Abortion
Emergency Contraception: Abortion Prevention
Conscious Conception and Contraception
Transforming Infertility
Pregnancy Loss
Adoption
Fertility as Metaphor

12 Pregnancy and Birthing 533
The Transforming Power of Pregnancy
Our Cultural Inheritance: Pregnancy
Preventing Premature Birth
Preventing Preeclampsia
Turning a Breech Presentation
Our Cultural Inheritance: Labor and Delivery
Birth Technologies
Mothering the Mother: A Solution Whose Time Has Come

How to Decrease Your Risk for a Cesarean Section
My Personal Story
Turning Labor into Personal Power

13 Motherhood: Bonding with Your Baby   605
Fourth Trimester
Formula Versus Breast Milk
Mothering in a Dominator Culture: The Hardest Job in the World

14 Menopause   637
Menopause: A Crossroads
Our Cultural Inheritance
Creating Health During Menopause
Adrenal Function: What Every Woman Should Know
Kinds of Menopause
The Hormone Therapy Question
A Hormone Primer
Symptoms of Menopause
Hot Flashes
Vaginal Dryness, Irritation, and Thinning
Osteoporosis
Sexuality in Menopause
Thinning Hair
Mood Swings and Depression
Fuzzy Thinking
Long-Term Health Concerns
Alzheimer's Disease
Deciding on Menopausal Treatment
Self-Care During Menopause
Menopause as a New Beginning

Part Three:

Women's Wisdom Program for
Flourishing and Healing

15 Steps for Flourishing   713
Imagine Your Future: Change Your Consciousness, Change Your Cells
Step One: Uncover and Update Your Legacy
Step Two: Sort Through Your Beliefs
Step Three: Respect and Release Your Emotions
Step Four: Learn to Listen to Your Body
Step Five: Learn to Respect Your Body
Step Six: Acknowledge a Higher Power or Inner Wisdom

Step Seven: Reclaim the Fullness of Your Mind
Step Eight: Get Help
Step Nine: Work with Your Body
Step Ten: Gather Information
Step Eleven: Forgive
Step Twelve: Actively Pursue Pleasure and Purpose

16 Getting the Most Out of Your Medical Care 796
Why You Must Take Responsibility for Your Healthcare
Choosing a Treatment: From Surgery to Acupuncture
Creating Health Through Surgery

17 Eat to Flourish 836
Creating Optimal Body Composition and Vibrant Health
The Wonders of Magnesium
Creating a Supplementation Program
Other Common Concerns
A Word About Smoking
Appreciate the Energy of Food

18 The Power of Movement 928
Our Cultural Inheritance
Benefits of Exercise
Exercise and Addiction
Exercise, Amenorrhea, and Bone Loss
Getting Started

19 Healing Ourselves, Healing Our World 954
Our Mothers: Our Cells
A Ritual of Reclaiming
Transforming Our Fear of Our Shaman Past
Our Dreams: Earth's Dreams
Making the World Safe for Women: Start with Yourself

Resources 979
Notes 1005
Index 1113

List of Figures

Fig. 1: Earth's Energy Going Upward   87

Fig. 2: Chakra Diagram with Female Figure   93

Fig. 3: Menstrual Cycle (Days)   123

Fig. 4: Lunar Chart for Menstrual Cycle   126

Fig. 5: The Female Mind-Body Continuum:
Interactions Between the Brain and the Pelvis   138

Fig. 6: Adhesions in Pelvic Organs   158

Fig. 7: Acupressure Points for Gynecological Problems   160

Fig. 8: Seasonal Affective Disorder (SAD) and PMS   168

Fig. 9: Uterus, Ovaries, and Cervix with Anatomic Labels   192

Fig. 10: Endometriosis   202

Fig. 11: Types of Fibroids   216

Fig. 12: The Clitoral System   273

Fig. 13: The Pineal Gland and the G-Spot/Sacred Spot   276

Fig. 14: The Microcosmic Orbit   286

Fig. 15: Vaginal Reflexology Zones   299

Fig. 16: Breast Anatomy   395

Fig. 17: Breast Self-Exam   396

Fig. 18: Fertility Awareness: Ovulation and Basal Body Temperature   488

Fig. 19: The Causes of Infertility   505

Fig. 20: Acupuncture or Acupressure Points to Turn a Breech   556

Fig. 21: Currents of Wisdom   645

Fig. 22: Hormone-Producing Body Sites   649

Fig. 23: Body Mass Index Chart   874

List of Tables

Table 1: Characteristics of an Addictive System   22

Table 2: The Body as a Process Versus Medical Worldview   27

Table 3: Sources of Guidance   57

Table 4: Energy Anatomy: Mental and Emotional Patterns,
the Chakras, and the Physical Body   94

Table 5: The Anatomy of Women's Wisdom   118

Table 6: Comparing Contraceptive Methods   496

Table 7: Potential Risk Factors in Childbirth   569

Table 8: The Effects of Hormone Therapy on Breast Cancer Risk   700

Table 9: Calculating Your Daily Protein Requirement   883

Table 10: Recommended Daily Supplementation   915

Acknowledgments

Great appreciation to Ned Leavitt, my literary agent, with whom I continue to share a rich history and spiritual kinship.

To Katy Koontz, scribe extraordinaire, whose innate feeling for this material and whose research and organizational ability have made yet another magnum opus a true pleasure to write.

To Pat McCabe for lovingly and skillfully keeping my home a place of beauty and order. All with a great sense of humor.

To Scott Leighton, for your outstanding medical illustrations—and for the joy of co-creating with you.

To Julie Hofheimer, for your healing bodywork skills.

To Hope Matthews, my Pilates instructor, for helping me transform my body and mind.

To Coulson Duerkson, my newsletter and website editor, for your intelligence, skill, and insight. You live the message on all levels.

To the late Louise Hay, Reid Tracy, Margarete Nielson, and all of the Hay House staff. You have shown me that work, pleasure, and prosperity go together beautifully. I give thanks every day for our association.

To Mike Brewer, for making me smile every time I drive into my driveway and see the lawn.

To Steve Meehan, for your incredible skill with my gardens and plants. You have created a personal paradise that blesses me daily.

To Paulina Carr, my girl Friday, for doing whatever needs to be done— always with a smile and willingness to help. I so appreciate it.

To Janet Lambert, for your incredible bookkeeping and business skills and also for being an incredible ageless goddess.

To Diane Grover, whose organizational skills, intuitive gifts, loyalty, friendship, and personal cheerleading on behalf of my business, personal health, happiness, and prosperity are divine gifts in my life and have been for more than forty years. Ours is a "marriage" that works. You are the CEO of

Everything and do the work of at least four people—all efficiently and with a lot of laughter. Thank you for being a cheerleader for the emerging tango dancer and courtesan within me. And also for doing regular Divine Love meditations with me. And for having the good sense to marry your charming husband, Charlie, so many years ago.

I thank my parents for the support they have always provided: my indomitable mother, Edna, and my late father, Wilbur, whose work I have carried forth in my own way. My heart is full of appreciation for my sister, Penny, her husband, Phil, my brother John and his wife, Annie, my brother Bill and his wife, Lori, and my nieces and nephews, who are a source of joy for me. You all create an incredibly strong first chakra that makes my immunity and sense of belonging really solid and secure. I appreciate you more now than ever before.

I acknowledge and thank my daughter Kate and her husband, Mike, and my granddaughters Ruby and Penelope—you are all living the legacy of this work, adding to it, and continuing to pass it on to the next generation. I am awed by this.

To my daughter Ann, whose intuitive abilities, sensitivity, and beauty are a gift to the world, you too are passing on this legacy in a way unique to you. Your being lights up the world and uplifts everyone you meet. What a gift you are to me.

Because of all of you, I can see the torch of women's wisdom burning brightly for years to come. I am filled with gratitude for your beauty, your vibrant good health, your enthusiasm for life, and your loud and boisterous laughter (which is not unlike my own!).

Christiane Northrup, M.D.

Introduction to the Fifth Edition

The Medicine of Empowerment

The female body was designed by our Creator to be a source of pleasure, fertility, movement, strength, and well-being. Our bodies connect us with the moon, the tides, and the seasons. They are the temples within which our souls dwell and experience life on earth. And they are profoundly impacted first and foremost by our beliefs about what is possible, by the culture in which we live, and then by the behaviors that stem from these beliefs. If you believe that it is a woman's lot in life to suffer and sacrifice, this will greatly influence your well-being. On the other hand, if you cherish your body and care for it well, you'll have the tools to be healthy. Each and every one of us has the capacity to flourish within a physical body. I suspected this when I wrote the first edition of *Women's Bodies, Women's Wisdom* in the early 1990s. Now, almost thirty years later, I have proved it to myself not only personally but also in the thousands of lives I have had the privilege to influence. And there is more research than ever before proving the unity of mind, body, and spirit. More than that, we now know how to take this research and apply it to our own lives to influence our health.

We, the human race, have now come to a crossroads, a turning point, when old, unsustainable ideas and behaviors are breaking down all over the planet. For example, the revelations about the Hollywood mogul Harvey Weinstein and his thirty-plus years of sexual abuse of countless women struck a deep chord within me when the news erupted. Not because this kind of abuse of power was anything new—I have witnessed the health effects of this for decades—but because, for the very first time in my lifetime, our society was no longer protecting a rich and powerful sexual predator, and neither was his wife or the mainstream media. It turned out that this was just the beginning of a huge cultural shift that we've been building toward for decades. Following the Weinstein scandal, countless other women and men came forth with their own stories of sexual abuse. And the careers of many famous and powerful men—cultural icons, really—ended overnight. I was stunned. How and why did this happen? Because women have finally become strong enough and empowered enough collectively to risk telling the truth. And instead of backing down, we are rising in support. The tide is really turning. And now it needs to turn when it comes to our healthcare.

Back in the 1980s, when I was starting out in my medical practice, I saw the toll that silence and abuse take on women's bodies. I noticed that many women with conditions such as chronic pelvic pain had been sexually abused. My colleagues denied this and told me my patients were "crazy" and that they only saw "normal" women. I persisted in telling the truth. And it cost me, just as it has cost every whistleblower and rape victim who has ever come forward and rocked the boat, because up until now, our society has been ruled by a belief system known as patriarchy—the rule of the fathers. And those who have challenged it have often paid dearly.

But that is all changing. Quickly. My observations have now become mainstream, and we have the data to support them. Long ago, Sonia Johnson, author of *From Housewife to Heretic,* wrote, "Women are rising like yeast all over the planet." And that yeast has just taken a quantum leap.

The current healthcare crisis is another example of this breakdown to breakthrough—an example with which I'm intimately familiar. You truly cannot create sustainable health through more prescription drugs, more disease screening, and more surgeries, all of which are the mainstay solutions of modern medicine. That's why there is no need to fear the crumbling of the old medical establishment, for this crumbling opens a space for the creation of new, more sustainable, and healthier systems and ideas in all aspects of the human experience on earth, including how we handle the experience of living in a female body.

Over the past four decades, my experiences as an ob-gyn physician, mother, midlife woman, and now grandmother have led me to put forth a revolutionary new approach to women's health and wellness that acknowledges the seamless unity of our bodies, minds, and spirits. Though this still isn't obvious within mainstream medicine, it is now abundantly clear that a woman's state of health is highly influenced by the culture in which she lives, her position within it, her experiences, and her day-to-day thoughts, beliefs, and behaviors.

It is possible to thrive in a female body instead of simply waiting for disease to happen. It boils down to this: Regardless of our individual circumstances, our pasts, or our ages, each of us has inner guidance available that we can tune in to in order to create vibrant health—now. Inner guidance is a second spiritual (and energetic) system that can override and influence physical reality. It is an innate intelligence that operates within us, one that we can learn to access in order to heal. It is the part of us that is capable of creating a spontaneous remission. We are born with this inner guidance, which comes in the form of the emotions and desires that lead us toward things (including thoughts) that feel good and are good for us, and away from things that feel bad and are bad for us. It is influenced by our conscious intent to be well. It's that simple. We are hardwired to seek love, joy, fulfillment—and health. Though we've too often been talked out of our desires as children, I've learned that we can trust those feelings that make us want to get up in the morning. Our desires are the way that the healing life force comes through us and replenishes our bodies. They are what make life worth living. They make up our hopes and dreams. And they invariably hold the keys to healing not only our bodies but also our entire lives.

As a physician, I've seen time and time again how our inner guidance also comes in the form of bodily symptoms and illnesses—especially when we are living lives devoid of pleasure, joy, and hope. Our illnesses are designed to stop us in our tracks, make us rest, and bring our attention back to the things that are really important and that give our lives meaning and joy—aspects of life we often put on the back burner until "someday."

The insights catalyzed by decades of medical practice as well as my own health problems challenged everything I learned in medical school and residency training about women's health. Over the years, it became abundantly clear to me that premenstrual syndrome (PMS), pelvic pain, fibroid tumors, chronic vaginitis, breast problems, and menstrual cramps were related to the contexts of an individual woman's life and her beliefs about herself and what she thought was possible in her life. All of these factors are associated with very real biochemical changes in our cells. Learning about their diets, work situations, and relationships often provided me with clues to the source of women's distress—and, more important, what steps needed to be taken to relieve that distress. Over the years, I have learned to appreciate the thoughts, beliefs, and behavioral patterns behind medical conditions in ways that simply aren't addressed in medical training. These insights are the missing link to optimal health on all levels.

As I have developed more sensitivity to these patterns of health and illness, I have come to the conclusion that without a commitment to looking at all aspects of our lives and accessing our power to change them, improving habits and diet alone is not enough to effect a permanent cure for conditions that have been present for a long time. I've worked with many women whose illnesses could not be ascribed simply to what they eat and could not be cured solely through medication or surgery. Following a special diet or running three miles a day won't make a woman feel well if her health is being adversely influenced by a subconscious belief that she isn't good enough, or that she is the wrong gender, or that it's a woman's lot in life to suffer. Or if she is living with a personality-disordered person who lacks empathy—individuals I refer to as energy vampires. If she has experienced incest and hasn't allowed herself to feel the emotions that are often associated with that history, or if she was unwanted or abused as a child, then no prescription drugs exist that will heal that wound and the physical aftereffects that often result.

Much of the degradation of the feminine, however, is far more subtle and pervasive than outright abuse. Examples include being made to feel uncomfortable breast-feeding your baby in public, being afraid to look and feel sensual for fear that you will attract unwanted attention (and then be blamed for it), and feeling the need to hide any evidence of your menstrual period and its effects. This is why the late feminist writer Adrienne Rich wrote, "I know of no woman . . . for whom the body is not a fundamental problem." Having internalized our bodies as a problem is at the heart of women's health. Changing our perception of this, one woman at a time, is, therefore, at the heart of the healing process. Still, trying dietary changes and alternatives to drugs and surgery for problems whose origins begin with our perceptions is often a very powerful, nontoxic, and health-enhancing first step—a step that opens us up to new, more holistic ways of addressing our symptoms. The secret to thriving is the knowledge that we are never simply victims of our bodies. It's very reassuring to know that we all have within us the ability to heal from anything and go on to live joy-filled lives.

This new edition of *Women's Bodies, Women's Wisdom* is designed to help you not only stay healthy but also thrive mentally, emotionally, and spiritually as well as physically. I want you to know that it is pleasure, not pain, that is your birthright, but that the path of pain is often the only way to get you back on the right track. When we finally make the connection between our thoughts, our heritage, our beliefs, and our physical health and life circumstances, we find that we are in the driver's seat of our lives and can make profound changes. Nothing is more exhilarating or empowering. You'll find stories of such healings and awakenings throughout this book.

One of my readers once wrote, "*Women's Bodies, Women's Wisdom* is a love letter to women and their bodies." I love that. And it's true. As you read this new edition, please know that it is designed to help you fall in love with your own body and to awaken to its divine processes. Let it help you become the physical embodiment of your soul so that you discover the woman you were always meant to be. Let it help you find the best possible solutions for your individual situation. But above all, let it fill you with the courage necessary to make radical and life-giving changes in your mind and body that will allow you to flourish on all levels. And remember, the most fundamental and radical of these changes is learning how to love and accept your precious body right now. It is, after all, the temple that houses your soul. This is the path not only for our individual healing but also for the healing of the planet and humankind.

Part One

From External Control to Inner Guidance

1

The Patriarchal Myth:
The Origin of the
Mind / Body / Emotion Split

The world we have created is a product of our thinking. It cannot be changed without changing our thinking.

—Albert Einstein

Belief becomes biology.

—Norman Cousins

Consciousness creates the body, pure and simple. Consciousness isn't just in the head. It is far more vast than our brains and bodies and exists beyond time and space. We can each use our intent and will to access this part of ourselves that is far greater than our intellects. This is where our true power lies. On a practical day-to-day level, our consciousness is the part of us that chooses and directs our thoughts. Thoughts that are uplifting, nurturing, and loving create healthy biochemistry and healthy cells, while thoughts that are destructive to self or others do just the opposite. We are born with innate love and acceptance of our bodies. Over time, our bodies and states of health are molded by the habitual thoughts and beliefs that guide our behavior, thoughts and beliefs usually laid down in childhood by the dictates of our cultures and families. To improve our lives and our health and truly flourish, we must acknowledge the seamless unity between our beliefs, behaviors, and physical bodies. Then we must critically examine, name, and change any health-eroding beliefs and assumptions that we have unconsciously inherited and internalized from our parents and our culture.

We must be willing to transcend what Gay Hendricks, Ph.D., calls our upper limits.

OUR CULTURAL INHERITANCE

Most modern civilizations are characterized by the belief that the intellect is superior to emotions, the mind and spirit are superior to and entirely separate from the body, masculinity is superior to femininity, and nature is something to be exploited for her resources. The work of cultural anthropologists and historians, such as Riane Eisler, J.D., and archeologist Marija Gimbutas, Ph.D., has documented that our current worldview is only about 5,000 years old. Before that, peaceful societies flourished for thousands of years. In these societies, women held high positions, art flourished, and religion included the worship of the Goddess.[1]

Over time, however, societies and the gods they worshipped changed. Dominator tribes in which authority was vested in men and fathers emerged. These societies were characterized by violence, warfare, and the subjugation of the masses by a relative few who were considered "chosen." Native American writer and anthropologist Jamake Highwater says, "All human beliefs and activities spring from an underlying mythology." Given this, it is easy to make the connection that if our culture over the last 5,000 years has been "ruled by a punishing authoritarian father," then our views of our female bodies and even our medical system have also followed male-oriented rules.[2] Yet patriarchy is only one of many systems of social organization.

I have been in the delivery room countless times, for example, when a female baby was born and the woman who had just given birth looked up at her husband and said, "Honey, I'm sorry"—apologizing because the baby was not a son. The self-rejection of the mother herself, apologizing for the product of her own nine-month gestation period, labor, and delivery, was staggering to experience. Yet when my own second daughter was born, I was shocked to hear those very words of apology to my husband come right up into my brain from the collective unconscious of the human race. I never said them out loud, and yet they were there in my head—completely unbidden. I realized then how old and ingrained is this rejection of the female by men and women alike. I also know that in the past four decades, our worldview has been rapidly changing, in large part because of the feminist, civil rights, and gay rights movements—and also because the Internet has decentralized and globalized communication. Individually and collectively, we are waking up to the ways in which we have been participating in and thus perpetuating our dominator culture. And finally we're taking action to change things.

At the time I wrote this, an unprecedented number of powerful men who have influenced the mainstream media for decades lost their jobs and their reputations overnight because of allegations of sexual abuse that had been going on for decades but had been hidden. It started with movie producer Harvey Weinstein, who not only paid off his victims to buy their silence but also hired former Secret Service agents to terrorize them. The fact that the culture finally believed the victims was a pivotal moment. These revelations were soon followed by the ouster of the much-respected Charlie Rose, a veteran PBS newsman; the über-popular comedian Louis C.K.; actor Kevin Spacey; and then Matt Lauer of the *Today* show, a popular media fixture for twenty years. Clearly the tide has turned. And to keep this healing trend going as the scales fall from our eyes about how those in power have exploited us, it is crucial for each of us to look at the ways in which we have individually participated in a culture that has, for centuries, undermined our universal need for nurturance, healthy food, safe and effective medical care, connection, touch, comfort, pleasure, and joy . . . all the values we associate with mothering, women, and the feminine. In this chapter, I lay out some of the beliefs that have been handed down to us for centuries and their consequences.

Far too often girls are given the message that their bodies, their lives, and their femaleness must be apologized for. As my friend Danielle Hendricksen pointed out in a recent Instagram post, "Girls don't just simply decide to hate their bodies, we teach them to." More than half of girls as young as six to eight years old think their ideal weight is less than they currently weigh, according to research by the child advocacy group Common Sense Media.[3] The group's research also showed that one in four children has engaged in some form of dieting behavior by age seven. So it shouldn't come as a surprise to read that nearly half of girls ages thirteen to seventeen say they look to fashion magazines for body images to strive for, wishing they were as skinny as the models they find there.

Have you noticed how often women apologize? I was walking down the street a while back when a man ran into a woman who was walking by, causing her to drop a package. *She* apologized profusely. Somewhere deep inside many of us is an apology for our very existence. As Anne Wilson Schaef, Ph.D., D.H.L., writes, "The original sin of being born female is not redeemable by works."[4] No matter how many degrees you get in college, no matter how many awards you earn, many women are left feeling that they can never measure up. If we must apologize for our very existence from the day we are born, we can assume that our society's medical system will deny us the wisdom of our "second-class" bodies. In essence, patriarchy blares out the message that women's bodies are inferior and must be controlled. And then we women internalize this message and become our own worst enemies.

This takes the form of Stockholm syndrome, in which women have tended to align with their abusers—the ones who have wielded power—while undermining other women. It's a form of internalized patriarchy. The famous novelist Alice Walker once wrote that slave owners knew exactly how to keep their slaves from organizing and rebelling: You get them to fight among themselves to keep each other down. This too is changing. Sisterhood is rising everywhere.

Our culture habitually denies the insidiousness and pervasiveness of sex-related issues. I first learned in my medical practice that abuse against women (and the feminine aspects of men, for that matter) is epidemic, whether subtle or overt. And I saw how abuse sets the stage for illness in our female bodies. At that time, back in the 1980s, when I suggested to my colleagues that chronic pelvic pain, for example, was associated with a history of sexual abuse, they often guffawed. One even said to me, "Well, maybe your patients have that history. I only see normal women." I soon came to realize that the women I was seeing were no different from those anywhere else—and they were perfectly "normal."

This culture of victim-shaming has finally been put under a glaring spotlight recently, as the #MeToo and #NeverAgain movements have caught fire. Women who have stepped forward to accuse their abusers have traditionally been not only summarily dismissed but also ridiculed and publicly shamed—sometimes even by their own families when the abuse happened at home. "Ignorance is the key reason people outside the relationship shame the victim," says Margaret Bayston, CEO and executive director of Laura's House, a nonprofit organization helping domestic violence survivors in Orange County, California.[5] Many more women suffering such abuse previously chose to stay silent for fear that no one would believe them, Bayston adds. Fortunately, the victim-shaming tide is now significantly receding. Yet plenty of women are still being victimized daily.

Consider the following: One in five women will be raped in her lifetime.[6] Almost 79 percent of women who've been raped experienced their first rape before the age of twenty-five, more than 40 percent before the age of eighteen, and more than 12 percent between eleven and seventeen.[7] (Believe it or not, in at least half a dozen states, rapists can claim parental rights to the children resulting from the rape.) In addition, not only has one in three woman been physically abused by an intimate partner,[8] but between 40 and 45 percent of women in abusive relationships will also be sexually assaulted during the course of the relationship.[9] Some 300,000 pregnant women experience violence during their pregnancies as well.[10] Even for those women who have not been the victim of abuse, the threat can loom large—one in six women report being stalked during their lifetime.[11] Despite this widespread violence against women, only 34 percent of those injured by intimate partners receive medical care,[12] and less than 10 percent of primary care physicians screen for domestic violence during routine office visits.[13] Even if they did, very few have the time to deal with the issue thoroughly.

Yet if the violence is not addressed, it is likely to escalate, putting victims at increased risk for committing suicide, being murdered, and suffering a host of serious injuries (such as brain damage) and chronic health conditions (including contracting sexually transmitted diseases and HIV/AIDS and abusing drugs and alcohol).[14] Abuse against girls has been connected not only with disability later in their lives and early death but also with such diseases as cancer, diabetes, and heart disease, according to research by the Southern California Kaiser Permanente Medical Group and the Centers for Disease Control and Prevention (CDC).[15] The relationship, the researchers report, is cumulative.

The United Nations reports that nearly two-thirds of the world's 781 million illiterates are women, and that when societies are faced with limited resources, females are more likely than males to be deprived of basic necessities, including food and medicine, increasing the risk of physical or mental impairment.[16]

Some of the abuse against women in other parts of the globe is even more shocking. Consider these findings:

~ Sex trafficking of women and children is the fastest-growing criminal enterprise in the world. At least 20.9 million adults and children are sold into commercial sexual servitude, forced labor, and bonded labor worldwide.[17] This includes about 2 million children who are exploited every year in the global commercial sex trade.[18]

~ The World Health Organization estimates that more than 200 million females alive today have undergone female genital mutilation worldwide and that each year an additional 3 million girls, mainly in Africa, are at risk for becoming victims of this practice.[19]

Unfortunately, this practice is even taking place in the United States now. Since 1990, the estimated number of females in this country who have undergone or are at risk of undergoing the practice has more than tripled to 500,000.[20] The increase is due to rapid growth in the number of immigrants to the United States from countries where the practice is common. In 2017, a U.S. doctor arrested in Michigan for performing female genital mutilation on two 7-year-old girls became the first person to be persecuted under a 1996 U.S. law banning the practice.[21] However, two U.S. gynecologists wrote a letter published in the *Journal of Medical Ethics* saying the law should allow for a less invasive procedure involving a small surgical nick to girls' genitalia as a compromise.[22] They likened the procedure to male circumcision—a ridiculous comparison, considering that male circumcision, unlike female genital mutilation, is *not* designed to reduce sexual pleasure (even though it does) nor to control boys' sexuality.

~ In India, the practice of sex-selective abortions in favor of male babies has become so widespread that the male-female balance has been dramatically thrown off (despite the fact that gender-based abortions have been illegal since 1994). Invisible Girl Project, a U.S.-based nonprofit organization devoted to ending gendercide in India, estimates that 700,000 girls are aborted every year in India. In 2001, India's census reported 93 girls to every 100 boys, a ratio that dropped to 89 girls per 100 boys by 2016, according to the World Economic Forum. The danger is greatest in urban areas with more access to amniocentesis and ultrasound, but laptop ultrasound units are now appearing in areas so remote that they don't yet have electricity or running water.[23] Although officially illegal in India, informing expectant parents of the sex of their unborn child is a common practice that is rarely punished.[24]

~ The United Nations estimates that 5,000 honor killings (murder at the hand of family members of women suspected of adultery) occur each year, most of them in Muslim countries (despite the fact that such killings are not condoned by Islamic law). Incest perpetrators have used such "honor killings" to cover up their crimes when their victims become pregnant, and others have used them to solve disputes over inheritance. Some victims of rape or sexual abuse have even been forced to commit suicide.[25]

~ In China, 39,000 girls under the age of one die every year specifically because their parents don't provide them with the same medical care and attention that they give to boys. For the same reason, girls in India between the ages of one and five are 50 percent more likely to die than boys of the same age.[26]

~ Globally, almost 100 million girls are vulnerable to being married before age eighteen because the laws in their countries allow marriage of underage girls if a parent or a judge consents. These legal exceptions account for 32 percent of child marriages—which means that 68 percent of child marriages are illegal. That's 7.5 million underage girls who are married illegally every year—20,000 per day.[27]

~ Some thirty-seven countries do not prosecute men for rape if they are married to (or subsequently marry) their victim.[28]

~ Globally, young women are twice as likely to acquire HIV as their male counterparts. In 2015, 7,500 young women between the ages of fifteen and twenty-four acquired HIV every week.[29] Young women in East and Southern Africa who acquire HIV typically do so five to seven years earlier than young men the same age.[30]

~ Worldwide, 225 million women who want to use contraception have no access to it, while 800 women die daily from preventable causes related to pregnancy and childbirth, according to the Global Fund for Women.

Riane Eisler, J.D., author of the bestselling book *The Chalice and the Blade* (Harper & Row, 1987) as well as *The Real Wealth of Nations: Creat-*

ing a Caring Economics (Berrett-Koehler, 2007), writes, "The world at large is finally waking up to the fact that we can no longer ignore the victims of intimate violence and the link between intimate violence and international violence, including terrorism." After much research, Eisler cofounded the nonprofit Center for Partnership Studies (with her husband, social psychologist and futurist David Loye, Ph.D.) to introduce a new partnership-based model of human rights, and "to show the link between 'women's and children's issues' and social violence, poverty, and other global problems, [as well as] to put an end to gender inequality and intimate violence." (For more information on how she is helping to effect global change, see the Spiritual Alliance to Stop Intimate Violence at www.saiv.org.)

Because of Eisler and others like her, the tide started turning. In 2009 alone, President Obama appointed a new White House Council on Women and Girls, the State Department created the new Office of Global Women's Issues, and the Senate Foreign Relations Committee formed a new subcommittee that deals with women's issues. And while it appears there may be setbacks to this progress during the Trump administration, we are at a tipping point when it comes to true partnership between men and women and between the masculine and feminine energies within us. As the hashtag so aptly puts it, #TimesUp—time really is up. The old patriarchal system is dying everywhere, despite its struggle to maintain control.

A particularly inspiring message comes from Pulitzer Prize–winning journalists and husband-and-wife team Nicholas D. Kristof and Sheryl WuDunn, coauthors of *Half the Sky: Turning Oppression into Opportunity for Women Worldwide* (Knopf, 2009). In a special issue of *The New York Times Magazine* devoted to women and girls in the developing world, Kristof and WuDunn wrote: "There's a growing recognition among everyone from the World Bank to the U.S. military's Joint Chiefs of Staff to aid organizations like CARE that focusing on women and girls is the most effective way to fight global poverty and extremism. That's why foreign aid is increasingly directed to women. The world is awakening to a powerful truth: Women and girls aren't the problem; they're the solution."[31]

PATRIARCHY RESULTS IN ADDICTION

The patriarchal organization of our society demands that women, its second-class citizens, ignore or turn away from their hopes and dreams in deference to men and the demands of their families. Instead of learning how to pay attention to the genius of our intuition and inner guidance, we instead internalize the belief that we are not worthy enough, smart enough, or good-looking enough to live lives of freedom, joy, and fulfillment. Lacking a compassionate language that acknowledges universal human needs, many women (and men) turn to addictions such as overwork, overcare, smoking, drugs and alcohol, and overeating to numb their pain. This results in an endless cycle of abuse that we ourselves help perpetuate. What I'm calling abuse might be as subtle as feeling guilty about getting enough sleep! Being abused or abusing ourselves, we become ill. Then we turn to a medical system that is set up to deliver mostly quick-fix pharmaceutical solutions to problems that can't be healed until we change our core beliefs and thoughts.

Anne Wilson Schaef writes that "anything can be used addictively, whether it be a substance (like alcohol) or a process (like work). This is because the purpose or function of an addiction is to put a buffer between ourselves and our awareness of our feelings—the key to accessing our inner guidance. An addiction serves to numb us so that we are out of touch with what we know and what we feel."[32] Dr. Schaef renamed patriarchy the "addictive system" and described the characteristics of societies that squelch people's inner knowing and emotions—thus favoring the use of addictive substances or processes to keep them going. (See table 1, "Characteristics of an Addictive System," page 22.)

This unhealthy buffering is also reflected in the rise in the incidence of self-harm—deliberately hurting the body by cutting or burning the surface of the skin—among younger girls, which can also turn into an addiction. Not meant as a suicide attempt, this behavior temporarily blunts emotional pain, frustration, and anger. But guilt and shame soon follow, along with the return of the painful emotions. Two million cases of self-harm are reported each year in this country, although the actual number is much higher because many cases go unreported. A recent study from the United Kingdom showed that the incidence of self-harm among girls ages thirteen to sixteen increased a whopping 68 percent from 2011 to 2014.[33]

Whether you call it patriarchy, the addictive system, the dominator society, or the mind/body split, it is abundantly clear that the way in which our society functions is harmful to both men and women (men die on average five years sooner than women and have four times the rate of suicide as women)[34] and that both genders participate fully in keeping it going. Yet the good news is that when we acknowledge our needs, listen to the dictates of our souls, and release the emotional pain that results from denial, we are put immediately in touch with our hearts, our feelings, and our inner guidance system. Our intellects and thoughts can now assume their rightful role: being of service to our hearts and our deepest knowing, not the other way around. This shift puts us in touch with the unmet needs behind our pain. And that is the first step toward healing.

FUNDAMENTAL BELIEFS OF THE DOMINATOR SYSTEM

Marshall Rosenberg, Ph.D., the founder of the Center for Nonviolent Communication (www.cnvc.org), says that all human behavior is an attempt to get a need met. I wholeheartedly agree. This begins by listening for our needs and the needs of others—and believing that it's okay to have needs in the first place! In order to flourish, we need to learn how to be in compassionate dialogue with ourselves. The first step in doing so is to get a handle on how we personally participate in the beliefs and behaviors characteristic of a dominator society. As you become more conscious of your own role in this feedback loop and then change your thoughts and behavior patterns, both your health as an individual and our health as a society will improve. See if the following descriptions of our cultural attitudes toward women and health ring true for you. They may help you become more conscious of your own body and health issues.

Belief One: Disease Is the Enemy

Dominator societies have been properly described as societies that are either preparing for war or recovering from war. Such societies elevate the values of destruction and violence over the values of nurturing and peace. We have only to look at what our society spends on defense to see where its values lie, since the amount of money spent on something is considered a measure of its worth. The sum spent on weapons every minute could feed 2,000 malnourished children for a year, while the price of one military tank could provide classrooms for 30,000 students.[35]

It's no mistake that the medical establishment describes our bodies not as natural systems homeostatically designed to tend toward health but rather as war zones. Military metaphors run rampant through the language of Western medical care. The disease or tumor is "the enemy," to be eliminated at all costs. It is rarely, if ever, seen as a messenger trying to get our attention. Even the immune system, which works to keep us in balance, is described in militaristic terms, with its "killer" T cells. At a hospital conference held to discuss a cancer case at our local medical center, one of the radiologists said, "The previous bullets we've fired at that area [the pelvis, in this case] have failed to sterilize it from disease."

The modern medical preference for drugs and surgery as treatments stems seamlessly from the ideology of our culture. That which is natural and nontoxic, such as the use of high-dose vitamin C as a well-studied and effective treatment for infection, is seen as inferior and ineffective compared with "real medicine"—the "big guns" of powerful antibiotics, drugs, chemotherapy, and radiation. Drug-free, natural methods of treatment with well-studied, well-documented benefits, such as massage, therapeutic touch, and prayer, are ignored at worst or tolerated as "probably not harmful" at best.[36]

A classic example of this in the field of obstetrics and gynecology is the impeccable research of Marshall Klaus, M.D., and John Kennell, M.D., on the effect of continuous labor support by doulas (women whose job is to sit with laboring mothers and provide emotional support). In a series of six different studies, Dr. Kennell found that the mere presence of a doula shortened laboring time in first-time mothers by an average of two hours and reduced the need for cesarean delivery by 50 percent. It also decreased the need for pain medication and increased the chances of successful breast-feeding.[37] Back in the early 1990s, Dr. Kennell estimated that having a doula to support birthing mothers would save the healthcare system more than $2 billion per year in unnecessary medical costs from epidurals, surgery, fevers, and so on. Dr. Kennell quipped, "If the doula effect were a drug, it would be considered unethical not to use it." But the effect of one caring human on another—which costs about $400—falls outside the paradigm of standard medicine, where the current rate of cesarean birth is about 32 percent.

The medical literature is loaded with similar examples. Given these benefits and the total absence of side effects, a true scientist would be fascinated and want to study the effects further. Bernie Siegel, M.D., the famous Yale pediatric surgeon and author of *Love, Medicine and Miracles* (Harper & Row, 1986), once told me that when he posted a study in the doctors' lounge about the beneficial effect of prayer on heart attack sufferers, within a few hours one of his colleagues had written "Bullshit" across the front page.

Keep in mind that our Western medical system has been in place for only about the last hundred years or so. But traditional systems of medicine, including Ayurveda (developed in India) and traditional Chinese medicine (TCM), have been used for thousands of years. The ancient Egyptians wrote a reference guide to more than 850 herbal medicines (many of which we still use today) around 1500 B.C.E., and even before that, the Sumerians are credited with creating the first written record of medicinal plants on clay tablets more than 5,000 years ago.[38]

Our culture considers the body to be inferior to the mind and its dictates of reason. It often teaches us to ignore fatigue, hunger, discomfort, and our need for caring and nurturing. It conditions us to see the body as an adversary, particularly when the body is giving us messages we don't want to hear. I once saw a T-shirt that said it all: "Pain is weakness leaving the body—U.S. Marine Corps." We're encouraged to try to kill the body—as messenger—along with the message. Though it's important to stretch and challenge the body to keep fit and healthy, it's also important to know the difference between stretching yourself and overextending. A dead giveaway that you are overextending, rather than stretching yourself, is the inability to nurture yourself or rest without a drink, a smoke, or overeating.

Belief Two: Medical Science Is Omnipotent

We have been taught that our disease-care system is supposed to keep us healthy. We have been socialized to turn to doctors whenever we have concerns about our bodies and our health. We have been taught the myth of the medical gods—that doctors know more than we do about our bodies, that the expert holds the cure. It's no wonder that when I ask women to tell me what's going on in their bodies, they sometimes reply, "You tell me—you're the doctor!" Doctors are authority figures for some women, right up there with their husbands and religious leaders.

Despite the fact that each woman is more knowledgeable about herself than anyone else could be, most women are trained to look outside themselves for answers. A glaring demonstration of this is the fact that everyone attending a laboring woman in a hospital setting—including the woman herself—looks at the fetal monitor when you ask her, "How are you doing?" instead of checking deep within, where the actual process of birth is taking place for both her and her baby. We live in a society in which so-called experts challenge and subordinate our own judgment and in which our ability to heal or stay healthy without constant outside help is not honored, encouraged, or even recognized.

As a physician, I was trained to be the paternalistic, all-knowing outside expert. The public, in turn, is conditioned to believe that doctors are paragons of healthy behavior who are entitled to judge them for their shortcomings. It always astounded me that my patients feared that I would yell at them for missing an annual Pap test or mammogram appointment when missing appointments is something I and my colleagues also have done!

Medicine itself has a very pathological focus. Scientists rarely study healthy people, and when people with chronic or terminal conditions manage to recover completely, defying the statistical medical prognosis, health professionals too often think that their initial diagnosis must have been wrong, instead of investigating why these people have done so well.[39] In medical school, I practiced on sick or dead people. I was trained in what could go wrong. I was taught to anticipate everything that could possibly go wrong and to plan for it. As an ob-gyn, I was taught that the normal process of labor and delivery was a "retrospective diagnosis" and that it could randomly become a disaster at any moment without warning. When this kind of training goes unquestioned by doctors, the fear and tension that the doctor carries into the room of a laboring woman can increase her anxiety, resulting in hormonal changes in her body that, if not interrupted, favor a cascade of physiological events that ultimately lead to a high rate of dysfunctional labors and cesarean deliveries.

Our culture and its conventional medical system believe that technology, testing, and more research will save us, that it is possible to control and quantify every variable, and that if we just had more data from more studies, we'd be able to improve our health, cure diseases, and live happily ever after. Back in the 1970s, the famous futurist Buckminster Fuller said that we had all the information we needed to wipe out poverty and hunger in the world, but what we lacked was the will to apply what we already know. Unfortunately, instead of applying what we already know, Americans and their doctors equate doing more with improving care. We believe that we can "buy" an answer by throwing money at it or doing more research. Again, we ignore or don't trust our inner guidance system and our own healing ability.

Physicians order lots of tests because we are taught to be uneasy about being uncertain. Healthcare consumers, for their part, are just as uncomfortable with uncertainty as their doctors are. They want to know things in absolute ways. When people ask me about genital herpes, for instance, they want to know, "How did I get it?" "How do I know I won't give it to anyone else?" These questions are essentially unanswerable with absolute certainty. And, of course, doctors also do a lot of procedures and testing for fear of lawsuits. This is one of the reasons why cesarean deliveries have skyrocketed.

Of the 15 million nuclear medicine scans, 100 million CT and MRI scans, and almost 10 billion laboratory tests performed annually in this country, many are "fishing expeditions" that will not improve outcome and may well do unnecessary harm, reports Atul Gawande, M.D., a surgeon, public health researcher, and Harvard professor, in a 2015 article in *The New Yorker*.[40] "For one thing, some diagnostic studies are harmful in themselves—we're doing so many CT scans and other forms of imaging that rely on radiation that they are believed to be increasing the population's cancer rates. These direct risks are often greater than we account for," he writes. Such overtesting leads to overdiagnosis. For example, he writes that although cancer screening has dramatically increased the number of breast, thyroid, and prostate cancer diagnoses during the past twenty-five years, "only a tiny reduction in death, if any, has resulted." The Institute of Medicine reports that such overtreatment costs the U.S. healthcare system at least $210 billion every year.[41]

When it comes to ourselves, doctors know all this. And it leads to a "Do as I say, not as I do" attitude. A very telling report from the University of California found that 50 percent of female physicians don't do monthly breast self-exams even though they tell their patients to do them (more on this in chapter 10, "Breasts"). The same thing is true with vaccinations. Many docs don't give their own children the same shots they feel compelled to recommend to everyone else. A 2014 study at Stanford University showed that most physicians tend to pursue aggressive, life-prolonging treatment for their terminally ill patients, even though they would not make the same choice for themselves in the same situation.[42]

My personal experience with both myself and my colleagues bears this out. I believe that the discrepancy between what doctors tell patients to do and what they themselves do is a matter of insider knowledge. We're far more clear on the limitations of medical science than are our patients. But we don't dare let on lest we destroy the placebo effect of our patients' faith in us! The answer to this dilemma is for both doctors and patients to acknowledge the unknown and also heed the message behind the symptom. This awakens inner guidance and is compatible with any and all treatment choices. It also takes courage.

Unfortunately, it's also true that an increasing amount of the medical research being published today involves financial conflicts of interest (see more about this in chapter 15). Medical policymakers are also not immune. A 2012 survey published in the *Archives of Internal Medicine* showed when it came to the leadership of the committees that write medical guidelines, 71 percent of the committee chairs and 91 percent of the co-chairs had financial conflicts of interest—that is, they had substantial financial connections to pharmaceutical companies.[43]

Belief Three: The Female Body Is Flawed

Because being male has always been considered the norm in our culture, most women internalize the idea that something is basically "wrong" with their bodies. They are led to believe that they must control many aspects of their bodies and that their natural odors, shapes, and processes such as menstruation are simply unacceptable. Women are socialized to think that their bodies are essentially dirty—requiring constant surveillance for "freshness" so that we don't "offend." Females naturally have more body fat than men, and because of better nutrition than in past decades, women today are also bigger than were their mothers and grandmothers. Yet the average fashion model, our cultural ideal, weighs 17 percent less than the average American woman. While the number of men diagnosed with anorexia nervosa or bulimia is on the rise, of the 30 million people in the United States with some form of eating disorder, 20 million of them are female.[44]

This denigration of the female body has made many women either afraid of their bodies and their natural processes or else disgusted by them. Many never touch or get to know what their breasts feel like, for instance, because they're afraid of what they might find. They may feel guilty for touching them, equating this with masturbation, since breasts are erotic for men—another sign of how thoroughly we have turned our bodies over to men. This also helps to explain why so many women feel uncomfortable breast-feeding their babies despite overwhelming evidence of the health benefits for both mothers and babies.

Healthcare practitioners and women alike have been acculturated to view even normal bodily functions such as menstruation, breast-feeding, menopause, and childbirth as medical conditions requiring treatment. The attitude that our bodies are accidents waiting to happen seems to get internalized at a young age and sets the stage for women's future relationships with their bodies. Given what we are taught, it is no wonder that so many women feel ill prepared to deal with and trust ourselves. Our bodies have been "medicalized" since before we were born. This process continues with the popular practice of "well baby" checks, which have become nothing more than an opportunity to give multiple vaccines at the same time—none of which have been thoroughly tested individually for safety against a placebo, let alone when they are all given at the same time. We are now at a point in which 43 percent of all children in the United States have a chronic disease, ranging from asthma and allergies to diabetes.[45]

Our culture fears all natural processes, including birthing and dying. Daily, we are taught to be afraid. When my older daughter was seven, she was out with her father chopping down some brush in our backyard. Suddenly she started to cry and came running into the house with a bleeding finger. She had cut herself on a blade of grass. As I calmly held her finger under some cold water and saw that it was only a tiny cut, she looked up at me and uttered what I consider a major healing principle: "It didn't hurt until I got scared."

Many procedures that have been routinely performed on women's bodies in particular are not based on scientific data at all but are rooted in prejudice against the body's innate wisdom and healing power. Some procedures have their origins in emotional views of women handed down from previous generations. Routine episiotomies at delivery (cutting of the tissue between the vagina and rectum to make more room for the baby's head) are an example. Despite the fact that studies have shown that episiotomy is usually unnecessary and increases blood loss, pain, and risk of long-term pelvic floor damage and tears (something that midwives have been saying for years), episiotomy is still too common. It wasn't until 2005 that a study published in the *Journal of the American Medical Association* on the outcomes of routine episiotomy was widely publicized, leading both women and their doctors to question the procedure more thoroughly.[46] The next year, the American College of Obstetricians and Gynecologists published new recommendations against routine use of the procedure. While the number of episiotomies has declined considerably since then, some hospitals inexplicably still have unacceptably high rates (including one in Los Angeles where episiotomies are performed in more than 60 percent of vaginal births).[47]

The reason this practice has persisted so long despite scientific data to the contrary is that obstetricians have truly believed that the birthing female body required the procedure to protect the pelvic floor and also to ensure a suitably "tight" vagina postpartum. One of the first things I was taught in my ob-gyn residency was how to place what was called the "husband's stitch" in the episiotomy incision. Yikes.

While this kind of biased thinking among medical professionals will change as more women become doctors (not to mention professors at medical schools), it simply can't change fast enough. In 1970, only 7 percent of gynecologists were women, compared to 57 percent today—yet overall, only 35 percent of all physicians are women.[48] And of the forty-four medical specialties, only six have more women than men (the highest percentage being in pediatrics). There's good news, though: Women represent more than 45 percent of medical residents today, so the balance is clearly shifting.

RECLAIMING THE AUTHORITY OF OUR OWN FEELINGS

Ultimately, I've found it enormously empowering to realize that no scientific study can explain exactly how and why my own particular body acts the way it does. That is because we each comprise a multitude of processes that have never existed before and never will again. In the end, our connection with our own inner guidance and emotions is the most reliable indicator of how well we're doing. Science must acknowledge truthfully how much it doesn't know and leave room for mystery, miracles, and the wisdom of nature.

My father used to say, "Feelings are facts. Pay attention to them." Yet in my scientific training I quickly learned that feelings, intuition, spirituality, and all experiences of life that cannot be explained by the logical, rational parts of our minds or measured by our five senses are suspect or discounted as "magical thinking." Because our culture places such emphasis on our intellects, we learn to fear our emotional responses. Women in particular are seen as emotional and thus in need of management. It took me years and years to break out of my own pattern of fearing emotional responses! In his groundbreaking book *The Biology of Belief* (Hay House, 2008), cellular biologist Bruce Lipton, Ph.D., who has done pioneering research on the effect of consciousness on cells, writes, "Bio-scientists are conventional Newtonians—if it isn't matter . . . it doesn't count. The 'mind' is a non-localized energy and therefore is not relevant to materialistic biology. Unfortunately, that perception is a 'belief' that has been proven to be patently incorrect in a quantum mechanical universe." Our entire society functions in ways that keep us out of touch with what we know and feel.

Remaining unconscious about our innate needs takes an enormous emotional and physical toll on our bodies and spirits. Not recognizing our needs for rest, intimacy, touch, good nutrition, acknowledgment, and so on—and not knowing how to get these needs met directly—prevents us from being connected with our inner guidance. This disconnection, in turn, keeps us in a state of pain that increases the longer we deny it. It takes a lot of energy to stay out of touch with our needs. And we often turn to acculturated habits, such as the use of addictive substances, to keep us from confronting the unhappiness and pain that result from unmet needs.

Almost everyone understands that physical destruction results from abusing alcohol and drugs. Fifty percent of the accident victims in most emergency rooms are there because of alcohol abuse. As one of our staff anesthesiologists once said, "If it weren't for cigarettes and alcohol, I'd be out of a job!" What many people don't appreciate, however, is the enormous and equally deadly toll taken by compulsive behaviors such as overwork and overeating, used to avoid or deny one's feelings.

Sexual and relationship addictions have gynecological implications and result in the epidemics of sexually transmitted diseases, such as venereal warts, herpes, and cervical cancer. A former patient of mine was married to a recovering alcoholic and was suffering from chronic vaginitis, for which I could find no cause. She finally came to the realization that her husband had been "medicating himself through sex with me every day for years. I saw that my body was his bottle—he was using it and sex the same way he had used alcohol, and I thought it was my duty as a wife to comply."

My experiences in my own practice and life have led me to believe that health promotion and education won't do a thing to decrease healthcare expenses unless we as individuals and as a society acknowledge our basic human needs and commit to fulfilling them compassionately. Only then can we begin to participate in our own recovery and truly flourish. Every overweight woman I know is clear about what she "should" eat. She doesn't need more nutrition information. She needs first to *feel* the pain of her unmet needs for intimacy, rest, recognition, grieving, and acceptance, which the excess food is a substitute for. This can happen only when she is encouraged to name those needs and learn how to meet them skillfully and compassionately. Her body and its state of health will always be a reliable barometer, letting her know how she's doing in this regard.

The Power of Naming

A first step toward making a positive change in your life or your health is to name your current experience and allow yourself to feel it fully—emotionally, spiritually, and physically. Back in the 1980s, it was crucial for me to see how often I used the caretaker and rescuer role as a way to get my need for recognition and reward met. It was crucial for me to name this behavior "relationship addiction." Before I did this, I looked to others to affirm me and tell me that I was okay. I took their cues for how to act, feel, and look; I was always seeing myself in terms of other people. I believed that if I said no to someone who needed me, I wouldn't be valued and loved. Looking back over my life, I see not only how persistent this pattern has been but also how much it has improved through insight and behavior change. My own life and health have improved enormously as a result of naming and changing this behavior, as well as coming to understand that I'm an empath, as are so many others. Simple. Not easy.

I came to see that my tendency to rescue people in need, my acquiescence to others, and my saying yes to everyone came out of my attempt to exercise a form of control, as well as from a sense that these were essential to my self-protection and survival. I believed that if I said yes, I would earn people's love and approval and would stay safe. This wasn't good either for me or for them, since by putting myself in the position of being other people's rescuer, a substitute for their own higher power or inner guidance, I allowed them to remain out of touch with their own strengths. My behavior actually helped to create victims who needed me. Of course, this behavior was completely in line with what our culture teaches women. All of those who are of lower status learn early on that to survive and protect themselves, they must pay more attention to meeting the needs and expectations of those in positions of authority and power than they pay to their own needs. Perfectly normal—and something to recover from nonetheless.

Now when someone says he or she needs me, a red flag immediately goes up. I wait, check out the situation, and see what my inner guidance tells me before I decide how to respond. I've learned that if my answer is not an immediate and joyful yes, then almost always it should be a no.

One of the most common characteristics of people in our addictive society is dependence. "Dependency is a state in which you assume that someone or something outside you will take care of you because you cannot take care of yourself," writes Dr. Schaef. "Dependent persons rely on others to meet their emotional, psychological, intellectual, and spiritual needs."[49] For centuries women have relied on men to meet their economic needs (not that they were given much choice, since in many cases they were owned like property), while men have relied on women to meet their emotional needs. As one patient of mine said about her former marriage, "Our agreement was, he would make the money and I would do the emotions." Clarissa Pinkola Estes, Ph.D., points out that one of the reasons women have not been more in touch with their creative instincts is that they have spent so much time succoring others who have been at war—either on the battlefield or in corporate America.[50]

The problem with this way of relating to others is that it prevents true intimacy. Intimacy can take place only in a partnership relationship, not in one based on intersecting dependencies. My parents once cautioned me, "If a man ever says, 'I need you,' run the other way." It's good advice.

Naming the ways in which we participate in the dominator/addictive culture offers us a way out of the culturally induced trance that affects almost all women. Far too often, the culture's definition of what it means to be a "good" woman is one who meets everyone's needs but her own. Though being self-sacrificing for others earns love and acceptance in the short run, it always backfires because our bodies were designed to be healthy to the extent that we follow our hearts' desires—not meet the needs of others at our own expense.

When you name an experience intellectually, be aware of how that experience actually feels in your body. Allow yourself to feel it physically. Otherwise, your own behavior—and your health—will not change. *Once an experience is consciously named and internalized, physically and emotionally, it can no longer influence us unconsciously.* When we change our perception, every cell in our body changes. We then begin to see how we have been influencing and perpetuating our own problems. Naming something that has affected us adversely—and also articulating the unmet need associated with it—is part of freeing ourselves from the negative influence of past trauma. Many times healing cannot begin until we allow ourselves to feel how bad things are (or were in the past). Doing this frees emotional and physical energy that has been stuffed, stuck, denied, or ignored for many years. When we can allow ourselves to feel exactly how we feel, without judgment, we begin to free our energy. Only then can we move toward what we want. Table 1 can help you name your addictive characteristics.

One of my former patients had a chronic and painful vaginal and vulva herpes condition that didn't respond to conventional drug therapy or even to alternatives such as dietary changes. After three years of unsuccessfully searching for a way to stop her recurrent outbreaks, she came to the following conclusion: "Maybe I just need to walk around for a while saying that my vagina hurts. I was never able to say that to my mother when I was little." From the moment she spoke this truth out loud, she began to heal. She told me that her father had sexually abused her for years and her mother hadn't believed her. Layer by layer, she began to uncover her wounds, name them, and heal. With great compassion for herself, she acknowledged the pain of her past, her unmet need to grieve and have her pain witnessed, and moved beyond judgment of herself and her parents. As she did this, her pain gradually decreased while her creative life as a writer began to blossom. Today, she no longer has herpes outbreaks.

Over time I have come to see that what society calls being a "good woman" or a "good doctor" or a "good mother" came dangerously close to an invitation for me to lose myself in serving others at my own expense. I was reminded recently of how insidious this message is when I read the obituary of a woman who had died in her early fifties. Among other things, it said: "She was a tireless worker for the rights of women." Anytime you see the word *tireless,* substitute *martyr* instead. We all get tired. And we're supposed to rest regularly. Thinking that *tireless* is the equivalent of *good* is a setup for resentment, anger, and eventually illness. I've learned that I am able to provide optimal service and friendship to others only to the degree that I'm also tuning in to what I need to do for me. Over time I've created a life in which my family, colleagues, and loved ones have all committed themselves to living in balance as well. As a result of learning how to care for myself and listen to my own inner guidance, I have become far more effective at helping others than I ever dreamed possible.

Part of flourishing is allowing others to go through their own learning processes. No one can create health for another person. I have realized that I don't have the answers for everyone—and neither does anyone else. Only the individual herself can gain access to her inner guidance when she is ready. After years of feeling that I was responsible for having all the answers for others at the expense of myself, I no longer try to convince anyone of anything (most of the time).

Many women are not in jobs and families that fully support their health. But if we can learn to value ourselves deeply, name our addictive behaviors, and commit to living our lives fully and joyfully, our jobs and circumstances will begin to change. Changing our thoughts and consciousness is always the first step toward healing. To help you in this, please read through the table on page 22 and honestly assess which of these characteristics apply to you.

Naming and Healing Emotional Pain and Its Physical Consequences

Our emotions and thoughts have such profound effects on us because they are physically and energetically linked to our bodies via our immune, endocrine, and central nervous systems. And new research has shown that the connective tissue throughout our bodies, which is called fascia, functions as a continuous liquid crystalline matrix in which a change in one area is immediately communicated throughout the entire system, because crystals are well-known energy transmitters and transducers. That means that the slumped shoulders associated with sadness and grief transmit the biochemistry of "sadness" instantaneously throughout the entire body. On the other hand, the very act of smiling sends the opposite message. Putting your arms up over your head in the V shape for victory, as many athletes do after they win, is associated with increased testosterone, which is why you see athletes do this after winning a race.[51] All emotions, even those that are suppressed and unexpressed, have physical effects. Unexpressed emotions tend to stay in the body like small ticking time bombs—they are illnesses in incubation.

A culture that is unsupportive of women and those attributes we call womanly sets the stage early on for health problems because the context of a woman's life contributes greatly to the state of her health. When I first got my period, for example, I developed astigmatism and myopia and had to get glasses. It is very common for girls to need glasses around puberty. The eyes are in what's called the "liver meridian" in traditional Chinese medicine, and the primary emotion associated with the liver meridian is anger. Because many young women lack the support necessary to identify the unmet needs fueling their anger, let alone a safe place to express anger in a healthy way, it's no wonder their eyesight is adversely affected. I myself truly resented having to get glasses—no one else in the family had them. I now know there was something I didn't want to see. I was unmistakably a girl in a family and a culture where male pursuits reigned supreme, and I was angry about this— but wasn't aware of it.

TABLE 1

CHARACTERISTICS OF AN ADDICTIVE SYSTEM

Characteristic	Definition	Examples
BLAME	Believing that someone or something outside of yourself is the cause of whatever is happening to you	"I can't help the way I am. My mother was an alcoholic." "I married a man who is completely incapable of having an intimate relationship."
DENIAL	Being out of touch with your feelings, needs, or other information	"My parents weren't alcoholics, they were heavy social drinkers." "There's a fine line between drinking too much and being an alcoholic." "I don't know why I've gained twenty pounds. I never eat a thing that isn't healthy."
CONFUSION	Lacking clarity about a situation or your emotions	"Nobody ever tells me anything." "I never know what's going on around here."
FORGETFULNESS	Putting out of your mind, ceasing to notice	Forgetting appointments, car keys, personal belongings, bodily needs

Characteristic	Definition	Examples
THE SCARCITY MODEL (ZERO-SUM MODEL)	Believing that there's a limited amount of everything that's desirable: love, money, intimacy, happiness	"If I am successful, someone else has to suffer." "It is not okay to spend time or money on oneself or to admit it."
PERFECTIONISM	Having an extreme need for external order to cover internal chaos	Relentless pursuit of a perfect body, home, mate, job
THE ILLUSION OF CONTROL OR OBJECTIVITY	Fearing your needs and feelings, and creating an illusion that you can somehow control yourself; separating yourself from your emotions, and believing that it is possible to be completely objective and unemotional	"If I could find the right drug, I could get rid of these panic attacks." "Premenstrually I become a different person. I'm like Dr. Jekyll and Mr. Hyde. I'm not myself." "The ozone level is high today. Please stay inside." (As though the inside air is disconnected from the rest of the environment!)
NEGATIVISM	Seeing life in terms of lack	"I always catch whatever is going around." "Now that I'm forty, everything is starting to fall apart." "You can't have that, it costs too much."
DEPENDENCY	Believing that someone or something outside of you will take care of you because you can't do it for yourself	"I can't leave my husband. Who would support me?" "I can't live without him."
CRISIS ORIENTATION	Using or creating an external crisis as a socially acceptable way to distract yourself from your feelings	"There's no question that we emergency-room nurses really look forward to the next multiple trauma. It gets the juices flowing."
DEFENSIVENESS	Being unable to accept feedback and make positive adjustments	"Who are you to tell me that PMS is related to my family? My childhood was perfect."
DISHONESTY	Not telling the truth	"Do I need a break? No, I'm fine." "It wasn't that bad. I can handle it."
DUALISTIC THINKING	Believing that there are only two choices: One is right or good, the other is wrong or bad	"Vitamins and herbs are good. Drugs and surgery are bad."

Sources: Anne Wilson Schaef, *When Society Becomes an Addict* (San Francisco: Harper & Row, 1987), p. 72; Anne Wilson Schaef and Diane Fassel, *The Addictive Organization* (San Francisco: Harper & Row, 1988).

Millions of women suffer from chronic pelvic pain, vaginitis, painful intercourse, ovarian cysts, genital warts, endometriosis, and cervical dysplasia (abnormal cells on the cervix that are picked up by a Pap test)—all diseases of organs that are unique to females. These conditions are the language through which our bodies speak to us. Often they are telling us that we need to heal from a deeper, often unconscious wounding—the ingrained belief that we are never enough and that we are somehow tainted.

A forty-one-year-old executive came to see me because she was having uncomfortable hot flashes. She was on four times the normal dose of estrogen and was still getting no relief. In addition to being related to decreased estrogen levels, hot flashes are a neuroendocrine problem and increase with stress. When a woman feels that she is under stress, the frequency and severity of her hot flashes increase both objectively and subjectively. My patient had already had a hysterectomy and removal of her ovaries for uncontrollable pelvic pain as a result of severe endometriosis two years before. Now she seemed beyond relief. It took this patient two years to tell me that when she was six, she had been sexually molested in the basement of a candy store by the man who ran the store. While this was happening to her, she had felt frozen, unable to speak. She said, "I just went numb. He told me never to tell anyone, because if I did they'd never like me. I felt completely ashamed." On the day she did tell me, she still felt that she had done something wrong and that she was bad. She later said that she drove away from the office certain that once I knew the truth about her, I'd never like her again.

My patient, trying to redeem her shame, had continually worked two jobs since high school and earned an MBA. Very successful in her career, she had used work, constant striving, and earning more degrees as a way to "prove herself" and to keep at bay that early emotional pain and the feeling that she was unworthy and bad. When I last saw her, she still hadn't shed a tear about her experience, an emotional release that I know will help her once she's ready.

The seeds of my patient's physical problems were planted by her childhood traumas. I am not saying that her childhood sexual abuse "caused" the endometriosis or chronic pelvic pain. What I'm suggesting is that her early abuse, common to so many women, inserted a set of destructive beliefs about her worth and her lovability that persisted well into adulthood, creating discomfort in both her mind and her body. Regardless of whether or not we've experienced childhood trauma, the truth is that every one of us was imprinted in the womb and in early childhood by our parents' beliefs and behaviors—as were their parents before them. This is inevitable. We become programmed with a set of upper limits for what we believe we deserve in life. That includes how healthy, how prosperous, and how well loved we can expect to be. These beliefs operate in our subconscious, under the radar of our everyday consciousness. But they unerringly attract to us experiences that reinforce what we already believe.

One of the primary ways of transcending those upper limits and starting the healing process is to consciously affirm our own worth and lovability while simultaneously allowing ourselves to feel the old unhealed emotional pain. The human heart has an almost endless capacity to transform emotional pain through the process of grieving, forgiving, and letting go. This isn't an intellectual process. It happens in the body. And, as Jungian analyst Marion Woodman, Ph.D., points out, the soul comes to us through the body. When one of my friends was going through a very difficult divorce, she started a meditation practice. One day, while in meditation, she had the realization that to doubt the beauty within herself was to doubt God. This was a turning point in her health and her healing.

Only by tuning in to how we feel in our bodies can we appreciate our inner guidance. Yet we look to our schools to tell us what is worth learning, our governments to take care of our communities, and our doctors to vaccinate us against the latest germ. We've been taught that we will be okay if we follow the rules. One of our patients who developed vulvar cancer said, "I can't understand how this happened. I've come in for an exam every year, had normal Pap tests, and yet I still got cancer." Like this patient, we've been misled into believing that screening tests alone will prevent us from getting ill.

In first grade my younger daughter was told on the first day of school what the acceptable times were for students to go to the bathroom. I went in and told her teacher that in my practice I regularly see adult women with constipation and urinary problems who cannot move their bowels in public restrooms because early "rules" from home and school like these had damaged their ability to know when their bodies needed to perform a normal function. I didn't want this to happen to my daughter. I made sure she heard my conversation with her teacher so that she felt supported in going to the bathroom when she needed to go.

Healing Means Leaving Wounding Behind

We can't make a new world for ourselves as long as we hold on to old self-destructive beliefs about ourselves and our worth—or about the worth of others. If we fail to notice the ways in which we daily cooperate with the system that's destroying us, we're in danger of operating in perpetual-victim mode, always blaming someone "out there" for our problems. Much like the battered woman who finally gets out because one day she realizes that if she stays she will die, each of us must recognize when and where we're cooperating with our own oppression.

One of my friends who was brought up Catholic in the 1950s describes the effect of confession on her body. "I remember having to go to confession," she says, "beginning at age seven, searching my conscience for crimes and misdemeanors, feeling caught in the horrible dilemma of being unable to speak the unspeakable—about sexual wonderings, masturbation. Who had the language for that? And were girls even capable of it? Was I the only one in this dilemma? It was suggested on a plastic card that guided the confessional process that these failings fall into the category of 'impure thoughts and deeds.' Even given this sanitized version, I could not confess to some man, semi-visible behind the confessional grille, whose breath smelled of cigarettes and alcohol, the sensual dimensions of myself. Without a complete confession, however, you were not allowed to take Holy Communion, or if you did, you would be condemned to hell, with a mortal sin on your soul. (They sort of had you coming and going.) This was my first encounter with an ethical dilemma.

"And so I unconsciously and ingeniously devised a way out. When I was at the entry of adolescence, around age eleven, I began systematically to faint during mass, right before Communion. I had to be carried out of church, and there on the entryway steps I remember being able to breathe, to hear the birds and feel the sun. This went on for over a year. I had no control over these fainting sessions. I was embarrassed by them and bewildered by what my body was doing—cold sweats, ringing in my ears, and the inevitable blackness closing in on me. (I have ever since felt oppressed in the confines of a church.) The intolerable and contradictory demands simply knocked me unconscious."[52]

Many women have been knocked unconscious by the conflicting demands of our culture. And women all over the world are waking up to it. Healing from conditions such as pelvic pain, PMS, and chronic fatigue syndrome is almost always enhanced when we realize that we are not alone in our suffering and that our problems occur in a cultural context that is often unsupportive of us. Recovering our health involves naming our experiences for what they are—no matter how painful—and then learning that the motor for our lives is within us, regardless of our past. Only then can we decide to truly flourish in spite of the health-eroding beliefs we've inherited from our culture and our parents.

Though it is extremely helpful to have a physician or healthcare provider who acknowledges the mind-body connection, it is even more important that we ourselves appreciate that our bodies and their symptoms are part of our inner guidance. They have a message for us. Always. We can free ourselves from our overdependence on the medical system by seeing the ways in which our own beliefs and behaviors perpetuate the parts of this system that do not help us create health. If we persist in thinking that our diseases and symptoms, such as endometriosis, fibroids, and PMS, are "just medical" and not related to the other parts of our lives, we are participating in and thus perpetuating the addictive system in medical care.

On the other hand, when we learn how to tune in to the language of our bodies, we're more able to make informed decisions about medical testing and technology, which can lead to more satisfactory relationships with our healthcare providers. We must begin to trust ourselves and our experience as much as we trust laboratory data. One of my patients who had infrequent periods came to see that she always got a period whenever she was "in love." She came to trust that she didn't need a lot of hormonal testing every time her period ceased for several months. Instead, she became interested in the meaning behind those periods and what emotions were associated with them.

TABLE 2

THE BODY AS A PROCESS VERSUS MEDICAL WORLDVIEW

The Body as a Process	Medical Worldview
~ The female body reflects nature and earth.	~ The female body and its processes are uncontrollable and unreliable. They require external control.
~ Thoughts and emotions are mediated via the immune, endocrine, and nervous systems. They are biochemical events.	~ Thoughts and emotions are entirely separate from the physical body.
~ The physical, emotional, spiritual, and psychological aspects of an individual are intimately intertwined and cannot be separated.	~ It is possible to separate an individual into entirely distinct, unrelated compartments.
~ Illness is part of the inner guidance system.	~ Illness is a random event that just happens. There is very little a woman can do to prevent illness.
~ The body creates health daily. It is inherently self-healing.	~ The body is always vulnerable to germs, disease, and decay.
~ Illness is best prevented by living fully according to one's inner guidance.	~ Illness prevention is not possible in this system. So-called prevention is really disease screening.

The Body as a Process	Medical Worldview
⁓ Life is best lived by embracing it, while accepting the inevitability of its end.	⁓ Life is all about avoiding death at all costs by focusing on all the things that can go wrong.
⁓ Our true selves don't die.	⁓ Death is seen as failure and final.

When doctor and patient acknowledge our respective areas of expertise, our areas of ignorance, and the unknown that lies beyond, a true partnership becomes possible, which is a joy for both.

As you read this book, remember that we all have choices—and we all have inner guidance and spiritual help available that can help us move toward optimal health and fulfillment. Recovery from the mind/body split means learning to live fully from the inside out in a culture that often negates this way of being in the world. Our bodies and their symptoms are our biggest allies in this endeavor, because nothing gets our attention as quickly. Our bodies never lie. They are impeccable barometers of how well we're living in the present and taking care of ourselves.

To become healthy and whole, you must have enough courage to be in touch with the wisdom of your female body, and to follow the desires of your heart. Nothing is more exciting than knowing that our bodies and our feelings are a clear, open pathway toward our destinies.

2
Feminine Intelligence and a New Mode of Healing

In the end I find I can't separate brain from body. Consciousness isn't just in the head. Nor is it a question of mind over body. If one takes into account the DNA directing the dance of the peptides [the] body is the outward manifestation of the mind.

—Candace Pert, Ph.D.

The mind and the body are intimately linked via the immune, endocrine, central nervous, and connective tissue systems. Today, mind-body research is confirming what ancient healing traditions have always known: that the body, the mind, the emotions, and the spirit are a unity. There is no disease that isn't mental, emotional, and spiritual as well as physical. Thoughts are the language of the mind. Emotions are the language of the body. Inspiration is the language of the spirit. We must become fluent in all of these different languages if we are to attain and maintain vibrant health.

ENERGY FIELDS AND ENERGY SYSTEMS

Humans are made out of energy and sustained by energy. Our bodies are ever-changing, dynamic fields of energy and vibration, not static physical structures. Cellular biologist Bruce Lipton, Ph.D., author of *The Biology of Belief* (Hay House, 2008), writes that when we truly understand the effect of thoughts, emotions, and energy on the body, "we will no longer fractiously debate the role of nurture and nature because we will realize that the fully conscious mind trumps both nature and nurture. And I believe we will also experience as profound a paradigmatic change to humanity as when a round-world reality was introduced to a flat-world civilization." I couldn't agree more.

The truth is that our bodies are holograms in which every part contains information about the whole. This can be appreciated by looking at the sheath of fascia that encases every muscle, nerve, and organ throughout the body. This connective tissue functions as a liquid crystalline matrix highly affected by your level of hydration. So, for example, the fascia on the bottom of your foot is connected both mechanically and electromagnetically (be-cause crystals are well-known energy transmitters and transducers) to the fascia that encases your brain, and everything in between. And it's the crys-talline properties of connective tissue (as well as of bones and teeth) that enable it to transmit information and energy instantaneously throughout the body. (This is thought to be the mechanism by which the meridian system used in acupuncture, a component of traditional Chinese medicine, works.)[1] Thus, everything your foot experiences also affects your brain. (Helene Lan-gevin, M.D., now director of the National Center for Complementary and Integrative Health, has published exciting research from when she was at the University of Vermont School of Medicine on a group of cells called integrins that are the physical link between cells and their surrounding tissues, thus providing further proof for the fascinating connection; see chapter 18 for more on this.)

Research has also shown that a gas known as nitric oxide is produced by the lining of every blood vessel in your body during exercise, sex, meditation, and the thinking of joyful or hopeful thoughts. Nitric oxide (not to be con-fused with nitrous oxide, commonly known as laughing gas) not only instan-taneously increases the circulation of blood throughout the body but also is the über-neurotransmitter, having the ability to balance all the other mood-enhancing neurotransmitters such as serotonin and dopamine.[2] I've come to believe that nitric oxide is the physical equivalent of the life force, *chi* (or *qi*), or *prana*. According to quantum physics, at the subatomic level, matter and energy—which can also be called spirit—are interchangeable. The best ex-pression of this that I have heard is that matter is the densest form of spirit and that spirit is the lightest form of matter. We can view our bodies as manifestations of spiritual energy. Our mind and daily thoughts are part of this energy, and they have a well-documented effect on matter and our bod-ies. Our daily thoughts and emotions, which are accompanied by a multitude of biochemical changes in our bodies, set up an electromagnetic field around us (and around every cell in our bodies) that attracts to us our vibratory equivalent. This tendency is known as the law of attraction and is the most fundamental law that governs the universe. Like is attracted to like. As we vibrate, so we attract. Or to state it more simply, birds of a feather flock together.

Psychological and emotional factors influence our physical health greatly because our emotions and thoughts are always accompanied by biochemical reactions in our bodies. These reactions are mediated by cell membranes, which are the actual "brains" of each cell. The mind-body continuum can be adequately understood only when we appreciate ourselves as an ever-changing energy system that is affected by, and also affects, the energy surrounding it. We don't end at our skins. This fact has been beautifully illustrated by the work of the late Masaru Emoto, a Japanese researcher who did groundbreaking work on the effect of emotions on the crystalline structure of water. In his book *The Hidden Messages in Water* (Beyond Words, 2004), and also in the movie *What the Bleep Do We Know!?*, Emoto documented the effects of different emotions on the structure of frozen water crystals, showing beyond a shadow of a doubt that the energy of loving appreciation creates the most profoundly beautiful crystalline patterns. Given that our bodies are 60 to 70 percent water, Emoto's research has profound implications for health. How we think about, talk to, and feel about ourselves creates an imprint on our cells that affects not only us but also everyone around us.

Though we cannot see this vibrational energy that makes up the body-mind and sustains us, it is nevertheless a vital part of us. It is the life force that keeps our hearts beating and our lungs breathing even when we are asleep. Anyone who has had the experience of being with a dying person will tell you that after the moment of death, something changes. Though the physical body is still present, the person we once knew is no longer there. His or her life force has gone elsewhere.

Vibrational fields interact within an individual person. They also interact between one person and another, and between one person and the world in general. These interactions, whose existence is well documented, are important for lifelong human growth and healthy development. A study at the University of Miami on premature babies, for example, found that babies who were stroked regularly gained weight 49 percent faster than did those of the same initial weight who weren't stroked. (Both groups of babies were fed exactly the same amount of food.) The stroked babies were longer and had larger heads and fewer neurological problems at eight months of age than did the controls.[3] Babies who are not touched and cuddled, even though they are fed and cared for physically, are at risk of death from the elusive diagnosis "failure to thrive."[4]

Even accidents, which we think of as random events, have been shown in a number of studies to be related to the emotional and psychological states (or vibrational fields) of the "victims." Several studies have indicated that accident-prone individuals have certain personality features, including impulsiveness, resentment, aggressiveness, unmet dependency needs, depression, sadness, loneliness, and unresolved grief. They tend to punish themselves when they feel anger toward others. In his book *Traffic Safety* (Science Serving Society, 2004), for example, Leonard Evans, president of Science Serving Society, presents exhaustive research on factors contributing to auto accidents, including safety standards, road conditions, and so on. One part of his analysis shows that drivers who are at higher risk for automobile accidents are, among other traits, less mature and intellectual, while they are more emotionally unstable, unhappy, antisocial, impulsive, openly hostile, and aggressive. They also have lower self-esteem and lower aspirations and are more likely to have had unhappy childhoods. In the language of vibrational systems, it appears that the vibrational field of certain individuals interacts with the environmental vibrational field in a way that increases the possibility of accidents.

Clearly, human interactions have profound effects on health. These effects can be either positive or negative, depending upon the state of mind of the people involved in those interactions. When we begin to appreciate ourselves as vibrational fields of energy with the ability to affect the quality of our own experience, we will be getting in touch with our innate ability to heal ourselves and create health every day of our lives.

Our bodies are influenced and actually structured by our thoughts and beliefs. Every thought is accompanied by an emotion or feeling, and every emotion creates a specific biochemical reality in our bodies. Thoughts that are reinforced over and over become beliefs. Beliefs drive our behavior. We inherit many of these beliefs from our parents and the circumstances of our upbringing. Scientific studies conducted by Leonard Sagan, M.D., a medical epidemiologist, underscore this and show that social class, education, life skills, and cohesiveness of family and community are key factors in determining life expectancy. Of all these factors, however, education has been shown to be the most important. A review of *all* the major epidemiological data on health makes clear that the major determinants of health are not immunization, diet, water supply, or antibiotics. In fact, the dramatic decline in death rates from infectious disease earlier in this century began long before the routine use of penicillin and antibiotics. *Hope, self-esteem, and education are the most important factors in creating health daily,* no matter what our background or the state of our health in the past.[5] All illnesses are affected by our emotional state. Jeanne Achterberg, Ph.D., has shown that the course of cancer can be better predicted by psychological variables such as hope than by medical measurements.[6] A striking 2012 study published in the *New England Journal of Medicine* analyzed public health records from 6 million adults in Sweden and found that those diagnosed with cancer were 5.6 times more likely to die of cardiovascular causes the week after getting the diagnosis than were those who were never diagnosed with cancer.[7] The stress of the cancer diagnosis caused a more immediate health crisis.

The huge Adverse Childhood Experiences (ACE) Study, begun in 1998, has documented the dramatic adult health consequences of childhood abuse and family dysfunction, and it has shown beyond a shadow of a doubt the health effects of our often inherited beliefs about our worthiness and lovability.[8] This study was initially triggered by observations made in the mid-1980s in the obesity program at the Kaiser Permanente Department of Preventive Medicine in San Diego. The program had a very high dropout rate—and, surprisingly, the people dropping out were successfully losing weight. Detailed life interviews with almost 200 such individuals unexpectedly revealed that childhood abuse was remarkably common and antedated the onset of their obesity. Many patients spoke openly about this. Obesity was not their problem; it was a protective solution to problems they had previously never discussed with anyone. For example, a woman who gained 105 pounds in the year after being raped said, "Overweight is overlooked. And that is exactly what I need to be."

The ACE study found that adverse childhood experiences are vastly more common than is recognized or acknowledged. Slightly more than half of the 17,000 middle-class, middle-aged participants in the ACE study had grown up in dysfunctional alcoholic homes, homes with a depressed or mentally ill person, or homes in which they had experienced sexual, physical, or emotional abuse. And these events were highly correlated with pharmacy costs, doctor visits, emergency-room visits, hospitalization, and premature death. A more recent long-term study from the Netherlands showed that stress in early childhood (up to age five) makes the brain mature faster during adolescence.[9] Faster maturation may be an effective survival mechanism, but it prevents the brain from learning how to adjust to current conditions in a healthy way. The study also found that children who experienced stress later on, between ages fourteen and seventeen, experienced slower brain maturation during these adolescent years, with a higher risk of developing antisocial personality traits. While the effects on the brain are different depending on when the stress was experienced, both sets of effects are extremely unhealthy and are a cause for major concern.

In reflecting on the enormous consequences of all this, ACE researcher Vincent Felitti, M.D., wrote: "If the treatment implications of what we found in the ACE study are far-reaching, the prevention aspects are positively daunting. The very nature of the material is such as to make one uncomfortable. Why would one want to leave the relative comfort of traditional organic disease and enter this area of threatening uncertainty that none of us has been trained to deal with?"

I know what Dr. Felitti is talking about. It's ever so much easier for both doctor and patient to ignore what's really going on; but it's ever so much more satisfying and effective to get to the heart of the matter. After all, our bodies never lie and they're always trying to get us to see the truth. So I suggest a middle ground. It's prudent to use symptomatic medical treatments as a bridge across the river to true health. But we must understand that in order to truly heal on the deepest level and give our cells the "live" message that creates health, we need to change and update our beliefs and behaviors. This includes releasing emotions that we have buried. Our past is not our destiny. Our power to change is now. This power within is engaged by affirming our worthiness and lovability, updating our beliefs, feeling our true feelings, and choosing thoughts that are more uplifting and healing.

One of my patients told me, "I had a flash of insight on the way to your office today. When I was little, the only way I could get my mother's attention was to be sick. So I've had a lot of broken bones, then cancer, and now an abnormal Pap test. I just realized today that I don't have to get sick to get her attention anymore!" She added that at the moment she had that insight in the car, the sun broke through the clouds, reinforcing her insight with its brilliance.

UNDERSTANDING THE BODYMIND

The science of the mind-body connection, or psychoneuroimmunology (PNI), helps explain how the circumstances of our lives can affect our bodies. PNI and related research show that the hormonal and neurological events within the body and the subtle electromagnetic fields around and within the body form a crucial link between cultural wounding, which we think of as "psychological" and "emotional," and the gynecological or other problems women have, which we think of as "physical."

Many women who've survived sexual abuse, for example, divorce themselves from their bodies. Some experience themselves in their bodies only from the neck up. As one of my patients with continual menstrual spotting said, "I don't want to think about anything below my waist. I hate that part of my body. I wish that part of me would just go away." This was an important understanding for her; it indicated where she needed to take a step toward healing. Her menstrual spotting continually drew her attention back to a disowned part of her body that needed healing. An associate of mine sometimes has patients draw pictures of themselves. She told me of a patient with chronic pelvic pain who drew a self-portrait only from the waist up. My associate pointed out to this woman that maybe her pelvis, which she was leaving out, was using pain to try to get her attention.

If the science of the mind-body connection helps explain how our emotional and psychological wounding becomes physical, it also supports our ability to heal from those conditions. All distress, all healing of distress, and all creation of health are simultaneously physical, psychological, emotional, and spiritual.

Up until fairly recently, scientists believed that information was passed linearly in the nervous system from nerve to nerve, just like in electrical wiring. But now we know that our body organs communicate directly with the brain and vice versa through chemical messengers known as neuropeptides, the release of which can be triggered by our thoughts and emotions. It used to be believed that receptor sites for neuropeptides were located only in the body's endocrine and immune system cells, as well as in nerve cells. Now we know that body organs such as the kidneys and bowel also have receptor sites for these so-called brain chemicals. It's the same with blood cells and all immune system cells. These chemicals are part of the way in which our feelings directly affect our physical bodies.

Not only do our physical organs contain receptor sites for the neurochemicals of thought and emotion, but our organs and immune system *can themselves manufacture these same chemicals*. What this means is that our entire body feels and expresses emotion—all parts of us "think" and "feel." It is well documented, for example, that the gut makes more neurotransmitters than the brain.[10] Moreover, white blood cells produce morphine-like pain-relieving substances, and those cells in turn contain receptor sites for the same substances. Thus we each have the ability to modulate pain without medication by virtue of the mind-body connection.

Herbert Benson, M.D., of the Benson-Henry Institute for Mind Body Medicine at Massachusetts General Hospital in Boston, believes that the gas nitric oxide is the key to the power of the placebo effect. The positive and hopeful emotions a patient feels when she's taking a medication she thinks might be beneficial trigger an increase in nitric oxide in her body, and the higher levels of nitric oxide in turn have a positive effect on her health—even if the medication contains no active ingredients. The effect of nitric oxide is experienced throughout the entire body instantaneously. Nitric oxide is also associated with lower blood pressure. Benson further suggests that higher levels of nitric oxide molecules in the brain can trigger yearnings that are linked with profound spiritual experiences.

Clearly the uterus, ovaries, and breasts are also profoundly influenced by nitric oxide and all the other neurochemicals of thoughts and emotion, which include hormones. The ovaries and adrenals are primary sites of hormone production. They, along with the uterus, vagina, and breasts, are loaded with hormone receptor sites to receive messages from the brain, immune system, and other organs. It's easy, then, to understand that when we are sad, our female organs "feel" sad and their functions are affected. And when we are happy, our female organs respond in kind.

Our thoughts, emotions, and brain communicate directly with our immune, nervous, and endocrine systems and with the organs of our bodies.

Moreover, although these bodily systems are conventionally studied and viewed as separate, they are, in fact, aspects of the *same* system. If the uterus, the ovaries, the white blood cells, and the heart all make the same chemicals as the brain makes when it thinks, then *where in the body is the mind*? The answer is, *the mind is located throughout the body* and even beyond.[11] In fact, an extensive body of research on prayer has documented that our minds are nonlocal and have profound effects at a distance from our bodies.[12]

Our entire concept of "the mind" needs to be expanded considerably. *The mind can no longer be thought of as being confined to the brain or to the intellect; it exists in every cell of our bodies.* Every thought we think has a biochemical equivalent. Every emotion we feel has a biochemical equivalent. One of my colleagues says, "The mind is the space between the cells." So when the part of your mind that is your uterus talks to you, through pain or excessive bleeding, are you prepared to listen to it?

When I asked a married thirty-five-year-old lawyer who had a sudden onset of bleeding between her periods what was going on in her life, she bristled. "I think this problem is medical," she said. By that, she meant that the problem was purely physical and was not related in any meaningful way to the rest of her life. I gently explained to her that I would have asked her the same question had she broken her leg, and I pointed out that all symptoms are "physical." My patient then calmed down and told me the truth: Recently she had had an extramarital affair and was feeling guilty, and she was terrified that she had acquired a sexually transmitted disease. Her irregular bleeding had started soon after her affair began. This additional history enabled me to give her better and more appropriate medical care, while she learned that she didn't have to separate herself into unrelated parts.

One of my patients went to see a biofeedback therapist about shoulder pain caused by chronic muscle tension. While she was learning to relax the muscles of her shoulder, she noticed that her muscle tension increased whenever she was thinking certain thoughts. One of these thoughts was of being spanked as a child. Another was of her husband's ill health and its possible implications for her. On the other hand, when she thought of the positive aspects of her life, her muscle tension lessened. She came to see that her fears and beliefs were encoded in her body. Through biofeedback, she learned that her muscle tissue had feelings, thoughts, and memories that were part of her body's wisdom.

The mind and the soul, which permeate our entire body, are much vaster than the intellect can possibly grasp. Our inner guidance comes to us first through our feelings and body wisdom—not through intellectual understanding. When we search for inner guidance with the intellect only—as though it exists outside of ourselves and our own deepest knowing—we get stuck in the search, and our inner guidance is effectively silenced. The intellect works best *in service* to our intuition, heart, inner guidance, soul, God, or higher power—whichever term we choose for the spiritual energy that animates life. Once we have acknowledged that we are *more* than our intellect and that guidance is available to us from the universal mind, we have accessed our inner healing ability. As William James once said, "The power to move the world is in the subconscious mind."

We Coauthor Each Other's Biology

Mario Martinez, Psy.D., author of *The Mind Body Code* (Sounds True, 2014) and founder of the Biocognitive Science Institute, takes the mind-body connection even further. He points out that each of us has a profound effect on the biology of others: We literally coauthor each other's biology. For example, if you are treated with respect and admiration, your biology will be positively affected. But if others consider your age, race, or sexual preference not acceptable, you may well be treated with derision and even violence—and made to feel as though something is inherently wrong with you.

We humans are herd creatures. We need social support in order to maintain a healthy immune system (more on this later). And that social support consists of our families, our coworkers, and our professions—our tribe. In order to fit into our tribe, we are expected to maintain certain standards of behavior, which are enforced and become internalized.

In the fourteenth century, certain groups lived in areas surrounded by a fence, known as a pale. The group was protected as long as it stayed inside the pale. Once anyone ventured outside of that enclosure, they had moved "beyond the pale," and their tribe would no longer protect them. Though we no longer have physical pales, every tribe does, in fact, have internalized, often unspoken standards of behavior and belief that it expects its members to embrace if they are to remain safe, included, and protected. An example is the tribe of conventional medicine, which expects its members to adhere to the guidelines of their various governing bodies, such as the American Heart Association or the American College of Obstetricians and Gynecologists—groups whose guidelines are often heavily influenced by outside financial interests like the pharmaceutical industry. If a physician questions this approach or suggests that there are healthier alternatives to drugs or surgery, he or she very often pays a price. The same is true for the millions of women who've been sexually abused in the workplace for decades but dared not say anything lest the power brokers in charge punish them in some way.

Dr. Martinez points out that tribes the world over use three archetypal forms of wounding to keep their members in line: shame, abandonment, and betrayal. Each of those three wounds is accompanied by the production of inflammatory chemicals in the body, such as interleukin 6, or IL-6 (which over time creates cellular inflammation—the root cause of all chronic degenerative disease). Given that we all need to feel a sense of safety, security, and belonging in order to maintain health and well-being, it is not surprising that these wounds so effectively keep so many stuck in less than optimal conditions. We feel damned if we do and damned if we don't.

The shared belief systems handed down to us in our families and cultures often trump our own inner wisdom—such as when we're told that all women need to have children in order to feel happy and whole, or that big boys don't cry. Thus the dictates of our souls and our inner wisdom, our innate power to get and stay well, often take a backseat to cultural convention—until an illness, injury, or developmental stage like menopause wakes us up out of our cultural or familial trance.

Beliefs and behaviors are passed down in families as directly as are eye color and skin tone. And all tribes—whether they be the tribe of one's profession, one's family, one's religion, or one's social status—profoundly influence our beliefs and behaviors. If you question those standards and that behavior, you are apt to be subjected to at least one of those three archetypal wounds, each of which adversely affects your immunity until you learn how to get support elsewhere. Consider this book one of those places.

FEMININE INTELLIGENCE: HOW THOUGHTS BECOME EMBODIED

Women (and many men) have the capacity to know with their bodies and with their brains at the same time, in part because their brains are set up in such a way that the information in both hemispheres and in the body is highly available to them when they communicate.

In school I was taught to distrust my own thinking process because it never fit with the dualistic way in which education is set up. On a multiple-choice test, for example, I could always find a reason why almost every choice given might be correct. I could always see "the big picture," and I could see how everything was related to everything else. In going over my wrong answers, my teachers often told me, "You're reading too much into it. The correct answer is obvious." It was not always obvious to me. Now that I have learned to appreciate how intimately my thoughts, emotions, and physical body are connected, I have begun to reclaim my full intelligence. It is staggering to realize how many highly intelligent women think that they are stupid because so much of their intelligence has been undervalued. Linda Metcalf, Ph.D., says, "Women think that their intellects are a male construct sitting inside their heads."

I have learned that like many women, I speak and think in a multimodal, spiral way, using both hemispheres of my brain and the intelligence of my body all at the same time. Anthropologist and visionary writer Jean Houston, Ph.D., describes the evolution of multimodal thinking like this: "For centuries, women stood in their caves, stirring the soup with one hand, bouncing the baby on one hip, and kicking the woolly mammoth out the door with the other foot." We evolved having to focus on more than one task at a time—understanding innately the consequences of our actions, not just for ourselves but for our entire family unit or tribe.

It makes sense that this way of thinking would evolve in the gender that had to balance so many different demands and responsibilities, and that the structure of women's brains would support this multimodal, multitasking approach to life.[13] In most women, the corpus callosum, the part of the brain that connects the right and left hemispheres, is thicker than it is in most men. That is, male and female brains are "wired" differently. Most men, most of the time, use their left hemispheres to think and to communicate their thoughts; their reasoning is usually linear and solution-oriented. It "gets to the point." Alison Armstrong, author of The Queen's Code (PAX Programs, 2013), teaches that most men are either in hunter mode (getting to the point) or warrior mode (concealing what they really feel so it won't be used to hurt them). Most women, in contrast, are gatherers. They seek connection and relatedness, thus recruiting more areas of the brain when they communicate than do most men. In addition, they use both the right and the left sides of their brain simultaneously. Because the right hemisphere has richer connections with the body than the left hemisphere, women have more access to their body wisdom when speaking and thinking than do most men.

This doesn't mean that male brains inherently lack this capacity. It's just that for centuries they haven't been encouraged to develop it. For the last 5,000 years, Western society has believed that a linear, left-brain approach is the superior mode of communication and that a woman's more embodied way of speaking and thinking is inferior and less evolved. Anne Moir, Ph.D., and David Jessel, the authors of the book Brain Sex (Viking Penguin, 1989), point out, "Men, it seems, are the sex who say the first thing that comes into their heads, while women communicate by calling on a much wider repertoire. Taken all together the evidence paints a comprehensive picture of a busier and wider interchange of information in the female brain."[14] Unfortunately, instead of developing embodied thinking deliberately, as an inherent strength, we learn to reject and denigrate this capacity.

In a dialogue with sociolinguist Deborah Tannen, Ph.D., Robert Bly said, "Words are in one lobe of the brain and feelings in the other. So that means women have an ability to mingle those much quicker than men can. Women have a superhighway going on there. And, as Michael Meade remarked, men have this little crooked country road, and you're lucky if a word gets over."[15]

My ex-husband used to say to me, "Can't you say that in fewer words? Can't you get to the point?" This expresses a stereotypically male communication style. When I think or speak, I use language to express the richness of what goes on in my mind and body while I'm communicating my thoughts. I like to hang out with language and wander around in it. I often come to understand how I'm feeling by talking about it for a while, letting my thoughts arise from my whole body and whole brain before speaking them. Processing ideas verbally or writing down my thoughts helps me to know more of myself.

In contrast, my ex-husband used as few words as possible. He and men like him want to get to the point, the product or solution, and everything has to have one, otherwise it is not worth talking about. Most men view and experience the *process* of getting to the point as tedious and worthless. George Keller, M.D., a colleague in holistic medicine, put it this way: "When men talk, they leave out the verbs. When women talk, they leave out the nouns." Alluding to quantum physics, which teaches that particles and waves are simply different aspects of matter, Dr. Keller observes, "Men speak particle language. Women speak wave language."

Multimodal, embodied thinking makes it possible for most women to go to the grocery store without a list and still remember everything they came to buy, plus other stuff that they suddenly remember they need. When my children were little and I was doing a lot of surgery, I was able to do the surgery and simultaneously know what my kids were doing and that I needed to pick up paper towels and bread on the way home. My husband, on the other hand, was able to hold only one or two thoughts and tasks in his mind simultaneously—and often forgot what he was going to the store for in the first place.

It's very healing and empowering for women to understand the fullness of their intelligence, appreciating the crucial role that inner guidance, intuition, and emotions all play in feminine intelligence. Once we embrace and celebrate these aspects of ourselves, our perception changes. We can then celebrate the differences between male and female intelligence without making men, or ourselves, wrong or inferior.

BELIEFS ARE PHYSICAL

Thoughts are an important part of our body's wisdom because we have the ability to change our minds (and our thoughts) as we learn and grow. This fact became the basis for the late Louise Hay's astoundingly successful *New York Times* bestseller *You Can Heal Your Life* (Hay House, 1987), which she self-published at the age of sixty and which has helped millions of people all over the planet to access their power to heal. A thought held long enough and repeated enough becomes a belief. The belief then becomes biology. Beliefs are vibrational forces that create the physical basis for our individual lives and our health. We actually do create our own reality—thought by thought, emotion by emotion. And once you realize the power inherent in this, you find that you actually have the keys to the ignition of your life. We become able to use the body as a playground for higher vibrational frequencies instead of simply waiting for something to go wrong. Simple. Not easy.

If we don't work through self-destructive, lower-vibrational thoughts and subsequent feelings ("I am worthless," "I'll never be good enough"), our destructive thoughts and suppressed emotions set us up for physical distress because of the biochemical effect that emotions have on our immune and endocrine systems. Diseases such as rheumatoid arthritis, multiple sclerosis, certain thyroid diseases, and lupus erythematosus, for example, are all called autoimmune diseases, meaning that the immune system allegedly attacks the body.

Medical medium Anthony William says this is categorically untrue and that our bodies are always working to help us heal—and that the very idea that our own immune system would attack us is, itself, very disempowering. I agree with this. Still, it is quite clear that cellular inflammation is the root cause of all these conditions, regardless of what's behind it. And so the key to healing is to replace any and all inflammatory thoughts (such as "I'm worthless" or "I'm unlovable") and behaviors ("Don't take my wine away from me—I need it to relax" or "Why bother even trying? Things never work out for me") with kinder, more compassionate ones (like "Wow! My blood pH is always in the right range. I don't have to do anything to maintain it. My body is amazing!" or "Just imagine—when I sleep at night, my heart keeps beating and I keep breathing. This happens all on its own. I am so grateful").

The literature linking specific thoughts and behaviors with disease is vast. Here are a few examples. Mental depression has been associated not only with self-destructive behaviors but also with depression of immune system functioning.[16] Depression is also an independent risk factor for heart disease and osteoporosis. Many women with autoimmune diseases suffer from depression as well. Studies have shown, for example, that stress and loneliness can help cause latent (inactive) herpesvirus to become active.[17] The same is true for those with Epstein-Barr virus, the virus linked with chronic fatigue syndrome and fibromyalgia, which William says is responsible for the symptoms of not only chronic fatigue but also Hashimoto's thyroiditis. The link between emotional stress and the flare-up of Epstein Barr is one reason why, even though over 90 percent of the population has been exposed to and has antibodies to Epstein-Barr virus, only a small percentage actually suffer from the disease. The same is true for those suffering from gastric ulcers associated with H. pylori bacteria and from yeast-related diseases. This information is especially relevant to women, since at least 80 percent of all so-called autoimmune disease occurs in us.[18] Even endometriosis, cancer, diabetes, epilepsy, premature menopause, infertility, and chronic vaginitis all have cellular inflammation in common.

What an individual believes is heavily influenced by the culture in which she lives. Beliefs held in common perpetuate the type of society in which we live. Given our society, it is not surprising that women feel so much stress. In several scientific studies, inescapable stress has been associated with a distinct form of immunosuppression (suppression of immune system response). Emotional shock is associated with the release of endogenous opiates (morphine-like substances) and corticosteroids (hormones from the adrenal glands), which prevent white blood cells from protecting the body from cancer and infection. One recent study of more than 54,000 civilian women showed a threefold higher risk of developing the autoimmune disease lupus among those suspected of having post-traumatic stress disorder and twice the risk among women who had experienced any traumatic event.[19]

People who have a sense of hopelessness or despair and who perceive their situation as being uncontrollably stressful have higher levels of corticosteroids and immune suppression than do those who have more resilient coping styles.[20] People who are exposed to what they perceive as inescapable stress actually release opioid-like substances (enkephalins) that literally numb the cells of their bodies (in stress-induced analgesia),[21] rendering those cells incapable of destroying cancer cells and bacteria if this goes on chronically.[22]

A young woman I know spent the summer doing volunteer work in a foreign country that was trying to recover from a natural disaster that had left it racked with severe economic challenges, serious health crises, and high levels of crime. Because of the dangerous conditions, this young woman was placed within a walled, guarded compound and told she could not leave unless she was with someone else. Soon after she arrived, she found that due to the inefficient infrastructure, she wouldn't be able to accomplish anywhere near as much as she had hoped to do to help. She felt trapped, isolated, extremely disappointed, and powerless to improve her situation.

Within the first few weeks, she had a bout of serious diarrhea that her digestive system never fully healed from. After she returned home, these difficulties continued. Another bad bout of diarrhea kept her in bed for a week. At that time, she also suffered a horrendous urinary tract infection and began having annoying neurological symptoms. An MRI indicated she had transverse myelitis, an inflammatory condition characterized by damage to the myelin, the layer of insulation that protects nerve cell fibers, in one section of the spinal cord. Several things can cause this condition, including infections and immune system disorders. After seeing no additional spots on subsequent MRIs, the woman's neurologist told her it seemed likely that her condition could be traced to the infection she had developed abroad. For some reason, the doctor told her, her immune system had overreacted to an infection her body normally would have been able to easily clear, attacking the myelin. To me, the reason seemed obvious: her sudden overwhelming feelings of being trapped, isolated, and powerless in a place far from her usual support network.

The most crucial thing to understand in such instances is this: It is not stress itself that creates immune system problems. It is, rather, the perception that the stress is inescapable—that there is nothing a person can do to prevent or change it—that is associated with immune system suppression. But perception can always be changed. And *that* is the key to getting and staying well.

It is important to understand that our beliefs go much deeper than our thoughts, and we cannot simply will them away or cover them over with affirmations or vision boards (though these actions can be helpful). Many beliefs are completely unconscious and are not readily available to the intellect. Some are even handed down in the DNA of families, which has been beautifully documented in Mark Wolynn's book *It Didn't Start with You* (Viking, 2016). Most of us aren't aware of the destructive beliefs that undermine our health. They don't come from the intellect alone, the part that thinks it's in control. They come from the other part that in the past became lodged and buried in the cell tissue.

Jean, a lovely dark-haired graphic designer, came to me for a consultation. At forty-five years old, she was concerned that her periods had changed over the years from a pattern of every twenty-eight days to every twenty-five to thirty-four days. She had no spotting in between and no other symptoms. This history sounded completely normal to me, but another doctor had told her that her cycle change might represent cancer. He had recommended a uterine biopsy. Because her cervical opening was too small to allow a biopsy instrument to enter, a D&C under general anesthesia was suggested. Jean decided to seek a second opinion. Her exam was normal, but she did in fact have a very small cervical opening and therefore could not have an office biopsy. Her ultrasound showed a normal uterine lining.

I told Jean that I thought she was a very unlikely candidate for uterine cancer and that I wouldn't recommend a D&C. If she was really worried and wanted one, I said, it could certainly be done to be sure she didn't have cancer. To help her make her decision, I asked her what her childhood experience of illness had been, since a woman's childhood experience tends to profoundly influence her beliefs around health and disease. Jean said, "I was an only child, and my mother was always sick. She constantly had bowel problems. I had to take care of her. As a result, I personally react to everything that happens in my body as though it's a catastrophe—just as my mother did."

Then I said, "If you decided to have a D&C and it turned out to be normal, would you be able to relax and stop obsessing over cancer?" She said that it wouldn't make any difference. She'd still worry. We agreed then that she had to change her belief system about her body and its vulnerability, which had been so firmly influenced by her early years.

To do this, Jean needs to understand that her fear is not entirely accessible to her intellect. Much of it is in her body and her subconscious mind. Telling Jean, or women with similar problems, to "just relax, you're fine, it's nothing" and that "it's all in your head" is not helpful or scientifically accurate. While Jean's belief is indeed in her mind, her mind is located throughout her body and in every organ in it.

For Jean to stop obsessing about cancer (or anything else), she will have to go through the same process that every one of us must go through to heal. To explain this process to patients, I used the first three steps of the twelve-step program, which originated with Alcoholics Anonymous. Since these twelve steps are based on spiritual truths, I've found them applicable to nearly every aspect of life about which I or my patients are seeking guidance. Step one is: "We admitted we were powerless over alcohol and that our lives had become unmanageable." Instead of the word *alcohol,* you can substitute anything that you currently are obsessing about or feel powerless over. In Jean's case, she must admit that she is powerless to change her belief and obsession about cancer with her intellect alone. She must also admit that this belief is not healthy and that it is making parts of her life unmanageable. Her belief won't go away if she beats herself up about it or tries to force herself to change it with her intellect alone. She must also understand that the obsessive thought is trying to keep her from feeling something she may not want to feel. (The intellect likes to think it's in control at all times.) But you have to feel in order to heal.

The second step is: "We came to see that a power greater than ourselves could restore us to sanity." This power "greater than ourselves" is a part of our inner guidance and bodily wisdom. You can even think of it as your soul—the part of you that lives beyond time and space. The word *sanity* means the same thing as inner peace or serenity. Acknowledging that we have access to guidance from a power greater than our own intellect is a very positive step toward actually accessing that guidance.

The third step is: "We made a decision to turn our will and our lives over to the care of God *as we understood Him.*" (You can change the word *Him* to *inner guidance* or *divine wisdom, higher self,* or *Divine Mother.*) This step bypasses the intellect entirely. It is a leap of faith that acknowledges the fact that all of us have inner guidance available within us and that this guidance has the power to remove our harmful beliefs. The words *made a decision* are very important. To create health, a woman needs to make a decision to do it. Then she must be willing to stay with the process. Participating in twelve-step meetings and working the steps around a fear, a belief, or even an illness that you've found your intellect to be powerless over can be very helpful and practical. As previously mentioned, I also love the affirming work of the late

Louise Hay, who wrote the classic *You Can Heal Your Life*. Of course, many other modalities can help rewrite our internalized negative scripts as well, including the Emotional Freedom Technique and eye movement desensitization and reprocessing (EMDR). (For more on this, see chapter 15.)

For Jean and thousands of women like her, the knowledge that she is not alone in her fears and obsessions is itself very helpful. I've never met anyone who didn't inherit at least some health-destroying beliefs either from her family or from the culture in general. By choosing to move forward into health and joy, we can uncover the deep programming of our bodies and change it to support health. The reason this works is that the very process of deciding to be happier or healthier will automatically bring up the thought patterns that have prevented greater happiness and health in the first place. Many women have been able to change their states of health and their lives once they understand that although their diseases are very real and physical, these diseases are often accompanied and reinforced by unconscious beliefs. Uncovering these and healing from them is a continuous, exciting, and empowering process. It is part of the process of creating health. It requires patience and compassion. And it works.

Beliefs and memories are actually biological constructs in the body. Think of your mind as an iceberg. The conscious part—the part that thinks it's in control—is what appears above the surface. But it amounts to only about 5 percent of the total iceberg. The so-called subconscious part of your mind is the much larger part—95 percent of it lies below the surface. Our personal histories are stored throughout our bodies, in muscles, organs, and other tissues. This information, like the submerged portion of the iceberg, is not generally recognized by the part of the iceberg on the surface, our conscious intellect. Our cells contain our memory banks—even when the conscious mind is not aware of them and actually battles to deny them.

Once when I called a bellman to my hotel room to help me with my bags, he noticed a bottle of Chinese cough syrup near the sink. He made a face, held his stomach, and said, "I thought that was castor oil, and I remember that my mother gave it to me often as a child. I used to have stomach pains after taking it. Just looking at the bottle now gives me a stomachache!" This man had no conscious control over his body's memory of his childhood pain. His body automatically reacted to the sight of a familiar-looking bottle even though the contents were entirely different.

On a different occasion, I was hiking with a woman who told me that two weeks before, she had gotten some sunscreen in her eye and her eye had watered all day from the irritation. Several days later, she merely smelled the same sunscreen when someone else was using it, and her eye started to water again. Her biological memory was already encoded in her eye. Her intellect had been bypassed entirely!

How Beliefs Become Physical

At any given time, our state of health reflects the sum total of our beliefs since birth. Our entire society functions under many shared and sometimes harmful beliefs. One that I hear regularly is, "Well, now that I'm thirty [or forty, or fifty], I suppose it's normal to have aches and pains." This is how our culture, not our biology, teaches us how to grow older. Mario Martinez, Psy.D., has studied 700 healthy centenarians on every continent. All of them are outliers who do not accept the common assumptions about getting older that are passed down in our cultures. I wrote my book *Goddesses Never Age: The Secret Prescription for Radiance, Vitality, and Well-Being* (Hay House, 2015), which was influenced by Dr. Martinez's work, to help women identify and overcome the ageism and expectation of deterioration that we all inherit from our culture.

All living things respond physically to the way they *think* reality is. Deepak Chopra, M.D., an authority on consciousness and medicine, uses the example of flies placed in a jar with a lid on top. Once the lid is removed, they will not leave the jar, except for a few brave pioneers. The rest of the flies have made a "commitment in their body-minds" that they are trapped. It has been shown in aquariums that if two schools of fish are separated with a glass partition for a certain amount of time, the fish will not swim into each other's space even after the partition is removed.

So it is that we can be sure the events of our childhood set the stage for our beliefs about ourselves and therefore our experience, including our health. For a woman to change or improve her reality and her state of health, she first has to change her beliefs about what is possible. This is a simple enough process. But it requires discipline and persistence.

That we have the wherewithal to overcome our destructive and unconscious patterns is a truth that I see proved daily. This power has also been documented experimentally in a study of the effects of beliefs on the aging process. Ellen Langer, Ph.D., studied a group of male volunteers over the age of seventy at a retreat center for five days. They all had to agree that they would live in the present as though it were 1959. Dr. Langer told them, "We are not asking you to 'act as if it were 1959' but to let yourself *be* just who you were in 1959." They had to dress as they had then, watch TV shows from 1959, read newspapers and magazines from that time, and talk as if 1959 were right now. They also brought pictures of themselves from that year and put them around the center. Dr. Langer then measured many of the parameters that often deteriorate with aging (but don't need to), such as physical strength, perception, cognition, taste, and hearing. The parameters reflected biological markers that experts in geriatric medicine often cite. Over the course of the five days, many of the chosen parameters actually improved. Serial photographs showed that the men looked about five years younger as well. Their hearing and memory improved. As they changed their mindsets about aging, their physical bodies changed as well.

In another of Dr. Langer's studies, hotel room attendants in seven different hotels were divided into two groups. In the informed group, room attendants were made aware that their housekeeping duties satisfied the Surgeon General's recommendation for optimal exercise. The control group did not receive any information about their work constituting healthy exercise. All participants were told that the experimenters were studying ways to improve the health and happiness of women in the hotel workplace, so everyone was weighed and had their percentage of body fat calculated and their blood pressure taken. Four weeks later, in a follow-up questionnaire, the perception of the amount of exercise they were doing had increased among the informed group while remaining the same among the control group, even though the level of exercise had not changed for either group. But the informed group's perception had changed, and that shift in perception produced remarkable improvements in health. After only one month, the group that was told that their job was good exercise had lost an average of two pounds each and had significantly reduced their percentage of body fat. The control group remained virtually unchanged. The informed group also showed significant drops in their blood pressure.[23] This is powerful evidence that changing our minds changes our bodies.

Yale researcher Becca Levy, Ph.D., a former student of Dr. Langer's, has also documented the profound effect that belief has on how we age. She found that older people with more positive self-perceptions of aging, as measured earlier, lived seven and a half years longer than those with less positive self-perceptions of aging. The most compelling part of this study is the fact that the increase in longevity for those with the more positive attitudes toward aging remained even after other factors were taken into account, including age, gender, socioeconomic status, loneliness, and overall health. The researchers used information from the 660 participants age fifty and older from a small town in Ohio who were part of the Ohio Longitudinal Study of Aging and Retirement. Dr. Levy and her coauthors compared mortality rates to responses made twenty-three years earlier by the participants (338 men and 322 women). The responses included agreeing or disagreeing with such statements as "As you get older, you are less useful." These beliefs often operate subconsciously, without our awareness, often beginning in childhood. Commenting on their research, the study's authors said, "The effect of more positive self-perceptions of aging on survival is greater than the physiological measures of low systolic blood pressure and cholesterol, each of which is associated with a longer lifespan of four years or less. It is also greater than the independent contributions of lower body mass index, no history of smoking, and a tendency to exercise; each of these factors has been found to contribute between one and three years of added life."[24]

There isn't a drug, exercise regimen, or vitamin that comes anywhere near the potential of our beliefs to add seven and a half years to our lives! And that's why examining our beliefs critically is crucial to getting and staying healthy. Dr. Langer writes, "The regular and 'irreversible' cycles of aging that we witness in the later stages of human life may be a product of certain assumptions about how one is supposed to grow old. *If we didn't feel compelled to carry out these limiting mindsets, we might have a greater chance of replacing years of decline with years of growth and purpose*" (emphasis mine).[25]

If we have the power to reverse the effects of aging, what might be possible with health? The hopefulness that these data raise cannot be overestimated. It suggests that if we can see beyond our collective cultural blindness, life holds possibilities that we've not imagined before. But before we get there, we must first acknowledge the dead ends that many of us keep falling into. Once we *see* the patterns we've been mindlessly repeating, we can create alternative routes.

HEALING VERSUS CURING

Freedom and fate embrace each other to form meaning; and given meaning, fate—with its eyes, hitherto severe, suddenly full of light—looks like grace itself.

—Martin Buber

There is a difference between healing and curing. Healing is a natural process and *within* the power of everyone. Curing, which is what doctors are called upon to do, usually consists of an *external* treatment; medication or surgery is used to mask or eliminate symptoms. *This external treatment doesn't necessarily address the factors that contributed to the symptoms in the first place.* Healing goes deeper than curing and must always come from within. It addresses the imbalance that underlies the symptoms. Healing brings together the often hidden aspects of a person's life as they relate to her illness. Healing is different from curing, though curing and the restoration of physical function may accompany healing. One can be healed completely and go on to die of her illness. This is a key understanding that is often missing from treatises on holistic medicine: Healing and death are not mutually exclusive. As a physician, I've been trained to improve and preserve life. But sometimes we need to let go of that training and accept death as a natural part of a process that is much bigger and more mysterious than we realize. Patricia Reis, who worked with many of my patients' dreams and body symptoms, put it this way: "The bigger meaning of healing is a 'wholeing,' a filling out of the missing pieces of a person's life. Sometimes this may even mean facing death in a more fully realized way. Certainly it is an opportunity to come more deeply and fully into life."

Although our entire bodies are affected by our thoughts and emotions and their various parts talk to one another, each individual's body language is unique. *No matter what has happened in her life, a woman has the power to change what that experience means to her and thus change her experience, both emotionally and physically. Therein lies her healing.* There are no simple formulas for deciphering the message behind a symptom, and only the patient herself can ultimately know what the message is about. Sometimes a woman's body, through chronic vaginitis, asks her to leave a relationship. Sometimes headaches that occur premenstrually are a sign that she needs to give up caffeine. In other women, these symptoms may be related to something entirely different. It is up to each woman to "sit with" her symptoms in a completely receptive, nonjudgmental way so that she can begin to appreciate the unique language of her body.

We don't yet understand completely why it is that one woman who has been abandoned by her husband, for example, will seem to deteriorate emotionally, mentally, and physically, blaming this particular trauma for a lifetime of woes, while another woman with a similar background will use this loss as a springboard for creating an entirely new and productive life. Some people can name an initially painful and traumatic circumstance as the stimulus from which major personal growth later arose. Childhood abuse, incest, loss of a parent, and other traumas are not absolutely linked in a cause-and-effect way with subsequent distress in adulthood. The effect of trauma on our physical, mental, and emotional bodies is determined largely by *how we interpret the event and give it meaning.*

Emotional factors are usually involved in common gynecological problems, along with diet, behavior, and heredity. I have found that most women with persistent genital warts, herpes, or ovarian cysts have experienced or are continuing to experience emotional and psychological stress or unrest. In these cases, a history of sexual abuse, abortions that haven't been resolved emotionally, or some conflict involving relationships or creativity is almost always present. These conflicts live in the body's vibrational field until they're resolved—they are healing opportunities simply waiting for our attention.

One of my ob-gyn colleagues, Maude Guerin, M.D., illustrates this beautifully by using the example of a woman named Joan who had severe endometriosis and pelvic pain. Dr. Guerin "cured" Joan with a total abdominal hysterectomy and removal of both ovaries and fallopian tubes—a standard treatment for her problem. Following surgery, however, Joan developed back pain, depression, and incapacitating hot flashes, requiring many times the regular dose of hormones. Although her pelvic pain had been "cured," in many ways she was no better off than she had been before. Instead of being healed, she had simply traded one group of symptoms for another. The surgical removal of her uterus and ovaries had not resolved the emotional con-flicts in her body's vibrational field that were the root cause of her problem.

Dr. Guerin discovered that Joan had been sexually abused at the age of six, had lived through the death of her sister at the age of sixteen, and had turned to workaholism to avoid her feelings. Despite these major traumas in her life, she had never been able to cry. Dr. Guerin writes, "This patient has been a wonderful teacher for me. Although I never discounted the concept that thoughts and feelings influence physical health, I had always perceived that influence to be relative. This patient taught me that consideration of the mind-body link is obligatory in the case of every patient, no matter how cut-and-dried their course seems to be.

"I certainly felt that I had cured this woman, and was proud of myself at her six-week checkup. It took the two of us years to learn that although she had been 'cured' by surgery, she was not healed by it.

"Looking back on her first visit with me, which I remember vividly, and her subsequent course, there were many, many clues to a much larger picture that I was unable to see at the time. On her initial office visit, she was sitting on the examination table while still wearing her pantyhose. Not only did she have trouble getting undressed for the exam, she also had a great deal of dif-ficulty even getting her body in the examination position. Once she was there, I found that placing the speculum in her vagina was nearly impossible because of her extreme anxiety and muscle tension. Since then my patients have continued to help me see the big picture, for each of them. I know that you can 'cure' many patients without acknowledging the mind-body link, but I also know that you will 'heal' very few."[26]

One of my own patients had an abnormal Pap test. She already knew that simply removing the abnormal cells from her cervix ("curing") would not address the underlying energy imbalance in her body that was at the root of the abnormality. She began working in her journal every morning with the intention of affirming her inherent ability to be whole and healthy. At the same time, she became receptive to what was necessary for her healing. She meditated on what this symptom was trying to teach her so that she could release any patterns that no longer served her. After she had been engaged in this inner healing work for several weeks, she uncovered a key belief that she felt was important to her. This belief was that the abnormal cervical cells were a punishment for her sexuality. Having discovered and named this be-lief, she proceeded to schedule standard medical therapy so that her healing and her curing would be in partnership. On her way to the appointment to have laser treatment for this condition, she experienced a wave of forgiveness toward herself and her sexuality that moved her to tears. She even felt a shift take place in her body. When she was examined at the office, all traces of the abnormality had gone, and she didn't require the surgery. She is very grateful for the physical cure, as well as the psychological and emotional healing that took place.

In this society, when a physician acknowledges a woman's innate healing ability, she or he often seems to be saying that the patient *caused* her illness to begin with. But our illnesses aren't based on simple cause and effect. It is simplistic and potentially harmful to believe that we consciously and intentionally create illness or any other painful life circumstance. Our illnesses often exist to get our attention and get us back on track. Feeling that we are to blame keeps us stuck and unable to move forward in our healing. The part of us that "creates an illness" is not a conscious part of us, but it can be affected by our consciousness once we put our healing process to work. When it comes to taking responsibility, there is a balance. We must learn to take responsibility for the things we caused or are perpetuating. On the other hand, it is equally important to let go of responsibility for those things that have nothing to do with us.

Many physicians, however, equate taking responsibility for illness with being to blame for it. Our culture in general assumes that taking responsibility means you are to blame. At the opposite extreme, other physicians feel that since their patients didn't cause their disease, they should not be overly involved in their own treatment. It is ideal, but not always possible, to have a doctor or healthcare practitioner whose beliefs can reinforce your healing. Studies have shown that the expectations that physicians have about their patients' healing potential are picked up consciously and unconsciously by their patients and do affect their ability to get well. This is how we coauthor each other's biology. Of course, all relationships, including those with our doctors, are two-way streets. As Phil McGraw, Ph.D., says, "We teach people how to treat us." When women become more empowered and able to ask for what they need, they find that they can evoke the healer that lives within the hearts of most doctors, whether conventional or alternative. And they get better care.

All relationships begin with how we treat ourselves. We can begin to heal our lives at the deepest levels when we begin to value our bodies and honor their messages instead of feeling victimized by them. Trusting the wisdom of the body is a leap of faith in a culture that fails to acknowledge how intimately the mind and body are connected. By *wisdom of the body* I mean that we must learn to trust that the symptoms in the body are often the only way that the soul can get our attention. Covering up our symptoms with external "cures" prevents us from healing the parts of our lives that need attention and change.

For healing to occur, we must come to see that we are not so much responsible for *our illnesses as responsible* to *them.* The healthiest people I know don't take their diseases or even their lives too personally. They spend very little time beating themselves up about their illnesses, their life circumstances, or anything else. They take their life one day at a time, as it unfolds in its own way and its own time. A young woman stated this attitude beautifully when she wrote, "I take full responsibility not for getting cancer in the first place, nor for ultimately surviving it, but rather for the quality of the way I am responding to this bit of chaos thrown into my life."

Healing and Mystery

The story of Martha, a close family friend, provides a most striking example of the mystery of illness and body symptoms. Though unusual in many ways, her story illustrates the range of experiences available to us when we are open to healing in whatever way it presents itself.

When Martha was in her late fifties, a series of painful childhood memories began to surface spontaneously. She allowed herself to feel fully how painful her childhood had been. She expressed and released these feelings through sobbing for hours over several days within the space of about a week. During this process she fully remembered the details of being taken to run-down bars by her bootlegger father. While she was at these places she had often watched him kissing women who were strangers. She recalled being left with an aunt for a few days while her mother broke her father out of jail. The aunt kept her and her younger sister in a cockroach-laden room with only crackers to eat and a single lightbulb hanging from the ceiling. As Martha let herself remember those and many other things that she had "deep-sixed" fifty-five years before, she was able to cry and wail for as long as she needed to as a trusted friend sat with her. This cleansing went on for several days, off and on. Afterward, she said, "I realized that there was nothing of beauty in my life when I was a child. It was worse than I ever let myself remember."

Once she was able to see this part of her life for what it really was and express her emotions around it, the chronic neck and shoulder pain that she'd had for years and that had been ascribed to "degenerative changes in her spine" went away completely. It has never come back.

One spring, Martha called me to say that she was experiencing terror of death to a degree she'd never known possible. Based on her past experience of trusting her symptoms, she decided to stay with her feelings and symptoms to see what they could teach her rather than running away from them or trying to suppress or "cure" them with drugs.

Martha is no stranger to death, having lived through the deaths of two of her children and her husband—two of these in the space of one year. Her fear of her own death, which she told me followed her to bed at night and confronted her in the morning, was accompanied by vague left-sided upper abdominal pains, which she at first misinterpreted as being related to taking penicillin for a dental infection. Her terror was so awful that she couldn't really talk about it for quite some time.

As her terror and the stomach pain became worse, her intuition suggested that she should drive across the country from New England to Taos, New Mexico, where one of her daughters lived. She wanted to be alone, and she felt that driving a long distance would be the right thing. I had never heard her so upset, but I was not worried. I trusted that she had something to work through and that I would hear from her afterward, when she was ready to talk to me. Several days later she called, still quite shaky. "It all started out on the prairie," she said. "For a couple hundred miles I drove, and then I felt this enormous emotional and physical pain. I was driving past the stockyards. There were all these cattle up to their bellies in the excrement. It hit me how we all live in all this crap and then gloss it over with scented toilet paper. I felt such sadness for the state of the world, for all the environmental problems. I thought of all the fear we always have. I found myself trudging across the prairie as a pioneer woman. I 'saw' thousands and thousands of women, of all races, all ages, trudging across the prairie, holding up the world through their labors. I felt the fear and the pain of all those women, the endless work." As these images were washing over her, she said, her stomach pain was getting worse and worse, and she had to stop the car and pull her legs up to her chest. She tasted blood in her mouth, but when she spat into a tissue, nothing was there.

"Then the flash came. I was a Viking, a male Viking. I had a huge sword. I killed a woman about to have a child. I killed them both with this sword. It was so awful to think of that. I just kept driving with tears and agony. To think that I was capable of doing such a thing! I felt such compassion for men because they were trained to do this. This pain in my stomach, the tears, the agony—this went on for about four hours. When I went over the mountain pass in the Rockies, the sun came out and I thought the pain would go away. But the horror still came. It was like some horrible dream that was real, but it wasn't.

"I needed to do this alone in an environment that wasn't 'home.' All night Friday on the day I left, the pain was on the left and seemed to be leaving. But on Saturday as I continued my trip, I'd get these waves of dread in the left side of my abdomen. That's exactly where I [the Viking] put the sword.

"When I got to Taos, I had a session with Mary, a gifted intuitive. She did a reading and felt it was not necessary for me to go any farther. This vision of the pioneer women and me as a Viking killing a pregnant woman has helped me to release my fear of death.

"I know I need to put a closure on this, I need to acknowledge it and close it. Perhaps it was necessary for the female to be killed. It was the worst thing I have ever done, the thing that I have tried to hide from God and from myself. The other thing I realized is that all of mankind has done this. We have all killed and murdered. I feel as though I have just died from another lifetime. Now I'm giving birth to myself. I can never go back to what I was before, because too much has happened to me. I can't be what I was before.

"I haven't felt my full physical energy for some time. I've always been at a physical high pitch. This experience helped me in a realization of my own death. The environment, the earth, and what we've done to it is very deep in me. I think that now I have also successfully dropped my ties to my children in the sense of holding on too tightly out of fear. I can move on now."

Martha realized that a full intellectual understanding of what had just happened to her was not necessary for her healing. She did not have to interpret the vision or experience of "being a Viking" as a past-life experience or anything else in order to heal. What was necessary was that she *feel* all of what was coming up from deep within her. After she acknowledged the act of murder, she felt freed of its burden and thus renewed. She also realized that she had to change the way she had been living. She needed to stop spending time with friends who contributed nothing to her life, in friendships that were based on habit, not mutual enrichment.

When Martha returned to her home a week later, she still felt some residual fear and dread from the experience and wanted to be free of it. She wrote down the whole thing, then went out into the backyard under a night sky full of stars, dug a hole, and burned her writing. She buried the ashes and stood up, and finally, after weeks of dread, she felt completely released.

About three weeks later, she was visiting her aunt and uncle in Ohio. Her uncle Roy took her aside and said that he didn't feel that he had much longer to live and that he had something he wanted to give her. He took her into a back room, reached up on a shelf, and handed down a bronze statue. It was a Viking with a sword.

We shared our amazement at this bit of synchronicity. ("Synchronicity is God's way of remaining anonymous," says Bernie Siegel, M.D.) Martha said, "I can have this statue in my house now. It is a symbol for me of healing. I know that if I had not allowed myself to experience this memory or dream or whatever it was, I would have developed a fatal stomach condition. I am certain of this."

This story illustrates profoundly that the notion that we are to blame for our illnesses in any conventional sense is irrelevant and narrow. In some mysterious way, our conscious intellect is *not* in control. Another part of us—our highest power, soul, or inner wisdom—is. The concept of the self needs to be expanded. Studies have documented the power of prayer to heal at a distance, instantaneously. Time and space are not absolute. We are acted upon by forces outside of our conscious control. We can be open to learning from all of life, from our inner selves, and from all that with which we are connected.

We have the body we have because it is precisely the vehicle in which we can best do what we came to do. Stevie Wonder has said that his blindness helped him feel the love that is all around him more than he would have if he were sighted. Perhaps he couldn't do the creative work he's doing if he were in a "normal" body. The late Elisabeth Kübler-Ross, M.D., pointed out that when our bodies are sick or nonfunctioning, our spiritual and mental capacities often expand way beyond what they would normally be. She used the example of children with leukemia who seem wise beyond their years.[27] I accept the truth of this on faith. We can't really hope to figure it out with our logical, intellectual selves. There are indeed more things in heaven and earth than are dreamt of in our philosophies.

Be open to the messages and mysteries of your body and its symptoms. Be eager to listen and slow to judge. What you learn can save your life.

3
Inner Guidance

To know what you prefer, instead of humbly saying "Amen" to what the world tells you you ought to prefer, is to have kept your soul alive.
—Robert Louis Stevenson

I call the high and light aspects of my being spirit and the dark and heavy aspects soul. Soul is at home in the deep, shaded valleys. Heavy torpid flowers saturated with black grow there. The rivers flow like warm syrup. Spirit is a land of high, white peaks and glittering jewel-like lakes and flowers. Life is sparse and sounds travel great distances.
—The Dalai Lama, as quoted by James Hillman in *A Blue Fire*

Right after Mary Lu was diagnosed with breast cancer, she called me to discuss her treatment options. I told her that part of her healing would be to learn how to trust herself to make her own decisions about her treatment after gathering information from a number of experts. She later wrote me, "I remember that I felt scared when I heard you affirm that in recovery, I would know what to do to deal with the cancer. I remember thinking that these were life-and-death choices and not on par with deciding how to spend some weekend. Then what flashed for me was that my soul has always been at stake all these years. My spiritual teacher at that time reminded me that I had come to my first group session with her concerned about my health. It was right after a diagnosis of ulcerative colitis and I was afraid I was killing myself. I do believe in the mind-body-soul connection. With decisions to make concerning my cancer treatment, *I had this sense that*

I would have a real chance to trust my inner guidance. Trusting myself at such a deep level was frightening to me, but I can gratefully say now, several months later, that this 'stuff' really does work, that I have trusted my process a lot through this. And each time that I have guided myself to my own healing, it gives me renewed courage to continue to trust."

Our inner guidance directs us toward that which is most life-enhancing and life-fulfilling for us. Following it can be lifesaving in medical situations as well as life-enhancing in daily situations, even those as minor as choosing what to wear. Mary Lu learned not only that she could find the surgeon she needed to work with and the treatment that worked best for her but also that she could enjoy her life at the same time, even while dealing with something as frightening as breast cancer. She did this by *allowing herself to be led by how she was feeling in each moment of the day.* Each step of the way, she moved toward the decision that felt best to her. When you move toward that which is most fulfilling and life-enhancing, healing follows.

Our inner guidance system is mediated via our thoughts, emotions, dreams, and bodily feelings. Our bodies are designed to act as receiving and transmitting stations for energy and information. Living in touch with our inner guidance involves feeling our way through life using *all* of ourselves: mind, body, emotions, and spirit. When I refer to this process in this book, I mean the various ways we listen and use our inner guidance to make conscious changes in our lives, behavior, relationships with others, and health.

TABLE 3

SOURCES OF GUIDANCE

External Guidance: Dominant Cultural View	Inner Guidance
⁓ The physical world is inferior to spirit.	⁓ Spirit informs everything.
⁓ Nature is inferior to God and must be controlled.	⁓ Nature is a reflection of divine spirit.
⁓ Human beings are superior to the natural world.	⁓ Human beings are co-creators with spirit and nature.
⁓ Behavior is based on fear and judgment.	⁓ Behavior is based on respect for self. Respect for self results in respect for others.
⁓ Difference is suspect and must be controlled.	⁓ Difference is celebrated as a reflection of the creativity of spirit.
⁓ There's only one right way to live and to be.	⁓ There are many paths to fulfillment and joy. None is superior.

External Guidance: Dominant Cultural View	Inner Guidance
Delay gratification; enjoyment and fulfillment must be earned.	Live in the moment and enjoy the process of creating.
The inherent worth of individuals is arranged in a hierarchy of superior to inferior.	Life is an interdependent, cooperative adventure with all beings connected holographically.
Guidance for behavior is dictated from external sources—by laws and institutions.	Guidance for behavior comes from connection with inner guidance.
There is such a thing as purely objective reality separate from consciousness.	The whole universe is a projection of consciousness.
Action and pushing against what we *don't* want is the only way to accomplish anything.	Consciousness creates all that is. Thoughts and feelings create reality. We can use them deliberately to improve our lives.
Support and nourishment must be earned from people and institutions outside oneself.	The individual is self-nourishing through her connection with her inner being and guidance system.
Approval from others is the basis for happiness.	Self-approval and self-acceptance are the keys to happiness.
God judges our worth.	The universe is continually unfolding. God is within every one of us and speaks through inner guidance.
It is possible to control everything and everyone.	Humans are not capable of understanding everything from a strictly physical viewpoint. Mystery is part of the wonder of life.

LISTENING TO YOUR BODY AND ITS NEEDS

We can generally trust our gut feeling about someone or something to be accurate information. This is because the solar plexus, the place in the body where we generally feel the gut reaction, is in fact a primitive brain. It is also a major intuitive center, the part of our body that lets us know whether we are safe and whether we are being lied to. Columbia researcher Michael Gershon, M.D., is a pioneer in the field of neurogastroenterology. In his book *The Second Brain* (HarperCollins, 1998), he details the discovery and gradual scientific acceptance of the enteric nervous system, which operates independently from the brain in the head. Dr. Gershon also points out that 95 percent of the body's serotonin is made in the gut.

Each of us must develop ways to tune in to our body's needs. We can start with simple things. When you're tired, rest. When you have to go to the bathroom, go. If you feel like crying when you read a certain passage in this book, let yourself cry. If you simply can't read certain parts of the text, notice them—they may refer to subjects that are painful to you. Just make a note of your reactions. Be aware of your breathing as you read: Does it speed up or slow down depending upon the material you're covering? What is your heart doing? Is it racing or is it slow? Does reading about the uterus or the menstrual cycle unearth any old memories of body feelings? Remember this: Only about 5 percent of our beliefs are conscious and readily available to our intellect. That means 95 percent of our beliefs reside in the subconscious mind. What we think we believe is only the tip of the iceberg. The rest of our beliefs operate below our radar, influencing our behavior and creating our biology.

I often ask women to pay attention to what their bodies feel like in the moment. In order to heal our bodies, we have to reenter them and experience them. (Right after I wrote that, I noticed that my legs were numb. I'd been sitting too long and had ignored my need for movement. After a ten-minute barefoot walk on the lawn and some deep breathing, my body felt much more alert and happy.)

We have to give our bodies credit for their innate wisdom. We also don't need to know exactly why something is happening in our bodies in order to respond to it. You don't need to know *why* your heart is racing or *why* you feel like crying. Understanding comes *after* you have allowed yourself to experience what you're feeling. Healing is an organic process that happens *in the body* as well as in the intellect. So if you are feeling out of sorts or off-balance, just be with that feeling; allow it to come up. After you have allowed yourself to experience it, take a moment and go back over the events of the last few hours or days. If you are feeling ill or having symptoms, reflecting on recent events may give you a clue about what preceded the symptoms.

Here's an example from my own experience. While writing this book, I woke up one morning with the visual signs and numbness of hand and face that are the symptoms of an impending migraine headache. I had developed classic migraines at the age of twelve, had one or sometimes two headaches approximately every month until my sophomore year in college, and then didn't get another one for twenty years. While growing up, I was a definite migraine personality, pushing myself mercilessly in school and in all my activities. Stress "shorted out" my body's electromagnetic system on a regular basis.

So when I began to get that old, familiar, sickening feeling, I immediately used it as an opportunity to learn. I put an ice pack under my neck, lay down, kept the room quiet, and concentrated on making my hands warm. (I had learned from a biofeedback therapist that migraines often can be aborted by relaxing totally and warming the hands.) By doing this I managed to avoid getting a full-blown headache that would have left me in pain, nauseated for most of the day, and very weak. After about one hour, I was able to resume my activities but felt very subdued. I thought back on the previous three days.

I had been tearing around the house, trying to pick up and organize years of clutter in two days. Toward the end of the weekend, my temper had been short, I had scarcely taken time to eat or go to the bathroom, and I hadn't taken a break from the bending and cleaning for hours. I had gone to bed with a dull headache. The next morning, I woke up with the migraine symptoms. It was clear to me that my ability to put my bodily needs for rest, recreation, and nurturing aside for long periods of time was intact. Only now my body wouldn't let me get away with it nearly as much as it used to. Hence the migraine. I took it as a warning, and I haven't had one since because I have finally learned how to rest and enjoy myself. It took decades.

The healing principle that summarizes this learning is this: *If you don't heed the message the first time, you get hit with a bigger hammer the next time.*

The purpose of emotions, regardless of what they are, is to help us identify and move toward the fulfillment of our needs, dreams, goals, and desires. When our needs for rest, touch, acceptance, and recognition (to name just a few) are satisfied, we feel good. And we thrive. When we feel left out, frightened, or angry, on the other hand, we can be sure that we have a need that we haven't identified, let alone figured out how to satisfy. (For an extensive list of feelings—and a separate list of the needs our feelings point to—go to www.cnvc.org or read *Nonviolent Communication: A Language of Life* [PuddleDancer Press, 2003] by Marshall Rosenberg, Ph.D.)

To become aware of our inner guidance system, we must first learn to trust our feelings. This isn't always so easy, because many of us have been taught to live our lives as though we were in a constant emergency situation. Remember that patriarchal societies are always either recovering from war or going to war. Rest is suspect and recreation is considered frivolous. They value "getting stuff done." We think, "Oh, I'll deal with that painful emotion later. Right now I don't have time. I have to get that report out [or cook dinner, or whatever it is]." This delay or denial requires our bodies to speak louder and louder to get our attention. The next time you feel moved to tears or moved to laughter, stop and experience it. It doesn't take that long. And it improves the quality of life enormously!

Many women have been taught to think—not feel—that we should be upbeat and happy all the time, an approach that inevitably results in squelching needs. Sadness and pain are natural parts of life. They are also great teachers. No one gets through life without experiencing sadness or pain. Yet our culture teaches us that there is something wrong with pain, that it must be drugged, denied, or otherwise avoided at all costs—and the costs are very high.

We are not taught that we have an innate ability to deal with pain, that our bodies know how to do this. The path is movement, sound, and tears. When a woman has just given birth, she often shakes uncontrollably—it's her body's way of recovering. When an antelope chased by a lion escapes, it shakes all over.

Crying is one of the ways in which we rid our bodies of toxins. Crying allows us to move energy around our body and sometimes to rechannel it or understand it in a different way. When we don't allow ourselves to feel our emotions and instead use addictive activities or substances such as running, alcohol, sugar, or recreational chemicals to get a high, we actually create hormones (enkephalins) that repress tears (and full emotional expression).[1] Tears contain toxins that the body needs to get rid of. When we allow ourselves a full emotional release, our body, mind, and spirit feel cleansed and free. Insight about what to do in a given situation often comes *only after* we feel our emotions about it and shed tears if necessary. Interestingly, tears of joy and tears of sorrow are physiologically and chemically distinct from each other, even though sadness and joy are very much related.[2] We cannot feel the height of our joy unless we have allowed ourselves to feel the depths of our sadness. Though joy and sadness express different emotions, both are natural parts of how our body processes and "digests" feelings. Making sounds (like moaning, crying, or singing), moving, and deep full breathing are also part of the body's emotional digestive system. They help us move through painful emotions quickly and efficiently. (See the four-cycle breathing exercise in chapter 15, page 759.)

Many illnesses are quite simply the end result of needs that have been buried, unacknowledged, and unexperienced for years—sometimes since birth or even before. One of my former patients with a long history of migraine headaches told me, "I finally hit bottom with my headaches when my neurologist wanted to put me on lithium. I knew I didn't want to deal with the effects of that drug on my body. I started biofeedback so that I could learn to relax. I had a childhood that was so painful, I had nowhere else to go but into the pain. Now I realize that I don't have to have the pain anymore. I notice that I start to get a headache the minute I stop taking care of myself. If I don't rest or get enough sleep, or if I don't stand up for myself with my family, the headaches start. I see that all along the headaches have been trying to show me something."

EMOTIONAL CLEANSING:
HEALING FROM THE PAST

Healing can occur in the present only when we allow ourselves to feel, express, and release emotions and unmet needs from the past that we have suppressed or tried to forget. I call this *emotional incision and drainage*. I've often likened this deep process to treatment of an abscess. Any surgeon knows that the treatment for an abscess is to cut it open, allowing the pus to drain. When this is done, the pain goes away almost immediately, and new healthy tissue can re-form where the abscess once was. That healthy tissue starts growing at the bottom of the abscess and works its way up to the surface. Keep that in mind, because it is the same with emotions: They, too, become walled off, causing pain and absorbing energy, if we do not experience and release them, going all the way down to their source and then bringing them all the way out by feeling them fully.

Children release emotion naturally and immediately, and each of us is born with the innate ability to do this. Unfortunately, for decades psychologists have taught parents to let their babies "cry it out" lest they become "dependent"—as though a newborn might become overly dependent on the human whose body it has just been formed in and which it must still remain in close contact with in order to learn how to regulate its breathing, heart rate, blood pressure, and temperature. Being left alone to cry it out is exactly the opposite of what human beings need, especially as children. To become emotionally secure, all of us (even adults) require attachments to other humans we can count on.

Yet because our culture worships emotional control and extols the virtues of suffering in silence, we learn early on how to suppress our natural emotional releases, and also to distance the messages behind them. When a woman is having panic attacks or crying spells, I know that some emotional material is coming to the surface to be processed. To observers who haven't experienced deep process (or emotional release), she may appear to be "losing it," "going off the deep end," or "getting out of control." She is not "out of control," however; she is simply allowing a healing process to arise within the body. Only the intellect and ego have lost control—they have taken a backseat to the innate wisdom of the body.

Too often, healthcare providers prescribe drugs in cases like this. As a result, a woman's natural healing process can get stagnated for months or years. And even if drugs are not prescribed, most people in our culture are uncomfortable with the emotions that arise when they are watching another person feel her emotions. They therefore rush to comfort the person who is beginning to cry or "lose it." This stops the person's emotional process and at the same time protects the comforter from feeling his or her own feelings. The healing process stops for both of them.

On the other hand, if a woman is encouraged to stay with what she's feeling, to go into it, to make the sounds she needs to make, and to cry or yell as long as necessary, staying completely with her innermost self, she'll often discover that her body has the innate ability to heal even very painful memories and events from her past. When we are willing to be with what is instead of running away from it, we will often be able to work through painful experiences that have lain dormant and taken up our energy for years. The late Stephen Levine, a meditation teacher and author of *Healing into Life and Death* (Anchor Press, 1987), called this experience "the pain that ends the pain."

When we have allowed ourselves a full emotional release, we end up experiencing compassion for the hurting part of us that has been crying out for acknowledgment and validation. As adults, we come to realize that we now have the skills and strength to get those unmet needs of long ago met directly. As a result, our body, mind, and spirit feel cleansed and free. Insights come up and long-buried self-understanding returns. I've watched people forgive themselves and others after deep process work because they are finally at peace with painful events in their pasts. This can happen even after years of intellectualizing that never really healed them. They naturally lighten up and are eventually able to laugh at themselves and their pasts.

One striking example of this was the deep process of an infertility surgeon I'll call Janine. Janine had found it very painful when she was not able to help a woman become pregnant, in spite of using all of the current technology at her disposal. Though the treatment of infertility is not an exact science, she took her couples' failures to conceive very personally. This made her emotional attitude toward her professional life fraught with sadness.

During a workshop I was leading, the discussion turned to the subject of mothers, and many of the participants began to cry. Janine got down on a mat and allowed herself to cry and wail. During this process she kept repeating, "I don't need to create any more mommies. I don't need to create any more mommies." When she was finished, she realized that she herself had never really had a mother in an emotional sense. Her mother had repeatedly beaten Janine when she was a child. Janine had chosen to be an infertility physician in part because of her unresolved early childhood pain: On an unconscious level, she was trying to "create mommies" in an attempt to create the mother she emotionally needed but never had. Following this deep insight, she was able to go back to her work refreshed and free, finally released from assuming complete responsibility for her patients' conceptions.

DREAMS: A DOORWAY TO THE UNCONSCIOUS

Dreams are another part of our inner guidance system. Scientific evidence shows that the amount of activity in our brain when we dream is identical to the amount when we are awake. During dreaming, our inner guidance works with our brain to lay down a map of the activities or goals that we desire or need for a healthy balanced future. Dreams also show us the beneficial and nonbeneficial directions toward which we are focusing our energy and how and where we need to make adjustments. Dream expert and clinical psychologist Doris E. Cohen, Ph.D., reminds us that every player in a dream is a part of our own unconscious.

One of my former patients who was healing from chronic pelvic pain related to me that as she healed, she became more and more competent and powerful in her dreams. She said it was fun to go to sleep at night to see what she'd be capable of next.

Another patient, recovering from incest, said, "I recently dreamed that a little four-year-old girl was trying to tell me about someone who hurt her. I know that I am that girl—and that I need to listen to her in my dreams."

Another woman, suffering from chronic vaginitis, asked her dreams for guidance about what to do, since none of our physical treatments was helping. She came back a week later and said, "I had the dream. Everything was black, and I heard a voice say, 'When you get rid of Larry, the problem will go away.'" She eventually was able to tend to her relationship problems, and her condition began to clear.

Years ago, I returned from a trip to Italy. When I arrived home, I dreamed that I was going to lunch at one of my favorite restaurants on the water. When I got there, I saw that a nearby store had a clothesline strung out front. On it were the two dresses that I had bought in Italy, from a line called Save the Queen! I couldn't believe that this local store not only had the very garments I'd thought were so special in Italy but also had a whole lot more of the same brand that I hadn't even seen while traveling. I began to try on other garments that were even better than the ones I had purchased abroad. And they all fit. In this dream, I was made aware of the fact that everything that I needed to present myself to the world in a royal fashion (the Save the Queen! label) was, in fact, right in my backyard. I didn't have to travel to find it— kind of like Dorothy when she wakes up back in Kansas in *The Wizard of Oz*. I found this dream very reassuring and fun.

Learn to pay attention to your dreams by writing them down first thing in the morning. Plan to remember them before you go to bed at night. Keep a notebook and pen beside your bed. Or dictate them into your mobile phone and transcribe them later.

STEP-BY-STEP PROCESS FOR
BRINGING DREAM WISDOM TO CONSCIOUSNESS

The following is the precise process I have used to glean wisdom from my dreams for many years. I learned it from Doris E. Cohen, Ph.D., with whom I have processed dreams regularly for nearly a decade.

1. Recall and record the dream. Do this the minute you awaken, or even in the middle of the night. Don't make the mistake of thinking you'll remember later; you most likely won't.

2. Give the dream a title, like the headline of a newspaper story. This will capture the essence of the guidance your unconscious is trying to convey.

3. Read the dream out loud. Hearing your own voice will make the message clearer.

4. Consider what is uppermost in your life right now.

5. Describe the objects in your dream or the qualities as though you were talking to someone from another planet. For example: You dream of a hotel room. What is a hotel room? It's temporary lodging. Or if you dream about your childhood home, you can be sure that the dream is letting you know about childhood issues.

6. Summarize the message from your unconscious.

7. Consider the dream's guidance for waking life.

If you dream about something or someone you've recently seen in a movie or on television, the dream is almost certainly *not* about them—and you didn't dream about them simply because you were just watching them in a movie. The unconscious is very efficient, simply using that actor or that situation to bring your attention to the issue at hand. For example, I had a dream about Jake, the assassin in the television show *Scandal* who was in love with the main character, Olivia Pope. Jake was a stand-in for something precious to me in a man—loyalty, skill, and commitment. And that was the message from my dream.

Here are a few other things to keep in mind: The hair on your head often represents the thoughts in your head. Shoes and clothes can represent the various roles we play in life. Airplanes, trains, and cars frequently signify the vehicles that take us through our lives. For more information, I highly recommend Dr. Cohen's book *Dreaming on Both Sides of the Brain: Discover the Secret Language of the Night* (Hampton Roads, 2017).

Another excellent reference is *Dreams That Can Save Your Life: Early Warning Signs of Cancer and Other Illnesses* (Findhorn Press, 2018) by Larry Burk, M.D., and Kathleen O'Keefe-Kanavos. The authors detail medical research on the diagnostic power of precognitive dreams and give information on keeping a dream journal and using it to interpret your dreams.

INTUITION AND INTUITIVE GUIDANCE

Intuition is the direct perception of truth or fact *independent of any reasoning process*. It is the ability to make the right decision with insufficient information. It is also our first sense, not our sixth sense. It's the one we're born with—and then get talked out of early on by a culture that favors left-brain reasoning.

A very good example of intuition is when you walk into a dark room and somehow know that someone is in there, even when you can't see anything and haven't been told anyone is there. Or when you know who is calling before the phone rings. We are all born with this ability, and all of us were highly intuitive as children. Most of us, however, were trained out of this way of knowing by the age of seven, when the frontal lobe reasoning centers come on board and tend to drown out the intuitive voice. The more education we get in this culture, in general, the less we trust our natural intuition. Because our society glorifies mostly logical, rational, left-brain thinking, we are taught to discount other forms of knowing as primitive or ignorant.

Thus, our intuitive capacity has become suspect and underutilized. Yet it is a skill that can be relearned at any time because it is a completely natural way of knowing. Although addictions keep us out of touch with what we know and what we feel, and although most of us are out of touch with our intuition much of the time, as we become more inner-directed and more in touch with our inner guidance system, we automatically gain access to our intuition. Our society admits that even the geniuses among us use only about 25 percent of their brain capacity. To use intuition is simply to use more of our intelligence than we are accustomed to using.

Intuitive guidance is the ability to read our own (or another's) energy field. Intuitive guidance is centuries old and has been part of many ancient healing systems. Every traditional shaman has worked in this way, as have healers in the Wicca tradition.[3] Intuitive guidance can help us detect energy blockages *before* they become physical. We can act on this information and keep ourselves healthy.

HOW INNER GUIDANCE WORKS

One of my medical student friends who has back issues has noticed that her back pain always emerges when she has to do something that she doesn't want to do. (This is true in spite of the fact that she has a so-called physical problem that should, by itself, explain her symptoms.) Not long ago she was contemplating writing a research paper. Whenever she even thought about writing this piece and about the colleagues with whom she would be involved, she got neck pain and felt sick to her stomach. All her training had taught her that publishing this research paper was what she *should* do for her career. Yet her inner guidance, speaking through her body's feelings, was telling her something quite different. She knew that if she was to remain healthy, she had to take the radical step of choosing between her inner guidance and what society was telling her was best. This friend eventually created a very satisfying career quite different from what she'd always thought she'd be doing—working in a hospital for a lab! Her body led her to it. My entire career in women's health began when I first saw a baby born when I was in medical school and nearly fell to the floor weeping with the wonder of it all. Talk about an intuitive message from my body!

Our bodies are designed to function best when we're doing work that feels exactly right to us. If we want to know God's will for us, all we have to do is look to our gifts and talents—that's where we will find it. Health is enhanced in women who engage in work that satisfies them. If a woman wants to know what her gifts and talents are, she can think back to when she was age nine to eleven, before the culture really put her into a trance. What did she love to do? What did she want to be? Who did she think she was? One of my close friends remembered that when she was about ten, she and her brothers often played around a junk car lot in a nearby field. Her brothers would help her pull the seats out of the cars. She then set them up as a "hospital" and had her brothers lie down as patients—a portent of her career as a nurse.

Another way to get in touch with our gifts and talents is to ask ourselves what we would do or be if we knew we had only six months to live. Would we stay at our current job? With our current partner?

We are meant to move toward whatever gives us fulfillment, personal growth, and freedom. We are born knowing what activities, things, thoughts, and feelings are associated with these qualities. We must learn to trust ourselves and know that we can naturally move toward that which is healing and fulfilling.

Many people have been taught that they can't have what they want and that a life full of struggle is somehow more honorable than one full of joy. We grow up believing that suffering buys us something. We have also been taught to distrust something if it is considered too fulfilling or if it is associated with too much pleasure or with having too much fun.

How many times have you been laughing in a restaurant or at home and had someone say, "You're having too much fun over there"? This belief is reflected in our bodies. An eminent hypnosis researcher once noted that negative effects, like blisters, were twice as easy to induce as positive outcomes.[4] Yet when we can clearly state what we want and why, we are instantly in alignment with our inner guidance. This is because it feels good in our bodies to think about and dwell upon what we want and why. We get excited and are inspired automatically by these thoughts and feelings, which in turn keep us in touch with our inner knowing and spiritual energy. The result is enthusiasm and joy—the feeling of heaven on earth.

Our culture has too often taught us that it is selfish to have our own wants and dreams and to enjoy ourselves. Many girls, when they are in touch with their inner power, have been told, "Who do you think you are, the Queen of Sheba?" Too many of us have heard "Don't break your arm patting yourself on the back" when we have done a job we're proud of or have given ourselves credit for something that we loved to do, just for us. All our lives, this kind of statement has stopped us dead in our tracks. We are accused of being selfish when we've given our own lives and interests priority. We have been brought up to avoid being seen as selfish at all costs. We learn to earn love and acceptance through self-sacrifice because we don't feel worthy of the best that life has to offer.

Please understand, I am not advocating self-indulgence and self-centeredness here. There is a vast difference between pursuing the things that call to you and expecting the world to serve you. Indeed, an estimated one in five people has what's called a character or personality disorder, which includes narcissistic personality disorder, borderline personality disorder, and antisocial personality disorder. One in twenty-five people is a full-blown psychopath with no conscience whatsoever.[5] These individuals wreak havoc in their families, in their other relationships, and in society in general and are a huge public health problem. I wrote an entire book on the subject, called *Dodging Energy Vampires: An Empath's Guide to Evading Relationships That Drain You and Restoring Your Health and Power* (Hay House, 2018). If you have one of these individuals in your life, you may find yourself trying very hard to make up for the damage they do by being über-conscientious and über-responsible—to your own detriment. I bring this up because too many women (and men) have spent a lifetime trying to please one of these individuals, and their health has suffered mightily as a result.

That said, most women in our culture have a difficult time going after what they personally want and need in an atmosphere in which it is assumed that they will be responsible for all of the tasks of daily living such as child rearing and housekeeping. On the other hand, if these activities are precisely what a woman wants to do the most, she may find that they are undervalued and underpaid. However, nothing will change in a woman's outer circumstances until she learns to value her own life and her own gifts as much as she has been taught to value and nurture the lives of others. As a friend of mine says, "If you want to be one of the chosen, all you have to do is choose yourself!"

Nearly every woman I know has been socialized to believe that putting everyone else before herself is the right thing to do. Just the opposite is true—we can't really be there for others unless we're there for ourselves first.

I love the way entrepreneur Danielle LaPorte once put it on her website (www.daniellelaporte.com):

> I notice this in myself, I see it in other people: the happiness muffle. We feel the sparkle, really we do. We feel rich with gratitude, we're keenly aware of a true smile curled in our cells. We tend to live on the light side of things. But we don't pronounce it. As a new friend just put it, "We butt back the joy because . . . happiness is a form of power."
>
> Is that any way to treat happiness?
>
> Happiness *is* power. Happiness is carbonated consciousness. It wants to spill out and radiate and be articulated. And every time we downplay our joy we confuse our synapses. Our brain is firing smiley neurons and our mouth is short-circuiting them. Repeated happiness muffling numbs our senses. If you keep it under the surface too long, it just might stay there—a light under a bushel.
>
> So do us all a favor. No matter what the weather, the odds, the circumstances, the company, if you're happy and you know it, by all means, say so!

I couldn't agree more. As a physician, I can assure you that happiness is also healing. Here's an example.

Dana Johnson, a researcher friend of mine and a registered nurse, recovered from Lou Gehrig's disease (amyotrophic lateral sclerosis, or ALS) by learning the power of love and happiness. After she had had the disease for some years, she began to lose control over her breathing muscles as well as the rest of her body. Her breathing difficulties made her think she was going to die. But she decided at that point that she wanted to experience unconditional love for herself at least once before dying. Describing herself as a "bowl of Jell-O in a wheelchair," she sat every day for fifteen minutes in front of a mirror and chose different parts of herself to love. She started with her hands because at that time they were the only parts of herself that she could appreciate unconditionally. Each day she went on to other body parts. Day by day, her physical body began to get better as she learned to appreciate it. She also wrote in a journal about insights she had during this process, and she came to see that since childhood she had believed that in order to be of service, acceptable to others, and worthy, she had to sacrifice her own needs. It took a life-threatening disease for her to learn that service through self-sacrifice is a dead end. In fact, the effect of psychological factors has been strongly correlated with the length of survival with ALS. Given that ALS has no known cause and no known cure, the importance of these factors can't be underestimated.[6] Although feeling good about being of service simply for its own sake is health-enhancing, far too many women bake cookies, make coffee, and clean up because it's expected of them and they would feel guilty (and unworthy) if they didn't do it. Service to others done under a sense of obligation creates exhaustion, burn out, and resentment.

Knowing What We Don't Want

In addition to knowing what we *do* want, we have the capacity to know what we *don't* want. Knowing what we don't want is inborn. Every baby knows what feels good and what doesn't feel good, and up until about the age of six, a child will automatically go toward what feels good and away from what feels bad. This capacity is seen in its purest form in a two-year-old child who has just learned how to say no. I laugh with delight when my two-year-old granddaughter says to me, "Lulu, stop it." She is learning to set her boundaries. But she is also learning good social skills like saying "please" and "thank you." (By the way, the only fears that a baby is born with are the fear of falling and the fear of loud noises. Every other fear is learned.)

The ability to say no to what doesn't support you is an essential part of your inner guidance system. It is never too late to start saying no to those things that drain you and yes to those that replenish you.

~ When a friend calls and asks for help, say to your friend, "Let me get back to you on that." Then stop for a moment and ask yourself, "Do I really want to help right now, or would I prefer to do something else?" If your answer to a request isn't an immediate yes, it's probably a no. If the answer is no and your friend gets resentful, it's time to question the validity of that friendship.

~ Check your body when someone asks you to do something. Are there areas of tension? Do you get a gut reaction of any kind? Does your body say, "Yes, this would be fun," or does it say, "No, doing this would be draining"?

~ If you find yourself tired or irritable at the end of a day, ask yourself what needs didn't get met. Also ask what thoughts, activities, or people drained your energy during the day.

~ On the days when you are feeling wonderful, ask yourself what thoughts, activities, or people enhance your energy flow.

~ Keep a journal and begin to notice and write down everything that contributes to a positive energy flow that replenishes you. Paying attention to these things will draw more of them into your experience.

~ Practice appreciation and gratitude, writing down all the blessings in your life. Remember that what we pay attention to expands.

~ Tap into the power of attention. Consciously directing our attention to thoughts, emotions, and circumstances that feel good and uplifting is powerful medicine. Paying attention to and appreciating what is working well in your life changes your vibration rate—the frequency at which you resonate. And you will attract more good things.

One of my former patients, a social worker, originally came to see me complaining of PMS and mild anxiety attacks. In going over her history, I noticed that she never had any time to herself and that her life was overrun with taking care of others' needs while neglecting her own. I told her that she must practice noticing what activities replenished her energy and which ones drained her. Then I told her that in order to reverse her symptoms, she had to spend at least one hour each day recharging her own energetic batteries by resting or doing something she liked. She did so, and a month later all her symptoms were gone. She told me that she was learning how she drained her energy in her daily life. She said, "When I lie down or sit down to write in my journal, I can literally *feel* the energy coming back into my body. Knowing how crucial this is to my physical and emotional well-being is a revelation."

Of course, the moment you say yes to yourself and no to what someone else has convinced you that you "should" do to be a "good" person, you will no doubt feel guilty. This kind of guilt gets passed down in families. One of my friends once called me over the holidays but had to cut the conversation short because she had to go with her parents to cut up fruit for the parishioners at her parents' church. I asked her why she had to do this over her brief vacation. She stopped short, then after a moment said, "Because we've always done it."

"Do you like to do it?" I asked.

"No," she answered.

"So why do you continue?" I responded. "You are no longer a child. And you don't live in your parents' town or go to their church anymore."

"It's expected," she told me. "We've always done it."

But, having realized that she didn't get any joy or satisfaction from it and was just blindly following along in the family trance, that was the last year she spent her holidays cutting up fruit. The next year she went to yoga class and got replenished.

All of us receive messages from our bodies regularly about what serves our health and well-being and what doesn't. Our bodies know immediately when we are doing something or even thinking about something that doesn't support us fully. One of my friends gets diarrhea and stomach cramps when she just thinks about going to visit her parents. She was abused both physically and emotionally throughout her entire childhood, and this abuse has continued into adulthood. Her body knows that visiting her parents will not be good for her, and it gives her symptoms as messages to stay away. When she gives herself permission to stay away, her stomach problems resolve immediately. (She has also had to learn how to soothe the anxiety that arises from the ingrained belief that not visiting or doing what her mother expects makes her a "bad" daughter.) In time, she may well be able to visit without it having to "cost" her anything. But that's Ph.D.-level healing work! I often tell people who think they've "evolved" enough to be around abusive people that it doesn't matter how forgiving and evolved you've become—eating ground glass still hurts and is harmful.

In order to flourish and stay healthy, we need to pay attention to the subtle signals from our bodies about what feels good and what doesn't. Foggy thinking, dizziness, heart palpitations, acne, headaches, and back, stomach, and pelvic pain are a few of the common but subtle symptoms that often signal that it is time for us to let go of what we don't want in life and start using our own power to improve things. Here's an example from my own life.

Back in the 1980s, when I had two young children, I was working too many hours, and I often felt that aspects of my work weren't respected by my colleagues. My face often broke out in large blemishes—cystic acne, really— which I had never had as an adolescent or at any other time in my life until then. I tried taking vitamins, changing my diet, and using a variety of skin creams. Nothing helped—until I left my place of work. Within six months the problem cleared and has never returned.

Clearly, my face was a barometer of my well-being during those years. Through my skin condition, my body had been telling me that my work setting was not supporting me optimally. My complexion had been registering my "thin-skinned" sensitivity and my anger at not being completely accepted by my colleagues. (I hadn't completely accepted myself, either, at this point, and my work environment was a reflection of that. Of course, it was way before anything holistic or natural was accepted by the medical profession.) All of these emotions lay just below the surface, though I couldn't appreciate this at the time. Once I faced my innermost needs and left the situation that simply was not supporting me, my complexion improved automatically. As my life cleared up, so did my face.

Negative emotions exist to let us know that we are not facing the clearest path to what we want. When we realize that our bodies and their symptoms—feelings—are our allies, pointing out what serves our highest good and what doesn't, we become free. Whenever you feel angry or upset, or have a head-ache or a bodily symptom, take a moment to reflect upon what unmet need the symptom is trying to bring to your attention. When I am caught up in a downward spiral of negative feelings, I instantly know that I am out of touch with my inner guidance and that I'm giving too much attention to what I don't want. I have learned to notice when I'm feeling bad, and I stop for a moment. If I can catch myself at the beginning of the bad mood, I can often get my energy flowing positively again by going through the following pro-cess:

1. I acknowledge what I am feeling *without making any judgment about it.* I avoid wallowing around in the negative emotions and prolonging them, but I definitely *feel* them fully. I stay with the feeling.

2. I acknowledge that there is a reason why I am feeling the way I am. And it's almost always an unmet need of some kind that the inner child has.

3. I spend twenty seconds or so identifying what is causing my energy to flow negatively. For example, a while back I was angry because a staff mem-ber didn't get an important message to me in time for me to return a phone call promptly.

4. Having identified the source of my negative emotion, I then ask myself what I need. Sometimes the need isn't immediately obvious, especially if you're in the middle of a downward emotional spiral that seems out of pro-portion to the situation. The reason for this is that any given event might trigger memories (even if not conscious) of a whole host of past events in which a similar need wasn't met. Given that, it can be very helpful to have a trusted friend present to help you home in on the actual need, rather than wallowing in the emotion.

5. I then state my need, which, in the example in step 3, is to be respected and acknowledged by my staff. I would say, "I want to receive my telephone messages on time so that I can respond to them promptly and efficiently." Stating our needs is powerful because it defines them clearly, allowing our creative energy to flow toward them. When we make a statement of pure positive energy with no negativity in it, it helps draw what we want into our experience. This turns the situation into something positive with an actual solution.

6. Finally, I affirm that I have the power within me, via my inner guidance and my power of intent, to get what I want.

Remember the law of attraction: The people and circumstances we attract to us are always a reflection of our own thoughts and beliefs. In my early days of practice and work, I quite often felt unsupported both at work and at home. I operated under the belief "If you want it done right, you have to do it yourself." Over the years, I slowly changed my beliefs about support and realized that I truly need it—and deserve it. I learned not to feel ashamed of that need. I learned that it is possible to ask for support and get it. As a result of this inner change, I now enjoy an amazing support system both at home and at work. I call it "assisted living."

Going through this process helps me acknowledge my emotions, feel them fully, and use them as guidance toward getting my needs met. I regularly sit down with a notebook and make a list of exactly what I want in a given situation. This aligns my thoughts with my inner guidance, and it feels good. Inspiration about what to do generally follows. Please note that I don't try to figure out what to *do* about a certain situation until I've gone through the entire process of looking in the direction of what I need and desire. And I don't try to figure out how to fight *against* something I don't want, because that just creates more of what isn't working. This is why I suggest you remove the notion of "fighting" cancer or other illness from your vocabulary.

In the past, for example, my former husband would often spend many hours at the hospital and wouldn't come home for dinner on time. I used to look out the window and wait for him, trying to keep the dinner warm, feeling angry with him and sorry for myself. The more I demanded that he show up on time, the more of a problem it became in our relationship. One day, I simply decided to go ahead and eat dinner myself and then get on with the evening's activities and enjoy myself. I did this whenever he wasn't home when he said he would be. Eventually, he began coming home on time spontaneously, or calling to say he'd be late. I realized that my attention to his continued absence was actually holding the painful pattern in place. I also realized that I was operating under the outdated notion that it was my job to provide a warm supper for him each night, even though we both were working in surgical specialties at the same hospital. When you acknowledge that you are attracting your experiences vibrationally, you have put yourself in the driver's seat of your life. You also have to be willing to let go of the notion that someone else is responsible for meeting your needs. That's your job. You must also stop making the behavior of others your excuse for unhappiness. Most of the time, your loved ones will be very happy to assist you when you learn how to make requests, not demands. (By the way, this is not true if you are dealing with an energy vampire.)

Unfortunately, instead of using our feelings as inner guidance, we're brought up to fear or deny our negative emotions and feelings or judge them as "bad." Though remaining emotionally calm and collected under pressure can be admirable and is often necessary, we cannot afford to allow this emotional control to become so ingrained that we lose touch with the richness of our emotional life. Men are even more at risk for being out of touch with their feelings than women, since they learn early on that "big boys don't cry." This has contributed to the "toxic masculinity" that is being addressed head-on in our culture right now, including by men such as Lewis Howes, author of *The Mask of Masculinity* (Rodale, 2017).

A friend of mine was taught that if she had to cry, she should bury her face in a pillow so that the rest of the family wouldn't have to hear it. Yet crying and making sounds are all a part of our emotional "digestive" system and a way to keep energy flowing evenly throughout our bodies.

I recently rewatched the movie *Sense and Sensibility,* based on the Jane Austen novel of the same name. Elinor, the main character, has spent her entire life being "sensible," attempting to keep a lid on her own needs and desires. One of those desires is to marry a particular man with whom she's in love. She never lets on about this, always waiting for him to approach her and bring up the subject. At the end of the story, when her beloved finally shows up to proclaim his love—after all kinds of plot twists and turns—the emotional dam within her bursts and she begins to sob uncontrollably. This scene is almost painful to watch when you realize that Elinor is not at all unusual. She is trying so hard to accept her lot in life and be sensible about her needs and desires. But underneath her calm exterior is a tornado of power and life force, just waiting to be unleashed. Luckily, none of us needs to have Mr. Right show up in order to unleash our inner guidance in the first place.

For thousands of years, our culture has had a kind of "nonliving" orientation that is now being transformed. This orientation has encouraged us to keep a lid on things, as in "Don't make waves." By learning very early on that emotions are bad or shameful, we learn not to trust our inner guidance or our bodies. When we are encouraged to be out of touch with what we know and what we feel, we are systematically trained out of moving toward the fulfillment of our innermost desires and needs. Even our religions teach us to squelch our innate joy and creativity and that feeling good is a sin. As Matthew Fox points out, "Our civilization has not done a good job with the energy called delight and joy."[7] We need to know that the very essence of a life based on inner guidance is abundant delight and joy. Anthropologist Richard Grossinger, Ph.D., puts it this way: "Guess what? God created beings not to act in a morality play but to experience what is unfathomable, to elicit what can become, to descend into the darkness of creation and reveal it to him [or her], to mourn and celebrate enigma and possibility. The universe is a whirling dervish, not a hanging judge in robes."[8]

Every smiling, laughing three-month-old baby I've ever met reflects the true, joyous nature with which we were all born. They also express their unmet needs vociferously. The late anthropologist and social biologist Ashley Montagu, Ph.D., once said that most adults are nothing more than "disintegrated children." Fortunately, our inner guidance is always available to remind us of our direction toward fulfillment. When we realign with our inner guidance and stop judging our bodies and our feelings as bad when they are offering us information, we are on the pathway to a life filled with growth and delight.

4
The Female Energy System

Look beneath the surface of the world—the world that includes your clothes, toaster ovens, philosophies, your skin—and you will discover a universe of swirling and subtle energies. While we do not know exactly what these energies are doing or how they are doing it, we do know that they are "here," forming the energies that underlie physical reality. They form *you*.

—Cyndi Dale

Understanding that thoughts and emotions affect how energy works in the female body can help us decipher our individual bodies' unique language. The location of disease within the body—where it occurs—has psychological and emotional meaning and significance. Specific mental and emotional patterns are associated with specific body locations. Our thoughts, emotions, and behaviors are reflected or patterned simultaneously in the brain, the heart, the spinal cord, the organs, the blood, and the lymphoid (immune) tissue, and the electromagnetic field that surrounds and penetrates all those areas. Understanding the different dynamic patterns of energy that our bodies give rise to and operate within can help you appreciate how positive or negative energies can manifest themselves in your individual body.

THE MATTER-ENERGY CONTINUUM

Our body's vibrational system is always changing, and the *potential* for healing or disease is present at all times. Precancerous cells, for example, arise regularly in our bodies. They form invasive cancers only when our own internal controls break down.[1] Unfortunately, a lot of today's disease screening—the sine qua non of so-called prevention—picks up too many conditions we would "die *with*" but not "die *from*." If you want to remain healthy in today's medical system, you need to keep this in mind.

Mental and emotional energy goes in and out of physical form regularly, bouncing on the continuum between energy and matter, particle and wave. Vibrational healer Deena Spear says, "Cancer moves in and out of physical reality constantly. But once you get a diagnosis, it really takes root and becomes established." Quite simply, emotional and mental energy can become physical in our bodies.

When we have unresolved chronic emotional stress in a particular area of our lives, this stress registers in our energy field as a disturbance that can manifest in physical illness. Here is how it happens: When we obsess about someone or something, or keep participating in self-destructive thoughts or behaviors, our life energy leaks away from our body. When we obsess, we tie up energy—*chi* or *prana*—in a negative process that diverts it from our cells. Vital cellular processes thereby become depleted. We leak energy in any situation in which our anger, fear, depression, or sadness is controlling our ability to move forward in our lives. While most doctors do not view the onset of disease in terms of these energy leaks, I have come to the conclusion that appreciating how thoughts and emotions affect our energy is a critical part of flourishing. It is interesting to note that more and more medical research supports this observation. In one study, for instance, cancerous cells were shown to "steal" energy (in the form of the ATP-like molecule DPN) from adjacent normal tissue.[2] Mira Kirshenbaum writes in her book *The Emotional Energy Factor* (Delacorte Press, 2003) that when she asked energy experts like endocrinologists, nutritionists, and sports medicine specialists how much energy we get from physical sources as opposed to emotional sources, the average of the answers was 30 percent. "Even if you had perfect physical health and ate the perfect diet and got the perfect amount of exercise," she writes, "all that would give you only 30 percent of the complete energy you need. The remaining 70 percent . . . must come from your emotional energy."[3]

Appreciating our bodies in terms of energy fields and energy leaks can help us understand and begin the healing process. When we persist in being angry with someone who has hurt us, for example, a part of our spirit is occupied with that person and is not available to us for healing. When a person has been severely abused, shamans believe, that part of the person's spirit

may flee in order to escape the abuse. One of the healing traditions of shamanism is called "soul retrieval," in which the missing spirit is called back.
Many women who have been sexually abused as children relate that they
"left" their bodies during the abuse. Some remember that a part of themselves actually left and went up to the ceiling and watched. This split-off part
of their spirit may not be available to them in the present for healing. This is,
in large part, what the Inner Child Rescue exercise mentioned later on in this
chapter (page 81) is designed to heal.

Many times we are not conscious of these energy leaks. But if these leaks
continue without being healed, bodily distress is often the result. Bodily
symptoms can serve to bring our attention to that area so that healing can
begin. One of my former menopausal patients who came to see me with insomnia and depression told me of her sexual abuse as a child—something she
had not been consciously aware of until a week before her visit with me. She
had gone through a painful divorce in her forties and had had a recent
breakup with her lover of seven years. She said, "I realize now that I've spent
my entire life trying *not* to remember that I was sexually abused. Now that I
know it happened, I realize why I've never had a satisfactory relationship.
I've always pushed people away. I didn't know how to be fully present in a
relationship. But I didn't know any better. I'm grieving for who I was in my
early life and the fact that it has taken me this long to remember and release
the past. But finally the chronic knot in my stomach is gone. I feel free. I am
so relieved." Her sleep problem and depression cleared up spontaneously as
her memories of abuse arose and were released from her energy field.

How to Heal Energy Leaks

To stay or become healthy, it is useful for each of us to notice where we
are leaking our energy. A good time to do this is when you go to bed each
night. To begin the process of healing your energy leaks, simply notice who
or what you are thinking about, worrying about, or obsessing about. What
thoughts, emotions, events, or people keep coming into your mind? Are there
any emotions or thoughts over which you are obsessing? See whom you're
holding resentments against. When you find these areas, you must call your
spirit back. One way to do this is by using your will and your power of intent
to call back the parts of you that are caught in past or present situations that
don't serve your highest good. It is helpful to do this out loud, using the following phrase or something similar: "I now call my Spirit and my power
back to me from all times and all places. I reclaim my own authority now."

As you're calling your spirit back, it also helps to affirm your spiritual
connection verbally. Repeat the following affirmation (or something similar),
really feeling the truth of it: "I am always being divinely guided toward my

highest good on all levels. Divine Love now dissolves everything that is not on my divinely designed path." The split-off parts of yourself are not used to this calling, but eventually they will respond to your efforts and your energy will return.

Most of the blockages in our vibrational systems are emotional in nature. And that is why merely understanding something intellectually is not enough. You need to truly feel to heal. And when the emotional stuff comes up, you're apt to be surprised by how powerful it is. For example, I recently had a session with my energy healer friend and colleague Melanie Ericksen (www.soulplay.us). She said, "I'm going to the back of your heart." She then put her hand on my back as I was lying down, and what came into my head was my baby sister Bonnie, who had died at age six months when I was about five years old. I don't recall grieving much for her because I was so young and she was in the hospital most of her life because she wouldn't eat. My mother had been on a high dose of streptomycin for the entire pregnancy for viral pneumonia, and it is likely that the antibiotic had an adverse effect on the baby. Anyway, as I lay there, I suddenly found myself sobbing in grief for the loss of my sister. I was astounded as I let the tears flow. I realized that my body—and my heart—had been holding on to those unshed tears for decades. After that, I felt a considerable lightening in my heart and chest. It has taken me many years to trust my own intuition and my own emotions as valid indicators of what is really going on and what needs to be done. And so when images come to mind as I'm having a healing session, or anytime deep feelings arise, I now know how to trust them and allow them to unfold. I want everyone to know how to trust themselves in this way because this is true preventive medicine.

It's helpful to think of your vibrational system as being like a stream of water flowing along. As long as this energy flow is healthy and you are feeling good about yourself, there's much less risk of disease. Environmental toxins, trans fats, and excess sugar or alcohol (to name a few) usually don't manifest in disease unless other factors have already set up the pattern of blockage in the body's energy system in the first place.[4] This is why some individuals who have smoked cigars and drunk whiskey daily and never exercised in their lives still live to a hundred and beyond. Environmental or dietary risk factors can be likened to debris carried along in the body's energy flow. This debris stays afloat unless there is a felled tree or other blockage to the water flowing in the stream. When there is, the debris collects in the branches of the felled tree and accumulates. Over time, similar accumulations in the body's energy flow can result in physical illness. In fact, scientific research has associated a failure of the flow of information between cells with the induction of cancer in those cells. A physical barrier of any kind that blocks communication between cells is a carcinogenic influence.[5] The fat and connective tissue that form a fibroid, for example, do so only when the energy flow around and through the uterus is already blocked in some way.

Our emotions are often stuck at the childhood level, when we were not allowed to experience them fully. Clinical psychologist Doris E. Cohen, Ph.D., explains that the child part of us actually takes over our adult nervous system, re-creating the same unhealed fears we were unable to fully work through as children. The purpose of this is to bring healing into the unhealed places. An example would be a woman who, at the age of three, was abandoned by her father. Whenever she begins a new relationship, she begins to feel a sense of impending doom—the work of her inner three-year-old. And then she ends up sabotaging the relationship and repeating her abandonment. Nothing changes until she catches herself engaging in this repetition and learns how to comfort the frightened child within her who has been unconsciously running the show. In this culture, which teaches us to split our adult intellectual knowledge from our emotional reality and needs, one can have a Ph.D. from Harvard but an emotional body that is only two years old. The emotions of a frightened or angry two-year-old, if unexpressed and unacknowledged, become energetically stuck in childish patterns. Emotions that are expressed, felt, and named, on the other hand, simply flow through our energy system, leaving no residual unfinished business. Once stuck emotions are expressed and released, we must also acknowledge that we are no longer children. It's time to put our adult selves in the driver's seat of our lives.

INNER CHILD RESCUE:
BRINGING YOUR CELLS UP TO DATE IN THE PRESENT

Many times when negative emotions and situations persist, an "inner child" is stuck at a certain age and stage—and she's running your central nervous system, your immune system, and your endocrine system. She needs to be acknowledged and "grown up." Otherwise, she will keep bringing you back to the scene of the crime, so to speak, until her unmet needs get acknowledged and met. To do that, follow these steps:

1. Close your eyes and visualize a stop sign. Say, "Stop! You're doing it again." Ask for a number between 1 and 10. The first number that comes into your mind is the age of the child inside whom you are dealing with.

2. Take a deep breath. Hold it for a count of three. This longer inhale engages the parasympathetic nervous system, which helps the body rest and restore.

3. Imagine entering a magical garden with flowers, a lake, and healing angels. Meet your inner child there. (Believe me, you will literally see her.) See what she is doing. Note it. What is she wearing? Ask her to come over to you. Will she let you hug her and comfort her? Either way, tell her you love her and that you won't ever abandon her again. Tell her you are leaving but that you'll be back. This leaving part is essential.

4. Take another deep breath. Exhale slowly.

5. Come back to the present and open your eyes. State your name, the date, and your location. This will reestablish you in the now as an adult who is no longer being adversely influenced by the unhealed child.

Repeat this process daily for forty days. If you miss a day, start all over. After the first visit to the garden, you can spend far less time on each visit. This whole exercise takes about two minutes, so everyone has time to do it, and it is so very powerful. I've done this exercise many, many times for many different situations and for many different ages—including my adult self. (Five years after my divorce, I went back and did forty days with my newly divorced self because the wounds were still there.)

This Inner Child Rescue is based on the work of Dr. Cohen and is available in far greater detail as "The 7 Steps of Rebirth" on her website, www.drdorisecohen.com.

We do not have to wait to develop cancer or other diseases in order to get the message that we need to change our vibrational point of attraction and begin creating health. None of us is completely free from the fear, anger, and stress that come and go as part of normal life. When these emotions become intense enough and chronic enough to affect our psychological and emotional well-being on a regular basis, we are heading for physical illness unless we resolve them in a healthy way. When our daily unresolved pain, anger, and frustration rob our bodies of vital health-producing energy, it is essential to bring healing and understanding into our daily thoughts, emotions, and actions.

Here is a crucial point: It is completely possible for a woman to go through her entire life free from physical illness even though she was abused, beaten, or neglected as a child. Early childhood problems do not *necessarily* cause energy disturbances and physical illness. Often these problems occur only after a woman begins to develop as an individual and form her own identity and opinions separate from those of her family and her tribe. From this vantage point, she often realizes that what happened to her as a child was not acceptable. However, she is realizing this from the perspective of a mature individual, not of the child she was then.

Hurts and wounds from a woman's past do not become potentially devastating to her, physically or emotionally, until she gets the idea that what happened to her in the past was wrong, that it shouldn't have happened, and that she was abused purposely and consciously by her family members. No one should be abused in any way. And anyone who was abused was entitled to better. No one would disagree with this. But very few of us had idyllic, pain-free childhoods. Abuse is remarkably common in part because the human race hasn't had much experience with allowing positive energy and joy into our lives for very long. We have a central nervous system that, for centuries, has been wired to expect and react to conflict—which we are also masters at creating until we recognize this pattern and change it. That's where our power lies, always.

Our families and those with whom we come into contact during childhood usually do the best they can with the hand they were dealt. They pass their dysfunctional patterns on to us unconsciously, not maliciously. If each of us was truly connected to our inner beings and souls and knew how to stand up for ourselves and our worth, the abuse would stop overnight. So regardless of what has happened to us in childhood, it's our job in adulthood to feel, transform, and heal our wounds. To thrive, we must become sources of health and healing so that we can break the chains of pain that run in our families. Part of thriving is avoiding toxic blame and resentment that goes on for years, and then removing ourselves, when possible, from the ongoing energy drainage that is inevitable when we are around toxic individuals. Energy disturbance and subsequent illness result from past abuse only if a woman is unable to work through her emotional and psychological pain, first with feeling her anger and sadness and then with forgiveness (especially of herself) and eventual understanding of herself and others—even for those who caused the abuse. However, it's important not to spend too much time trying to understand abusers. You don't want to rush to forgiveness as a way to avoid feeling the pain and anger of the abuse. And always remember that forgiveness does not mean that you are condoning the behavior of the person who hurt you. Forgiveness is, instead, a way to free yourself from the past. Howard Brody, M.D., Ph.D., director of the Institute for the Medical Humanities at the University of Texas Medical Branch, put it this way: "Suffering is produced or alleviated primarily by the meaning that one attaches to one's experience."

Forgiveness doesn't preclude anger, however. Feeling rage and anger from past violations is a necessary first step toward healing. Anger mobilizes and energizes us to make long-overdue, life-enhancing changes. It's far preferable to the stasis of depression. The key is to feel that anger and then move on. This is a process, not an event. Anger and blame are a necessary stop on the road of life, but they make a lousy destination. The longer we stay in this mode, searching for a perpetrator to blame for what happened to us—be it men, our mothers, the government, or doctors—the more our bodies are energetically depleted. I've learned how to recognize the poisonous effects of righteous indignation in my own body. Getting stuck in this energy for a long time becomes self-destructive. However, as Mario Martinez, Psy.D., so brilliantly points out, righteous anger—when one's innocence or that of another is threatened—is an actual cause of health. That's right. Allowing oneself to feel anger, at least temporarily, at being violated actually contributes to health. An example would be when you see a waitress being treated poorly at a restaurant. If you say something to support her, your immunity will be enhanced. Just as if you saw your child being abused by a teacher, you would jump in and say something. Failure to do so could adversely affect your own health.

Our early family life clearly has a profound influence on our character and health. A famous prospective study by Caroline Thomas, M.D., for example, indicates that a man's lack of closeness to his parents, or having a father who was physically and emotionally less involved, could predict early disability and death from suicide, hypertension, coronary artery disease, and tumors.[6] This certainly corroborates the ACE Study findings discussed in chapter 2. Nevertheless, our bodies and minds are self-renewing. Writing a new script for ourselves changes our biology. We can decide to heal ourselves and move on.

EARTH'S ENERGY

Traditional Eastern philosophies describe the profound interaction between the earth's energy and that of the physical human body, and the strong connection between female energy and the earth's own natural pull. Understanding women's nature, with its natural ebbs and flows, as positive and powerful gives us a chance to heal and live in a balanced, healthy way.

According to some Eastern traditions, women's bodies are different from men's in that the earth's energy moves up through our bodies and inward. I'm talking about most males and most females here, recognizing that this energy flow may differ with transgender or binary individuals. This female energy is "drawing-in" energy, or centripetal force. This centripetal female energy is irresistible. It is so powerful that if one lives in a family setting, most of the household will want to be around the person with the most centripetal energy—usually the mother—and will be acutely aware when she is gone. Children will save up their complaints for their mother at the end of the day if she hasn't been around. My children always needed to know where I was in the house. If I walked out of a room, they called, "Mom, where are you?" after about one minute. When they were younger, they always had to be in the same room with me. I couldn't take a bath alone until the older one was about nine. In contrast, when the children were small, my former husband could have been away for much longer before they'd notice. A woman's inward-pulling energy is at work when she puts the baby to the breast, accepts the penis into the vagina (if she is heterosexual), and sends chemical signals to encourage sperm to swim toward the egg. You'll also notice it when your dog insists on lying in the efficiency triangle of your kitchen when you're trying to make supper.

This powerful attracting energy is present not only in our biology but also in our hearts and minds in the form of our unique dreams and desires. When a woman finds the courage to articulate her heart's desires and share them with others, she will soon find that her irresistible drawing-in energy will help her to fulfill them. Part of the reason for this is the fact that the heart has an electromagnetic energy field that is 5,000 times stronger than that of the brain.[7]

Michio Kushi, the macrobiotic teacher who first discussed and illustrated this energy pattern for Western readers, points out that the earth's centripetal force, coming up through the feet, is present in men as well as women, just as heaven's force, coming downward from the sky through the head and the body (centrifugal force), is present in women as well as men. What differs is the degree to which each energy is present. In women, in general, more "earth's energy moving up," or centripetal force, is present. I've been told that Navajo women wear skirts because doing so increases the body's access to this earth energy through the circle that the skirt creates on the earth in relationship to the body (see figure 1). The Lakota tradition holds that the energy of women during menstruation (called "moon time") spirals counter-clockwise and downward, into the earth. (Because of this, menstruating women don't participate in sweat lodges because their energy conflicts with the upward-spiraling energy of the sweat lodge ceremony.)[8]

Centripetal energy is a grounding force that affects everyone around us because women tend to be the centers of their households, taking on psychological responsibility for the well-being of other family members. Therefore, when a woman changes her life for the better, her entire family (whether or not she has children) generally benefits. She sets the tone. The well-being of the family and of society itself depends upon women becoming and remaining healthy. Part of creating health is understanding the power of female energy and its implications. The health of a woman's loved ones is directly linked to her own personal health. So we owe it to ourselves to take the time we need to heal and to become healthy, happy, and whole. You can't quench another's thirst if your own cup is empty. Or as the energy called Abraham (who is channeled by Esther Hicks) puts it, "You cannot get poor enough to help poor people thrive or sick enough to help sick people get well. You only ever uplift from your position of strength and clarity and alignment." Truer words were never spoken.

THE CHAKRAS

Centripetal or "drawing-in" force is only one way to characterize female energy. We also have seven specific vibrational centers in our bodies, known as *chakras*. Chakras are the primary organs of your body's subtle energy system that correspond with and affect specific areas of your physical body. The word *chakra* derives from the Sanskrit for "wheel of light." Cyndi Dale, the author of *The Subtle Body: An Encyclopedia of Your Energetic Anatomy* (Sounds True, 2009), refers to chakras as the "power centers that run the 'you inside of you.'" Every human being, male or female, has the same chakras, and each of them is affected by specific emotional and psychological issues. These energy centers connect our nerves, hormones, and emotions. Their locations run parallel to the body's neuroendocrine-immune system and form a link between our vibrational anatomy and our physical anatomy. Chakras act as transformers that take refined emotional and spiritual information and distribute it to the cells of the physical body.

The vibrational system of the human body is a holographic field that carries information for the growth, development, and reproduction of the physical body. This holographic field guides the unfolding of the genetic process that transforms the molecules of our bodies into functioning organs and tissues. Though standard Western medicine has not recognized chakras yet, Eastern cultures have long appreciated them.

If we look at the chakras as the key areas in which emotions manifest in the physical body, we can begin to grasp how cultural experiences of wounding or affirmation may have psychological and emotional consequences that set us up either for health or for subsequent gynecological, obstetrical, or other health problems. Whether you perceive chakras as literal places in the body or as metaphoric ones, they can help you activate mind-body connections to help you heal.

Each of the seven chakras of the human body is associated with specific organ systems and specific emotional states. Each is also either enlivened or weakened by one's beliefs and feelings. In other words, specific fears and emotions actually target specific areas of the body (see figure 2, page 93). The location and naming of the chakras and their functioning vary somewhat in different texts and different traditions.

The system I have used here is a compilation of my clinical observations

FIGURE 1: EARTH'S ENERGY GOING UPWARD

Female energy = centripetal or "drawing-in" force. Earth's energy coming upward through the feet, then spiraling around the uterus, breasts, and tonsils.

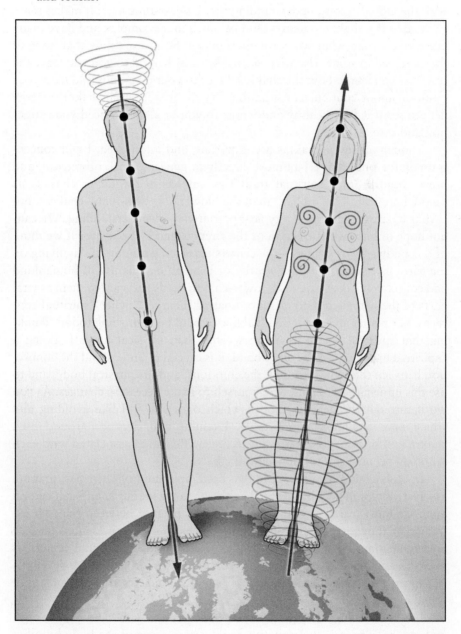

Source: Adapted from Michio Kushi

combined with the work of Arthur Avalon, a Western authority on tantric and kundalini yoga; Norman Shealy, M.D., Ph.D., a neurosurgeon; and medical intuitive Caroline Myss.[9] According to Sanskrit scholars, the original depiction of the chakras was highly variable and not necessarily in alignment with the more Western understanding that I will outline here. It makes sense to me that the chakra system would be much more complex and have many more layers than what we normally think of. So please know that none of this is etched in stone. Use what seems the most helpful to you and leave the rest.[10] As you learn about the chakras, listen to your own body and trust your intuition about your current situation. Try to visualize each chakra's energy field to see if it feels healthy and whole to you or seems to need your attention and care.

Though all seven chakras are important and interlinked, I will concentrate on the ones that relate most directly to gynecological, obstetrical, and breast health. Some spiritual traditions emphasize the upper chakras as "more important" or "holier" than the "lower" or "less-than" chakras, but I want to stress that this is a typical patriarchal misunderstanding. We cannot hope to improve our health or the circumstances of our lives if we think of our body's lower centers—the centers involved with day-to-day living on the earth as humans—as less worthy or beneath our dignity. If humankind had collectively taken care of its lower-chakra needs and viewed them as vital parts of the whole, instead of subordinating them to "higher" spiritual concerns, our planet and our individual lives would be flourishing today. Thinking that spiritual needs are more worthy than physical needs is doing a "spiritual bypass." On the other hand, it is crucial to understand the connection between the soul, the mind, the emotions, and the physical body, and to use this information to empower yourself to make necessary changes. As you work through the chakras, notice which ones you feel like avoiding and which ones feel most comfortable. Examine your feelings around each chakra's emotions. You may want to review the issues associated with each until you become comfortable with them.

In each chakra area there are two basic polarities, or extremes, that are associated with ill health. To stay healthy or to regain our health in a certain area, we must learn how to strike a healthy balance between the two extremes of thought patterns and emotional expression represented in each area. Our inner body wisdom, through each of these emotional centers, is always leading us toward health and balance by requiring that we develop a full repertory of skills encompassing the entire range of thought and emotional expression.

One more thing: Though the energies associated with blame, guilt, rage, and loss have been associated only with certain areas of the body by other authors, a thorough search of the psychosomatic medical literature indicates that this view is incomplete. These energies affect each area of the body simultaneously, though they may be expressed as health problems in the area of your body that is most vulnerable. The same is true for the health-enhancing energies associated with love, appreciation, hope, and forgiveness.

THE LOWER FEMALE CENTERS: CHAKRAS ONE TO THREE

The bottom three chakras are related to our physical life: the people, events, memories, experiences, and physical objects within our environment, past and present. They are particularly influenced and imprinted by our parents and extended families. All three of the lower female centers are inextricably linked and interacting. Therefore, although I address each one separately, understand that they all affect one another. (Ultimately, all seven chakras affect one another and are interactive.)

The *first-chakra* area is affected by our feeling of safety and security in the world as well as by our sense of belonging. First-chakra health is determined by how well we can balance trust versus mistrust, independence versus dependence, and standing alone versus belonging to groups. It's important to remember that all humans are designed by nature and evolution to be healthiest and happiest when they have secure attachments to other humans whom they can count on. For far too long, Western culture (especially in the United States) has emphasized the virtues of independence and standing on one's own two feet over our need for intimate bonds. This is reflected in the child-rearing advice that parents have received for decades, including separating babies from their mothers and letting infants "cry it out" lest they become "spoiled." Keep that in mind. We can get talked out of our need for secure attachments starting in infancy, which in turn can lead to chronic illness.

The first chakra is also affected by the balance we strike between feeling fearless and allowing ourselves to feel our fear fully. The first-chakra area is, quite literally, affected by how connected we feel to the earth and the processes of the earth. The body areas that correlate with this chakra are the spine, the rectum, the hip joints, the blood, and the immune system. The foundation for our sense of safety, security, and belonging usually is formed in childhood, when we get a sense about whether or not this planet is a safe place to be and whether or not we're accepted for who we are. Therefore, unresolved family and physical survival issues—such as problems concerning one's house, family, sexual identity, and race—are represented in the first chakra. A person with a first-chakra issue would be likely to say or think regularly: "No one is here for me"; "I'm all alone"; "I just don't fit in"; "Nobody cares"; "I'll starve."

The health of the *second-chakra* area has to do with two separate issues.

The first involves our outer drives in the world and includes both how we go about getting what we want and the actual things we go after. Do we actively go after what we want, or do we allow things to come to us? Finally, when we do go after what we want, do we do so wholeheartedly with a sense of deserving the fulfillment of our desires or are we filled with shame and guilt, believing that we're not worthy to have what we desire?

The other second-chakra issue has to do with how we get our needs met within a relationship. Are we dependent or independent? Do we take more in relationships, or do we give more?

Attachment Styles Are First- and Second-Chakra Issues

In their groundbreaking book *Attached: The New Science of Adult Attachment and How It Can Help You Find—and Keep—Love* (Tarcher, 2010), authors Amir Levine, M.D., and Rachel S. F. Heller discovered that our attachment style begins in infancy and continues to influence how we bond right up to adulthood. There are three overall attachment styles, each highly predictive of how successful our most intimate bonds are likely to be: the anxious style (25 percent of the population—these individuals desire closeness and intimacy and are often unsure about their lovability), the avoidant style (25 percent of the population—these individuals tend to push intimacy away even though they need it as much as everyone else), and the secure style (50 percent of the population—these people have the ability to uplevel both the anxious and the avoidant types). All too often, the anxious types end up dating avoidant types, and this creates a huge amount of anxiety and stress for the anxious types. All of this could be avoided if the anxious bonders knew that their job was to simply state their need for reassurance and intimacy from the very beginning of any relationship (see the discussion of nonviolent communication in the section on fundamental beliefs of the dominator system in chapter 1). It's also important to realize that these bonding types need not define us. If you are an anxious or avoidant type, there is a lot you can do to change—but first you have to be aware of your general tendencies. What is our balance between relying on others to fulfill our needs versus relying solely on ourselves? Do we give to others unconditionally, or do we give in order to get something, such as love, recognition, touch, sex, or money? Do we know how to receive and accept support? Do we have well-defined boundaries, or are they poorly defined? Are we assertive or submissive? Do we protect others, or do others protect us? Do we tend to oppose others, or do we acquiesce to their opinions or actions?

The pelvic and reproductive organs (vulva, vagina, uterus, cervix, and ovaries) are associated with the second chakra, and so are the bladder and the appendix. The health of this area is affected by the degree to which our relationships are based on feelings of trust or, alternatively, control, blame, and guilt. If we use sex, money, blame, or guilt to control the dynamics of our relationships (including our relationship with ourselves), then the organs of the second chakra may be adversely affected. A person with a second-chakra issue might often say or think: "If you loved me, you'd come to visit more often"; "He doesn't write, he doesn't call"; "What do I have to do to earn your love (or respect or recognition)?"; "You're never there for me." As you can see, those with an anxious attachment style are more likely than others to suffer from second-chakra issues until they learn how to get their innate needs for security and intimacy met directly and healthfully.

The *third chakra* is associated with a person's self-esteem, self-confidence, self-respect, and sense of responsibility. In other words, how do we balance our feelings of adequacy or worthiness with inferiority in what we do in the outer world of work or achievement? Are we hyper-responsible or irresponsible? Are we aggressive, or do we tend to be defensive? Are we prone to threatening and intimidating others? Are we territorial? Or do we feel trapped and want to escape? In our work, are we overly dependent upon boundaries, or do we have issues around limitations? Finally, do we know how to balance our competitiveness? Do we know how to both win and lose with grace? How do we handle gains and losses? All of these issues affect the health of this area. Addictions are generally third-chakra issues. For example, people who abuse alcohol or food often suffer from painful feelings of inadequacy. But the abuse of alcohol or food is also an abdication of responsibility to self and others. It's little wonder that eating disorders or overdrinking often adversely affect the third-chakra organs: gallbladder, liver, pancreas, stomach, and small bowel. Familiar health-damaging statements here would be: "If I don't do it, it won't get done"; "I'll never be good enough"; "It's okay, I'll do it myself."

All of the unresolved stresses of our early life related to people, events, memories, and experiences pull energy *primarily* from the three lower power centers, the first three chakras, and have the potential to affect the organs "below the belt."

STRESS IN WOMEN IN THE FIRST THREE CHAKRAS

~ Any unresolved anger

~ Resentments and feelings of rejection

~ The need for revenge

- ⁓ Wanting to leave a relationship but fearing the financial consequences
- ⁓ Shame about one's body
- ⁓ Shame about one's family background or one's mate's social status
- ⁓ Being either a child abuser or an abused child
- ⁓ A history of incest or rape
- ⁓ Guilt over an abortion
- ⁓ Inability to conceive
- ⁓ Inability to launch one's creations

FIGURE 2: CHAKRA DIAGRAM WITH FEMALE FIGURE

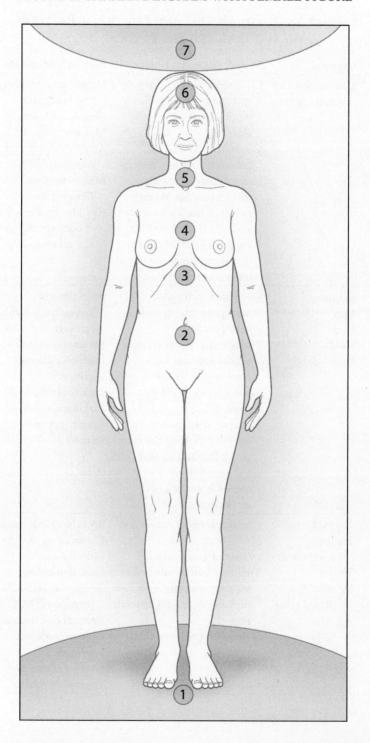

TABLE 4

ENERGY ANATOMY: MENTAL AND EMOTIONAL PATTERNS,
THE CHAKRAS, AND THE PHYSICAL BODY

Chakra	Organs	Mental, Emotional Issues	Physical Dysfunctions
7	Can involve any organ system	Clear sense of life's purpose vs. trusting that life has a purpose that may not be clear Connection to God or universal source of energy Understanding the paradox that an individual can influence her life's events and also trust that things happen as they should and that some things are out of one's control	Developmental disorders (cerebral palsy) Genetic disorders Multiple sclerosis Amyotrophic lateral sclerosis (ALS) Multiple-system abnormalities Any life-threatening illness or accident that serves as a wake-up call
6	Brain Eyes Ears Nose Pineal gland	Perception: clarity vs. ambiguity (ability to live with paradox) Thought: left brain vs. right brain—rational vs. nonrational, linear vs. holographic, rigid vs. flexible Morality: conservative vs. liberal, following the rules vs. understanding that rules have exceptions Repression vs. lack of inhibition	Brain tumors/hemorrhages/stroke Neurological disturbances Blindness/deafness Ménière's disease Dizziness Tinnitus (ringing in ears) Parkinson's disease Learning disabilities Seizures
5	Thyroid Trachea Neck vertebrae Throat Mouth Teeth and gums	Communication: expression vs. comprehension (speaking vs. listening) Timing: pushing forward vs. waiting; constant time pressure vs. having enough time Will: willful vs. compliant	Bronchitis/hoarseness Chronic sore throats Mouth ulcers Gum difficulties Temporomandibular joint problems (TMJ) Cervical disc disease Chronic neck pain Laryngitis Swollen glands in neck Thyroid problems

Chakra	Organs	Mental, Emotional Issues	Physical Dysfunctions

4	Heart/lungs
	Blood vessels
	Shoulders
	Ribs/breasts
	Diaphragm
	Upper esophagus
		Passion and compassion
		Emotional expression,
		  including capacity to feel
		  fully, express, and resolve
		  anger, hostility, joy, love,
		  grief, forgiveness
		Capacity to form mutual,
		  reciprocal partnerships
		  with balance of giving,
		  receiving, nurturing of self
		  vs. nurturing of others,
		  intimacy with others vs.
		  capacity to be alone
		  (intimacy with self)
			Coronary artery disease
			Myocardial infarction
			  (heart attack)
			Hypertension
			Cardiac arrhythmias
			Chest pain
			Mitral valve prolapse
			Cardiomegaly
			Congestive heart failure
			Asthma/allergy
			Lung cancer
			Pneumonia
			Upper back, shoulder
			  problems
			Breast problems, including
			  cancer

3	Abdomen
	Upper intestines
	Liver, gall
	  bladder
	Lower esophagus
	Stomach
	Kidney, pancreas
	Adrenal gland
	Spleen
	Middle spine
		Self-esteem, self-confidence,
		  or self-respect
		Adequacy vs. inferiority
		  relating to competence and
		  skills in the outer world
		Substance abuse
		Responsibility vs.
		  irresponsibility
		Aggression vs. defensiveness
		Competitiveness vs.
		  noncompetitiveness;
		  winning vs. losing
		Territoriality/too many
		  boundaries
		Fear of assuming
		  responsibility or making
		  decisions for self
		Feeling overly responsible vs.
		  abdicating responsibility to
		  self and others
			Gastric or duodenal ulcers
			Colon/intestinal problems
			Ulcerative colitis, irritable
			  bowel syndrome
			Heartburn/gastritis
			Pancreatitis/diabetes
			Constipation and diarrhea
			Indigestion, chronic or
			  acute
			Anorexia and bulimia
			Liver dysfunction
			Hepatitis
			Adrenal dysfunction

Chakra	Organs	Mental, Emotional Issues	Physical Dysfunctions
2	Uterus, ovaries Vulva, vagina, cervix Large intestine Lower vertebrae Pelvis Appendix Bladder	Balanced drives in the outer world toward sex, money, power, and relationships Capacity to co-create with others Fertility and generativity Relationship dynamics: dependency vs. independence, giving and taking, defined boundaries vs. poor boundaries, assertiveness vs. passivity	Ob-gyn problems Pelvic/lower back pain Creativity Sexual potency Urinary problems Appendicitis
1	Physical body support Hip joints Spine Blood Immune system	Safety/security in the world; knowing when to trust or mistrust Sense of belonging Knowing when to feel fear and when not to Balance between independence and dependence	Chronic spinal problems Back pain Sciatica Scoliosis Rectal tumors/cancer Chronic fatigue Fibromyalgia Autoimmune diseases Arthritis Skin problems

Sources: C. Dale, *The Subtle Body: An Encyclopedia of Your Energetic Anatomy* (Boulder, CO: Sounds True, 2009), and C. N. Shealy and C. M. Myss, *The Creation of Health: Merging Traditional Medicine with Intuitive Diagnosis* (Walpole, NH: Stillpoint Publications, 1988). Scientific documentation of the human energy system and updated information from Mona Lisa Schulz, M.D., Ph.D., *Awakening Intuition: Using Your Mind-Body Network for Insight and Healing* (New York: Harmony Books, 1998).

Now that you've looked at the table and gotten an overview of the physical problems that can be associated with the various chakras, I'll discuss the issues of each chakra in more detail.

The First Chakra:
How Family Wounds Are Stored in the Body

Our first-chakra health is related to our upbringing and early life. This includes our immediate and extended family, race, social status, educational level, family legacy, and family expectations as these were handed down through the generations. To describe the breadth of the issues involved in the first chakra, Caroline Myss uses the word *tribe*. For example, we all learn very early what it means to be a member of a defined group: a Smith or a Jones, a Catholic or a Jew. Another first-chakra "inheritance" is the tribal programming of many first- and second-generation immigrant families in the United States, who often pass on the belief that to accomplish anything worthwhile, one must suffer and sacrifice personal happiness and pleasure for the benefit of the next generation. Family scars and the social and familial information that form a person's idea of reality are connected to the first-chakra area. An example provided to me by a friend from New York City involves a famous man whose lifelong sense of inferiority (covered up with bragging and bullying) stemmed from the fact that he came from Queens and could never be as tough as those who were from Brooklyn.

The tribal mind is not an individual's mind. The tribal mind is primarily a collective brain that seeks to hold on to its own and fight for its own survival in the world. The tribal mind is concerned with *loyalty,* not love, kindness, or tenderness. A current example of this is the call for "due process" by men who have been fired and have lost their status because of past sexual abuse of women (and sometimes men). "Due process" is a legal term that suggests equal treatment before the law. But in the case of sexual predators, who have been protected for centuries, the call for due process for the abusers fails to take into account the due process that is finally owed to the countless victims these men have left behind, including the many whose lives they have destroyed.

What the tribe refers to as "love" is really obligation to the tribe. An example of this is a family member who says to another, "If you really loved me, you'd come to church with me every Sunday." Tribal consciousness, then, is not a high-level, highly evolved consciousness. Yet we all share it to some degree, and many women admit that as they get older, they can hear that tribal mind within themselves. Many women say, "I sometimes hear my mother's words coming right out of my mouth, and I can't believe it." Above all, the tribal mind seeks stability by keeping everything the same; for example, family holidays and birthdays become obligations, not joyful times of sharing. Recall what I wrote earlier about how all tribes the world over keep their members in line through the three primal wounds of betrayal, abandonment, and shame. That's what I'm referring to here. The age-old conflicts in the Middle East provide additional examples of entrenched first-chakra beliefs about who is worthy and who isn't.

The tribal mind can be likened to "crabs in the bucket." If you have a bunch of crabs in a bucket and one crab tries to escape over the edge, the other crabs will always pull the escapee back down with the rest of them. The same sort of thing often happens to women and their families as the women decide to break free from limiting patterns. Almost invariably, family or community members try to sabotage the women's efforts—at least initially. This is how society keeps its members in line.

Countless women have had the experience of confronting their parents about abuse or incest soon after remembering these events, only to find that their parents deny these allegations outright. The unconscious motive to preserve the tribe is the reason so many parents deny having ever violated a tribe member. At some level, their tribal memory bank has absorbed the memory very differently from the way the individual member records the same event. The person who is waking up from the tribal trance is almost invariably seen as a "traitor" to the family, the church, or other social group.

FIRST-CHAKRA ISSUES THAT CAN SET THE STAGE FOR ILLNESS

~ Unfinished business with parents, such as anger or resentment about childhood wounding

~ Incest (this is a second-chakra issue as well)

~ Abuse or neglect in childhood

~ Psychological programming from one's early years that is limiting, such as:

> ~ "You're stupid"
>
> ~ "You're useless"
>
> ~ "You're a bad girl"
>
> ~ "Only Catholics go to heaven"
>
> ~ "Your body is something to hide out of shame"
>
> ~ "Sex is dirty—save it for your husband"
>
> ~ "Girls are meant to serve men"
>
> ~ "Men always come first" (for example, in many families the men get the best cuts of meat, and the women get what is left over)
>
> ~ "Girls should not be ambitious or bright"
>
> ~ "Women can't make money—they must marry it"

Most tribes or families do not deliberately try to poison their members—they are merely handing down what they recognize as tribal wisdom, even in the form of limiting and painful ideas. It is useful to think of yesterday's tribe as today's dysfunctional family.

My friend Carla recently realized, after resolving her many physical illnesses, that the seeds for these illnesses had been planted in her childhood. Her mother had repeatedly beaten her, not out of malice or lack of love but simply following her own tribal programming of how to love and prepare a daughter for life. She had told Carla that the beatings were how she showed her love. Whenever Carla's mother saw another woman beating a child in the supermarket or elsewhere, she used to remark to Carla that obviously that woman really loved her child. Carla's mother, a first-generation immigrant from southern Europe, deeply believed that life is very difficult and filled with pain and that to accomplish anything, Carla would have to suffer. Later, each time Carla reached a cherished goal, she developed a serious illness. She eventually realized that she could reach her goals joyfully by using her innate gifts and talents and her inner guidance, and that repeated illness and suffering need not be part of her experience. Carla is an extreme example, of course. Most childhood wounds are far more subtle, but potent nonetheless.

The Second Chakra: Symbolic Creative Space

The second chakra is concerned with the day-to-day physical aspects of living, with the people to whom we relate, and with the quality of our relationships. The second chakra also relates to everything we own: money, relationships, and passions. Since most of our early programming is to serve the tribe, most men and women automatically move into the roles of their second chakras in an unconscious way. They choose the partners that fulfill the needs of their second chakra. Women thus tend to marry for physical security, money, children, and social status, and out of fear of abandonment. We then carry out our roles accordingly. We are programmed to tend to the needs of our personal tribe and often become completely controlled by the fears of the second chakra.

SECOND-CHAKRA ISSUES:
HOW RELATIONSHIP WOUNDS MANIFEST IN THE BODY

~ Fear of abandonment

~ Not feeling sexually desirable or lovable

~ Financial security

~ Feeling incapable of supporting yourself financially

~ Social status

~ Children

~ Fertility issues

~ Creativity

The uterus and ovaries are the major organs in the second chakra. This area is both literally and figuratively creative space, out of which women can produce babies, relationships, money, careers, novels, insights, and other creative or artistic works. When our energy is not flowing smoothly in this area of the body, gynecological problems, such as fibroid tumors, can result.

When I think of the uterus as potential space, I also think of what we as women are usually expected to "store" in there. A slang term for the uterus is "the bag," and as humans who have or have had a uterus, we are also the ones who carry all the stuff that others don't want to carry. Women who are married and have children often notice that their children give them—not their husband—the half-eaten food, gum wrappers, and other garbage that they no longer want to carry. We have all heard older women referred to as "old bags." When I was pregnant, nursing, and caring for small children, I felt like a "multiple-bag lady."

Not only do women carry physical excess, we are also expected to carry emotional excess for others—usually for men, but not always. One sixty-year-old former patient of mine with three grown children was living alone with her husband, who had recently retired. She told me she was now chomping at the bit to do other things in her life that she had long wanted to do, such as traveling and writing. But her husband was not enthusiastic about her endeavors. He wasn't sure what to do with his newly acquired freedom from work. My patient said, "But my husband still wants me to carry his anima—his moods, his enthusiasm, his fun. And when I let down and allow any of my own feelings to show, other than enthusiasm, *he* gets depressed." *Anima,* a term coined by the famous psychologist Carl Jung, is a man's inner feminine aspect, which often gets projected onto the women in his life when he is unwilling to feel his own emotions and work through them. What unconscious material do we store in our body centers that neither we nor anyone else really wants to carry around? When unresolved second-chakra-related issues surrounding relationships, creativity, and/or a sense of security exist, the pelvic area of the body as well as the lower back can become vulnerable to disease.

A number of second-chakra experiences can set the stage for illness. The studies of Gloria Bachmann, M.D., indicate that childhood sexual abuse is associated with eating disorders, obesity, and somatic complaints in the genitourinary system, as well as substance abuse and other self-destructive behaviors.[11] Studies by Robert Reiter, M.D., Astrid Lampe, M.D., Pallavi Latthe, M.D., and others have found that previous sexual abuse is a significant predisposing risk factor for chronic pelvic pain.[12]

Whenever I see a woman with a uterine problem such as fibroid tumors—which are present in 40 percent of American women—I ask her to meditate upon her relationships, creativity, and sense of security. Is her creative energy being routed into any dead-end jobs or relationships? What is her fibroid telling her about these areas? Fibroids, endometriosis, diseases of the ovaries, and other pelvic disorders are manifestations of blocked energy in the pelvis. In a misogynist culture in which at least 18 percent of women are sexual abuse survivors and approximately one in five gets physically raped, it's not hard to figure out how this happens.

During her annual exam, I found a small fibroid in Gina, a patient who was thirty-eight years old at the time. I asked her to meditate on blocked energy in her pelvis, and she later told me, "When I got home and took some time with this question, I realized that when my brother died in an accident, I was furious with him for leaving. I was twenty-five and really couldn't allow myself to feel that rage. So I just stuffed it in my pelvis. I hadn't thought about that for years." On a follow-up exam three months later, I found that her fibroid was gone. I believe that by expressing and experiencing the full impact of her anger for the first time, she changed the energy pattern in her pelvis and actually dematerialized the fibroid, transforming it from matter into energy. She told me, "I had a feeling that when I came in today, you'd say it was gone. I literally felt it let go." I've seen other women decrease or eliminate their fibroids when they remembered and released old experiences.

Third Chakra: Self-Esteem and Personal Power

The foundation for a woman's sense of herself, her self-esteem and personal power (third chakra), is formed by her sense of security and safety in the world (first chakra) combined with the quality of her relationships, especially in the areas of money, sex, and power (second chakra). If we feel safe and secure and have supportive relationships that help us secure resources and power, we will be in a good position to achieve our goals in the outer world and to complete tasks that help us develop a sense of self-esteem and self-worth. Third-chakra strength or weakness is related to feelings of adequacy and competence in the world versus inferiority, and to our ability to assume responsibility for our lives and our choices versus the degree to which we relinquish this power to others. Self-esteem and vibrant third-chakra health are always enhanced by doing useful work that is recognized by society, not just by our immediate families. On the other hand, workaholism depletes the third chakra and is a setup for overeating or other addictions. The ability to learn from both winning *and* losing creates health in this area. On the other hand, excessive competitiveness and needing to win all the time can weaken the third chakra. It is also affected by the balance one strikes between being aggressive and being defensive.

As a result of their collective and individual histories, most women have low self-esteem. For centuries women haven't been validated or valued except in their capacity as servers and pleasers of others. Our natural desire to create and achieve in the outer world has often been thwarted at an early age. Thus, as women have become individuals in their own right, their families, at least until fairly recently, have often not supported them in becoming all they can be. (Remember, women still make only 85 cents for every dollar that men earn doing the same job, according to the Pew Research Center; women of color make even less.)

All of this happens, in part, because families usually hold an unconscious tribal fear that their female members will abandon them to serve their own needs and live out their personal dreams without the family. This unconscious fear is, I believe, why voluntary termination of pregnancy is such a polarizing issue, and also why so few women are willing to reveal publicly that they've had abortions. The ability to freely and deliberately choose one's own life over the inevitable sacrifices required to meet the needs of others strikes at the very heart of patriarchal conditioning. We've all inherited the belief that a woman cannot develop herself fully without simultaneously sacrificing her ability to serve her family. You will notice that at a job interview, few if any men are asked how they plan to balance being fathers with showing up for their careers. Yet we still question a woman's ability to have both children and a career, and precious few mothers go about their careers without worrying they're shortchanging their children. This is because we've been socialized to see the family as a woman's primary job. Many women have great difficulty expecting and getting the support they need. (This is especially true in the United States, where paid maternity leave—beyond a meager six weeks—is essentially nonexistent.)

One of my friends, a talented art teacher, would really like to hire someone to care for her three-year-old daughter a few hours a week so that she can paint. But her husband, a doctor, is the one making all the money. And he likes to have her home with their child. So she's afraid to even bring it up with him, even though she put him through medical school and paid all the bills. Talk about deep and obsolete programming!

Besides undertaking the classic struggle to balance our personal desires and our responsibilities, women often pace our self-esteem to our mate's cycle. If a woman's partner becomes highly successful, she may become depressed because she can't keep pace with him (or her), or she may not back her partner's new adventure into different thoughts or creative new territories for fear that he (or she) will leave. On the other hand, when a mate is unsuccessful in the outside world and becomes depressed or abusive, this too affects the woman in her third chakra (and also the first and second). Conflicts such as these cause energy system dysfunction in the third chakra and can result in eating disorders (anorexia nervosa and bulimia) or physical illness in the stomach (ulcers), gallbladder, small intestine (irritable bowel), liver, and pancreas (diabetes).

Archetypes and the First Three Chakras

When a woman feels that she is being forced to participate in an activity she doesn't like, her body, mind, and spirit are at risk for harm.[13] When she unwittingly participates in a pattern of self-abuse and abuse from others, she is acting under the influence of what in vibrational medicine is called the rape archetype.

Archetypes are psychological and emotional patterns that influence us unconsciously until we become aware of their power. Archetypes are universal ideas, images, and patterns of thought that we all share in our subconscious. Though the concept of archetypes may at first seem elusive, these unconscious patterns of thought and behavior have a very real effect on our bodies and emotions.

To help you understand the concept of archetype more clearly, I'll use an example—the mother archetype. A woman who is unconsciously operating under the influence of the mother archetype (as it currently exists in this culture) thinks obsessively about the needs of her children while forgoing her own. Even when her children are old enough to care for most of their physical needs themselves, the woman under the influence of the mother archetype focuses her thoughts on whether they've had enough to eat, whether they are happy, and whether they are warm enough or cool enough, ignoring or suppressing her own needs in order to do something for them. I know this one well. Up until very recently, I've felt bad about myself if one of my daughters asked for a tissue and I didn't have one! Let me be clear here. Caregiving to those I love is deeply rewarding and satisfying to me. The issue here is overcaring about others at the expense of my own needs. The culturally encouraged behavior of worrying about the needs of others without caring for our own needs can become a damaging stereotype. Another example of an archetype is the hero. When we see the word *hero*, we instantly think of a person who is strong, bold, and brave. A hero is one who may fearlessly rescue others and neglect his or her own safety and needs because of a compulsion to save someone else. If unconscious, this kind of behavior, too, can be detrimental to health. I have a good friend, a man, who routinely sacrifices his own free time and his need for rest and recreation by being a hero who rescues everyone else—fixing their cars, cutting down fallen trees in their yards, shoveling snow, and so on. These are all good deeds. But he continually puts his own well-being on the back burner.

When we are unconsciously participating in archetypal patterns of behavior, we lose touch with our deepest selves and our inner needs. When a woman is not following her own heart's desires and instead acts only to fulfill others' needs, she may be under the influence of either the rape archetype, the prostitute archetype, or the mother archetype, depending upon the circumstances.

The rape and prostitute archetypes are very closely related. When a woman engages in sexual activity that she doesn't really want but feels unable to do anything to prevent, she is under the influence of the rape archetype. The same archetype is present if she denies herself sexual pleasure because she feels that this is what her partner wants—and again feels unable to alter her situation. The rape archetype may occur when a woman participates in her own violation, such as having an abortion that her mate wants but that she doesn't. A woman who resents her partner but stays in the relationship anyway for financial or other reasons is not acting from her individual strength but is under the spell of the prostitute archetype. Women often handle this archetype by blaming ourselves or by absorbing our own anger and rage, lest telling of these feelings results in being abandoned.

A woman's second-chakra organs are also put at risk when she herself becomes an aggressor or victimizer. Women participate in the rape archetype, for example, when they violate their children's physical and psychological boundaries. Giving daily enemas and rough washing of the genitalia are other common examples of the ways women may act as violators. Women use emotional weaponry, while men add to that their fists. Women who victimize pay for it not only through disruption in the energy of their female organs in the second chakra but through problems with organs in the first and third chakras as well. According to Caroline Myss, aggressive behavior can be associated with cancer in the organs of the first three chakras.

It is important for us to understand and accept that women do have the potential for aggression. When we refuse to acknowledge a problem, we simply perpetuate it. Recovering from patriarchal influences isn't about blaming men, because in our culture we're all potential victims and potential perpetrators. When I first had a reading with Caroline Myss, for example, she told me that my body registered a rape between the ages of twenty-one and twenty-nine—the years that I was in medical school and doing my residency. Though I had not been physically raped, my body's energy system had been emotionally and psychologically "raped" by my medical training—something I had not been consciously aware of at the time. Myss states that almost everyone in this culture has suffered from a psychological or emotional rape of their innermost self at least once. That is one reason why so many women who have not suffered from overt sexual abuse nonetheless have chronic pelvic pain and other second-chakra problems. Many women feel stuck in jobs in which the rape or prostitute archetype is a daily reality.

When we continually see women only as victims, we do not acknowledge the damage women do to themselves and to others. If you've ever borne the brunt of female abuse or been an abuser yourself, you'll understand the significance of this point of view.

Shame and the First Three Chakras

Another issue for many women is shame. Shame hits the first three female centers and the associated interior organs, including the uterus and ovaries. Shame can be a result of social programming that tells a woman she's inferior or that her genitalia themselves are shameful. This point of view is embedded deeply in our culture. The major nerve to the vulva is called the pudendal nerve. The root word from which *pudendal* is taken means "shame." Shame over a rape, whether it was physical, emotional, or psychological rape, affects the vaginal area. Shame about one's sexuality can be a setup for vaginitis, pelvic pain, and so on. Shame can also come from family relationships, such as shame about a father's alcoholism or a mate's social status. Shame is associated with the production of an inflammatory chemical in the body known as interleukin 6 (IL-6). Keep in mind that almost all chronic degenerative diseases, such as cancer, arthritis, and heart disease begin as tissue inflammation.[14]

Research supports the idea that energy dysfunctions cause disease. Henry Dreher, author of *Mind-Body Unity: A New Vision for Mind-Body Science and Medicine* (Johns Hopkins University Press, 2003), points to a very large body of research showing that women who have experienced sexual abuse are significantly more likely to develop gastrointestinal disorders, including irritable bowel syndrome.[15]

Other research points to differences in personality between women who develop interior cancers and those who develop exterior cancers.[16] An individual's perception of whether her body is permeable and easily penetrated by external influences, either physical or emotional, is related to whether she is susceptible to cancer. Those women who perceive their bodies as permeable are subject to cancers that are located more deeply in their bodies—for example, in the ovaries or uterus. Those women who believe that their bodies are strong and protected against external influences are more prone to cancers in the external genital areas.

Research by Lydia Temoshok, Ph.D., author with Dreher of *The Type C Connection: The Mind-Body Link to Cancer and Your Health* (Plume, 1992), found that women with more aggressive and life-threatening cancers (including both breast and cervical cancer) tend to be more self-sacrificing and less aware of their needs and feelings, including physical sensations, than other women.

The Fourth Chakra

The bodily areas associated with the *fourth chakra* are the heart, breast, lungs, ribs, upper back, and shoulders. The fourth chakra is related to our capacity to feel, to express ourselves emotionally, and to participate in true partnerships in which both members are equally powerful and equally vulnerable. Giving and receiving equally from an open heart with no agenda other than appreciation strengthens all the organs of the fourth chakra. Our culture is loaded with references to the function of the fourth chakra: "When I heard that symphony, my heart soared"; "I wept for joy"; "I thought my heart would burst with joy"; "Watching that little girl cry broke my heart."

Our fourth-chakra health requires a balance between anger and love, joy and serenity, sadness and happiness. Can we be stoic at times and at other times lose it emotionally? Can we allow ourselves to feel grief and loss fully? In partnership, can we allow ourselves times of intimacy balanced with time alone? Can we both nurture others and allow others to nurture us? The unmet emotional and psychological needs associated with ill health in the fourth-chakra area are an inability to give or receive love from self or others (nurturance), lack of forgiveness, unresolved grief, and/or hostility stemming from the inability to express and release anger or resentment. (It's not surprising that right after the events of 9/11, the heart attack rate in our local hospital doubled.)

The second and fourth chakras have a unique interrelationship. The uterus is sometimes called the "low heart," while the heart in the chest is the "high heart." It's been said that if the low heart has been closed, through rape, incest, abuse, or shame, a woman cannot truly open her high heart. In this culture, women also tend to shut down their low hearts, or their sexuality and erotic needs, because we're taught that "nice" girls aren't sexual. The opposite is also true. The younger generation of girls is now part of the "hookup" culture, in which it's deemed perfectly acceptable to have sex with boys—or provide them with oral sex—even when neither of them has any affection or love for the other. In cases like this, the high heart is most often shut down. And this is precisely why girls who have been sexually abused in childhood or adolescence quite often become sexually promiscuous. Whether you believe that it's fine to be in touch with your emotions and feelings but not with your sexuality, or you believe the opposite—that sexual activity is perfectly acceptable with no emotional connection whatsoever—either way, we're set up for second- and fourth-chakra conflicts.

In addition, women are taught that if we are powerful and successful financially (second chakra), we'll be isolated from others and won't be able to experience intimacy fully (fourth chakra). As a result, too many women end up with unbalanced relationships in which they provide not only the finances but also the emotional support, housework, sex, and everything else. Many successful women have what researcher and psychologist Sandra L. Brown, author of *Women Who Love Psychopaths* (Mask Publishing, 2009), calls "super traits." These super traits include unusually strong resourcefulness, self-reliance, loyalty, self-directedness, optimism, and low harm avoidance (they don't think they will get hurt). These same women often become doctors, lawyers, CEOs, judges, and über-effective mothers. In other words, they have what it takes to be highly successful in the outer world. The same traits, however, make them targets for energy vampires—people who display the dramatic behavior associated with a particular cluster of personality disorders.[17] Given our cultural programming, this vulnerability makes sense. Women have been told for centuries that men don't want a woman to be "too successful" or make too much money, lest they outshine their male partner. And so, rather than risk being alone, these same women often become targets of those who feed off the energy of others and contribute very little to the relationship. This explains why so many successful women fail in the intimacy department.

Men, on the other hand, have been socialized to believe that their masculinity depends upon being able to bring home the bacon and make the major financial decisions in a relationship. We're now at a historic crossroads as men and women learn how to renegotiate these inherited (and often obsolete) partnership and intimacy beliefs and behaviors. Understanding the energy dynamics at play is key to remaining healthy.

High Heart and Low Heart Yin/Yang Balance

Saida Désilets, Ph.D., founder of the Désilets Method (a form of qi gong; for more information, visit www.thedesiletsmethod.com) and author of *Emergence of the Sensual Woman: Awakening Our Erotic Innocence* (Jade Goddess, 2006), has articulated a very useful way to think about the energy difference between men and women. Men have genitalia on the outside and visible erections when aroused. Their genitalia are dominant, yang, and active. Hence, they are comfortable going out in the world of money, sex, and power to pursue what they want. Men's hearts, on the other hand, are yin, hidden, and difficult to access directly. In women, it's the other way around. A woman tends to lead with her heart—which is very yang. It's far easier for most women to express their feelings openly than it is for most men. Women freely cry, hug, and emote in public. Evidence of a yang fourth chakra is the fact that a woman's breasts protrude from her chest. Her genitalia, on the other hand, are inside and hidden. They are yin. To get a woman to open to a man sexually, he must use a slow yin approach that involves tenderness, earning trust, and praise. A woman gets into a man's heart in the same way.

Though it's clear that men rape women with their genitals, it's equally true that women abuse men (or boys) with their yang hearts—by being cold, withholding, critical, or impossible to please. Boys and men feel very, very deeply, though they often won't talk about it. And the wounds they suffer at the hands of women can last a lifetime. When a woman becomes conscious of her power within a relationship and takes steps to heal herself, the men in her life do much better as a result—unless the men are narcissists, in which case the best course of action is to cut your losses and get out, because no amount of supporting and healing will change them. And they will do whatever it takes to get your energy, known as "narcissistic supply."

Energy dysfunctions often arise when a woman is confused about how to use both her loving energies (fourth chakra) and her creative power drive energies (second chakra) optimally. The major conflict within women is that most of us have been taught that in order to be loved, to receive love, and to guarantee that someone will be there for us, we must care for our loved ones' external physical needs—usually at the expense of our own, which we deny. Over time this leads to inevitable burnout and resentment, which results in cellular inflammation, which in turn is a setup for disease. Such so-called love relationships, dependent upon ties of family obligations ("If you loved me, you would [fill in the blank]") and tribal tradition, are recognized as relationship addictions once a woman begins to individuate and become conscious of her patterns. Energy dysfunctions that arise in the second- and fourth-chakra areas at the same time are very common in our culture. They often result when women unconsciously participate simultaneously in both the rape archetype and the mother archetype. And all too often, these second- and fourth-chakra dysfunctions involve someone with narcissistic tendencies, often beginning with a parent who sets the pattern.

Sally, a twenty-six-year-old waitress, had very-early-stage cervical cancer (second chakra) and multiple breast cysts (fourth chakra). When she was a girl, her father had been both emotionally and physically distant. In her early teenage years, to fill up this emptiness, she had multiple sexual partners, boys whom she neither loved nor respected. This addictive pattern of behavior (the rape and prostitute archetypes) disrupted the energetic patterns of her second-chakra area, depressing her immunity. She suffered from very painful and frequent herpes outbreaks in her vagina. She also had recurrent genital warts.

Like Sally's distant father, Sally's mother took care of neither her own nor her daughter's physical or emotional needs. Sally never learned how to care for her own emotional needs, in that no one ever demonstrated this behavior to her. Both Sally and her mother had energy disruptions in their fourth-chakra areas related to lack of self-respect and self-nurturance. Both mother and daughter had breast problems. Sally's mother had already had breast cancer, and Sally had had two breast biopsies for benign lumps.

Neither Sally nor her mother is unique in our culture. I've seen many women like them. When a woman neglects her own inner needs, when she addictively cooks, cleans, and cares for the physical needs of her family to earn love, when she works obsessively at her job to prove her self-worth, and when she provides sex on demand because of feelings of obligation or guilt, she becomes susceptible to disease in both her second and fourth chakras. Quelling her insecurities about abandonment or about being good enough, about self-esteem, uses up her emotional energy. Her life force gets drained by her fear of abandonment and her belief that she's not good enough.

Supporting these theories of energy system dysfunctions, research has shown that the personality patterns of women who have disease only in the second chakra differ from those of women with disease only in the fourth chakra. (An extensive literature search reveals no studies on the personality patterns of women who have malignancy in *both* the second- and fourth-chakra areas.) In one study, 50 percent of patients with cervical cancer (a second-chakra disease) had physically lost their fathers due to death or desertion during their early years (a second-chakra-related emotion). In contrast, in the homes of those with breast cancer (a fourth-chakra disease), the father was emotionally distant (a fourth-chakra-related pattern).[18] Other studies have shown that significantly more cervical cancer patients have behaviors that suggest a second-chakra energy imbalance: They had married multiple times, had a high incidence of sexual activity with partners whom they neither loved nor respected, and were very concerned with body shape and size. They also had a feeling that they had been neglected as children. In contrast, studies of breast cancer patients suggest behavior patterns associated with fourth-chakra dysfunction: They had a greater tendency to stay in a loveless marriage, had a relatively high likelihood of carrying a heavy load of responsibility for younger siblings during childhood, and had a greater chance of denying themselves medical care and physical nurturance.[19]

My observations further substantiate the research above. In general, medical intuitives such as Caroline Myss and Belinda Womack find that emotions that are of the raging variety hit below the belt. Sadness that cannot be expressed, on the other hand, is associated with disease above the belt. I will be covering this in more detail in chapters 5 through 10.

How to Heal Lower-Chakra Wounding

Lower-chakra wounds *don't heal until they're witnessed*. Someone has to say, "Yes, this happened to you." Right now our culture is in the midst of a huge witnessing moment, with the #MeToo movement and sexually harassed and abused women who have broken the silence about sexual predators like Harvey Weinstein. (Collectively, these "Silence Breakers" were named Person of the Year by *Time* magazine in 2017.) As a result, thousands of women all over the world are breaking the silence, telling their stories, and seeing others stand with them.

One of the key functions of this book from the time of its first edition in 1994 has been this witnessing process. As a physician, I represent an authority figure. When I or another person validates a woman's woundings, she can use that as a very powerful catalyst for healing. But it is even more important that the *woman herself* acknowledge her wounding and need for healing. As long as a woman is stuck in denial ("It wasn't really all that bad, he never hit me" or "My family loved me very much—my father would never have done that"), she won't be able to tell the truth to herself. Her secrets will remain locked in her cells, unavailable for witnessing and healing.

After the witnessing of her wounds, a woman must then investigate how these wounds have affected her life. This is the naming stage—the stage when she realizes that her life has indeed been adversely affected by someone or something. Denial has now left. The recovery movement that characterized the 1970s and 1980s marked the beginning of this stage for many women. And it is now going on in full force.

But the final stage required for healing and the optimal functioning of a woman's energy system involves releasing the power of the wound to control her life. This is the stage in which many of us now find ourselves, or soon will, as we move from #MeToo to #NowWhat? Forgiveness, releasing the past, and acceptance are required, for both herself and others. Once she understands and moves beyond the past, she is ready to assume personal dominion over her life and her choices for the future. She is now in a position to stop repeating the wounding and truly begin to flourish.

OTHER CHAKRA ISSUES

The *fifth chakra* is related to communication, timing, and will. When you communicate your ideas in the outer world, do you talk as much as you listen? Do you express yourself as well as you comprehend others? As far as timing goes, do you push forward or do you wait? I believe that the epidemic of thyroid problems in our society right now is energetically related to the perception that we have too much to do and never enough time in which to do it. We're constantly rushed. But this perception itself is the chief problem. My colleague Gay Hendricks, Ph.D., has a unique solution to this, which he calls "Einstein time"—and which I'll cover in chapter 15, "Steps for Flourishing."

Finally, the thyroid has to do with one's will. Do you tend toward willfulness or are you overly compliant? Associated with this chakra are the throat, mouth, teeth, gums, thyroid, trachea, and neck vertebrae. Dysfunctions in this chakra include chronic sore throats, throat and mouth ulcers, gum disease, neck pain, temporomandibular joint disease (TMJ), thyroid disease, cervical disc problems, swollen neck glands, and laryngitis. Women with fifth-chakra problems such as hypothyroidism often have difficulty speaking up for themselves and holding their own point of view, and may have overly soft voices, making it difficult for them to be heard. The fifth chakra is associated with the ability (or inability) to speak your truth. A friend of mine who has had hypothyroid problems for years recently broke one of her teeth right after she finally broke up with a man who seemed very supportive at first—telling her how much he enjoyed her ebullient energy—but then slowly, inexorably started to criticize that same energy. She finally got up the courage to tell him the truth about his behavior and her reaction, something she had never had the courage to do in her previous marriage. Her tooth broke shortly thereafter—a reminder that, in breaking her tooth, she had also broken her pattern of staying silent! A recent thyroid test showed that her thyroid function is also returning to normal.

Conversely, there are women who have an overdeveloped will that is not connected to their inner wisdom. This can result in disease such as hyperthyroidism and the exertion of one's intellectual will without acknowledging a higher will or higher power—for example, "I don't care what my body is telling me, I'm going to do it anyway" or "I'm going to will my way through this no matter what."

The *sixth chakra,* sometimes known as the third eye, is related to perception, thought, and morality. When we perceive the outer world, do we have the capacity to see clearly while also tolerating ambiguity? Can we allow ourselves to have razor-sharp focus sometimes and at other times become relaxed and unfocused? Do we know when to be unreceptive to the ideas of others and when to be receptive? Can we accumulate knowledge but also allow ourselves to be open to what we still need to learn? Can we acknowledge our areas of ignorance? Can we appreciate rational and logical thought from the brain's left hemisphere but also acknowledge the gift of the right hemisphere: the nonrational and the nonlinear? Are our thought processes rigid, obsessive, and ruminating, or do we have flexibility in our thinking? Finally, how do we apply our moral beliefs to ourselves and others? Do we tend to be repressed and overly conscientious model citizens who judge ourselves and others according to rigid standards, or do we allow ourselves, in some cases, to be more liberal, risk-taking, and uninhibited?

This chakra is located between the eyes, near the ears, nose, brain, and pineal gland. Dysfunctions associated with this chakra are vision problems, brain tumors, blood clots (blood clot formation is related to stopping the flow of intuitive information), neurological disorders, blindness, deafness, seizures, and learning disabilities. Health-detracting statements associated with losing energy in this area are: "I don't care how you feel. Tell me what you think"; "I don't have enough information to make a decision"; "Can't you see that I know what I'm talking about? Why are you arguing with me?"; "I'm surprised that you believe in that mind-body nonsense, given that you are an intellectual, educated person."

The *seventh chakra* is related to seeing the larger purpose in our lives. It's also related to our attitudes, faith, values, conscience, courage, and humanitarianism. Do we have a clear sense of purpose? Do we acknowledge that we as individuals have the power to create our lives, while simultaneously acknowledging the larger forces of the divine at work in the universe? Do we understand the paradox of knowing that we can influence some events, while also knowing that things happen that we can't control, which we may not like, but that may ultimately serve a purpose we don't understand at the time? This chakra is located near the crown of the head. The seventh chakra is the metaphysical framework around which you build your morals, your values, and your conscience.

Any life-threatening event in your life or any serious illness holds the potential to awaken wisdom in this area by connecting you with a larger view of the universe and your purpose in it. Those individuals who've undergone a near-death experience often relate how this changed their lives on every level and left them with a deep certainty about how best to spend the rest of their lives. Although all life-threatening illness can have seventh-chakra meaning, those that are specifically related to awakening wisdom in this chakra include paralysis and multisystem disease affecting the muscular and nervous systems, such as multiple sclerosis and Lou Gehrig's disease. An individual may be born with a seventh-chakra challenge such as genetic disease. Genetic disorders or birth defects are conditions that the spirit of the individual was in agreement with before birth. In other words, the issue goes far beyond our ability to understand why it happened and how. (This soul knowledge does not preclude investigating purely physical reasons why these things might have happened, such as in-utero exposure to toxins or drugs.) Life-threatening accidents are also related to this chakra and can be major wake-up calls.

Understanding vibrational/energetic anatomy and the law of attraction holds the key to true healing, rather than just masking our symptoms, because it offers a comprehensive and holistic view of how each of us co-creates health or disease. Regardless of our past, our power to heal and stay healthy is in the present moment, right now. When we're truly present, we can heal almost anything. But most people tie up the bulk of their energy in woundings from their past, while the rest of it is consumed by worrying about the future. You cannot heal anything unless a significant amount of your energy and spirit is available in the present moment.

The late Lewis Thomas, M.D., the former president of the Memorial Sloan Kettering Cancer Center in New York City, once said that he had come to believe that cancer was the physical metaphor for the extreme need to grow. Healthy growth involves getting as many parts of yourself as possible available in the present moment, the now—the only place that healing can happen. Rarely is a person always present right now, today. Living in the now is a skill that is developed through introspection, meditation, and taking leaps of faith into freedom and joy—one small leap at a time, one day at a time.

Part Two

The Anatomy of Women's Wisdom

5

The Menstrual Cycle

How might it have been different for you if on your first menstrual day,
your mother had given you a bouquet of flowers and taken you to
lunch, and then the two of you had gone to meet your father at the jew-
eler, where your ears were pierced, and your father bought you your
first pair of earrings, and then you went with a few of your friends and
your mother's friends to get your first lip coloring; then you went,
for the very first time,
   to the Women's lodge,
     to learn
       the wisdom of women?
How might your life be different?

—Judith Duerk

We can reclaim the wisdom of the menstrual cycle by tuning in to our cyclic nature and celebrating it as a source of our female power. Astrologer Sioux Rose put it this way in her book *Moon Dance: The Feminine Dimensions of Time* (iUniverse, 2009): "Since women are biologically clocked to the moon, we are destined to feel her cycle changes via our monthly menses. This rhythmic correspondence represents the un-charted feminine realm of time. A Divine heritage bequeathed to women." The ebb and flow of dreams, creativity, and hormones associated with differ-ent parts of the cycle offer us a profound opportunity to deepen our connec-tion with our inner knowing, our cyclic energy, and our creativity. I am profoundly moved by the fact that since the first edition of this book was released, scores of women all over the world are now making this connection in their own lives. For example, my daughter Kate Northrup Watts runs a global online community, known as the Origin Collective, for entrepreneurs who are looking for new and innovative ways to balance motherhood and creative work. They use the phases of their moon cycles to plan their work and rest time most effectively and in tune with their inner wisdom. Her community is just one of many examples of thinking differently about our cycles and consciously working with their magic and wisdom.

TABLE 5

THE ANATOMY OF WOMEN'S WISDOM

Body Organ or Process	Encoded Wisdom	Energy Dysfunction	Physical Manifestation
MENSTRUAL CYCLE	Cyclic intuitive wisdom and emotional recycling and processing	Refusal to embrace both difficult and pleasant emotions: the dark and the light Not allowing shadow side to be seen and worked through Belief that menstrual cycle is bad or shameful	Lack of periods Heavy periods Irregular periods Painful periods PMS
UTERUS	Creative center in relationship to self	Bondage to the emotions of others Unable to birth most creative self Shunting one's creative energy into a dead-end job or relationship	Fibroids Adenomyosis
OVARIES	Creative drives in outer world Assertiveness in outer world Excessive, insufficient, or imbalanced drive toward financial, creative, or relationship goals	Addiction to external authority or approval Disbelief in creative ability Inability to create financial support on one's own Being awash in the anger or criticism of another without being able to escape Sexual or emotional abuse	Ovulation abnormalities Ovarian cysts Ovarian cancer Endometriosis

Body Organ or Process	Encoded Wisdom	Energy Dysfunction	Physical Manifestation
BREASTS	Balancing giving with wholehearted receiving	Inability to name, feel, express, and resolve resentment, anger, sadness, or loneliness Feeling unlovable and undeserving of love Difficulty asking for and receiving love and support Inability to participate in balanced partnerships Imbalance between intimacy with self (time alone) and with others	Breast cysts, pain Breast cancer Lung problems Shoulder problems
PREGNANCY	Capacity to conceive an idea or a life with another, hold it, nurture it, and allow it to be born and live independently	Insufficient energy to create and maintain new life Inability to trust the process of giving birth Ambivalence about effect of pregnancy and childcare on work life, body image, and personal needs Hanging on to grief and loss Intergenerational fear of dying in childbirth or losing a baby	Infertility Miscarriage Dysfunctional labor

Body Organ or Process	Encoded Wisdom	Energy Dysfunction	Physical Manifestation
CERVIX/VAGINA, VULVA	Discretion about intimacy Ability to create healthy boundaries	Poorly defined boundaries in relationships Sexual or other relationships (e.g., work) that detract from well-being Guilt or shame about sexual pleasure or sexuality Unresolved trauma from rape (either physical or psychological)	Herpes Warts Chronic vulvar pain (vulvodynia) Vaginal infections: yeast or dysbiosis Abnormal Pap tests Cervical cancer
URINARY TRACT, BLADDER	Capacity to feel emotions (especially anger) fully, heed their message, and then discharge them completely	Being chronically "pissed off" at life in general Stagnated flow of emotions in relationships Dependency in relationships Inability to release outmoded thoughts Inability to "go with the flow"	Chronic urinary tract infection Interstitial cystitis
MENOPAUSE	Passage into the wisdom years Capacity to be open to constant intuitive knowing Reseeding the community	Unfinished business from past that is unaddressed Fear of growing older Fear of owning one's power Living from the dictates of societal expectations instead of one's soul	Incapacitating hot flashes Melancholia Depression Palpitations Anxiety Forgetfulness Heart disease Loss of libido

OUR CYCLICAL NATURE

The menstrual cycle is the most basic, earthy cycle we have. Our moon cycles and our blood are our connection to the archetypal feminine. The macrocosmic cycles of nature—the waxing and waning of the moon, the ebb and flow of the tides, the changes of the seasons—are reflected on a smaller scale in the menstrual cycle of the individual female body. The monthly ripening of an egg and subsequent pregnancy or release of menstrual blood mirror the process of creation as it occurs not only in nature but in human endeavor. In many cultures, the menstrual cycle has been viewed as a sacred source of insight and renewal. (These cultures weren't far off. One day in the not-too-distant future, menstrual blood may even save lives. Research reveals that it's a potential new source of stem cells, which can be used to treat a variety of diseases, including cancer.[1] It also makes an amazing fertilizer for houseplants.)

Even in modern society, where we are cut off from the rhythms of nature, the cycle of ovulation is influenced by the moon. Studies have shown that peak rates of conception and probably ovulation appear to occur at the full moon or the day before. During the new moon, ovulation and conception rates are decreased overall, and an increased number of women start their menstrual bleeding. Scientific research has documented that the moon rules the flow of fluids (ocean tides as well as individual body fluids) and affects the unconscious mind and dreams.[2] The timing of the menstrual cycle, the fertility cycle, and labor also follows the moon-dominated tides of the ocean. Environmental cues such as light, the moon, and the tides play a documented role in regulating women's menstrual cycles and fertility. In one study of nearly 2,000 women with irregular menstrual cycles, more than half of the subjects achieved regular menstrual cycles of twenty-nine days' length by sleeping with a light on near their beds during the three days around ovulation.[3]

The menstrual cycle governs the flow not only of fluids but of information and creativity. Astrologer Sioux Rose refers to this as our moon dance—our initiation into the feminine dimensions of time. We receive and process information differently at different times in our cycles. I like to describe menstrual cycle wisdom this way: From the onset of menstruation until ovulation, we're ripening an egg and—symbolically, at least—preparing to give birth to someone (or something) else, a role that society honors. Many women find that they are at their peak of expression in the outer world from the onset of their menstrual cycle until ovulation. Their energy is outgoing and upbeat. They are filled with enthusiasm and new ideas as well as being quite willing to fold the towels and fulfill their perceived role of helping others. At midcycle, we are naturally more receptive to others and to new ideas—more "fertile." Sexual desire also peaks for many women at midcycle, and our bodies secrete into the air pheromones that increase our sexual attractiveness to others.[4] (Our male-dominated society values this very highly, and we internalize it as a "good" stage of our cycle.) One woman, a waitress who works in a diner where many truckers stop to eat, has reported to me that her tips are highest at midcycle, around ovulation. Another man described his wife as "very vital and electric" during this time of her cycle. Women find that they attract far more attention from men in public as they pass by—even when they are in baggy clothes and devoid of makeup. This biology is powerful and reminds us that, on some level, no matter our intellectual prowess, we are still mammals.

The Follicular and Luteal Phases

The menstrual cycle itself mirrors how consciousness becomes matter and how thought creates reality. On the strictly physical level, during the time between menses and ovulation (known as the follicular phase) an egg grows and develops, while deep within the wall of the uterus circular collections of immune system cells, known as lymphoid aggregates, also begin to develop.[5] On the expanded level of ideas and creativity, this first half of the cycle is a very good time to initiate new projects. A researcher friend of mine tells me that she has the most energy to act on ideas for new experiments during this part of her cycle. This is when my daughter's community members schedule their brainstorming sessions for maximal effect. Ovulation, which occurs at midcycle, is accompanied by an abrupt rise in the neuropeptides FSH (follicle-stimulating hormone) and LH (luteinizing hormone). The rise in estrogen levels that accompanies this has been associated with a rise in left-hemisphere activity (verbal fluency) and a decline in right-hemisphere activity (visual-spatial ability, such as the ability to draw a cube or read a map).[6] But this may be offset by the simultaneous peak in testosterone production, which enhances visual-spatial ability while also increasing libido. Ovulation represents mental and emotional creativity at its peak; the FSH-LH surge and the subsequent rise in hormone production that accompanies ovulation may be the biological basis for this. The weeks following ovulation lead up to the menses; this is evaluative and reflective time, looking back upon what has been created and on the negative or difficult aspects of our lives that need to be changed or adjusted. My researcher friend notes that during this part of her cycle, she prefers to do routine tasks that do not require much input from others or expansive thought on her part. It's a perfect time, for example, to simply rest more or to clean out a closet slowly and mindfully.

Our creative biological and psychological cycle parallels the phases of the moon; recent research has found that the immune system of the reproductive tract is cyclic as well, reaching its peak at ovulation and then beginning to wane. From ancient times, some cultures have referred to women having their menstrual periods as being "on their moon." When women live together in natural settings, their ovulations tend to occur at the time of the full moon, with menses and self-reflection at the dark of the moon. Scientific evidence suggests that biological cycles as well as dreams and emotional rhythms are keyed into the moon and tides as well as the planets. Specifically, the moon and tides interact with the electromagnetic fields of our bodies, subsequently affecting our internal physiological processes. The moon itself has a period when it is covered with darkness, and then slowly, beginning at the time of the new moon, it becomes visible to us again, gradually waxing to fullness. Women, too, go through a period of darkness each month, when the life force may seem to disappear for a while (premenstrual and menstrual phases).[7] We need not be afraid or think we are sick if our energies and moods naturally ebb for a few days each month. In many parts of India, it's perfectly acceptable for women to slow down during their periods and rest more. I have come to see that all kinds of stress-related disease, ranging from PMS to osteoporosis, could be lessened a great deal if we simply followed our body's wisdom once per month. Demetra George writes that it is here, at the dark of the moon, that "life cleanses, revitalizes, and transforms itself in its evolutionary development, spiraling toward attunement with its essential nature."[8] Studies have shown that most women begin their menstrual periods during the dark of the moon (new moon) and begin bleeding between

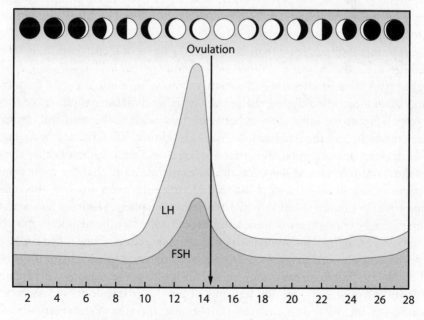

FIGURE 3: MENSTRUAL CYCLE (DAYS)

four and six A.M.—the darkest part of the day.[9] Many women have noticed that on the first day or two of their periods, they feel an urge to organize their homes or workspaces, cleaning out their closets—and their lives. Our natural biological cleansing is accompanied by a psychological cleansing as well. Before I went through menopause, I experienced this regularly myself.

If we do not become biologically pregnant at ovulation, we move into the second half of the cycle, the luteal phase—ovulation through the onset of menstruation. During this phase, we quite naturally retreat from outward activity to a more reflective mode. During the luteal phase we turn more inward, *preparing to develop or give birth to something that comes from deep within ourselves.* Society is not nearly as keen on this as it is on the follicular phase. Thus many women still judge their premenstrual energy, emotions, and inward mood as "bad" and "unproductive." (See figure 4, page 126.)

Since our culture generally appreciates only what we can understand rationally, many women tend to block at every opportunity the flow of unconscious "lunar" information that comes to them premenstrually or during their menstrual cycle. Lunar information is reflective and intuitive. It comes to us in our dreams, our emotions, and our hungers. It comes under cover of darkness. When we routinely block the information that is coming to us in the second half of our menstrual cycles, it has no choice but to come back as PMS or menopausal madness, in the same way that our other feelings and bodily symptoms, if ignored, often result in illness.[10] Or as my physician friend Paulanne Balch, M.D., puts it, "The longest relationship you'll have in your life is the one with your body. It's time I exchanged phone numbers with my body and became willing to take the call. Tumors, illness, and injury are all signs that your voicemail is full."

The luteal phase, from ovulation until the onset of menstruation, is when women are *most in tune with their inner knowing and with what isn't working in their lives.* Studies have shown that women's dreams are more frequent and often more vivid during the premenstrual and menstrual phases of their cycles.[11] Premenstrually, the veil between the worlds of the seen and unseen, the conscious and the unconscious, is much thinner. We have access to parts of our often unconscious selves that are less available to us at all other times of the month. In fact, it has been shown experimentally that the right hemisphere of the brain—the part associated with intuitive knowing—becomes more active premenstrually, while the left hemisphere becomes less active. Interestingly enough, communication between the two hemispheres may be increased as well.[12] The premenstrual phase is therefore a time when we have greater access to our magic—our ability to recognize and transform the more difficult and painful areas of our lives. This is one of the reasons why dreams of overflowing toilets, muddy bottoms of ponds, or trapdoors in basements leading to unexplored rooms are so common at this time. Premenstrually, we are quite naturally more in tune with what is most meaningful in our lives.

We're more apt to cry—but our tears are always related to something that holds meaning for us. The many studies done by the late Katharina Dalton, M.D., have documented that women are more emotional premenstrually, more apt to act out their anger, and more prone to headaches and fatigue, and they may even experience exacerbations of ongoing illnesses such as arthritis. To the extent that we are out of touch with the hidden parts of ourselves, we will suffer premenstrually. Years of personal and clinical experience have taught me that the painful or uncomfortable issues that arise premenstrually are always real and must be addressed. Only then will they resolve completely.

Women need to believe in the importance of the issues that come up premenstrually. Even though our bodies and minds may not express these needs and concerns as they would in the first part of our cycle—on our so-called good days—our inner wisdom is clearly asking for our attention. One woman told me, for example, that whenever she becomes premenstrual, she worries that the house, car, and investments are in her husband's name only. When she mentions this to her husband, he replies, "What's wrong? Don't you trust me?" I'd call that a premenstrual reality check that needs attention! One husband reported that in the follicular phase of his wife's cycle, she was great—she was always cheery, kept the house in order, and did the cooking. But after ovulation she "let herself go" and talked about wanting to go back to college and get out of the house more. I told him that these issues which arise premenstrually should be treated seriously, and I asked him to consider that his wife's needs were for her full personal development. I pointed out that her difficult behavior premenstrually was her way of expressing those needs. She, of course, also needs to learn how to articulate her needs directly.

There is an intimate relationship between a woman's psyche and her ovarian function throughout the menstrual cycle. Before we ovulate we are outgoing and upbeat, while ovulating we are very receptive to others, and after ovulation (premenstrually) we are more inward and reflective. An astounding study done in the 1930s supports my observations. The psychoanalyst Therese Benedek, M.D., studied the psychotherapy records of a group of patients, while her colleague Boris Rubenstein, M.D., studied the ovarian hormonal cycles of the same women. By looking at a woman's emotional content, Dr. Benedek was able to predict where she was in her menstrual cycle with incredible accuracy. The authors wrote, "We were pleased and surprised to find an exact correspondence of the ovulative dates as independently determined by the two methods"—that is, psychoanalytic material compared with physiological findings. They found that before ovulation, when estrogen levels were at their highest, women's emotions and behavior were directed toward the outer world. During ovulation, however, women were more relaxed and content and quite receptive to being cared for and loved by others. During the postovulatory and premenstrual phase, when progesterone is at its highest, women were more likely to be focused on themselves and more involved in inward-directed activity. Interestingly, in women who had periods but did not ovulate, the authors saw similar cycles of emotions and behavior, except that around the time when ovulation should have occurred, these women missed not only ovulation but the accompanying emotions; that is, they were not relaxed, content, or receptive to being cared for by others.[13]

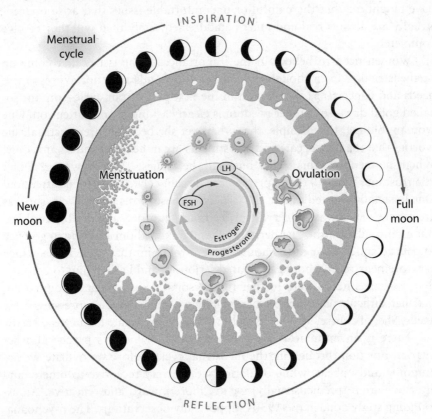

FIGURE 4: LUNAR CHART FOR MENSTRUAL CYCLE

Given our cultural heritage and beliefs about illness in general and the menstrual cycle in particular, it is not difficult to understand how women have come to see their premenstrual phase not as a time for reflection and renewal but as a disease or a curse. In fact, the language that our culture uses regarding the uterus and ovaries has been experimentally shown to affect women's menstrual cycles. Under hypnosis, a woman who is given positive suggestions about her menstrual cycle will be much less apt to suffer from menstruation-related symptoms.[14] On the other hand, one study found that women who were led to believe that they were premenstrual when they weren't reported more adverse physical symptoms, such as water retention, cramps, and irritability, than another group who were led to believe they were not premenstrual.[15] These studies are excellent examples of how our thoughts and beliefs have the power to affect our hormones, our biochemistry, and our subsequent experience.

Healing Through Our Cycles

Once we begin to appreciate our menstrual cycle as part of our inner guidance system, we begin to heal both hormonally and emotionally. There is no doubt that premenstrually, many women feel more inward-directed and more connected to their personal pain and the pain of the world. Eckhart Tolle in his famous book *The Power of Now* (New World Library, 2004) says that a woman's "pain body" arises premenstrually and that the best way to dissolve it is to be present with it—instead of projecting it onto others (which is what gives PMS its bad name). Many naturally empathic women pick up and absorb the emotions of others, and the pain of the world, like human lint rollers. As I explain in my book *Dodging Energy Vampires: An Empath's Guide to Evading Relationships That Drain You and Restoring Your Health and Power* (Hay House, 2018), these individuals are natural light workers who need to know that their bodies are naturally clearing darkness from the collective. Nothing more needs to be done. This is what it means to dissolve your pain body—whether that pain body is actually yours or something you are unwittingly carrying. Doing so allows a woman to be more in touch with her own creativity, though she may not act on the ideas that surface at this time until later because during the premenstrual phase, she needs time to be alone, time to rest, and time away from her daily duties. Taking this time is a new idea and practice for many women. And many will, at first, feel guilty for doing so. That's part of the process.

Premenstrual syndrome results when we don't honor our need to ebb and flow like the tides. This society likes action, so we often don't appreciate our need for rest and replenishment. We would do well to remember that all the functions of our bodies have both an active (yang) phase and a receptive (yin) phase. For example, the heart actively contracts during systole, sending the blood out into the vessels. (This is the top number we measure when taking blood pressure.) The space between heart contractions, known as diastole (the lower number of blood pressure), is equally important. Without adequate relaxation in this phase, the entire cardiovascular system suffers under too much strain. The same is true in our lives and during our menstrual cycles. The menstrual cycle is set up to teach us about the need for both the in-breath and the out-breath of life's processes. When we are premenstrual and feeling fragile, we need to rest and take care of ourselves for a day or two. In the Native American moon lodge, bleeding women came together for renewal and visioning and emerged afterward inspired and also inspiring to others. I think that the majority of PMS cases would disappear if every modern woman retreated from her duties for three or four days each month and had her meals brought to her by someone else.

I personally found that simply and *unapologetically* stating my needs for a monthly slowdown to my former husband was all that was needed. When I showed respect for myself and the processes of my body, he showed respect as well, and my body responded with comfort and gratitude. Indeed, my experience of my own menstrual cycle began to change after I noticed that my most meaningful insights about myself, my life, and my writing came on the day or two just before my period. In my mid-thirties, I began to look forward to my periods, understanding them to be sacred time that our culture didn't honor. When I was premenstrual, the things that made me feel teary were the things that were most important to me, things that I knew tuned me in to my power and my deepest truths. My increased sensitivity felt like a gift of insight. I usually didn't become angry, though if I did, I knew to pay attention and not chalk it up to "my stupid hormones." I liked to keep track of the phases of the moon in my daily calendar to see if I was ovulating at the full moon, the dark of the moon, or in between. When I ovulated at the full moon and menstruated at the dark of the moon, my inner reflective time was synchronized with the moon's darkness. Getting my period at the time of the full moon resulted in a more intense period: I was more emotionally charged than usual, and my bleeding was often heavier than normal. I found that sometimes simply intending to bleed at the dark of the moon might move my cycles in this direction, though not always. (I didn't try to control this.) My daughters have discovered the same thing. Noting your individual cycle in relationship to the moon's cycle consciously connects you with the earth and helps you to feel connected with women past and present. Truly welcoming and appreciating your cycles in this way also makes the transition into menopause much easier. Having been truly present with inner wisdom during your cycling years, you will not mourn when you move into your wisdom years. In addition, you will have used all those hundreds of opportunities given to you by your monthly cycle to upgrade your thinking, your behavior, and your life.

AN INCONVENIENT TRUTH

Throughout the world, too many menstruating girls and women must leave school or work simply because they do not have access to or cannot afford to buy menstrual products to deal with their bleeding times—a situation activists have named "period poverty." For example, 65 percent of the women and girls in Kenya cannot afford period products. Even in the United States, women living below the poverty line often struggle to buy menstrual products because they are not covered by food stamps.

Happily, this issue is more and more often being addressed by organizations like Period.org, which have as their mission the distribution of "period packs" to those who do not have access to conventional pads and tampons. Other such organizations include I Support the Girls (www.isupportthegirls.org), which provides bras and underwear in addition to menstrual products; Days for Girls (www.daysforgirls.org); and Dignity Period (www.dignityperiod.org).

In addition, women's health advocates are creating more eco-friendly menstrual products like the menstrual cup, which simply catches the blood as it comes out of the cervix. A good example is the medical-grade, silicone-free menstrual cup made by Femme-Tasse (www.femme-tasse.com), which can be washed and reused for years, helping to eliminate thousands of pounds of pad and tampon waste from landfills. For each cup purchased from Femme-Tasse, the company donates one to women around the world who don't have access to menstrual hygiene products.

Finally, organic and nontoxic menstrual pads and tampons are also now available from companies like Cora (www.cora.life). With each purchase, Cora provides menstrual pads and health education to a girl in need.

OUR CULTURAL INHERITANCE

The menstrual cycle and the female body were seen as sacred until 5,000 years ago, when the peaceful matrilineal cultures of Old Europe were overturned.[16] The original meaning of the word *taboo* was "sacred," and women having their periods were considered sacred; now in some societies they are considered unclean. Often their dreams and visions were used to guide the tribe. The Yurok people of Northern California, for example, believe that a menstruating woman should isolate herself from mundane duties during her period because she is at the height of her spiritual power at this time. So instead of wasting these precious days, she is supposed to devote herself to meditation, purification, and turning inward to address her life's purpose and to gather spiritual energy.[17] Native cultures the world over have honored young women with coming-of-age ceremonies. First menstruation has meant being initiated into the "offices of womanhood" by mothers, aunts, and other initiated women.[18] The Kinaalda coming-of-age puberty rite of the traditional Navajo, for example, is considered one of the most important of the tribal rituals because the young girl is now of an age to bring new life to the tribe. In the month after a girl gets her first period, her entire extended family gathers together for a four-day ceremony. During this time, the girl wears a traditional buckskin dress and has her hair braided in a special style. Every morning she gets up at dawn and is expected to run into the rising sun, running faster and farther each day. When she returns, an older female relative instructs her in how to be a woman. She also enjoys traditional massage. The entire tribe participates in a special feast. And during this time she is expected to take on more and more responsibility. On the last night, the tribe stays up all night and, led by the shaman, prays for the girl and her family. The emphasis is on both physical strength and upstanding character.[19]

Archaeological evidence from more than 6,000 years ago points to the fact that the original calendars were bones with small marks on them that women used to keep track of their cycles.[20] Yet throughout much of written Western history, and even in religious codes, the menstrual cycle has been associated with shame and degradation, with women's dark, uncontrollable nature. Menstruating women were thought of as unclean. In A.D. 65, in his encyclopedia *Natural History*, Pliny the Elder wrote:

> But nothing could easily be found that is more remarkable [note the ambivalent word choice] than the monthly flux of women. Contact with it turns new wine sour, crops touched by it become barren, seeds in gardens dry up, the fruit of trees falls off. The bright surface of mirrors in which it is merely reflected is dimmed, the edge of steel and the gleam of ivory are dulled. Hives of bees will die. Even bronze and iron are at once seized by rust and a horrible smell fills the air. To taste it drives dogs mad and affects their bite with an incurable poison.[21]

The taboo associated with the menstrual cycle has continued to this day. Generations of women have been taught that we are more physically vulnerable during our periods—that we shouldn't swim, have sex, bathe, or even wash our hair during this time. In the Victorian era, it was believed that bathing, shampooing hair, or swimming might "back up" menstrual flow, resulting in stroke, insanity, or rapid onset of tuberculosis.[22] Though these notions have served to keep women afraid of their natural body processes for generations, there is a kernel of truth in these outdated notions that can be a source of wisdom and strength when put into proper perspective. I asked Sandra Chiu, a licensed acupuncturist and a practitioner of traditional Chinese medicine, to explain this from a TCM point of view (see box opposite).

This information rounds out all of the myths about menstruation. And it's also very validating to women everywhere who would prefer a hot bath and a cup of tea to going out in the cold during their periods.

TRADITIONAL CHINESE MEDICINE AND MENSTRUATION
By Sandra Lanshin Chiu, L.Ac.

Understood simply, the ultimate goal of healing in traditional Chinese medicine is to restore well-being by removing all the obstructions to healthful and proper movement (or flow) in all the body's systems. This usually refers to circulation of *chi* (or *qi*), a term that means life force or vital energy, as well as of blood and vital fluids. But it also includes the movement within organs, whose healthy function depends on proper flow and movement within their systems.

Blockage of movement equates with disrupted function, which is at the core of all diseases and pain. Translated through a Western lens, this is not unlike the concept of inflammation. In TCM understanding, many factors create blockage in the body, and one of them is the energy of coldness.

The nature of cold is to contract and slow down. Think of how coldness of temperature applied to water slows its movement. If you drop the temperature enough, it will altogether halt fluid movement, to the point where a solid mass of ice forms. This same principle of nature occurs within your body just as it does in the external environment. (Think how testicles shrink into the body when exposed to the cold.)

So why is this concept important to a menstruating woman? During menstruation, a woman's body is focused on discharging menstrual blood, what TCM refers to as her "heavenly waters." If this process is healthy, she will have a smooth, painless, and unimpeded flow without painful cramps, mood swings, fatigue, acne, or other discomforts.

TCM places great importance on supporting the strong and healthy movement of blood during this monthly discharge. This is why it is almost sacrilegious for a menstruating woman to eat ice cream or have iced drinks, go swimming, or wear clothing such as a crop top that might expose her naked abdomen to the external environment. All these things have the effect of cooling down her body, thus slowing circulatory movement.

In a menstruating woman, impeding circulatory flow can aggravate pain, among other distressing symptoms. When TCM practitioners treat dysmenorrhea (painful periods) they often use warming moxibustion or herbal medicines that are hot in nature to expel cold in the womb. Many menstruating women intuitively do something similar when they apply a heating pad or hot water bottle to a cramping abdomen.

Opposite to cold, the nature of heat generates movement and quickens flow. Think of heat applied to ice: At first the ice thaws into liquid form, and eventually, with high enough temperatures, can reach a rolling boil. Supporting the healthy heat of the body is thus an important practice for a woman's reproductive health.

In modern life, this translates to practices such as avoiding cold or iced food and drinks (this includes smoothies), making sure your belly is always warm and covered, wearing slippers on cold tile, and abstaining from swimming and water sports (because the water is usually much cooler than body temperature).

It wasn't only the Chinese who recognized this phenomenon, by the way. Folk medicine during Victorian times also held that bathing, shampooing, and swimming could "back up" or obstruct proper menstrual flow. In this time before modern heating and hair dryers, taking a bath or washing the hair was understood to make the body susceptible to cold—and therefore illness. If this concept is difficult to understand, just imagine stepping out of a bath with wet hair in the middle of winter, with no electricity (let alone electric appliances like hair dryers) and the only heating in your home being the wood-burning oven in the kitchen. Maintaining a healthy warmth internally would no doubt be challenging.

Though this concept of how cold impacts menstruation may require some getting used to for the Western mind, it's worth highlighting how the sheer existence of such a concept reflects the importance TCM places on supporting the health of a woman's menstruation. Rather than seeing menstruation as a dirty, annoying, or terrible time of the month, it's regarded as a natural process that requires and deserves special care and supportive practices.

(For more information from Sandra on TCM, visit www.lanshin .com.)

If we are to reclaim and embrace our menstrual wisdom and honor our cyclic natures, we must at the same time acknowledge the negative attitudes that most of us have internalized concerning our menstrual cycles. We must acknowledge the pain and discomfort that many women experience monthly.

Our cyclic nature has borne the brunt of all kinds of jokes about being "on the rag" or having "the curse." Puberty and the first menstruation for many women have been saturated with shame and humiliation. Nothing in our society—with the exception of violence and fear—has been more effective in keeping women "in their place" than the degradation of the menstrual cycle. It's gratifying to see that this attitude is now changing as our culture realizes that the first menses is an important rite of passage.

Replacing the harmful inherited myths about our menstrual cycles with accurate information is part of women's healing. After menarche (the first menstruation), which in this society generally occurs around the age of twelve, give or take a couple of years, a young woman reaches sexual maturity—though it's likely to be many years before she attains the emotional and psychological maturity necessary to truly embrace her sexuality as a source of power, joy, and renewal. A certain body composition is required for the onset of menarche. Usually the body mass must be about 17 percent fat for a young woman to start having periods. Studies have indicated that a body fat level averaging about 22 percent is necessary for sustained ovulatory cycles in most females.[23] The obesity rate in children is one of the factors (along with environmental toxins) that has caused earlier puberty—with first signs of puberty beginning as early as age eight or even younger—in so many young girls. On the other side of the coin, anorexic young women and female dancers and athletes who have very little body fat don't have regular periods, though emotional factors that affect the hypothalamus of the brain also play a key role in these situations. Though a young woman's first cycles are usually not ovulatory, she gradually becomes fertile over the next several years, producing an egg each month from her ovaries. If the monthly egg is not fertilized at midcycle, this results in a menstrual period about fourteen days after ovulation. In the flow, the lining of the uterus (the endometrium) is shed. Each month, the lining, or endometrium, builds up and is shed cyclically, stimulated by a complex and amazing interaction between hormones produced by the ovaries, the pituitary gland, and the hypothalamus. (See figure 5, page 138.) Because of the complexity of this hormonal interaction, many areas of a woman's life affect the menstrual cycle. The cycle in turn affects many areas of a woman's life.

Too many girls still learn about the menstrual cycle in a sterile, clinical way, without respect for their female bodies and their own sexuality. How their bodies, their sexuality, and their creativity are linked to the menstrual cycle and the moon has, up until the last generation or so, rarely been discussed, let alone celebrated. In the past, very few girls were introduced to menstruation as a positive rite of passage. My mother told me the "facts of life" and explained eggs and sperm to me when I was in the fourth grade. I recall being very upset by this information. My sister, eleven months younger than I, had said earlier that day, "Mom, I know where babies come from, but how do they get there?" My mother took us into her bedroom and read us a book that said that girls get a menstrual period around the age of twelve, and that after they get their period they could have a baby if they had sex.

I was not happy with this information. I continued to hope that women could get pregnant by kissing rather than by the disgusting act my mother described. Why I found the whole thing so disgusting might have had something to do with my own mother's initiation into puberty. She was not concerned with the meaning of the menstrual cycle and the sacredness of the female body, though she was and is a woman who is truly wise and ahead of her time. My mother had learned that once she got her period, somehow she could no longer enjoy herself in the same way. Her favorite girlhood activities had been playing baseball and climbing trees with the boys. But once she "became a woman," she was no longer allowed to play with the boys. Years later, she told me that she begged her mother to take her to the hospital to get her "fixed" so that she wouldn't have periods anymore and could go back to baseball. Because my mother didn't completely resolve her adolescent feelings about her menstrual cycle until she was in her sixties, I absorbed many of her unconscious feelings around menstruation, even though she presented it to me as a normal part of life. Like thousands of baby boomer mothers, I attempted to pass a more positive message on to my daughters. But to do that effectively, I first had to acknowledge the depth of my own pain around the menstrual cycle.

Instead of celebrating our cyclic nature as a positive aspect of our female being, up until very recently we've been taught that we shouldn't acknowledge our periods at all, lest we neglect the needs of our spouses and children. Consider this excerpt from a 1963 insert inside a tampon box:

WHEN YOU'RE A WIFE

Don't take advantage of your husband. That's an old rule of good marriage behavior that's just as sensible now as it ever was. Of course, you'll not try to take advantage, but sometimes ways of taking advantage aren't obvious.

You wouldn't connect it with menstruation, for instance. Yet, if you neglect the simple rules that make menstruation a normal time of month, and retire for a few days each month, as though you were ill, you're taking advantage of your husband's good nature. He married a full-time wife, not a part-time one. So you should be active, peppy, and cheerful every day.[24]

Always cheery—just like June Cleaver in those old *Leave It to Beaver* reruns. No wonder so many women have PMS! When I think of the indoctrination represented by that 1963 insert, from the year I got my first period,

I marvel at how far we've come in such a short time. But I'm constantly amused at how market forces continue to shape our experience of our cycles, for better or for worse. At a 2009 conference of the Society for Menstrual Cycle Research in Spokane, Washington, David Linton, Ph.D., gave a keynote address entitled "The Rise of the Happy Period: From Shame to Humor in Mediated Menses." He pointed out that advertising has led to decreasing shame around monthly bleeding. This more upbeat approach to a woman's period has been driven, in part, by the pad and tampon industry, which, in the face of so many women taking menstrual suppression birth control pills (such as Seasonale; see below), wants to keep women bleeding![25] On the other end of the spectrum is the newer practice of inserting synthetic progestin implants into the arms of girls and women to prevent them from having periods altogether. One or two flexible plastic rods are inserted by a clinician under the skin of the inner arm, just above the elbow. They slowly release a low dose of progestin (a synthetic progesterone) at a steady, sustained rate, preventing pregnancy for up to five years (depending on which brand you use), although your doctor can remove the implants at any time and you could get pregnant right away. The Mirena IUD also can eliminate periods because of the effect of the synthetic progestin it contains.

The Menstrual Cycle, Birth Control Pills, and Women's Intuition

Our intuition works differently during the various phases of our menstrual cycle. It changes again after menopause. One of my colleagues, an osteopathic physician, noticed this connection between intuition and the menstrual cycle when he referred a patient to me for a change in birth control method. She had been on the pill for a number of years, but he felt that continued use of the pill was interfering with her ability to know what her next steps in life should be. The referral note to me read: "Birth control pills are interfering with intuitive function. Suggest alternatives." This was one of my all-time favorite referrals from a very insightful man.

In an age in which millions of women's bodies, due to the use of birth control pills, are more in tune with pharmaceutical companies than with the moon, it is no small task to rethink a medication that has offered so many women such highly touted advantages. After all, the pill provides women with periods that need never ruin their weekends, it often decreases menstrual cramps, and it is associated with a decreased risk of ovarian and endometrial cancer. Many women are sold on the benefits of Seasonale, a birth control pill that results in only four periods per year. One for each season! But no one is sure whether this or other birth control pills increase the risk of breast cancer (studies show a slightly increased risk, yet researchers couldn't rule out other factors that may have caused the increase),[26] although studies have shown that it can increase the risk of cervical cancer.[27] (It's also possible to suppress menses entirely using many other brands of birth control pills. Doctors have been prescribing them in this way for years. For more information on this approach, visit www.noperiod.com.)

Laurie, one of my colleagues in ob-gyn, was on the pill for more than nine years before she changed her mind about its advantages. She had routinely pushed the pill as a panacea for all her patients, using her own experience as coercion. When she lectured them on why they should all be on the pill, she always ended her talk with the statement "They'll never get my pills away from me." Only after Laurie began to see her own illnesses as physical manifestations of the diseases in her spirit was she able to reevaluate her position on the pill. The breakthrough for her happened in part because her relationship with her husband had begun to deteriorate. They were having frequent arguments around the subject of sex. "It drove me crazy," she said, "that he seemed to separate it completely from everything else that was going on in our relationship. At the same time, my own confusion about my body, my feelings of discomfort with its size and shape, my inhibitions about noise and awkwardness during sex, and mixed messages from my childhood about sex and seduction made sex something fraught with negative connotation and sometimes insurmountable obstacles."

Laurie was learning about how different parts of our bodies talk to us through symptoms as part of our inner guidance system. As she did, she realized that remaining on birth control pills might prevent her female organs from optimally communicating with her, especially in a personal crisis around her own sexuality. She began to awaken to how she had inadvertently become separated from her body by following the dictates of the culture instead of her inner guidance. This awakening was accompanied by an interest in feminism for the first time in her life. Up until then, she had considered herself highly successful and functional, which is how she seems on the surface. Yet she had had a benign ovarian cyst, operated on several years before, and during her ob-gyn residency she had been operated on for thyroid cancer. Her emerging inner wisdom showed her that these conditions had been her body's way of trying to get her attention and let her know that something was out of balance in her life. Now she was willing and eager to pay attention to what her body was saying.

"I felt sadness," Laurie says, "that I had taken for granted, drugged away, or labeled a 'curse' all the wondrous workings of my brain, my hormones, my uterus, and my ovaries. No one ever celebrated my first period. No one had helped me connect the power of giving birth to my sexuality. I longed to recapture some of that lost magic and mystery. But it took me almost two years of pulling down the curtains of my life and dusting away the cobwebs before I felt that I could tentatively trust my body."

After these two years of personal struggle, Laurie decided to take a year off from her busy obstetrical practice in a large city. She was exhausted from the demands of three children, her practice, and a marriage that was now ending. She knew that she needed to reflect on her life and explore some new directions. She said that when she finally got around to doing it, going off the pill was "something of an act of celebration and rebellion." It was clear to her that a divorce was imminent. "Since I did not need contraception any-more," she observed, "it occurred to me that now might be the time to allow myself the luxury of my hormones. So I threw away the last dial-pack and waited. I was pretty sure that after nine years of instruction from Ortho Pharmaceutical, my ovaries would be totally confused, so I was willing to be patient. I was prepared for swelling, irritability, wild emotions, and confusion. I was not prepared for what happened."

Two weeks after stopping the pill, Laurie was sitting with a group of women and relating the events of the past two years. She noted, "Suddenly, I was in tears and I could hardly speak. I remember thinking, 'Now isn't this strange?'" It took her a while to realize that even though she did indeed feel sadness about the changes under way in her life, she had in fact told others about these changes and feelings before, while she was on the pill, without any emotional or physiological reaction whatsoever. She discovered that for her, ovulation was associated with an increased ability to feel and express her deepest emotions. She wrote, "I didn't realize for two more days that the excessive cervical mucus [a very common sign of ovulation] and the sudden opening of the emotional floodgate were signs of ovulation. Even when I did put it together, I refused to trust my body. 'Well,' I thought, 'I'll just wait two weeks and see.' Two weeks later, there I was in my red dress—my first spontaneous period in over nine years, never a more welcome sight. I felt as though I had been given a wondrous gift from a long-lost friend. This body, which I had abused for so long and in so many ways, was suddenly talking to me again, giving me encouragement and reassurance. All was not lost."

In addition to finding that her emotions were now more available to her, Laurie found that she was more in touch with anger that she would have previously denied. She related that shortly after her own periods resumed, "I found my anger. My righteous, fiery, white-hot anger. Of course, my husband was the unwitting recipient of what felt like twenty years of suppressed emotions. I don't know if he deserved all of it—certainly not all at once. But as it came pouring out, I remember thinking, 'This is amazing! This is really me. My hormones. My magic!' I think now that if I had been feeling that anger as it came up all those years, I might still be married—or I would have divorced much sooner. Either way would have been better than what had happened. It was not okay that I had missed so much of myself."

Laurie knew to honor and pay attention to what was happening to her, even though some of it was painful. She later reflected, "Since then I have learned to expect to hear regularly from my hormones. They teach me where I still need to put my attention. When I am suddenly in tears, I know to pause and consider what emotional work I still have to do in that area. When anger comes, I remind myself that being able to push it down inside myself is not a gift. Anger unexpressed produces disease. It belongs outside my body."

The other thing that Laurie noticed was the connection between her menstrual cycle and her inherent sexuality. I have heard similar stories from

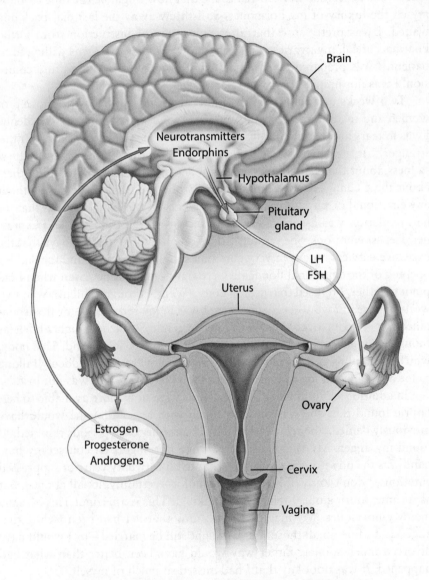

FIGURE 5: THE FEMALE MIND-BODY CONTINUUM:
INTERACTIONS BETWEEN THE BRAIN AND THE PELVIS

many women. She told me, "There is this wild desire racing around in my brain for several days every month around ovulation. My friends told me about it, but this is amazing. And I thought all those years that the pill was helping my sex life by getting rid of all those messy barrier contraceptives!" (The pill suppresses the midcycle testosterone surge, thus decreasing sex drive in many women. And unfortunately, this suppression can last even after a woman has come off the pill.)[28] She had used the diaphragm only while breast-feeding, and she realized she had blamed her lack of sexual desire on the messiness of diaphragm use. But now she understood that her lack of desire was most likely related to breast-feeding hormones and energy drain, not the diaphragm. Many nursing mothers simply are not interested in sexual intercourse, for complex reasons related to lack of support and sleep as well as conventional birth practices that lower oxytocin and endorphin levels. This needn't be the case. Sexual desire tends to resume gradually as the baby gets older, but this is not inevitable, either.[29] (See chapter 13.)

Laurie noted another change that is very common. After going off the pill, her body tended to make up for lost time, with ovulations coming more frequently for a while, then adjusting to approximately once per month. "When I first reclaimed my cycles," she wrote, "they were very short, about every three weeks. Although the thought flashed through my head briefly that it would be a pain to be bleeding one week out of every three, I realized that the thought was a conditioned one. How many forty-year-old women had complained to me about the increasing frequency of their periods and begged me to 'do something' about it? Now I realized that I had been given a gift of short cycles to 'catch up.' I loved getting to cycle more often. I got to ovulate every three weeks. I got more lessons about my body. It was like a crash course in female physiology—my own. I began to celebrate getting my periods every three weeks and hoped that menopause would not come until I was sixty-five. Having given myself permission to enjoy all these new lessons, I once again learned that I was not in control—my cycles began to spread out to three and a half, then four weeks. I think it was just a test, having three-week cycles. It was to see if I really wanted this part of my body back. I do."

Laurie's story illustrates what reclaiming our menstrual wisdom and power feels like. Though the pill has been a boon to many women, it has also taken them out of touch with some essential parts of their female wisdom. When people are in close contact with one another, for example, one way they communicate is via pheromones. Oral contraceptives, however, have been shown to eliminate part of our pheromonal communication pathway, including our sexual communication with men. It has now been well established that women secrete pheromones around ovulation that are definitely associated with greater romantic interest from men. The birth control pill blocks these.[30] Women who live together often cycle together, in a process one of my friends calls "becoming ovarian sisters." This doesn't happen to women on the pill. Studies have shown that women who have close relationships with other people have shorter and more regular cycles, whereas women who isolate themselves are more likely to have irregular cycles.[31]

MENSTRUAL CRAMPS (DYSMENORRHEA)

As many as 60 percent of all women suffer from menstrual cramps. A smaller percentage are unable to function for one or more days each month because of the severity of their pain. The fact that the majority of women in our culture suffer from menstrual cramps is a very clear indication that we have something wrong with our lifestyles and our relationship to our bodies. It testifies that we have lost much of our connection to our menstrual wisdom and the behaviors that would enhance it. The psychological gynecological literature of the 1950s was filled with studies that suggested that menstrual cramps were mainly psychological, related to being unhappy about being a woman. Caroline Myss says that cramps and PMS are classic indications that a woman is in some kind of conflict with being a woman, with her role in the tribe, and with the tribal expectations of her. Given our current society's traditional expectations for women, it's amazing that 100 percent of us don't have cramps and PMS.

Cramps are not the same as PMS, although women often suffer from both. Dysmenorrhea is divided into two types. Primary dysmenorrhea is cramps that are not secondary to another organic disease in the pelvis. Secondary dysmenorrhea is cramps that are caused by endometriosis or other pelvic disease. Treatments that help primary dysmenorrhea usually help secondary dysmenorrhea as well.

I had primary dysmenorrhea in my teens and up until after the birth of my first child. I sometimes had to call my mother from school and leave class because of the pain. Once during my residency I even had to leave a major surgical case because of menstrual cramps. One of my fellow residents said to me, "Gee, Chris, you have cramps? Maybe it's not all in women's heads!" (Remember, I was "one of the guys" back then and was doing everything in my power to maintain that position. You can imagine what a blow it was to have to leave the operating room because of that dreaded female weakness, cramps!)

Beginning in the late 1970s, studies showed that women with cramps have high levels of the hormone prostaglandin F2 alpha (PGF2 alpha) in their menstrual blood. When this hormone is released into the bloodstream as the endometrial lining breaks down, the uterus goes into spasm, resulting in cramping pain.[32] (Menstrual cramps are not in the head after all—they're in the uterus! Actually, it's not either/or. What goes on in the head does affect what goes on in the uterus.)

When I first got my period, I was conflicted about growing up in general and growing up as a girl in particular, just as my mother had been. The increased stress of puberty produced high levels of the stress hormones cortisol and norepinephrine and subsequently of insulin, the hormone that helps the body process glucose. High stress hormone levels, in combination with my diet of too many refined carbohydrates and sugar, resulted in an overproduction of insulin, and the overproduction of the inflammatory chemical PGF2 alpha in the lining of my uterus. Bad cramps were the result! The cramps disappeared for a while after the birth of my first child, but they came back, though much milder and not with every period, when my second daughter was about five. This time of no cramps taught me that when my life was in balance, I didn't have cramps. When I became too busy or stressed out, producing too much cortisol, norepinephrine, and insulin, my body produced too many inflammatory chemicals and I'd have a few hours of cramps on the first day of my period. They slowed me right down and were a good reminder that I needed to make some adjustments and to tune in to the wisdom of my body.

Medication. Nonsteroidal anti-inflammatory drugs, such as Advil, Nuprin, Anaprox, and Motrin, block the synthesis of prostaglandin F2 alpha when taken just at the onset of periods, *before* the pain starts, or as soon after as possible. Once the endometrial lining begins to shed and prostaglandin F2 alpha (and other inflammatory chemicals) gets released into the bloodstream, it's much harder to interrupt the resulting uterine spasms that cause the pain.

Birth control pills, which eliminate ovulation and therefore the hormonal changes associated with cramps, work well for many women who are not interested in making lifestyle or dietary changes. Some women, however, get cramps even on oral contraceptives. The newer pills can be safely used by most women over thirty-five, as long as they do not smoke.

Traditional women's herbs such as *Pueraria mirifica,* when taken cyclically (on days seven through twenty-one of your cycle), will often eliminate both cramps and PMS after about three months or even sooner in some. This approach can then be continued indefinitely as long as a woman isn't pregnant or wanting to conceive. (See Resources.)

Women's Stories

Ann: Healing Menstrual Cramps by Going Within

Ann, a woman in her mid-twenties, had had a history of cramps, nausea, and vomiting, off and on, since she first got her period at age fourteen. She'd gone for stretches when the symptoms were very mild, and then at other times they would become severe. From time to time, she tried many of the treatments mentioned elsewhere in this chapter, and they helped to one degree or another. But nothing seemed to make a huge difference.

She had always rested during her period, she told me, but that was mostly by default or because her body was forcing her to do so. Then after reading Lara Owen's *Her Blood Is Gold* (Archive, 2009), Ann decided to try Owen's suggestion to consciously plan to rest, be still, and go inward during her bleeding time. Here's what she wrote me about her experience:

> The first time I did this, I let nearly everyone with whom I was in regular contact know ahead of time that I might be incommunicado for a day or two, as I was going inward for my moon time. And I didn't even turn on my computer until about four or five in the afternoon that day, which was absolutely revelatory for me. I felt like I was walking in this magical, powerful energy within my cocoon all day. I wrote in my journal, meditated, listened to music, and rested. That month I had almost no cramping at all, and no nausea whatsoever—this after a couple of months in a row of some of my worst symptoms yet. I thought to myself, *Aha!*
>
> I can't say that I have always succeeded in replicating that powerful cocoon/retreat day that I created for myself that first time after reading Lara's book. But I had that experience of what it could do for me—physically *and* spiritually and emotionally. And I will always know that, in my body and in mind. So now I am on the path of doing my best to deliberately create that space for myself during my moon time—a space to go inward, to feel my feelings, to be in my creativity, to rest and be still. The difference is that I am doing my best to choose this in partnership with my body, instead of being a victim of my body forcing me to lie down because I'm in such terrible pain that I can't function.
>
> My period has been telling me to slow down, be still, and listen to my inner voice every month, faithfully and patiently, since I first started menstruating. She is always there, always communicating to me. And the more I listen and take the space I need for my dance with her each month, the better I feel, both physically and otherwise. I have had amazing creative ideas come through me during my moon time. Lots of emotions come through and release, and lots of clarity comes in as well, often during meditation or journaling. I also find my period to be a very grounding time. It's such a relief when I feel tired the way I do during my period. It's a soft, cozy kind of tired that I don't feel the compulsion to resist. My period brings me *into* my body—an invaluable gift.
>
> Now I've come to look forward to my moon time, and I continue to experiment with how to best create the time and space to really com-

mune with myself during that time. Some months are easier than others. But when I am able to do it, the benefits are immense on so many levels, and the insights, rejuvenation, and creativity I receive during moon time actually make me happier, healthier, and more productive during the rest of the month—not to mention more grounded. I know I'm not alone in this challenge and that taking that monthly retreat, even for a few hours or a day or two, is still quite revolutionary because in our culture, women usually have to be sick before they'll take time alone to rest and be still. I wonder what might happen if every woman took that time and space that her moon time offers and requests of her. Maybe the entire concept of menstrual cramps would disappear and start to sound like a nonsensical utterance in a foreign language. Until then, I'm happy to carry the torch with my very own cocoon revolution each month.

Master Program for Optimal Hormonal Balance and Pelvic Health

The following program is effective not only for eliminating menstrual cramps but also for balancing hormones, alleviating PMS, and reestablishing normal periods in women with abnormal, heavy, or irregular periods. This program is also the mainstay of natural treatment for polycystic ovary syndrome and fibroids (both of which are addressed separately later in this chapter) as well as endometriosis (which is discussed in the next chapter).

Diet
~ To balance your hormones, the number one thing that has to happen is getting your insulin levels down to normal by following a low-glycemic-index diet. A nutrient-poor diet that contains too many refined carbohydrates that raise blood sugar levels too quickly (high-glycemic-index foods) increases insulin levels and favors the production of inflammatory chemicals throughout the body that result in pain and tissue damage. These inflammatory chemicals (also known as eicosanoids) go by a wide variety of names, including cytokines, bradykinins, interleukins, prostaglandins (including PGF2 alpha), and prostacyclins. Many of the most common drugs on the market, including aspirin, block the effects of these substances. When high-glycemic-index foods are consumed by an individual who also has high circulating levels of stress hormones, the amount of inflammatory chemicals produced is even higher. Menstrual cramps are just one manifestation of this vicious cycle. Others include fluid retention, headaches, insomnia, and muscle aches and pains. In fact, all of the symptoms of PMS (see page 162) are caused, in part, by cellular inflammation from the overproduction of inflammatory chemicals.

Therefore, a nutrient-rich, whole-food diet that balances insulin and glucagon and also decreases the production of inflammatory chemicals is the backbone for treatment of cramps and many other health problems. (For a full discussion, see chapter 17.) The basic approach is the following: Eliminate or greatly reduce refined carbohydrates (including products with refined sugar and/or refined flour, such as cookies, cake, chips, crackers, and so on).[33] Decrease grain products to no more than two or three servings per day or eliminate them completely. Most dry cereals, for example, contain far too much refined carbohydrate to justify their fiber content, so stick with oatmeal and shredded wheat. The diet should consist mostly of fresh vegetables and fruits along with legumes and protein either from vegetarian sources like soy foods (such as tofu, tempeh, and natto) or from free-range chicken, grass-fed beef, naturally raised pork, wild-caught salmon or other seafood, and eggs from free-range chickens. Healthy fats, which can include some saturated fat (depending on what the source is), are also important, although they have gotten a bad rap for the last forty years or so—a big mistake that we are only now rectifying. Healthy fats also include avocado, ghee, and coconut oil. Some women do best on a diet that severely limits carbohydrates (a modified ketogenic diet), while others do best on a more vegan diet that includes lots of fruits and vegetables, some whole grains, and some healthy fats. There is no one diet that is appropriate for everyone. A great deal depends upon your genetic heritage and your environment. In general, though, the key is keeping insulin levels down.

Regardless of one's dietary approach, however, everyone should eat more cruciferous vegetables. These include kale, collard greens, mustard greens, broccoli, cabbage, and turnips and have been shown to modulate estrogen levels (helpful for conditions such as endometriosis and fibroids). Try for one or two servings of these daily (or take a supplement containing indole-3-carbinol, the active ingredient in these vegetables). Also note that a diet high in fiber can decrease total circulating estrogens. Try for 25 grams per day in the form of whole grains, chia seeds, psyllium husks, beans, brown rice, vegetables, and fruits. Remember that with nutritional approaches, it's important to give them at least two to three months to achieve optimal results.

If you are overweight, loss of excess body fat increases insulin sensitivity and normalizes insulin secretion, which results in normalization of blood sugar and insulin and a reduction in excess androgens. Women with type 2 diabetes often greatly improve their health by this approach.[34] In fact, type 2 diabetes can be completely reversed with dietary management. (See chapter 17.)

~ Stop eating conventionally produced dairy foods, especially ice cream, cottage cheese, and yogurt—even low-fat versions of these products. It has been my clinical experience that many women get relief of symptoms such as menstrual cramps, heavy bleeding, breast pain, and endometriosis pain when they stop consuming dairy foods. This is not true for everyone, but it works often enough to be worth a try. (When I was in clinical practice, one of my patients who had endometriosis for many years decided to eliminate dairy products from her diet after unsuccessfully trying prescription drugs and surgery. Her symptoms disappeared for more than ten years, and she was able to conceive her first child without difficulty, even though another doctor told her that she probably wouldn't be able to get pregnant.)

Though it's not clear why conventionally produced pasteurized dairy foods seem to be associated with women's pelvic symptoms, I have a few theories. One possible explanation is that most milk today is produced by cows treated with rBST (recombinant bovine somatotropin, also called bovine growth hormone, or bGH), which overstimulates the cow's udder. These cows are more likely to have infected udders and thus require antibiotics. Both hormone and antibiotic residues in the milk may stimulate the female hormonal system in some way we are not yet able to pinpoint. We do know that antibiotics fed to livestock make their way into the human food chain. Antibiotics change the way hormones are metabolized in the bowel and thus can change hormonal levels. Other research suggests that lactose (milk sugar) may have a toxic effect on the ovaries. The research of Daniel Cramer, M.D., Sc.D., at Brigham and Women's Hospital in Boston has linked lactose consumption with increased risk of ovarian cancer. He found that women who consume one or more servings of skim or low-fat milk daily had a 32 percent higher risk of epithelial ovarian cancer compared with those who consumed three or fewer servings monthly.[35] This research has now been replicated by others. One large study done in the United States in 2013 showed that a high intake of low-fat and skim milk, yogurt, and cheese was associated with lower ovarian cancer risk, while high intake of other dairy foods such as whole milk and cream cheese was associated with increased risk.[36] A similar study in Denmark in 2012 showed parallel results.[37]

This doesn't prove that daily consumption of certain types of dairy causes ovarian cancer. There might be other confounding variables that are part of the equation. Rarely are things this simple when it comes to what causes what. Dairy foods produced organically, without rBST, antibiotics, or pesticides in the cow's feed, don't seem to have the same adverse effect on uterine and breast tissue, though this has never been studied systematically. Many women have noted that when they change to organically produced dairy foods—or, better yet, raw milk products—their symptoms go away.

THE BENEFITS OF RAW MILK AND DAIRY

Raw milk (fresh milk that is not pasteurized or homogenized) is an entirely different food from the processed milk you see in grocery stores. In fact, it's one of the most nutrient-dense foods available. It is considered a whole or complete food, meaning that it retains all of its natural enzymes, fatty acids, vitamins, and minerals, many of which are destroyed by the high heat used in the pasteurization process.

Unlike pasteurized milk, for example, raw milk is rich in enzymes like lactase (which helps the body absorb and digest milk's natural sugars and fats) and phosphatase (which allows the body to absorb calcium). This superfood also contains beneficial bacteria and lactic acid (necessary for these beneficial bacteria to live in the gut). Also important is what raw milk *doesn't* contain: additives such as the thickening agents, like carrageenan, often mixed into low-fat milk to improve texture. Raw milk is collected in clean stainless steel containers and then filtered, rapidly cooled, and bottled—that's it.

Ironically, pasteurization was developed in the late nineteenth century to kill harmful bacteria that can cause various diseases and foodborne illnesses. But medical researcher Ted Beals, M.D., has shown that the risk of this happening is extremely low; you are 35,000 times more likely to get sick from other foods than from raw milk![38] Even so, keep in mind that the risk is greater for infants and young children, the elderly, pregnant women, and those with a weakened immune system.

Another advantage raw milk offers is that it usually comes from grass-fed cows (or goats, sheep, or other mammals) that don't eat the heavy grain diets commonly given to cows in commercial dairy operations. A mostly grain diet changes the composition of the milk the cows produce, and not for the better. For example, milk from grass-fed animals has natural antibiotic and antimicrobial properties that help protect it from the kinds of bacteria that make you ill.[39] Milk from grass-fed animals is also rich in conjugated linoleic acid (CLA), a beneficial fatty acid.[40] Grain-fed cows produce milk with as little as one-fifth the CLA found in milk from grass-fed cows.[41]

Many people have been told they are allergic to milk or at least have difficulty digesting it. But this reaction can often have more to do with the pasteurization process than the milk itself. In fact, naturopathic doctors often recommend raw milk for their patients with allergies or lactose intolerance. A study involving more than 8,000 children who ate various diets showed that those who drank raw milk were 50 percent less likely to develop allergies and 41 percent less likely to develop asthma due to raw milk's "naturally immunizing" effects.[42] Additional benefits of drinking raw milk include stronger immunity; healthier skin, hair, and nails; increased bone density; and improved digestion. It also can help build lean muscle mass.

Although the U.S. Food and Drug Administration (FDA) requires all milk sold across state lines to be pasteurized, many states allow the sale of raw milk within the state in which it is produced. The best places to look for raw milk include farmers' markets, grocery stores specializing in healthy or natural foods, or online. To find where you can purchase raw milk in your state, visit the Real Milk Finder website (www.realmilk.com/real-milk-finder), operated by the Weston A. Price Foundation.

Remember that the nutritional content of any raw milk varies, depending on many factors (including the grass and soil quality where the cows grazed, the breed of cow, and the health of the animal). Always buy raw milk (and dairy products made from raw milk) from a reputable distributor. Ask at your local farmers' market for recommendations, and read customer reviews online. As with all milk, keep it refrigerated and use it before the expiration date.

Experiment and discover what works for you. But be willing to stop consuming conventionally produced dairy foods just for a couple of weeks as an experiment to see if you notice any benefits. You can get your calcium from other sources. (And besides, calcium intake is not the answer to osteoporosis prevention that we've been led to believe it is—see chapter 17.)

～ Limit red meat and egg yolks to no more than two servings per week, or eliminate them. If you do eat red meat, use cuts from grass-fed animals. Red meat and egg yolks are very rich in arachidonic acid (AA), which can result in increased cellular inflammation and uterine cramps in susceptible individuals. Not all individuals are sensitive to AA, so this recommendation will not apply to everyone; to find out if you are sensitive to AA, avoid all red meat and egg yolks for at least two weeks, then eat several servings in one day and see if your symptoms return. In general, meat from grass-fed cattle and eggs from free-range chickens are entirely different foods—with different effects—from food raised in factory farms.

～ Eliminate partially hydrogenated fats (trans fats) because they increase the production of inflammatory chemicals. Check labels on all prepared foods. Partially hydrogenated fats have a very long shelf life. That is why food manufacturers use them. But this type of fat can insert itself in the cell membranes of your body—particularly your brain—and cause dysfunction. Avoid them!

~ Eliminate or limit caffeine. As I've learned through the years, just getting off caffeine, even if consumption has been as little as one cup of coffee or one can of cola per day, can have a dramatic effect on PMS for some women (although not for all).

Nutritional Supplements and Herbal Support

~ Take a pharmaceutical-grade multivitamin-mineral supplement daily, all month long. (Look for "GMP," which stands for "good manufacturing practice," on the label.) A dietary approach that nourishes the body fully will also help a woman attune herself to her spiritual, intuitive side. This helps reestablish emotional flow and can often help normalize a woman's hormonal levels. Choose a comprehensive supplement rich in B complex, zinc, selenium, vitamin E, and magnesium—you need about 50 to 100 mg of each of the B vitamins (vitamin B_6 in particular has been shown to decrease the intensity and duration of menstrual cramps)[43] and 300 to 800 mg of magnesium. Dian Shepperson Mills, a nutritionist in London and a former trustee of the British Endometriosis Society, reported a double-blind study of dietary supplements that resulted in a 98 percent improvement in endometriosis symptoms over those not on the supplement. The supplements used were thiamine (vitamin B_1), riboflavin (B_2), and pyridoxine (B_6), 100 mg each; zinc citrate, 20 mg; and magnesium aminochelate, 300 mg.[44]

Vitamin A (5,000 to 10,000 IU per day) is important because it appears to help regulate excessive estrogen levels.[45] Doses of vitamin A as high as 100,000 IU per day can be given if limited to three months—otherwise, there is a risk of toxicity. (Though 5,000–10,000 IU of vitamin A is well within the safe range, it's best not to use this if you're trying to get pregnant.) Beta-carotene is a safe form of vitamin A that does not reach toxic levels. Vitamin A as well as vitamin C with bioflavonoids (500 mg per day) have also been shown to decrease menstrual blood loss.[46]

If you have particular problems with cramps and PMS, you may find it helpful to divide your dosage of vitamin E and magnesium throughout the day. Take your vitamin E three times a day during your entire cycle (for a total of 100 to 400 IU).[47] Make sure it's in the form of d-alpha-tocopherol or it won't have any biological effect. Vitamin E works because it prevents excessive clotting and helps maintain a more normal menstrual flow. With magnesium, you can take as much as 100 mg every two hours during the menstrual cycle itself, and three or four times per day during the rest of the cycle. (Use a chelated form.) Magnesium relaxes smooth muscle tissue, and a deficiency of this mineral is common in PMS.[48] (See chapter 17.)

~ Get enough iodine. Though most physicians know very little about the extrathyroidal role of iodine, a large and robust body of research has shown that iodine at amounts far greater than the RDA is necessary for the optimal health of the breasts, ovaries, and the uterus. The ovaries, breasts, muscles, joints, and bones actually have cellular pumps in them to concentrate iodine. The optimal amount to take daily is 6–12.5 mg/day, though some women need less and some more. (For a full discussion, see chapter 10.)

~ Take essential fatty acids. Omega-3 fatty acids in the form of fish oil or marine algae, which contains DHA (docosahexaenoic acid) and EPA (eicosapentaenoic acid), have been shown to work well for menstrual cramps even in those who didn't change other aspects of their diets. One study suggested a dosage of 1,080 mg EPA and 720 mg DHA, together with 500 IU of vitamin E; you can use any amount that approximates this. Because fish oil degenerates with exposure to oxygen, take capsules that have added vitamin E (to prevent oxidation). A much cheaper and often healthier alternative is to eat sardines packed in their own oil or in olive oil two to three times per week. Other cold-water fish such as mackerel, salmon, and swordfish are also good sources of fish oil.[49] DHA made from marine algae is also available (the brand name is Neuromins, and the usual dose is 400 mg one or two times per day). Flaxseed oil—500 mg two to four times per day—as well as sesame, sunflower, safflower, macadamia nut, and walnut oils can also be used if fish oil is not available or if it is unacceptable. You can also buy fresh flaxseed and grind it in a coffee grinder just before adding it to soups, salads, or cereals. Usually one to two tablespoons per day of the freshly ground seeds will be enough.

~ Try *Pueraria mirifica,* 80–100 mg twice per day during days seven through twenty-one of each cycle. Most women get significant relief from cramps, PMS, and menstrual problems after three months of cyclic use, which is then continued for maintenance. This herb contains a very special phytoestrogen known as miroestrol that acts as an adaptogen in the body— protecting estrogen-sensitive tissues from overstimulation or having an estrogenic effect for balance if the body is low on estrogen. *Pueraria mirifica* has been used for more than 700 years in Thailand to address all manner of menstrual, menopausal, and reproductive issues. (See Resources.)

~ Take black cohosh, or "cramp bark," as a preventive. This herb is available in tablet or tincture form in natural food stores. Follow directions on the bottle.

⁓ Try Menastil, a roll-on product made from calendula oil, for cramps. It's widely available online.

⁓ Consider a TENS (transcutaneous electrical nerve stimulation) unit. Of the several brands currently on the market, Livia has done a particularly good job of creating a user-friendly product.

SEED ROTATION FOR MENSTRUAL REGULATION

Some women find that period problems resolve beautifully when they try seed rotation for several months. Seed rotation is based on the unique nutritional and hormonal properties of four different types of freshly ground seeds—flax, pumpkin, sesame, and sunflower—which you can eat in smoothies, soups, or salads.

Here's what you do: For days one through fourteen of your cycle (the follicular phase, when an egg is maturing), take the following each day to support estrogen production:

1 tablespoon freshly ground flaxseeds
1 tablespoon freshly ground pumpkin seeds

For days fifteen through twenty-eight of your cycle (the luteal phase following ovulation), take the following to support progesterone production:

1 tablespoon ground sesame seeds
1 tablespoon ground sunflower seeds

Women with irregular periods or perimenopausal women can pick any day as day one of their cycle. (I prefer the new moon in these cases, given the moon's effect on the menstrual cycle. Why not align with it?)

You can grind a half cup of each seed in advance and keep it in the refrigerator, but be sure to use it within one week.

For more information, read *Cooking for Hormone Balance* (HarperOne, 2018) by Magdalena Wszelaki or visit her website at www.hormonesbalance.com.

Reestablish Cyclic Emotional Flow

⁓ Allow yourself a full range of emotional responses to the events in your life. Try recording these in a journal to discover the natural rhythm of your emotions and moods. Are they related to the seasons, the time of day, and other cycles? Keep track of the phases of the moon on a calendar and in your date book. It is well known that the menstrual cycle is affected by the cyclic waxing and waning of the moon. If you live near the ocean, keep track of the tides. Simply paying attention to environmental cues including the light, the moon, and the tides may regulate a woman's menstrual cycle and fertility.[50]

Reestablish Cyclic Ovulatory Flow

~ Get in tune with your body's daily cycles, regulated by a kind of internal body clock located in the part of the brain known as the hypothalamus. This is true whether or not you are having menstrual periods. These daily cycles follow the day-and-night rhythms of nature, relying on light and darkness to time the release of various hormones and neurotransmitters that make us sleepy or wakeful (among other things).

The daily cycles and rhythms of dark and light actually become imprinted on our genes over time. But because our modern lives with electric lights, smartphones, and fast-paced schedules are out of sync with natural rhythms, we find it harder if not downright impossible to stay in tune with our bodies' natural cycles. Unless we make an effort to become conscious of them, it becomes increasingly difficult to tune in to the ticking of our internal clock.

With small changes, however, we can help reset our genetic clocks and get our bodies back in sync so we have more energy, we get more sleep, and our lives flow more smoothly. Here are a few suggestions:

~ Go for regular walks outside during the day, preferably in nature. Natural light is a nutrient, so you'll find that this practice will energize you. At the very least, sit by a window whenever possible, especially at work. Open it when weather permits.

~ Get up at the same time each day, no matter what time you go to bed the night before.

~ Create an "electronic sundown" every night around 9:30 P.M. by turning off your computer, television, cellphone, and any other piece of electronic equipment.

The blue background light from cellphones and computers is very bright and activates the brain, making it much more difficult to get to sleep. Download f.lux (www.justgetflux.com) on your computer and cellphone to change the wavelength of light coming off your computer screen to be warmer and more calming at night.

~ Make your bedroom completely dark, covering or turning off any of the blinking or glowing lights from your alarm clock, cellphone, computer, DVD timer, and other devices. (Or, if you can't do that, wear an eye mask.) Even these tiny bits of light can affect your melatonin levels, which are important for restful and restorative sleep.

~ Allow mealtime to follow your body's natural rhythms. Your metabolism peaks around noon, so try to make lunch your biggest meal of the day and have a smaller dinner. Start the day with a smoothie for breakfast (or even lunch if you're doing intermittent fasting) containing a good protein and healthy fats instead of a sugary, carb-heavy meal. I recommend a smoothie developed by Kelly Brogan, M.D., for its brain-boosting qualities (see chapter 17).

~ Use light therapy. Determine what the first day of your last period was, as nearly as possible. (You may need to guess.) From days fourteen to seventeen of your cycle, sleep with a 100-watt lightbulb in a common bedside-table lamp (one that has a shade that disperses light onto the ceiling and wall but is minimally disturbing to sleep) on the floor next to your bed. Do this for six months. In one study of 2,000 women, more than 50 percent regulated their previously irregular periods to a regular cycle of twenty-nine days by doing this.[51]

An alternative method is to take a walk outdoors daily for twenty to thirty minutes without sunglasses. Or use full-spectrum lightbulbs in a spot in your home where you can see the ambient full-spectrum light (2,500 to 10,000 lux) out of the corner of your eye for at least thirty to sixty minutes (and up to two hours) each evening or each morning.[52] (A lux, by the way, is a measure of light intensity; a cloudy day in northern Europe provides 10,000 lux, while a sunny day near the equator provides 80,000 lux.) A light box is another good choice. These types of light therapy are especially helpful during the fall and winter months, when the sun is less intense. (See Resources, as well as www.sunshinesciences.com.)

Energy Medicine

~ Try traditional Chinese medicine, which includes both herbs and acupuncture. TCM has been shown to eliminate or greatly decrease many gynecological problems. The usual course of acupuncture is ten treatments, but many women feel relief after as few as three treatments.[53] (Something like shrinking a very large fibroid, however, could, according to some studies, require a major commitment to having daily treatments for a while.) Just as many emotional settings and energy dysfunctions are responsible for setting the scene for a woman's menstrual disorders, many appropriate and specific Oriental herbal and acupuncture treatments may be prescribed.

You may receive one of numerous diagnoses, including (but not limited to) deficient blood of the heart, spleen, or liver; deficient *chi*; stagnant blood; and stagnant *chi*. Depending upon your history or physical symptoms, as well as your physical examination, specific acupuncture points and/or herbs will be selected that are appropriate for your condition. Each woman who is drawn to this approach must find an appropriately trained practitioner of TCM with whom she feels safe.

One of the most common TCM diagnoses for women with gynecological problems is something called "liver stagnation." The Chinese herbal formula bupleurum (xiao yao wan, also known as hsiao yao wan) may help, and many of my patients have done very well with it.[54] Take four or five of the tiny tablets four times per day two weeks before the period is due and continue through the first day of bleeding. It may take two or three months to experience optimal results.

~ Follow the TCM principle of staying warm during your period. Enjoying warm baths, saunas, heating pads, and warm foods helps keep the menstrual flow normal and healthy. Avoid iced beverages, cold foods, and overexposure to cold and drafts. (See the box "Traditional Chinese Medicine and Menstruation" on page 131.)

Stress Reduction

~ Meditate. Women who practice meditation or other methods of deep relaxation are able to alleviate many of their symptoms. Relaxation of all kinds decreases cortisol and epinephrine levels in the blood and helps to balance your biochemistry, including the reduction of inflammatory chemicals. There are numerous types of meditation that work. Each woman should choose the type of meditation that she feels most drawn to and incorporate this discipline into her daily routine.

For example, the relaxation response suggested by Herbert Benson, M.D., is practiced fifteen to twenty minutes twice per day. This meditation involves: (1) sitting quietly in a comfortable position with eyes closed; (2) deeply relaxing all muscles, beginning with the face and progressing down to the feet; (3) breathing through the nose and becoming aware of the breath; and (4) saying the word *one* (or *rose*, or *peace*) silently on exhaling. One study showed significant relief of PMS within three months of regular practice.[55]

~ Do some inner work. Ask yourself the following questions and answer them honestly:

~ What are my emotional needs?

~ What would I like to see happen in my job or my life that would nourish me fully?

~ Am I getting enough rest?

~ Do I believe that I have the power to change the conditions of my life?

Consider journaling the answers. As you do so, also write down everything that you'd like to create in your life. See how much enthusiasm and energy you can muster simply by imagining what it would be like to let your creative talents or secret selves manifest fully. Note where you have any blocks to this process. They will usually be identifiable as "yes, but . . ." statements, such as "Yes, I'd love to sew beautiful clothing regularly, but there's no way I can get the time." You will soon be able to identify the limiting beliefs that are blocking your creativity.

Realize that this inner work is a vital part of any plan to promote pelvic health, because while any one of the components of this plan (including dietary changes and supplements) will help, none is likely to completely cure pelvic problems if you do not also address the energetic cause and release the energy blockages in the pelvis. In fact, I've seen fibroid patients go on very strict macrobiotic diets, only to find that their fibroids have actually grown. These women usually had unresolved childhood issues, such as incest, or were married to abusive partners.

⁓ Use affirmations. Regularly affirm your power to change your life for the better by saying this affirmation out loud in the mirror twice per day for a month: "The healing power that created the universe is now working in and through me, creating quickly and easily the perfect outcome—the perfect result." Remember, as Rev. Michael Bernard Beckwith, founder of the Agape International Spiritual Center near Los Angeles, says, "Affirmations don't make something happen. They make something welcome."

Homeopathy

⁓ Try homeopathy. Although I have not been trained in it, I wholeheartedly embrace homeopathic medicine, which addresses the vibratory nature of life at its deepest levels. Practitioners report that fibroids shrink or disappear and many gynecological symptoms can be alleviated with the right homeopathic remedy. Homeopathic medicine is a type of natural medicine that was very popular at the turn of the twentieth century. In fact, the very first placebo-controlled, double-blind clinical trials were designed by homeopaths to prove the efficacy of homeopathic remedies, which must be individually prescribed. A variety of homeopathic remedies are available specifically for gynecological problems. (See Resources.)

Castor Oil Packs

⁓ Use castor oil packs to improve immune system functioning and decrease stress and adrenaline levels. Also known as palma Christi (the palm of Christ), castor oil has been used for healing for hundreds of years. The medical intuitive Edgar Cayce often prescribed this treatment for many different conditions. I was introduced to it by Gladys McGarey, M.D., who has used the packs in her general practice for more than forty years.

The packs are made by saturating a piece of wool or cotton flannel, folded so that it is four thicknesses, with cold-pressed castor oil. The oil-saturated flannel is then placed directly on the skin of the lower abdomen and covered with a piece of plastic, such as a plastic bag. Heat, in the form of a hot water bottle or heating pad, is then applied over the pack and the plastic. A blanket or towel can be placed over the heat source to keep everything in place. I prefer a nonelectric heat source and often recommend a hot water bottle or a Fomentek bag. (See Resources for everything you need to make a castor oil pack.)

Recline with a castor oil pack applied to your lower abdomen at least three times per week for one hour each time, except during times of heavy bleeding. During this treatment, I suggest that you pay attention to thoughts, images, and feelings that arise and make note of them in a journal. This regimen should be followed for at least three months and then can be tapered down to once a week. (A good alternative is taking warm baths for twenty to thirty minutes; add a few drops of rose oil, an aromatherapy treatment known for its soothing effects.)

Natural Progesterone

~ Consider natural progesterone, which in combination with lifestyle changes often produces profound improvement in PMS symptoms.[56] In their capacity as neurotransmitters, estrogen and progesterone clearly affect mood. Estrogen, if unopposed by progesterone, tends to irritate the nervous system. Progesterone, on the other hand, is associated with tranquility and is a central nervous system relaxant. It binds to the same receptors in the brain as Valium and has a soothing and relaxing effect.[57]

I recommend natural progesterone for women who have moderate to severe PMS that doesn't respond to simple lifestyle changes or the modalities I've already mentioned. Progesterone is for those women who often describe a Jekyll-and-Hyde personality change premenstrually. Studies show that in women who suffer from PMS, progesterone levels decline sharply during the three days before their periods begin (while in women who don't report PMS symptoms the levels decline more gradually during this time), so supplementing makes good sense.[58] Natural progesterone also works well for women whose major premenstrual symptom is a migraine-type headache. These headaches often start with the gradual change in estrogen and progesterone levels that tends to occur in the years leading up to menopause.

Natural progesterone is not the same thing as the synthetic progesterones (progestins), such as medroxyprogesterone acetate (Provera) and norethindrone (commonly used in birth control pills). There are no serious side effects with natural progesterone at the usual doses. Sometimes it might cause intermenstrual spotting or delay the period. This usually resolves itself in one to two months. Extremely high doses—much higher than I recommend—have been associated with euphoria and occasional dizziness in rare cases. Oral natural progesterone is available by prescription from your doctor. The dosage depends on the symptoms; usually it is 50 to 200 mg orally on a daily basis from midcycle to the onset of menses (usually days fourteen to twenty-eight of the cycle), for at least three months. Natural progesterone can also be given vaginally for thirty days or more, depending on the patient. Again, it's available by prescription.

It's also available in the form of skin creams. Note that while natural progesterone is synthesized from wild Mexican yams, creams that contain only yam extract, though helpful for some women, are not the same as those that contain adequate amounts of natural progesterone. Formulary pharmacies always carry natural progesterone.

For application to the skin, you can use one of several natural progesterone creams available over the counter, or have your doctor prescribe one for you from a pharmacy that specializes in individualized prescriptions. I have recommended a 2 percent progesterone cream such as Pro-Gest from Emerita for many years. These 2 percent creams contain at least 375 mg of natural progesterone per ounce. One-quarter to one-half teaspoon applied to the skin once or twice per day has been shown to result in physiological levels of progesterone that match those found in the normal luteal phase.[59]

General instructions are to apply one-quarter to one-half teaspoon (approximately 30–60 mg) on the soft areas of skin (breasts, abdomen, neck, face, inner arms, or hands) in the morning and again in the evening. Apply on days fourteen through twenty-eight of your menstrual cycle for at least three months. The precise timing and dosage will vary from woman to woman, however. It is important to get the progesterone into your system *before* you normally experience your mood change. You need to apply the cream a day or two before ovulation or a day or two before your symptoms usually start. For some women, this will be on day twenty-one; for others, day twelve or thirteen. Continue through the first day of menstrual bleeding (day one of the cycle). This will often prevent symptoms or greatly alleviate them. Waiting until you are symptomatic to start treatment often doesn't work. Increase or decrease the dosage depending on the severity of the symptoms; most women have to experiment to find a level that works for them. You may safely use natural progesterone for more than two weeks of your cycle provided that you interrupt use in each cycle for at least twelve hours.

Synthetic progestins, as opposed to natural progesterone, have many known side effects, such as bloating, headache, and weight gain. Unfortunately, many women are told that synthetic progestin is the same as natural progesterone. But synthetic progestins can actually increase PMS symptoms, because taking a synthetic progestin decreases the body's natural progesterone levels.

Women who do well on progesterone are often those who experience a rapid change in mood that begins after ovulation and ends just as the menstrual flow starts. They describe feeling fine and then within several hours having a "black cloud" come over them.[60] When their periods start, they feel as though "a light has gone on." These women are describing a biochemical change in their bodyminds that is very real and not just "in their heads."

The possible relative imbalance between estrogen, progesterone, and other hormones that is associated with PMS appears to be a dynamic, changing phenomenon that currently cannot be documented with existing laboratory tests. A subtle hormonal imbalance is also associated with irregular periods and emotional stress. Emotional stress increases levels of the hormone ACTH, often resulting in anovulatory cycles (cycles in which an egg is not released) characterized by inadequate levels of progesterone.[61]

The use of natural progesterone over time helps rebalance the estrogen-progesterone ratio. Using natural progesterone produces a gradual improvement of symptoms with each cycle. Many women are able to decrease or eliminate their dosages over time once their symptoms have been completely relieved (though progesterone has many beneficial effects, and some may want to stay on it even after PMS symptoms are gone). It is much more effective, however, to start out with dosages that are on the high end of usual and stay with these for several months. Many women are able to reestablish hormonal balance without this hormone, but it can be very helpful in the beginning.

The use of the herb *Pueraria mirifica* also helps rebalance estrogen and progesterone over time. Many women find that when they switch to this herb and continue to take it, they experience the same benefits offered by progesterone.

Manual Therapies

~ Get a total body massage at least once every other week for two months. Notice how you feel after the massage.

~ Find a physical therapist trained in the Wurn technique, a noninvasive, nonsurgical type of deep tissue massage developed by Larry and Belinda Wurn that's performed by specially trained physical therapists. The treatment is done over a series of five consecutive days and breaks up pelvic and abdominal adhesions caused by injury, surgery, or infection. It often eliminates menstrual cramps and also helps in a wide variety of other conditions, including infertility from blocked tubes, chronic pelvic pain, pain with intercourse, and even small bowel obstruction. (See figure 6.) All of this is described in detail in their book *Miracle Moms, Better Sex, Less Pain* (Med-Art, 2009). (For more information, contact Clear Passage Therapies at 352-336-1433 or visit www.clearpassage.com.)

~ Consider Maya traditional massage. Indigenous Mayan healers in Central America have long used a technique called Maya abdominal massage to treat many conditions of the pelvic organs, including painful periods, endometriosis, bladder infections, and more. Though this treatment is not as extensive as the Wurn technique, it can also be very effective—and less expensive. Maya abdominal massage practitioners report that this technique reduces adhesions from old surgeries, endometriosis, fibroid tumors, and ovarian cysts. (For more information, including a directory of certified practitioners of Maya abdominal massage, visit www.arvigotherapy.com/arvigo-practitioners.)

~ Get reflexology. Treatment involving specific pressure points on the ear, hand, and foot has been shown to relieve PMS symptoms. The usual length of treatment with a trained reflexologist is thirty minutes once per week for eight weeks. An entire program of pressure point therapy to relieve

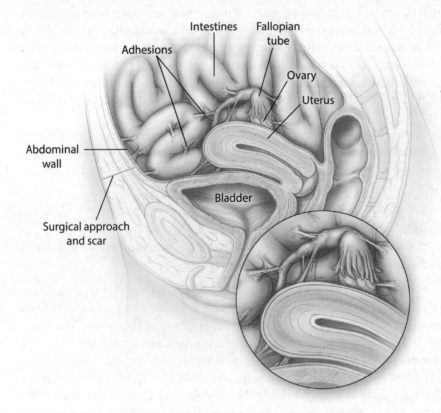

FIGURE 6: ADHESIONS IN PELVIC ORGANS

Adhesions are filmy areas of connective tissue resulting from surgery, trauma, or infection that can cause pain and infertility.

PMS, dysmenorrhea, and endometriosis symptoms can be found in Jeanne Blum's book *Woman Heal Thyself* (Charles Tuttle, 1995).[62]

⁓ Try acupressure. Licensed acupuncturist and TCM practitioner Sandra Chiu recommends massaging the following four points with good, strong pressure for premenstrual problems or cramps:

  ⁓ Large intestine 4 (he gu)

  ⁓ Spleen 6 (san yin jiao)

  ⁓ Spleen 8 (di ji)

  ⁓ Kidney 5 (shui quan)

When looking for a point, she advises, you will often find it by the tender, sore, or even bruise-like sensation you feel when you press on it. This is a sign of congestion at the point, and using massage can help promote movement in the channel and improve your symptoms. Massage into each point for a good three to five minutes, even if it's sensitive or slightly painful at first. The tenderness will go away after several strokes.

Chiu also recommends heat and massage on the lower abdomen/pelvis area for a day or two before you expect your period, or when you start to feel its impending onset. Hot water bottles and heat packs are soothing when placed on the abdomen for fifteen to twenty minutes a day.

Detoxification

⁓ Do something every day to work up a sweat. Get at least twenty to thirty minutes of aerobic-type exercise five times a week.[63] Brisk walking is all that is necessary. This is beneficial for several reasons, including the fact that sweating is a natural way to detoxify. Also, exercise increases levels of endorphins (naturally occurring morphine-like substances that help the body deal with depression and physical pain) and lowers levels of stress hormones, which decreases cellular inflammation. It is estimated that half of all depression cases can be helped through exercise alone. (See chapter 18.) (By the way, yoga is also helpful for a number of reasons, including the fact that it often relieves cramps.) Exercise hydrates the fascia, thus optimizing tissue and organ function. Fascia is a semisolid secondary nervous system of connective tissue that encapsulates every organ and muscle in the body. It is the place in the body in which acupuncture meridians run.

⁓ Take saunas. Japanese researchers recently found that spending fifteen minutes in a sauna every day for two weeks was good for heart health, improving the function of the endothelial cells lining the arteries by 40 percent.[64] Researchers in Finland who followed more than 2,315 middle-aged

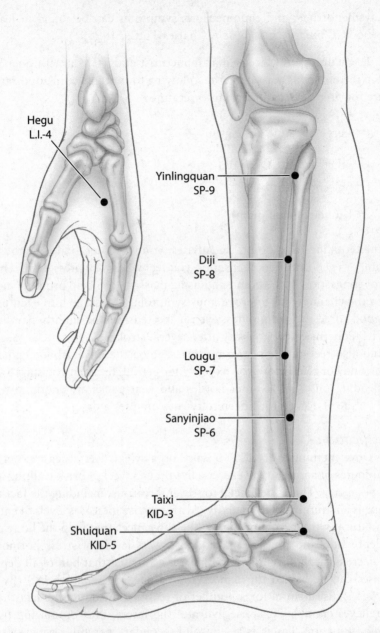

FIGURE 7: ACUPRESSURE POINTS FOR GYNECOLOGICAL PROBLEMS

These are some of the major acupressure points that you can massage to prevent or relieve menstrual cramps. They will often be tender to the touch at first.

men for about twenty years found that the more frequently the men went to the sauna and the longer they stayed, the lower their risk for sudden cardiac death, fatal coronary heart disease, and fatal cardiovascular disease. Those who took saunas two to three times a week had a 24 percent lower risk of all causes of mortality than those who went only once a week, while those who took saunas four to seven times a week had a 40 percent lower risk.[65]

One of the huge benefits of taking saunas is that they allow you to sweat out toxins.[66] As long as you drink plenty of water to stay hydrated, the more you sweat, the more toxins you'll expel. Far-infrared saunas are believed to have a greater detoxifying effect than traditional saunas because the radiant energy of the infrared light penetrates more deeply—to a depth of 1.5 inches—so your body heats up from the inside out, instead of the reverse, as in a traditional sauna. (This also means the temperature of an infrared sauna can be cooler than a traditional sauna—typically 120–140 degrees, as compared to the 180–200 degrees of traditional saunas.) Also, in traditional saunas, 95 to 97 percent of the sweat produced is water, the rest being salt. In infrared saunas, only 80 to 85 percent of the sweat produced is water, the rest being cholesterol, fat-soluble toxins, toxic heavy metals, sulfuric acid, sodium, ammonia, and uric acid. (One good brand of far-infrared saunas is Sunlighten; see www.sunlighten.com.)

~ Use a dry brush on skin regularly to help shed old skin and stimulate lymph flow. Brush in the direction of the heart. (These brushes are available at natural food stores.)

~ Take a fiber supplement containing both soluble and insoluble fiber, which helps the body excrete excess estrogen and other substances. One of the best such supplements is one to two tablespoons of whole psyllium seed husks in liquid every morning (which are much milder than wheat bran); oat bran or slippery elm is also excellent.

PREMENSTRUAL SYNDROME (PMS)

No modern disorder points to the need to rethink our ideas about menstruation and reclaim the wisdom of our cycles more directly than the common malady known as premenstrual syndrome, or PMS. Having treated hundreds of women with PMS, I know that such a rethinking is needed to get to the root causes of PMS. Dietary change, exercise, vitamins, herbs, and/or progesterone therapy are all useful in treating PMS, and I initially recommend them for many women. But in persistent cases of PMS, a deeper imbalance exists that lifestyle changes alone won't help. As studies have confirmed, unresolved emotional problems may disrupt the menstrual rhythm and the normal hormonal milieu.[67] The reason for this is the intimate connection between our thoughts, emotions, and hypothalamus—the part of the brain that governs the master gland, the pituitary.

Up to 80 percent of all women suffer from PMS.[68] It is most likely to occur in women in their thirties, though it can occur as early as adolescence and as late as the premenopausal years. PMS has been known since ancient times, but it was popularized in the 1980s by an article in *Family Circle* magazine, which articulated the monthly suffering of millions of women. The media picked up on this, and within a few months PMS became a nationally known problem and a household word.[69] It also became a hot topic with feminists, who argued that the diagnosis would be used against women. Doctors worried that it would become a "wastebasket" diagnosis that women or their families would use as an excuse when no one could figure out what was really going on. Meanwhile, scores of women finally had a name for their monthly suffering and sought medical help for it.

The demand created by women and the media for treatment of PMS had become such that by the mid-1980s, PMS was a lecture topic at many major ob-gyn specialty meetings, and research began appearing in the journals. Just as the desire for natural childbirth forced doctors to reform their patriarchal approach to obstetrical practice, women's desire to understand PMS influenced the practice of medicine and helped move it toward a more enlightened attitude toward the female body.

Diagnosis

A wide variety of symptoms can be present with PMS. In making the diagnosis, it doesn't matter what specific symptoms a woman has premenstrually. *What is important is the cyclic fashion in which they occur.* Women who chart their symptoms for three months or more often see a pattern and are able to predict when in their cycle their symptoms are likely to start. Most women will have at least three days during the month when they are entirely free from the symptoms listed here, except in very severe cases. In the second half of the menstrual cycle many underlying conditions are exacerbated, such as glaucoma, arthritis, and depression. Exacerbation of underlying conditions is not defined as PMS, though it is related to PMS. There are more than 100 known symptoms of PMS.[70] Every one of these symptoms is related to cellular inflammation, resulting from a complex interaction of emotional, physical, and genetic factors.

PMS SYMPTOMS

Abdominal bloating	Accident proneness
Abdominal cramping	Acne

Aggression	Hemorrhoids
Alcohol intolerance	Herpes
Anxiety	Hives
Asthma	Insomnia (sleeplessness)
Back pain	Irritability
Breast swelling and pain	Joint swelling and pain
Bruising	Lethargy
Confusion	Migraine
Coordination difficulties	Nausea
Depression	Rage
Edema	Salt craving
Emotional lability	Seizures
Exacerbation of preexisting	Sex drive changes
conditions (arthritis, ulcers,	Sinus problems
lupus, etc.)	Sore throat
Eye difficulties	Styes
Fainting	Suicidal thoughts
Fatigue	Sweet cravings
Food binges	Urinary difficulties
Headache	Withdrawal from others
Heart palpitations (heart pounding)	

If nothing is done to interrupt PMS, it often gets worse over time. In the early stages of PMS, women describe symptoms that arise a few days before their menstrual period and then stop abruptly when the bleeding starts. Then the symptoms gradually begin to appear one to two weeks before the onset of menses. Some women experience a cluster of symptoms at ovulation, followed by a symptom-free week, then a recurrence of the symptoms a week before menses. Over time, a woman may have only two or three days of the month that are symptom-free. Eventually, no discernible pattern of "good" days and "bad" days is left: She feels as if she has PMS virtually all the time.

Some women equate menstrual cramps and PMS, but PMS is different from menstrual cramps (dysmenorrhea). This difference is not always clearly stated in writings on PMS. Many women with PMS have completely pain-free periods. Many women with severe cramping have *no* premenstrual distress. Menstrual cramps are caused by uterine contractions and cramping that results from excess prostaglandin F2 alpha, a hormone produced as the lining of the uterus breaks down during the menstrual cycle. Prostaglandins and other inflammatory chemicals are also involved in PMS symptoms. For that reason, dietary change, vitamin and mineral supplements, and antiprostaglandin medication (usually nonsteroidal anti-inflammatory drugs such as Advil) are often useful both for cramps and for PMS.[71]

Though some doctors are still looking for a "biochemical lesion" that causes PMS and hundreds of scientific papers have been published on the topic, no one has been able to find such a lesion or a magic-bullet drug to cure it. A reductionistic approach—looking for the chemical "cause" and "cure"—simply doesn't work because the causes of PMS are multifactorial and must be approached holistically. (This is why using drugs such as SSRIs— like Prozac or Paxil—does women a true disservice.) The effects of the mind, emotions, diet, light, exercise, relationships, heredity, and childhood traumas must all be taken into account when treating PMS. All combine to create the end result of cellular inflammation, which manifests in many different ways.

All of the following events result in hormonal changes in the body. PMS is apt to be initiated or exacerbated by these changes unless treatment is initiated.

EVENTS ASSOCIATED WITH PMS ONSET

~ Onset of menses or the year or two before menopause

~ Coming off birth control pills

~ After a time of no periods (amenorrhea)

~ The birth of a child or the termination of a pregnancy

~ Pregnancies complicated by toxemia

~ Tubal ligation, especially when done in such a way that the major blood supply to the tube is interrupted (an increasingly rare procedure, as the latest tubal ligation techniques no longer destroy large areas of the tubes and their blood supply)

~ Unusual trauma, such as a death in the family

~ Decreased light associated with autumn and winter and also lack of exposure to natural, full-spectrum light

A variety of nutritional factors contribute to PMS. Studies have shown that women with PMS tend to have the following nutritional and physiological characteristics.

FACTORS CONTRIBUTING TO PMS

~ High consumption of conventionally produced dairy products.[72]

~ Excessive consumption of caffeine, in the form of soft drinks, coffee, or chocolate.[73]

~ Excessive consumption of foods that raise blood sugar too quickly, resulting in elevated insulin levels, hormonal imbalance, and subsequent cellular inflammation.

~ A relatively high blood level of estrogen, resulting either from overproduction from dietary and body fat or from the decreased breakdown of estrogen in the liver. High estrogen levels are associated with deficiencies of the vitamin B complex, especially B_6 and B_{12}. The liver requires these vitamins in order to break down and inactivate estrogen.[74]

~ A relatively low blood level of progesterone, the hormone that works to balance excess estrogen. This decreased level is felt to be secondary either to lack of production or to excessive breakdown of this hormone in the body.[75] Studies in this area are inconsistent.

~ A diet that leads to increased levels of the hormone prostaglandin F2 alpha and also contributes to high levels of estrogen in conjunction with low levels of progesterone.[76] Vegetarians with a whole-food, high-fiber diet are known to excrete two to three times more estrogen in their feces than nonvegetarians. They also have 50 percent lower blood plasma levels of unconjugated estrogens (a type of metabolized estrogen) than women who eat the standard American diet, and as a result, they have a decreased incidence of PMS.[77] (It has been my experience that vegetarians tend to eat more fruits and vegetables and fewer trans fatty acids than do nonvegetarians. Evidence is mounting that meat is not the culprit we once thought it was as long as it is consumed in moderate amounts and accompanied by an abundant intake of green leafy vegetables, whole grains, fruits, and other whole foods—and as long as one's diet doesn't contain excessive amounts of high-glycemic-index foods or those that contain trans fatty acids.)

~ Excessive body weight, which increases the chances of excessive levels of estrogen and PMS.[78] Body fat manufactures estrone (one of the estrogens) and is also associated with an increase in inflammatory chemicals.

~ Low levels of vitamins C and E and selenium. As with the B vitamins, the liver also requires these substances to metabolize estrogen properly.[79]

~ A deficiency of magnesium, which is very common.[80] Chocolate cravings have been linked to low magnesium levels. The liver needs magnesium, along with B vitamins, to metabolize estrogen optimally.

~ Lack of exercise.

SAD and PMS: Shedding Light on the Link

Many women with PMS notice that their symptoms get worse in the fall, when the days get shorter. Many of the symptoms associated with PMS are precisely the same as those associated with the form of depression known as seasonal affective disorder (SAD). Light acts as a nutrient in the body. When it hits the retina, it directly influences the entire neuroendocrine system via the hypothalamus and the pineal gland. In one study, patients with PMS responded significantly to treatment with bright light. Their weight gain, depression, carbohydrate craving, social withdrawal, fatigue, and irritability were reversed with two hours of full-spectrum bright light in the evening.[81] This is not surprising, because both natural light and carbohydrate consumption increase serotonin levels, which ease depression. Living under artificial light much of the time, without regular exposure to natural light, not only can profoundly affect the regularity of the menstrual cycle but also can create PMS.[82]

The link between PMS and SAD is a profound example of how women's wisdom is simultaneously encoded in both the cycle of the seasons and our monthly cycles. Figure 4 (page 126) illustrates how the phases of the moon are linked to the phases of the menstrual cycle. In figure 8 (page 168), I've added the seasons to this diagram, so that one can clearly see that the time of the monthly cycle when PMS is most common parallels the calendrical period when SAD occurs. The natural tendency to turn inward during the premenstrual time of our monthly cycle is reflected in the natural tendency to turn inward during the autumn of the year. All of nature reflects this wisdom back to us. In fall and winter, the trees send their energy down into their roots, where profound activity and revitalization go on even though it is not obvious to us. The early luteal phase of the menstrual cycle, following ovulation, is when our energies go deep into our roots so that we can take stock and then prepare for the next cycle of outer growth in the world. Because our culture doesn't understand this cyclic wisdom, we have been taught to be afraid of both the times in our cycles and the seasons of year when wisdom demands that we go into darkness, withdraw, and take stock of our lives.

We have been taught to be suspicious of these natural energies—and too many women see them as a weakness that needs to be overridden and ignored. Heaven forbid we should follow our body's wisdom and take a break from getting it all done!

The second half of the menstrual cycle and autumn are times when the tide is out and everything that you don't want to see on the muddy bottom of the bay is uncovered for all to see. Women need to learn to pay attention to the information available to them at these times of the month and of the year. Think of this information as compost that you'll be using to create new growth in your life once the light comes back. Remember Eckhart Tolle's teaching that a woman's "pain body" arises premenstrually (and also during the autumn and early winter of the year). It is our individual responsibility to recognize and do what we can to dissolve our pain bodies with our presence. To do that, we simply feel the discomfort in our bodies and witness it with the part of ourselves that exists beyond time and space. We should also resist the urge to tell ourselves a story about why it's there. Instead, ask: What shape is it? Where is it located? Simply stay present with the pain body and breathe. It will eventually go away on its own—and you will have helped heal the planet by letting more light and a higher vibration into your body.

Treatment

Many women are given symptomatic treatments for PMS that over the long run don't work. Treating a woman's bloating with diuretics, her headaches with painkillers, and her anxiety with a drug such as Prozac often serves to create new side effects from the drugs themselves and ignores the underlying imbalances that lead to PMS in the first place. In the past, psychotherapy was often prescribed for women with PMS. Although it may provide insights about stress, it ignores the nutritional and biochemical aspects of this disorder. Many women with PMS are now given drugs that increase serotonin levels, such as Prozac. Studies have shown that these can be very helpful for alleviating symptoms of PMS in severe cases. These medications are best taken in low doses only during the luteal phase of the cycle.[83] But as mentioned previously, if they are not used with the insight that PMS is part of a much bigger imbalance, they do not help a woman truly learn from, and create health through, her PMS. And besides, after a couple of years they stop working and, worse, may deplete the body's own ability to make serotonin. Ultimately, when women are willing to be present with the emotions behind their PMS and heed their messages, they are eventually able to change their internal hormonal status *without* outside hormones. The process of addressing our emotional and psychological stresses directly results in biochemical changes in our bodies.

Women's Stories

Gwendolyn: Transforming Premenstrual Rage

Gwendolyn was thirty-six when she first came to see me. She was tall, thin, dramatic, and articulate, with a great sense of humor, but her PMS was so bad that she routinely flew into rages and became manic. In one high-energy premenstrual manic phase, she stayed up all night painting her kitchen and then, without any rest, put in a full day of work. This was followed by several days of depression and fatigue so severe that she was unable to get out of bed. At one point her family was so concerned about this behavior that they considered removing her children from her care and called me for my advice. Her PMS and severe mood swings had begun early in her teenage years and were often accompanied by self-destructive behavior that led her into some dangerous situations. During one of these times, she had been gang-raped. On another occasion, she had become pregnant and later got an abortion.

By the time of her first visit with me, Gwendolyn had divorced and was meditating regularly and eating a whole-foods, macrobiotic type of diet, which was helping her to some extent. She was exercising regularly and tak-

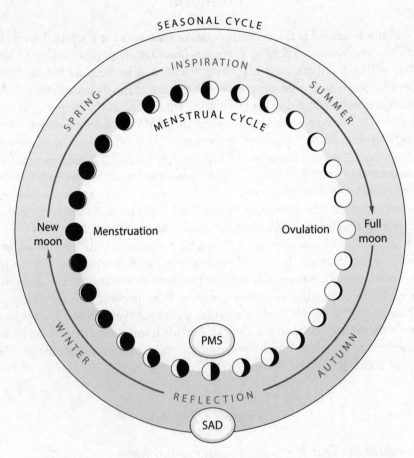

FIGURE 8: SEASONAL AFFECTIVE DISORDER (SAD) AND PMS

PMS is to the monthly cycle as SAD is to the annual cycle. Both conditions respond to the same treatment while asking us to deepen our connection to our cyclic wisdom. We must also become comfortable with darkness, rest, and being versus doing.

ing the appropriate food supplements. These dietary and lifestyle practices are often enough to cure PMS in its mild stages. Despite these adjustments, however, she still went through an emotional hell each month. She had so much unfinished emotional business in her life that her premenstrual wisdom was forcing her to look even deeper at the imbalances in her life. Because of the severity of Gwendolyn's symptoms, I initially prescribed high-dose progesterone therapy.

When Gwendolyn began her progesterone treatment, many aspects of her life were totally out of control. She came to see that the emotional crash that she experienced premenstrually each month actually was forcing her to peel off all the layers of denial in her life. Looking back, she came to see that this process was essential for her healing. A significant factor in her healing was joining a twelve-step program known as Sex and Love Addicts Anonymous (SLAA). She realized that she had a history of moving from one abusive relationship to the next, never finding the "right" man but always obsessing about whomever she was with. Once when a boyfriend expressed his need to leave the relationship, Gwendolyn was premenstrual and flew into a rage, during which she beat him physically with a vengeance that both surprised and scared her. She realized that she had a significant relationship problem and went into counseling to explore and heal her abuse issues. She learned how a sex and love addiction is often the result of childhood sexual abuse, and she began to connect an early abuse experience and the rape with her current self-destructive behavior. She began to appreciate that her premenstrual rages were those of an unhealed child and that they needed to be addressed now that she was an adult. Meanwhile, she continued to meditate, exercise, eat well, go to counseling, and attend twelve-step meetings. As she began to recover, she told me, "In my premenstrual times, every ounce of anger, bitterness, and sense of betrayal erupted—often at such a rate that it became increasingly difficult to stay in my marriage and to continue to care for my autistic daughter and two younger children."

Through supporting her physical body with natural progesterone, good nutrition, and the regular deep rest of meditation, Gwendolyn developed the inner strength necessary to "handle all that had to erupt and clear out of my body." During her office visits, no matter how bad she felt, I repeatedly reminded her to stay with what she was feeling, that anger and rage were okay and a natural part of the healing process. She needed to feel her anger, even pound a pillow if necessary. Though it wasn't okay to attack a person with her anger, she did need to respect it as a message telling her about her unmet need to express emotions that hadn't been allowed in childhood. As her healing process continued, she found that underneath her premenstrual rage and anger, the wisdom and the truth lay waiting. By feeling her anger and staying with it, she discovered tears and a profound sense of abandonment left over from the abuses. "The feelings of abandonment are overwhelming sometimes," she told me. "But if I allow the sadness to come, in the end I come out stronger." After nine months of progesterone therapy, Gwendolyn was able to cut way back on her dosages. At that time, she said, "I continue on the progesterone only two days a month and only because of mild irritability. I hit an occasional emotional wall, but the difference now is that I am able to cope much better knowing where it is all coming from. I believe that when a woman has PMS, the physical, emotional, and spiritual all have to be addressed so that a human being can feel whole again."

It has been a number of years since Gwendolyn first began to listen to and understand her menstrual wisdom through learning to trust and transform her rage. When I last spoke with her, she was doing better than ever. She said that if she had to describe her life in one word, it would be *empowerment*. She's taking care of old business, making amends to those she's hurt, and telling the truth to those who have hurt her. She is thrilled that "the talents I was born with are flourishing: my voice, music, and art. I believe that we all have these talents. But we aren't made to feel that we have anything worthwhile." She wrote me a note that said, "When I become angry at all, I give myself quiet space, go within, and ask myself, 'What is it that you're afraid of or what pain are you trying to escape?' I simply stay present with the feeling in my body until something shifts. Then I almost always get an answer that I can then work with."

PMS and "Othering"

There is a strong correlation between PMS and growing up in an alcoholic family system, in which the parents or grandparents were alcoholic. The correlation between PMS and giving your life away to meet other people's needs—which I used to call relationship addiction—is very high. In her groundbreaking book *Unshakable Confidence: The Freedom to Be Our Authentic Selves—Mindfulness for Women* (CreateSpace, 2017), author and mindfulness teacher Mare Chapman points out that the terms "codependence" and "relationship addiction" are wholly inadequate in describing what happens to women in situations in which they are treated as second-class citizens, much like servants who, in order to survive, must be on constant alert for intuiting the needs of their masters so they won't lose their jobs and means of support. Mare writes that many women—perhaps the majority—have been brought up in situations in which their value and worth are determined by how well they are able to ignore their own needs to meet the needs of those with more power. Generally speaking, men have had far more power to pursue their own destinies than have women. In dysfunctional homes, the needs of the alcoholic, food addict, workaholic, or drug addict often set the tone for the entire family system (or even work situation), so abandoning yourself to the needs and desires of others becomes a very effective survival strategy that makes perfect sense. Chapman calls this "othering," and I find the term far more palatable and accurate than the more pejorative labels "codependent" or "relationship addiction." "Othering" is simply a conditioned response to being in an environment in which one's innate needs have been systemically ignored in favor of the needs of others who have more power.

In my experience, in families in which the men have a tendency to become alcoholics, the females tend to develop PMS. Children of alcoholics have a 40 percent chance of becoming alcoholic, not only because they have a genetic predisposition toward it but also because they've learned that alcohol is the way to deaden their emotions and not feel. This behavior is frequently passed on to them, along with genes that predispose them to drinking. Women in alcoholic families or with alcoholic partners develop PMS as a result of cutting off their feelings. I've worked with countless women who have decided to break the chain of PMS experience by generations of women in their families. (Hypoglycemia [low blood sugar] and a resulting tendency toward sugar craving are also very common in women from alcoholic families who have PMS. This condition tends to be much worse premenstrually and can be easily treated with the dietary recommendations I've already covered.)

Leslie, a forty-nine-year-old homemaker and former teacher with PMS, came to see me with severe premenstrual mood swings, sugar cravings, and fatigue. As I read through her history, I noted that her husband was an alcoholic and that she had been in a teaching position that she hated. She had had an alcoholic mother and sister and had never addressed any of these family issues. During the initial visit, I counseled her about supporting her body during the menstrual cycle through nutrition and exercise, and stressed that she wouldn't "cure" her premenstrual discomfort until she was willing to look at the messages it was sending her about her own family situation. I could tell that she wasn't ready to hear this information, and she did not return for a follow-up.

Seven years later, however, Leslie made an appointment. She told me, "When I was in to see you the first time, you told me that I needed to check out my codependence [a term I now readily replace with "othering"] and that my PMS and decreased energy were related to that. I left thinking, 'Dr. Northrup's a nice woman, but she doesn't know what she's talking about, and in fact I think she's crazy. How could codependence ["othering"] and PMS be related?' But now I realize the connection between what was happening in my life and my PMS. I finally realized that my husband has been verbally abusive for years. I am in the middle of a divorce, and I see now that I had totally 'de-selfed' myself." ("De-selfing" is simply another term for "othering.")

Leslie told me that she had joined a twelve-step group and was picking up the pieces of her life and learning about the effects of living with verbal abuse and alcoholism for so many years. Leslie's feelings are no longer deadened. She's becoming her own person and determining what she will and will not tolerate in her family's behavior. She no longer has PMS most months, but when she does, she pays attention to it, slows down, and makes the necessary adjustments in her life, so that she gets her needs met. She has learned that her menstrual cycle is loaded with wisdom and information, and that she can trust herself and the signals her body and menstrual cycle are providing for her.

IRREGULAR PERIODS

After nearly forty years as a physician, I continue to be amazed by how clearly menstrual cycles and bleeding are connected to the contexts of our lives. Abnormal uterine bleeding is nearly always connected to family issues in some way. As Caroline Myss says, blood is family—always. One woman told me that she and her two sisters, who were living in different parts of the country, skipped periods in the same month when a fourth sister had a miscarriage, although they didn't realize it until they talked at their next get-together. One of my patients, age fifty-five, who had her last menstrual period at the age of fifty-two and went through a classic menopause with hot flashes and lab tests confirming "change of life," nevertheless got a completely normal period right after her mother died. When a menopausal woman develops postmenopausal bleeding, I always ask her what is going on with her and her family. She will often tell me that an emotionally significant family event preceded the bleeding. I had my final menstrual period on the day my younger child left home for college. I hadn't had any bleeding for eleven months prior to this.

Menstrual blood, especially when it comes at an unscheduled time, is a message. It carries wisdom of some kind. Myss points out that most bleeding problems originate from an imbalance in our system: too much emotion and not enough mental, intellectual energy to balance it. She notes that bleeding abnormalities are exacerbated when a woman internalizes confusing signals from her family or society about her own sexual pleasure and sexual needs. A woman may, for example, desire sexual pleasure but feel guilty about it or be unable to ask directly for what she desires. She may not be consciously aware of this inner conflict.

Most practicing physicians have seen the profound effect that the psyche can have on the menstrual cycle. Way back in 1949, S. Zuckerman recognized that emotional disturbances could disorganize menstrual rhythm, accelerate uterine bleeding, and also influence the time of ovulation. Diffuse

networks of nerves connecting the brain with the ovaries (called pregangli-
onic autonomic pathways) are one of the ways the connection between emotions and uterine and ovarian function is mediated.[84] It is also well documented
that the thoughts arising in the prefrontal cortex of our brains result in feelings associated with neurotransmitters that directly influence the hypothalamus and pituitary—the parts of the brain that are intimately connected with
all the organs and functions of the body.

What Are Regular Periods?

Before I examine the subject of menstrual period irregularity, it's necessary to explain what is normal. Women are sometimes taught that their periods are irregular if they do not occur every twenty-eight days. I consider
periods regular when they occur roughly every twenty-four to thirty-five
days. Having a period every twenty-eight days like clockwork happens for
some women but not all. Thousands of women who don't fit the every-
twenty-eight-day pattern are under the impression that their periods are irregular, when in fact they are completely normal.

Period regularity is determined by a complex interaction between the
brain (hypothalamus, pituitary gland, and temporal lobes), the ovaries, and
the uterus. Period patterns can shift with changes in seasons, lighting conditions, diet, or travel, or during times of family stress. Irregular and anovulatory menstrual cycles are associated with premature bone loss. Often
women can tell when they have ovulated because they have a clear discharge
twelve to sixteen days from the first day of their last menstrual period. (This
is discussed in more detail in chapter 11.) Cycles in which a woman has ovulated are also characterized by what is called premenstrual molimina, a group
of "symptoms" resulting from normal cyclic hormonal changes in the body.
These include a slight premenstrual redistribution of body fluid, often experienced as "bloating" or slightly tender breasts, slight abdominal cramping,
and mood changes associated with being in a more reflective, less active state.
Women who don't ovulate usually don't have these changes and will often
get a period out of the blue, without having any idea that one is due. Periods
in which there is no ovulation tend to be more irregular.

EXCESSIVE BUILDUP OF THE UTERINE LINING (ENDOMETRIAL HYPERPLASIA, CYSTIC AND ADENOMATOUS HYPERPLASIA)

In some women with irregular periods, a biopsy of the inside of the
uterus (endometrial biopsy) reveals a condition in which the normal lining of

the uterus has been replaced by an overgrowth of glandular tissue. Under the microscope, the endometrial glands look as if they are piled on top of each other and packed too closely. This overgrowth results from overstimulation of the uterine lining by estrogen without the balance of progesterone. It is known as cystic and adenomatous hyperplasia (meaning too many glands) of the endometrium.[85] (It is not to be confused with endometriosis, which will be discussed at length in chapter 6.) Hyperplasia results when a woman's ovaries haven't produced eggs regularly. Instead of a uniform thickening and then sloughing off of the uterine lining (the endometrium), caused by the hormones associated with regular ovulation, the endometrium gets out of sync. Some parts of the lining "think" it's day seven, while others "think" it's day twenty-eight. This results in irregular and intermittent bleeding.

Cystic and adenomatous hyperplasia or simple endometrial hyperplasia is not considered dangerous unless abnormal cells are present in the biopsy of the uterine lining. Finding some simple endometrial hyperplasia on the biopsy is fairly normal and is not a cause for alarm if it happens only once or twice. Many women in their forties and fifties skip an ovulation every now and then as their ovaries undergo the changes leading up to menopause. When a woman's periods become irregular, she does not necessarily require a uterine biopsy, though this decision must be made on a case-by-case basis depending on her history and examination findings.

Treatment

Please note that for this and other conditions, I will be discussing the treatments that are most commonly prescribed in the United States. These treatments do not address the issues underlying symptoms. The underlying issues and what a woman can learn from them are covered in the individual stories throughout this chapter.

Many cases of simple endometrial hyperplasia go away on their own. However, a very small percentage of women with this condition have atypical cells on their biopsies. Endometrial hyperplasia needs to be monitored and followed to be sure it is going away rather than progressing. Women with chronic anovulation over many years do have a statistically higher incidence of uterine cancer, especially if they are also obese or have been diagnosed with polycystic ovary syndrome (see below as well as chapter 7). Gynecologists are trained to treat everybody as though there were a potential cancer risk. Therefore initial conventional treatment of endometrial hyperplasia consists of giving a synthetic progestin such as Provera or Aygestin for one to three months and then repeating the endometrial biopsy to make sure that the condition has cleared. I often recommend natural progesterone for this purpose, especially in those women who have adverse side effects from synthetic progestin. (See page 155 for the difference between synthetic and natural progesterone.) Physicians vary widely on how much of the drug they give and for how long they give it. Prescribing a progestin drug is sometimes called a "medical D&C" (dilation and curettage of the uterine lining), because it causes the endometrial lining to slough off in a uniform manner all at once and helps the uterus get rid of the tissue buildup. Natural progesterone, on the other hand, has the ability to downregulate estrogen receptors, meaning that it reduces the cells' sensitivity to estrogen; this often clears up benign endometrial hyperplasia. The same is true for many women's herbs, including chasteberry and *Pueraria mirifica*.

Some women with persistent endometrial hyperplasia do not respond to treatment with progestin, progesterone, dietary change, or herbs and may require a surgical D&C in the operating room. In extremely rare instances, they may need a hysterectomy if this condition does not go away or if it progresses to the stage of producing abnormal cells.

DYSFUNCTIONAL UTERINE BLEEDING (DUB)

Skipping periods more than just occasionally, frequent bleeding between periods, or spotting between periods is known as dysfunctional uterine bleeding, or DUB. (See also the section on polycystic ovaries on page 247.) Women who have had cesarean sections may occasionally have abnormal bleeding patterns because of disruptions of the uterine lining caused by the scar on the uterus. Many abnormal patterns are hypothalamic in origin, meaning that they are related to the complex interaction between the brain, ovaries, and uterus. Severe anxiety and depression change neurotransmitter levels in the brain and can affect hypothalamic function. Dysfunctional uterine bleeding is often associated with anovulatory cycles and too much estrogen relative to progesterone. It is also related to the hormonal imbalance that results from elevated cortisol and insulin levels, which change the way estrogen is metabolized. Though doctors are trained to look for endocrine abnormalities—such as thyroid problems or pituitary problems—that can cause menstrual abnormalities, these tests almost always come back normal. Because DUB is sometimes (though rarely) related to high prolactin levels caused by small pituitary tumors known as pituitary microadenomas, a blood test for this hormone is also indicated. However, prolactin hormone levels that are too high, a condition known as hyperprolactinemia, is not common. Moreover, the tiny pituitary tumors that cause it have often been found to go away on their own.

A diagnosis of DUB is made on the basis of history, blood tests that check pituitary and thyroid hormone levels, and sometimes a biopsy from inside the uterus to see if the uterine lining shows signs of anovulation or abnormal cells.

Conventional Treatment

The conventional treatment of DUB consists of giving hormones such as birth control pills to regulate the periods. This common treatment is now given even up until menopause in women who don't smoke. Birth control pills do result in reliable periods every month, and taking them may be the first choice for women whose lives are too busy to change their diets, take supplements, or exercise. But pills don't heal anything—they simply mask the underlying issues in the body or put an imbalance to sleep for a while. Taking birth control pills to regulate a woman's period is like shooting out the indicator light on the dashboard of your car that tells you the engine needs attention. Nevertheless, like most gynecologists, I have prescribed birth control pills for many women, both for contraception and for DUB, because taking the pill is the easiest way for a woman to eliminate her symptoms without doing the work of changing aspects of her life that are contributing to the problem. Sometimes this is appropriate, but a woman should be very clear that this is what she's doing when she takes period-regulating hormones.

Women with DUB who are in their forties and older are statistically at greater risk for endometrial hyperplasia, and most physicians will do an endometrial biopsy before they initiate hormonal treatment. Progestin hormone (synthetic progesterone such as Provera or Aygestin) is often the treatment of choice, both to clear up the hyperplasia if it is present and to stop the abnormal bleeding.

Natural Treatments

My first recommendation for DUB once an endometrial biopsy has shown no abnormalities would be the herb *Pueraria mirifica*, taken either cyclically (on days seven through twenty-one of your cycle) or daily depending upon the circumstances and whether or not a woman has other perimenopausal symptoms. (See Resources.)

Natural progesterone (Crinone or Prochieve vaginal gel or Prometrium capsules) could also be used. Over-the-counter 2 percent progesterone creams (one-quarter to one-half teaspoon applied to the skin daily) have also been shown to achieve adequate serum levels and help protect the endometrium.[86] If a woman is skipping periods and wants to get pregnant, the fertility drug

Clomid, which tricks the brain and ovaries into ovulation, will often be prescribed.[87]

DUB and Polycystic Ovary Syndrome (PCOS)

A subgroup of women with DUB don't ovulate regularly. Many of these women are overweight, with body fat that produces too much estrogen. The estrogen overstimulates the uterine lining and can result in anovulation. These women sometimes have a condition known as polycystic ovary syndrome, in which their ovaries develop a thickened outer wall, just under which many unreleased, partially stimulated eggs form cysts. On ultrasound examinations, the ovaries show up as being enlarged and having multiple small cysts in them. (Interestingly, medical intuitives report exactly the same appearance when they do readings on these women.) Studies have shown that the risk of menstrual irregularities is two to three times greater in obese women than in women of average body size.[88] Dietary change to decrease excess body fat and stabilize blood sugar and insulin levels can help create hormonal balance as well as lower estrogen levels. These women also have elevated androgen levels, which contribute to their problems. Androgens are a group of hormones that include testosterone and are produced in the ovaries, the adrenal glands, and body fat. Not all women with PCOS are overweight, however.

As with PMS and menstrual cramps, unabated stress, a diet high in refined foods and low in nutrients that raises blood sugar and insulin, and a lack of exposure to natural light can *all* result in DUB and/or PCOS. Many women with DUB and/or PCOS have been helped by lifestyle and dietary changes alone. In fact, PCOS is almost always associated with insulin levels that are too high. The moment those go back to normal with dietary change, the PCOS goes away. (See Resources.)

Women's Stories

Deborah: Breaking Family Ties

Deborah was seventeen when she left her family to go to college. She described her family as "lower-middle-class and not oriented to a college education." In fact, Deborah was the first person from her family ever to leave home for any reason except to marry. Her family was not supportive of her living away from home, and they wanted her to visit every weekend.

During her first year in college, Deborah met many people who were interesting and exciting to her, and a whole new world of intellectual challenge and career possibilities began opening up for her. She was happier and felt more fulfilled than at any other time in her life. Unfortunately, her mother, fearing that she would lose Deborah, began to call her on the phone every evening, telling her that she was a failure and that she would never succeed at anything if she stayed in college. She threatened to call the dean of the college and have Deborah's scholarships rescinded so that she would have no choice but to come home.

Deborah became depressed, and her periods became irregular for the first time since menarche. They came two or three times per month, or not at all for two or three months at a time. To feel better about herself, she began to run as a form of exercise. At first, this made her feel physically stronger, more independent, and more in control of her body—which seemed to be out of control for the first time in her life. But the exercise didn't help her irregular periods. In fact, it contributed to long periods of amenorrhea (no periods at all). She saw a gynecologist, who told her that her pelvic exam was completely normal. The reason for her problem, he said, was that she was "fooling around with too many guys." Since she was not involved with any men at this time, she was not helped by this physician and avoided gynecologists for the next eleven years.

Deborah did, however, consult with an acupuncturist, who prescribed Chinese herbs for her in addition to acupuncture. These treatments helped regulate her periods within two months, but she discovered that her periods went right back to their abnormal pattern as soon as she stopped her acupuncture and herb treatments, and she found that she had to deal with the source of her depression, which returned when she had to stop running because of an injury. She came to see that her relationship with her mother was the source of her problems, and she eventually moved out of state to break her mother's control over her life.

When I first saw Deborah, she was recovering from an addiction to exercise. She had begun psychotherapy and was exploring her relationship to her mother. I recommended a mindfulness workshop to help Deborah learn how to be present with the sensations in her body without getting caught up in her mental story. I also recommended a whole-food diet, *Pueraria* on days seven through twenty-one of each cycle, and a calcium-magnesium supplement. Over the next six months, her periods became regular, every twenty-eight to twenty-nine days, and she was no longer depressed. She finished college and completed her Ph.D. She has broken the original family ties that were at the root of her problem, and her life is becoming balanced on all levels.

Donna: Dysfunctional Family and Dysfunctional Bleeding

Donna, a forty-two-year-old professor, came into my office with a six-month history of irregular periods—bleeding for two weeks, then nothing for six weeks, then a few days of spotting, and so on. She also had bouts of severe anxiety and depression that lasted for three weeks straight, at just about the time the irregularity started. An endometrial biopsy revealed cystic and adenomatous hyperplasia, an abnormality associated with anovulation (failure to ovulate).

Donna's mother had also gone through abnormal periods and mood swings in her forties but had decided that it was all her hormones, and she was just going to have to live with it. Donna was quite sure that her mother had unresolved issues with her own father, since Donna remembers her grandfather as someone who was very scary to be around when she was a child.

Donna told me that she'd been having some dreams about and memories of sexual abuse by her uncles. "I've been terrified that if I tell anyone what happened or what I think happened, God will get me," she told me. "Can I force myself to deal with this stuff any faster?" Like many women, she was under the impression that merely having the facts—who, what, where, and when—would help her deal with her discomfort and get on with her life once and for all. But getting the facts satisfies only the intellect—which always wants more facts. The intellect is the part of us that keeps telling the same story over and over again—thus re-creating the biology of conflict. Healing happens in the body, not the intellect. We have to let healing work its way through us—gently, gradually, and respectfully.

Donna's upbringing had led her to claim, "Everything in life is my fault. I keep thinking that I must be crazy and must be making this stuff up." I reassured her that in this culture women have been labeled crazy for centuries for telling the truth and that what she was going through was quite normal, given her history. She decided to do some work with an incest survivors' group to help her break through her own and her family's denial. After several months of work, she had another endometrial biopsy—to check for abnormal cells—and it was perfectly normal, as were her pituitary hormones. Her periods had gradually become more regular.

Dealing with her emotional trauma was what actually cured Donna's period problems. Her periods, through their irregularity, had communicated to her a bodily wisdom. Her menstrual blood turned her attention to the healing that was required in her relationship with her family, her bloodline.

Darlene: Irregular Periods Since Menarche

I first saw Darlene, a teacher, as a patient when she was thirty years old. She was married, had no children, and had a very long history of dysfunctional uterine bleeding since puberty. She experienced long stretches of time with no periods, followed by bleeding almost continuously for a month at a time, then spotting infrequently. Darlene had ongoing anxiety issues and had panic attacks if she had to leave the house for a long period of time. Her marriage was a source of unhappiness to her rather than comfort. She was generally anxious, had trouble sleeping, and had frequent headaches.

Darlene's upbringing had been stressful. Her father and at least one grandfather were alcoholics—although, she said, there was a lot of family denial around this. Her mother, her maternal grandmother, and her cousin had had lifelong problems with irregular bleeding that led to hysterectomies. Her aunt and another cousin had uterine cancer and also had hysterectomies.

Darlene originally came to my office for a fertility workup. Because of her bleeding pattern, we did an endometrial biopsy, which showed endometrial hyperplasia. For treatment of this condition, she was placed on large doses of synthetic progestin. In contrast to most women on this therapy, however, her bleeding didn't stop. A repeat biopsy after the progestin treatment again showed the abnormality of cystic and adenomatous hyperplasia. The next step would be a surgical dilation and curettage (D&C) to be certain that she didn't have uterine cancer.

But Darlene was terrified of the procedure and begged me for an alternative. Because of her strong reaction, I compromised and recommended a low-glycemic-index diet to stabilize blood sugar plus castor oil packs on her lower abdomen three or four times a week to help restore her immune system. I knew this would give her a chance to reflect at least three times per week on her condition and any messages it might hold for her. We agreed that if this didn't change her cells, we would go ahead with the D&C.

Two weeks later, I did another endometrial biopsy. The tissue was normal endometrium, consistent with the first phase of her menstrual cycle. Darlene was ecstatic and cried with relief. She then went on to have a completely normal period. In the ensuing months her periods were normal, too, and have remained that way. During these months she changed her biochemistry through biofeedback, which she practiced for her insomnia, headaches, and intense anxiety. Realizing that her marriage had not been healthy for her, she separated from her husband, began divorce proceedings, and entered into a love affair where her sexual needs were addressed, which turned out to be deeply healing for her.

Three years later, when Darlene came in for her annual exam, she told me that she was developing a feeling of power around her menstrual cycle that was new and very exciting for her. "My breasts get bigger," she said, "I feel powerful, and I walk around like I know the secrets of the universe. I think my family has been terrified of my power for years. I can remember feeling it even when I was a little girl. Although having this power seems new, it also seems like something I've known for a long time." Darlene has reclaimed her connection to the universal feminine and her sexuality. By doing so, she has broken a cycle of irregular bleeding that was generations deep within her family.

HEAVY PERIODS (MENORRHAGIA)

Some women bleed so heavily during their periods that they routinely bleed through one or two tampons and a pad worn at the same time. Their blood may even soak through their clothing. Some are unable to leave the house during certain days of their periods because the bleeding is so heavy. One of my patients decided to have a hysterectomy after she bled through her clothes into the upholstery of her airplane seat on two different business trips to Europe.

This kind of heavy bleeding is called menorrhagia. Women with menorrhagia have periods at regular intervals, but the periods are heavy. Over time, menorrhagia may lead to anemia (a low red blood cell count) if a woman doesn't get enough iron in her diet or if her body can't replace the blood she loses each month. Menorrhagia can be caused by fibroids, endometriosis, or adenomyosis. Rarely, it is associated with a thyroid problem. Some women bleed heavily for no obvious reason.

Chronically heavy periods can be related to chronic stress over second-chakra issues, including creativity, relationships, money, and control of others. One of my patients who sometimes had very heavy periods noted that her periods became heavy when she was upset and needed to weep. "When I bleed like that," she said, "I feel like it's the lower part of my body weeping for the losses I have suffered in my life." When she took the time to pay attention to the different problems she was having and let herself feel her disappointments and pain, her periods were normal. Another patient, who had bad cramps every month and bled profusely, began to think of the uterine pain as related to her strong need for creative space in her own life. She began to set aside one hour a day to do sculpture. Each time she did, she got in touch with the sheer joy of creating for its own sake, and her pelvic pain and bleeding gradually lessened each month.

Adenomyosis, a common cause of pain and heavy bleeding, is a condition in which the glands that normally grow in only the lining of the uterus—the endometrium—grow deeply into the walls of the uterus. (Sometimes called "internal endometriosis," adenomyosis is often present along with fibroids and/or endometriosis, but not always.) This condition can result in bleeding into the uterine wall with each menstrual period. The uterine wall becomes spongy and engorged with blood, producing a condition in which the uterine muscles can't contract normally to decrease the bleeding.

A diagnosis of adenomyosis is usually suspected from a woman's history and from a characteristic boggy-feeling uterus on pelvic examination. A definitive diagnosis can be made, however, only by magnetic resonance imaging (MRI) or by a biopsy of the uterine wall, which entails surgically removing a piece of the uterus or the entire uterus.

Young girls with heavy periods should be screened for von Willebrand disease, an inherited bleeding disorder that causes blood not to clot very well. Although this is the most common bleeding disorder among young girls with heavy periods, doctors frequently overlook it. Up to 20 percent of girls with heavy menstrual bleeding have an underlying bleeding disorder such as this.[89]

Treatment

Women whose menorrhagia does not respond to diet or herbs such as *Pueraria mirifica* can often be helped by a synthetic progestin to keep the bleeding under control. The usual regimen is 5 to 10 mg of Provera or Aygestin taken once or twice per day during the last two weeks of each menstrual cycle. Birth control pills also can work well in many cases. Natural progesterone, either applied as a skin cream or taken orally or vaginally, can also be used. The dosage depends upon the severity of the problem: For oral progesterone, I recommend 100 mg four times per day for the most severe cases, 50 mg two times per day for milder cases, from days fourteen to twenty-eight of the cycle. For progesterone cream (400 mg/ounce), I suggest half a teaspoon twice per day on the soft areas of the skin—breasts, neck, face, abdomen, inner thighs, inner arms, or hands. Vaginal gels of micronized progesterone are also available. The usual starting dose is 45 mg, either daily or every other day on days fourteen through twenty-eight of your cycle. Following the diet outlined in chapter 17 often decreases or eliminates the need for the progestin or progesterone over time. Some women have used this treatment for months or even years as an alternative to hysterectomy.

Prostaglandin inhibitors, such as ibuprofen (Advil or Motrin) or naproxen sodium (Aleve or Naprosyn), have also helped some women decrease menstrual bleeding.[90] These are best taken one or two times per day for three to four days before the menstrual cycle is due and continuing through the days of the period that are usually the heaviest.

Endometrial ablation, in which the lining of the uterus is removed either by electrocautery or by laser, is a surgical treatment for heavy bleeding in women whose menorrhagia has failed to respond to other treatments. This is an excellent alternative to hysterectomy and effectively controls heavy bleeding in more than 85 percent of cases. It can be done on an outpatient or overnight basis in the hospital.[91] Women who opt for this procedure must be carefully screened beforehand to make sure that their condition is likely to respond, because it doesn't work for all women. NovaSure is one type of endometrial ablation that has worked well for many (see www.novasure.com). Hysterectomy is also an option.

HEALING OUR MENSTRUAL HISTORY:
PREPARING OUR DAUGHTERS

Many women, like those about whom you've read in this chapter, have turned around their painful menstrual experiences and begun to reclaim their rightful heritage: their bodily, lunar, and cyclic creative wisdom. As a woman does this, she passes on to the next generation a more positive body image and relationship to her body. In this way, she frees herself and others from the patriarchal degradation of the feminine, and the possibility of healing all women's cycles is greatly enhanced.

For too long, young girls have been introduced to the menstrual cycle solely in terms of sexual intercourse and the possibility of getting pregnant inadvertently. Most girls are not emotionally prepared to grasp the full responsibility and impact of their female sexuality until they know about and understand the workings of their own uterus, fallopian tubes, ovaries, and cyclic menstrual nature. Unfortunately, our culture's advertising, merchandising, and media are saturated with sexualized images of young women and girls that undermine a girl's healthy sexual self-image.

The American Psychological Association's Task Force on the Sexualization of Girls has issued a full report on this damaging trend.[92] Eileen Zurbriggen, chair of the task force, said, "We have ample evidence to conclude that sexualization has negative effects in a variety of domains, including cognitive functioning, physical and mental health, and healthy sexual development." According to the report, the sexualization of girls undermines their confidence, making girls feel dissatisfied with their bodies, which leads to feelings of shame and anxiety about their appearance. It's also linked to eating disorders, low self-esteem, and depression. The report also found that in various forms of media, girls are portrayed in a sexual manner more often than boys, dressed in revealing clothing and shown in postures or facial expressions implying sexual readiness.

Social media and smartphones have only fanned the fire. A systematic review published in 2014 found that an estimated 10 to 25 percent of adolescents have sent photos or text messages of a sexual nature, while 15 to 35 percent have received such communications.[93]

In her bestselling book *American Girls: Social Media and the Secret Lives of Teenagers* (Alfred A. Knopf, 2016), author Nancy Jo Sales reports after interviewing more than 200 adolescent girls that social media often reinforces a culture of sexism and misogyny. Being pressured by boys to text nude or semi-nude photos of themselves and then being shamed and sometimes even blackmailed for sending them has become a serious problem among teenage girls today. To make things even worse, other girls often spread rumors about and belittle the victims, adding exponentially to the shaming.

Indeed, in one recent study, Stephanie V. Ng, M.D., wrote that "while sexualization of females is rewarded online (usually by males), females are also punished for these same displays and are quick to be labeled by other female peers as 'sluts' or 'skanks.' This perpetuates sexual double standards that reinforce gender stereotypes."[94] Dr. Ng also notes that "because social media features peers (rather than celebrities), exposure may generate even more social comparison and body shame than traditional media."

The situation doesn't get much better when girls get to college. Yet another study reports that 94 percent of undergraduate women (of all races and sexual orientations) reported experiencing unwanted objectifying sexual comments and behaviors at least once over a semester.[95]

This is unlikely to change as long as images of women in advertising continue to sexually objectify them. A study at Wesleyan University that analyzed 1,988 ads in fifty-eight popular U.S. magazines found that 51.8 percent of the ads that featured women portrayed those women as sex objects.[96] Three out of four such ads in men's magazines did so, compared with approximately two out of three such ads in women's fashion magazines and publications targeted at adolescent girls.

The study's authors hypothesized that the pervasiveness of such images of highly sexualized women reinforces the status quo of male dominance "by designating women's bodies as property that can be evaluated, ogled, and touched at the whim of men's desire."[97] They continue, "In a cultural climate defined by increasing possibilities, in which women have earned advanced degrees and have infiltrated careers traditionally dominated by men, society has demanded that women become servants to popular images of beauty and sexuality." The researchers then quote Naomi Wolf, author of *The Beauty Myth: How Images of Beauty Are Used Against Women* (William Morrow, 1991), in saying that this objectification has become ubiquitous in images seen in the media, because during a time in which "many women have guilt feelings and uncertainties about their entry into public life, and many men have fears about women's empowerment, those images or articles that show women being put, or putting themselves, back under control are most likely to get a strong audience reaction."[98] In other words, the Wesleyan researchers suggest, the pervasive nature of these sexually objectifying images in the media may be a means for society to (consciously or subconsciously) compensate for images of women's increased independence. Clearly, while this situation is rapidly changing, it cannot change quickly enough. Awareness, as always, is the first step toward change.

We must educate ourselves and others about female sexuality. Fathers, too, can help. Though the primal need that fathers feel to protect their daughters from other men and boys stems directly from a patriarchal worldview in which men assume ownership over the women in their lives, it's also true that knowing she is protected by a strong, loving father or father figure can be a boon to a young girl or woman if it helps her feel secure in her body and in her sexuality. Women who have or had adoring and supportive fathers are definitely given a leg up on thriving in the world. Far too often, however, this is not a woman's experience. Many times her father was not around. And other times he was not supportive. Many women have told me about their fathers' response when they reached menarche: "As soon as I got my period, things changed between us. He never hugged or cuddled me again. Our relationship was never the same." One woman with a uterine fibroid suddenly recalled her father yelling at her across the room when she was fourteen and all dressed up to go on a date, "You slut, you whore!" She hadn't remembered this for years. She said that it had felt as if his words went right into her body and stayed there, affecting the way she felt about herself as a woman for the next twenty years. A lot has changed in the last two decades.

Reclaiming menstrual wisdom starts with women of all ages envisioning a new and more positive way of thinking and talking about the menstrual experience to ourselves, our daughters, our nieces, our loved ones, and the men in our families. Women who are attuned to their cyclic wisdom and who embrace it without shame or embarrassment go a long way toward helping the next generation move into their womanhood.

For many girls in this society, puberty has been a time of loss. When my oldest daughter was eleven and I was tucking her into bed one night, she told me that she was worried about something. She had a sore growth on her chest that was scaring her. She wanted me to check it. I did and found a small nipple budding on the left—the first sign of puberty. I told her that it was normal and that she had nothing to worry about. I congratulated her!

Later, unable to sleep, she came into my room and said, "Can we talk?" I said, "Of course," and asked what was troubling her. She burst into tears and said, "I don't want to grow up." I held her and told her that I remembered feeling the same way. I hadn't thought about it for years. But now, with her in my arms, perched on the brink of puberty, I remembered the deep sadness I had felt about growing up. I recalled never wanting to leave home and never wanting my life to change. We sat on my bed while I shared this with her and held her.

After a while, I asked her if she wanted to talk about this with her father, and she said yes. She asked, "Dad, were you ever sad about growing up?" He responded, "Not until the last few years." All of us laughed together at his reply. After a few more minutes of acknowledging my daughter's feelings about puberty, she thanked us and went happily off to bed. This experience was a great example for me of how our emotions, when we respect and express them, quite naturally move through the body and are released.

My daughter didn't bring up the subject again but knew that she could.

When she got her period at the age of fourteen she was well prepared and enjoyed getting flowers from her father and a special doll and book from me. Our celebration of our daughter's coming-of-age could not have taken place if I hadn't appreciated the fact that at some deep, inarticulate level, she knew that moving from the innocence of girlhood to puberty was not an entirely happy prospect in a culture in which the female body is a commodity. As we work together to create new rites of passage for women, we must acknowledge that moving forward also means letting go and grieving over what we are losing.

Clearly we cannot take our daughters into a space where we have never been. We cannot provide healing for them in areas in which we're still deeply wounded ourselves. If we still carry generations of shame about the processes of our female bodies, we cannot hope to pass on to our daughters a genuine sense of love for our own bodies. But the minute we decide to address this whole area, think about it in new ways, and begin the process of reclaiming our menstrual wisdom, the entire map changes. We can begin to create new ceremonies and new rites of passage for ourselves and for our daughters while at this same time working through our old programming and pain.

The good news is that this is now happening all over the planet. In the United States, for example, a group of menstrual health advocates has founded the member-run Red Web Foundation (www.theredweb.org), which is dedicated to supporting a positive societal view of girls' and women's bodies and menstrual cycles, first bleeding through last, and creating physical, emotional, and spiritual well-being. This foundation provides a wide range of resources for introducing girls to their first menstrual cycle in an empowering way as well as educating women of all ages about the positive aspects of their cycles.

The Red Web Foundation was inspired by the pioneering work of the late Tamara Slayton, founder of the Menstrual Health Foundation. Tamara taught me that most girls are not emotionally prepared for a full-fledged understanding of their sexuality until they have first connected their own creativity to their menstrual cycles. To that end, she often taught menstrual empowerment through doll making and other creative arts. Though there are dozens of ways to celebrate a girl's coming-of-age within her own family, there's nothing more powerful than doing this in community—with other girls and their families. This gives the celebration clout and meaning that it otherwise lacks. When a girl is surrounded by her ever-important peer group for a coming-of-age celebration (by the way, it's not necessary that she have her first period to do this), her own hesitancy and embarrassment fall away and she feels embraced by the larger community in a powerful way. Remember, adolescence is all about learning how to fit in with peers. Nothing is more important to an adolescent girl. (For a full curriculum on how to deliver a workshop for girls on menstruation empowerment, go to www

.roadtoracialjustice.org/about-kesa and scroll down to "Moon Magic Work-shop on Puberty.")

A woman commenting on my Facebook page shared the following story:

My daughter was eleven and I celebrated the momentous occasion by throwing her a "period party," to which the key women in her life were invited. Each brought a small gift, such as red heart earrings, light pink cupcakes, her first lacy undies, and a card with womanly advice from each of us. Back then, she said it was weird and now, at seventeen, she brags to her friends about how special it was to be welcomed into sister-hood by all the women she loved.

Such "period parties" can be just as special for the adults who gather to celebrate the guest of honor. A friend and colleague told me the story of at-tending such an event for the granddaughter of her yoga teacher:

About fifteen of us from our yoga class brought presents wrapped in red and sat around in a circle with candles in the center. One by one, we each spoke to the young woman and her best friend, who sat right next to her the whole time. Each of us offered a piece of advice or told a story or somehow shared something meaningful about when we started our periods or about having periods in general. Then she opened her pres-ents and we all had great party refreshments—including some surpris-ingly delicious beet juice!

What amazed me was that even with that many of us present, every single woman had something genuinely wonderful to share—some were downright hysterical and others were poignant, but no one overlapped at all. Each of us had something unique to contribute. Consequently, we all felt an amazing kinship that night, as though we'd indeed created and witnessed something incredibly personal and sacred. We all felt truly blessed to be women, and the beautiful girl in whose honor we were gathering truly felt part of that powerful vibe in a way I'm sure she didn't expect.

Not all girls will appreciate a large event, of course. Another woman commenting on my Facebook page wrote about having planned a whole ceremony for her oldest daughter, including the important women in her life, out in the woods, where they would drum together:

Luckily, one day before this happened, I had the realization that the ceremony I had planned was really for me, and my daughter would not be so keen on it. So I changed the plan. I bought small diamond stud earrings, and I arranged a mom-daughter spa day with massages and pedicures. We then met her father at a little French bistro he and I frequently visited. We had champagne, escargots, and crème brûlée. We gave her the earrings and welcomed her to the next stage of her life.

The next morning, she and I went to get her ears pierced. One of her friends came along, and I was happy as a bee, buzzing about her entrance into womanhood. My daughter was mortified I was talking about "it." I was sad and a little hurt. I told her I was mothering her as I wished I had been mothered. Since we are two different people, she would have to let me know what she needed from me. All in all, it was a beautiful memory for me, and she also speaks of it fondly. I'm so glad I nixed the drumming in the woods!

Yet another woman posted this story on my Facebook page:

When my daughter got her period, I did a "big deal" day with her to celebrate. I woke her with a dozen roses to Alice Cooper's "Only Women Bleed" and took her for a massage and mani-pedi. I gave her a book of stories on first blood traditions from around the world and a pearl necklace, and we had lunch and then I had a small ritual during which I presented her with a large bloodstone egg, telling her that she would give birth to so many hopes, dreams, and desires throughout her life, as well as perhaps some little humans (which she did—three).

Most of us will not have the opportunity to participate in a coming-of-age celebration with a large group. But we can still honor our daughter's (or another young woman's) first period with a special dinner, shopping trip, flowers, or special gift. It's also important to include her father, if possible. All of us have an innate need for ritual and recognition. (I've come to the conclusion that the fiftieth birthday is really a belated coming-of-age ceremony for the baby boom women who were never celebrated during their adolescence but for whom, at fifty, all the passion, power, and ebullience of adolescence come roaring back.)

Creative ways abound for making this a special time for young women and for teaching them the truth about their periods. For example, *Menstrupedia Comic: The Friendly Guide to Periods for Girls* (www.menstrupedia .com) is a comic book published in India that presents information about menstruation in an easy-to-understand and entertaining way. Menstrupedia founder Aditi Gupta designed the book to shatter the myths and misunderstandings about the subject. The book is available in print (through Amazon) as well as in digital form.

Of course, menstrual empowerment doesn't end with a coming-of-age ceremony. Learning to embrace our bodies, our cycles, and our sexuality is an ongoing process. Many of today's teenage girls are precocious "fertile time bombs" because they have no knowledge of their own cycles and use sexuality and intercourse as a rite of passage.[99] I advocate teaching all teenage girls how to make love to themselves, so that they don't feel the need for teenage boys for an outlet. When we teach our young women respect for their bodies and for their cycles, and when we heal ourselves in these areas as well, we help break the cycles of abuse that have gone on for centuries.

After reading a newspaper article on Patricia Reis's work with the Goddess and women's bodies, Marge Rosenthal remembered that she had introduced the menstrual cycle to her daughter by creating a myth. In a letter to Reis she wrote, "When my daughter was four or five and I was premenstrual and searching for something positive about cramps, grouchiness, and all the other pleasures of being a woman, I created the Goddess Menses. She came out of a spontaneous situation: Mama grouchy, a kid wondering why, and me grasping for a believable answer.

"I told her that once a month the Goddess Menses visited a woman's body, and that she was a very mysterious goddess. Sometimes she sneaked in without us knowing, and sometimes she announced herself with powerful tuggings inside our bodies. I told her that when men bleed it is always a sign of illness or injury, but that the bleeding the goddess brought was a reaffirmation of life. A cleansing of our body. I told her that the goddess's arrival is a time of celebration, a time to buy flowers or something small and special, just for us women.

"I told her the grouchiness was because I wasn't listening to my body. Had I felt the tuggings, I would have known to be extra loving to myself (and perhaps taken a couple of aspirin). As a result of my doing this, I saw all the positive value of creating our own goddesses. I created a little goddess to make positive association with the menstrual cycle. She is a high-spirited, energetic goddess who plays tricks with our bodies, arriving early or late, quiet or stormy, tagging or rolling over us, but once her presence is acknowledged she is very happy to quietly settle down and wait—until next time.

"As I approach menopause I will miss the goddess. It will be a time of her holding on to the youth we shared and me letting go to let the next spirit enter my body. I wonder what her name will be?"

Creating Health Through the Menstrual Cycle

Sitting quietly, ask yourself, "What is my personal truth about the menstrual cycle? How am I feeling about this information? What messages about menstruation and hormones have I learned from my family? What information have I handed down to the younger women in my life? What do I tell myself about my menstrual period? What can it teach me?" Regardless of where you are, be gentle with yourself.

For the next three months, keep a moon journal specifically for noticing the effects of your menstrual cycle on your life. In her book *Do Less: A Revolutionary Approach to Time and Energy Management for Busy Moms* (Hay House, 2019), my daughter Kate Northrup documents the power of our connection with the different phases of our menstrual cycles, which we can use to create more healthful and profitable lives.

Keep track of the phases of the moon. (There is a wide variety of apps available for this.) See if you notice any correlation between your cycle and the phases of the moon. See if you crave certain foods premenstrually. What are they? Would taking a long bath feel as good as eating that hot fudge sundae? When are you feeling the most energy? The most libido? Consider scheduling lots of your "to-dos" on those days—and reserve the days when you are bleeding for more restful activities.

Give yourself time to tune in to and reclaim your cyclic nature. Write a short journal entry every day. The rewards of doing this will be beyond measure. You'll feel connected to life in a whole new way, with increased respect for yourself and your magnificent hormones.

Celebrate the Goddess Menses in your own unique way, knowing that doing so will improve your life on all levels.

6

The Uterus

The oldest oracle in Greece, sacred to the Great Mother of earth, sea, and sky, was named Delphi, from *delphos,* meaning "womb."

—Barbara Walker

The uterus is located in the low center of the pelvis, in the middle of the pelvic bowl. Also known as the *hara,* this low-belly body center (which includes the ovaries, too) is associated with power, passion, and creativity. This makes sense because the uterus is the vessel in which new life is nourished and brought to fruition. The uterus is connected to the vagina by the cervix and to the pelvic side walls by the broad and cardinal ligaments. The back portion of the bladder attaches to the lower front part of the uterus—the lower uterine segment. The fallopian tubes come off each side of the upper portion of the uterus, known as the fundus. The ovaries are located below the ends of the tubes, known as the fimbria. The fimbria look like delicate fern fronds. (See figure 9, page 192.)

The ovaries, tubes, and uterus are all part of the female hormonal system. Each of these structures is intimately connected to the others. The circulation of blood to the ovaries depends in part on the intact uterus. Following a hysterectomy, changes in the blood supply to the ovaries result in an earlier menopause in many women. The uterus itself is very sensitive to the effects of hormones. As the central organ in the pelvis, the uterus and its attachments to the pelvic side walls, the cardinal ligaments, are important but underrated components of the entire pelvic anatomy.

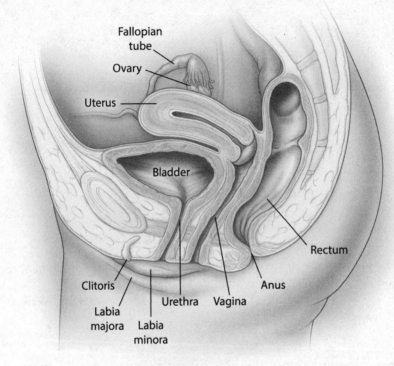

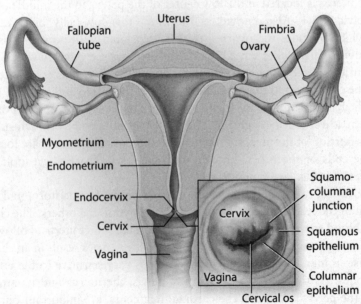

FIGURE 9: UTERUS, OVARIES, AND CERVIX WITH ANATOMIC LABELS

OUR CULTURAL INHERITANCE

The uterus has hardly been studied separate from its role in childbearing, a fact that reflects this society's baseline cultural biases.[1] The uterus is seen as someone else's potential home and is valued when it can potentially play that role. After the uterus's childbearing function has been completed or when a woman chooses not to have a child, modern medicine considers the uterus to have no inherent value. The ovaries usually have been viewed in much the same way because medical science believes that hormonal replacement from artificial sources can perform their functions as well as or even better than a woman's own organs. For centuries, women have been taught to view themselves in the same way, too—valuable as someone's mother or mate, with no inherent value of their own.

When I was in my residency training, one of our oncology fellows (a doctor doing specialty training in gynecological cancer) taught us, "There's no room in the tomb for the womb." Another slogan from my training was: "The uterus is for growing babies or for growing cancer." Occasionally, during my training, when one of our staff physician teachers removed a uterus that looked perfectly normal, we'd jokingly call the diagnosis CPU, a medicalized acronym for "chronic persistent uterus." These attitudes have pervaded conventional medicine for years but are finally changing quite rapidly.

The possibility that the uterus might have any function other than childbearing or tumor production has only recently begun to be addressed in conventional ob-gyn training. Traditionally, if a woman with a fibroid wanted to keep her uterus even though she had no interest in childbearing, her medical team might have viewed her as overly emotional or sentimental, a bit superstitious, and not well educated about that organ. The general dismissive tone of some doctors was that if such a woman were more sophisticated, she would know that the uterus is useless to her except for childbearing.

For example, I once did a fibroid removal from the uterus of a forty-eight-year-old woman who didn't want a hysterectomy. The chief resident who assisted me said, "Why don't you just do a hysterectomy? They can have my uterus anytime they want. Now that I've had my children, it's only good for growing cancer." I told her she'd been brainwashed.

In truth, the uterus plays a role in hormonal regulation, sexual satisfaction, and also bowel and bladder function (see the section later in this chapter on hysterectomy, page 228). Its removal is not advisable unless absolutely necessary.

This undervaluing of the uterus by doctors and the public alike has contributed to the fact that, after cesarean section, hysterectomy remains the second most commonly performed major surgical operation for reproductive-age women in the United States. About 600,000 such surgeries are performed every year in the United States.[2] The average age of a woman undergoing hysterectomy is 46.1 years.[3]

The rate of hysterectomy varies by region of the country, with the South having the highest overall rate of this procedure and the Northeast the lowest. Hysterectomy historically has been performed more commonly on African American women than on Caucasian women and more frequently by male gynecologists than by female gynecologists. The number of hysterectomies performed peaked in 1985, when 724,000 operations were reported.[4] Since then the number has declined. Between 2006 and 2010, 11.7 percent of women ages forty to forty-four had a hysterectomy, according to the CDC.[5] Even though the overall hysterectomy rate has gone down since 1985, rates have remained largely unchanged in the past decade, and more than one-third of all American women will have this procedure by the time they reach sixty.[6] A total of 20 million have had this operation already.

Clearly, hysterectomy is still performed too often when other options are available. Nine out of ten hysterectomies are performed for noncancerous conditions that are not life-threatening.[7] The incidence of hysterectomy for such benign conditions is five times higher in the United States than in Europe.[8] The number of hysterectomies won't change significantly until women and their healthcare providers incorporate alternative methods of healing that don't involve surgery. Since our thoughts affect our bodies, the negative messages about the uterus that are reflected in the current statistics and which we internalize over a lifetime are associated with a large number of problems that women experience in this area. Thus, to change our experience, we first have to address our beliefs about our pelvic organs and their role in our lives.

ENERGY ANATOMY

Though there are distinct differences between the energies of the ovaries and those of the uterus, many women have problems in both at the same time. For example, many women whose ovaries are affected by endometriosis also have fibroid tumors in the uterus. It is helpful, therefore, to discuss in general the overall nature of the emotional and psychological energy patterns that create health and disease in the pelvic organs.

The *internal* pelvic organs (ovaries, tubes, and uterus) are related to second-chakra issues. And second-chakra issues are always related to money, sex, and power. Thus the health of the pelvic organs depends upon a woman's feeling able, competent, or powerful enough to create both financial and emotional abundance and stability and to express her creativity and sexuality fully. She must be able to feel good about herself and about her relationships with other people in her life. Relationships that she finds stressful and limiting, and which she feels she has no control over, on the other hand, may adversely affect her internal pelvic organs. Thus, if a woman stays in an unhealthy relationship or job because she feels she cannot support herself economically or emotionally, her internal pelvic organs may be at increased risk for disease. Given our cultural history of being conditioned to care more about the needs of others than ourselves, it is certainly not surprising that so many women have pelvic problems.

Disease is not created until a woman feels frustrated in her attempts to effect changes that she needs to make in her life. The likelihood and severity of disease in this area are related to how well the various other areas of her life are functioning. A supportive marriage and family life, for example, can partially compensate for a stressful job. A classic psychological pattern associated with physical problems in the pelvis is that of a woman who wants to break free from limiting behaviors in her relationships (with her husband or job, for example) but who cannot confront her fears about the independence that making that change would bring. Though she may perceive that *others* are limiting her ability to break free, her major conflict is actually within herself around her *own* fears. One of my patients developed a fibroid tumor of the uterus and an ovarian cyst when she was forty. I asked her if her need for creativity was being met, and she told me that she very much wanted to leave her job and begin a florist business. She'd been interested in flowers since childhood, but her parents always discouraged her interest, since they considered it "frivolous." She had dutifully gone along with their suggestion that she learn typing and secretarial skills instead. She eventually became an executive secretary in an accounting firm. Though this work was not satisfying to her, she stayed at her job because it provided her with a steady income and good benefits, and she was afraid of the risks of striking out on her own. As her fortieth birthday approached, she felt the need to pursue her childhood passion and had recurrent dreams about fields of flowers that she couldn't get to because they were fenced in by barbed wire. She came to see that through her ovarian cyst and fibroid uterus, her body's birthing center was trying to tell her something.

Another issue that affects a woman's pelvic organs is competition among her various needs. When her innermost needs for companionship, sexual and/or creative expression, and emotional support are in competition with her outer needs for success, autonomy, and approval, this situation may manifest in her inner pelvic organs, the ovaries and the uterus. For centuries, our culture has taught women that we can't be both emotionally fulfilled and financially successful; we can't have it all. Historically, women have not been taught how to be competent in handling economic and financial assets because the patriarchal system has depended upon the unpaid labor of women to keep it functioning. The work of nurturing and caring doesn't figure into what is considered valuable and is, therefore, not reflected in the gross national product, an index of a country's wealth.

While women made up only one-third of the workforce in 1969, they make up nearly half the workforce today—although overall, they earn 85 cents for every dollar men earn. A 2016 study published by the American Association of University Women called *The Simple Truth About the Gender Pay Gap* points out that there are marked differences in this pay gap between states and also between racial groups. In Utah and Louisiana, for example, women earn 70 cents for every dollar men earn; in New York it's 89 cents. Asian women earn 87 cents for every dollar white men earn, while Latinx women make only 54 cents for every dollar white men earn. These lower wages contribute significantly to a lower standard of living for many women and their families given that slightly more than 42 percent of American women are their family's primary breadwinners, and another 22.4 percent bring home at least a quarter of the family's bacon.[9]

In her illuminating book *All the Single Ladies* (Simon & Schuster, 2016), Rebecca Traister reports that in 2009 the proportion of American women who were married dropped below 50 percent. In fact, currently only 20 percent of Americans between the ages of eighteen and twenty-nine are married, compared to nearly 60 percent in 1960. This has enormous social, political, and economic implications, as women now have potentially more freedom than ever before to pursue their own dreams and desires. At the same time, however, many women—married or not—still struggle with balancing paid work with caring for family members (whether children or aging parents), unpaid and unacknowledged work that still falls mostly to women.

The Pelvic Bowl

Rather than thinking about the pelvic organs separately, it is useful to think of everything that is in the pelvic bowl—the center in the body that is associated with creativity and birthing.

Physical therapist Tami Lynn Kent, author of *Wild Feminine* (Atria Books, 2011), specializes in training others in how to approach and strengthen this area. I have worked with her personally and have experienced directly how our relationships with our mothers and our children (if we have them) profoundly affect the health of this area of our bodies. I have also observed what happens to the function of the pelvic floor when a woman doesn't feel safe or supported. In fact, I was working with Tami shortly after the Boston Marathon bombing in April 2013 when a client arrived who had a close friend who had run in the marathon that day, and she had not yet heard whether or not he was safe. Her pelvic floor registered this as profound weakness. Quite literally, it was as though the bottom had fallen out. In other words, her fear and dread led to a direct (though temporary) weakness in her pelvic floor.

More recently a good friend of mine lost her younger brother. The two of them were like soul mates, and she had taken care of him throughout his life—more so even than their mother. Six months after his death, she began to have symptoms of uterine prolapse. She too was feeling the effects of the bottom falling out of her life as she went through this loss and grief. Like many, she was able to reverse the situation once she understood what was happening and started to work with a physical therapist who understood the pelvic bowl. I asked Tami to further explain this mind-body connection. Here is her account:

> I have learned from experience that when trauma happens, the stress registers in the root chakra and can be felt in physical symptoms. The first time I saw this in a striking way was the day after the tragedy of 9/11 in 2001. I was preparing to discharge eight clients from my care because we had already worked together for several visits and they were doing well. However, as I saw each one that day, their bodies reflected what I call "trauma imprints." They had multiple trigger points in their pelvic muscles, a high level of tension, and an energetic sense of dissonance that is similar to static on the radio. None of them had family members directly involved in the terrorist attacks, but just the knowledge of the events of that day, being a part of the collective trauma, registered in a common way in their bodies.
>
> Likewise, when women come to my office after a personal tragedy— the death of a loved one, a car accident, or an emergency with a child, for example—I have learned to address the stress in the pelvic bowl. This stress manifests in the root of the body, the root chakra, because this area registers any threat to our safety or security.
>
> After making this discovery on that day in 2001, I vowed to be part of the collective healing. We never want to have trauma, but trauma plus healing makes a powerful medicine. That night, I began writing what eventually became *Wild Feminine* as a piece of the healing response. Though our female bodies record trauma events, we can change the way we hold the trauma imprint so that it includes the medicine of healing. In this way we heal ourselves and resource ourselves for the future.

The pelvic bowl is also the center in the body that contains what Tami refers to as "the birthing field," an energetic imprint of our own birth and also that of anything we have birthed, including not only babies but also anything else that has required our creative energy, such as books, art, a home, a relationship—absolutely anything. I learned through working with

Tami that it is possible to go back in time and "repair" that birthing field. I did this in a guided meditation with both of my daughters. The following exercise shows how to do it.

ATTUNING YOUR PELVIC BOWL

The pelvic bowl is a source of energy medicine for every woman. Learning how to attune to the energy in this area of the body is vital because it is a portal to the sacred feminine. Attuning to this energy allows creating, healing, and manifesting to flow effortlessly. The five-step exercise below, designed by holistic women's healthcare visionary Tami Lynn Kent, will teach you how to work with the potent energy of this area.

Bowl: Find the outline of your pelvic bones, your own pelvic bowl. Energetically drop down to this place within yourself. Take note of how you are feeling in this space and sense the present state of your creative energy. Notice what changes as you attune to the energy in your bowl.

Clear: Feel the base of your pelvic bowl, the place where you are sitting, and imagine a line of energy running from there to the earth. Our female bodies need this connection to the earth in order to clear the energy within. Clarify your bowl by using your inner awareness to sweep the energy around your bowl and then down to the earth. Give permission for your body to clear old energies or anything that no longer serves you. The bowl energy is meant to flow, so be sure to move any stagnation. On each inhale, imagine fresh energy replenishing the core of your bowl. Let it bring in new inspiration and perspective. With each exhale, invite a full release.

Balance: Balance the ovarian fires within your bowl, the left (feminine) and the right (masculine). Focusing on the left ovary, send your breath toward it as if blowing on a small coal. As you breathe with this ovary, imagine the light of your feminine fire expanding. Ask your body what is needed to tend to your feminine essence. Receive its answer. The feminine is connected to your dreams, your intuition, and your ability to receive and gestate. Know how to engage with this essence by communicating with your feminine light within.

Now focus on the right ovary, sending your breath toward it in the same way. As you breathe with this ovary, imagine the light of your masculine fire expanding. Ask your body what is needed to tend to your masculine essence. Receive its answer. The masculine is connected to physical action and the adventures you direct your energy toward. Ideally, it receives guidance from your feminine knowing. Align these inner fires to benefit the full expression of your creative life.

Center: Find the center of your pelvic bowl, the womb space. Take a moment to acknowledge this portal within. Our first heartbeat begins in the womb, the doorway between spirit and form. It contains the energy of the Great Mother, but it is not just for making babies. Think of your womb as an altar where you can place questions, intentions, or prayers for yourself as a woman. This is an inner sanctuary, where you may rest and receive guidance. Whatever dream seeds you have in your heart, place them here to activate your creative field. You are inherently creative. Your body is designed to co-create with the divine. Receive this powerful energy into your body and your life.

Bless: Energetically walk around your bowl now and bless this space. Invite the radiance of spirit to fill your bowl. Imagine these words as you tend to your bowl: "I am sacred. I am blessed." Let the light pour into your center as healing, inspiration, love, or whatever is needed. Take this vibration and embody your brilliance. This is the energy medicine of your female body—*your pelvic bowl sings.*

The uterus is related energetically to a woman's innermost sense of self and her inner world. It is symbolic of her dreams and the selves to which she would like to give birth. Its state of health reflects her inner emotional reality and her belief in herself at the deepest level. The health of the uterus is at risk if a woman doesn't believe in herself, is excessively self-critical, or is putting too much of her energy into a dead-end job or relationship. Given how society has treated women for the last 5,000 years or so, it's easy to see why so many women have problems in this area.

CHRONIC PELVIC PAIN

Pelvic pain can occur in one pelvic organ such as an ovary, in several pelvic organs, or throughout the pelvis, even if all the pelvic organs have been removed. A certain percentage of women with chronic pelvic pain are not helped by surgery or medical treatment. Though hysterectomy can relieve chronic pelvic pain in some, almost one-quarter of women who undergo hysterectomy for this condition fail to get pain relief.[10] Women who have chronic pelvic pain often have complex psychological and emotional histories. Studies have found that they are more likely to have sought treatment for unrelated somatic complaints, have a higher total number of sexual partners, and are significantly more likely to have experienced previous significant psychosexual trauma.[11] Their physical pain is also related to unfinished emotional pain in either past or current relationships with partners or with jobs, sexual abuse, emotional abuse, or rape (on any level). Emotional stress in a woman's personal or professional life that she perceives to be unresolvable is a big contributor to pelvic pain. Unresolved traumatic events from the past live in the energy system of the body, even after the pelvic organs have been removed surgically. I commonly see pelvic pain flare-ups in women who uncover incest memories, visit the place in which the incest occurred, or work at jobs that control them but in which they feel they must continue to work. I tell these women that, through their pain, the body is asking them to pay attention to it and begin to make changes. The body, in its wisdom, wants to bring their attention back to the physical site of their emotional pain so that they can begin the healing process.

In many cases of chronic pelvic pain, no physical cause can be found and therefore the medical profession does not take it seriously. But chronic pelvic pain that comes from unresolved, past emotional pain is real—it is not just "in the head." Pain is patterned or stored physically and chemically in our nervous, immune, and endocrine systems; it is in the bodymind. It cannot simply be cut out surgically.

Physical therapists Belinda and Larry Wurn have discovered that women who've had infections, trauma, or multiple surgeries often have adhesions that pull on nerves and glue organs together, so pelvic pain with intercourse or with one's period is common. The Wurn technique has been shown to decrease pain significantly when adhesions are the problem. (See chapter 5.)

ENDOMETRIOSIS

Endometriosis is a mysterious but increasingly common condition. The tissue that forms the lining of the uterus, the endometrial lining, normally grows inside the uterine cavity (and is responsible for monthly menstrual cycles). In endometriosis, for some reason, this tissue grows in other areas of the pelvis and sometimes even outside the pelvis entirely. (There are documented cases of endometriosis in the lining of the lungs and even in the brain.) The most common site for endometriosis is in the pelvic organs, especially behind the uterus, but it can also occur on the pelvic side walls (which surround the internal organs in the pelvic cavity), and sometimes on the bowel.

Endometriosis is sometimes associated with infertility and pelvic pain, though not always. Since fibroids and endometriosis are often present in the same individuals at the same time, everything I say about fibroids often applies to endometriosis as well. Like fibroids, endometriosis is related to diet, immunity, genetics, hormone levels, and blocked pelvic energy.

Endometriosis is, energetically speaking, an illness of competition.[12] It comes about when a woman's emotional needs are competing with her functioning in the outside world. When a woman feels that her innermost emotional needs are in direct conflict with what the world is demanding of her, endometriosis is one of the ways in which her body tries to draw her attention to the problem.

Alycia's case illustrates this point well. When she first came to see me with pelvic pain and endometriosis, she related that she'd become pregnant in college and had had an abortion. Though she had felt torn over this decision, and though at some level she had really wanted to have the baby, she also felt compelled to finish college and go to law school. She told me that she had never been able to resolve the conflict between her desire to have a baby and her competing desire to be creative in the outer world of law and business. It is this conflict that can be associated with chronic endometriosis and pain. The conflict articulated by Alycia is almost archetypal, and I see it regularly. Women are now part of the traditionally male world of competition and business. And many do not get emotional support in their homes or personal lives. Others have abandoned the notion that they even have emotional requirements. A great many of the women I've seen who have endometriosis drive themselves relentlessly in the outer world, rarely resting, rarely tuning in to their innermost needs and deepest desires. It makes perfect sense that so many women would have this disease at this time in our history. One Jungian analyst has referred to endometriosis as "a blood sacrifice to the Goddess." It is our bodies trying not to let us forget our feminine nature, our need for self-nurturance, and our connection with other women.

Historically, endometriosis was called the "career woman's disease," which is clearly an outmoded notion now. In the past, women who delayed childbearing were felt to be at greatest risk for it. In the recent past, many women with endometriosis were told that if they'd stay home and have babies, they would be okay. This is a controversial assertion—besides being an offensive one—since some recent studies show that there is no difference in the incidence of endometriosis in women who have been pregnant and those who have not. David Redwine, M.D., an internationally known pioneer in the identification and surgical treatment of endometriosis, concluded that pregnancy offers no protection against endometriosis. What would protect against the disease would be business and personal environments that don't require a mental-emotional split. This split is why so many women are dropping out of the corporate world to work at home or start their own busi-

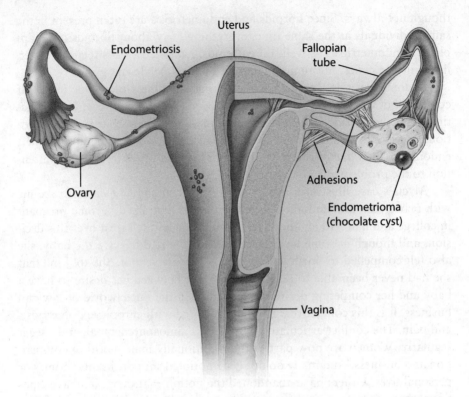

FIGURE 10: ENDOMETRIOSIS

Endometriosis, which can grow virtually anywhere in the body, is usually limited to the pelvis lining, the uterine surface, and the ovaries, where it shows up as endometriomas (also called chocolate cysts).

nesses. Regardless of what she chooses, a woman with endometriosis can work toward healing herself immediately, starting with a willingness to listen to her body.

Symptoms

Endometriosis, which is present in about 10 percent of women, is classically associated with pelvic pain, abnormal menstrual cycles, and infertility. These symptoms vary a great deal from woman to woman.

Some women with advanced endometriosis have never had any symptoms at all and don't even know that they have the disease until their doctor diagnoses it. Others, with only minimal endometriosis, may nonetheless have debilitating pelvic pain and cramps almost continuously. Most women are somewhere in between these two extremes. The most common area for endometriosis to occur is behind the uterus in the area between the uterus and rectum, known as the cul-de-sac of Douglas. Endometriosis in this area can cause painful intercourse, rectal pressure, and pain with bowel movements, especially before a period.

Diagnosis

Endometriosis of the pelvic cavity can be diagnosed definitively only via laparoscopy, though I often suspect it in women whose symptoms are consistent with endometriosis, such as a history of pelvic pain and intermenstrual spotting. In a few rare cases, it can be seen during a pelvic exam if endometrial lesions are present on the cervix, vagina, or vulva.

Unfortunately, studies show that the average woman with endometriosis goes to about five doctors before the diagnosis is made because many other medical conditions, such as irritable bowel syndrome, mimic endometriosis. Even among those who have been properly diagnosed, many are given treatments that don't work. Andrew Cook, M.D., an expert on all aspects of endometriosis including surgical excision, had this to say when he was a guest on my Hay House Radio show: "Endometriosis is the story of the invalidation of women." In his California practice, he has seen countless women from all over the world who have had the wrong diagnosis, the wrong surgery, and the wrong treatment in general before finally having their problem taken seriously and being treated properly.

Some authorities believe that you can find endometriosis in anyone if you look hard enough.[13] I agree with this. I've found endometriosis in a surprising number of completely asymptomatic women at the time of laparoscopic tubal ligation. Neither they nor I would have suspected it.

What I'd like to know is the incidence of endometriosis in women who have no problems. I believe that all women probably have embryonic cells in their pelvic cavities that could grow into endometrial tissue. But if all of us have the potential for endometriosis, why do some women develop symptoms while others do not? Until further research clarifies this, the answers lie within the individual woman. It is up to her to decipher what her symptoms are trying to tell her and to take steps to change the factors that favor the growth of endometriosis.

Common Concerns

Why Do So Many Women Have Endometriosis?

When I was in training, we didn't see nearly as much endometriosis as we're seeing now. There are a number of reasons for the perceived increase in the disease. First, with the advent of laparoscopy, we are diagnosing it more frequently. The patient is in and out of the hospital on the same day. The ease of looking into the pelvis without doing major surgery results in laparoscopy being offered rather routinely to patients who have pelvic pain.

Another factor in the apparent increase in the incidence of endometriosis is that women today are delaying childbearing. When they do have children, they are having fewer of them—which means they have a greater number of menstrual cycles than women did in the past. Since endometriosis is a hormone-dependent disorder, when the body has relatively high circulating estrogen levels without the break that occurs during pregnancy and nursing, endometriosis becomes more likely.

Probably the most relevant factor in the rising incidence of endometriosis is the fact that the majority of women are now overweight—an increasingly global problem resulting from the fact that food manufacturers have successfully manipulated the food supply to include too many refined, nutrient-depleted carbohydrates plus partially hydrogenated fats (think packaged cookies, chips, and convenience foods). Nutrient-poor refined carbohydrates, which raise blood sugar and insulin, combine with partially hydrogenated fats to result in excess body fat and estrogen dominance—all of which favor the growth of estrogen-sensitive tissues, like embryonic endometrial cells that may be present at birth but which grow into endometriosis only when the environment supports this growth.

Is Endometriosis Hereditary?

Endometriosis often runs in families, so there is some hereditary link. I've seen patients whose sisters and mothers all had it. But having a close relative with endometriosis does not guarantee that you'll have it, too, especially if you live your lives in different ways. The genetic potential for endometriosis does not have to manifest unless your environment and health habits promote it. The standard nutrient-poor American diet, which favors cellular inflammation and hormone imbalance in susceptible individuals, contributes to endometriosis and is often the type eaten by families who have endometriosis. In my clinical experience, intake of conventionally produced dairy foods and a refined-food diet are especially associated with exacerbating the pain of endometriosis.

Will Endometriosis Interfere with My Fertility?

Many endometriosis patients are fertile women whose main problem is pain. Endometriosis does not cause infertility, but it is felt to be a major contributing factor. Currently, 40 to 50 percent of women who have a laparoscopy to determine the cause of their problems with infertility are found to have endometriosis.[14] Many women with endometriosis have the massive pelvic scarring usually associated with infertility. Dr. Redwine says, "Studying the disease among predominantly infertile women only serves to confuse the issue."[15] Whatever is causing the endometriosis symptoms may also be responsible for the infertility, but one doesn't cause the other.[16]

So What Causes Endometriosis?

Medical theories about endometriosis abound, but no one really knows what it is and why so many women seem to have it now. The classic theory is that endometriosis results from retrograde menstruation, or menstruating backward, so that some of the menstrual blood and tissue that line the uterus go back up the fallopian tubes, then implant in the pelvic tissue and begin to grow.[17] Since retrograde menstruation probably occurs in every menstruating woman at some point, this doesn't explain why some women get the disease and others don't. Another theory is that pelvic tissues spontaneously convert to endometrial tissue, possibly due to irritation or hormonal activity from environmental toxins such as dioxin, which can have estrogen-like activity.

The pain associated with endometriosis clearly results from an increased production of inflammatory chemicals such as cytokines and prostaglandins that are produced by the endometriosis lesions, which also, interestingly enough, produce additional estrogen. And in the face of excess stress hormones such as cortisol, that additional estrogen itself acts like an inflammatory hormone. Endometriosis lesions are also stimulated in part by the hormones of the female cycle, and the pain is worse at ovulation and during the premenstrual and menstrual times of the cycle. Since endometrial lesions are the same as the tissue inside the uterus, it is understandable that when a woman bleeds with her menstrual cycle, her endometriosis implants bleed microscopically inside her body, too. Some experts feel that the endometrial lesions also secrete some kind of chemical that results in bleeding from surrounding capillaries in the peritoneum (the Saran Wrap–like lining of the pelvic cavity, where endometriosis is found). Over time, this recurrent monthly bleeding into the pelvic cavity is believed to cause painful cysts and adhesions that tend to flare up under the right circumstances.

The theory that makes the most sense to me is that endometriosis is a congenital condition that is present at birth.[18] According to this theory, endometriosis arises from embryonic female genital tissue that never made it to the inside of the uterus during development. This helps explain why endometriosis can run in families and why some girls have severe pelvic pain from endometriosis *as soon as* they start their periods. Yet in this theory all fe-males have the capacity to develop endometriosis if embryonic cells in their pelvis get stimulated by the right set of circumstances.

Though most gynecologists have been taught that endometriosis is a pro-gressive disease that gets worse over time, some studies, including those of Dr. Cook as well as Dr. Redwine, show that endometriosis doesn't spread or get worse over time (though its appearance changes) and won't recur if all of it is removed surgically or if the conditions that stimulate it are no longer present.

When performing laparoscopies to diagnose the cause of pelvic pain, many gynecologists miss the diagnosis of endometriosis in its early stages because they were taught to look only for the characteristic black "powder burn" lesions. In fact, endometrial lesions come in a range of colors: clear, white, yellow, blue, and red. Many of these early lesions are very subtle and difficult to see without the proper equipment.[19]

The color of endometrial lesions may be related to blood leaking from nearby capillaries. Over time, the lesions progress from clear to black, de-pending upon the amount of scarring present. The older the woman with endometriosis, the greater her chances of having "classic" endometriosis with black "powder burn" lesions and "chocolate" cysts of the ovaries. (En-dometriosis in the ovaries can result in large ovarian cysts filled with old blood. When these are operated on, the contents of the cysts look just like chocolate syrup.)

The Neuroendocrine-Immune Connection

The intimate interactions between our thoughts, emotions, and immu-nity hold the key to interpreting the message that endometriosis has for the individual woman as well as helping her heal it. Studies on the immune sys-tems of women with symptomatic endometriosis show that these women's bodies produce inflammatory chemicals.

These inflammatory factors can interfere with various processes of human reproduction, including sperm function, fertilization, and normal progression of pregnancy. Their presence may explain the association be-tween infertility and endometriosis in those women who have both problems at the same time. Endometriosis has been clearly associated with decreased egg fertilization, decreased success rates for in vitro fertilization ("test tube" fertilization), and increased miscarriages. The clinical experience of the late therapist Niravi Payne with women with infertility and endometriosis shows clearly that at an unconscious level, these women may have an ambivalence about becoming pregnant. Their minds may desire it, while their hearts aren't sure. The cellular inflammation present in women with endometriosis holds the key to understanding many characteristics of the disease that scientists have been unable to explain when they have looked at it as a structural problem only, as if it were a tumor to be removed.[20]

A new body of research is documenting the intimate link between a healthy immune system and a healthy bacterial ecosystem in the places in our bodies that interface with the environment. These include the vagina, the mouth, the lungs, and also the entire surface of the gut. When the bacterial ecosystem balance is lost, then immune system function suffers. It is well documented, for example, that antibiotic usage destroys health-promoting bacteria in all those areas, leading to an overgrowth of yeast and mold. This yeast and mold have been shown to trigger allergic responses in the lungs when they are exposed to mold spores, which is one of the reasons why there is so much more asthma and allergies in children now than in the past. Children are put on too many antibiotics and there is an ever-increasing use of household disinfectants.[21] The immune system imbalance that results could help explain the immune components of endometriosis. When a woman stops taking antibiotics, gets on a good probiotic to replenish her bowel and vaginal flora (normal bacterial life in this area), takes immune-enhancing supplements such as vitamin D (2,000–5,000 IU per day, depending on blood levels), and also follows a diet that halts cellular inflammation, the endometriosis pain often disappears in a few weeks.

Treatment

Women with symptomatic endometriosis do best with a comprehensive treatment program that fully supports their immune systems while they remain open to finding out what they need to change about their lives. My patients have healed endometriosis symptoms through a variety of treatments. Most important, many of them have come to a greater understanding of what they need to learn for true healing, not just masking of their physical symptoms.

Hormones

The most common treatment for endometriosis, once diagnosed, is hormonal therapy, in the form of birth control pills, synthetic progestin, danazol (Danocrine), or the GnRH (gonadotropin-releasing hormones) agonists, such as Synarel and Lupron. These drugs act on the pituitary gland to make a woman temporarily menopausal, thereby allowing the endometriosis to regress by stopping its cyclic hormonal stimulation.

All of these hormonal therapies change the amount of estrogen and other hormones in the system, so that endometriosis is not activated. When hormone levels are decreased, symptoms often disappear and the disease itself becomes inactive. Danazol and the GnRH agonists are also used to decrease the amount of endometriosis prior to surgery—in some cases so that surgical removal is easier. The problem with these approaches is that they don't really cure the disease; they simply shut down the hormonal stimulation of it for a while. In addition, there are significant side effects from these treatments. Danazol is expensive—it costs at least $1.50 dose, depending on the strength—and it can have masculinizing side effects, such as hair growth and voice deepening. Most women gain some weight while they are on it. GnRH agonist therapy results in hot flashes, thinning of the vaginal tissue, and bone loss. Yet other women badly need these hormonal treatments as a respite from pain, even though the pain often recurs once the drug is discontinued.

I once saw a patient who had been on Synarel (a GnRH agonist) all summer. "It was so wonderful to go camping, water-skiing, and hang gliding and not have to worry about the pain," she told me. "I felt just wonderful. I know I can't stay on it forever, but I sure felt great." She had been off it for two weeks when I saw her, and her pain was beginning to recur. As we talked about her options, she said that when she was having the pain before she went on the drug, she would often get complete pain relief from a massage. She was surprised by that, but she felt that massage was too expensive and that dietary change was too difficult due to her schedule. Yet Synarel cost nearly $400 per month at that time.[22] Once she thought it all through, however, she decided to try to change her schedule to eat better, and she became willing to try a few nondrug approaches for a trial period of three months. She knew that surgery was an option. When I last saw her, she was doing well with lifestyle changes.

Even though the menopausal symptoms associated with GnRH agonists are reversible once the drug is stopped, this type of therapy, if used longer than a few months, is not appropriate for everyone. I'd be particularly wary of using it in anyone who has had a problem with irregular periods or central nervous system disorders, since it has been associated with memory problems in some. The lifestyle of a patient who may need it is characterized by a very high-pressure job, long work hours, a lot of travel, almost no time to herself, and lack of desire or ability to change her career. Using drugs in this type of situation makes it easier for the woman to continue activities that may nonetheless be harming her at some level. Lifestyle and dietary changes are always the first things I recommend. On the other hand, I know that many women are not ready for this approach and will therefore choose drug treatment. I have learned over the years that whatever option a woman chooses, she will learn something. What brought her to the doctor will eventually open her to learning about her body. The body is innately self-healing, and when there's a genuine desire to be well, the patient almost always finds the modality that suits her best.

Natural progesterone or *Pueraria mirifica* often works very well to relieve endometriosis symptoms. These are my treatment choices in addition to dietary improvement.

Progesterone. The usual way is to use a 2 percent progesterone cream such as Emerita Pro-Gest, one-quarter to one-half teaspoon on the skin twice a day. (See page 156.) Natural progesterone helps counteract endometriosis by decreasing the effects of estrogen on the endometrial lesions. Natural progesterone is free from side effects and is very well tolerated. Use it on days seven to twenty-eight of each cycle; some women may need to use it daily. Sometimes the dose of progesterone needs to be increased beyond what is available in 2 percent progesterone cream. In these cases, a prescription transdermal cream can be compounded by a formulary pharmacist. (See Resources for how to locate one in your area.) Natural progesterone capsules taken orally are another choice; the usual dosage is 50 to 200 mg per day, taken on days ten to twenty-eight of each cycle. Progesterone vaginal gels are also available by prescription.

Pueraria mirifica. *Pueraria mirifica* has been used for centuries in Thailand for its beneficial hormonal effects. It contains a potent phytoestrogen known as miroestrol that binds to the beta estrogen receptor on estrogen-sensitive tissues, thus blocking them from being overstimulated by the estrogen produced by the ovaries and body fat. The end result is less estrogen stimulation and lower inflammatory response in endometrial tissue. Dose is 80–100 mg twice per day (see Resources).

Surgery

Many women with severe endometriosis, having tried hormones and pain medication for years, often end up at a very young age with complete hysterectomies, including removal of their ovaries. This should be a last resort, since even this can leave endometriosis lesions behind, which means the pain won't be eliminated. If your ob-gyn has suggested this, please get a second opinion to make sure you are under the care of someone who knows exactly how to perform the right kind of surgery.

More conservative surgery that removes only the endometriosis and preserves the pelvic organs can be very helpful. More and more gynecologists (but by no means all) are skilled at this pelviscopic surgery and have learned how to remove endometriosis without missing any lesions. If any endometriosis is left behind after this conservative surgery, the pain is likely to recur. Dr. Cook reports an average improvement of 75 percent after proper surgery. In these women, the pain is frequently associated not with endometriosis but with fibroids, adhesions, or adenomyosis. (See chapter 5.)

I suggest that every woman research the work of Dr. Cook and schedule a consultation by phone, which he is willing to do once he reviews your records. Also check out Dr. Cook's other resources (www.vitalhealth.com), as he and his team work with endometriosis patients from all over the world and are well versed not only in the proper surgery, if necessary, but also in promising nutritional and functional medicine approaches.

Natural Healing Program for Endometriosis

See the Master Program for Optimal Hormonal Balance and Pelvic Health in chapter 5, page 143.

Women's Stories

Doris: Learning from Endometriosis

Doris was forty-one when she first came to see me. She was a highly successful professional who spent lots of time traveling and working but had little time for herself and her personal, emotional needs. She had heavy periods that got worse at night and sometimes would soak through the sheets. She complained of fluid retention, bloating, and severe menstrual cramps. Her uterus was enlarged to ten-to-twelve-week-pregnancy size from fibroids. She had a history of infertility, several miscarriages, and an abortion. A laparoscopy by another physician had confirmed the presence of endometriosis as well as fibroids, and he felt that these were associated with her miscarriages. Her gynecologist had suggested a hysterectomy because he said that her periods would continue to be difficult and that she would eventually end up with the surgery anyway. She was not happy with this diagnosis, however, and came to see me about her alternatives.

When I first saw her, she had a great deal of tenderness behind her uterus, which is very common in women with endometriosis. I asked her questions about her lifestyle, diet, miscarriages, abortion, exercise, and stress levels. I agreed that surgery was not something we needed to consider right then and suggested several alternative treatments. Among them were eliminating dairy products from her diet, applying castor oil packs to her lower abdomen, taking vitamin supplements, and reading about perfectionism, addiction, and whole foods. From what Doris had told me about herself, I felt that she needed to heal her feelings about her miscarriages and her abortion. She decided to follow my suggestions. To unlock her feelings about her fertility, she decided to write letters to the unborn potential beings who had been in her body. As she wrote me later, "Obviously they were still there in some form in my mind and had taken form as fibroids and maybe endometriosis in my body. The most incredible experience occurred after I wrote the letters. I had been remembering my dreams with great regularity through visualization techniques. One night in a dream, I was fully aware of my body, and I dreamed that thousands of white doves were flying out of my uterus. An unbelievable feeling of lightness came over me, and I awoke crying with joy."

Three months after Doris's dream experience, I examined her and found that many of her fibroids were gone and so was all of her uterine tenderness. The remaining fibroids seemed to have solidified into a smooth mass that was definitely smaller than it had been at the time of her earlier examination. Doris found that when she takes care of herself and follows her diet, gets exercise, and does some things just for herself, she feels fine and has no pelvic symptoms of any kind. Though her fibroids didn't disappear entirely, they didn't grow for years. The last time I saw her she had no tenderness on examination, a testimony to the fact that her endometriosis became very inactive.

Doris used the wisdom of her body to heal some very painful experiences about which she had not allowed herself to grieve. She was willing to risk completely changing the way she saw herself in the world, a change that often needs to be made if women are to heal at the deepest level. This often involves examining with microscopic honesty how we really feel about being female while also affirming our worth and our inherent goodness. It also may involve cutting way back on our worldly activities and creating a healthful balance between our inner and outer selves.

UTERINE PROLAPSE

Uterine prolapse refers to a condition in which the fibromuscular tissue, fascia, and ligaments that normally hold the uterus in place become damaged or relaxed, thus allowing the organ to drop from its normal position in the pelvis. In severe cases, the uterine cervix and the uterus itself may actually protrude from the vaginal opening.

You could liken the pelvic floor supports for the uterus, vagina, and rectum to a floor in a building. In order to support the weight of whatever is on it, the floor must be firmly attached to the structural beams and supports that suspend it. The same is true of the pelvic floor. It relaxes or sags when pelvic muscles have become weak, when the pelvis is tilted improperly, when there is a genetic weakness in the collagen of the connective tissue, or when the pelvic floor and muscles become damaged from delivering a large baby or from having multiple babies (although if laboring women are properly supported and not encouraged to push too hard, most do not have this problem after delivery). Pelvic floor dysfunction can show up as prolapse of the uterus (sometimes known as procidentia), prolapse of the bladder (cystocele), prolapse of the rectum (rectocele), or prolapse of all three. If a loop of bowel prolapses into a rectocele, it is known as an enterocele. Sometimes the vagina itself will prolapse following a hysterectomy, resulting in a vaginal vault prolapse.

In moderate cases of prolapse, women experience pressure in the lower pelvis and vaginal area. Sometimes they will feel the cervix moving down their vagina. Others may experience difficulty emptying their bowels completely because of the enterocele.

About half of women between the ages of fifty and seventy-nine may have prolapse, according to the American Urogynecologic Society. Prolapses of all kinds are more common in women of northern European heritage and in those with red hair. The reason for this is that blondes and redheads have a collagen layer that is thinner than those who have darker skin. (This is also why those of northern European heritage are more apt to have osteoporosis.) African Americans and those with darker skin are the least likely to experience prolapse.

Treatment

Although approximately 15 percent of the hysterectomies done in the United States are for pelvic organ prolapse, many nonsurgical approaches exist. Mild to moderate pelvic floor sagging can be treated effectively by strengthening and toning the pelvic floor through exercises such as classic Pilates. In fact, many physical therapists now specialize in pelvic floor rehabilitation using Pilates exercises, including what is known as a reformer. My Pilates teacher, Hope Matthews, reports that many of her clients enjoy complete recovery from urinary stress incontinence (inability to hold urine when laughing, coughing, or exercising) after just a few months of regular Pilates.

The position of the pelvis is also a factor. Esther Gokhale is a pioneer in what she calls Primal Posture—the posture we were all born with but which our modern lifestyle erodes. She has studied many indigenous peoples throughout the world and notes that these groups must use their bodies well since there are no wheelchairs, anti-inflammatory drugs, or other fallback fixes available for those with back pain and so on. Many of these people bend, lift, and walk around with eighty pounds on their heads—and also sit for long periods of time—but they don't have the same problems with prolapse and back pain that are so common in industrialized countries. This is because their alignment and pelvic position support health and pain-free living. Hence there is no undue pressure on their joints or their backs. In these cultures, people sit and walk with their "tails" behind them and their backs straight except for a curve at the segment of the spine between the fifth lumbar vertebra (the lowest vertebra in the low back) and the first sacral vertebra (the highest of the vertebrae in the sacrum, the triangular bone at the base of the spine just above the tailbone). This area is known as the J-spine. If you go to an art museum and look at classical painting or sculpture, you will see this normal human anatomy over and over. Gokhale points out that people in modern civilizations lost their original human posture starting around 1920, when it became fashionable to slouch and also to tuck your pelvis under your body. When the pelvis is tucked under, the pubic bone—which is meant to keep the contents of the pelvic bowl in place—gets tilted upward in the wrong position and is not available to hold the pelvic organs in properly. The popular Kegel exercises are designed to strengthen only one relatively small muscle—the pubococcygeus muscle, the one you would use to stop the flow of urine. Unfortunately, strengthening this muscle alone is nowhere near as effective as learning how to sit and walk properly using your gluteus maximus muscle and keeping your pelvis tipped forward (think pouring water out of a bowl in front of you). You can easily learn how to put your pelvis in the right position by sitting on a folded-up towel under your sitz bones so that your pelvis tips correctly. A Gokhale chair is also available that keeps your pelvis in the proper position when sitting—it features a slightly downward tilt in front. This chair has been one of the best investments I've ever made for my health. (See Resources.)

Biomechanics expert Katy Bowman also points out that doing regular squats to strengthen the gluteus muscles helps tone and stretch the pelvic floor muscles, making prolapse and incontinence far less likely. Begin with ten squats twice per day, and work up to fifty per day. You don't have to go all the way down—just stick your butt out and bend your knees as low as is comfortable. I like to use a yoga ball against the wall and slide down with the ball behind me at the small of my back. This helps with alignment.

Pessaries are also available to hold the organs in place during the day, and most such products are made by the Milex company. Not all gynecologists are familiar with fitting pessaries, so go to one who is well trained in their use. I fitted them for years, especially a soft pessary known as a cube pessary. A woman can easily learn how to insert this pessary herself. It will provide comfort and repositioning of her pelvic organs while strengthening her pelvic floor. Women with more severe prolapses can use larger pessaries. For very mild prolapse, a diaphragm—or sometimes just a tampon inserted in the vagina—can hold things in place.

Hormone Therapy

Women with thinned vaginal tissue secondary to lack of hormones may experience worsening prolapse. A small amount of vaginal estrogen cream or regular use of *Pueraria mirifica* vaginal moisturizer along with the exercises listed above will often arrest the prolapse while it's in the mild stage so that surgery can be avoided. Many healthcare practitioners tell their patients that the prolapse will definitely get worse over the years. But in women who maintain pelvic floor tone (and replenish vaginal tissue thickness via plant hormones, mammalian hormones, or laser treatments), this needn't be the case.

Surgical Approaches

All pelvic floor prolapses are highly amenable to surgery. And over the years, a number of procedures have been developed that allow a woman to keep her uterus by having it surgically suspended in the pelvis rather than removed. This is commonly done via laparoscopy. Surgeons trained in urogynecology often do this type of procedure. I recommend that all women who are suffering from uterine prolapse consult with a surgeon who is well versed in prolapse corrections that allow the pelvic organs to remain intact. If you opt for a hysterectomy, make sure your surgeon does the surgery in such a way that avoids future vaginal vault prolapse, if possible.

Many women with prolapse have received pelvic mesh implants, also referred to as slings, designed to physically support and reposition the weakened organs. In 2016, the FDA reclassified the use of this mesh from moderate risk to high risk, stating that such surgeries yield no better results than traditional pelvic organ prolapse surgery that does not use mesh, and that in fact these surgeries may expose the 75,000 women who annually receive mesh implants to greater risk.[23] Complications can include pain, urinary problems, sexual dysfunction, infection, organ perforation, and hemorrhage (sometimes even resulting in death). The most common such complication reported was vaginal mesh erosion, which happens when the mesh dislodges from the vaginal wall where it was implanted and moves into the surrounding tissues and organs, sometimes even protruding from the opening of the vagina. Based on data from 110 studies including 11,785 women, approximately 10 percent of women undergoing transvaginal pelvic organ prolapse repair with mesh experienced mesh erosion within one year of surgery.[24] Mesh erosion can require several surgeries to repair, and pain can continue even after the mesh is removed. Not surprisingly, many class-action suits have been filed as a result.

A 2016 British study that looked at data from thirty-five hospitals in the United Kingdom came to a conclusion similar to the FDA's, finding that there was "no benefit to women having their first prolapse repair from the use of transvaginal synthetic mesh."[25] The researchers reported that more than 10 percent of women having such surgeries had complications, and 30 percent needed additional surgery.

The National Association for Continence has a good website about prolapse (www.nafc.org/pelvic-organ-prolapse). I also recommend the website for Miklos & Moore Urogynecology, previously known as the Atlanta Center for Laparoscopic Urogynecology (www.miklosandmoore.com), which offers excellent illustrations, explanations, and information about the various treatments under the Procedures/Treatments tab on the drop-down menu.

Laser or Thermal Treatments

A number of unique nonsurgical treatments for vaginal rejuvenation that are also effective for early-stage prolapse and even mild urinary incontinence have become available in recent years. These include the MonaLisa Touch laser (www.monalisatouch.com) and ThermIva radiofrequency treatment (www.thermiva.com). Both require patients to receive three treatments, spaced about four to six weeks apart. An annual maintenance treatment is recommended. Both methods restore vaginal thickness and elasticity by stimulating the production of collagen and elastin. Both also improve the blood flow to vaginal tissue, restoring vaginal moisture. In tightening this tissue, the bladder neck can be lifted back into position. Many women report improvement in urinary incontinence after this procedure, but I know of no long-term studies supporting this treatment, which is currently not covered by insurance.

MonaLisa Touch uses a carbon dioxide laser administered through a probe inserted into the vagina. The procedure is painless and lasts only about five minutes, and downtime is minimal. ThermIva uses a thin wand to gently heat tissue in and around the vagina. The procedure takes between 30 and 45 minutes. Unlike MonaLisa Touch, this procedure can also decrease the size of the labia for those women who are concerned about this. The procedure is almost painless, with no downtime. It is far superior to the increasingly popular vaginal plastic surgeries (see chapter 9). Please note that the FDA has not approved any of these energy-based treatments for vaginal rejuvenation. And there is no question that inappropriate use can cause burns or pain during intercourse. Still, the treatments help enough women to make them worth considering.

To maintain the vaginal moisture and thickness restored by these treatments, I recommend using a topical herbal moisturizer like *Pueraria mirifica* vaginal moisturizer or a hormonal cream.

FIBROID TUMORS

Fibroids are benign tumors of the uterus. They grow in various locations on and within the uterine wall itself or in the uterine cavity. (See figure 11.) Standard medical practice to gauge the size of a fibroid is to compare the size of a uterus with a fibroid with the size of the uterus at various stages of pregnancy. Thus, a woman will be told that she has a fourteen-week-size fibroid if her uterus is as big as it would be if she was fourteen weeks pregnant. Fibroids are made of collagen, a type of connective tissue, and they are hard, white gristly masses with a whorl-like pattern. They are present in 70 percent of all women.[26] One of my patients, who watched her fibroid removal via a mirror, later said, "The appearance of the fibroid surprised me. I expected it to be messy-looking. A fibroid looks like a piece of high-density polyethylene plastic, the stuff cutting boards are made of."

Fibroids are responsible for as many as 33 percent of all gynecological hospital admissions, and they are the number one reason for hysterectomy in this country. They are three to nine times more common in African American women than in Caucasians, and premenopausal women have a three to five times higher risk than postmenopausal women. Many women with fibroids are unaware that they have them until they are discovered during a routine pelvic examination. No one knows, from a conventional medical standpoint, what causes them, although some risk factors have been identified. Family history is associated with a threefold higher risk, and hypertension with a fivefold higher risk. Currently taking birth control pills or using injectable contraception reduces risk by two-thirds, and having three or more children reduces risk by 80 percent compared to women who have not given birth.

Caroline Myss teaches that fibroid tumors represent our creativity that was never birthed, including "fantasy" images of ourselves that have never seen the light of day and creative secrets of our other "selves." Fibroids also

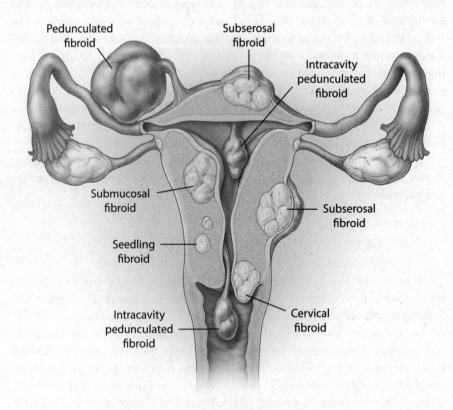

FIGURE 11: TYPES OF FIBROIDS

result when we are flowing life energy into dead ends, such as jobs or relationships that we have outgrown. I ask women with fibroids to meditate on their relationships with other people and how they express their creativity. Fibroids are often associated with conflicts about creativity, reproduction, and relationships.[27] I certainly can relate, having developed a large fibroid about five years prior to my divorce. I realized that I had been pouring lots of energy into trying to make a dead-end relationship work. In our rapidly changing culture, where women's roles are in flux, it is quite obvious to me that conflicts about child rearing, personal expressions of creativity, and changing roles in relationships are a cultural phenomenon, not just an individual one. The fact that so many women have these growths is perhaps evidence of our collective blocked creative energy in this culture. How could it not be, given that women have had the right to vote only since 1920? Talk about culturally blocking women's creativity and destiny!

Symptoms

Most women do not have symptoms from their fibroids. These uterine growths usually come to a woman's attention on routine pelvic examination. Whether a fibroid is symptomatic has to do with its size and location within the uterus. Those that are located in the muscle wall of the uterus just under the surface (subserosal) may not be symptomatic. But those growing into the uterine lining itself (submucosal) often cause heavy or irregular bleeding. Some fibroids are attached to the inside or even the outside of the uterus by a thin stalk. These are known as pedunculated fibroids. If they are on the outside of the uterus, they are sometimes confused with ovarian tumors. I've had two patients who "delivered" pedunculated six-centimeter fibroids through the cervical opening. I simply removed these fibroids by suturing and then severing the stalk. Neither of these women had any further problems.

Women who have both fibroids and endometriosis may experience menstrual cramps, pelvic pain, or both. Most fibroids can be treated conservatively by letting them be and having an examination every six months to a year or so to monitor their growth.

Bleeding

Some women with fibroids have extremely heavy periods, resulting in anemia, fatigue, and even an inability to leave the house during the heaviest days. If the fibroids are growing quickly, if a woman's hormones are in flux (which is common around the time of menopause), or if she's been under a great deal of stress, she can even develop hemorrhaging from uterine fibroids. Some women grow so accustomed to their large monthly blood loss that they don't even realize how a normal flow would feel. Some may become severely anemic without knowing it.

Fibroid tumors can cause a lot of bleeding because the uterus is endowed with a very rich blood supply. If the fibroid is submucosal, located just under the uterine lining, the body has an especially difficult time with the usual mechanism that stops menstrual flow. Menstrual flow is stopped, in part, by muscular contraction of the uterus, and fibroids may interfere with this mechanism. An endometrial biopsy (taking a sample of tissue from inside the uterus) or sometimes a D&C is necessary in cases of abnormal bleeding to be certain that the bleeding is caused by fibroids and not cancer (though cancer is rarely found). This is especially true for those women who have bleeding at irregular intervals throughout the month.

Fibroid Degeneration

A fibroid may start to degenerate following its rapid growth. This can happen, for instance, during a particularly stressful or emotionally demanding time, during pregnancy, or during the year or so before menopause. Fibroid degeneration can occur when the fibroid outgrows its blood supply. When this happens, the center of the fibroid is deprived of oxygen from the blood, and the nerves deep inside this tissue register a lack of oxygen as pain, in the same way that frostbitten toes do. The pain can be a nuisance, but the condition is not usually dangerous. The degeneration in the center of the fibroid often causes some shrinkage in fibroid size, and on occasion the fibroid disappears. The pain usually goes away after a week or so as the nerves adjust.

Pelvic Pressure and Urinary Frequency

Sometimes the position of a fibroid causes symptoms because the fibroid pushes into another organ, such as the rectum or the bladder. Pressure or a sense of fullness in the rectum, lower back, or abdomen may result. If the fibroid is in the front of the uterus and relatively low, the pressure on the bladder can decrease the bladder's ability to hold urine, resulting in urinary frequency (having to void in frequent small amounts). These symptoms are annoying but not harmful to the body in general. I've never seen an organ contiguous to a benign fibroid that was harmed by the fibroid. An occasional very large fibroid can partially block the ureter (the tube going from the kidney to the bladder) when a woman is lying down. Neither urologists nor gynecologists know for certain whether this situation can eventually cause kidney problems. I have never seen this happen or even heard of it in actual practice! Most women with fibroids large enough to cause urethral pressure prefer surgery simply because they don't like looking pregnant. Several of my patients, however, have done very well without surgery, and their kidneys are fine. One of these women, who had a very large fibroid uterus for at least

ten years and whose ureter had occasionally shown some blockage from fibroids, began to experience rapid shrinking of her fibroids as she went
through menopause. This is common.

Common Concerns

What If I Have a Fibroid?

When fibroids are felt for the first time, I recommend a pelvic ultrasound
to measure them and to check out the status of the ovaries. Sometimes it's
impossible on a pelvic exam to tell the difference between an ovarian growth
and a fibroid on the uterus. I also recommend not feeling rushed to do anything about the fibroid. They are not an emergency. And most never cause
any problems.

Can Fibroids Be Cancerous?

Fibroids are almost never cancerous. Fewer than one in a thousand turns
into a uterine sarcoma, a very rare type of cancer of the uterine muscle. The
only way to tell for sure, however, is to take them out and look at them
under the microscope. Since the mortality rate for hysterectomy itself is one
in a thousand, the risk of surgery is actually greater than the risk of the fibroid being malignant.

The most common problem with fibroids is their tendency to grow and
to cause bleeding. But, as many women I've worked with have discovered, if
the underlying energy patterns, life questions, conflicts, and emotional issues
associated with the fibroids are addressed and changed, the fibroids usually
do not grow or cause problems. Sometimes they go away completely on their
own.

Are Fibroids Genetic?

Fibroids can run in families. One of my fibroid patients told me that
every female in her family for three generations had fibroids. She is planning
to be the first woman in her tribe to get to menopause with her uterus intact.
She has changed her diet and now is completely free from symptoms.

Just as in a strong family history of alcoholism, in a strong family history
of fibroids the individual woman is up against a family belief system, from
which it is very difficult to break free. I once read an article about familial
ovarian cancer entitled "My Mother, My Cells," in which the author articulated her difficulty with inheriting a tendency toward a disease that terrified
her and over which she felt she had no control.

In this country, we tend to think of a genetic predisposition as an inevitable "sentence" that we *will* get the disease. However, environmental factors play a much bigger role than genetics in whether that predisposition ever

gets expressed. When it comes to how a gene gets expressed, it is generally accepted that 90 percent of what happens to us is environmental (our thoughts, beliefs, and behavior) and only 10 percent is genetic.

Even with severe genetic disorders like cystic fibrosis, some individuals have managed to keep the disease under control and live well into their fifties. This was unheard of several decades ago. And many women with very strong family histories of breast cancer never get the disease.

Some women who have strong family histories of fibroids, ovarian cysts, or endometriosis have developed these conditions themselves but have healed from them. One patient summarized a necessary part of this healing when she said, "I've finally realized that I am not my mother. I don't have to live out her life in my body." In families in which there is a genetic disease, we should study those members who *don't* get the disease. Most likely they are the individuals who broke the family mold, the ones who did not live out family expectations on a cellular or other level.

Will My Fibroids Interfere with Pregnancy?

During pregnancy, hormone levels are very high and preexisting fibroids can grow rapidly. If they begin to degenerate, fibroids can sometimes cause uterine contractions that can result in premature delivery. This doesn't happen with all fibroids, however. I've seen women with large fourteen-week-size fibroids get pregnant, carry to term, and go through normal labor and delivery without *any* problem.

One twenty-nine-year-old woman who came to me was already twelve weeks pregnant, and she had a large fibroid in the posterior portion of her uterus. The pregnancy had been unplanned, but she was thrilled about it. Her doctor had told her to have an abortion and then have the fibroid removed before conceiving again. He told her that the fibroid would probably cause the early delivery of a baby who would be so premature that it wouldn't live. She was very upset about her dilemma and needed a physician who was willing to go along with the pregnancy, knowing that there might be a problem while being open to the possibility that all could go well. Her pregnancy proceeded normally, going to full term without pain, bleeding, or premature labor. She delivered a seven-pound, three-ounce girl after an eight-hour labor. Her fibroid had shrunk to an eight-week size by the time of her six-week postpartum checkup.

Fibroids can result in miscarriage or even infertility, particularly if they've distorted the uterine cavity enough. Whether there are problems seems to depend on the location of the fibroid within the uterus and how close it is to the developing baby and placenta. An ultrasound or hysterosalpingogram (an X-ray study in which dye is injected into the uterus and tubes) can give you some idea of fibroid location before pregnancy, as can an MRI.

Some pregnant women have fibroids that start degenerating. They end up in the hospital to be watched closely while they rest in bed on pain medication. Generally, fibroids don't hurt the developing baby unless they cause so much uterine irritability that the uterus starts contracting and premature labor results. There are no guarantees against developing problems with fibroids during pregnancy because the entire uterus grows, including the fibroid wall. The farther away from the uterine cavity the fibroid is located, the less likely that a woman will have problems. Some doctors are willing to take a wait-and-see attitude about fibroids and pregnancy, suggesting that a woman try to get pregnant and see what happens. Others will suggest that she have the fibroids removed before attempting pregnancy.

Will the Fibroids Grow? Will They Go Away?

Many women with fibroids are told that hysterectomy should be performed when their fibroids are relatively small so that a more risky and complicated hysterectomy in the future, should the fibroids grow, will not be necessary. Studies have shown that there is little or no justification for this.[28] Fibroids do grow sometimes, but not always. They tend to grow quite briskly during the years just before menopause, when hormonal levels fluctuate widely, then shrink dramatically after menopause. One of my perimenopausal, or "almost menopausal," patients, age forty-nine, whom I followed for more than twenty years, could easily feel her fibroids through her abdominal wall by pressing down with her fingers. She said that her fibroids grew up to her belly button just before her period and shrank down to just above her pubic bone within three days after her period was over. Fibroids often change size during each menstrual cycle, reaching their peak during ovulation and just before the menstrual period begins. They can also grow during periods of stress. Fibroids can be followed by a physician or other qualified healthcare provider with an exam every six months to a year. There's no reason to rush into surgery, unless you have repeated episodes of severe bleeding that cannot be controlled with hormonal treatments or other measures.

Sometimes fibroids go away completely. A religious woman who had been scheduled for hysterectomy because of fibroids prayed about them daily. Six weeks later, when she went back to her doctor, the fibroids were gone and she didn't require the surgery. I recently met another woman who works as an esthetician. While she was doing a facial for me, she told me that she had recently been diagnosed with a fibroid. Her doctor suggested a hysterectomy. I told her to read my book and also taught her how to do a Divine Love meditation (see page 757). Three months later her fibroid was gone.

One of my patients, a forty-three-year-old musician and sound healer named Persis, first came to see me with a fibroid the size of a four-to-five-month pregnancy. After two years of a strict diet, reflective inner work, massages, and therapeutic sound, her very large fibroid uterus returned almost to normal.[29] I rarely see fibroids shrink as much as hers did. This shrinkage was not because of menopause. She is still having normal periods. Here is her story.

In the summer of 1988, I was diagnosed with endometriosis and a grapefruit-size fibroid tumor. The preceding years had been filled with increasingly excruciating pain that left me almost blacking out while driving. I had gotten used to being in pain for two weeks, then recovering from the exhaustion in the next two weeks, and had become terrified of getting my period.

The doctor I was seeing at the time told me about all the alternatives for correcting the problem. His favorite was hysterectomy—"At your age you don't need your uterus anyway," he said. Then there was hormone therapy to stop the periods for one to two years: "Your voice will drop, and you will lose your sexual desire." And the last offer he made was that I could continue with the pain and bleeding until menopause.

Since I wanted to keep my body whole, didn't particularly like the idea of giving up my womanhood to hormone therapy, and couldn't tolerate the pain, I looked for other treatment. I made a commitment to my life. I accepted the responsibility for taking care of myself. I accepted the loving help of others. I began a very strict regimen of macrobiotic diet, sitz baths, exercise, and meditation. Looking back, I don't know how I fit all that into my busy life. I do know that I am a changed person.

I also began gently to search out the reasons behind my "woman's troubles." I accepted my codependent nature and began opening up to the pain of my childhood and young adulthood. The pain in my belly was a culmination of a lifetime of pains. I knew just cutting it out wouldn't "fix" all the other pains in my life.

I now have little pain and feel extraordinarily well. I am and always will be in process throughout my life. Through meditation and sound healing on myself, I have renewed my inner faith. I accept my life and my ability to heal myself as well as to help others heal. As I do for others, I do for myself.

If I Undergo Fibroid Removal Treatment, Will the Fibroids Grow Back?

The answer to this question must be individualized. In general, a woman who is within five years of menopause when she has her fibroids treated is not likely to have them grow back, because her estrogen levels will be decreasing naturally. If the underlying energy pattern, emotional issues, or hormonal levels associated with the fibroids haven't changed, then other so-called seedling fibroids can start to grow. Women who change their diets dramatically, however, decrease the likelihood that the fibroids will return. In the women whose fibroids I have treated, I have rarely seen them recur or get worse. This is probably because of the law of attraction. Women who resonate with my approach are highly motivated to take responsibility for their own healing. I recommend dietary change, bodywork, homeopathy, and other alternative methods, even for those women who choose fibroid removal as their treatment. Surgery or fibroid ablation alone will not change the fundamental pattern in their bodies that encouraged the fibroids to grow. It is vital to listen to what our bodies are trying to teach us and affirm our ability to be whole.

Treatment

At no point is it appropriate for a doctor to make dictatorial treatment recommendations about what any woman should do with her uterus. There is no right and wrong. Instead, it's best to offer women ways to think about their uterus, ovaries, and body, so that when they need to make a decision about hormones, drugs, surgery, or fibroid ablation, they'll know what their personal truth is regarding those organs. More treatments for fibroids are now available than ever before. Once a woman has gathered the facts about treatment choices, she can tune in to her own inner guidance to decide which is the best for her.

For many women, just knowing that they have a choice in the matter is a huge relief. Some women interpret surgery, for example, as further abuse, when they have not freely chosen to undergo it. Incest survivors sometimes tell me that the very thought of an invasive procedure in their body, particularly of a gynecological nature, feels just like rape. Obviously, alternative modes of treatment should be tried in these cases, rather than allowing the abuse cycle to once again be ignited.

The following section illustrates different treatment approaches to problems in the uterus. There is no one right way to treat uterine problems. Each of these women mentioned in this section needed help for fairly straightforward and common symptoms, and each chose a different treatment. Only one woman wanted a hysterectomy. Each woman was able to arrange treatment that respected her individual choice. Medical technology, when consciously used in an individualized treatment, can be a major aid in healing women's lives. To claim that hysterectomy is always the wrong or inferior choice is as dualistic and harmful as claiming that all natural remedies are quackery. I do not address the specific psychological and emotional issues connected with "blocked energy in the pelvis" for any of these cases. Not all women are open or ready to explore their deep issues, and I respect their choice to wait for the right time.

Conservative: Watch and Wait

If a woman's fibroids aren't causing her any problems, I recommend a pelvic exam every six months to a year, depending upon her situation. I also recommend a sonogram (ultrasound) initially to be sure that the problem is a fibroid and not an ovarian cyst or tumor. Sonograms can measure fibroid size and check the ovaries. Conservative treatment is sometimes called "benign neglect" or the "tincture of time." Very often it's the best therapy. By the way, one often cannot see the ovaries when an enlarged uterus is blocking the view. This doesn't necessarily mean that there is something wrong with the ovaries and that you need a procedure to find out.

Hormone Therapy: Synthetic Progestin or Natural Progesterone

To women whose primary symptom is bleeding, I suggest synthetic progestin, natural progesterone, or the herb *Pueraria mirifica* to keep the lining of the uterus from building up too much. In many cases this therapy works very well to control bleeding and is much more benign than major abdominal surgery. Progesterone, progestin, or herbs are an option for women who are unable to change their diets or whose symptoms aren't alleviated by dietary changes. Some women become depressed while they are on synthetic progestin; others feel bloated or premenstrual or get headaches. Bioidentical (or natural) progesterone is generally free of these side effects, as is *Pueraria mirifica*. I'd much rather use these than a synthetic progestin. Since each woman's life situation is different, her medical treatment needs to be individualized.

GnRH Agonists

GnRH (gonadotropin-releasing hormone) agonists such as Lupron and Synarel are synthetic hormones that cause the pituitary gland to shut down the function of the ovaries. After about one month on these drugs, a woman's body becomes artificially menopausal. Her estrogen levels fall very low, and her periods cease. The cyclic stimulation of her fibroid tissue ceases, and in most cases the fibroids shrink in size. GnRH agonists are used in select cases to shrink fibroids before surgery or to shrink them enough so that surgery is not necessary. Some physicians use these drugs to keep a woman's fibroids asymptomatic until she reaches menopausal age, at which point the fibroids naturally shrink. In this way, she can avoid surgery. It takes about three months to get the maximum effect from these drugs, but most women need to be on them for only two months in order to get significant shrinking before surgical removal. Not everyone gets the same result because not all fibroids are created equal.[30] Unfortunately, because GnRH agonists put a woman into artificial menopause, the resulting hot flashes and sleep disturbances can be very disruptive, and these drugs are associated with an increased risk for osteoporosis.

GnRH agonists are very expensive, and they are not recommended for use longer than six months. Once use of the drug has stopped, the fibroids grow back quite rapidly unless a woman becomes naturally menopausal during the time she is on the drug.

Many women are understandably hesitant to use such synthetic hormones. Baby-boom-generation women remember that diethylstilbestrol (DES) was enthusiastically used for more than thirty years to prevent miscarriage. In 1971, the drug was withdrawn after it was linked to certain rare vaginal cancers and other genital tract abnormalities in some of the female (and even male) offspring of the women who used it. Having said that, it is clear that GnRH agonists do have a place in the treatment of fibroids. They can be used to shrink fibroids while administering enough "add back" hormones to lessen their menopausal side effects without compromising their effectiveness. This approach can save some women from undergoing perimenopausal hysterectomies.

Endometrial Ablation

Christine had heavy periods for years—she had to use two super tampons at a time, as well as a pad. Sometimes these needed to be changed every half hour during day two of her period, making it very difficult for her to travel or even leave the house to grocery shop. The minimal dietary changes she made had not worked. Further testing revealed that she had multiple, very small fibroids in the uterine wall.

Christine very much wanted to avoid hysterectomy, so we tried synthetic progestin therapy for the last two weeks of each month for three months.[31] Even though this treatment almost always decreases bleeding, it didn't work in her case. A D&C also failed to alleviate her bleeding. I referred her for a procedure called endometrial ablation using hysteroscopy. Hysteroscopy is a surgical technique in which the lining of the uterus can be visualized and operated on by passing a scope through the cervix from the vagina. Various techniques are available, including cautery and laser. The technique used depends on the patient's condition and the choice of the surgeon. Submucosal fibroids can sometimes be removed this way by surgeons skilled in this technique. This procedure, done under anesthesia in the operating room, cauterizes and obliterates the endometrial lining—the part of the uterus that bleeds every month. When it works, menstrual periods cease or become very light. For Christine, the procedure worked beautifully. Instead of recuperating for a month from the removal of her uterus, she went into the hospital the day of her surgery and left the next. Though this type of surgery isn't appropriate for everyone, it is a great option for some. It cannot be done in some cases, depending upon the position of the fibroids.[32]

Fibroid Embolization

Uterine fibroid embolization (UFE), also referred to as uterine artery embolization, involves injecting a substance such as polyvinyl alcohol particles into the uterine artery, blocking the fibroid's blood supply and shrinking the fibroid. Interventional radiologists specifically trained in this technique thread a catheter into the femoral vein of the thigh to reach the uterine arteries. The patient is usually conscious during the procedure (although sedated and in no pain) and typically spends one night in the hospital afterward. Most women resume normal activities within seven to ten days.

The results are encouraging. The Society of Interventional Radiology reports that 85 to 90 percent of women who have this procedure experience significant or total relief of their symptoms, including heavy or irregular bleeding, pain, uterine enlargement, and symptoms like increased urinary frequency that relate to the size of the fibroid. Recent data presented at the society's annual meeting show that this procedure is vastly underused (especially in rural and smaller hospitals), even two decades after its introduction, despite the fact that it's been shown to be safe and effective, with fewer complications and a shorter hospital stay (at significantly less cost) than hysterectomy.[33] Even so, some serious complications do exist, including renal failure or an allergic reaction to the clotting agent.[34] Recurrence within ten years of the procedure is rare, although long-term follow-up data aren't yet available.

One of my ob-gyn colleagues had the procedure done and was very happy with her result. Given that she has spent her career doing lots of hysterectomies and surgical fibroid removals, this speaks volumes in my mind. If this procedure appeals to you, seek out the advice of a specialist at a center where UFE is frequently done, call the Society of Interventional Radiology at 800-488-7284, or visit their website, www.scvir.org.

MR-Guided Focused Ultrasound Treatment for Fibroids

In the fall of 2004, the FDA approved a new device that combines MRI imaging to map out uterine fibroids followed by high-intensity focused ultrasound that heats up and destroys fibroid tissue. Fibroid tissue is very well suited to this treatment because the blood vessels in fibroids help the body dissipate the excess heat that is generated. The procedure is called MR-guided focused ultrasound (MRgFUS) and is done on an outpatient basis. It is noninvasive, leaving the uterus and ovaries intact. It involves lying on your abdomen in an MRI tube for up to three hours while ultrasound heats up and destroys the uterine tissue. Side effects may include blisters on the abdominal skin, cramping, nausea, and some pain that is alleviated by over-the-counter pain medication.

Studies show that the treatment successfully reduces fibroid symptoms in about 70 percent of women, but 20 percent will require additional surgery within a year. The FDA reports that though the MRgFUS treatment success-fully reduces symptoms in the majority of women who undergo the proce-dure, those symptoms will return in some women. And so will the fibroids. This is why I recommend that *all* women suffering from fibroids also do their best to employ the kind of lifestyle changes mentioned above that change the metabolism of hormones to reduce fibroid symptoms naturally. Still, I feel this treatment is a major step forward and a very exciting use of technology. If it had been available when I had my fibroid (mine was very large), I would have strongly considered this treatment. Note: When this technology first came out, women who hoped to eventually become pregnant were warned against using it because not enough data existed to determine what happens to the uterine wall and uterine lining following the procedure. More recently, however, the FDA has approved labeling on MRgFUS equipment stating that it is safe for women wishing to retain their fertility. For more information about MRgFUS, call 214-630-2000 or check out the website for InSightec, the company that developed the technology, at www.uterine-fibroids.org.

Myomectomy (Surgical Removal of Fibroids)

Myomectomy is a surgical procedure in which the fibroid tumors are removed, but the uterus is repaired and left in place. Advances in surgical techniques over the past twenty years have made this a very nice option for women who want to keep their pelvic organs intact or have children.

Many of my patients elected to have myomectomies even after they'd eliminated all of their symptoms with dietary changes. The presence of the fibroid can still cause an enlarged abdomen that affects how they look and feel about themselves. (I felt the same way.) More and more myomectomies are being done through the laparoscope (a telescopic instrument that is in-serted through the abdominal wall into the pelvic cavity, thus making a large abdominal incision unnecessary). Typically this procedure is reserved for fi-broids that are six centimeters or smaller, but that depends upon the sur-geon. Many physicians prescribe a GnRH agonist to shrink the fibroid(s) first so that the surgery will be easier. The smaller the fibroid, the better the chance that it can be removed through the laparoscope.

Gloria was forty-five when she first came to see me. She had borne two children, and her husband had had a vasectomy. Gloria had a large fibroid that was pressing on her bladder, causing urinary frequency that kept her up at night. Her periods were regular, and she had no pain. Her gynecologist had recommended a hysterectomy, but this choice felt entirely too drastic to her. Instead, she opted for a myomectomy. (Today I would have offered her the choices of uterine artery embolization or MRgFUS.) At the time, her gy-necologist wouldn't do this procedure "because of her age," an ageist atti-tude on his part. Like many conventionally trained gynecologists, this one felt that Gloria's uterus was useless, since she was over forty and didn't want more children. The myomectomy that Gloria ultimately had completely relieved her urinary symptoms, and she started sleeping through the night. She is very glad to have kept her uterus.

When the position or size of a fibroid makes childbearing an issue, myomectomy is a good choice. (Note that uterine artery embolization is not recommended for women who wish to become pregnant because we don't yet know how this procedure affects fertility, although MRgFUS has been cleared for women who still want to become pregnant.) Before they undergo myomectomy, some women are told that once they are in surgery the surgeon may find it necessary to turn the procedure into a hysterectomy. I never saw a single case in which this was necessary, either in my own experience or in the experience of those patients whom I referred out for the procedure. In general, myomectomies are best done by those gynecologists who have specialty training in infertility surgery. This type of surgery focuses on repairing the pelvis, not on removing organs. Dedicated fibroid centers exist at major medical centers around the country, where you will find the right surgeons for the job. (See Resources.)

Hysterectomy

Hysterectomy is probably the option most commonly offered to American women who have fibroids. This option is often chosen when a woman has been bleeding for months or even years, is anemic from the blood loss, has an abdomen that looks pregnant, can't leave home for fear of bleeding through her clothes, and has urinary frequency from a fibroid pushing on her bladder.

Studies have shown that a hysterectomy can improve the quality of a woman's life if she is given the choice of options other than surgery and decides that hysterectomy is right for her.[35] If, however, a woman has surgery for which she isn't really ready, without adequately exploring the alternatives, the results can be devastating. Over the years, I've come to see that women who give their options a great deal of consideration before deciding on surgery are much happier with the outcome. (On how to prepare for surgery and the recovery process, see chapter 16.) Unfortunately, there's often a tendency in medicine to create a crisis situation and rush in. Sometimes a woman who has had a single frightening episode of bleeding with a fibroid will be told to have a hysterectomy as soon as possible. Because of her fear and the sense of being pushed by her doctor or family, she will often go along, when she could have waited. The women who often regret their decisions later, I believe, are the ones who did not feel that they had any choice except surgery, usually hysterectomy. Before embarking upon any course of treatment, a woman should allow herself the time to gather all necessary information and weigh all her options.

Fran, a teacher with one daughter, came to see me when she was forty-two. Over the previous six months, she had developed bleeding between periods, increasing cramps, and some pain during intercourse. When I examined her, I found that she had a fibroid the size of a large grapefruit (about eleven centimeters in diameter). I had known Fran for many years before this, and I had delivered her daughter. She traveled to many different schools during the course of her teaching day and had always found it difficult to maintain a healthful diet. She was significantly overweight and married to a man who hated his job and was somewhat depressed. Given her life situation, her treatment choice was hysterectomy with preservation of her ovaries. She knew that although I could remove the fibroid and leave the uterus intact, this would not guarantee that she'd be rid of her cramps and irregular bleeding.

Fran wasn't interested in taking the time to pursue alternative treatment modes, nor was she interested in learning about what her fibroids might be saying to her. The idea of being free from periods, cramps, and the fear of pregnancy was very appealing to her. She had her surgery without complications and returned to her normal routine within one month. She has never had second thoughts or regrets. Fran is a good example of a woman who knew she had options and was very clear about her choice.

Sexual Response. About half of women who have their ovaries surgically removed (most often accompanying hysterectomy), no matter their age, will develop testosterone deficiency rather suddenly due to the total loss of ovarian testosterone production and the subsequent reduction in adrenal androgens.[36] In general, the incidence of sexual dysfunction following hysterectomy is anywhere between 10 and 40 percent. In studies conducted in the United Kingdom, for example, 33 to 46 percent of women reported a decreased sexual response after a hysterectomy-oophorectomy (removal of the uterus and the ovaries).[37] But the Maine Women's Health Study, done in 1994, failed to show a rate that high.[38] And some women actually report *increased* sexual response after hysterectomy. For example, Dutch researchers reported that among women who underwent hysterectomies for reasons other than cancer, postsurgical sexual pleasure increased. The results held true regardless of the type of hysterectomy. Of the women studied who were not sexually active before surgery, 53 percent became sexually active after the procedure.[39] Doctors haven't paid nearly enough attention to the connection between hysterectomy and sexual response and have regarded changes in sexual response or loss of interest in sex following hysterectomy as psychogenic only, or "all in the head." Though the brain is clearly the biggest sex organ in the body, it is also true that hysterectomy can and does affect pelvic nerves and blood supply, which are important for sexual response. One of my patients came to me for a second opinion when her doctor asked her why she was so attached to her ovaries (he wanted to remove them at the time of her hysterectomy). To put it into perspective for him, she asked him why he was so attached to his testicles. As most women know, the mind and the body are a unity. Quite simply, if a woman feels positively connected to her sexual organs, then their removal can affect her sex life for both biological and psychological reasons.

We now know that there is a physiological basis for decreased sexual response in *some* women following hysterectomy-oophorectomy. For example, the androgenic hormone loss associated with the removal of the ovaries is a factor in loss of libido following surgery. Even if the ovaries are left intact, some women experience orgasm differently after hysterectomy, probably because the cervix and uterus act as a trigger point for orgasm. These women feel the deep, rhythmic contractions of the uterus as a very satisfying part of orgasm. Once the uterus is gone, they sometimes experience the loss as a change, an actual decrease in orgasmic depth. Women who experience orgasm mainly through clitoral stimulation may not have this same experience. In a review article of sexual functioning following cervical cancer treatment, a group of European sex researchers concluded that there was considerable vaginal and urinary nerve disruption following surgical treatment for cervical cancer. It is unknown to what extent pelvic surgery for benign disease might be cutting nerves important for female orgasm. Though the nerve pathways for female orgasm historically haven't been well worked out, animal studies provide some clues. In 1986, British primate researcher Alan F. Dixson, Ph.D., D.Sc., studied the genital sensory feedback in marmosets (small monkeys) and showed that two separate sensory pathways existed in the female: one that was fired by either clitoral or labial stimulation and a separate neural pathway for vaginal and cervical stimulation. On the other hand, for women who have experienced pain with intercourse for years or who have had pelvic pain from uterine or ovarian problems, a hysterectomy can greatly enhance the quality of their sexual experiences and the overall quality of their lives. (The Wurns report that many women with chronic pelvic pain who've undergone their treatment of manual adhesion removal end up experiencing far more pleasurable sex lives. Belinda Wurn's own situation was what led the couple to their current approach. Following hysterectomy and radiation for cervical cancer, Belinda had a great deal of pelvic pain and difficulty with sex. This led the couple on a worldwide search for therapies that would help her. The end result is the Wurn technique, which has undergone rigorous documentation of its effectiveness (see chapter 5, page 157).

Women who suffer from loss of sexual desire or general loss of energy following hysterectomy can often restore their libido through the use of natural hormones (estrogen, progesterone, and/or testosterone) or herbs such as *Pueraria mirifica* or maca. Natural testosterone can be administered in a skin cream base. The usual dose is 1 to 2 mg every day or every other day. This must be prescribed by a healthcare practitioner and prepared by a formulary pharmacist. Some women, but not all, are helped by DHEA; the usual dose is 5 to 10 mg once or twice per day. A few women feel best on 25 to 50 mg per day. The dose of *Pueraria mirifica* is 80 to 100 mg twice per day. This herb works best when iodine, vitamin B_{12}, and methylated folic acid supplementation is included (see Resources).

Menopause. Removal of the uterus alone does not necessarily result in menopausal hormone levels in a woman who is still ovulating. It always results in cessation of menstruation. Even if the ovaries remain, however, their blood supply will be altered. This changes the hormonal milieu of the body and may result in menopausal symptoms and an earlier menopause. In one study this occurred in about 50 percent of the sample.[40] (Many women report hot flashes for several months following hysterectomy, even when the ovaries are left in place. The same thing can happen after removal of an ovary alone, with no other surgery. It sometimes takes a while for an ovary to recover function postoperatively or for one ovary to take over the function of two.) There is some evidence that women who have had hysterectomies have an earlier onset of osteoporosis than other women, even when the ovaries are left in. And clearly, anything that impairs ovarian function in any way can result in decreased libido.

Urinary Problems. Women who have had hysterectomies are more likely to develop stress urinary incontinence later in life. The reason for this is that the nerves innervating the bladder are very close to the uterus. Some of the nerve fibers may be damaged during hysterectomy.[41]

Heart Disease. Recent studies have shown an increased risk of cardiovascular disease when both of a woman's ovaries are removed prior to her natural menopause (the average age of natural menopause is fifty-one).[42] Although removing the ovaries obviously prevents the subsequent occurrence of ovarian cancer, the same studies show that it nonetheless increases the chance of developing other, more prevalent cancers, and it also leads to higher overall mortality. Since the ovaries continue to contribute hormones even after menopause, it is possible that there are adverse effects from ovarian removal even after menopause.[43]

After Menopause: Nature's Hormonal Treatment

Fibroids often shrink dramatically once a woman reaches menopause (usually between fifty and fifty-two). Women with fibroids frequently experience symptoms only when they are in their mid- to late forties, the age when hysterectomy is most often performed. If a woman prefers it, hysterectomy can be avoided by keeping the fibroids manageable until they naturally shrink during menopause. This can usually be accomplished by a combination of dietary change, progesterone therapy, stress reduction, exercise, and watchful waiting.

After menopause, any hormone replacement therapy may theoretically cause a woman's fibroids to grow again, but the low levels of hormones used in such therapy generally do not cause problems.

Natural Healing Program for Fibroids

See the Master Program for Optimal Hormonal Balance and Pelvic Health in chapter 5, page 143.

Women's Stories

Fibroids, like other disorders, don't just come out of nowhere and land on your uterus. When you become willing to be in a relationship with your uterus by letting its messages speak to you, you have taken the first steps toward healing, instead of just masking or eliminating symptoms. After you get in touch with the messages from your uterus, you can choose the treatment that works best for you, whether it's surgery, diet, acupuncture, or a combination of these.

Many women can correlate the onset of their fibroids with the onset of verbal abuse from their mates, job stress, or other problems in their relationships with the outside world. Inner work is often very useful for finding new ways to deal with these hurtful or limiting situations.

Shirley: Fibroids and Creativity

Shirley, a nurse in her mid-forties, had been experiencing irregular periods and heavy menstrual flow when she was diagnosed with a small fibroid at the time of her annual exam. Shirley had been in treatment for an eating disorder and codependency a year before this. When I diagnosed her fibroids, she was in the midst of a career change, trying to decide whether to leave a stifling but lucrative management job.

I suggested she go on a whole-food diet and supplementation program and use castor oil packs. I also asked her to think about what she really wanted to do, what she would find truly satisfying. As she thought about it, she realized that her creativity had been stifled at work. She asked her body what it was telling her and to reveal it to her in dreams or meditations. Several months later, she told me, "I learned to surround myself with healing energy and love through the use of castor oil packs, meditation, and therapy."

She used Reiki treatments, a type of energy treatment similar to therapeutic touch, involving healing with the hands. Two weeks after her office visit with me, she reported, "I had a vision of the masseuse lifting a bowling-ball-shaped apparition from my abdomen. She had me draw it, and I drew what looked like a burr that you would find on your socks in the woods. It had exactly forty-five spikes on it. [Shirley was forty-five years old.] My apparition, the burr, represented me and how I cling to things in an unhealthy way. It symbolized clinging to work and people through whom I try to find fulfillment. From my dreams and meditation, I learned that my uterine growth was a physical manifestation of my own stifled creativity that could never be expressed fully through depending upon others. Through my emotional and physical healing process, my fibroid reduced in size, and I was led to a more creative, satisfying job in direct patient care." Her follow-up exam three months later showed that her uterus was much smaller, and I could find no fibroid.

Marsha: Unsupportive Relationships

Marsha, a massage therapist from out of state, first came to see me in 1986, when she was forty-one years old, to get a second opinion about her fibroids. Though her uterus was only moderately enlarged, to the size of a twelve-week pregnancy, and she was having no symptoms, she had been told that she should have a hysterectomy. Her mother had also had fibroids and had had a hysterectomy, but Marsha wanted to avoid surgery. She had mistreated herself for years by overeating and getting involved in harmful relationships with abusive men. She had undergone three abortions and had no children. When she came for her first visit, she had already started a macrobiotic diet to keep her fibroids from growing.

Since everything else was normal on ultrasound testing, I affirmed Marsha's choice to treat her fibroids with dietary changes and suggested that she visit her gynecologist back home every six months. Given her insight into her own patterns of behavior, I felt she should work with alternatives to surgery. She followed the treatment plan in her home area.

Four years later, she returned to see me because she had had several episodes of very heavy bleeding and her gynecologist had strongly suggested surgery. Marsha, who was in the twelve-step program Sex and Love Addicts Anonymous, told me that she had just gotten out of a very unhealthy, addictive four-year relationship. She was still completely consumed by the relationship, even though both of them had agreed that it was over. She told me that she had begun to appreciate that "all the anger I've felt toward my old boyfriend has been a way to avoid doing my work on myself, my emotions, and my past." Now she began to take responsibility for her life and her situation and to get on with self-healing. Through her recovery work, she was finding that every relationship she'd ever been in since her childhood, with an alcoholic father, had been dysfunctional. She admitted that she was very good at creating drama in her life to fill the void of deadened feelings within herself and to compensate for her lack of connection with her own body.

Marsha was just starting to realize the profound connection between her relationship and her sense of self, and how they manifested in her body. She knew that not all the aspects of her fibroid were related specifically to food, yet she used food to cover up her emotions. Her recovery, one day at a time, has gradually put her in touch with her inner wisdom. When I saw her for a checkup in 1992, her fibroid size was stable and she was having regular periods. She had entered a stage of healing that is sometimes necessary for many women, though not all: She felt the need to withdraw from men for a time and be mostly with women. Each time I saw her, she was more centered, more positive, and stronger. She realized that her fibroids were a signal, calling her back to herself and her own life.

Louise: Children and Loss

Louise is a woman who is willing to assume partnership in her healthcare and who is not afraid to express her views. A producer for a radio station, she came to see me for a second surgical opinion regarding her fibroid uterus. Her fibroid had developed shortly after her second daughter had decided to leave home for boarding school. After her visit to me, Louise wrote the following letter to her gynecologist, who had suggested a hysterectomy.

Dear Dr. _____,
On your recommendation I went to get a second opinion for hysterectomy because of my uterine fibroids. Let me tell the story behind my process, in hopes that you can incorporate a broader, less conventional approach to other women who present with fibroids in the future.

First, I was struck by how powerless I felt by your recommendation for surgery. Suddenly, I began to think of myself as sick, diseased. But my heart was telling me, "No, there's nothing the matter with you!" So I followed my heart's voice. I got my hands on everything I could read about fibroids, especially books and articles presenting alternatives to surgery.[44] I have learned how many unnecessary hysterectomies are performed each year in this country, and I learned of the significant, often long-term postoperative problems.

Even the small amount of research I did on the function of the uterus, especially postmenopausally, suggests that it is integral to overall good health. Chemical hormones cannot substitute for the magnificent functioning of the female organs.

So I became determined to keep my uterus—and not just for physical reasons. You didn't ask me anything about my feelings, about my family or lifestyle, or about how a hysterectomy might affect all that.

My two beautiful daughters have both left home within a year's time. My nineteen-year-old is in her second year of college, and my fifteen-year-old has gone away to private school in Vermont, at *her* insistence. Though I am supportive of them, at the same time it is a major life adjustment for a mother to have them both leave home so close in time. My children are gone, the offspring of my uterus, and then you tell me I should have my uterus removed as well. No, thank you. I'll hold on to it for the time being and, I expect, always. If I had a life-threatening disease of the uterus, I might feel differently.

All of this may sound bizarre to you, but I firmly believe that we contribute to illness in our bodies. The flip side is that we can contribute to healing our bodies as well. I urge you to take a little extra time with your patients to hear their full story. If I had not questioned what you were telling me, I might have been one of those unnecessary hysterectomies. It would have been a convenience, perhaps, to be rid of the heavy periods, but it would have been at such a cost—in dollars, lost work, long-term hormone replacement therapy, and long-term psychological damage.

Please give your patients all the options, and the time to consider them.

Sincerely,

Louise T.

Louise's gynecologist is not unusual. We doctors are not trained to listen to our patients' feelings about what their diseases mean to them. Larry Dossey, M.D., in his book *Meaning and Medicine,* tells the story of Frank, a patient with chest pain whom he admitted to the coronary intensive care unit. Frank was able to change his heart rate at will by thinking about what his chest pain *meant* to him. He told Dr. Dossey that if he let the pain mean a heart attack, he immediately got anxious thinking about his damaged heart, clogged vessels, the loss of his job, and the possibility of another heart attack. But if he let the chest pain mean just a muscle ache or indigestion, he felt relieved and his heart rate came down. Dr. Dossey discovered that Frank's heart monitor acted as a "meaning meter." The same is true for fibroids.

When I saw Louise seven months after her initial visit to me, she had taken a job in another state, at a radio station where her work was truly appreciated. She had realized the degree of loss associated with her daughters' leaving home and had taken the time to grieve that. While she was interviewing in the new city, she had realized that her relationship with her husband had been unfulfilling for years—that they had really stayed together only for the children. She saw it clearly and began plans for a divorce, which was accomplished mutually. She then met a new lover, something she had never dreamed would happen and hadn't been seeking. This relationship proved very sensual and meaningful to her. She had changed her diet significantly and stopped eating dairy foods. When I examined her, the fibroid was almost completely gone. She had basically changed her entire first- and second-chakra energy.

Paula: Fibroids and Abortion

I occasionally see women whose fibroids appear to be related to an abortion or abortions. When I say "related" I don't mean "caused by." Abortion, in study after study, has not been associated with adverse physical effects on the body. The problems that women have after abortion, if any, are related to the *meaning* of abortion in their lives and in the society in which they live.

Paula came to see me for an annual exam at the age of thirty-six. She had had three abortions when she was in her teens and her twenties and had no children. I do not know the circumstances of her abortions except that she was matter-of-fact about them. She developed fibroids in her early thirties and had suffered from pelvic pain for at least five years. When I saw her, she was feeling well and healthy and believed that her well-being was related to the following story: "I was having increasing problems with bleeding between my periods and pelvic pain. Not happy with the prospect of surgery or hormones, I went to a Native American healer. He told me that I had to release the spirits of the beings who had been with me before my abortions. He performed a releasing ritual with me in which I literally saw and felt white wings flying out of my lower pelvis and away. I cried for hours with grief and relief. After that my periods went back to normal, and I've never had a day of pain since."

Paula's story is a dramatic example of the power of emotional release for healing. Though I could still feel an enlarged fibroid uterus of about eight-week size in her, this was not a problem that required more than regular checkups. She told me that it was a relief to be able to tell her story to a doctor, since she was certain that most doctors would laugh at her and think she was nuts. That, of course, is why doctors rarely hear these stories of wonder and healing from their patients. The stories are common, and yet they are kept secret because they are too often discounted or patronized by medical professionals.

True healing, not just curing our body or soothing our mental anxiety, involves transformation of our energy field and consciousness. In the women I've just described, the healing came in part because each woman created meaning from the messages and symptoms her uterus was sending her about how she was using her creative power in the world. And then she took the next step. She affirmed her innate wholeness and followed an action plan to manifest it in the here and now. You can do the same!

7
The Ovaries

She sings from the knowing of *los ovaries,* a knowing from deep within
the body, deep within the mind, deep within the soul.

—Clarissa Pinkola Estes

From an energy medicine standpoint, ovaries are the female equivalent
of male testicles. They can be thought of as "female balls" because they
represent exactly the same thing in the world. When a man goes out
into the world to perform acts of difficulty or courage that require manipulating the external world of things or people, he's said to "have balls." For a
female, going out into the world, particularly a male-oriented world, also
"takes balls," but she must use her ovarian energy. She should not try to
imitate a man, because her ovaries and their energy field can be adversely
affected by an overly masculine relationship with the outside world. To
maintain health, she needs to understand how to use her "balls" in a life-
enhancing way.

Our ovarian wisdom represents our deepest creativity, that which waits
to be born from within us, that which can be born only through us, our
unique creative potential—especially as it relates to what we create in the
world outside of ourselves. Biologically, when a woman ovulates, the egg
attracts the sperm to it by sending out a signal to the sperm. The egg simply
waits for the sperm to arrive; it does not go actively seeking sperm. The resulting biological creation, a baby, has its own life and consciousness connected to, but also separate from, that of its mother. Although its growth and
development are influenced profoundly by the mother, they are at the same
time separate from her. She cannot use her will to force her baby to develop

faster; nor can she use her will to determine when her child will be born. (However, planned inductions and C-sections are increasingly interrupting this natural flow—which is sometimes prudent but also has a downside. See chapter 12.) And once the child is born, a mother must acknowledge that her creation has and always will have a life and personality of its own, even though it was created from her own flesh and blood.

Similarly, all of the creations that come from deep within us, from our ovarian wisdom—whether they be babies, books, or works of art—have a life of their own that we have a responsibility to initiate and allow but ultimately not to control. Just so, our deepest creativity cannot be forced. It must be allowed the time and space to grow and develop in tune with its own internal rhythm. Like biological mothers, we as women must be open to the uniqueness of our creations and their own energies and impulses, without trying to force them into predetermined forms. Our ability to *yield* to our creativity and to acknowledge that we cannot control it solely with our intellect is the key to understanding ovarian power. We must *allow* this power to come through us. This doesn't mean that we passively sit by and wait for our creativity to "happen" to us, however. We are meant to use our second-chakra power drive to attract or go after the people, places, and circumstances that will help ensure the safety and nourishment of our creations (including children).

Society tries to overly control creativity through the imposition of deadlines (note the connotation of the word—sometimes the time factor literally kills our creativity), quotas, and productivity ratings. One of my colleagues, who has always maintained very healthy ovaries, used to do scientific research as an assistant in laboratories. The lab director would always tell her exactly what he wanted her to produce. Once, for example, he wanted her to manufacture an artificial cell called a liposome. Whenever she tried to create this cell model by running the experimental design according to his predetermined directions, using her will and intellect to try to control the setup and force the process, the attempt failed and the artificial cell was nonfunctional. She felt miserable. She then looked beyond the lab director's specific demand and asked herself, "What do I want to know in this situation? How can I find out more about an aspect of life by doing this experiment? What can this teach me about cells in general?" At these times she connected with the broadest possibilities inherent in the experiment, which she described as like "touching the hand of God." Invariably, in the liposome experiment and in others, she would design an experiment that yielded far more information than had been originally expected of her. The end result was never exactly what the lab director had asked for, but it was usually far more valuable and enriching. In the liposome experiment, my colleague ended up creating not only an artificial cell model but an experimental design that could potentially be used to produce a vaccine against a serious disease. A by-product of this was that the lab director was always thrilled with her results and eventually learned to allow her to design her own experiments without interference. Her scientific work was brilliant. By remaining true to her deepest creative wisdom, her end results benefited everyone concerned. This is feminine creativity at its finest. (And of course it's also present in men—they just use the term "gut feeling," not intuition.) We can do this in our own lives and jobs by always considering how one task is connected to others and by remembering our interconnections and how one act can give birth to or build bridges to others.

Because many women get both ovarian and uterine problems simultaneously, as the previous chapter mentioned, the relationship between the different issues they signal is worth underscoring. Basically, ovarian energy is more dynamic and changes more quickly than uterine energy. That's because the biological gestation time for an egg is only one lunar month, while the biological gestation time for the fetus is nine lunar months. In the reproductive years, healthy ovaries release new seeds monthly in a dynamic way—and when this dynamic ovarian energy needs to get our attention, the ovaries are capable of changing very quickly. A large ovarian cyst, for example, can grow in a matter of days under the right circumstances.

While uterine health is directly related to a woman's belief in herself at the deepest inner level, ovarian health is related to the quality of a woman's relationships with the people and things outside herself. Ovaries are at risk when women feel controlled or criticized by others or when they themselves control and criticize others.

ANATOMY

Ovaries are the small, oblong, pearl-colored organs that lie just below the fallopian tubes on each side of the uterus. They are located in a thin sheet of connective tissue known as the broad ligament. Ovaries produce eggs. A woman has the greatest number of eggs in her ovaries that she'll ever have—about 20 million—when she is a twenty-week fetus inside her mother. Although the number of eggs starts to decrease from that point on, all females continue to have far more eggs than they ever need.

Though it has long been believed that the mammalian ovary loses the ability to create new eggs after fetal life, new research may indicate otherwise. In 2017, a research team led by Evelyn Telfer, Ph.D., at the University of Edinburgh discovered that ovarian biopsies taken from young women with Hodgkin's lymphoma who had taken the chemotherapy drug AVBD had two to four times the density of eggs than did healthy women of the same age—even though chemotherapy in general often causes fertility problems.[1] The scientists noted that the eggs appeared younger, indicating that the ovaries may have formed new eggs (although this was not conclusively proven). To me, this relates to something we see in nature quite frequently. When you prune a tree or disturb the roots of a flowering wisteria, for example, the plant very often puts forth a lot of new leaves or blossoms the next season. It may be that the threat of death (chemo in a young woman, pruning in a tree) releases a survival signal that causes the organism to do what is necessary to reproduce itself quickly.

Dr. Telfer and her team also made another important discovery when they were able to develop fully mature human eggs in the laboratory for the first time.[2] The researchers took ovarian biopsies from ten young adult women undergoing elective cesareans. The tissue biopsied was embedded with immature eggs that the researchers then nurtured in the lab through a series of steps over the next three weeks. This resulted in the development of thirty-two fully mature eggs, although further research is needed to determine if the resulting eggs remain normal and can indeed be fertilized. Researchers are hopeful, however, because this has already been achieved in studies with mice. In 2016, scientists in Japan reported the first birth of healthy baby mice originating from lab-grown artificial eggs.[3] The researchers took stem cells from mice and used them to grow mature mouse eggs in the lab. Then they fertilized the eggs and implanted the resulting embryos into female mice, resulting in several healthy live births, although the overall success rate was low. The implications of all this are remarkable. Not only may women undergoing chemotherapy eventually be able to recover their fertility, but a variety of new fertility treatments may result from what we are now learning about the ovary and how it functions.

Other research on human eggs by Joe Nadeau, Ph.D., principal scientist at the Pacific Northwest Research Institute, has shown early evidence that eggs may choose which sperm will fertilize them, screening out sperm with unsuitable genes, so the sperm with the best genes remain.[4] Semen, on the other hand, does not seem to have the same ability to detect bad genes. Developments like these certainly inspire us to think about our ovaries and our eggs in a whole new, more positive way!

Ovaries release eggs about once a month, from about age fourteen or fifteen onward—sometimes earlier, sometimes later. After a girl's first period, it takes two or three years for ovulation to get going regularly, just as at menopause it takes a number of years for ovulation to cease altogether. Because ovulation always produces a small cyst in the ovary, it's very common for ovaries to have small cystic areas in them that are either the result of newly developing eggs or ovulations that have already occurred. As the egg begins to develop each month, a nourishing fluid-filled area forms around it, so that it is encapsulated or walled off from the rest of the ovary. This fluid-filled area, known as a cyst, is physiologically and completely normal, a fact that many women don't appreciate. At ovulation, when the egg is released and picked up by the fallopian tube, the cyst actually bursts as part of the ovulatory process, and the surrounding fluid, known as the liquor folliculi, is released into the pelvic cavity along with the egg.

After ovulation, in the space where the egg used to be, a second small cystic area, known as the corpus luteum, develops and begins to secrete progesterone. The corpus luteum eventually gets reabsorbed by the ovary. Frequently the process of egg development begins and a small cyst forms, but ovulation doesn't occur in that particular site. In this case, a small cyst will be left in that area of the ovary for a while. Because of this monthly process of egg development and cyst formation, it is perfectly normal for a woman to have small fluid-filled ovarian cysts at almost any time throughout her reproductive life. In fact, ovaries almost always have small cysts in them.

Whenever a woman gets a pelvic ultrasound for chronic pelvic pain, a fibroid, or any other reason, her ovaries are also scanned and these cysts show. Small 1-to-3-centimeter cysts are almost always normal, because producing small physiological cysts that come and go is part of what normal ovaries do. They gestate little eggs, little cysts—or, in energy medicine terms, young ideas ripe with potential.

Ovaries also produce hormones—including estrogen, progesterone, and androgens—throughout the life cycle, though the amounts they produce change (not necessarily declining), depending upon a woman's age. Androgens, the hormone type associated with libido, were thought in the past to be produced almost entirely by the adrenals, which are the endocrine glands located at the top of the kidneys. However, various studies have established that both premenopausal and postmenopausal ovaries produce a significant quantity of androgens, perhaps as much as 50 percent of the body's supply.[5]

It has been commonly thought that ovaries become essentially nonfunctional after a woman stops having periods, but the role of the ovary in the second half of life is now being reevaluated. We now know that the normal ovary should not be surgically removed because it maintains its ability to produce steroid hormones for several decades after menopause.[6] Parts of the ovaries do start to decrease in size when a woman is in her thirties, and they do lose mass more rapidly after age forty-five on average, but they are *not* the inert fibrous tissue masses they've been thought to be.

As women age, only part of our ovaries regresses, the part known as the *theca*. The theca is the outermost covering of the ovary where the eggs grow and develop and where physiological cysts form. In midlife the theca regresses, but the innermost part of the ovary, known as the inner stroma, becomes quite active for the first time in our lives.[7] In other words, as one function is winding down, another one is starting up. This process deserves much more study than it has heretofore received. In the second half of life, women's ovaries still produce significant amounts of a hormone known as androstenedione, a type of androgen. This substance is often converted to estrone (a type of estrogen) in our body fat deposits. Studies have shown that our ovaries can produce progesterone and estradiol even after menopause. These hormones are significant in preventing osteoporosis and heart disease and also in maintaining energy and libido.[8]

Up until fairly recently, menopause has been studied mostly as a "deficiency disease." Because of this cultural attitude toward menopause, scientists have studied this natural process only to find what is lacking. If we were to design studies of postmenopausal women in which the ovary was viewed as active and useful, we would find out more and more about the ovary's role in maintaining normal balance in our bodies as time goes on. The truth is that our ovaries are dynamic organs that are part of our body's wisdom throughout life, not something useless or potentially harmful to us when we are over forty.

Some ancient traditions have supported this view. In Taoist cultures the ovaries are thought to contain large amounts of the life force that constantly produces sexual energy. Special "ovarian breathing" exercises can be learned to release the life force energy produced by the ovaries and "store" it to revitalize other organs of the body, while the person achieves a higher state of consciousness. Ovarian sexual energy is thus transformed into *chi* (life-force energy) and *shen* (sheer spiritual energy).[9] In the fascinating book *The Sexual Teachings of the White Tigress* (Destiny Books, 2005), author Hsi Lai presents ancient teachings from Japan that suggest that women can maintain their sexual attractiveness far into old age by consciously working with this energy. (See also chapter 8, "Reclaiming the Erotic.")

When a woman does not heed her innermost creative wisdom because of her fears or insecurities about the world outside herself, ovarian problems can arise. They may arise in situations in which she perceives herself as being controlled by or criticized by forces outside herself. Financial or physical threats in the outer world affect the ovaries, particularly if a woman believes that she has no way to alleviate the threats. Thus, a woman who is abandoned by her mate or feels stressed on the job may develop ovarian problems if she feels that she has no means of escape from her situation and that the outer world (usually in the form of limited finances) is preventing her from changing. Just as life stresses may cause uterine problems, they may also cause ovarian problems. Uterine and ovarian problems are often intimately related, but there are also differences. The primary energy involved in uterine problems is a woman's perception in her innermost self that she can't or shouldn't or doesn't deserve to free herself from a limiting situation or create solutions that can support her. The uterus is very intimately linked with the third chakra and self-esteem. Uterine problems result when a woman's personal and emotional insecurities keep her from expressing her creativity fully. In these cases, she believes that she herself lacks the inner resources to do so; in other words, she is doing it to herself.

Ovarian problems, on the other hand, result from a woman's perception that people and circumstances *outside of herself* are preventing her from being true to herself and living from her center: They are doing it to her. An additional energy affects only the ovaries and not the uterus—the energy of vengeance and resentment, or the desire to get even. The second-chakra area is the part of the body where we traditionally wear weapons, such as guns, knives, and wallets. When a woman uses her emotional weaponry to indulge in being highly critical or wanting to get even, it is her ovaries that are at risk, not her uterus.

Benign ovarian growths differ from cancer only in the degree of emotional energy involved. Cancer in a woman's ovarian area is also related to an extreme need for male authority or approval, as she gives her own emotional needs last priority.

Note: This so-called male approval may come not from an outside source but from a critical thought pattern she has internalized and which causes her to drive herself relentlessly. Alison Armstrong, author of *The Queen's Code* (Pax Programs, 2013) and internationally known teacher of courses such as "Understanding Men" and "Understanding Women," teaches that most all women have an internalized "ideal woman" to whom they relentlessly compare themselves (and also other women and even men). She calls this a "weapon of mass destruction," and I certainly agree with her. Living up to the standards of this ideal woman can wreak havoc in our lives and with our health.

I once saw an outstanding example of this. I was exercising in a hotel gym where the woman beside me on another elliptical trainer was talking incessantly on her cellphone. This went on for thirty minutes, rendering her unable to use her arms or her breath to get the full benefit of the workout. When she was finally finished, she limped—yes, limped—out of the gym, still on the phone. She hadn't bothered to stretch or cool down. And her limp (on her right leg; the right represents the male side) suggested that she had perfected the art of ignoring her body and need for balance completely. Though I had no way of knowing what the health of this woman's ovaries was like, it was very clear to me that if her behavior in the gym was any indication of the overall balance of her life, she was heading for a health crisis (or at least an orthopedic injury that would force her to get off her feet). So many women expect themselves to have a perfect home, prepare organic whole-food lunches for their children each day, maintain the perfect weight, and be perfectly dressed every day. This is completely unrealistic, of course.

A woman at risk for ovarian cancer may feel that she doesn't have enough power, financial or otherwise, to move or to change even an abusive situation. In contrast to cervical cancer, which may incubate for years, ovarian cancer usually develops rather quickly due to a precipitating psychosocial trauma, such as a mate announcing that he or she is leaving.[10]

A friend of mine developed an ovarian cyst when she began to realize that her job was not good for her and that her relationship with her husband was not mutually supportive. During the same period, her husband began having an affair. Dealing with her cyst helped her to realize that there were real problems in her day-to-day life that she had to deal with. Her body was concretizing her emotional dissatisfactions and, in its wisdom, drawing her attention to her need to care for herself.

One of my patients, Beverly, had a long history of endometriosis, and her right ovary had been removed because of a benign growth four years before I met her. When she first came to see me, she was complaining of intermittent pain associated with her left ovary. She was worried that she might have to have this ovary removed as well, but she did not want to do this. She was only thirty-two and didn't want to be on hormones to replace her body's own supply. She was ready to work toward the deepest level of inner healing. On ultrasound, her remaining ovary had some small cysts in it consistent with endometriosis of the ovary. A skilled medical intuitive did a reading that revealed that Beverly had a lifelong history of truncating her own creative needs in order to meet the demands of her family, who lived close by. She also hated her high-powered executive job, which took up about seventy hours of her time per week.

The intuitive told Beverly that she was not likely to get well until she allowed her creativity to flow. Beverly settled on allowing herself at least one hour a day of creative time just for her. During this time, she decided to release all expectations of productivity. She would simply allow her creativity to flow in whatever way it needed to. Beverly had always enjoyed working with fabric and was accomplished at needlecraft. She began to sit each day and create small, very magical-appearing dolls that, she said, "seemed to have a life of their own." She told me that the dolls themselves dictated to her how they would look and what they would wear. When she first brought a few into my office, I was enchanted by them and purchased two for my daughters for Christmas. As she allowed herself this creative time, her pelvic pain eventually disappeared. It returned intermittently when she got caught up in the demands of the external world at the expense of her own creative work. Her ovary, through its persistent voice, became a personal barometer for her of how well she was allowing her innate creativity to flow. As she changed her entire "male" approach to life, the dolls that birthed through her continued to change and evolve as well.

OVARIAN CYSTS

We women are meant to express our creative natures throughout our lives. Our creations will change and evolve as we ourselves grow and develop. Our ovaries, too, are always changing, forming, and reabsorbing those small physiological cysts. As long as we express the creative flow deep within us, our ovaries remain normal. When our creative energy is blocked in some way, abnormally large cysts may occur and persist. Energy blockages that create ovarian cysts may result from stress. Such stress is not necessarily negative; for example, a woman may have a job that she loves but may sometimes simply neglect her need for rest. A cyst may be the result.

The left side of the body represents the female, receptive, yin side, while the right side is the male, more analytic, action-oriented yang side. And amazingly, these differences are reflected in the differing connections of each ovary in the brain.[11] Most of the ovarian cysts I've seen are on the left side— symbolic, I feel, of the wounded feminine in this culture. Many women try to imitate male ways of being in the world that don't always fit their inner needs. When I had my first intuitive medical reading with the world-renowned medical intuitive Caroline Myss, she told me that if I had stayed in my former medical group, I would have developed a pathological ovarian cyst within the next year that probably would have required surgery. It had already been forming in my body's energy field! When I heard this, I realized that my inner guidance and decision to leave that practice proactively had averted a health crisis.

In premenopausal women in general, cysts that are less than four centimeters in diameter are considered normal. An ovarian cyst is called a *functional cyst* when it arises as part of the ovulation process. A cyst larger than four centimeters may be watched for a few months to see if it goes away. An abnormal cyst may contain fluid, blood, and cellular debris under the surface covering the ovary or within the body of the ovary itself.

Symptomatic Functional Ovarian Cysts

Follicular Cysts. Many ovarian cysts that grow bigger than four centimeters and persist after two or three menstrual cycles are actually functional. Such cysts form when the follicle, the physiological cyst in which the egg develops, fails to grow and discharge the egg in the normal way. When this happens, the ovarian follicle may continue to grow beyond the time when ovulation should have taken place. It sometimes grows as big as seven or eight centimeters in diameter and can be painful. These cysts are described on ultrasound as unilocular and thin-walled, meaning that they consist of just a single collection of fluid contained within a thin membrane. They usually go away on their own, but some persist and require surgery. Although some physicians prescribe birth control pills to stop the ovulation process and allow the cyst to regress, the newer low-dose-estrogen birth control pills do not contain enough hormone to shut down the ovary and influence the cyst.

Luteal Cysts. Another type of functional cyst is known as the corpus luteum. A corpus luteum, or luteal cyst, forms when the mature egg is discharged from its follicle at ovulation. This process is sometimes accompanied by a small amount of bleeding into the ovulation site on the capsule of the ovary—and sometimes into the pelvic cavity as well—at the time when the egg erupts from the ovary.

Some ovarian cysts are completely asymptomatic, while others cause pain. The pain can be sharp and knife-like if, for example, the cyst bursts and spills its contents into the pelvic cavity. Or the pain can be dull and aching if the condition is more chronic, as in many cases of endometriosis of the ovary. A small pain sometimes accompanies ovulation, caused by the release of blood into the pelvic cavity. It is known as mittelschmerz (middle pain). Bleeding into a cyst cavity or the pelvic cavity often causes pain because it stretches the ovarian capsule (the tissue on the surface of the ovary). This pain can last from a few minutes to a few days. If the bleeding continues into the cyst wall for longer than a few hours, the corpus luteum becomes known as a *corpus hemorrhagicum,* which simply means "a body that bleeds." Bleeding from a corpus hemorrhagicum can last for several hours or even days and sometimes mimics an ectopic (tubal) pregnancy. It may be accompanied by vaginal bleeding. Hemorrhagic cysts usually go away on their own, but they can cause several days of pain. Very occasionally, the bleeding doesn't stop and surgical intervention, usually through the laparoscope, becomes necessary. Most often, this procedure stops the bleeding and removal of the ovary isn't necessary.

Most functional ovarian cysts are diagnosed by a pelvic examination, followed by an ultrasound evaluation. Both ovaries are examined and compared to be sure that it is an ovarian cyst and not something else, such as a fibroid, that is being felt.

Neither type of functional ovarian cyst—follicular or luteal—leads to cancer. Some women have symptoms from them repeatedly, while others have them only once in a lifetime. The important point to keep in mind is that these cysts can arise in only a matter of days or hours because our bodies are able to produce ovarian cysts rapidly. They can also go away rapidly.

Benign Neoplastic Cysts. Because ovaries contain cells that are capable of growing into complete human beings, they also contain cells that are capable of growing into a wide variety of cysts and growths, reflecting our enormous creative potential. When our creative expression is frustrated, this creative energy calls our attention to it through our body and physically manifests itself in the ovary rather than moving through us smoothly into the outer world. Conventional medical training teaches that the cause of ovarian cysts is not known unless they are of the "functional" variety and related to ovulation.

Benign, nonfunctional ovarian cysts occur when those cells of the ovary that are not associated with ovulation begin reproducing. The term *neoplastic* is often used in discussing these and other growths, both benign and malignant. *Neoplasia* means "new growth."

Other Cysts. Besides follicular, luteal, hemorrhagic, and benign neoplastic cysts, some ovarian cysts are solid in character and don't go away after two or three menstrual cycles. This kind of cyst is assumed to be an ovarian growth arising from something other than ovulation. They require further investigation and treatment via surgery, because until a doctor has surgically removed tissue and examined it under the microscope, it is not certain whether the cyst is benign. I've occasionally had patients with ovarian cysts that were present on pelvic exam and visible with ultrasound for many years but that did not change in any way or cause any symptoms. These women knew that they were taking a risk, in the conventional sense, by not having surgery. Some were willing to take that risk and live with their ovaries untouched and undiagnosed for years. Though this approach is not advocated by my training, I also respect the decisions of well-informed adults to avoid surgery after all the options have been thoroughly explained. In my experience, many, many women are tuned in to their innate wisdom and know how to be healthy with the right support.

POLYCYSTIC OVARY SYNDROME (PCOS)

As mentioned in chapter 5, many women have a condition known as polycystic ovary syndrome. So-called polycystic ovaries are a sign of hormonal malfunction. PCOS is a complex disorder because it is so affected by a woman's emotions, thoughts, diet, and personal history.

Doctors used to call PCOS "polycystic ovary disease," but currently PCOS is considered not a disease but a sign of an underlying imbalance. It is the end result of a complex series of subtle hormonal interactions. A few cases are genetic and therefore run in families, but most cases have no known genetic link. Conventional medicine cannot explain why or how PCOS occurs, but we do know that it is strongly associated with insulin resistance—which often results in excess body fat. About 50 percent of women with PCOS have excess body fat. Women with a high waist-to-hip ratio (apple-shaped figures) are more likely to experience ovarian dysfunction.[12] Jason Fung, M.D., a leading expert on intermittent fasting, has demonstrated that weight-loss programs that decrease insulin levels (including intermittent fasting and low-carb, moderate-fat diets) can often reverse PCOS. (See chapter 17, on nutrition.) The work of David Ludwig, M.D., Ph.D., an endocrinologist at Boston Children's Hospital, has shown the same thing.

The major problems associated with polycystic ovaries are that the woman's ovaries do not produce eggs, and her body produces too many hormones known as androgens. As a result, her periods may cease or become very irregular. Androgens occur naturally in both men and women, but in women with PCOS, they are present at higher levels than normal, often because of high levels of circulating insulin.[13] And high circulating insulin is a direct result of a refined-food diet that raises blood sugar too quickly. This is a crucial link for women to understand because high insulin levels are associated with so many other diseases. High blood insulin levels increase circulating androgen levels, change the way estrogen is metabolized, and are directly linked with obesity, diabetes, heart disease, hypertension, and hirsutism (excess facial hair).[14] High levels of testosterone also alter the gut microbiome, and since recent research at the University of California at San Diego has shown that PCOS sufferers have less diverse gut bacteria than women without the syndrome, this is of major concern.[15]

Chronically high levels of androgens also prevent normal cyclic egg development in the ovary, blocking the growth and development of eggs before they reach full maturity. When a woman's hormonal cycle is blocked by chronic androgen overproduction, neither she nor her ovaries will experience the natural cyclic changes associated with normal ovarian function. Her hormonal levels remain static. Thus, a woman's ovaries contain many small cysts from underdeveloped eggs. On ultrasound, the ovaries look enlarged, with multiple small cysts just below the entire surface of the ovaries (hence the name "polycystic ovaries"). Dietary change often produces amazingly fast improvements. (See Master Program for Optimal Hormonal Balance and Pelvic Health in chapter 5, and also chapter 17, on nutrition.)

The Mind-Body Connection in Amenorrhea

Whenever a woman has a problem with something as complex as the ovulation process, we know that there may be a problem with the regulatory mechanism of the menstrual cycle in the brain. The hypothalamus is affected by emotional and psychological factors, such as stress and repressed pain from the past, which can cause menstrual cycle dysfunction. Because most causes of amenorrhea are hypothalamic in nature, which means they are somehow associated with alterations in the fine-tuning of brain neuropeptide levels that are poorly understood, it is possible that the hypothalamus may have something to do with PCOS. In women with PCOS, the normal cyclic release of hypothalamic hormones from the brain is altered. It is not known whether this change is the result of the ovarian problem or the cause of it. It is well documented that the stress hormone cortisol also increases insulin levels. So both diet and emotional or other stresses can and do affect ovarian function.

Stresses that have been found to suppress ovarian and menstrual cycle functioning include negative feelings about being female and also feeling subordinate or inferior. I have found that when a woman has grown up being told that women are inferior, on some level she wants no part of becoming or being a woman. In some women, these negative feelings may work in the body to cause it to stop ovulating and become more "androgynous."[16] In fact, studies in female monkeys have shown that those who are in a position of social subordination will often undergo ovulation difficulties.[17]

Studies have also shown that women who don't ovulate may be tense, anxious, more dependent, and less productive mentally compared to ovulatory women. They may also have suppressed rage at their mothers. Some feel guilt and fear about their need for parental care and protection and also fear losing this protection. As they grow up, this can manifest as amenorrhea—an attempt to "halt" becoming fully mature women.[18] All of this is completely understandable (albeit often unconscious) given women's history as second-class citizens.

Treatment of PCOS

Since standard medicine doesn't know or acknowledge the cause of most cases of PCOS, treatment is aimed at quelling the symptoms only. Therefore, most women are currently placed on birth control pills, antiandrogenic drugs such as spironolactone, aromatase inhibitors that change the way hormones are metabolized, insulin-lowering drugs such as metformin, and/or progestin to create cyclic menstrual periods. These treatments do not address lack of ovulation or the hormonal status of the brain, though they can be helpful. Birth control pills and progestin also prevent excess hormonal stimulation of the uterine lining. Herbs such as *Pueraria mirifica* can also help when taken cyclically. These agents, therefore, decrease the risk of uterine cancer, which may result from years of buildup of the uterine lining if a woman doesn't have her period. Though birth control pills and other hormonal therapies do prevent some of the risks and symptoms associated with PCOS, they only partially mask the problem and never address the baseline cause.

In those women who desire pregnancy, ovulation can sometimes be induced with drugs. The most common one is clomiphene citrate (Clomid). Of course I've also seen many women get pregnant despite PCOS when they implement lifestyle changes.

If you have PCOS, you can help restore cyclic ovulatory function through looking carefully at any negative childhood messages you may have internalized about being a fertile woman. Commit to bringing these messages to consciousness so that they no longer control your body and your ovaries. One of my patients who had been diagnosed with PCOS three years before I first saw her realized that she had internalized feeling bad about herself as a woman because of being raped by her father. She unconsciously blamed her mother for not protecting her and so saw women as powerless. When she became aware of these messages, got off birth control pills (for PCOS), and began to celebrate her female nature, her periods and her ovulations reestablished themselves in about six months. (She also needed to hear from me that PCOS did not need to be a lifelong, chronic condition for her. Unfortunately, many doctors still mistakenly tell their patients that it is.) One of the fastest ways to uncover and transform old negative messages is by affirming new, healthier ones. Paste the following affirmation on your bathroom mirror or other obvious place and say it out loud looking into your own eyes every morning and every night for at least thirty days: "I now give thanks for my fertility and my femininity. I am completely safe to be all of who I am." (See also Master Program for Optimal Hormonal Balance and Pelvic Health in chapter 5.)

Women's Stories

The following stories illustrate how several of my patients have used their ovarian cysts to change and improve their lives. These stories show women waking up to the messages their bodies were sending them and then changing their lives. The message to all of us is particularly clear: to see the ways in which we participate in the dominator system and allow ourselves to be swayed by outside authorities rather than following our inner guidance. And then to appreciate how we can change our point of attraction by changing our perception and redirecting our thoughts.

Gail: Crystallized Overdrive

Gail has been a friend of mine for years. She first consulted me about a persistent ovarian cyst, and eventually, when she was in her late thirties, it required surgery. Here is her story.

"In 1984, during a routine gynecological exam, a woman doctor found a large ovarian cyst on my left side. This sleek doctor in New York's SoHo district announced to me that this was dangerous and that I should have surgery to remove it as quickly as possible. I should then expect to be completely laid up for about four to six weeks, she said. She, of course, would be glad to perform the surgery. All of this transpired in about fifteen minutes.

"I was terrified, completely blown away. At the time I didn't know enough about myself to know why I was so scared by this information. As was my pattern in those days, I covered the terror by increasing my activity and going into high gear. This was supremely easy for me to do in 1984, as I was directing a massive global peace initiative that had me traveling to several different continents a month. Besides covering my feelings by going into action, I had a strong intuitive sense that this ovarian cyst was neither as urgent nor as serious as this doctor seemed to think. I did not have the surgery.

"Several years went past, and I didn't really think about the cyst too much. I was in warrior overdrive, changing the world and lots of people's lives while ignoring my own. Though much of this activity was positive and deeply meaningful to me, I was out of balance in my life.

"In late 1987 my father died. Though he was well into his eighties and had led a full life, I had had no idea of the impact this would have on me. I experienced a kind of spiritual crisis. Through what I consider pure grace, a friend recommended a therapist who might help me. My journey with this wonderful man changed my life. With consummate skill and rare gentleness, he empowered me to recognize and heal much about myself that I had been afraid to look at. A pattern that was enormously important to my healing was my understanding that I had betrayed my feminine/mother and sided with my masculine/father. For much of my life this had resulted in my absolute allegiance to doing over being, thinking over feeling, and the outer world over the inner world. For me, this was a deeply personal betrayal, as well as a symbol of the collective societal betrayal of the feminine that has so profoundly wounded our culture.

"I began to experience my ovarian cyst as a physical manifestation of the warrior/masculine part of my personality that caused me to be so driven all the time. I called it 'crystallized overdrive.' I had betrayed my deep feminine side to such a degree that this warrior cyst was literally taking up much of the room in the feminine creative center of my body. It had grown to the size of a large grapefruit.

"Though I began to have more spiritual and emotional clarity about my cyst, I still struggled with how to deal with it on the physical level. I never felt it—I had absolutely no pain. Rather, it had a kind of looming presence, reminding me that something in me was out of balance."

In the fall of 1991 Gail came to see me. Her most recent ultrasounds showed that the cyst had begun to grow again and that the inside was changing, becoming more solid and dense. When a cyst becomes more solid, it means that its fluid parts are being replaced by more cells and growth within it. It was becoming more substantial. I felt that she had watched it long enough and that these changes signified the potential for the cells to become precancerous. (If an individual does not heed the body's wisdom that is announced by a bodily growth, the growth often needs to speak louder and more clearly. Thus, it may grow more quickly and become symptomatic. Nonphysiological ovarian cysts have the capacity to become large very quickly, depending upon the circumstances.) Gail was also starting to get some pressure on her bladder. I suggested surgery, since I felt that the persistent and now-changing cyst was a drain on her energy. As we have seen, unhealthy tissue literally "drains" the molecules needed for cellular metabolism from adjacent healthy tissue. (See chapter 4.)

A consultation with Caroline Myss confirmed my suspicions. She said that the cyst was now "waking up" and becoming active. It had the capacity to undergo rapid growth under the right circumstances. She felt that it should come out within three months. She confirmed that the growth had developed because of Gail's conflict between her personal inner needs and the demands of her outer world. Myss also said that the energy difference between Gail and her husband was at its most extreme ever; Gail felt drawn toward the quiet, reflective archetypal feminine, just as her husband (her partner in work as well as marriage) was reaching his peak in recognition and activity in the outer world. This was recognition in which Gail could share if she wished. She felt acutely the competition between this drawing inward toward the core of her being and the demands of success in the outer world, for which she had worked for years. If she didn't participate in this worldly success, the culture would judge that she was now "throwing it all away." Despite this conflict between her inner and outer worlds, Gail's ovarian wisdom was drawing her more inward than ever before in her life. This is a classic example of the type of competition in energy and body language that hits women in their ovaries.

Gail agreed to have the surgery, performed by me, whom she trusted. As part of her preparation, she worked with a spiritual studies group. The process included a kind of guided meditation in which she experienced her surgery in archetypal images, her warrior/masculine aspect standing behind her hospital bed protecting her emerging mystic/feminine aspect. As she remembered it, "The warrior reached to stroke gently the mystic's forehead. At the conclusion of the surgery my mystic held the cyst and handed it to the warrior. The warrior took the cyst and bowed deeply to the mystic. This was a profound image for me. I knew at that moment that through this surgery something very old, at my very essence, would come into balance.

"In partnership with this mythic changing of the guard, another friend led me through a meditation several days before my surgery. I had a dialogue with my cyst. I visualized it as being like the inside of a golf ball. I told it I was ready to release its 'crystallized overdrive.' I was ready to balance my outer warrior side and my inner reflective mystical side. I truly yearned for this as a healing for me.

"During this second meditation, I gave Chris [Northrup] permission to cut open my body and remove the cyst. I meditated about the removal of the cyst. I experienced vast space in my body, the turquoise color of the Caribbean Sea healing and cleansing me. Into that infinite turquoise, the female lineage of my family appeared—a long line of sisters, mothers, grandmothers, and on and on back. They acknowledged me for reclaiming my feminine self for myself and for them."

With these healing images instilled in her mind and heart, Gail created a medicine pouch of items of significance to her. It included some crystals that had been given to her, some special stones from a beach she loved, pictures of her mother and grandmother, and some childhood toys. She packed her bag and left for Maine, to have her surgery at the hospital where I performed surgery. As she later said, "My husband and two of my dearest friends were with me before and after my surgery. Their presence created a calm, loving, and joyful center from which my surgery/initiation could unfold.

"The surgery went smoothly and gracefully. Chris removed the benign cyst that had replaced my left ovary. She reported to me that I had a gorgeous and healthy uterus and right tube and ovary. When she showed my dear friends the cyst she had removed, one of my friends said that it looked like the bulging red muscles in the neck of a runner who is overexerting. Overdrive itself.

"I felt only a small amount of pain from the surgery and only mild effects from the anesthesia. I left the hospital after two days with an enormously positive feeling about my adventure there. My body then began the miraculous process of healing itself.

"I am enjoying my time of healing retreat. It's too soon to understand all of what has changed and transpired in me. What I do know is that I have faced one of my scariest dragons, and for that I am a fuller, richer person. I know that I can ask for support when I am afraid, and I know that I am loved and cared for by many dear ones. I know that I have shifted and balanced an ancient partnership within myself where the warrior waltzes with the mystic."

In many cases of large, complex ovarian cysts like Gail's, the healthy ovarian tissue is replaced almost entirely by that of the cyst, and there is almost no way to distinguish healthy from unhealthy tissue. Therefore, the entire ovary requires removal.[19] Gail continues to do well, however. The very way in which she approached her cyst, her hospitalization, and her postoperative care are good examples of allowing more feminine, intuitive, nurturing energy into her life, part of the lesson she learned from her left ovary.

Mary Jane: Married to the Job

Mary Jane is a molecular biologist who has spent her entire career working in male-dominated institutions. When she was in high school, she wanted to take physics and advanced mathematics, but her father, a physics professor, told her that she should take typing instead, because it would be much more useful to her. Like many men of his generation, he felt that his daughter would only get married and have children and that higher education would be wasted on her. Ironically, Mary Jane eventually went on to get an advanced degree in science, and she published many more research papers than her father. Though she was once married and has one child, her marriage was unsatisfying to her almost from the beginning. She divorced, and then became married to her job.

Mary Jane had been a patient of mine for a few years, always traveling from out of state to my office in Maine for her annual exam. At one of these exams, I felt a seven-centimeter left ovarian cyst, which was confirmed by ultrasound. Because she was very open to working with the symptoms in her body in a conscious way, I told her that this manifestation was there to teach her something about second-chakra issues, specifically her relationships and her creativity. I told her to talk with her ovary and see what it was telling her. My plan was to reevaluate her in three months or less.

An intuitive reading by Caroline Myss revealed that the cyst was filled with anger, the anger of violation. It also had "cancer energy." This isn't the same as physical cancer but is moving toward it, and Caroline felt the cyst would have to be removed soon. Although there was no cancer now, the angry energy in the cyst was very strong.

After Myss's intuitive reading, Mary Jane started a dialogue with her ovary. As she discovered, "I found that it was filled with anger, a sense of abandonment, and also jealousy. But there was love there as well. Though I had felt this love on occasion, I couldn't express it. I had needed a place to put all of this—it went into my ovary."

Mary Jane took a leave of absence from work. She had decided to have the surgery because of Myss's warning. I affirmed her decision and told her that she should not look at surgery as a giving-up on her self-healing capabilities. Surgery can be a very healing choice, and it would allow her to move forward quickly with healing her life on all levels. Mary Jane's personal healing issues would mean working to heal her relationship with her father and her work.

Mary Jane had her surgery and all went well. The cyst was benign. During her immediate postoperative period, she went through a process of deep grieving and let go of the unattainable vision of the relationship with her father that she had always wanted but could not have. She realized that her longing for paternal approval that never came had set up a lifelong pattern of unsatisfactory relationships with men that also affected her work and work relationships. She came to understand that she had to release her father from her expectations and demands. She saw that she had used her research as a method to win the approval of her peers, not simply for the joy of scientific discovery. Four weeks later, at the time of her checkup, she was doing beautifully—grateful to her ovary for showing her a truth about her life that was not obvious to her intellect. Mary Jane used her ovarian growth as a transformational journey that reconnected her body's wisdom and joy in her life's work.

Conny: Truncated Creativity and Need for Outer Approval

Conny was thirty-eight when she developed a six-centimeter benign left ovarian cyst. It was removed surgically, leaving some normal left ovarian tissue behind. During the time she was developing this cyst, she had been trying to decide whether to have a child. At the time of her surgery we had discussed how she could best maximize her cyst experience for change and growth. She knew that her job was stifling her. She very much wanted to pursue making pottery and was, in fact, very good at it—she was always able to sell what she had time to make. But her job had great benefits. I told her to check out whether it was worthwhile to kill herself for her "benefits."

A year after her surgery, Conny was back in my office, reexperiencing the pain in her left side that had been there when she had the ovarian cyst. This time there was no cyst, but the pain was the same. She found that as soon as she arrived at work, the pain started, and it was getting worse. Her body was speaking loudly to her this time. She had already had one surgery. The conditions leading to the cyst in the first place—the energy pattern in her body—hadn't really changed.

Conny understood her dilemma intellectually, and she knew that something had to change. But somewhere deep inside, whenever she thought about leaving work to pursue her creative instincts, she heard her father's voice in her head saying, "You're a fool to leave your job security. Making art is not a job. That's a hobby. That's what you do when you've finished your work." She'd been carrying this belief from her father since childhood. Her job represented his approval in her life. She thus allowed forces outside herself to control her inherent creativity. Meanwhile she was denying the anger and rage associated with this situation.

I asked Conny to consider what she would do if she were given six months to live. She gave it a great deal of thought. Finally, exhausted, depressed, and in pain, she took a three-month leave of absence from work with the blessing of her company in order to sort out her priorities. The pain went away almost immediately, her energy returned, and her artistic side began blossoming. Her challenge was to balance her creative needs with her job.

When she first returned to work after her leave, her company put her in a different location, one in which she didn't have to deal directly with the public. Instead, she worked behind the scenes processing paperwork and invoices. This change fit her needs only temporarily. It was not satisfying work, and she was still allowing many aspects of her life to be controlled by her need for approval from her parents and her bosses. Within three months of a completely normal pelvic exam, she developed a very large precancerous tumor of the left ovary. It was growing so fast that she noticed a bulge in her abdominal wall that hadn't been there the week before. At surgery, the tumor was found to be a "borderline tumor"—halfway between benign and malignant. The tumor growth at the time of surgery appeared confined to the left ovary only, and after consultation with a gynecological oncologist, only the left ovary was removed—leaving Conny with a normal uterus and a normal right ovary. (Borderline ovarian tumors often grow so slowly that it's possible to remove only the abnormality, leaving a woman's other pelvic organs—and physical fertility—intact.)

However, she knew at a deep cellular level that her creativity was desperate for expression and that her body would not settle for anything less than her complete yielding to her innermost wisdom. She quit her job and spent as much time as she could making pots. She eventually planned to return to school to study holistic medicine. When I last saw her, the veil of depression that had surrounded her for the previous three years had lifted. She was blossoming into the fullness of her creative self. Her relationship with her parents had never been better. She was making peace with the fact that they might never understand her creative needs fully, but that didn't mean she couldn't have a relationship with them. She also learned that she could not hold her parents responsible for the years when she chose to curtail her creativity. She regarded her ovarian message as a "kick in the pants" that she really needed. She was grateful.

OVARIAN CANCER

Many American gynecologists are trained to remove the ovaries after the age of forty if a woman has pelvic surgery of any kind. The reason for this is to prevent ovarian cancer. Yet the American Cancer Society reports that ovarian cancer affects only one in seventy-eight women in the United States. This means that thousands of women throughout the country are having normal organs removed to prevent a condition that will actually affect very few of them. Thousands will be deprived of the essential benefits that these hormone-producing organs provide.

In fact, several studies, including a 2009 study of 29,000 women who had their ovaries removed before the age of forty-five and who were followed for twenty-four years, have shown that women who have this procedure have numerous increased risks:

- Double the risk of lung cancer—even if they don't smoke[20]

- Increased chance of coronary heart disease and stroke[21]

- Increased risk of dying from any form of cancer (although risk decreases for breast and, of course, ovarian cancer)[22]

- Fivefold higher risk of mortality for neurological or mental diseases[23]

~ Increased risk of getting Parkinson's disease[24]

~ Increased chances of cognitive impairment and dementia[25]

~ Increased risk of hip fracture[26]

~ More self-reported depression and anxiety later in life[27]

~ Decreased skin thickness, which results in a more aged appearance and possible increase in bruising[28]

Hormone therapy can help prevent several of these outcomes, although research shows that even long-term supplemental hormone use does not make up for the impact of hormone deficiency following the surgery.[29]

Other problems that occur after having both ovaries removed include decreased sex drive and decreased sexual attention. The research of Winnifred Cutler, Ph.D., has shown that hysterectomy with ovarian removal decreases or eliminates a woman's ability to produce sex-attractant pheromones, rendering her less attractive to appropriate partners.[30] The good news is that the use of commercially available pheromones reverses this. (See chapter 8, "Reclaiming the Erotic.")

Medicine in this culture, however, focuses on ovarian removal for its potential cancer-prevention benefits and downplays any adverse factors possibly associated with it. Removal of the ovaries to prevent ovarian cancer is based on the assumptions that (1) prophylactic removal of the ovaries during hysterectomy is associated with a lower incidence of ovarian cancer, and (2) a woman's own hormones can be easily replaced with hormone medication. But studies have shown that neither of these assumptions is always true.[31]

In the absence of ovarian disease, the ovaries are best left in place unless a very clear genetic risk has been identified: That is, a woman has one or more first-degree female relatives who have had ovarian cancer. And even then, the burgeoning field of epigenetics has shown that 90 percent of what happens to our health is not genetic but a direct result of how our environment (which includes thoughts, nutrients, and so on) influences gene expression. We have far more control over our gene expression than we've been led to believe. (See Resources for information on genetic counseling.) Neither synthetic nor bioidentical hormones can match the complex mix of androgens, progesterone, and estrogen that the normal ovary produces. When the actual drug-taking behavior of patients is considered, including their lapses in taking medication and other erratic factors that impede a drug's absorption and performance, retaining the ovaries results in longer survival.[32]

We need another approach to prevent the needless sacrifice of our ovaries. Understanding ovarian wisdom and energy holds the key to this approach. Ovarian cancer may result from the energy of unexpressed rage or resentment, encoded in the second-chakra area of the body. A woman may not be consciously aware of this encoding. But this energy may be present in a woman whose mate or boss is always angry with her and who may be otherwise abusive. A woman can be in an abusive partnership with her work or even with herself, and it may affect the ovaries in the same way. A woman who continues this pattern because of her fear of physical, emotional, or financial abandonment does not believe in her own inner ability to change her circumstances. She is out of touch with her innate power, and sometimes her body will try to get her attention via the ovaries, especially if she feels resentment or anger or blames others for her circumstances. (Remember that the uterus has a more passive energy than the ovaries.)

Though other choices may be available to her, such a woman consciously believes that she is being *forced* to keep her life as it is. She is being controlled unconsciously by the pattern of behavior I discussed in chapter 4 as the rape archetype. If the woman continues to participate in an abusive relationship in which she is continually violated either emotionally or physically (or in which she continually violates or abuses herself), she is, in energy terms, being raped. Neither she nor her abusive partner or abusive work situation recognizes her inherent dignity and inner creative power, and so her dignity, too, is raped. Such a woman often feels paralyzed by her rage—an energy that, if it were recognized and expressed, could help her create change. Another part of her paralysis is the belief that her job, husband, or other external source has control over her. Finally, her emotional wound may not have been validated or witnessed on some level and in some way. Yet in most abusive situations in which women feel powerless, husbands, bosses, or other external authorities rarely assume any responsibility for their part in the continued abuse—they, too, are unable to validate the wounding. Many of these women are highly intuitive and skilled empaths. They have what Sandra L. Brown, the author of *Women Who Love Psychopaths: Inside the Relationships of Inevitable Harm with Psychopaths, Sociopaths, and Narcissists* (Mask Publishing, 2010), calls "super traits," which include being self-directed, loyal, empathic, nurturing, organized, and effective in every situation except their most intimate relationships. Unfortunately, these traits are a setup for being taken advantage of by what I call energy vampires (popularly known as narcissists). I've written extensively about this in my book *Dodging Energy Vampires: An Empath's Guide to Evading Relationships That Drain You and Restoring Your Health and Power* (Hay House, 2018).

When a woman doesn't understand the dynamics of a vampire relationship, she will often blame herself or bury her own anger and rage deep within herself. She is often afraid that if she ever let her feelings be known, she would be abandoned (and if she is in a relationship with a narcissist, she likely would be abandoned, given that energy vampires move on very quickly to other sources of "narcissistic supply" once their tactics are identified).

It's important for women in this situation (and in any other situation) to begin to listen to their bodies' wisdom and their inner guidance systems, which can help them create the changes needed in their lives. Recall that the second chakra is compromised to the degree that a woman despises her job or her mate but believes that she cannot survive without these financial resources (money is, after all, a second-chakra issue).

The Golden Handcuff Syndrome

Ovarian cancer is linked epidemiologically with high socioeconomic status. Women of higher socioeconomic status may suffer from the "golden handcuff" syndrome—that is, a situation in which a woman is unhappy with her marriage or work, even despises her husband or job, yet that same husband or job provides her with the financial wherewithal to take expensive vacations, live in a beautiful home, and belong to an exclusive country club. Fearing that she would lose all these "benefits" if she left her situation, the woman stays—meanwhile stuffing her emotions into her body and feeling miserable and trapped on some level.

I've seen several women with ovarian cancer whose husbands have accompanied them into the office. The energy of criticism coming from these men has been palpable. I recall feeling suddenly vulnerable, guarded, and defensive in their presence. Though they said nothing, I was sure that they were silently criticizing everything about me and my office. One man shook my hand at the end of the visit without looking at me! When this man and his wife left, I said to my nurse, "How could any woman live with that energy day in and day out? I felt battered simply being in his presence."

Possible Contributors

Such a wide variety of types of ovarian cancer exists that a full discussion of them all is beyond the scope of this book. Basically, ovarian cancer occurs when some kind of ovarian cell begins to grow abnormal tissue. Ovarian cancer can grow very rapidly. Almost every gynecologist I know has had the experience of seeing a woman with a normal pelvic exam who three to six months later had a pelvis full of ovarian cancer that had spread rapidly and widely.

Although conventional medicine doesn't know what causes ovarian cancer, it's linked epidemiologically to a diet high in saturated fat and the consumption of dairy foods. Studies have shown that ovarian cancer patients consume 7 percent more animal fat in the form of butter, whole milk, and red meat than do healthy controls, and they eat more yogurt, cottage cheese, and ice cream.[33] Quite frankly, I don't think there is any direct causation there. Remember, the vast majority of women—no matter what their diet is like—will not get ovarian cancer. Here's how I see it. Once energy blockages in the second chakra are already present, environmental factors can clog the system and swing the body's cells into disease. (Regardless of what studies suggest about diet and ovarian cancer, the case can be made for everyone following a real-food diet rich in antioxidants and nutrients [see chapter 17].)

Several studies have linked the most common types of ovarian cancer, known as epithelial cancer, with the use of talcum powder applied either to the external genitalia or to sanitary pads. The largest such study so far looked at 8,525 women with ovarian cancer and 9,859 who didn't have it and found that women who use talcum powder on their genitals were about 24 percent more likely to have ovarian cancer.[34] These studies don't prove causality, of course, just an association. The idea is that the talc (and possibly other substances) can migrate into the pelvic cavity via the cervix and vagina, and then out to the fallopian tubes, where it might act as an irritant to the covering of the ovary and thus be a risk factor for ovarian cancer.[35] It has been shown experimentally, for example, that carbon particles applied to the vulvar area can migrate into the pelvic cavity via the pelvic organs in a rather short period of time.[36] In my view, you'd have to have other emotional factors going on as well for talc to result in ovarian cancer.

That said, so far more than 9,000 women with ovarian cancer and their families have sued Johnson & Johnson for not warning them about the cancer risks of using its talcum powder. In 2018, the company was ordered to pay $4.14 billion in punitive damages (the biggest single verdict yet in such cases brought against Johnson & Johnson) and $550 million in compensatory damages to a group of twenty-two plaintiffs. Similarly, the year before, a sixty-three-year-old ovarian cancer patient who had used talc daily for fifty years was awarded $417 million—although Johnson & Johnson was later granted a new trial.

Even though, as I said, other factors may have preceded the cancer and talc wasn't the sole culprit, in my opinion it's not a good idea to use any product like talc or douche in the genital area every day for many years. (The vagina is self-cleaning and needs no help from any such products except perhaps a bit of mild soap and water on the vulva if needed.)

Other factors linked to ovarian cancer include:

- A variety of toxins that poison the oocytes (the eggs of the ovary) may increase a woman's risk of having ovarian cancer.

- Radiation, mumps, virus, polycyclic hydrocarbons (which are present in cigarette smoke, caffeine, and tannic acid).

- High levels of gonadotropins. Though not all studies support this, it has been hypothesized that the reason birth control pills lower the risk of ovarian cancer is because they lower gonadotropin levels and thus decrease ovarian stimulation.[37] Conversely, fertility drugs increase gonadotropin levels, which has been hypothesized as the reason that these drugs have been associated with ovarian cancer.[38]

~ Chronically high levels of the androgen androstenedione. The researchers who discovered this link failed to show any association between high gonadotropin levels and ovarian cancer but found a relatively strong link between androgens and ovarian cancer.[39] Androgens are increased by chronically high insulin levels from diet and/or chronic stress.

Several studies have demonstrated a significant reduction in ovarian cancer risk, up to 37 percent, following either tubal ligation or hysterectomy.[40] The explanation for this might be, in part, because after either of these procedures, the passageway from the external genital organs to the inner pelvic cavity is permanently blocked.

Diagnosis

One of the biggest problems with diagnosing ovarian cancer in the early stages is that there are very few symptoms. Vague abdominal complaints such as indigestion are often cited. Unfortunately, a number of other problems can cause such pains, too.

Ovarian cancer is most often diagnosed in the late stages, but by then it is far less curable. We still do not have any well-tested screening methods to diagnose ovarian cancer in the early stages, let alone prevent it. In 2018, the U.S. Preventive Services Task Force concluded that not only does screening for ovarian cancer not reduce ovarian cancer mortality, but also the potential harm of screening (including complications from unnecessary surgery in women who receive false-positive screening test results) outweighs the benefits.[41]

Genetic or molecular biomarkers such as BRCA1 may indicate if a woman has a particularly high risk of ovarian cancer, yet their use as a screening tool is still experimental and currently limited to research purposes.[42]

Hundreds of women are now asking for sonogram screening and the blood test known as CA-125, which checks for tumor antigens—proteins that are shed from the surface of cancer cells. Unfortunately, neither test can give a guaranteed yes-or-no answer to the question "Do I have ovarian cancer?"[43] Despite initial optimism that this test would be a good screening tool, it has not lived up to its promise and may do more harm than good.

A high CA-125 reading in an otherwise normal woman creates a great deal of anxiety and fear (and may subject her to unneeded and possibly harmful testing)—yet it doesn't necessarily mean ovarian cancer. Endometriosis, fibroids, liver disease, and other unknown factors can also give high readings. At the same time, if a woman's CA-125 level is normal, it doesn't guarantee that she doesn't have ovarian cancer. In fact, only about 3 percent of women with elevated CA-125 levels actually have ovarian cancer, and no evidence shows that CA-125 screening decreases the chance of death from ovarian cancer.[44] Having this screening is recommended only for monitoring current cancer patients, to check for cancer recurrence, or to screen certain patients who are at high risk. None of the major professional organizations recommend using CA-125 as a screening test for those with an average risk of ovarian cancer.

Ultrasound doesn't give a definitive answer, either. One study estimates that using ultrasound screening in 100,000 women over the age of forty-five would uncover 40 cases of ovarian cancer—along with 5,398 false-positive results.[45] And here's the problem: False-positive tests must be investigated, because a false positive isn't false until so proven. And that means that far too often, those with false-positive results will be subjected to invasive surgeries in order to get a tissue sample and biopsy (at the very least). Such tests are often not benign because of the risks associated with anesthesia and the potential for excessive bleeding and infection.

No one can guarantee that everything is all right until laparoscopic surgery is performed and the pelvis is explored, a procedure requiring general anesthesia. Even among women generally considered at high risk who have laparotomies, relatively few cancers are diagnosed as a result. In one study of 805 high-risk women, thirty-nine laparotomies uncovered only one case of ovarian cancer (plus eight other benign tumors).[46]

In 2009, the FDA approved a new blood test known as OVA1 to be used to screen women who have pelvic tumors and are known to need surgery.[47] OVA1 tests for five different proteins that are known to undergo change when ovarian cancer is present, although the test is not diagnostic for ovarian cancer. Since women with ovarian cancer do better when their surgeries are performed by gynecologic oncologists, having this test prior to surgery allows the right team of surgeons to be assembled beforehand. Recent studies on the use of this type of test to screen for early ovarian cancer have shown disappointing results, however, and research on improving such testing is ongoing.

While screening isn't a reliable tool, paying attention to subtle physical symptoms has proven to be a valuable practice. A 2009 study of women diagnosed with ovarian cancer in thirty-nine primary care centers in England found that these women do, in fact, have early symptoms for which they seek medical attention. But the symptoms are nonspecific and so are not investigated thoroughly. The most common are abdominal distention (bloating), abdominal pain, and urinary frequency. This led to the authors admitting that "ovarian cancer is not silent, rather its sound is going unheard."[48] This study may raise awareness among healthcare practitioners and patients of the possibility that these symptoms signal cancer. In the meantime, ovarian cancer challenges us to explore the interface between the immune system, the emotions, nutrition, and genetics in new and creative ways. It's also important to remember that even women with very advanced disease have experienced total healing.

Familial Ovarian Cancer

A woman who has a sister, mother, maternal first cousin, maternal aunt, or other first-degree female relative with ovarian cancer has a higher-than-average risk of getting the disease herself. Familial ovarian cancer was first brought to general public awareness by the Gilda Radner story,[49] and by the well-publicized case of actress Angelina Jolie, who in 2013 chose to have both breasts removed and two years later had her ovaries and fallopian tubes removed (even though no sign of cancer had been detected in any of these organs) because she carries the BRCA1 gene. Some women who have a very strong family history of ovarian cancer (and thus have a 20 to 30 percent chance of getting the disease) opt for prophylactic oophorectomy. Prophylactic removal of the ovaries after childbearing is over is often recommended for these women. Yet even in women who have family histories of ovarian cancer, this does not necessarily prevent the disease. Even after prophylactic removal, cancers indistinguishable from ovarian cancer can still occur from cells in the lining of the pelvic cavity.[50]

I've noticed that women who have seen a close friend die of ovarian cancer are more inclined to have their ovaries removed because of fear. Though this might be unscientific, I find that most of our major life decisions are based on our emotional realities and not on statistics.

When a disease runs in families, we need to realize that we're not dealing solely with a simple matter of genetics. Attitudes also run in families, and attitudes translate to biochemical realities in the body, which influence how genes get expressed. It would be very interesting to study only those females in families with a history of ovarian cancer who did not get the disease. Most likely these would be the women who have broken the family mold and left their tribe, on both an energetic level and a physical level.

Oophorectomy During Other Pelvic Surgery

When a woman chooses to have a hysterectomy, to remove a fibroid uterus or for any other benign condition, she must also decide whether to remove the ovaries. I ask each individual woman before surgery how high her fear level of ovarian cancer is, and I ask her to check out how she feels about her ovaries. I tell her that it's not possible to discern the condition of the ovaries until the surgeon visualizes them directly during surgery. If there's a problem at that time, they may need to be removed. Before just handing them over, however, it's very helpful to review all the benefits of keeping your ovaries. Remember, very few men are willing to subject themselves to removal of the testicles. In my view, women should be just as protective.

If the patient decides to preserve the ovaries, she must defer to her surgeon's judgment if the ovaries look abnormal during surgery. It's best to find a doctor who is "ovary friendly." The ultimate decision about what to do with the ovaries must be left to the patient following informed consent. There are many factors, conscious and unconscious, that come into play when each of us makes major decisions about our bodies.

As you might imagine, the women who are drawn to my approach usually choose to keep their ovaries during hysterectomy because—like me—they value their female organs. Though my training led me to believe that ovaries should be removed as early as age thirty-five, I'm well past that age now, and I value my ovaries as a part of my body that will continue to function and support me as long as I live. I know that they are part of my inner guidance system and they will let me know if adjustments are required for their health. As I mentioned earlier in this chapter, numerous research studies lend weight to the idea that removing your ovaries isn't always the best option and can be risky. Taking hormones helps, but it doesn't completely negate these risks. (See "Artificial Menopause" in chapter 14, page 664, for more details.)

Most gynecologists train in large university centers that, because of their focus on certain specialties, treat more women with ovarian cancer in a week than the average practicing gynecologist sees in a decade. Thus, gynecologists tend to see more ovarian cancer in their training years than they ever see again. This creates a bias against the ovaries. An ovarian cancer death is difficult to watch; it can be associated with pain, recurrent bowel obstruction, huge amounts of fluid collecting in the abdomen, and a variety of other extremely uncomfortable symptoms. A doctor who has seen someone die of ovarian cancer is apt to be prejudiced in his or her relationship to ovaries from that point on, even though the vast majority of women will not get ovarian cancer.

One of the hospitals in which I worked in the past is the major referral center for our state. The gyn pathologist at that time said, "I'm scared to death of ovarian cancer. I'm having my wife have her ovaries removed when she's forty, and I even think she should have her breasts removed prophylactically." He was not completely serious about this recommendation, but this physician spent his days doing autopsies on women from all over the Northeast who had died of breast and ovarian cancer. He saw the devastation of these diseases as a daily part of his work. He cut into huge tumors and received surgical specimens in which a woman's uterus, tubes, ovaries, and even vagina, bladder, and rectum had been replaced by tumor. He saw the devastation of breast tumors that had eroded into the chest wall. It is little wonder that he felt the way he did, or that routine ovarian removal at the time of hysterectomy is still advocated by many.

Conventional Treatment

When diagnosed at advanced stages, ovarian cancer is considered a difficult disease to treat. Conventional treatment is surgical, sometimes followed by chemotherapy and radiation, depending upon how far it has spread. The diagnosis itself is usually made definitively at the time of surgery for some kind of pelvic growth. Despite advances in treatment and attempts at early diagnosis, long-term survival has been statistically unfavorable. According to American Cancer Society statistics, only 47 percent of ovarian cancer patients survive five or more years after diagnosis (with those under age sixty-five having the highest rates of survival). The five-year survival rate jumps to 92 percent if ovarian cancer is caught before it spreads outside the ovary, but this is the case only 15 percent of the time.

Without looking in the abdomen and taking a biopsy, there is no way to tell whether an ovarian growth is benign or malignant. If an ovarian growth is malignant, treatment usually consists of removing the ovaries, tubes, uterus, omentum (the apron of fat covering the bowel), and any tumor that has spread into the pelvis. This is followed by chemotherapy. Pumping two cancer drugs—paclitaxel and cisplatin—directly into the pelvic cavity in patients with advanced ovarian cancer who meet certain criteria has been shown to improve survival by an average of sixteen months. This treatment—called intraperitoneal (IP) chemotherapy—is, though not a cure, clearly a major breakthrough. The National Cancer Institute issued a clinical announcement early in 2006 to encourage doctors to use the abdominal treatment or refer their patients to medical centers that do it,[51] although a 2015 study showed that, unfortunately, fewer than half of eligible patients receive it.[52] For further information, visit the NCI website (www.cancer.gov) or call 800-4-CANCER. In the very early stages of ovarian cancer, surgery can be curative. Let me hasten to add that there have been well-documented cases of so-called spontaneous remission even in advanced cases of ovarian cancer.[53] That means there's always hope.

Women's Stories

One of my patients who died of ovarian cancer healed her life and her emotional issues more in her last month of life than in all her prior years. She had gone through extensive surgery and had also followed a dietary approach to her problem. She had done all the "right" things. But still her tumors grew. A physical cure was not part of her healing, though her healing came in the course of her search for a physical cure.

A doctor friend of mine who was working with her for her pain took her through a process of meditation during deep relaxation in which he asked her body to tell him what was feeding her tumors. She replied, "Fear and sadness." He then asked her to remember and reexperience a time when she did not have this fear and sadness. She went back to a time when she was a twelve-week fetus in her mother's uterus. Her mother had tried to abort her with a red-and-white pill. In her final days she was able to bring this information to consciousness and share it with her mother, who herself was in need of healing around this incident from many years before. My patient died in her mother's arms, free from pain, and finally free from a lifelong burden.

CARING FOR YOUR UTERUS AND OVARIES, OR PELVIC SPACE

~ Know that the inherent creativity symbolized by your ovaries is always present for you, regardless of whether they are still physically present in your body.

~ Find a creative endeavor that makes time stand still for you. Immerse yourself in something so absorbing that you forget to eat. If you don't know what that is, ask your higher power to guide you to it. What you are seeking is also seeking you!

~ Make time each day to do something of creative value that has meaning for you. Let it come through you. This could be as simple as organizing your underwear drawer beautifully!

~ Write down a list of your past creations. Notice how many of them have a life of their own now.

~ If you're still hanging on to and trying to control someone or something you've created, see if you can manage to let go and trust. (I know, I know. This takes a lot of courage—especially if, deep inside, there is a scared little girl who is desperately trying to control everything so she won't be abandoned or hurt.)

~ Know that your creative power is sorely needed in the outer world now. This power can serve you and others very well when you access it fully and don't try to control or force it. The late African American writer and civil rights leader Howard Thurman articulated this perfectly: "Don't ask yourself what the world needs; ask yourself what makes you come alive. And then go and do that. Because what the world needs is people who have come alive."

8

Reclaiming the Erotic

If you cannot face directly into your sexuality,
You will never discover your true spirituality.
Your earthly spirit leads to discovering your heavenly spirit.
Look at what created you to discover what will immortalize you.

—Hsi Lai

When I speak of the erotic, I speak of it as an assertion of the lifeforce
of women; of that creative energy empowered, the knowledge and use of
which we are now reclaiming in our language, our history, our dancing,
our loving, our work, our lives.

—Audre Lorde

WE ARE SEXUAL BEINGS

Appreciating and embracing our sexuality is a key part of flourishing.
All life is, after all, sexually transmitted. Most of us were conceived
with an orgasm, even if it was just your father's. I'm out to change all
that—physically, mentally, and spiritually—so that all women are finally free
to reclaim their erotic nature without shame or exploitation. This starts by
understanding the potency of eros and noticing how it works. The main reason why sex sells everything from cars to shampoo is that we are naturally
drawn to life-sustaining and pleasurable energy. Our cells recognize it just as
instinctively as a bee recognizes honey. Sure, you can sublimate sexual energy into other areas of life besides actually having sex. But your body will
respond to the erotic until the day you die. We are hardwired from birth for

sexual pleasure. It is our birthright. Humans are the only primates whose sexual desire and functioning are not necessarily related to the reproductive cycle. Women's ability to enjoy sexual pleasure is virtually limitless, which is why marriage and family therapist Pat Allen, Ph.D., refers to women as "orgasmatrons." Women's sexuality is involved in both giving and receiving sexual pleasure, as well as in reproduction. Even the act of giving birth can be orgasmic. (See chapter 12.)

Sexuality is an organic, normal, physical, and emotional function of human life, and we are capable of sexual pleasure and function for our entire lives. The research of the late Gina Ogden, Ph.D., a well-known sexuality researcher and author of the groundbreaking book *The Heart and Soul of Sex* (Trumpeter Books, 2006), points out that it is women in their sixties and seventies who are having the best sex of their lives.[1] Research studies have shown that regular sex with a partner is associated with more regular and fertile menstrual cycles, lighter periods, better moods, pain relief, better bladder control, fewer colds and fevers, reduced stress, staying in shape, increased estrogen and testosterone, and better weight control.[2] For those without a partner, take heart. Regular sexual expression with yourself is also very fulfilling and healthy. This is true even for those in relationships.

One of the main reasons for the health benefits of sex is that pleasurable sex causes a huge outpouring of the gas nitric oxide from the lining of our blood vessels. This not only increases circulation throughout the body but also balances hormones and neurotransmitters. Nitric oxide has been referred to as the fountain of youth, which is probably the reason why David Weeks, Ph.D., found that people who engage in sex on a regular basis look much younger than their chronological age. Dr. Weeks, a neuropsychologist at Scotland's Royal Edinburgh Hospital, studied 3,500 people ranging in age from 18 to 102.[3]

Women's Erogenous Anatomy: The Clitoral System

The external portion of the clitoris that most of us are familiar with is simply the tip of what is actually a much larger (mostly internal) organ, the anatomy of which has only recently been fully understood and appreciated by the medical profession. Australian urologist Helen O'Connell, M.D., who headed a team that took MRI scans showing the size and complexity of the clitoris in an aroused state for the first time, refers to the entire system as the "clitoral complex."[4] This complex, she reports, has at least eighteen distinct interacting functional parts, including muscular, erectile, and sensitive tissues, most of which expand during arousal. Taken in its entirety, the clitoris is actually larger than the average unerect penis!

The entire organ is shaped somewhat like a wishbone. At the top (in the front of the body) is the external part of the clitoris (the glans clitoris), a relatively small bud-like protrusion just above the vaginal opening. The glans of the clitoris is partly covered by the clitoral hood or foreskin. The clitoral shaft in an unexcited state is less than an inch long and mostly hidden from view. When excited, however, it may swell to twice its normal diameter. From the glans and shaft, two arms or branches called the corpus caverno-sum extend on either side within the lips of the vulva, wrapping around the vaginal opening. At the base of each of these branches is an extension called the crus clitoris that points toward your thighs when not aroused and toward your spine during arousal. The total length of the corpus cavernosum and crus clitoris (on each side) is about four inches. Nestled between each of these branches and the vaginal opening are bulbs (these are commonly called vestibular bulbs but are more correctly referred to as clitoral bulbs). During arousal, the corpus cavernosum, the crus, and the bulbs, as well as the spongy erectile tissue surrounding the urethra (aptly known as the urethral sponge), all swell. As they swell, the bulbs "hug" the vagina. The vagina elongates, and the innermost third of the vagina balloons out, lifting the uterus and cervix. If intercourse occurs after full female sexual response, the changed shape of the vagina will help bring sperm to the cervix, facilitating concep-tion. As is obvious from this description, female sexual response is far more internal than external. (Also, because of the extensiveness of the clitoral sys-tem, some surgeons have been able to restore orgasmic response to victims of genital mutilation by removing the scar tissue and exposing a small part of the clitoris that was previously internal, a procedure formally known as cli-toroplasty. The surgery is complicated, the recovery takes time, and results are not guaranteed. Even so, it can give back a measure of the control that was taken away from these women against their will.)

Until very recently, most medical textbooks haven't included diagrams of the entire clitoral system, and many of those that have attempted this aren't accurate (while the penis, in contrast, is always shown in full and ac-curate detail). Even so, it's difficult to fully understand the details of this anatomy in a two-dimensional drawing. As Dr. O'Connell noted in a 2005 paper in the *Journal of Urology*, "It is impossible to convey clitoral anatomy in a single diagram."[5] That said, the illustration on page 273 is a good start.

In 2016, French sociomedical researcher Odile Fillod created a three-dimensional anatomically correct model that anyone with access to a 3-D printer can create for free. Fillod, who specializes in sex and gender issues in biomedical science, originally intended for the model to be used in French classrooms, although sex therapists, sex educators, school nurses, biology teachers, and sex-information institutions have all begun using Fillod's model in their work. (Note that the webpage where you can access the instructions for printing your own model—http://carrefour-numerique.cite-sciences.fr/

fablab/wiki/doku.php?id=projets:clitoris—is currently available only in French.)

Even without the aid of a three-dimensional model, you can learn to appreciate how your own clitoral anatomy works with a little personal experience. The external tip of the clitoris, which contains 8,000 nerve endings whose sole function is pleasure, is extremely sensitive to the touch. The clitoris will easily emerge from underneath its hood under pleasurable conditions of all kinds, including being admired by a lover, or simply when a woman sends positive thoughts and feelings to this area of her body. The inner lips of the vulva will also begin to engorge and the vagina will begin to lubricate when a woman so much as thinks about her genitals in a positive way. Stop right now and just feel your clitoris and the erotic anatomy connected to it deep inside. See what happens. Also try this: Get a magnifying hand mirror and sit down in a place with good light. Examine your vulva, clitoris, and vagina. Now send loving, admiring thoughts to the area. Watch what happens. (This is also a wonderful exercise to do with a lover.) You'll notice that your genitals begin to engorge and become rosier. The clitoris begins to enlarge and emerge from its hood. The more you admire this area and talk nicely to it, the more it "wakes up."

The clitoris is also anatomically connected to the G-spot (the sacred spot in tantric texts). In 2009, Pierre Foldès, M.D., and Odile Buisson, M.D., used cutting-edge two- and three-dimensional sonography in mapping the clitoral system and found that the G-spot is actually the ends of the branches of the clitoris's wishbone shape.[6] I think of the external glans of the clitoris as the north pole and the internal G-spot as the south pole. The recognition of the clitoris as an organ much vaster than what we see externally has led to the growing understanding that there aren't really two kinds of female orgasms, clitoral and vaginal. (Freud, for example, rather famously dubbed clitoral orgasms as "immature.") Orgasm reached during vaginal penetration that does not directly involve stimulation of the external tip of the clitoris is actually still a clitoral orgasm; it just results from stimulation of a different part—the internal part—of the clitoris. So, thankfully, we can finally put *that* debate to rest.

Nipple sensation also leads directly to strong clitoral stimulation and pelvic muscle contractions. So does kissing. The level of sensitivity can be very clearly understood by looking at a sensory homunculus, which is a kind of body map that illustrates by the relative size of the lips, tongue, and genitals, as well as hands and feet, which parts of the body have the most sensory connections—via nerve endings—to the brain, and therefore which have the greatest sensitivity to sensation.

All in all, women have more pelvic blood flow than men and just as much pelvic erogenous erectile tissue. That, combined with stronger and longer pelvic floor muscles, argues for an even greater capacity for sexual response in women than in men. In her book *Vagina: A New Biography* (Ecco, 2012), Naomi Wolf cites research showing that vaginal blood flow increases when a woman is turned on by people, places, or things. In other words, women's erotic anatomy responds (whether consciously or not) to life force in all its many forms. This can include a sunset, a flower, seeing your partner being nice to your grandmother, or the sight of your strong husband throwing an old couch off the truck at the dump. Once you begin to notice this turn-on, you will find that your erotic anatomy functions as a kind of guidance system leading you to a more fulfilling life.

Most women, however, have never been taught about their clitoral system and erotic anatomy. Many don't even have a name for their genitals other than "vagina" (which refers to only one part of the pelvic anatomy). Men, on the other hand, have dozens of names for their penises, and not one is "down there." It's little wonder that so many women have yet to experience the fullness of their erotic potential.

Amrita: Female Ejaculation

During sexual arousal (or turn-on), the vagina produces lubrication from a number of sources. The glands (Bartholin's and Skene's glands) at the junction of the vulva and the vaginal opening (the introitus) secrete fluid. The walls of the vagina itself produce a fluid known as transudate during sexual stimulation. Some women experience a gush of fluid from their vaginas during orgasm, called female ejaculate. The female ejaculate is actually made up of different fluids from different parts of the urogenital system, including a female "prostatic" gland.[7] This fluid has also been called *amrita,* or divine nectar. Many women mistake this female ejaculation for loss of urine at the time of orgasm, but this fluid is not urine, even though it does come in part through the urethra. This fluid release, which may amount to a cupful or more at a time and may occur more than once during lovemaking, is a normal component of female sexual response. Knowing its true nature is very reassuring for women.[8]

Release of the *amrita* may occur even without an orgasm, such as when a woman "loses it" during laughter, joy, or love. In such a case, the woman is not "losing it"—she is actually *becoming* the energy of joy or love and, far from losing anything, is *gaining* the essence of these ecstatic feelings.[9] Though every woman has the potential for experiencing this outpouring of her divine nectar, she can do so only by learning to surrender herself to deep happiness—which may or may not be sexual.

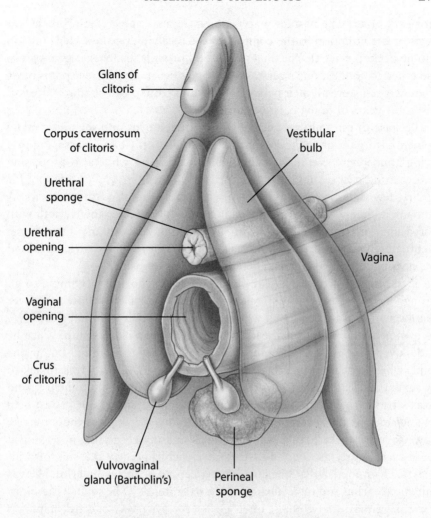

Glans of
clitoris

Corpus cavernosum
of clitoris

Vestibular
bulb

Urethral
sponge

Urethral
opening

Vaginal
opening

Vagina

Crus
of clitoris

Vulvovaginal
gland (Bartholin's)

Perineal
sponge

FIGURE 12: THE CLITORAL SYSTEM

The clitoral system is a rich network of erectile, erogenous tissue in the pelvis that is as extensive as that found in the male penis. The clitoris is the only part that is easily visible from the outside.

Awakening the Sacred Spot

Charles Muir and Caroline Muir, authors of *Tantra: The Art of Conscious Loving* (Mercury House, 1989), have helped many individuals and couples learn how to connect their sexuality and spirituality by teaching a technique that involves massaging the sacred spot very, very gently (starting with the little finger) while also breathing together and keeping eye contact with each other. The partner who is doing the massaging gives 100 percent of his or her attention to the comfort of the receiving partner. Her only job is to lie back, receive this healing touch, and provide feedback. Great care is also taken to connect one's genitals with one's heart. The sacred spot is often where women store all their personal hurts and pain. (I can certainly attest to this in my years of doing pelvic exams.)

Because of our cultural and individual heritage around sexuality, many women have pain or numbness in their sacred spot. Gentle massaging in a loving atmosphere eventually causes this to dissipate while also processing and releasing past sexual trauma. For many women, arousal of this spot for the first few times is often associated with pain or unpleasant memories. A woman and her partner who understand this will proceed slowly, both with sacred spot massage and also with lovemaking, particularly intercourse. Eventually this process can awaken a woman to more bliss than she realized was possible. It will also strengthen and prolong orgasms.

Elizabeth, a forty-seven-year-old accountant who was beginning to go through menopause, came in for a checkup and told me the following: "Over Thanksgiving vacation, I met a wonderful man through a mutual friend. We were immediately attracted to each other and began a relationship. When he made love to me for the first time, it was such a beautiful thing. But at one point, when he was stimulating me deep in my vagina, I had a flashback to my sexual abuse. I began to shake and to cry. I couldn't seem to help it, and I was worried that he'd think he'd done something wrong. But he just held me and told me that everything was all right and that he was there for me. Now when we make love, I still sometimes find myself getting upset, but it doesn't last nearly as long and I feel safer each time. My pleasure also increases. I had no idea that being with a man could be this wonderful. He was gentle and caring and took his time. I am so grateful." The sexual attentions of a caring man (or woman) often go a very long way toward helping a woman achieve her true sexual potential.

THE G-SPOT/SACRED SPOT

To find your G-spot, it's best to start after you're fairly aroused because this tissue deep in the vaginal wall is easier to find if it is already swollen, which happens with sexual stimulation. Use plenty of lubricant, and you also might want to trim your nails so you won't scratch yourself. (By the way, diaphragm users may find the diaphragm can interfere with this sensation in some women, so you might want to experiment before you insert the diaphragm.)

If you're exploring on your own, it's easier if you're upright (on your knees is ideal) rather than lying down. If you and your partner are exploring, you can lie on your belly with your hips slightly elevated or on your back. Insert one or two fingers or have your partner insert his fingers about two inches (usually up to the knuckles) into your vagina, palm facing up. The fingers should then press lightly on the front wall of the vagina, looking for a slightly swollen spot. Experiment with a few different ways of stroking and different amounts of pressure. Some women prefer a tapping motion. Others prefer pulling the fingers in and out of the vagina, while curving them as if making the "come here" gesture during the out motion. Keep up the stimulation. The area will continue to swell (to about the size of a walnut) and become spongy. It may feel slightly ribbed, sort of like corduroy.

Because the G-spot is located along the urethra and near the neck of the bladder, women often feel the urge to urinate when this spot is stimulated. If you're worried about leaking as you are exploring, know that you probably won't and that the urge will pass. (You can urinate before you start, if you want to reassure yourself that your bladder is empty.)

The most important thing is to relax and take your time. Maintain a curious attitude, rather than being performance-oriented. Don't have any goal other than to feel and see what happens. Some experts believe that women in their forties and beyond get more pleasure from G-spot stimulation than younger women because their lower estrogen levels make the vaginal lining thinner, which makes the G-spot more prominent when stimulated. Have fun with this.

The G-spot is connected energetically by an acupuncture pathway called a *nadi* to the pineal gland, which secretes a potent neuropeptide known as DMT. (See figure 13.) The pineal gland is known as the third eye in sacred texts and is our connection with the divine. DMT floods the body during orgasm and also during near-death experiences. Perhaps this is why in French an orgasm is sometimes called *la petite mort*—"the little death." This anatomic connection also explains the strong connection between spirituality and sexuality. So while stimulating your G-spot, simply visualize this energy going right up to your brain. You may even experience a kind of burst-of-light feeling.

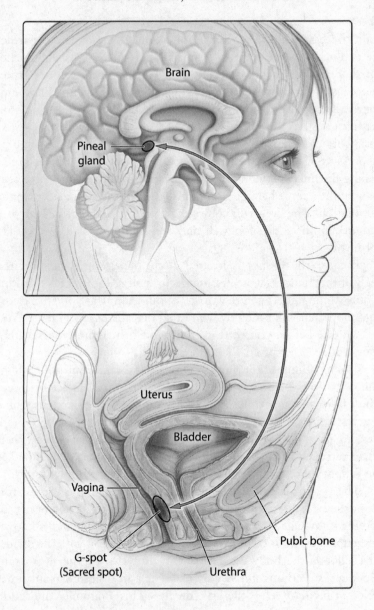

FIGURE 13: THE PINEAL GLAND AND THE G-SPOT/SACRED SPOT

How to Strengthen Your Pelvic Floor for Better Sex

Most women—and their doctors—have been taught that Kegel exercises are the key to optimal pelvic floor health. Classic Kegels involve strengthening and toning the pelvic floor muscles, particularly the pubococcygeous (PC) muscle (the same muscle you use to stop the stream of urine). The problem is this: The PC muscle is relatively small, and it's only one muscle out of an entire system of muscles that constitute the pelvic floor. Moreover, just strengthening that one small muscle won't do anything to align the sacrum or pelvis properly. If any part of the pelvis is out of alignment, it doesn't matter how much you strengthen that one PC muscle—it won't produce true pelvic floor strength and function.

As biomechanical expert Katy Bowman points out, "The pelvic floor is not supposed to be a muscle you 'train.'" In fact, compromised pelvic floor health is the end result of problems with alignment and how we habitually use our bodies. According to Bowman, about 80 percent of the population now has some kind of pelvic floor dysfunction. From my clinical experience, I would concur. The pelvic floor is an entire group of muscles and ligaments connected to the bony pelvis that is designed for continuous electrical flow based on the correct use of the legs and muscles of the trunk. This includes the diaphragm, the psoas muscle, the intercostals—actually the entire body. (One particularly telling example: Physical therapist and pelvic floor specialist Isa Herrera reports that 85 percent of women who suffer from low back pain have compromised pelvic floor muscles.) For most women, years of misalignment and incorrect leg muscle development leads to not having enough space and support for the pelvic floor muscles to maintain proper tension. As Bowman points out, a Kegel is a good way to "fake it," but the PC muscle is too small to do the work of the larger, slacking muscle groups.

If a woman has pelvic floor dysfunction, it is a sign that her entire body is collapsing from the inside. The condition results from weakness of all the muscles that attach to the bony pelvis, not just the PC muscle. That's why a Kegel contraction simply cannot do everything that needs to be done to heal all pelvic floor dysfunction. Most important, nothing about the process of growing older requires surgery or organ removal to do what proper alignment and strength are designed to do for a lifetime.

Here's what to do instead. First, most women have been taught to tuck their pelvis, but this results in excessive strain on the pelvic floor and also the low back. We are designed to have our tails out behind us. If you are in the right position, your pubic bone should be located at the bottom of your pelvis when you are standing—thus helping to hold in your pelvic organs.

To facilitate this when you're sitting, fold a towel in half lengthwise and then once again. Place this towel under your sitz bones (the bones at the very bottom of your pelvis that you literally sit on). This will help tilt your pelvis forward. Think of the pelvis as a bowl that works best when tilted forward, not backward.

When you walk, do not tuck your pelvis under. In fact, stick your tail out slightly so that you have a slight curve between the last lumbar vertebra and the first sacral vertebra, as mentioned earlier. This is what Esther Gokhale in her ingenious book *8 Steps to a Pain-Free Back* (Pendo Press, 2008) calls a J-spine. It is the normal physiologic position in which our buttocks are *behind* us (which is why we call it a "behind"); otherwise the back is straight. This is the position that little children normally assume until they learn to tuck their pelvis under and hunch their shoulders forward. It is in this physiologic position that all organs, including those in the pelvis, function optimally. (For a free online presentation of the Gokhale Method, go to www.gokhalemethod.com.)

A MORE HOLISTIC MOVEMENT PROGRAM FOR A HEALTHY PELVIS AND PELVIC FLOOR
By Katy Bowman

Just as your body dwells in the ecosystem of the planet, your pelvis lives within the ecosystem of your body. So the state of your pelvic floor depends on the state of all your body parts that attach to it. Women with pelvic floor disorders are often told to start doing Kegel exercises to strengthen their pelvic floor. This exercise prescription can tighten their pelvic floor muscles, but it overlooks the fact that pelvic floor issues can also stem from pelvic floors that are already *too* tight.

If you enjoy doing Kegels, that's fine, but consider a more whole-body approach with the exercises below. They're designed to improve the movement of the many parts surrounding and connecting to the soft tissues of your pelvis and to help you create healthy pelvic floor movement—a responsive pelvic floor that can tense *and* relax as necessary (depending on what you're doing).

Bonus: These moves don't change only the way you load your pelvis. They also change how you load your feet, knees, hips, and low back all day long.

HIPS OVER HEELS

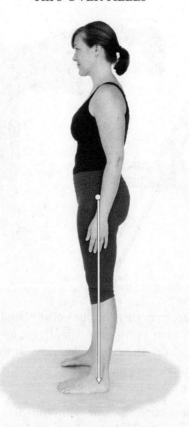

Stand sideways to a mirror and imagine a line going straight from the center of your hip to the floor (better yet, use a plumb line). Does it drop over the front of your foot? This means you're wearing your pelvis forward.

Shift your hips back until that line stacks over your ankles. You can do this move hundreds of times each day. Whenever you're just standing around, move your weight back over your heels.

You'll soon find that wearing heeled footwear of any kind makes it virtually impossible for you to get your lower body lined up in this way. (Note that even most athletic shoes have raised heels.) This is one of the reasons I suggest slowly transitioning to wearing minimalist footwear that doesn't have a heel at all—your footwear can directly limit the movements of your knees, hips, low back, and pelvis.

DOUBLE CALF STRETCH

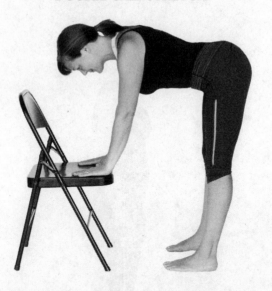

Pelvic issues are prevalent in our culture, and so is sitting. One way to strengthen your pelvis is to simply get up out of your chair more often. Once you're up, try this next exercise using your chair—it targets muscle tension you might have in your calves and hamstrings that can be pulling on your pelvis.

~ Stand facing the seat of a chair with your feet pointing forward and your legs straight. Then bend forward from your hips (without bending your knees) until your palms rest on the chair. If you can't reach the chair without bending your knees or rounding your back, add a pillow or stack of books to the seat, or move to a counter or desktop.

~ Once your arms are supported, relax your spine toward the floor, lifting your tailbone toward the ceiling. Don't force your ribs to the floor or arch your back—just relax the spine toward the ground as much as you can.

The more you lift your tailbone, the more you'll feel the tension down the back of your legs. Hold this stretch up to a minute.

LEGS ON THE WALL

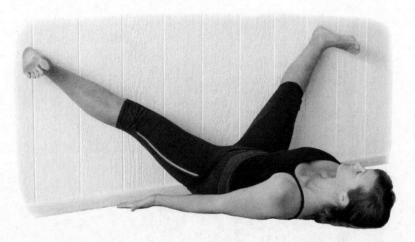

Tight inner thigh muscles can limit the motion and strength of the pelvic muscles (or perhaps vice versa). This exercise will help you introduce new movement into this area of your body.

~ Lying on your back, place your straight legs up against a wall and then back yourself away just enough to allow your pelvis to relax into a level position. There should be a little space under your waistband—if not, scoot back until that happens.

~ Keeping your legs straight, relax them away from each other until you feel a stretch in your inner thigh.

This move can be difficult, so come out of it as necessary (bringing your knees into your chest or to the side) and then return to it when you feel ready.

RECLINED SOLE-TO-SOLE SIT

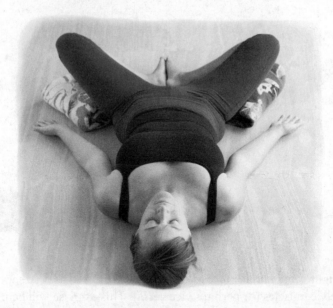

- Lie on your back on a pillow, with your knees bent, feet flat on the floor. Slowly drop your knees away from each other, placing the soles of your feet together.

- Place pillows under each knee to support yourself in this position as necessary. (You might need more pillows under one knee than under the other.) Lower the support bolsters as the position becomes more comfortable.

- Relax for at least one minute. (I'll often do my evening or morning reading in this position.) Once you've done this for a while, you can vary the move by sliding your feet farther away from or closer to your bottom (making sure the soles of your feet are still touching).

BUTT BUILDER

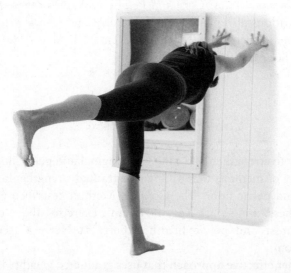

Many women are surprised to learn their butt strength matters to their pelvic health, but I've found over and over again that the function of the pelvic floor is improved by strengthening the glutes—which makes sense because they're connected to each other via the sacrum (the triangular bone at the base of your vertebral column). Be sure to do this exercise a few times a day.

~ Stand barefoot in front of a wall and place your hands on it.

~ With your hands still touching the wall, walk back and lift your left leg so all your weight is on your right leg.

~ Keeping the right leg straight (make sure you're not bending your knee), shift your weight back into your heel. Use your hands on the wall to help find the position.

~ Lower the left (floating) side of your pelvis toward the floor. This will engage the glutes on your standing leg, especially if your weight is back over your heels and the knee is straight. Again, use the wall to help you find this position. Over time, the muscles of your pelvis, hips, and legs will become stronger, and you'll be able to make this move more challenging by using your arms less.

For more pelvic floor moves, see Katy Bowman's DVD, *Nutritious Movement for a Healthy Pelvis,* and her in-depth video course,

Whole Body Biomechanics: Core and Pelvis, available on her website, www.nutritiousmovement.com. You'll also find several articles and instructional videos about better movement as a way to improved pelvic floor health.

Yoni Egg Exercises

It is quite easy to strengthen and tone your vaginal and pelvic floor muscles using a variety of methods that all involve gradual strengthening of the vaginal muscles and pelvic floor. The Gokhale Method described earlier is certainly one of these, and so are Katy Bowman's exercises above or those of physical therapist and pelvic health expert Isa Herrera (see www .pelvicpainrelief.com).

There is another effective approach that uses graduated weighted vaginal cones, which are available by prescription and act as biofeedback devices. You simply insert one and hold it in for a couple of hours, then gradually increase the weight until you can easily hold in the heaviest weight. A device known as an ApexM Pelvic Floor stimulator (see www.incontrolmedical .com) uses electrical signals and biofeedback to help strengthen the pelvic floor. My all-time favorite approach, however, is the ancient practice of using a gemstone egg with a hole drilled in it so that you can attach silk thread, dental floss, or organic hemp string with beeswax (my favorite) to it and then attach that string to various weights (like a small bag of marbles or crystals that you can add to as your strength increases) for vaginal weight lifting or exercises done lying down and pulling on the string while you hold in the egg. (See Resources.)

The use of smooth gemstone eggs for vaginal strengthening and the cultivation of sexual energy is a practice that is thousands of years old and was originally used exclusively by the royal concubines of the ancient Chinese emperors. According to ancient Taoist teachings, the toning and strengthening of the vaginal muscles and pelvic floor were powerful ways to maintain sexual energy and stamina. Today the practice has become more widely known as a way for modern women to maintain vaginal tone and enhance sexual and vital life-force energy.

Yoni Egg Practice

Yoni eggs are made from polished crystals and, like all crystals, hold and transmit energy. Rose quartz holds the energy of love, for example, while jade is an all-round healing stone. Choose the type of crystal that speaks to you.

Before using your yoni egg, program it for maximum love and healing on your behalf. Crystals can be cleansed and programmed in many ways. One of the easiest is to put the crystal in a bowl of salt water and place it in the sun for a couple of hours, although you can also cleanse the crystal by burning some sage and smudging it—which just means making sure the smoke from the burning sage goes around the egg. The easiest way to cleanse and program a crystal is with your breath, using your intention and the energy of Divine Love (see page 757). Simply hold the crystal in your palm and say, "I now imbue this crystal with Divine Love so that it functions to bring health, healing, and pleasure to my body." Then take a deep breath in. Hold it for a count of four. Then pulse your breath out through your nose or mouth into the crystal. This out-breath puts your intention into the crystal. You are now ready to use it.

Take a ten- to twelve-inch piece of silk thread, dental floss, or waxed hemp string and insert it through the hole in the egg. Tie it so that the knot is at the bottom of the egg, in a spot where it won't irritate your vaginal wall. Then lie down with your knees propped up on two pillows. Place the egg just above your pubic bone. Take some slow, deep breaths. Relax completely. Imagine your breath running energy up the back of your spine from your perineum to the top of your head and then down the front of your body and back to your perineum. This circuit is called the microcosmic orbit (see figure 14). Do two more breaths through your microcosmic orbit.

Now take your egg and wet the widest part of it with saliva (or use any kind of lubricant, including coconut oil). Hold the egg right at the opening of your vagina, and slowly insert the egg. See if you can move it up to the very top of your vagina—where the cervix is. When you have it there, squeeze the egg for a count of three while you exhale. Then inhale and relax for a count of three. Repeat three times.

Now push the egg down to the middle part of your vagina. Again, squeeze the egg for a count of three on an exhale. Relax for a count of three on an inhale. Repeat nine times.

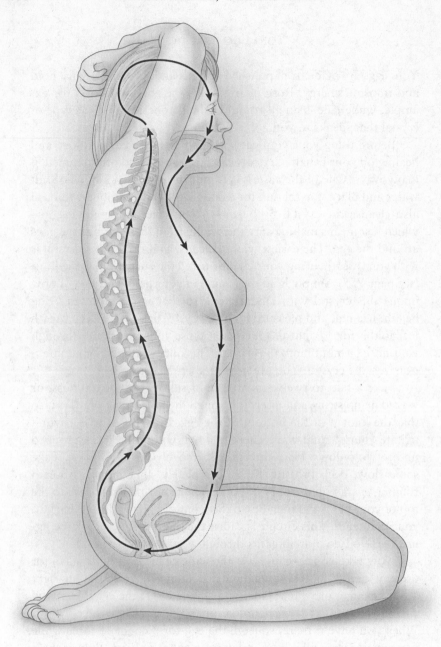

FIGURE 14: THE MICROCOSMIC ORBIT

Finally, push your egg down to the lowest part of your vagina, near the opening. Squeeze for a count of three and then relax for a count of three. Repeat nine times. (You may have to hold the egg in to keep it from popping out, but that's fine.) Now inhale deeply and imagine your breath going up the back of your spine, like a serpent, and then exhale as you imagine your breath going down the front of your body to your perineum. Repeat one time, and you're done.

Notice how you feel. With practice you will be able to sense your muscles strengthening. You will also notice better orgasms and more lubrication.

There are many, many more ways to use your yoni egg. You can also insert the egg while standing and see if you can easily move it up and down. When you can, try tying a little weight on it—like a small silk bag holding a couple of small crystals. Practice this weight lifting in each of the three segments of your vagina.

Aim for three yoni-egg exercise sessions per week. You will be amazed at how quickly your vagina and pelvic floor strengthen as well as how turned on with life force this practice will make you. (See www.rosierees.com, www.jadeegg.com, or www.kimanami.com.)

The Brain Is the Biggest Sex Organ in the Body

Although the clitoral system is clearly the most obvious erogenous area of the female body, female sexuality is not limited simply to the genitalia. Daniel Amen, M.D., author of *Sex on the Brain* (Harmony Books, 2007), writes, "Even though it feels genital, the vast majority of love and sex occurs in the brain. Your brain decides who is attractive to you, how to get a date, how well you do on the date, what to do with the feelings that develop. How long those feelings last, when to commit, and how well you do as a mate and a parent." The brain is also the seat of orgasms, which is why women with spinal cord injuries who can't feel anything below the waist can still have orgasms—and why a friend of mine had her first orgasm when she first heard the Beatles sing "Michelle." Sex researcher Gina Ogden, Ph.D., has found that some women can reach orgasm just from thinking about things that are erotically stimulating to them.[10] This is why Isabel Allende quipped, "For women, the best aphrodisiacs are words. The G-spot is in the ears. He who looks for it below there is wasting his time."

OUR CULTURAL INHERITANCE

The functioning of our sexual organs and our sexual response are determined in large part by our cultural conditioning concerning sexuality, usually programmed in childhood and also by the culture in which we live. To understand female sexual response and the workings of the organs involved in it, we must also understand women's cultural inheritance.

Naomi Wolf writes about this in her *New York Times* bestselling book *Vagina: A New Biography* (Ecco, 2012). "When a woman feels threatened or unsafe," she explains, "the sympathetic nervous system . . . kicks in. This system regulates the 'fight or flight' response." Research shows, she continues, "that a threatening environment—which can include even vague verbal threats centered on the vagina or dismissive language about the vagina—can close down female sexual response." Evidence suggests that if a woman is raped or suffers early sexual trauma, the effects stay in the body, potentially permanently altering the sympathetic nervous system—including breathing, heart rate, blood pressure, and sexual response. Because of this, Wolf says, rape and sexual assault should be considered a form of injury to the brain and body, even a "variant of castration." She adds that the same physiological changes (including problems with arousal) can happen when a woman feels diminished or unsafe in any other setting, including at work or at school—and the effect begins even before she is consciously aware of feeling unsafe. If this goes on long enough, it also affects her ability to effectively perform her work (whether in school or in her job) as well as her overall capacity for joy, hopefulness, and creativity. We are seeing evidence of this over and over again with women speaking out in the #MeToo movement, telling their stories of how sexual mistreatment—from harassment to rape—has greatly affected their health and their lives.

Furthermore, in this society, sexuality is closely linked with body image and self-esteem. There's a saying, "Men and women will never be equal until a woman can be bald and have a potbelly and still be considered good-looking." Women are brought up to feel that they deserve sexual pleasure only if they look a certain way or weigh a certain amount. Therefore, many women feel that they don't look "good" enough to fully receive sexual pleasure—because their breasts aren't big enough, their genitals don't look like those of a porn star, and so on. Not only that, there's also the fear of getting pregnant.

There is reason to believe that in ancient pre-patriarchal times, women knew how to control their fertility naturally and understood the importance of sexual pleasure as a natural part of human experience. It is also entirely possible that female sexuality existed then in an entirely different mindset that was free from the stigma of shame or even free of monogamy. Indeed, women at that time were not controlled by men. In their groundbreaking book *Sex at Dawn: The Prehistoric Origins of Modern Sexuality* (Harper-Collins, 2010), authors Christopher Ryan and Cacilda Jetha posit that monogamy is a more recent approach to sexuality that didn't exist in prehistoric times. They hypothesize that one of the reasons women are so vocal during sex (unless programmed not to be) is that historically speaking, it was a way of attracting potential mates. Back then, before anything was known about paternity (in other words, before patriarchy), women had sex with those men whose qualities they most wanted to have in a child. So if a man was a good musician and that was what she valued, she'd have sex with him. And then, perhaps in the same session (for her), she'd have sex with someone else who was particularly strong, or kind. It was believed that having sex with a man imbued your potential child with that man's qualities. One can scarcely imagine this kind of approach in modern patriarchy.

Our current culture also believes in the "big bang" theory of heterosexual pleasure, which holds that the thrusting of the penis into the vagina is the most important part of sexuality. Though this is true for some women, it is not true for others. Naomi Wolf's *Vagina,* mentioned earlier in this chapter, further points out that the pelvic nerve anatomy is different in different women—making it easier for some to experience orgasm with intercourse, while others will require different types of stimulation. The truth is that intercourse is only one aspect of sexuality and pleasure (even though it is quite often the only part of sex that has, until recently, been shown in the mainstream media), and women who do not enjoy it or who don't reach orgasm through it need not feel abnormal in any way. For some women, penis-in-vagina intercourse—the kind that we're taught is the "real" thing—is not particularly satisfying. Therefore, many women fake orgasm to make their male partners feel that they are good lovers. This is a shame and robs both members of the couple of true pleasure and intimacy. Research demonstrates that clitoral, vaginal, and uterine stimulation, or a combination of these, leads to orgasm—along with the proper mindset, of course.[11] Only 25 percent of women regularly reach orgasm through intercourse, though a woman can train herself to experience this more regularly.

Unfortunately, it is not uncommon for *frequency of intercourse* to be the sole measure by which the quality of a sexual relationship is judged—especially in medical circles.[12] It is clear, however, that many other factors determine actual relationship quality besides the number of times per week that a couple has intercourse.

The quality of a person's sex life should also not be judged by the number of sexual partners he or she has or has had. An unhealthy, potentially destructive sex life is one in which a woman medicates her fears of loneliness and abandonment by having sex with people she does not love or respect, using sex addictively. On the other hand, having multiple sex partners is not necessarily a bad thing, either, so long as neither of the partners in a given sexual relationship is using the other in a dishonest or hurtful way, and both partners are getting pleasure. But women who had childhoods associated with sexual abuse, either subtle or blatant, often have unhealthy, degrading sexual relationships that make them feel bad about themselves and do not give them pleasure.

It's worth noting that several ancient spiritual traditions, tantra among them, teach that having sex is not only an intimate physical coupling but also an intimate energetic one. We literally take into ourselves the energies of our partners, and the more we have sex with a particular person, the greater the effect their energy field will have on ours. When we have sex with partners with whom we are more energetically and spiritually aligned, this energetic exchange benefits both parties. But when we feel pressured for whatever reason to have sex with those we do not feel energetically aligned with—especially when those partners feel free to direct their negative energy toward us even outside the bedroom—the effect can be detrimental. Lisa Chase Patterson sums it up this way: "Never sleep with someone you wouldn't want to be."

Alexandra D'Amour, founder of the website On Our Moon (www .onourmoon.com), wrote about having to forgive herself for not heeding her intuition about a creepy acquaintance who eventually raped her after she blacked out from drinking at a party: "I thought of all the times I've had sex because I was uncomfortable. The times I've had sex to please a new boy. The times I told myself that sex was how I could get someone to like me. Of all the times I felt loved by a man when what he was really feeling was lust. Of the times I've had sex to keep a relationship from ending. I thought of all the times I walked into a bar knowing that sex was my power. Crying uncontrollably, I realized I've been giving away my power for years. I've handed my body and my soul over to someone not worthy too many times."[13]

The cultural imperative that judges a woman's worth by her attachment to a man and by her sexual attractiveness to men—all men—runs very deep. And that cultural imperative is aided and abetted by the fact that what we deem valuable in our media and everywhere else is what appeals mostly to men. An example of this is the rating site Rotten Tomatoes, which people often consult when deciding what movie to watch, either in the theater or on TV. In a press conference at the 2015 London Film Festival, before the U.K. premiere of the movie *Suffragette,* Academy Award–winning actress Meryl Streep reported that at that time, Rotten Tomatoes included reviews from only 168 women along with 760 men, skewing the "perceived wisdom" of what we consider worth watching in a way she described as being not just unfair but infuriating. She also reported her discovery that the New York Film Critics Circle, an organization of film reviewers from New York City–based publications whose annual awards are often considered harbingers of Oscar nominations, at that time consisted of two women and thirty-seven men. Men and women often differ on what they enjoy or think is worth watching. While there's nothing wrong with that, you can see the problem when one gender so overwhelmingly gets to represent (and therefore shape) public opinion. (By the way, a Rotten Tomatoes–style movie review website called CherryPicks that features only female critics launched in 2018; see www.thecherrypicks.com.)

As a result of this and other factors, far too many women turn themselves into pretzels trying to become what they think men want. This is the basis for all those women's magazine articles on "must-know techniques that will blow his mind!" Clearly many women believe that it is their duty to fulfill their partner's sexual desires and frequently ignore their own erotic or physical needs. The key to pleasurable sex for heterosexual couples is the knowledge that it takes the average woman about thirty minutes of lovemaking before reaching orgasm. The average man can have an orgasm only five to ten minutes after lovemaking begins. Women too often engage in sexual behavior from which they receive very little more than an unwanted pregnancy, discomfort, or various diseases. A study on dyspareunia (painful sexual intercourse), for example, found that of 324 women surveyed, only 39 percent had never had it, while 27.5 percent had suffered from it at some point in their lives. Fully 33.5 percent (105 women) still had painful intercourse at the time of the study at least some of the time, while 25 percent of them had the problem virtually all the time. Yet the frequency of intercourse among all of the groups of women was virtually the same. The study also found that most of the women had never discussed the problem with their healthcare practitioner. This means that a very large number of women are suffering during sex and not saying anything about it. Since the transmission of sexually acquired diseases in women is increased by any break in the integrity of the vaginal mucosa, not only is dyspareunia painful, but it can also put a woman at risk from the trauma to her tissues.[14]

How to Avoid Painful Intercourse

Most women experience pain during intercourse if penetration occurs before their arousal has been sufficient to lift and move the uterus and cervix out of the way. In these cases, the ovaries may be hit during repeated thrusting, resulting in pain. This generally doesn't occur when a couple allows enough time for full female sexual arousal prior to actual intercourse.

Women who have persistent painful intercourse should be checked for scar tissue from old infections or endometriosis. For those who do have adhesions from old infections, injury, or prior surgery, the Wurn technique improves sexual pleasure in over 80 percent of the women who use it to treat pelvic pain or infertility. (See chapter 5, page 157.)

Scar tissue in the pelvis can cause adhesions that interfere with the normal range of motion for pelvic organs during sex. It can also interfere with blood flow to the pelvic floor, reducing lubrication and thereby resulting in painful sex (which also affects desire). Women can develop scar tissue in the pelvis from accidents, infection, abdominal surgery, radiation, and childbirth (including cesarean sections). Ellen Heed, a pioneer in therapeutic sexological bodywork, notes that 70 percent of women have problems with some type of scar tissue after birthing. Heed has helped hundreds of women heal pain and discomfort caused by pelvic floor trauma and injury. She and fellow sexological bodyworker Kimberly Johnson (author of *The Fourth Trimester: A Postpartum Guide to Healing Your Body, Balancing Your Emotions, and Restoring Your Vitality* [Shambhala, 2017]), recently cofounded a school called STREAM (Scar Tissue Remediation Education and Management) to train bodyworkers and somatic professionals in helping both women and men suffering from various scar-tissue-related problems using hands-on manipulation (including therapeutic genital touch), trauma counseling, self-care protocols, support for lifestyle and nutritional changes, and active relaxation tools. STREAM's cutting-edge therapy not only helps manage (and often repair) scar tissue but also works to minimize inflammation and engage the nervous system to change a client's relationship to pain. It's the first multidimensional hands-on training for professionals that addresses scar tissue in a way that can improve sexual, reproductive, and overall health. (For more information, see www.scartissueremediation.com/stream.)

In addition to enduring pain, some women put their very lives at risk when they have sex. This is obviously true for those who have no other way to make a living other than sex work. But sometimes a woman's self-esteem and sense of worth are so low that she uses the only thing that she has been taught is worthwhile—her sexuality—as a way to gain status. And at other times—as in the case of the Hollywood "casting couch," when having sex with a director or producer is the only way for a woman to get a particular role—women are coerced into sex as a condition of getting or keeping a job. This point was brought home to me years ago when the news came out that basketball star Magic Johnson had AIDS. A November 1991 article in *Time* magazine pointed out, "Sex and sports have almost become synonymous." The article reported that "Wilt Chamberlain boasts having slept with 20,000 women—an average of 1.4 per day for 40 years." It quoted another basketball player: "After I arrived in L.A. in 1979, I did my best to accommodate as many women as I could—most of them through unprotected sex."[15] This problem is significant. In the United States, one in four people who have HIV/AIDS is a woman, and of those women, 89 percent got it from heterosexual contact (and one in eight doesn't even know she's infected).

The *Time* article went on to say that "for women, many of whom don't have meaningful work, the only way to identify themselves is to say whom they have slept with."[16] In their own eyes, these women weren't *nobody* any longer: They had had sex with a sports star. Even though this man didn't care for them at all or even remember them, they had achieved some perverse kind of status by letting their bodies be used in this way. One need only listen to the lyrics of popular rap songs to see that this attitude is still too common.

Women who have experienced rape and incest have even greater trouble than non-abused women in establishing fulfilling sexual relationships that are free of abusive elements and victimized behavior. Many of these women have never had a sexual encounter that was supportive and pleasurable. Given all this, it's no surprise that in a 2008 study on female sexual dysfunction, Harvard researcher Jan Shifren, M.D., found that 43 percent of the 32,000 respondents, age eighteen and up, reported sexual problems. However, only 12 percent were upset by them.[17] I found that part particularly ironic because funding for this study came from Boehringer Ingelheim, the drug company that developed flibanserin (sold under the brand name Addyi), a drug for female sexual dysfunction (FSD). Drug companies have repeatedly tried to come up with the "female Viagra," and, after much controversy, the drug was finally approved by the FDA in 2015. What's amazing about this drug is the fact that its very common side effects (mild to moderate dizziness, drowsiness, nausea, and fatigue) can interact with alcohol to produce severely low blood pressure and loss of consciousness. So much for a romantic dinner and a glass of wine followed by lovemaking. For all these side effects, the "benefit" was reported to be one-half of one additional sexually satisfying encounter per month.[18] And in 2019, the FDA approved another drug, Vylessi, for premenopausal women with low sex drive. In clinical trials 40 percent of women who took the drug experienced nausea! I hate to break the news, fellas, but female sexuality is simply too complex to be reduced to a quick pharmacologic fix. What we currently call FSD is simply a reaction to our cultural programming about sexuality.

Patricia Reis, a therapist who worked at my former office for a number of years, counseled one of my patients, Lydia, for several years concerning her chronic vaginitis. Reis learned that Lydia's husband liked oral sex a great deal and rented numerous pornographic movies to try to stimulate her to perform oral sex. Lydia had been raped as a teenager. During the rape she had had to perform oral sex on her assailant. She recalled that the odor and the trauma of the event were so bad that the thought of oral sex had disgusted her ever since. Fortunately for her, after two years of therapy she was finally able to tell her husband firmly that oral sex was not something she could cooperate with willingly at that point. She had felt used by him sexually for years and needed to distance herself from this kind of sex for a while and reestablish comfort with her own sexual desires before she would be ready to consider the possibility of lovingly providing oral sex.

Whenever people use sex to diminish, control, or harm others, it does not contribute to the health of either participant. Many women have experienced the controlling attitudes and negative effects of certain religions on female sexuality. The tenets of the Roman Catholic and other Christian churches degrade sexuality—a normal human function—and subordinate it to reproduction. The consequences of such repression are seen in the problems women have in expressing their sexuality as well as in the sexual deviancy of some church representatives, such as priests who have sexually abused children. The Academy Award–winning movie *Spotlight* highlighted how common this abuse of power is worldwide.

Many women are so invested in their sexual relationship at the expense of themselves that they repeatedly put themselves at risk for pregnancy or sexually transmitted diseases rather than jeopardize the relationship. The pattern often starts early, in the teen years. A teenage girl wrote a letter to Ann Landers in which she complained that all her boyfriend wanted to do was have sex. He barely even talked to her anymore, and they no longer did much of anything together except have sex. She was afraid to say anything to him, however, for fear of losing him!

Writer Peggy Orenstein, author of *Don't Call Me Princess* (HarperCollins, 2018), spent three years talking to girls ages fifteen to twenty about their experiences with sex and how they felt about it. In her 2016 TED Talk, she says she found that while young women may feel entitled to engage in sexual behavior, they don't necessarily feel entitled to *enjoy* it.[19] Citing a study published the year before in the *Journal of Sexual Medicine,* she notes, "In the largest study ever conducted on American sexual behavior, young women reported pain in their sexual encounters 30 percent of the time. They also used words like 'depressing,' 'humiliating,' and 'degrading.' Young men never used that language."[20]

She adds poignantly, "Girls' early sexual experience shouldn't be something that they get over." Orenstein also mentions University of Michigan psychologist Sara McClelland, Ph.D., who found young women are more likely than young men to use their partner's pleasure as a measure of their satisfaction. Young women report sexual satisfaction levels equal to or greater than young men's, she says, noting that this is deceptive because, as she puts it, "the absence of pain is a very low bar for your own sexual fulfill-ment."

While I find this alarming, it doesn't surprise me. I lectured at a local private high school several years ago on pro-choice issues. Afterward, several young men came up to me and told me that the girls they were having sex with didn't ask them to use condoms—in fact, they had even told these boys, "It's okay—you don't have to use anything." These girls (they were upper-middle-class and mostly white) perceived discussing contraception with their boyfriends as putting their social worth at stake. Some of today's middle-school girls are providing oral and even anal sex as a way to win the atten-tion of boys. Women have been socialized for centuries to put their physical bodies at risk in order to sustain interpersonal relationships that really don't support them or their well-being. Although the birth rate for teens in the United States is now at its lowest point in seventy years, that rate is still higher than it is in other developed nations.[21] Every year, nearly 2 in every 100 teenage girls in the United States has a child. Condom use by young people has increased from just over 46 percent in 1991 to just over 60 per-cent in 2011, but that still leaves almost 30 percent of teens unprotected.[22] Since a sexually active teen who does not use contraceptives has a 90 percent chance of getting pregnant within one year,[23] failure to use protection, against both pregnancy and disease, is still a serious concern in this country.

RECLAIMING OUR EROTIC SELVES

Here's the good news. Regardless of what has happened to us as children or what we've learned from our culture, our brains and bodies have the abil-ity to change. This is known as plasticity. And when it comes to experiencing a fulfilling sex life at any age, this is great news. When we reclaim our own sexuality on our own terms, the whole world changes. When we learn how to turn ourselves on to life, instead of waiting for a Prince Charming to come along and do it for us, then we hold the reins of fulfillment in our own hands.

The most important thing to know is that a turned-on woman turns on the whole world. Think of the opening line to the old *Mary Tyler Moore Show* theme song ("Who can turn the world on with her smile?"). It's the truth. A turned-on woman is what turns on a man (or another woman). An angry, resentful woman does just the opposite. A business executive col-league of mine recently came up to me to thank me for helping his wife. It turns out that she had overheard me say that men like to please women and that a turned-on woman is what turns on a man. She went home and asked him if this was true. He said, "Absolutely!" From that moment on, their sex life reached a whole new level of satisfaction for both of them.

I first learned of this effect while teaching at Mama Gena's School of Womanly Arts in New York City. I met a woman in her sixties who told me that her husband no longer needed to take Viagra to get erections. This was a direct result of her getting in touch with her own pleasure through participating in the School of Womanly Arts. A lightbulb went off for me. Increasing nitric oxide is the mechanism through which the erection-enhancing drugs work to increase blood flow to the penis. This woman had become "virtual Viagra" for her husband. Her turn-on had transferred to him and resulted in higher levels of nitric oxide and better erections. The implications of this are vast. The number one sexual dysfunction in women right now is lack of desire. This is the FSD referred to earlier. If a woman doesn't know how to turn herself on, she won't be able to turn her mate on, either. He may then turn to an erection-enhancing drug. Imagine how much healthier the world would be if women knew, in the words of Regena Thomashauer (Mama Gena), "how to put the key in their own ignition, and then drive down the road." (I've written extensively about this in *The Secret Pleasures of Menopause* [Hay House, 2008] and *The Secret Pleasures of Menopause Playbook* [Hay House, 2009].)

Program for Consciously Reclaiming the Erotic in Your Life

Sexual energy, or eros, is life force that permeates all of creation and is part of the joyfulness of life. It is exactly the opposite of thanatos—the force leading to death. For too long, our culture has dwelt on thanatos, without a balance from eros. It has taught us to fear, denigrate, and suppress our own eroticism, instead of using our erotic feelings as a sure sign that we are getting in the flow of a healthy and fulfilled life. Your body will tell you when you are heading in the direction of life-giving pleasure. You will actually feel it right in your genitals!

Before you get to the steps below, I want to stress that every man and woman I know has been, to one degree or another, adversely affected by our culture's view of sex and the way it exploits and objectifies both men and women. Almost no women look the way our culture's sex symbols look. Most of us don't accept and love our bodies fully. Many women have been sexually abused in some way. Others have endured very hurtful comments from partners that have damaged their self-esteem. Men have also been harmed by our culture's view of dominator sex. (See "A Word About Pornography," later in this chapter.) Many feel inadequate and worry about being acceptable to women.

In the end, both men and women are looking for unconditional love and acceptance as well as sensual pleasure. Carl Jung called eros "relatedness" because eros is all about relationships as well. But most of us were never taught to be good lovers.

Here's the good news. If you want to experience your birthright of glorious, healing sex, you can begin right now, with yourself. Whether you are single or in a relationship, or whether you're gay, straight, bisexual, or transgender, when you change yourself and your relationship to your sexuality, then your outer experience of sexual relationships with others will change and improve as well. Guaranteed.

Consciously Decide to Allow Pleasure and Life Force to Flow Through You. Start affirming yourself as sexy. I don't care how old you are or what you look like. Trust me. This is an inside job. Say the following out loud to yourself at least twice a day: "I am a sexy, irresistible woman." Or my favorite: "I am Aphrodite. I make love with wild, unleashed abandon. I am an irresistible force of nature." Make up your own affirmations. Remember, it all begins in your mind. Let the power of words and your mind consciously shape your sexual experience. Steve Bodansky, Ph.D., and Vera Bodansky, Ph.D., teach that a woman's desire is an enormously powerful force for creating a more pleasurable life. I agree. When a woman feels sexy and consciously knows how to turn herself on by feeling sexy and exuding sexuality (just to please herself), she sends out a signal to the world that changes what and whom she attracts. She emulates the egg that sends the signal to the sperm.

An intriguing study recently done in Belgium illustrates this perfectly. Trained sexologists were able to discern with 80 percent accuracy if a woman has vaginal orgasms merely by observing the way she walks in public. Researchers found that vaginally orgasmic women have a more fluid, energetic, sensual walk with a longer stride and greater spinal rotation. This, they concluded, could reflect "the free, unblocked energetic flow from the legs through the pelvis to the spine."[24]

Here's another suggestion. In her playful book *Life Magic: The 7 Keys to Unlocking Your Magical Life* (Miramax, 2005), gifted clairvoyant Laura Bushnell recommends the following: Imagine that a person you consider very sexy (e.g., Sophia Loren, Salma Hayek—your choice) is pressed against your left side (the feminine receptive side). Breathe in her essence for about two minutes, imagining her sexy qualities permeating your body. Do this twice per day for about six weeks. You will notice a change. Consciously decide to do things that make you feel sexy. Wear sexy underwear under your business suit. Take more sensual baths. Read sexy romance novels (a male friend of mine jokingly refers to these as "clitoriture"). Fantasize more. (I know this is difficult when you have little kids and are working full-time. But, as with all good things, you have to consciously decide to have a good sex life.)

Focus on Sex and the Erotic More. If you want your sex life to improve, you have to spend time thinking about sex and the things that turn you on.

Though it is true that our culture is obsessed with sex and uses it to sell everything, few people actually make it a priority in their lives. We become voyeurs, not direct participants. It's time for that to change. Developing the capacity for sexual pleasure is a skill that can be learned like any other skill. The more you practice, the better you become. It's a delightful feedback loop, and the health benefits are well worth it.

Get Fit and Healthy. A sexy person is a healthy person. Many women find that the healthier they become, the more libido they have. Take a good multivitamin and do aerobic exercise three times a week for twenty minutes. Strengthen and tone your pelvic floor using a yoni egg. Reclaim your posture—read *8 Steps to a Pain-Free Back* (Pendo Press, 2008) by Esther Gokhale with Susan Adams. You can't be at your sexual best without good blood flow to the pelvis; the right movement patterns and right nutrients help with this. Make sure you are getting adequate sunlight exposure and that your vitamin D levels are optimal. There is a very direct correlation between sun exposure, vitamin D, and testosterone levels. One recent study on testosterone-deficient men showed that vitamin D supplements increased testosterone levels by more than 25 percent.[25] Another study showed a linear relationship between testosterone levels and vitamin D levels (up to a point).[26] While most such studies have been done on men, the same is inevitably true for women, as at least one study so far indicates.[27]

Ancient Taoist practices, still taught today, view sexual energy as life energy. When it is consciously directed during meditation, this energy can help rebuild organs within the body. Sexual energy is one of our most powerful energies for creating health. By using sexual energy consciously, whether we are in a relationship or not, we can tap into a true source of youth and vitality. One of my favorite ways of doing this involves using a yoni egg for strength, flexibility, dexterity, and tone, which I have already mentioned.

The vagina, like the sole of the foot, the ear, and the palm of the hand, also has reflexology points that correspond to the major organs. The use of the yoni egg stimulates these areas in a healthful way.[28]

Although it takes time to learn these techniques, every woman's health can benefit from developing her pelvic floor and vaginal muscles. Women who have healthy, strong pelvic muscles are less prone to vaginal problems and urinary stress incontinence, and they tend to have more fulfilling sexual functioning with better pelvic blood flow, better vaginal lubrication, and stronger orgasms. (For women who have experienced sexual or other pelvic trauma, I highly recommend seeing a physical therapist who specializes in pelvic floor rehabilitation. A good alternative would be a physical therapist who is skilled at the Wurn technique; see page 157.)

A note about medications: It is well known that certain antidepressant medications decrease libido. Ironically, new research is also showing that oral contraceptives, the effectiveness of which has long made women feel

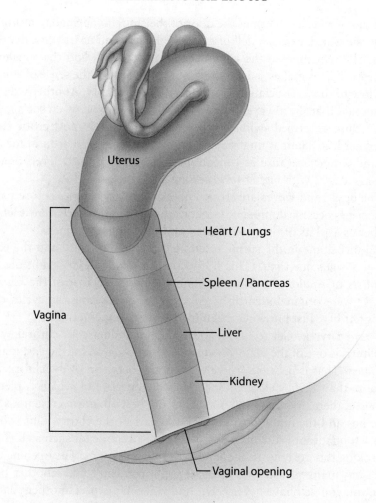

Uterus

Heart / Lungs

Spleen / Pancreas

Liver

Vagina

Kidney

Vaginal opening

FIGURE 15: VAGINAL REFLEXOLOGY ZONES

freer to have sex without worrying about pregnancy, might actually contribute to long-term sexual dysfunction because the pill lowers testosterone levels—even after women discontinue taking it. (See the section on oral contraceptives in chapter 11, "Our Fertility," for more information.) If you are on either of these medications, you can still experience very satisfying sex by using my suggestions to help develop more robust pleasure pathways in the brain.

Connect with Nature. They don't call it the "birds and the bees" for nothing. Sexuality is abundantly reflected in nature. One of my friends recalled that when she went out the door of the church one Sunday morning in spring, the warm, earthy smell of a newly plowed field nearby awakened her senses. She remembered the combination of the smell and the sunshine as very erotic.[29] This makes sense—the brain pathways for the sense of smell are very close to those associated with arousal and sexuality. Another woman, a lesbian, said that she always thinks of the Grand Canyon when she's making love. A third described swimming with dolphins as the most erotic experience of her life.[30] Sunbathing is also associated with sexual arousal for many men and women because as I mentioned earlier, vitamin D levels are positively associated with higher testosterone levels.

The ocean and waves are erotic images for many people. Before patriarchal societies became dominant, fertility, sexuality, and nature were celebrated together as aspects of the same energy and the same phenomena. The pagan festival of Beltane in the spring celebrated human sexuality and the earth's fertility at the same time. (This festival is beautifully described in the book *The Mists of Avalon*, by Marion Zimmer Bradley.) Most of the Christian holidays were originally earth-based festivals, celebrating the cycles of the earth's fertility. Just knowing this information is empowering.

Know Thyself. Get to know your body, including your clitoral system. The clitoris is one of the main keys to sexual satisfaction for the vast majority of women. That is because, as we've seen, the outer tip of the clitoris alone has more than 8,000 nerve endings, the sole purpose of which is pleasure. Of course, there are many other areas of the body that are erogenous, such as the lips and the nipples. In general, the part of the clitoris that is on the upper left quadrant is the most sensitive. Using a lubricant such as K-Y Jelly, try stroking this area, noticing the pleasurable sensations. The opening of the vagina has many pleasurable areas as well. You can't take another person where you yourself have never been. And you can't expect another person to know how to please you if you can't please yourself. So commit to self-pleasuring (which the Taoists call self-cultivation) twice per week for thirty minutes each time in order to learn exactly what kinds of strokes you like. Then you can teach your partner.

In her book *Five Minutes to Orgasm Every Time You Make Love: Female Orgasm Made Simple* (JPS Publications, 2000), author D. Claire Hutchins makes the point that the most sexually satisfied women are those who know what to do to please themselves—and then do it even with a partner, including stimulating their own clitorises so that they reach orgasm every time. Taking responsibility for one's own pleasure takes the onus off the partner to "make it happen." In the case of heterosexual partnerships, it's as much of a burden for a guy to feel that it's his job to bring a woman to orgasm as it would be for a woman to believe that it is her job to bring a guy to orgasm. (Can you imagine the pressure of that?)

Noting that both men and women take about the same amount of time to reach orgasm through self-pleasuring (about four minutes), Hutchins explodes the myth that it always takes women much longer than men. The reason it takes longer for women during sex (thirty minutes as opposed to about ten minutes for men) is because women are socialized to be more inhibited in bed than males. We worry far more about how we look. And if we don't look like *Playboy* centerfolds, we're not sure we deserve sexual pleasure or attention. Note that most men who have potbellies or who are bald don't worry at all about deserving a good sex life! Hutchins also points out that a missing link for many women is using some good fantasies to turn them on. Interestingly, studies have shown that women are as aroused by visually erotic material as men are. But we've been led to believe that we're not supposed to be. Remember, a fantasy doesn't hurt anyone. It doesn't have to be about something you would actually do. But if the thought of having sex with a gorgeous stranger in an elevator (or whatever does it for you) works, then use it! The range of sexual desires and fantasies that satisfy people are as varied as our fingerprints. You shouldn't be ashamed of asking for what turns you on from a partner, including acting out a fantasy, as long as the activity is consensual and doesn't involve the degradation or harming of another. Sometimes what a woman desires sexually may be far removed from what our society considers "normal," but as long as no one gets hurt, that's fine.

When you use your imagination to turn yourself on, your body will respond in kind because of the power of the mind-body connection. Frankly, one of the very best fantasies for every woman is to imagine herself as sexy and irresistible. Here's a fantasy affirmation that really helps: "I love the pleasure that my body gives me and I always experience orgasm quickly and easily."

In addition to fantasy, I also recommend using the woman-on-top position for intercourse so that the clitoris is maximally stimulated. Just as a man knows exactly how to move during intercourse to get maximal pleasure from the sensations, a woman on top can do exactly the same thing. And if she needs help, she can also use her finger (or a vibrator) to give her clitoris extra stimulation while in the on-top position.

Consciously Increase Your Capacity for Pleasure. Understand that we humans are capable of far more pleasure than we've been led to believe. It's now common knowledge, for example, that many women are multiorgasmic. What most people don't know is that men can be, too. It is possible to learn how to reprogram your central nervous system so that you literally feel more and more with less and less stimulation. You can train your body to become multiorgasmic simply by learning how to relax and "wake up" to more erotic feeling throughout your body. Sex educator Jack Johnston has put together a very effective process to teach you how to retrain the nervous system to experience more pleasure through the use of deep relaxation and a very specific sound (see www.multiples.com). I've tried it. It works. You can also learn how to extend your orgasms. This is done by relaxing fully, opening your throat, and making a sound that starts low and gets higher the closer you get to orgasm, becoming a high-pitched singing sound the moment an orgasm begins. Men can learn how to have an orgasm without ejaculating (these two reflexes are actually separate). All of these approaches also increase nitric oxide throughout the body.

A WORD ABOUT PORNOGRAPHY

Explicit sexual images are as old as humanity. However, the Internet has created an entirely new problem for human sexuality—the ability to see thousands of explicit images in a short period of time, each of which creates a quick hit of the feel-good neurochemical dopamine. With each additional "hit" of dopamine, there is the desire for more—and more. In his book *The Hacking of the American Mind* (Avery, 2017), Robert H. Lustig, M.D., points out that dopamine (whether from sugar, alcohol, pornography, or "likes" on social media) results in fleeting but unsustainable happiness. What brings true peace and a sustainable quality of life is more serotonin in the brain. And this comes only through fulfilling relationships, eye-to-eye contact with loved ones, meditation, and making a contribution. You can't buy it.

In his book *The Brain That Changes Itself: Stories of Personal Triumph from the Frontiers of Brain Science,* neuropsychiatrist Norman Doidge, M.D., points out that our brains have two pleasure systems. One regulates "appetitive" pleasure, the pleasure of desire, and the other one regulates what is called "consummatory" pleasure, the pleasure of satisfying a desire. Doidge points out that our brains are quite malleable when it comes to using pornography. We have the ability to create new brain maps that reinforce the pathways connecting pornographic viewing with excitatory pleasure—the kind that releases dopamine. More and more research is discovering that pornography is not a healthy and pleasurable outlet for sexual tension—in fact, it increases and exacerbates it. Doidge notes that many of his male patients often craved pornography but didn't actually like it. Worse yet, exposure to pornography (for both men and women) decreases sexual satisfaction with one's partner. What it delivers is addiction, tolerance, and an eventual decrease in pleasure. Journalist Pamela Paul reached similar conclusions in her survey of pornography users, detailed in her book *Pornified: How*

Pornography Is Transforming Our Lives, Our Relationships, and Our Families (Henry Holt, 2005). She found that for many pornography users, viewing porn can quickly become a slippery slope where viewers seek out and become inured to things they have previously found disgusting, such as group sex, bestiality, child pornography, and genital torturing. In some, this can lead to addiction.

In today's world, most young people—especially boys—are getting their sexual education through pornography. This means that boys as young as twelve are already being set up for sexual addiction and difficulty with future relationships. One of my urologist friends points out that he is seeing young men in their twenties with erectile dysfunction—they can't get it up during sex because their brain and body arousal circuits have been co-opted by habitual porn viewing. And as a result, they are unable to have healthy sustainable sexual relationships with actual human beings. One of my former patients, recently married, was wondering why her new husband—whom she was deeply in love with—kept putting off having sex with her. She later discovered the porn on his computer. When she confronted him, he said, "All men do this. Back off." Tragic.

I have a clinical psychologist friend who counsels priests. One of his jobs is to try to get them off porn. Here's what he tells them: "Those who create pornography are not your friends. Do not consume these images to become sexually aroused. They are not healthy in any way. I am not your spiritual counselor, so I won't tell you not to self-pleasure. What I will tell you is that it's far healthier for you to use your own imagination when you do—not porn." He told me that this approach is working quite well.

Bottom line: Be very, very careful when it comes to viewing porn. It is not harmless. It harms society at many levels, robbing us of true intimacy and pleasure. It also has enormous adverse implications for families and children—especially if it is violent or degrading. (For details on this, read *The Social Costs of Pornography: A Statement of Findings and Recommendations* [The Witherspoon Institute, 2010] by Mary Eberstadt and Mary Anne Layden.) The good news is that despite the enormous amount of porn consumed on the Internet, only one in four Internet users actually logs on to a porn site regularly. So despite what we see in movies and television, where it is "hip" to use porn, many people know better.

There is a quiet revolution going on as women discover sexual pleasure on their own terms and then teach it to the men in their lives. I heard the following story from one of my newsletter subscribers. "For years my sex life has been influenced by my belief that men's sexual needs come first. Though I can reach orgasm most of the time, I have really focused on my husband, not myself. To tell you the truth, sex had become pretty ordinary in my marriage. I used to joke that my husband and I were in a same-sex marriage—the same sex over and over again. Then a friend gave me the book *It's My Pleasure* (Free Press, 2005) by Maria and Maya Rodale and I started to think more and more about the importance of adding more pleasure to my life. I was also drawn to the book *Extended Massive Orgasm: How You Can Give and Receive Intense Sexual Pleasure* (Hunter House, 2000) by Steve Bodansky, Ph.D., and Vera Bodansky, Ph.D. I know from my work as a biofeedback therapist that we have the capacity to change our perception of pain simply by focusing on our bodies differently. Well, the same thing is true with pleasure. I followed the directions in the Bodanskys' book about learning how to take the time to turn myself on. I started to feel my body differently—not just my genitals, my entire body. The deliberate pursuit of pleasure has revolutionized my entire life, both in the bedroom and out."

In their book, the Bodanskys describe a technique called Extended Massive Orgasm (EMO), which is designed to enhance orgasmic pleasure and make it last far longer than the usual sixty seconds. This book has the best instructions I've ever read for getting out of your head and feeling more sensations in your body. So it's helpful even for those who don't have partners yet. (I also like *The Passion Prescription: 10 Weeks to Your Best Sex—Ever!* [Hyperion, 2006] by Laura Berman, Ph.D.) Learning EMO requires time and commitment to giving and receiving pleasure. Pleasure is given with the hands (which makes this technique ideal for men with erection problems). You have to practice. But the health-giving benefits of sexual pleasure are well worth the time and effort.

A WORD ABOUT VIBRATORS

In her book *The Technology of Orgasm: "Hysteria," the Vibrator, and Women's Sexual Satisfaction* (Johns Hopkins University Press, 1998), historian Rachel Maines, Ph.D., documents the amazing fact that the first steam-powered vibrators were used in the 1860s by doctors to bring women to orgasm in their offices. This method was faster and required less skill than the manual method that doctors had previously employed for the treatment for all kinds of female problems including hysteria, depression, and listlessness. When electric vibrators showed up in blue movies in the early 1900s, the respectability of this treatment fell from grace. Dr.

Maines and her colleagues also made a very entertaining and eye-opening movie about this called *Passion and Power* (www .passionandpowerthemovie.com), which is women's history at its finest.

Nowadays, vibrators are available everywhere, and many women enjoy using them. Dr. Ruth Westheimer has even endorsed a particularly interesting device known as the Eroscillator, with all kinds of different attachments. Some women require vibrators to reach orgasm. I have a caveat about their use, however. We have the ability to train our nervous systems to experience more and more pleasure with less and less stimulation (the exact opposite of what happens with porn). We have already discussed the nitric-oxide-increasing health benefits of this approach. Vibrators, by contrast, provide so much stimulation that they reduce sensation over time, so eventually you may find yourself requiring more and more stimulation to feel less and less. This can become addictive. That said, enjoy your vibrator. But also experiment with other ways of feeling more with less.

Understand the Sexuality-Spirituality Connection. The human experiences that provide us with the greatest ecstasy and the greatest pain are sex, love, and religion. In her book *Sacred Pleasure* (HarperSanFrancisco, 1995), Riane Eisler writes, "Candles, music, flowers, and wine—these we all know are the stuff of romance, of sex, and of love. But candles, flowers, music, and wine are also the stuff of religious ritual, of our most sacred rites. Why is there this striking, though seldom noted, commonality? Is it just accidental that passion is the word we use for both sexual and mystical experiences? Or is there here some long-forgotten but still powerful connection? Could it be that the yearning of so many women and men for sex as something beautiful and magical is our long-repressed impulse toward a more spiritual, and at the same time more intensely passionate, way of expressing sex and love?"[31]

It is important to understand that the human capacity for ecstasy is a normal part of who we are and that the ecstatic sensual experience can be a spiritual one. We can experience the uplifting ecstatic energy through art, through intense feelings of love, and during experiences such as religious worship or meditation in which we partake of an ecstatic energy that can be erotic in nature. I interviewed physician-turned-healer Sarah Bamford Seidelmann, M.D., author of *Swimming with Elephants* (Conari Press, 2017), on my Hay House Radio show a few years ago. She told me that at their initial visit, she asks depressed, sick, or dispirited clients, "When did you stop singing? When did you stop dancing?" This is a question asked by shamans the world over. We would each do well to ask ourselves the same question.

Only by recognizing that ecstasy and spirituality are part of human nature can we generate ways to provide and experience ecstasy and connections with one another that are nondestructive and nonaddictive. We must feed our souls as well as our bodies.

Create Community. It's challenging to embrace sustainable pleasure as a lifestyle in a community that is addicted to suffering. That's why it's crucial to have support for the shift you are making. My daughters and I did the Mastery Program at Mama Gena's School of Womanly Arts in New York City when they had just finished college and I was a few years postdivorce. This was a turning point for us as a family. We stopped criticizing other women, ourselves, men, and each other and instead learned how to make optimism and pleasure a priority. Many, many resources are available to guide you. Read *Pussy: A Reclamation* (Hay House, 2016) by Regena Thomashauer. Follow the work of Deborah Kern, Ph.D., who does group and individual sessions focused on reclaiming your bliss. Deb's dance classes are legendary, and you can follow along online at www.drdebkern.com.

The deliberate pursuit of sustainable pleasure is not the same as sugarcoating problems. (When you meet someone who is doing that, you know immediately. They do not radiate pleasure and well-being. They are simply pasting a false smile over pain.) Instead, you are fueling your life with eros— life force. You become a gardener instead of someone who is always looking for weeds to pull or pests to kill. It is the essence of being a woman, and it uplifts everyone around you (except toxic people, who will consider it annoying, although you'll find that they'll eventually leave your experience if you don't lower yourself to their level; for more on this, read my book *Dodging Energy Vampires: An Empath's Guide to Evading Relationships that Drain You and Restoring Your Health and Power*).

You have the ability to create a sustainable circle of good friends and flourishing community. But you'll most likely have to make the first move. I sure did. I remember back then telling my daughters, "Everyone is looking for a good gig." And it's true. We all crave community—where we cook together, dance together, and watch movies together. I went from a time of thinking that all the "fun" people were in California or elsewhere on the West Coast to now being surrounded by a wide circle of friends, a fantastic tango community, and a body that now experiences more pleasure of all kinds—including sexual pleasure—than at any other time in my life. You can do the same.

Expect Resistance. One reason sex, love, and religion cause so much pain is that our dominator culture has brainwashed us into believing that it is holy to suffer and sinful to experience pleasure. We've been taught that if we get "too happy" or feel "too good," the boom will drop! That's why we have phrases such as "No good deed goes unpunished." And because our beliefs shape our reality, that's exactly what happens. But it's natural for humans to seek out joy and pleasure. We're born that way and then get talked out of it. And so many seek the experience of ecstasy through addictive means such as food, cigarettes, alcohol, drugs, or even degrading sexual practices, which over time actually serve to further numb us. Bringing more joy and pleasure into your life is guaranteed to push your upper limits. Expect this. One of my colleagues did some one-on-one work with the Bodanskys a couple of years ago. During her time there, as she was learning how to experience more pleasure, she got the worst cold and sore throat of her life. She knew that this was simply resistance. And she didn't let it stop her. She says that her experience was a turning point in enjoying life (and sex) more than ever.

Help Your Partner Become a Good Lover. Neither men nor women (nor monkeys, for that matter) are born knowing how to be good lovers. You have to learn. Men are often under a great deal of pressure to perform. They've been taught that it's their job to bring a woman to orgasm. But this is difficult if a woman doesn't know what pleases her and can't talk about what she wants. Please remember that his ability to really please a woman makes a man feel good about himself. Most men will want to please you if you continually give them feedback about what they're doing right. One of my guy friends said he learned how to please women by watching lesbian erotic films. He said, "Men know nothing about pleasing women." I thought his approach was brilliant.

Make an effort to learn more about sex. Get videos (for a very thorough couples' guide to erotic videos, visit www.clitical.com/sensual-senses/porn-for-couples); read books. Talk about sexy things—this can be very erotic. Notice how your clitoris responds. I love Olivia St. Claire's book *227 Ways to Unleash the Sex Goddess Within* (Harmony Books, 1996). In addition, *Healing Love Through the Tao: Cultivating Female Sexual Energy* (Destiny Books, 2005) by Mantak Chia and Maneewan Chia, *The Multiorgasmic Man* (HarperOne, 2009) by Mantak Chia and Douglas Abrams, and *The Multiorgasmic Couple* (HarperCollins, 2000) by Mantak Chia, Maneewan Chia, Douglas Abrams, and Rachel Carlton Abrams, M.D., belong in everyone's library.

Steve and Vera Bodansky point out, however, that most women are angry with men at some level because we women have been second-class citizens for so long. And though this anger is justified, the problem with it in an individual relationship is that it interferes with your ability to experience sensual pleasure. Anger and pleasure are mutually exclusive. You can't have pleasure when you're angry. Learn how to discharge your anger effectively without blame. (See part three, "Women's Wisdom Program for Flourishing and Healing.") Though this isn't easy, please make every effort to leave your resentments at the bedroom door. Let your partner know when he's doing it right. Most men are performance oriented. When you let them know when they *are* doing it right, they will go out of their way to do it right every time. When they are able to give you pleasure, they feel good about themselves.

In the process, lose the goal orientation. Nothing is more elusive than the orgasm that you are "trying" to get to. And nothing is less sensual than the goal orientation of today's hurried couple. One of the best parts of the Bodanskys' work is that they teach that orgasm begins at the first sign of a pelvic floor muscle contraction. Instead of contracting your muscles and striving to reach an orgasm, you do just the opposite. You learn how to relax all your pelvic floor and buttock muscles so that you feel more and more. Any other approach limits your erotic potential. It's okay to have a "quickie" now and then. But make sure you have some uninterrupted afternoons or evenings when the only goal is to explore each other and not try to reach a finish line. Remember, orgasm doesn't have to be the ultimate goal.

In fact, once you know how to have an orgasm, you don't have to worry about it. Now you're free to lose yourself in the sensation of your partner's skin, scent, and kisses. This is what's really missing from many couples' lovemaking. And it's why lack of desire is so common. We literally have to train ourselves to stay in the moment and bask in the delicious sensation of being touched or kissed, without any other goal in mind. It's like being seventeen again, when you weren't ready for intercourse and spent hours and hours necking and petting instead. The amount of desire and fulfillment you can build up is wonderful.

Give Nature a Hand if Necessary. It is very well documented that humans secrete sexual attractant pheromones in their sweat. These are particularly potent in women at ovulation, which, when women lived together under natural light, tended to occur at the full moon. One example of the power of pheromones is their effect on mosquitoes. It's also well documented that the biting activity of female mosquitoes increases 500 times at the full moon. At ovulation, women are also more likely to be bitten by mosquitoes, and blondes are more likely to be bitten than brunettes.[32] According to the research of Winnifred Cutler, Ph.D., and others, external application of specially formulated pheromones can mimic the sexual attractant properties of naturally occurring pheromones, thus rendering the wearer more attractive to potential sexual partners. In her research on women who had had hysterectomies and who were using pheromones, the researchers stopped the study because it was so obvious that the women who were using the pheromones were attracting more attention than the control group.[33]

We're just beginning to appreciate this new and exciting area of human biology. For example, there is evidence that when the hormone oxytocin is given to people via nasal spray, they become more trusting.[34] Oxytocin is the bonding hormone and is produced in the body in large amounts during childbirth and breast-feeding and in lesser amounts during pleasurable social interactions and also during sex. (A word of caution: Pat Allen, Ph.D., points out that having intercourse with a man you've recently met and are attracted to produces a lot of oxytocin in a woman—so much so that she can become addicted to him. Then if "he doesn't write, he doesn't call," she has to go through a painful oxytocin withdrawal that can take up to two years. It's worse than crack cocaine! Most women know exactly what I'm talking about. So if you are looking for a committed mate, you should be careful about having intercourse before you are clear about your potential partner's intentions. See Dr. Allen's website at www.drpatallen.com.)

Pheromones are a different class of hormones than oxytocin, but I use the example simply to document the powerful effect that small molecules can have on our brains and behavior. Pheromones are available from Winnifred Cutler's Athena Institute (see www.athenainstitute.com) and also from www .love-scent.com.

By the way, a little help from herbal or hormone therapy can also boost a low libido if you've already tried the other suggestions outlined here (including practicing self-cultivation twice per week, as mentioned on page 300). If the problem is vaginal dryness or painful intercourse, using a bit of *Pueraria mirifica* cream (see Resources) or some estrogen may work wonders. Be sure to use lots of lubrication. Note that if you practice regularly with a yoni egg plus a bit of herbal or hormonal help at the beginning, you may well get to a point at which your own lubrication increases naturally. If that doesn't work, try systemic *Pueraria mirifica* or estrogen for a month or so.

For postmenopausal women taking aromatase inhibitors for the treatment of early-stage breast cancer, vaginal testosterone cream and the estradiol vaginal ring have been shown to be effective for vaginal dryness and decreased libido.[35]

Get Creative. Don't be afraid to try new things, step out of the box a little, and expand your ideas about who you are. Adding some spice keeps your sex life exciting, and a little creativity can go a long way. For example, a colleague of mine takes turns reading erotic fiction out loud with her boyfriend in bed. "The book we're reading, part of the Herotica series of women's erotic fiction, has almost seventy stories, so if one doesn't appeal we just flip to another that does. I love these stories because they're written for women, which is better for couples than the male-oriented material out there (much of which is a turn-off for me)." She finds that reading such stories out loud works because it's far less intimidating to speak someone else's words than to come up with her own.

She's also experimented with using a silk scarf as a blindfold. "It doesn't have to be kinky," she says. "It just heightens your senses (when you're the one who is wearing it) and builds anticipation in a major way. When we did this the first time, in front of a wonderful fire on a cold winter night, my boyfriend gave me a fabulous massage with essential oils. What we did wasn't necessarily so amazing, but using the blindfold dialed up the excitement so it felt pretty amazing. A side benefit is that this also fosters trust, because the person being blindfolded is trusting his or her partner, and the partner is honored by being the recipient of that trust."

Of course, every woman needs to find what works for her, and the variations are endless. I personally like the erotic literature edited by Lonnie Barbach, such as *Erotic Interludes* (Plume, 1995). The *Emmanuelle* movies from the 1970s are also very erotic, as is the movie *Two Moon Junction*.

CIRCUMCISION AND SEXUALITY: THE CRUCIAL LINK

If we are to reclaim the erotic in our lives and move toward a partnership society in which the sexuality of males and females is celebrated equally, we must be willing to look at our participation in practices that are as harmful to the sexuality of men as they are to women. In other words, women aren't the only ones who have suffered sexually in our dominator society. Routine male infant circumcision, done within the first three days of life and often without anesthesia, is a form of massive, societally approved male sexual abuse that removes a very important erotic tissue in men. Few people would disagree that routine female circumcision—the removal of the clitoris and labia—is completely unacceptable. In fact, the United Nations has issued a resolution calling for its elimination. Happily, the rate of male circumcision continues to fall in the United States.

Uncircumcised Is the Norm. The vast majority of the world's men, including most Europeans and Scandinavians, are uncircumcised. And before 1900, circumcision was virtually nonexistent in the United States as well—except for Jewish and Muslim people, who've been performing circumcisions for hundreds of years for religious reasons. Believe it or not, circumcision was introduced in English-speaking countries in the late 1800s to control or prevent masturbation, similar to the way that female circumcision was promoted and continues to be advocated in some Muslim and African countries to control women's sexuality.[36] As the absurdity of this position became apparent, new justifications, such as the prevention of cervical and penile cancers, received the blessing of the medical establishment. But these are justifications that science has been unable to support. Nor is there any scientific proof that circumcision prevents sexually transmitted diseases.

The Pleasures of Natural Sex. The male foreskin, one of the most richly innervated and hyperelastic pieces of tissue in the male body, is there for a reason. In her well-researched book, *Sex as Nature Intended*

It (Turning Point Press, 2001), author Kristen O'Hara documents why the design of an intact penis not only ensures maximal sexual sensation for the male but also satisfies the female need for clitoral stimulation at the same time. Most American women have not personally experienced the sensation of sex with an uncircumcised man because the majority of men in this country, especially those born before 1980, have been circumcised. But O'Hara's long-ago affair with an uncircumcised man was the spark that touched off years of research, the result of which is her eye-opening book. Consider the following:

~ The primary pleasure zones of the natural (uncircumcised) penis are located in the upper penis, which includes the penis head, the foreskin's inner lining, and the frenulum—the hinge of skin that connects the foreskin to the head of the penis. When a male is circumcised, some of the most erotically sensitive areas of the penis are removed: the foreskin that normally covers the head of the penis (the glans) and some or all of the frenulum.

~ The frenulum contains high concentrations of nerve endings that are sensitive to fine touch. The glans was designed by nature to be covered all the time except during sexual activity. Upon erection, both foreskin layers unfold onto the upper penile shaft, leaving the highly innervated frenulum, glans, and inner lining exposed and readied for sexual activity. This is one of the reasons why the penile tip is the focus of sexual excitement.

~ Scientific evidence shows that highly erogenous tissue equivalent to the female clitoris is located in the core of the penis, beneath the corona (the hook-like head of the penis) and coronal tip. This sensitive tissue extends all the way down the length of the penile shaft to the pubic mound, and onto the pelvic bone in a manner analogous to the anatomy of the female clitoris. Though the penis contains nerves that are sexually excited by pressure, its tip contains the greatest density of these nerves and is therefore the most sexually responsive part, just as the tip of the clitoris is the most sensitive part in the female. And like the tip of the female clitoris, the tip of the penis is sexually stimulated by the pleasurable sensations created by the massaging actions of the movement of the foreskin upon it during intercourse.[37] During intercourse, these exquisitely sensitive nerves of the upper penis both excite a man sexually and control the rhythm of penile thrusting. "When the natural penis thrusts inward, the vaginal walls brush against the erotically sensitive nerves of the glans, the foreskin's inner lining, and the frenulum, causing these nerves to fire off sensations of pleasure," writes O'Hara. "The inward thrust of the penis keeps these pleasure sensations ongoing, but after these nerves have fired, the penis senses a reduction in pleasurable feelings, so it stops its inward thrust and begins its outward stroke in search of stronger sensations. During the outward stroke, the foreskin's outer layer slides forward to cloak the nerves of its inner lining, while the inner lining itself covers the frenulum," she continues. "Once covered, these nerves are allowed to rest from stimulation until the next inward thrust. As the foreskin moves forward on the shaft, it bunches up behind the coronal ridge, and may sometimes roll forward over the corona, depending upon the length of the stroke. This applies pressure to the interior tissue of the corona and coronal ridge where nerves that are excited by pressure send a wave of sexual excitement throughout the upper penis. The natural penis receives pleasure sensations from one set of sensory nerves on the inward thrust and a different set of nerves on the outward stroke. It can maintain a continuous stream of highly pleasurable sensations by maintaining the right rhythm." And intriguingly, because the area of sexual sensation is so localized in the tip, the penis only has to travel a short distance to excite one set of nerves or another. In other words, it doesn't have to withdraw very far to receive pleasure on the outward stroke. This allows the penis to stay deep inside the vagina, keeping the man's pubic mound in close and frequent contact with a woman's clitoral area, which increases her pleasure and a sense of closeness. Most women really enjoy the sense of melting into their mates that this position enhances.

O'Hara surveyed approximately 150 women—enough to make her study statistically reliable. Here's how one survey respondent described sex with an uncircumcised partner: "Sex with a natural partner has been to me like the gentle rhythm of a peaceful but powerful ocean—waves build, then subside and soothe. It felt so natural, as if it were filling a deep need within me, not necessarily for the act of sex, but more in order to experience the rhythm of a man and woman as they were created to respond to each other."

The Sexual Consequences of Male Circumcision. After circumcision, the exposed head (or glans) of the penis thickens like a callus and becomes less sensitive.[38] Men who have been circumcised later in life and who therefore know the difference report a decrease in their sexual sensations. In addition, research shows that the most sensitive region of the penis (the transitional region from the external part of the foreskin to the internal part) is removed with circumcision—and that this region is also more sensitive than the most sensitive region of the circumcised penis.[39]

Because of this, the circumcised penis must thrust more vigorously with a much longer stroke in order to reach orgasm through stimulating the less sensitive penile shaft. In her study of women who have had sexual experiences with both natural and circumcised men, O'Hara notes that respondents overwhelmingly concurred that the mechanics of coitus were different for the two groups of men. Seventy-three percent of the women reported that circumcised men tended to thrust harder, using elongated strokes, while uncircumcised men tended to thrust more gently, to have shorter strokes, and to maintain more contact between the mons pubis and clitoris.

What if You're with a Circumcised Man? As with the millions of women who've suffered from genital mutilation, it's important for all of us to acknowledge the damage that has been done by circumcision on the body, mind, and spirit of men—even though men "don't remember the procedure." Believe me, their bodies do! Obviously, despite this wound, men are capable of a great deal of sexual pleasure. And though I've no doubt that nature designed our genitalia to facilitate the kind of physical intimacy so many women crave, it's important to know that it's possible to experience deeply satisfying sex with any kind of penis when you have true intimacy with and respect for each other.

Reclaiming the Erotic: Concluding Thoughts

As women, we need to consider becoming "virgin" again by being true to our deepest selves. We must do and be what is true for us—not to please someone else but for the sake of our own truth. The original meaning of the word *virgin* had nothing to do with sexuality. It referred instead to a woman who was whole and complete unto herself, belonging to no man.[40] It's time for all of us women to reestablish our virginity in that sense.

~ Acknowledge that you have access to eros, to the life force—the erotic, ecstatic energy of your being. It is part of being human.

~ Imagine what your sexuality would be like if you thought of it as holy and sacred, a gift from the same source that created the ocean, the waves, and the stars.

~ Reconnect with your sexuality simply as the expression of this creative life force.

~ Learn to experience and then direct your sexual energy (with or without actually having sex) for your greatest possible pleasure and good. Secondarily, imagine how you can use it to benefit other people in their lives as well.

~ Think of yourself as a goddess. Allow your life to change by completely embracing your innate sexuality without guilt, shame, or fear. There. Isn't that a relief?

9

Vulva, Vagina, Cervix, and Lower Urinary Tract

This . . . is dedicated with tenderness and respect to the blameless vulva.
—Alice Walker

The vulva is known in Sanskrit as the *yoni,* which means "gateway to life." It consists of all the parts that make up the external female genitalia. As an essential gateway to life, symbolic of a sacred portal, the vulva should be celebrated, not maligned, mutilated, or considered shameful in any way. After all, this is the area of the body through which the seeds of human life are planted and later harvested through birth. It is also the area associated with the most exquisite pleasure that women are capable of experiencing.

More than 80 percent of the human immune system cells are at the mucosal openings in the body, including the vulva, vagina, cervix, and urethral openings. When this area is intact and healthy, it affords effective protection against sexually transmitted disease, including AIDS. Keeping the genitals healthy is also essential for optimal fertility, sexual functioning, and elimination. The very first step that a woman must take to achieve this is to lovingly accept this area of her body.

OUR CULTURAL INHERITANCE

It's crucial that we tell the truth about the cultural programming that makes the lower genital areas so problematic for so many women. Western culture has considered the genital area "dirty" and defiles it by this attitude.

Every function associated with the genitals—birthing, bleeding, sex, and elimination—is *highly* charged emotionally and psychologically. Since childhood, most of us have picked up the idea that this part of our body is different from other parts: It is taboo, dirty, and unworthy. Over the years, many patients of all ages and backgrounds have asked me during their pelvic exams, "How can you do this job? It's so disgusting." One woman recalled visiting her college health service to be treated for a yeast infection and being told by a young male M.D., "The female genitalia are like a cesspool." The most common reason that women douche, moreover, is their mistaken belief, handed down from mother to daughter, that this area of the body is offensive and requires special cleaning. It is now well documented that douching is not necessary and can even be harmful (it can irritate tissues, making them more susceptible to infection). The practice is on the decline. Still, the promotion and sale of feminine hygiene deodorants and deodorant-impregnated tampons and sanitary pads give women the impression that the vagina in its natural state is unacceptable, that it must be sanitized and deodorized.

The very word *vagina* comes from Latin and originally meant "sheath for a sword"—or the sheath for a penis, an example of a woman's body being defined only in reference to men.[1] In prehistoric egalitarian societies, vulvas and pubic triangles were frequently drawn or inscribed on cave walls to symbolize a sacred place, a gateway to life. We further see that the doorway to Gothic cathedrals also mirrors the external female genitalia, with the archways coming up to a point, and often with an oval window or decoration above that. There is also ample evidence that these cathedrals were often built over ancient Goddess sites. The sacred vesica piscis symbol of two intersecting circles is also said to represent—among other things—the vulvar opening of the goddess. For centuries, sexuality and spirituality have been appreciated as two aspects of the same thing—an idea that is now reawakening in our culture.

Perhaps the most shocking and extreme evidence in our global culture today of blatant disrespect for the vulva is the practice of female genital mutilation (euphemistically called circumcision), which is routinely carried out by elder women in cultures in which it is practiced. As I noted in chapter 1, more than 200 million women globally are victims of this practice, with numbers actually growing in the United States due to immigrants from countries where this is common. The tribal wisdom is that the young girl will be considered "tainted goods" if she hasn't been circumcised. The entire tribe shares in this belief system, so those who have had it done don't necessarily feel abused. From our Western cultural standpoint, this is barbaric. Because consciousness of the physical, psychological, and spiritual effects of female circumcision is now growing, the entire subject is being brought out into the open, discussed, and reevaluated. Incest and other human rights abuses have been the norm for the last 5,000 years. "These did not become the crimes they are today," says theologian and medical intuitive Caroline Myss, "until we began to reevaluate our personal boundaries within our tribal settings." In my view, this collective reevaluation constitutes recovery from the addictive system in which we have been caught up.

Given our collective history, then, it is little wonder that the entry points to the female body are associated with problems for so many women. Problems in the vulva, vagina, cervix, and lower urinary tract are primarily associated with a woman's feelings of violation in her one-on-one relationship with another individual or in her job. Given the substantial number of immune cells at the mucosal surfaces, such as our vagina, urethra, cervix, and bladder, and given that the function of these cells is highly influenced by stress hormones such as cortisol, it is not difficult to see how a perception of violation and the subsequent biological cascade of hormones that results in response to this perception might well impair optimal function in this area of the body.

Indeed, it has now been well documented that psychosocial stress increases both the prevalence and incidence of bacterial vaginosis (BV), a type of vaginal infection caused by an imbalance in the normal vaginal bacterial environment. BV raises the risk of postoperative infections, HIV shedding and acquisition, and premature labor in pregnant women. BV is difficult to eradicate and often recurs. Though this infection is also associated with douching, oral sex, and multiple sexual partners, psychosocial stress has now been found to be an independent risk factor for it, probably because of the adverse effect of stress hormones on the immune function of the vaginal mucosa.[2]

Energy Issues and the Lower Genital Tract

The inability to say no to a boundary violation can lead to increased susceptibility to infection secondary to decreased levels of immunoglobulin type A or immunoglobulin type M. Think of it this way: Any perception of invasion in one's emotional life can result in increased permeability of one's immune system boundary, both on the surface areas of the body and internally. This is especially true in those women with a history of psychosexual trauma in early life. A woman who has been in a sexually active love relationship and is rejected may perceive her rejection as a violation, and vulvar or vaginal problems can result. If she can't feel and release her anger over this, she may develop recurrent urinary symptoms. Incest memories, sexual violation, and guilt feelings about sexuality can also result in repeated episodes of vaginitis.

A woman who has a health problem in the vagina, vulva, or cervix may be involved in a situation in which she is being used sexually or in a job without her complete conscious cooperation and consent. Or she may be feeling forced to do something against her consent or to act in a sexual way about which her emotions are divided. In such a situation her body is likely to respond with problems that we associate with sexual violation. These physical problems can appear if, for instance, she is using sex to obtain financial, physical, or emotional security or to manipulate another person, rather than to bring mutual pleasure. Feelings of being used or raped are associated with chronic vaginitis, chronic vulvar pain, recurrent venereal warts, recurrent herpes, cervical cancer, and associated abnormal Pap tests (cervical dysplasia).

Women with episodic urinary symptoms often find that the episodes are accompanied by anger or feeling "pissed off." Getting a urinary tract infection (UTI) may be the body's way of releasing anger. Women with recurrent UTIs should pay attention to what happened in their lives and relationships twenty-four to forty-eight hours before the onset of the symptoms. With practice, we can often become aware of the offending situation and take steps to change either the situation or our response to it. When the anger becomes more chronic and less available on a conscious level, the symptoms may take the form of continual urinary urgency and frequency. (Of course, it's also necessary to replenish the microbiome in the area; see page 345.)

Studies have shown that women with chronic bladder infections have more free-floating anxiety and more obsessive personality traits and tend to experience emotions only through their bodily symptoms (somatoform disorder) compared to women without this problem. In one study, in fact, women with chronic cystitis had scores comparable to those of psychiatric patients for levels of obsessionality. They were also prone to emotional states that were not balanced by their intellect.[3] Several researchers have found that women who feel the need to urinate frequently but who don't have infections are more anxious and neurotic than those without the problem. It has also been found that symptoms of anxiety correlate with urinary urgency (feeling as if she can't make it to the bathroom in time), needing to get up at night to urinate, and frequent urination.[4] Many women can relate to urinary frequency around exam time at school or when trying to get to sleep at night while worried about something.

Chronic vulvar problems such as pain and itching are associated with stress from anxiety and irritation related to being controlled either by a partner or by a situation that in energy terms is equivalent to a partner. An example would be a woman who feels so "married" to a job that totally controls her that, unconsciously, she is not free to experience her life on her own terms. Caroline Myss suggests that we might think of this external control as a modern-day "chastity belt." A woman's mate may control her either by forcing her to have sex or by withholding sexual activity that she desires.

Ruth came to see me with a history of recurrent vaginitis and urinary tract infections that had not responded to the usual treatments, such as antifungal creams and antibiotics. Her husband wanted sex every night, and she believed that filling his sexual needs was part of her "job." She did love him, but she was often too tired to have sex in the evening and his desires irritated her. Nevertheless, she forced herself to do it, even as her unconscious resentment grew. Like many women, Ruth equated having a lot of sex with having a "satisfactory" sex life. At first she denied to me that her sex life had any problems. I pointed out to Ruth that when she had sex she didn't want, the normal lubrication associated with female sexual desire was not present, and this, coupled with the friction of intercourse, set the scene for vaginal and urethral irritation and inflammation. (It is very clear that when women engage in any sex that is traumatic to their tissues, infection and inflammation can result.) When tissue trauma is combined with a lack of receptivity and a feeling of not being able to refuse, then the immune system will be affected adversely, making healing from the trauma that much more difficult. Eventually, as part of her treatment, Ruth sought help through therapy and learned how to express her needs in a positive way that enhanced her marriage.

The sexual imperative of our culture—that desirable women serve men sexually—is largely what gets women into trouble in the first place: in other words, into sexual situations that don't serve their needs and that are in fact harmful. Many women are conflicted between needing to be loved and needing sexual pleasure, on the one hand, and wanting to say no to intercourse, on the other. Gynecological problems in the vulva, vagina, and cervix are often related to a woman's inability to say no to entry into this area of her body when she wants to refuse but doesn't believe she should. These problems are quite literally related to allowing herself to "get screwed." One of my patients developed chronic vaginitis, for example, when her college (illegally) refused to award her credit for courses that she had completed. At first, she decided that she had no choice but to accept their mistreatment because she didn't want to "make waves." Despite many external remedies for vulvovaginitis, however, she did not get better until she appealed her college's decision about her credits and then refused to back down. She was eventually awarded the credits due her, and her vaginitis cleared up.

Besides frustration and anger, another emotion that generally tends to affect our health adversely is guilt. When our guilt is centered on our sexuality, it can become associated with problems specific to our entry points. The sexual revolution of the 1960s and 1970s broke down some of our culture's puritanical views about sexuality, but a sexually repressed culture cannot be healed just by taking off its clothes. Now, nearly half a century later, it is even more important for women to be clear about their sexuality and their choice of sexual partners. It is especially important that women consciously use their freedom to understand what their bodies really want and not be led by the blandishments of partners who equate freedom with irresponsible behavior.

Scientific research supports the premise that certain emotional factors are associated with chronic urinary, vaginal, vulvar, or cervical problems, including cervical cancer.[5] One study showed that, compared with women with other types of cancer, women with cervical cancer are more likely to have sexual ambivalence, lower incidence of orgasm during sexual intercourse, and a dislike of sexual intercourse amounting to an actual aversion. They have more marital conflict, as evidenced by the increased incidence of divorce, desertion, or separation.[6] Another study was done on women who had severely abnormal Pap tests that required further evaluation to assess whether the woman had progressed to actual cervical cancer. The authors found that they could predict which women had progressed to cervical cancer based on the women's responses to their questions about recent stressful life events. If a husband or boyfriend had been unfaithful, was drinking, or was having sex with other women (or men), for example, a woman with cervical cancer would always say something like, "I should have left him, but I couldn't because of the kids" or "I thought he needed me." When responding to the same situation in their own lives, the women without cervical cancer would say, "I can't trust him—he wants more than he gives." In this same study, if a family member got a major illness or died, the women with cervical cancer would say, "I should have worked harder and taken better care of him [or her]." The women without cervical cancer, on the other hand, were more realistic about the limits of their responsibility to others and about their ability to change the natural course of events.[7] One could argue that because these studies were done in the 1950s and 1960s, their conclusions are no longer valid. However, a 1988 study revealed the same thing—that cervical neoplasia and subsequent risk for invasive cancer were more likely to develop in those women who were passive in their relationships, avoided an active coping style, and were more socially conforming and appeasing when compared with a control group whose Pap tests were more benign.[8] A 1986 study showed that women scoring high on scales of helplessness, pessimism, and social alienation had a higher incidence of disease involving the cervix. These personality characteristics were measured before the diagnosis of cervical cancer was made, thus minimizing the possibility that it was the diagnosis of the cancer that caused the personality characteristics.[9] On the other hand, those women who were resilient, optimistic, and had active coping styles tended to have Pap tests that did not reflect abnormal and invasive cells. A 2003 study at the University of Texas School of Public Health found that relationship stress (in women who experienced divorce, infidelity, increase in arguments, and psychological and physical partner violence) but not other forms of stress (from loss, violence, or financial problems) was associated with higher incidence of cervical cancer in white women (but not in African American women).[10]

Most women with chronic vaginal, urinary, or vulvar problems have had them for years. These problems are usually associated with unexpressed complaints about a situation in their lives that has been accumulating for an equally long period. Clinically, it is well known that treatment for chronic problems of this nature is often unsuccessful if the psychological and emotional aspects of the problem are ignored. Unfortunately, many such women have been to scores of doctors, looking in vain for the physical cure for their problem.

In energy terms, a woman sets the stage in her body for chronic vulvar, vaginal, or urinary problems when she *lacks the courage or the agency to change* the negative aspects of an unhealthy relationship. Women with these problems have often had boundary violations early in their childhoods, and so they confuse violation with love. In adulthood, when a woman stays in a relationship with someone she doesn't respect or even like because she is afraid to leave—for whatever reason, be it fears about financial or physical insecurity, about being single, or about her own dependence—she is participating in a prostitute archetype. If she continues to have sex with someone whom she doesn't respect or love, she is participating in an energy pattern that is associated with chronic vaginal, cervical, or vulvar problems.

ANATOMY

The vulva is the outermost point of entry into the female genital system, leading to the vagina, which ends at the cervix and its opening, known as the cervical os (*os* is an anatomical word for "entrance" or "mouth"). The cervix forms the entryway into the uterus and inner pelvic organs—the tubes and ovaries. (See figure 9, page 192.) The vulva comprises the labia majora (outer lips) and labia minora (inner lips). The outer entrance from the vulva to the vagina is known as the introitus. The pubic hair on the vulva forms a protective barrier to the more delicate tissues of the vagina and the cervix. The vulvar skin contains apocrine sweat glands, identical to those under the arms. Apocrine sweat glands differ from regular sweat glands in that their secretions are triggered by emotional situations, not just by physical exertion. The vulva sweats more than any other part of the body.

The bladder is located just above the vagina, while the urethra, the structure that leads from the bladder to the outside, can be felt as the protruding tube-like ridge that runs down the top part of the vagina to just above the vaginal opening. The clitoris is just above the urethral opening. The anus lies just below and in back of the vagina.

The vagina constitutes a passageway to the cervix, which is actually the lowermost part of the uterus (and is sometimes called the uterine cervix). The cervix protrudes into the uppermost part of the vagina and is covered by the same type of cells as the vaginal lining.

The Pap test (previously referred to as a Pap smear), a screening test for abnormal cervical cells, is taken from the opening in the center of the cervix, where the squamous cell covering of the outer cervix meets the inside of the cervical canal. (*Squamous* refers to a flattened type of epithelial cell that covers mucous membranes of the body—for example, inside the vulva, vagina, and mouth.) This area is known as the squamocolumnar junction (SCJ), a very dynamic location in which the mucus-producing endocervical gland cells are constantly changing into the tougher squamous cells. As a result, the normal secretions from the endocervix sometimes get trapped, causing mucus-filled cysts (nabothian cysts). These feel like little bumps on the cervix and can sometimes grow to one or two centimeters in diameter. Though many women who feel these bumps think they have an abnormality, they are completely normal and don't require treatment.

In some women and most teenagers the SCJ is located way out on the outer part of the cervix, with the inner, redder-appearing cells of the endocervix extending outward onto the cervix. In the past many physicians have confused this normal anatomy with pathology, referring to this red glandular area out on the cervix as "cervical erosion" or "chronic cervicitis." Many women have had normal cervical tissue cauterized because of this misunderstanding.

The current recommendation, made by the U.S. Preventive Services Task Force in 2018, is that most women should have their first Pap test at age twenty-one, and then repeat Pap tests every three years. However, most women between the ages of thirty and sixty-five can choose the type of screening that works best for them: a Pap test every three years, an HPV DNA test every five years, or a combination of an HPV DNA test plus a Pap test (called co-testing and involving just one swab) every five years.[11] Currently, the American College of Obstetricians and Gynecologists recommends that women ages thirty to sixty-five have either the Pap or co-screening every five years, but not just the HPV test alone. In one study of 250,000 women, HPV testing overlooked 19 percent of cervical cancers and Pap tests missed 12 percent, while co-screening missed only 5.5 percent.[12] Yet other research favorably compares HPV testing to Pap tests.[13] While some doctors wonder if Pap tests may eventually become obsolete, they are not yet in serious danger of being dismissed.

At this time in our history, chronic vaginitis, sexually transmitted diseases such as venereal warts and herpes, and abnormal Pap tests (also considered a sexually transmitted disorder) are virtually epidemic. These disorders can affect the vulva, vagina, and cervix all at the same time. And because the urethra and bladder are contiguous to this area, they are often affected as well. Though these disorders are often blamed on certain viruses, countless women who do not develop symptoms also have these same viruses present in their bodies.

Gynecologists work right in the middle of women's most secret and painful issues. To be healers, they must recognize that a woman's sexual vulnerability often hovers around her gynecological exam. When a woman is diagnosed with a sexually transmitted disease, has an abnormal Pap test, or discovers she is HPV positive, all her fears, beliefs, and misconceptions about her sexuality and body may well come up. It's vital for healers to be sensitive to these emotions and help their patients articulate their distress and grief, as well as their questions. If you do not think that your feelings about an exam or diagnosis are being treated with concern, tell your practitioner that your feelings are important to you and that you've learned to respect them as a necessary key to eventually understanding yourself better. Ask her or him for help and compassion during the pelvic exam. Though strong emotions may occur during a pelvic exam, don't expect your practitioner or yourself to know exactly why at the moment they first arise. Simply stay with what you are feeling, with the intent to heal the situation. Then relax and allow the healing to come, by turning the situation over to your inner guidance. Eventually, when you are ready, you will get the insight you need about the situation.

A Healing Pelvic Exam

Pelvic exams used to be considered a vital part of a woman's annual visit to the gynecologist, but no longer. For women having no symptoms (no abnormal vaginal discharge, no pelvic pain, no unexpected bleeding, no urinary issues, and no sexual dysfunction), annual pelvic exams are now recommended only every three to five years, in conjunction with cervical cancer screening.

Even if you don't need a pelvic examination every year, when you do need one, it's an ideal time to become acquainted with your lower genital tract in a positive and healthy way. Here's how: Ask your healthcare provider to push the back of the exam table into an upright position so that you can watch the entire exam. Ask him or her to explain to you exactly what they are examining and why. If you are nervous about the exam, request that your healthcare provider tell you what he or she is about to do—and get your permission before proceeding with each subsequent step of the exam.

A pelvic exam begins with close examination of the labia majora (the large outer lips) and then the labia minora (the small inner lips) of the vulva. The urethral opening and clitoris are also examined, and so is the perineum—the area between the vagina and the anus. It's a good idea to ask for a mirror so that you can see these parts of your body and recognize exactly what "normal" looks like. After that, a warmed speculum is inserted into the vagina and opened so that the vaginal side walls and the cervix can be seen. (It should be routine for the doctor to use a warmed speculum. But we have a ways to go—when my daughters had their first pelvic exams by a female gynecologist in New York City several years ago, both the speculums and the doctor were very cold!) Many different speculum shapes and sizes are available (and some promising new types, including one covered with silicone, are currently being developed), so this part of the exam should be comfortable. Your doctor can also show you what your cervix looks like and where the Pap test or HPV sample is taken.

The part of the exam before the speculum is the perfect time to learn where your PC muscle is and how to contract it. Your healthcare provider can point out the muscle and then teach you exactly how to contract it. He or she will usually put one gloved finger in the vagina so you can tighten around it. Contracting and releasing the muscle several times before the speculum is inserted makes this part of the exam much more comfortable. After the speculum exam is completed and the Pap test is taken from the cervix, the speculum will be removed and your doctor will do what's called a bimanual exam, meaning that he or she will insert one or two fingers in your vagina and, with the other hand, palpate your lower abdomen above the pubic bone in order to feel the uterus and ovaries. This will be followed by a rectovaginal exam with one finger in the vagina and one in the rectum to feel the area behind the uterus. This part of the exam is simply not comfortable, though it doesn't cause pain.

It's perfectly acceptable for you to ask that the exam be stopped before it is complete. Some women with a history of trauma or adverse childhood programming about their genitals may find that going through a complete exam is too much for them until they get to know their practitioner better and feel more comfortable. This is fine. Many women feel uncomfortable during pelvic exams. But as you learn to accept and appreciate your lower genital tract, and also to contract and relax your PC muscle at will, you will be well on your way toward better gyn health and also sail through your pelvic exam!

HUMAN PAPILLOMA VIRUS (HPV)

Human papilloma virus (HPV) is a very common virus with more than a hundred different DNA subtypes that can cause venereal warts and cervical dysplasia. It is associated with abnormal Pap tests. The CDC estimates that nearly 80 million Americans are currently infected with this virus, with an additional 14 million people becoming newly infected each year. The virus is now so common that nearly all sexually active Americans will become infected with HPV at some point in their lives. For the vast majority of women, this viral infection will spontaneously clear from the immune system within one to two years without any symptoms at all. Others will develop warts or cervical dysplasia. And some who have been exposed to certain high-risk subtypes of HPV will be at risk of developing cervical cancer.[14]

The DNA of HPV has been found in the cells of virtually all abnormal Pap tests and cervical cancers. In 2009, doctors began using HPV DNA diagnostic tests to identify certain types of HPV that have been associated with cervical dysplasia. More recently, available tests have been expanded to include those that detect the RNA of high-risk HPV. Though these tests have their place (see below), here's what all women should know: The majority of women who have been exposed to even the most virulent strains of HPV do *not* get cervical dysplasia. HPV should be thought of as an important risk factor for cervical dysplasia but shouldn't be seen as the single cause of it.

We don't really know, in a conventional sense, who will develop abnormalities from the virus and who won't, unless we look at the factors that can contribute to decreased immunity. Abnormalities start to grow and cause damage only when the immune system has already been weakened in that area of the body and is unable to maintain the health of the tissue. The good news is that even though HPV is quite common in women under thirty, it usually clears up by itself in six to eight months. Because of this, the American College of Obstetricians and Gynecologists recommends HPV DNA screening only in women age thirty and over. And this doesn't need to be done annually. (See Pap test recommendations on page 322.)

Chronic stress and specific attitudes about sex actually change the blood flow to cervical tissue and affect its secretions. Studies suggest a link between stress and the subsequent development of disease in this area of the body.[15] Suppression of the immune system as a result of chronic emotional or other stress can lead to changes in immunity that allow increased virus production in the first place. The link between abnormal Pap tests and deficient immune system functioning is well known: Women who have organ transplants and are on drugs that suppress the immune system (such as prednisone) have a much greater chance than normal of developing abnormal Pap tests. They also frequently have recurrent wart and herpes outbreaks. (Emotional reactions to the diagnosis of venereal warts can be similar to those that accompany a diagnosis of herpes. If you have concerns about either condition, please read through both sections.)

If our bodies are a hologram in which each part contains the whole (see chapter 2), then the HPV virus and the abnormal cells associated with the virus are two interrelated aspects of a greater whole that is not as yet entirely understood. For a variety of reasons, depressed immunity makes it much more likely that any HPV present on the cervix or in the vagina will attack already weakened cells. I think of the HPV virus as an opportunist at the scene. The virus doesn't "cause" cervical dysplasia, and it doesn't "cause" cervical cancer, either. Most women who have the HPV virus don't go on to develop cervical cancer, because most viral activity and infections are halted by good immune functioning. But in about 10 percent of women with high-risk HPV on their cervix, the HPV infections will be long-lasting and may put them at risk for cancer.

Symptoms

Most women with HPV have *no* symptoms. In those who do, the most common symptom is warty growths (condylomata acuminata) on the outside of the vulva that are painless but can be seen and felt. These can grow and multiply during pregnancy, when the hormones associated with pregnancy stimulate their growth. They often disappear on their own following delivery, when the hormones once again change. Warts can vary in appearance from plaque-like growths to pointy, spiky lesions. Some women have only a few, while others have many all over the vulva. The virus can also cause warty growths on the tongue, the lips, and in the throat, though these sites are rare. Sometimes a woman has no obvious warts on the vulva but has them in the vagina or on the cervix. She may not be aware of these.

HPV infection is sometimes associated with chronic vulvar pain, chronic vaginitis, and chronic inflammation of the cervix (cervicitis). A vaginal discharge is usually not present, although it can be. Because some women have HPV infection in association with vaginal infections from yeast or from an imbalance in the vaginal flora known as bacterial vaginosis, it is not always possible to tell exactly what virus or bacteria is causing what symptom. Unless a woman has actual warty growths on her vulva or has chronic vulvar or vaginal irritation associated with HPV, she won't know that she has it, which, given the fact that the vast majority of infections resolve on their own, is not such a bad thing.

Diagnosis

Warty growths on the vulva, vagina, or cervix and abnormal cells on a Pap test or cervical biopsy are usually associated with HPV. If these appearances are a first occurrence, a biopsy is taken and sent to the lab to confirm the diagnosis. Sometimes HPV is diagnosed by a colposcopy, an examination of the cervix and vagina through a magnifying lens, or a cervigram, a screening test in which a photograph of the cervix is made after applying dilute acetic acid (vinegar) to the tissue. When vinegar is applied to the vulva, cervix, or vagina and HPV is present in the tissue, the tissue often turns white. (This tissue is then called acetowhite epithelium, or white skin cells.) Biopsies of the white area often reveal HPV.

Common Concerns About HPV

Why Do So Many Women Have It? HPV has probably always been present in the human genitals. You can certainly find it on old slides of Pap tests from more than forty years ago. Back then, HPV simply wasn't recognized or studied as much as it is today. Several factors have contributed to its more frequent diagnosis now. One is the advent of colposcopy, a diagnostic technique developed in the 1970s as a follow-up to abnormal Pap tests. If any abnormal areas show up under examination by colposcopy, biopsies of those areas of the vagina or cervix will be done for further evaluation in the lab. (See page 352 for more details.) Because colposcopy and follow-up biopsies have allowed us to diagnose cervical abnormalities in their earlier stages, pathologists are now more likely to make the connection between cellular changes and HPV.

The sexual revolution and multiple sexual partners have increased the number of women who have been exposed to the HPV virus. Condoms don't always prevent the transmission of HPV because the virus can exist in areas other than the penis, such as the scrotum; they do help, however. And monogamy is no guarantee against HPV if your partner is not monogamous, too. Of course, even if you are both monogamous, you could have been exposed to HPV by past sexual partners. Factors implicated in HPV leading to abnormal growths include a depressed immune system from suboptimal nutrition, emotionally unhealthy relationships, excessive amounts of alcohol, cigarette smoking, a high-sugar pro-inflammatory diet, and a microbiome that is not balanced. Therefore, it's not simply the viruses from our past sexual partners that we bring to our current sexual partners. We also bring our current state of emotional health, which in part determines whether those viruses will become active.

How Did I Get This? Who Gave It to Me? This is one of the big questions for most women. The truth is that HPV inserts itself into the DNA of the tissue it infects, and once it does this, it may lie dormant for years. That means theoretically that a virus a woman "caught" in 2010 may not express itself in any visible way until 2020. This also means that whoever "gave" it to her may well not have known that he or she even had it. I've seen couples who have been monogamous for twenty or more years in which one partner has developed warts or herpes. And even though the couple has not been using condoms, the other person in the relationship may never develop the same problems. Very often, then, it's difficult if not impossible to assess "blame" for HPV infections. Which doesn't stop a lot of people from pointing fingers at others, or feeling horribly guilty themselves if they develop one—especially if they are from strict, male-dominated religious backgrounds. The resulting shame, combined with the fear fueled by media stories linking HPV with cervical cancer, can be a deadly combination for the immune system. Later in this chapter, I will give some recommendations for dealing emotionally and mentally with these conditions and for boosting your immune system.

Will HPV Interfere with Pregnancy? Vulvar warts are often stimulated to grow by the hormones associated with pregnancy. In rare instances, a woman's warts will cause bleeding at the time of delivery, especially if an episiotomy is made through an area of the vulva that is affected by warts. In general, however, warts do not interfere with pregnancy. They often disappear without treatment once a woman has delivered. A woman with HPV can theoretically transmit it to her baby at delivery, and some babies can theoretically get vocal cord papilloma (which can be treated with surgery) from HPV. This is very rare, however; I have never seen a case of it, and it is not a reason to do a cesarean section in a woman with HPV. The immune system of the baby protects it almost every time.

Treatment

Treatment is aimed at removing the visible warts and making sure the woman doesn't have any of the abnormal or precancerous cells that are sometimes associated with the warts. Once the bulk of a wart is removed, the immune system can deal with and remove the remainder more easily. Removal or disappearance of a wart, however, doesn't necessarily prevent recurrence or the possibility of transmission.

I've seen all manner of treatments "work" for warts. Warts on the hands, for instance, are known to disappear after a variety of treatments ranging from hypnosis to applying cold potato or even duct tape.[16] We just don't know what makes warts go away, even after thousands of years of observing that warts are responsive to suggestion and folk remedies.

Even though removal of warts doesn't really "cure" anything, it does help the body fight HPV. One reason for this is that treatment reduces the amount of virus that the warty growth sheds. Another reason is that the immune system is enhanced by the feeling that we're "doing something." We live in a very action-oriented culture, and Americans want to get things done. When we treat a wart and get rid of it, the patient at some level feels that it's been "taken care of." The immune system gets the message and continues to "take care of it."

It is controversial as to whether it's important for males to get treated for warts. Many doctors downplay the male role in HPV, and many men are infected without visible warts. Therefore, many men don't know that they have HPV, and no consistent effort is made to diagnose them.[17] The female cervix is a unique environment and appears to be more susceptible to virus-associated abnormalities than male penile or scrotal skin.

Laser Treatment. Laser treatment, very popular for warts back in the 1990s, has not lived up to the medical profession's initial expectations, though it is still performed. If a physician is highly skilled in the use of the laser, it can be a good way to remove persistent warts, but a few studies have shown that once warts have been lasered off the cervix or the vulva, they come back faster after laser treatment than after other treatments. Perhaps this is because the laser vaporizes tissue and spreads the wart virus into the surrounding areas. HPV on the mucous membranes of the vagina and cervix can be compared with the virus that causes the common cold in the respiratory tract. We would never think of using a laser to denude the surfaces of the trachea and bronchial tree of the cold virus. But using a laser to remove warts from the genital tract is really no different—we know that ultimately we can't eradicate the wart virus, any more than we can eradicate the common cold virus. I have not been impressed with the effectiveness of laser treatment over the long term and prefer other treatment.

Podophyllin. Podophyllin is a chemical resin derived from the mayapple. It interferes with cell division and therefore stops genital warts from growing. It can be effective in some people, but it is for use with external warts only, because it can have toxic effects on surrounding tissues whose cell division is normal. Podophyllin is used only on the wart itself and must be washed off within several hours.

Podofilox (Condylox) is a topical 0.5 percent antiviral treatment that a woman can apply herself to external warts after an initial treatment from her healthcare provider. This convenient treatment may decrease the number of office visits she must make for recurrent warts. This medication is related to podophyllin and is available by prescription.[18]

Aldara (Imiquimod). This is an immune response modifier that comes as a topical cream for use on HPV warts, among other things. It can take several weeks to work but is more effective than placebo. It can cause skin irritation.

Acids. Many doctors use trichloroacetic acid (TCA) to treat warts on the cervix, vagina, and vulva. This acid is very effective but doesn't "cure" the warts—it just burns away the visible ones. This acid must be applied in minute amounts and only to the warty areas themselves because it causes painful burns to healthy tissue. (It also can burn through clothing.) Even on warty areas, it can cause immediate stinging, followed later by ulceration of the skin. If the acid gets on any area other than the wart (and it often does), it takes from one to two weeks for the skin to heal. It also takes about that long for the ulceration of the wart to slough off. The treatment may need to be done more than once.

Cryocautery. Warts can be frozen with a cryocautery device in the office. Freezing a wart causes it to disappear over a one-to-two-week period. I have found this treatment to be time-consuming and often painful for the patient. I don't recommend it.

Electrocautery. Removal of very large collections of warts is possible using electrocautery. In this treatment the wart is burned off by a heated electrical device. This procedure is usually done under anesthesia in the operating room. It is used only when all other methods haven't worked.

LEEP. Loop electrosurgical excision procedure (LEEP), also called large loop excision of transformation zone (LLETZ), can be used to remove warts and wart-affected tissue on the vulva, cervix, and vagina. It removes warts by electrocautery, using an electrically charged wire loop. It is also used to treat cervical dysplasia. It can be very beneficial. The problem is that a LEEP procedure on the cervix doubles the risk for premature rupture of the membranes during subsequent pregnancy. This increases the risk for prematurity.[19]

Natural Escharotic Treatment. For women whose doctors suggest LEEP but who are concerned about the risks for obstetrical complications, escharotic treatment by a naturopathic doctor together with an oral, anticarcinogenic HPV protocol of vitamins and botanical medicine (for one year) and a vaginal suppository protocol (for twelve weeks after the escharotic), may be a good alternative.[20] Escharotic treatment is an ablative therapy that involves applying bromelain, a natural enzyme found in pineapple, to the surface of the cervix to break down the walls of the abnormal cells, destroying them. After fifteen minutes, the bromelain is washed away with an herbal solution designed to stimulate the regrowth of normal tissue, followed by the application of bloodroot tincture mixed with zinc chloride, which is left on the cervix for about a minute. After this is washed away, herbal vaginal suppositories with antiviral properties (typically containing magnesium sulfate, glycerin, goldenseal tincture, thuja oil, tea tree oil, bitter orange oil, vitamin A, ferric sulfate, and ferrous sulfate) are inserted and left in overnight. A scab, known as an eschar, forms. This is typically done twice a week for five weeks (though the treatment is personalized), and the suppositories are continued for twelve weeks after the escharotic treatment concludes. An oral anticarcinogenic protocol of vitamins and botanicals is begun with the escharotic treatments and continued for one year; it includes folic acid, indole-3-carbinol, antioxidants (such as vitamin C, vitamin E, and CoQ_{10}), green tea extract, and a mushroom known as turkeytail (*Coliolus versicolor*). Repeat Pap tests are conducted to evaluate whether the treatment was effective.

Nutritional Approach. The effectiveness of wart removal treatment can be enhanced with dietary change and supplements. Studies have shown that foods high in antioxidants, such as vitamin C, folic acid, vitamin A, vitamin E, beta-carotene, and selenium—or supplements containing these—help heal and prevent cervical dysplasia.[21] The antioxidant class known as the proanthocyanidins, found in pine bark and grape seeds, have proven to be very helpful in some cases. (For dose instructions, see the section on cervical dysplasia, page 347, and see Resources for reliable sources.) Regularly eating cruciferous vegetables can also help—particularly land cress and watercress. When researchers at South Dakota State University added a compound found in them to a petri dish with human cervical cancer stem cells, about 75 percent of the stem cells died within twenty-four hours.[22] Because of the connection between HPV, cervical dysplasia, and cervical cancer, I recommend that a woman diagnosed with HPV support her immunity by following the Master Program for Optimal Hormonal Balance and Pelvic Health in chapter 5.

Energy Medicine. Of course, none of us has complete control over whether a virus inserts itself into our DNA or whether it gets expressed once it has done that. Especially in persistent cases of warts or herpes, however, tuning in to oneself with love, forgiveness, good nutrition, and a good multivitamin can work wonders to keep the warts or herpes from showing up again. I also suggest meditating on the following affirmation from the late Louise Hay daily: "I rejoice in my sexuality. It is normal and natural and perfect for me. My genitals are beautiful and normal and natural and perfect for me. I am good enough and beautiful enough exactly as I am, right here and right now. I appreciate the pleasure my body gives me. It is safe for me to enjoy my body. I choose the thoughts that allow me to love and approve of myself at all times. I love and appreciate my beautiful genitals!"[23]

HPV Vaccine: Is It Worth the Risks?

In the summer of 2006, Merck Pharmaceuticals received FDA approval to market the first HPV vaccine, Gardasil, a genetically engineered drug designed to prevent the most common HPV infections implicated in cervical cancer. With the unbelievably rapid approval of Gardasil, HPV and its link to cervical cancer suddenly became front-page news, with remarkably effective media ads marketing the vaccine to all young women. The CDC and many other groups quickly recommended that all girls start the two- or three-shot vaccine series by age eleven or twelve, although girls as young as nine could also be vaccinated, as could women up to age twenty-six.

Overnight, women with virtually no risk for cervical cancer (the vast majority) were suddenly made to feel vulnerable ("I could be one less statistic," says the cool teenage girl on the skateboard), thus creating a huge market for a vaccine that most healthy women and girls simply don't need and that is dangerous for some. Although Merck continues to promise that Gardasil is safe, the National Vaccine Information Center (NVIC), an independent organization and vaccine safety group, has documented cases of seizure, stroke, cardiovascular disease, paralysis, autoimmune diseases such as rheumatoid arthritis, and even death connected to the vaccine. According to the NVIC's data, Gardasil causes serious side effects about thirty times more frequently than the meningitis vaccine, which is given to a similar cohort.[24] (For more information, see the NVIC website, www.nvic.org.)

This isn't all that surprising considering that Merck's clinical trials for Gardasil followed more than 20,000 women, half of whom received the vaccine, for an average of three and a half years—yet that group included fewer than 1,200 girls younger than sixteen and only about 100 who were age nine, with the younger girls followed for only eighteen months.[25]

Reports of problems with Gardasil began to surface at medical meetings. At the October 2008 meeting of the American Neurological Association, researchers presented a report of a fatal case of motor neuron disease that occurred after a fourteen-year-old girl received three doses of Gardasil.[26] The month before, researchers presenting papers at the annual meeting of the European Committee for Treatment and Research in Multiple Sclerosis reported one case of multiple sclerosis (MS) and another of neuromyelitis optica (an autoimmune disorder in which the immune system attacks the optic nerve and spinal cord) following Gardasil immunization.[27] In 2009, Australian researchers reported five cases of MS, with symptoms appearing within twenty-one days of Gardasil immunization.[28] To ramp up the concern about safety even further, Spanish health authorities made headlines in 2009 when they withdrew 76,000 doses of Gardasil after two teenagers got seriously ill just hours after receiving the vaccine. In August of that year, an article in the *Journal of the American Medical Association* noted that the government had so far received more than 12,000 reports of adverse events associated with Gardasil immunizations—772 of them considered serious, including 32 deaths.[29]

A 2009 Medscape article pointed out that the death rate from cervical cancer in the United States (then 3 out of every 100,000 women) and the rate of serious adverse events from Gardasil (3.4 of 100,000 doses distributed) were roughly equal. (Currently, the death rate from cervical cancer has dropped even lower, to 2.3 in 100,000.)[30] The story quoted Diane Harper, M.D., of the University of Missouri–Kansas City School of Medicine and one of the principal investigators in the initial Gardasil trials, as saying, "This is a sobering reality. Would a parent accept such a rate of serious adverse events if the same cancer prevention can occur with continued Pap screening? Is there any acceptable level of risk of serious adverse events, including death, to prevent genital warts?"[31]

In 2009, the FDA approved a second HPV vaccine, this one manufactured by GlaxoSmithKline and named Cervarix, which promised protection against only two of the four HPV types Gardasil targeted. In the same year, the FDA approved Gardasil for boys ages nine through twenty-six. In 2014, the agency approved a new HPV vaccine from Merck called Gardasil 9, which targets five additional HPV types. Gardasil 9 is now the only HPV vaccine available in the United States. Yet even though the Gardasil 9 package insert reports the rate of serious adverse events to be slightly lower than its previous vaccine at 2.3 to 2.5 percent—meaning for every 100,000 people receiving the vaccine, there will be at least 2,300 serious adverse events—the fact remains that only 7.4 women in 100,000 get cervical cancer in the United States.[32] Let me put this into plain English: 2,300 out of every 100,000 young women are placed at risk for serious adverse events from the HPV vaccine in order to possibly prevent 7.4 cases of cervical cancer per 100,000 women (we do not yet have actual prevention statistics).

The vaccine may not even be fully effective, depending on the recipient's health status. If a girl who receives Gardasil already has HPV, for example, the vaccine not only is useless against that particular strain but also won't give her full protection against the other HPV strains. Given that CDC data report that 25 percent of females between the ages of fifteen and nineteen and 45 percent of females between the ages of twenty and twenty-four show evidence of HPV infection, that's not a minor point.[33] Merck's own clinical studies show that Gardasil actually *increases* the risk of cervical cancer by 44.6 percent among women who were exposed to HPV infection prior to receiving the vaccination.[34] There's also evidence now that those who've had the vaccine are becoming infected later on with other strains of HPV that the vaccine doesn't target. The danger is that these strains could become even more virulent. In 2012, researchers at Columbia University published the results of their ATHENA Human Papillomavirus Study, which followed more than 47,000 women. They discovered that vaccinated women reduced their chances of becoming infected with HPV type 16 (one of the types Gardasil targets) by only 0.6 percent, while they increased their chances of becoming infected with additional high-risk HPV types Gardasil doesn't target by 2.6 to 6.2 percent.[35] A study at the University of Texas several years later showed similar results.[36]

Even when the vaccine is effective, we're not sure how long it will continue to work. Clayton Young, M.D., a fellow of the American College of Obstetricians and Gynecologists (ACOG), wrote a letter of protest to ACOG's professional journal, *Obstetrics and Gynecology,* noting that the maximum median follow-up in the studies done on Gardasil is four years (and even in the latest studies, HPV prevention has been shown to last only five to six years),[37] although it typically takes cancer anywhere from eight to almost thirteen years to show up. What that could mean is that preteens receiving the vaccination may unexpectedly be left unprotected when they later become sexually active and need protection the most. "Claiming this vaccine prevents cervical cancer," Dr. Young writes, "is inappropriate."[38]

Let's put the whole discussion of risks and benefits into perspective by looking not just at percentages but at absolute numbers. There are 13,240 new diagnoses of cervical cancer and 4,170 deaths from the disease in the United States each year, according to the American Cancer Society, with somewhere between 90 and 100 percent of them associated with HPV. More than fourteen types of HPV are associated with cervical cancer. Gardasil 9 is thought to protect against the four most common ones plus five other high-risk types that together are implicated in about 90 percent of HPV-associated cases—which means the number of cervical cancer cases that it might potentially prevent against is fewer than 12,000.

The key word there is *potentially*. The figures for effectiveness in the clinical trials looked for absence of cervical dysplasia (an abnormal Pap test) and precursors for cancer as proof the vaccine was effective.[39] But most dysplasia does not develop into cancer, so preventing infection with HPV and subsequent dysplasia is not at all the same thing as preventing cancer, thus making the vaccine's claims misleading.

In video clips of interviews available on YouTube conducted for the as-yet-unreleased documentary *One More Girl* from ThinkExist Films, Dr. Harper (mentioned previously and one of the researchers who conducted the original clinical trials on Gardasil) laid it out like this: About 70 percent of all women who are infected with HPV will clear that infection in the first year, and 90 percent will clear the infection within two years—with no intervention whatsoever. Of the 10 percent left with an infection, only 5 percent will develop a precancerous lesion. It takes five years for about 20 percent and thirty years for 40 percent of precancerous lesions to become invasive carcinomas—which would happen only if those women were not followed by routine Pap tests and subsequently treated.[40]

So the majority of those women supposedly "saved" from cancer by the vaccine would not have gone on to develop cancer anyway, again making the vaccine's claims misleading. (Those who develop cervical cancer typically have a weakened immune system.) Allow me to restate the obvious: The vast majority of cervical cancer cases could be prevented with routine screening, safe-sex practices, and early treatment measures that are already in place.

In a 2008 interview with *The New York Times,* Dr. Harper said, "Merck lobbied every opinion leader, women's group, medical society, politicians, and went directly to the people—it created a sense of panic that says you have to have this vaccine now. Because Merck was so aggressive, it went too fast. I would have liked to see it go much slower."[41] She further noted that the FDA expedited the process, approving Gardasil only six months after Merck's application, and that the CDC came out with its recommendations for the vaccine weeks later. Most vaccines, she notes, take three years to get that sort of endorsement, and then five to ten additional years for universal acceptance. It's worth noting that both Gardasil vaccines and Cervarix, which is no longer available in the United States but is given in other countries, provide Merck and GlaxoSmithKline with more than $2.5 billion in annual sales around the globe.[42]

Drug companies have also successfully lobbied some state governments to mandate that their students receive the vaccine. The latest figures from the National Conference of State Legislatures report that at least forty-two states and territories have introduced legislation to require the vaccine, fund the vaccine, or educate the public or schoolchildren about the vaccine since its introduction in 2006, with twenty-five states and territories having enacted such legislation. Michigan and Ohio were the first two states to try to require that the vaccine be given, although the legislation failed in both cases. Texas was the first state to actually enact a mandate (not by legislation but by executive order from the governor, whose former chief of staff was at that time a Merck lobbyist), although the Texas legislature overturned the governor's order. Currently, three jurisdictions require HPV vaccines for school attendance—Rhode Island, Virginia, and the District of Columbia—and at least eight states proposed HPV-related legislation for the 2017–18 sessions.

As Thomas Nolan, M.D., chair of obstetrics and gynecology at Louisiana State University Health Science Center, a renowned expert on HPV, and a critic of the HPV vaccine, writes in *The Female Patient,* "I have seen billions of dollars spent on HPV research over the last 25 years. . . . The statistics show that we have done an excellent job. The number of new cervical cancer cases and the mortality from this disease have declined by 4 percent annually over the past 20 years, with the death rate falling by 74 percent between 1955 and 1992."[43] Indeed, while cervical cancer was one of the most common cancers in the United States before the advent of Pap tests, today the majority of precancerous lesions found through testing can be successfully treated before they develop into cancer.

The debate now includes a slightly older population. In October 2018, the FDA extended its HPV vaccine recommendation to cover adults ages twenty-seven to forty-five. Even so, the American Cancer Society recommends those older than twenty-six not receive the vaccine, noting on its website that it is "unlikely to provide much, if any, benefit as people get older."[44]

The quality of the initial safety trials on the HPV vaccine has also recently come into question. In 2017, researchers from the National Institute of Cardiology in Mexico examined twenty-eight studies on three HPV vaccines that received FDA approval. In the sixteen randomized trials—where a placebo is tested against the active drug—only two used an inert saline solution for the placebo (a true placebo), while the other fourteen used a saline solution that also contained aluminum—increasing the chances that those receiving it would react.[45] Aluminum has long been a common adjuvant added to many vaccines because it creates a stronger immune system response. Yet adding aluminum to the placebo in a trial can make the drug being tested appear safer than it really is since the difference between those receiving the active drug and those receiving the placebo will not be as great as if the placebo did not contain a potentially reactive ingredient. Gardasil and Gardasil 9 contain amorphous aluminum hydroxyphosphate sulfate (AAHS), a relatively new form of aluminum that causes the immune system to become 104 times more powerfully stimulated than would occur naturally. A 2016 study comparing Gardasil to a true placebo showed that this aluminum adjuvant and the HPV antigens in the vaccine caused neuroinflammation, autoimmune reactions, and behavioral changes in mice.[46] In 2012, a systematic review of HPV vaccine pre- and post-licensure trials found evidence of selective reporting of results and highly flawed design, concluding that "optimism regarding HPV vaccines' long-term benefits appears to rest on a number of unproven assumptions (or such which are at odds with factual evidence) and significant misinterpretation of available data."[47]

After eight months of investigative research, *Slate* published a cover story in December 2017 taking Merck to task for major flaws in design in their clinical trials for Gardasil.[48] The story reported, for example, that trial investigators were allowed to use personal judgment when reporting medical problems as an adverse event, allowing them to decide which symptoms were and were not related to the vaccine. They also reported new health issues that occurred after subjects had been vaccinated as being part of their medical history instead of as adverse events from receiving the vaccine, and they followed subjects for only fourteen days after each dose was administered. Yet another issue in this debate focuses on conflicts of interest involving government policymakers. In 2000, the U.S. House Committee on Government Reform conducted an investigation on this, determining that "conflict of interest rules employed by the FDA and the CDC have been weak, enforcement has been lax, and committee members with substantial ties to pharmaceutical companies have been given waivers to participate in committee proceedings."[49]

Meanwhile, reports of adverse effects keep coming in, and several countries (including Japan, France, and India) have banned Gardasil or filed criminal lawsuits about the vaccine. In January 2016, Sin Hang Lee, M.D., director at the Milford Molecular Diagnostics Laboratory in Milford, Connecticut, sent an open letter of complaint to the director-general of the World Health Organization charging a group of WHO officials and government employees with manipulating data and suppressing scientific evidence.[50]As proof, Dr. Lee referred to a series of emails (obtained via an Official Information Act request submitted in New Zealand) among health officials from the United States, Canada, Japan, and the WHO discussing the existence of research showing that HPV vaccines cause a greater inflammatory reaction than other vaccines, yet choosing to ignore that data in official hearings and statements about vaccine safety.[51] The emails had been sent in preparation for a 2014 hearing in which the officials would be advising the Japanese government on HPV vaccination safety. Despite this, Japan became the first country to suspend its recommendation of HPV vaccines pending further investigation.

A partial list of adverse events related to HPV vaccinations that have been reported to the CDC's Vaccine Adverse Event Reporting System (VAERS) include Bell's palsy, Guillain-Barré syndrome, seizures, paralysis, blindness, pancreatitis, speech problems, short-term memory loss, ovarian cysts, blood clotting and heart problems, miscarriages and fetal abnormalities, cardiac arrest, and sudden death. Actual numbers are undoubtedly higher because reporting to VAERS is voluntary for doctors, not mandatory.

As of February 2018, VAERS has also received reports of fifty-three cases of multiple sclerosis after vaccination with Gardasil and two after vaccination with Gardasil 9. VigiAccess, WHO's database of adverse events (see www.vigiaccess.org), reports 38,527 nervous system disorders following Gardasil vaccination as of November 2018. At a forum on multiple sclerosis in September of the same year, University of Miami researchers presented two cases of teenagers who developed the disease within two weeks of receiving the Gardasil vaccine.[52] Their study concludes that despite a large Swedish study published in 2015 showing no relationship,[53] "these 2 cases and the others that have been previously reported suggest a temporal association between HPV vaccination and onset of MS."

Though some women might benefit from this vaccine, you have to ask yourself: Who really benefits by vaccinating millions of girls and women with a vaccine that costs about $360 per dose, isn't always safe, may not always work, and doesn't guarantee immunity for longer than six years? The evidence against Gardasil is so damning that in 2018 Mary Holland, J.D., a faculty member at the New York University School of Law, and her colleagues Kim Mack Rosenberg, J.D., and Eileen Iorio published a compelling history of the Gardasil vaccine, *The HPV Vaccine on Trial: Seeking Justice for a Generation Betrayed* (Skyhorse Publishing, 2018). Anyone considering giving their daughter or son this vaccine should read this evidence first. As Katharine Hikel, M.D., author of Medscape's Green Mountain Doc blog, put it, "It is shameful that this has happened largely at the unopposed instigation of Big Pharma. Perhaps what we really need is a vaccine to protect doctors from the adverse effects of marketing."[54]

HELP FOR SIDE EFFECTS FROM GARDASIL

If you (or someone you know) experience side effects after receiving a Gardasil immunization, report that experience to a healthcare professional immediately. Also know that there are many ways you can naturally detoxify your body after exposure to all sorts of environmental toxins, including not only the heavy metals and chemicals found in vaccines but also toxins from air pollution and pesticides.

One of the most effective and well-studied detox regimens includes simply taking enough vitamin C (either regular ascorbic acid or buffered ascorbic acid) to reach what is called "bowel tolerance" (in other words, you will get loose stools once your tissues are saturated). Individual bowel tolerance is so varied that some people will reach it by taking 500 mg three times a day, while others will be able to take 2,000–3,000 mg (2–3 grams) every hour. Just keep taking the vitamin C until bowel tolerance is reached; then back off until you stop having loose bowels, and keep taking that slightly lower amount for the next couple of days. Then gradually taper the dose until you're on a maintenance level of about 1,000–2,000 mg per day. I personally find that this regimen almost always prevents the onset of a cold if I start pushing the vitamin C as soon as symptoms arise.

Magnesium is also a powerful antioxidant. The best way I've found to benefit from its detox properties is with a supplement known as ReMag, created by magnesium expert Carolyn Dean, M.D., N.D. Start with one-quarter to one-half teaspoon in a quart of water to which one-eighth teaspoon of Celtic sea salt or Himalayan sea salt has been added. Drink slowly over the course of the day. Increase as needed according to the instructions that come with the product. Continue daily as long as needed.

Dr. Dean has created a very effective detox regimen to help with any adverse effects from vaccines, which are far more common than most people realize. For example, the National Center for Health Statistics (NCHS) reports that one in thirty-six children is now autistic,[55] and some health experts, myself and Dr. Dean included, believe it's from all the neurotoxins in vaccines given to increasingly susceptible individuals. Obviously other environmental factors such as the herbicide glyphosate, found in so much of our food, is also a culprit. Dr. Dean recommends taking vitamin C to bowel tolerance (as described above), as well as taking two to three teaspoons of ReMag in sea-salted water plus, if a live vaccine was given, Pico-Silver Solution (a dietary supplement that is a stabilized ion of nontoxic silver, used to boost immunity).

Better yet, Dr. Dean suggests not waiting for a reaction after receiving a vaccination and instead prophylactically taking vitamin C, ReMag, and another supplement called ReAline (a formula that contains l-methionine, the building block for an important antioxidant that assists in the detox process). In her ebook *Future Health Now Encyclopedia* (last updated in 2017), Dr. Dean gives instructions for how to make a homeopathic remedy to combat vaccines' toxicity from whatever tiny drops of vaccine are left in the bottle the vaccine dose comes in.

Many plants also have powerful detox properties. These include Hawaiian spirulina, Atlantic dulse, parsley, wild Maine blueberries, turmeric, and cilantro. Adding these to your diet regularly (conveniently accomplished by adding them to smoothies) is a very easy way to benefit from regular detox. In addition, maintain a diet that includes optimal nutrition (see chapter 17), take pharmaceutical-grade multivitamin-mineral and antioxidant supplements, and use vibrational healing, such as the advanced protocol for applying Divine Love as outlined by the World Service Institute (see www .worldserviceinstitute.org) or working with a good medical intuitive.

For health problems that persist after following simple detox regimens, consider seeing a healthcare practitioner who is familiar with oral chelation, which can be very effective for ridding the body of toxic heavy metals (including those often found in vaccines, such as aluminum and mercury). To find such a healthcare practitioner, visit the website for the Institute for Functional Medicine at www .functionalmedicine.org.

HPV Prevention

Condoms. Although condoms can't prevent all cases of HPV because the virus can live in cells not covered by the condom, they do greatly reduce the chances of infection—even more than previously believed. A University of Washington study showed that women whose partners *always* used condoms were 70 percent less likely to be infected with the HPV virus, while those whose partners used condoms half the time reduced their risk by 50 percent.[56]

Additional Means of Prevention. Any and all modalities that shore up your immunity will help prevent HPV infection and transmission. These include making sure your vitamin D level is optimal (see page 435). Studies have shown that curcumin, an antioxidant found in turmeric, can slow or limit the activity of the HPV virus.[57] Following the Master Program for Optimal Hormonal Balance and Pelvic Health (see chapter 5) is prevention at its finest. And the suggestions in nutritional and energy medicine approaches to HPV can also be used for prevention.

HERPES

Herpesviridae is a large family of DNA viruses that are implicated in diseases of animals and humans. All are called herpesviruses. The word *herpes* comes from the Greek word *herpein* ("to creep"), which refers to the fact that these viruses are implicated in recurrent lesions but can be dormant for long periods of time. Herpesviruses include the chicken pox and shingles virus (varicella zoster), the Epstein-Barr virus (which is implicated in mononucleosis), and cytomegalovirus. More than 90 percent of all adults have evidence of some kind of herpes infection.[58] When we think of herpes, however, we're generally referring to genital herpes.

Herpes genitalis virus can cause small, painful ulcers on the vulva, in the vagina, or on the cervix. Herpesviruses can also cause cold sores on the mouth. These herpesviruses are divided into several types. Type 1 (HSV-1), the kind that causes cold sores, tends to live "above the belt," but it can also cause genital herpes. In fact, herpes simplex type 1 has now emerged as a major cause of genital herpes among populations in which oral-genital contact is common. It explains why, in the past couple of decades, up to 80 percent of new cases of genital HSV infections are type 1.

Type 2 tends to live "below the belt" and up until very recently has been the most common herpesvirus associated with genital herpes. Type 2 can occasionally live "above the belt," too, and cause oral infections. Once a person has herpes, he or she has it for life. A herpesvirus that is dormant (or latent) resides in the infected tissue around the lips (either genital or oral) or in the spinal nerves.

One out of eight people ages fourteen to forty-nine in the United States has had a genital HSV infection.[59] While the percentage of those infected rose about 30 percent from the late 1970s to the early 1990s, that number has decreased some over the past decade. Even so, as many as 776,000 new cases of genital herpes occur annually. Genital HSV-2 infection is more common in women. The CDC reports that about one out of six women have HSV-2, while in men, the figure is closer to one out of twelve. This may be because male-to-female transmission is more likely than female-to-male transmission.

Both HSV-1 and HSV-2 have the same symptoms. But the frequency of genital reactivation is much less with HSV-1, which rarely recurs after the first year of infection.[60] In contrast, type 2 (HSV-2) can continue to recur for many years.[61] This difference in prognosis is a good reason to have a blood test if you suspect you have been infected.

Symptoms

As with HPV, most women who have been exposed to herpes never get sores and therefore have no reason to suspect that they have the virus. Research shows that fewer than 10 percent of people who tested positive for herpes knew that they were infected.[62] Many women attribute their mild genital symptoms to something else, such as a yeast infection or irritation from pantyhose. In fact, in one study of women at high risk for sexually transmitted diseases, 47 percent had evidence of the virus on testing, though only one-half of these had ever had any symptoms.[63] When the virus becomes active, however, it causes very characteristic small ulcers on the genital organs. The first episode of herpes outbreak that a person has (known as a primary herpes infection) can be extremely painful, resulting in a fever, systemic illness, swollen lymph nodes in the groin, genital pain, and even an inability to urinate secondary to pain and herpes infection in the bladder or urethra. Herpesvirus can also cause urinary retention by temporarily paralyzing the motor nerves to the bladder. This is rare and also self-limiting. After a primary herpes outbreak, a person will almost never have symptoms this severe again, since the body produces antibodies to the herpes.

Subsequent outbreaks are known as secondary herpes. These usually start with a sensation of tingling in the affected area, prior to the outbreak of an actual sore. Some women will feel pain down their legs as well, because the herpesvirus lives in the spinal nerves that innervate both the genitals and the inner thighs. Emotional factors, such as depression, anxiety, or hostility, may allow increased production of the herpesvirus and subsequent chronic vaginal irritation.[64]

However, herpes tends to "burn itself out" after a number of years. That means that a person may get outbreaks frequently for a year or two, but they usually don't continue. One of my patients had only one outbreak. At the time of this outbreak she had found out her husband was having an affair. She eventually divorced him, is now in another relationship, and has *never* had a recurrence. Her immune system has kept the herpesvirus inactive, even though her lifestyle includes behaviors that are often associated with immune system depression, such as heavy smoking and the stress of constant dieting. In this woman's case, her immune system in the genital area is keeping her herpes in remission—further evidence that the immunity of our entry points is enhanced when our one-on-one relationships are going well.

Diagnosis

Given the high number of women (and men) who don't know they have herpes, the most accurate way to diagnose it is through testing.

If you have an active herpes sore, or have developed herpes for the first time, cultures can be taken by a healthcare practitioner to determine whether you have the virus as well as to determine which type (HSV-1 or HSV-2) you may have. The newer DNA test (nucleic acid amplification testing, NAAT) gives fewer false-negative results, so if you do get tested, ask for that.

Cultures can also be taken even when you are asymptomatic to determine whether or not you are shedding virus, although one negative test on a given day doesn't guarantee that you won't be shedding virus at another time. Although blood tests don't identify the herpesvirus itself, they can determine if you have antibodies against it, but both the CDC and ACOG do not recommend that asymptomatic people be tested for herpes because of the possibility of false-positive results. In 2016, the U.S. Preventive Services Task Force released recommendations against screening for genital herpes in asymptomatic adolescents and adults, including pregnant women, because the harms outweigh the benefits.[65]

Common Concerns About Herpes

Where Did I Get Herpes? Can I Give It to Someone Else? How Can I Minimize My Chances of Recurrence? The answer to the first question is the same as for HPV: The virus can be dormant for years, so a person who has a primary outbreak may have "caught" it twenty or more years ago! I've seen first-time genital herpes outbreaks in eighty-five-year-old women who've been celibate and widowed for twenty years.

Most sexual transmission of HSV occurs when the virus is reactivated but asymptomatic among people with unrecognized infections. Recent studies indicate that virtually all HSV-2 seropositive persons shed the virus intermittently from mucosal surfaces, and it can be spread by either intercourse or oral-genital contact.[66] In response to the second question, it is generally recommended that people with herpes use condoms to cut the risk of infecting someone else.

In general, herpes outbreaks are associated with the following stressors: anxiety and depression, lack of sleep, overexertion, microabrasions of the vagina from sexual intercourse, and an unbalanced genital microbiome. These outbreaks can be greatly decreased or eliminated by following the nutritional and herbal advice below. The emotional ramifications of having a herpes diagnosis are usually far more troubling than the actual infection. If you've been diagnosed with herpes and are feeling bad about it, there's good information and advice on this website: www.datingwithherpes.org.

You can find labs offering confidential testing for herpes and other STDs at www.stdcheck.com.

What Are the Risks of Herpes If I'm Pregnant? Neonatal herpes is the most severe complication of genital herpes and is caused by the newborn's contact with infected genital secretions at the time of labor. Herpes does not pose any risk for the baby during pregnancy itself unless a woman is first exposed to it when she is pregnant and the virus reaches high enough levels in the blood (known as viremia) and also crosses the placenta to infect the baby. Getting herpes for the very first time during the last four months of pregnancy carries the biggest risk for neonatal herpes because the mother's body hasn't yet had a chance to produce antibodies to the virus.

Though no one actually knows how many babies are exposed to the herpesvirus during labor, we do know that neonatal herpes occurs in up to 1 in 3,200 live births, with an estimated incidence of 1,500 cases annually in the United States.[67] To give you an idea of how rare it is for a baby to actually get herpes, consider the fact that there are a little over 4 million births per year in the United States. And given the large number of women with undiagnosed herpes infections at the time of labor, it's clear that the immune system of mothers offers protection most of the time.

Here's the problem, however: When a newborn does get infected with herpes, it can cause disseminated or central nervous system disease about 50 percent of the time. Of these cases, up to 30 percent will die and up to 40 percent will have some kind of long-term neurological damage. And that's why it's important to do everything possible to minimize the risk of a baby getting infected with herpes during labor. This is why most women with active herpes lesions who are in labor almost always deliver by C-section, which doesn't prevent all cases of neonatal herpes but does decrease the risk by 85 percent.[68] Since there are ways to greatly decrease herpes outbreaks during pregnancy, especially before the onset of labor, the best approach is prevention (see below).

If You Are Pregnant or Considering Pregnancy. If you are considering getting pregnant, it's a good idea for both you and your partner to be tested for herpes. (About 2 percent of pregnant women will become infected during pregnancy.) If you know that your partner is seropositive for herpes and you aren't, then you can use condoms during intercourse or rubber dams during oral sex to prevent genital transmission.

Make every effort to remain as well nourished and healthy as possible during your pregnancy. Worrying for an entire pregnancy about having an active herpes sore at the time of labor may, in my view, increase the chances for an outbreak.

Follow the steps in this section on treatment to prevent an outbreak, such as taking supplements like garlic, a good probiotic, and a good multivitamin.

Note: Antivirals such as valacyclovir and acyclovir (see below) can be used in pregnancy for those with severe or recurrent lesions. No significant adverse effects have been found in newborns exposed to this drug.[69]

Herpes Doesn't Mean an Automatic C-section. If you have a history of herpes but have no lesions during labor, then you can safely deliver vaginally. The major sites of entry of the virus into the newborn include the skin, so any procedure that damages the baby's skin could increase the risk of transmission. Among newborns exposed to herpes at delivery, studies have shown that 10 percent of those delivered with the use of fetal scalp electrode, vacuum, or forceps were infected, compared to only 2 percent of those who did not have invasive obstetrical procedures.[70]

Because the risk of transmitting the virus to the baby is so low even for HSV-2 seropositive women with active herpes lesions, some experts are suggesting that it's safe for these women to deliver vaginally.[71] I certainly agree with this. After all, once you've been exposed to herpes, your body makes antibodies against herpes that cross the placenta and help protect the baby. Despite this evidence, however, the current standard of care in most centers is delivery by C-section for those who have active herpes lesions when they go into labor. The main reason for this is fear of litigation.

Treatment

Medication. A variety of antivirals (e.g., acyclovir [Zovirax] and valacyclovir [Valtrex]) are widely available for treatment of herpes. Acyclovir comes in both pill and ointment form, and some people take it on a long-term basis (for two to three years). When taken orally, this antiviral medication works like any antibiotic in the system. Within twenty-four hours of taking the pills, the virus is inactivated. The topical ointment for actual outbreaks takes a bit longer to work. Antivirals are available only by prescription.

Though antivirals are very helpful in primary (first-time) outbreaks, I'm concerned that chronic use of them may result in resistant viral strains that will be even stronger and harder to treat later. This has happened with other disease-causing organisms over the fifty years that doctors have been prescribing antibiotics and antivirals. Routinely giving antibiotics or antivirals when they are not indicated and failing to look at other ways to support the immune system's own ability to fight germs has resulted in our current battle against "superbug" strains of tuberculosis, pneumonia, and staphylococcus.

For that reason, I prefer an approach that bolsters a woman's inherent ability to keep the virus under control.

Nutritional and Herbal Treatments. Garlic is a highly effective remedy for herpes recurrence, and it has no known side effects. It also works for cold sores. Garlic has been shown to have a number of antiviral, antibacterial, and antifungal properties.[72] For women with recurrent herpes, I recommend the following: When the familiar tingling sensation starts, signaling that an outbreak is about to occur, take twelve capsules of deodorized garlic (available in health food stores) immediately.[73] Then take three capsules every four hours while you are awake, for the next three days. In almost every case, the herpes outbreak will be prevented. Take the deodorized variety of garlic, to prevent the bad breath that is the only downside to garlic's use. I generally recommend brands that contain allicin (such as Garlitrin 4000 and Kyolic, both widely available from most health food stores).

For women with a history of herpes who are planning a pregnancy or who are already pregnant, I recommend they take two garlic capsules every day. This can be increased to six to eight capsules per day if they are under more stress than usual. In my clinical experience, women who do this don't get herpes outbreaks.

Other Herpes Treatments

Monolaurin is made from nontoxic glycerin and lauric acid found naturally in coconuts and breast milk. It is a potent antiviral and immune system booster that works very well to prevent or attenuate herpes outbreaks. Because of its oil base, it is thought to work by disintegrating the cell wall of the herpesvirus before it can replicate. Lauricidin is a good brand that is widely available, but coconut oil is mostly made up of lauric acid, so you can use that topically as well. I recommend putting a couple of drops of tea tree oil in some coconut oil and applying it to the affected area.

Melissa extract (*Melissa officinalis*), also known as lemon balm, has been scientifically shown to have antiviral activity against herpes infections. It can prevent ulcers and speed healing if used at the onset of symptoms.[74] A cream form of this extract, PhytoPharmica's Cold Sore Relief (formerly called Herpalieve), can be purchased at natural food stores. It should be applied to the affected area two to four times daily for five to ten days.

Tea tree oil, from the Australian tea tree, can be applied directly to the tingling area just prior to a herpes outbreak, using either a Q-tip or your finger. In most cases, this topical treatment will prevent an outbreak.[75]

Shoring up your microbiome is also helpful. The microbiome of the genital area is a complex community of bacteria, viruses, and fungi that remain in symbiotic balance. Some of the "good bacteria" are actually able to kill off the pathologic ones with what are known as bacteriocins, peptides that seek out and kill pathogens. The problem is that when microbiome health is compromised through a diet high in sugar or alcohol, or a lifestyle marred by the effect of stress (including lack of sleep), the microbiome balance can go awry. That's why it's helpful to make sure you are regularly eating foods that keep the microbiome healthy—including fermented foods such as yogurt, sauerkraut, and pickles—but also, if necessary, through the regular use of a probiotic. Good examples include Fem-Dophilus and *Saccharomyces boulardii*.

To get a good picture of the health of your vaginal microbiome, I also recommend SmartJane, a screening test from uBiome (see www.ubiome.com) that you can order with a prescription from your healthcare provider. SmartJane measures twenty-three vaginal flora (and also tests for fourteen high-risk and five low-risk HPV strains and four common sexually transmitted infections, including chlamydia, gonorrhea, and syphilis). (By the way, uBiome also offers SmartGut, a test that evaluates gut bacteria and how it affects your health.)

Finally, it also helps to change your perception. Neither herpes nor genital warts need be a big deal. In the vast majority of cases your immune system will take care of them and they won't cause you or anyone else any harm. The problem is the perception that you are somehow bad or tainted if you get them. You can "cure" this through celebrating your genitals and your sexuality as something good. (See Louise Hay's affirmation on page 331.) Here's an example from one of my newsletter subscribers who took my advice and subsequently healed her herpes—in both mind and body—simultaneously.

> I went through a divorce five years ago after a monogamous marriage that lasted twenty-three years. It took me about four years to even have a date. I finally found a guy I really liked. We both got ourselves tested for AIDS before having sex. And neither of us had a history of anything else. So we had sex. It felt so good to be making love again with someone I like and trust. But four days later, I came down with herpes. At first I was horrified. I felt like such a fool. How could I have let this happen? My lover also felt so badly that he had "made me sick," especially since he didn't even know he had herpes. But then I read your book and realized that my attitude and shame weren't helping my immunity a bit. So I took your advice. I started to eat better and take a good multivitamin every day. I also started to affirm the goodness of my own sexuality. I realized that I hadn't done anything wrong. I wasn't bad or tainted—and neither was my lover. The herpes sores healed in about ten days. And now my lovemaking is more pleasurable than ever. I found a guy who really cares, is a wonderful lover, and who affirms my beauty and

desirability every day. Believe me, herpes was a small price to pay. I'm certain that it will never recur now that I feel better about my genitals and my sexuality than ever before!

I applaud my reader for her courageous turnaround of a situation that is devastating to many women. And it is my fervent hope that she really never does get a recurrence! If she does, she'll know what to do about it.

CERVICITIS

True cervicitis is an inflammation of the cervix caused by the same infectious agents that cause vaginitis, such as trichomonas or yeast. Cervicitis and vaginitis are usually present at the same time, and treatment for them is the same. (See the section on vaginitis, page 360.)

In some women, the mucus-secreting cells of the endocervix sometimes extend out onto the outer cervix (the exocervix). This is a normal anatomical variation and is not true cervicitis. Though these women sometimes experience a bit more vaginal discharge than usual, this only rarely requires treatment. In cases in which the discharge is truly a problem, cryocautery (freezing) of the cervix or LEEP cautery can be done. (See page 330.)

CERVICAL DYSPLASIA (ABNORMAL PAP TESTS)

Cervical dysplasia is the name given to cellular abnormalities that arise in the endocervical canal or on the cervix itself: *Dysplasia* simply means "abnormal." It is diagnosed by a Pap test, and the cells are then classified, according to nationally agreed-upon standards, as either *cervical intraepithelial neoplasia* (CIN), which means abnormal cells in the epithelial layer of cells covering the cervix, or *squamous intraepithelial lesions* (SIL), which means abnormal cells in the squamous layer covering the cervix, vagina, or vulva. (Some medical centers don't distinguish between SIL and CIN and use SIL as the all-purpose term.) The pathologist who reads the Pap test ranks these cells numerically, according to the degree of the cellular change. Thus CIN 1 or SIL 1 is considered mild, while CIN 3 or 4 or SIL 3 or 4 is severe.

When a Pap test or other cytology comes back as abnormal, I know that a woman is likely to immediately jump to the worst-case scenario: "Oh, no, I have cancer!" Prompt investigation of the abnormal Pap test generally results in her being reassured. Most abnormal Pap tests *do not* mean cervical cancer, though a certain percentage of dysplasias will go on to become cervical cancer if they are not diagnosed and treated. Some CIN abnormalities, particularly the mild ones, will go away by themselves. This is because the majority of mild dysplasias are actually HPV infections that are self-limiting. Self-limiting infections are those that the body's immune system takes care of on its own.

Symptoms

Cervical dysplasias are not usually associated with symptoms, though some women who have had abnormal Pap tests have told me that they knew something was wrong because they felt a "burning" sensation in the cervical area. (Cervical cancer can be asymptomatic as well, but its symptoms usually include bleeding between periods, pelvic pain, foul-smelling discharge, and/or bleeding after intercourse.)

Pap Test Screening

The Pap test is the single most cost-effective disease screening test known to modern medicine. Ever since the Pap smear (as it was first called) was introduced by George Papanicolaou, M.D., in the late 1940s, the incidence of invasive cervical cancer and the death rates from this disease have gone down dramatically. In fact, it is estimated that 70 percent of cervical cancer deaths are actually prevented because of this inexpensive and noninvasive test. The results are so impressive that I've often joked about the need for a drive-through Pap test center that would make the test as easy to obtain as a McDonald's meal.[76]

A Pap test takes a sample of cells from the transformation zone in the squamocolumnar junction of the cervix, up inside the cervical opening. The cervical cells are then placed in a test tube of liquid media to keep them from drying out and to filter out debris before the cells are placed on a slide and analyzed for abnormalities. Having this information doesn't necessarily change the treatment. In fact, Pap tests often find abnormalities that are benign.

Pap testing is not perfect: Cervical cancer has not yet been completely eradicated. But we're gaining. About 4,170 women still die from this condition annually in the United States—not all of whom failed to get a regular Pap test. Let me put this figure into perspective: Every year 435,000 people die from alcohol use, 365,000 die from poor diet and inactivity, and 7,600 die from aspirin and nonsteroidal anti-inflammatory drug use.[77] The number of deaths from cervical cancer every year in the United States is very low (in developing countries, the rate is much higher)—especially compared with the amount of worry about abnormal Pap tests.

Abnormalities from the upper genital tract, the endometrium, the fallopian tubes, and occasionally the ovaries may show up on Pap tests, but only rarely. The Pap test screens for cervical abnormalities only. Many women don't understand this limitation in their healthcare practitioner's ability to diagnose problems.

The U.S. Preventive Services Task Force updated its Pap test screening recommendations in 2018, as mentioned earlier in this chapter. Here are the current recommendations:

~ **Ages twenty-one to twenty-nine.** Women should have their first cervical cancer screening at age twenty-one, regardless of when they begin having sex. After that, they should have subsequent screenings every three years until they reach age thirty. Note that the HPV DNA test is not recommended in women younger than thirty. That's because any HPV changes in their cervix generally resolve on their own by the age of thirty.

~ **Ages thirty to sixty-five.** Women in this age group can continue to have Pap tests every three years or they can switch to having either an HPV test alone or co-screening (a combined Pap plus HPV test) every five years.

~ **Over age sixty-five.** Most women may stop having cervical cancer screenings once they pass age sixty-five if they do not have a history of moderate or severe abnormal cervical cells or cervical cancer and if they have had three negative Pap tests in a row, or two negative co-screening tests in a row within the past ten years (with the most recent test performed within the past five years).

~ **Special cases.** (1) Women of any age who have been diagnosed with a high-grade precancerous cervical lesion or cancer, are immunocompromised, or were exposed in utero to DES may require more frequent cervical cancer screenings. (2) Most women who have not had abnormal cervical cell growth but who have had a hysterectomy with removal of the cervix for other reasons may discontinue routine cervical screening. However, even if they have had a hysterectomy, women who have had a history of abnormal cell growth (classified as CIN 2 or 3) should continue to have cervical cancer screening for twenty years after their surgery.

ACOG still recommends that women have annual gynecological healthcare visits, even in years when they do not have pelvic exams for Pap tests. Furthermore, it is very important for women who have had the HPV vaccine to continue to follow the same screening guidelines as unvaccinated women since the HPV vaccine does not protect against all forms of HPV, and women who have had it can still get cervical cancer. There is even disturbing evidence that those who've had the vaccine are more susceptible to other, more virulent forms of HPV, from which they're not protected at all.[78] An article published in *Pediatrics* in 2016 reported that while rates of HPV have decreased for the types of HPV the vaccine is designed to protect against since its introduction, the prevalence of all types of HPV has increased 3.7 percent.[79] The danger is that these newly common strains will eventually become even more virulent than those the vaccine protects against now. (See the discussion of the HPV vaccine on page 331.)

ACOG previously recommended that cervical screening begin three years after the first time a woman starts having sexual intercourse or by age twenty-one, whichever came first. But statistics show that women under age twenty-one rarely get cervical cancer. If they are sexually active, however, their rates of HPV infection and dysplasia are high. Numerous studies show that women who have a LEEP procedure to treat dysplasia are more likely to have a subsequent preterm delivery. (Not only is the Pap not necessary in this age group, then, but LEEP is also overkill here because the immune system usually clears 90 percent of HPV infections within one to two years.) The bottom line is that young women were being overtreated for dysplasia showing up in Pap tests, potentially compromising the health of their future children. I applaud these changes and concur with them.

I'd recommend a yearly Pap test if you have had any of the following:

~ Infection with HIV (human immunodeficiency virus)

~ Immunosuppression secondary to organ transplantation (e.g., kidney transplant)

~ Smoking or regular use of alcohol, cocaine, or other similar substances

~ A history of abnormal Pap tests, cervical cancer, or uterine, vaginal, or vulvar cancer

~ Low socioeconomic status (the American College of Obstetricians and Gynecologists points out that this factor appears to be a surrogate for a number of closely related factors that often place these women at greater risk)

How Reliable Is the Pap Test? No test is 100 percent reliable, and the Pap test is no different. Studies have shown that the false-negative rate of the test runs from 5 to 50 percent, depending upon the practitioner and the lab used. Occasionally a Pap test will come back negative even though abnormal cells are present. About two-thirds of these false-negative tests are the result of errors made by the healthcare practitioner in the collecting of the cells (known as sampling errors). About one-third of false negatives are due to laboratory error. There are also times when the abnormal cervical cells are located in areas of the cervix that simply can't be reached by a Pap test. So even under ideal circumstances, when everything is done perfectly, some cervical cancers will not be picked up early with a routine Pap test.

What If My Pap Test Isn't Negative? Sometimes you'll get a Pap test result that is scary or confusing. Here are the basic categories of Pap test results and how to deal with them.

~ Sometimes a Pap test will come back labeled "unsatisfactory for interpretation" or "limited." This is not a cause for alarm. It just means that there were not enough cells present on the slide to interpret the test adequately. An "unsatisfactory" reading doesn't necessarily mean that your practitioner took a bad Pap or did it wrong. It just means that you need to get it repeated.

~ Another designation used on Pap test reports is "limited interpretation secondary to inflammation." Sometimes a yeast, trichomonal, or bacterial infection will result in inflammation being present in the cells taken on a Pap test. Inflammation is also sometimes associated with thinned cervical and vaginal tissue (called *atrophy*) that occurs after pregnancy, after menopause, or during other times of low estrogen. Inflamed cells on a Pap test are almost never a cause for alarm. Just get your Pap test repeated after getting the infection or atrophic tissue treated. In many cases, the inflammation simply clears up by itself without treatment, especially if you improve your diet and lifestyle when necessary.

~ A Pap test category that is often very confusing for practitioners and patients alike is known as ASCUS (atypical squamous cells of undetermined significance), present in 10 percent of Pap tests. Most of the time when the Pap test comes back with this designation, it means that the cells of the cervix are atypical-looking because of some kind of reaction—healing, inflammation, atrophy, and so on. In 75 percent of cases of ASCUS, no actual cervical disease is present. This is when an HPV DNA test is helpful. If it's negative, the cellular abnormality is pretty much guaranteed not to be because of precancerous changes. If it's positive, current guidelines recommend getting a colposcopy and having a biopsy done on any areas of abnormality that the test finds; the abnormal tissue can often be removed immediately. I'd also recommend antioxidant supplements.

If you have inflammation present and your practitioner can find a cause, get it treated and then have your Pap repeated. ASCUS associated with atrophic changes in a postmenopausal woman will disappear with topical estrogen treatment or treatment that nourishes and replenishes vaginal mucosa such as *Pueraria mirifica* orally or vaginally. Remifemin, a standardized extract of black cohosh, has been shown to thicken vaginal tissues after four to six weeks. So has *Pueraria mirifica*. So either of these is a good choice for women who want to avoid estrogen. Estriol is another good choice. (See chapter 14.)

⁓ Sometimes ASCUS Pap tests are associated with what is called LGSIL (low-grade squamous intraepithelial lesion). When LGSIL is suspected, you'll want to be sure to get close follow-up, with repeat Pap tests and HPV DNA testing every four to six months until your results come back normal. Statistics have shown that up to 50 percent of these abnormalities go away on their own—which is very good news. In some cases, your healthcare practitioner may recommend (or you may prefer) further investigation of your cervix through a colposcopy.

⁓ Finally, if your Pap comes back as HGSIL (high-grade squamous intraepithelial lesion), your healthcare provider will schedule a colposcopy and directed biopsies of your cervix and possibly even a LEEP (loop electrosurgical excision procedure) to be absolutely certain about the extent of your abnormality. LEEP removes abnormal tissue from the cervix for diagnostic and treatment purposes while preserving normal cervical function. It can be done in the office and often can be used instead of surgical cone biopsy, a treatment for precancerous changes in the cervix that must be done in the operating room under anesthesia. Be aware, though, that, as explained above, there are some risks with LEEP because it can weaken the cervix and increase the chances of having a subsequent premature birth.

Whether or not you have LEEP, I recommend that you follow the Master Program for Optimal Hormonal Balance and Pelvic Health outlined in chapter 5, with additional high doses of folic acid to support your immune system (see below).

Other Technologies for Testing Cervical Cells

Colposcopy. If an HPV DNA test finds one of the higher-risk subtypes of HPV, the next step is to further delineate the extent of the problem by a test known as colposcopy. In this test, the doctor observes the cervix through a magnifying lens to check the blood vessels and tissue patterns, taking biopsies from areas that appear abnormal, and sending them to the lab. Special attention is paid to the SCJ, making sure that this entire region is seen. Sometimes the abnormal cervical cells extend up into the endocervix, where they cannot be seen or tested. In these cases, a cone biopsy (a biopsy of the internal cervix in the shape of a cone) or LEEP procedure (see page 330) is recommended to further test the tissue in the endocervix. This procedure is not only diagnostic but also often curative. Local anesthetic is available that can be sprayed on the cervix (or vagina) before the biopsies are taken, making this procedure virtually painless. Ask your doctor about it.

Common Concerns About Cervical Dysplasia

How Did I Get It? No one knows precisely why one woman develops cervical dysplasia and another doesn't. Like HPV, cervical dysplasia is related to the functioning of the immune system. In one study, women who were on immunosuppressive drugs for kidney transplants had a sevenfold greater chance of an abnormal Pap test than did a control group of non-immunosuppressed patients. Smoking is a definite risk factor for cervical abnormalities leading to cervical cancer. Women with cervical abnormalities have been found to have lower levels of antioxidants and folic acid in their blood. There is a known link between birth control pills and certain kinds of cervical dysplasias.[80] This may be in part because the pill decreases blood levels of nutrients such as the B vitamins.

Can Smoking Affect My Risk for Cervical Dysplasia? Many studies have documented the link between smoking and cervical dysplasia. Cotinine, a toxic by-product of tobacco, has been found in the cervical mucus of cigarette smokers. If you smoke, your mucosal immunity will be adversely affected in the cervical and vaginal areas.

Treatment

Women need to know that up to 50 percent of mild cervical abnormalities return to normal without treatment. A smaller percentage of the more severe abnormalities also regress. Follow-up Pap tests can help determine whether or not you need treatment.

When dysplasias don't regress on their own, the treatment goal is to eradicate all the abnormal tissue. Standard gynecological medicine has excellent tools to treat both cervical dysplasia and early cervical cancer. The cure rate by standard methods is over 90 percent. Everyone who has an abnormal Pap should follow the nutritional recommendations in chapter 17 and in the Master Program for Optimal Hormonal Balance and Pelvic Health in chapter 5.

Methods to destroy abnormal cervical tissue include laser, cryocautery, trichloroacetic acid, and LEEP. LEEP is used to diagnose and treat some cases of SIL that in the past required cone biopsy under anesthesia in the hospital. Some practitioners use laser in the same way. The cervix heals well after a LEEP procedure, but it does increase the risk for subsequent prematurity in pregnancy.

Regular follow-up with a Pap test every three months for one year, and every six months thereafter, is necessary to be sure that the abnormality doesn't return. After several years of normal Pap tests at six-month intervals, many women can be tested yearly. This decision is made on an individual basis. As one of my colleagues says, "No one ever died from close follow-up." Women who have had moderate to severe cervical dysplasia are likely to get into trouble if the disease progresses, which is why more frequent screening seems appropriate.

Nutritional Approach. Numerous studies have linked low levels of vitamins A and B with cervical dysplasia. Oral contraceptives can increase a woman's chances of having an abnormal Pap test, though the data supporting this are not well known by gynecologists; the pill lowers B vitamin levels in the blood. In women whose diets are already low in nutrients, the pill can set up a slight deficiency state. High doses of folic acid have been used to reverse cervical dysplasias in women who developed them while on the pill. That's why every woman who is on the pill (or HRT) needs to take a good multivitamin rich in B vitamins, including folic acid.

If you have a Pap in the LGSIL or another abnormal category, add 5 mg of folic acid to your diet every day with a good B complex vitamin and multivitamin-mineral supplement. (The usual recommended intake of folic acid is 400 mcg per day, so this is a much higher dose.) Also add antioxidants to your diet. One of the best is from a group of plant substances known as proanthocyanidins, found in grape pips or pine bark. Popular brand names are Pycnogenol and Proflavanol. Initially, take 1 mg per pound of body weight, in two to three divided doses, daily for one week. Then decrease your dose to 20 mg two or three times per day. Anecdotally, I have seen many cases of mild to moderate cervical dysplasia greatly improved with a multivitamin-mineral supplement plus added antioxidants.[81] One more thing: If you smoke, stop!

Cervical dysplasia, if left untreated, can progress to cervical cancer, which traditionally has been treated with hysterectomy. While a full discussion of the treatment of cervical cancer is beyond the scope of this book, let me say at least this much here: I've seen several women who had the beginning stages of cancer on their Pap tests—microinvasive cervical cancer, confirmed by cone biopsy—who have refused hysterectomy. In those women who desire children, this choice is increasingly being supported—along with close follow-up. Depending on the situation, the prognosis can be very good.

Women's Stories

When a woman is willing to look at the stress points in her life, then combines this inner work with standard medical techniques as well as immune support, she is almost guaranteed a successful outcome. Three women's stories of their reactions to cervical and vulvar abnormalities and to cervical cancer, and their struggles to understand and deal with their emotional issues, follow.

Sylvia: A Wake-up Call

Sylvia was thirty-nine when she first came to see me. Two years earlier, she had been diagnosed with the beginning stages of cervical cancer and underwent a cone biopsy treatment. She had had normal Pap tests for two years, but a follow-up test came back with the rating CIN 2. Following that diagnosis, as she was going out of the room, the nurse had remarked, "Too bad this is going to keep recurring every two years."

Sylvia later said that that remark finally galvanized her into action. She had always intended to get around to stopping cigarettes, alcohol, and caffeine, but this time she realized that it was a matter of life or death and that she had to clean up her act. She also said, "I realized, too, that it was time to stop hating my mother. I was a typical 'bad' girl until about a year ago. I then began doing healing visualizations and meditating. I realized through my healing work that I came from a family in which many generations of women have hated themselves. My sister-in-law died of lung cancer from smoking four packs per day, and at her funeral my mother was more abusive to me than I can ever remember. About two days after that, I was diagnosed with cervical cancer. I'm grateful, because I feel like I'm alive now and I hardly was before." Sylvia also told me that her sisters had all had hysterectomies and that one had had a breast removed for breast cancer. She said, "My mother has had her uterus removed, and she is a woman who is filled with self-loathing. Now suddenly I'm realizing that all of these women in my family just hate themselves and have done so for years."

Sylvia decided to break this pattern. To do so, she improved her diet, stopped smoking, and began to keep a journal in which she recorded any insights that arose about beliefs that no longer served her. She began to treat herself with more respect on every level. Her Pap tests have all remained normal since the abnormality was excised.

Faith: Healing Cervical and Vulvar Dysplasias

Faith, a woman in her early thirties, was a nurse and was taking art classes. She had been diagnosed the year before with CIN 1 of the cervix, VIN 1 of the vulva (vulvar intraepithelial neoplasia), and VAIN 1 (vaginal intraepithelial neoplasia). All of these abnormalities were felt to be secondary to HPV infection and had been treated with laser a year before. Now the same abnormalities had returned. Faith's doctor had recommended laser treatment again, but she was reluctant to proceed. It had been quite painful, and there were no guarantees of success.

By the time Faith came to see me, she had already made some dietary improvements. I explained to her the viral nature of the HPV infection and the subsequent cellular abnormalities, and I told her that she could improve her immune system by further improving her diet and by using the healing practices for a while. She understood the importance of careful follow-up.

Then I didn't hear from her again until three years later, when she came in for a consultation. She told me that within six months of her dietary changes and meditation practice, all her HPV abnormalities had gone away. Her doctor couldn't believe it. Her Pap tests had remained normal. But now she was contemplating entering a sexual relationship once again, and she was worried about the HPV. Would it flare up again? She had already done a great deal of inner work around her sexuality through reading and going to twelve-step groups, particularly Sex and Love Addicts Anonymous. She realized that in the past she had had sex when she didn't want it and had participated in it almost automatically, as a way to stave off her fears of abandonment. She had been brought up in a religion that made her feel guilty about her sexuality. Her brothers had been taught by her parents not to get anyone pregnant, while she had been taught that she wasn't supposed to be sexual at all—or at least not until marriage. Having gone through a period of celibacy, she felt that she was once again ready to explore her sexuality with another person. At the time I saw her, she had developed a supportive and loving relationship with a man that did not yet include sex.

Faith and her potential lover had both had HIV tests that were negative. I suggested that he be checked for HPV and herpes, though both of us agreed that the results wouldn't affect the course of their relationship. I asked her to consider whether the relationship would be a source of nourishment and joy for her. When I last saw her, she was in the midst of deciding and didn't plan to proceed until she and her inner guidance were in complete agreement about her next steps.

Barbara: When Surgery Failed

Barbara was thirty-nine when I first saw her. Her story illustrates beautifully the connection between a woman's past, her social situation, her body's "entry points," and her ability to heal.

The first time I saw Barbara, she was blond, petite, perfectly dressed, and had a smile on her face that looked permanently glued in place—a mask to cover what was going on underneath. Though she loved her work as a teacher, her body was giving her a lot of warning signals. Her mother had died at sixty-three of ovarian cancer. Her maternal grandmother had had the same disease. Over the previous nine years, she herself had had over fifteen different surgeries for early-stage cancer, first of the cervix and later of the vagina.

She said of her earlier history, "As time passed, subsequent doctors' reports continued to show precancerous cells. Biopsy after biopsy led to one surgery and then another. Laser treatments proved ineffective. Finally a total hysterectomy, with removal of the ovaries, was done nine years after the first signs of abnormal cells appeared. I was advised not to worry. There was still some normal tissue. I was grateful."

Barbara's hysterectomy was done when she was thirty-six, three years before she came to see me. At her first visit, we took a Pap test of her vagina, which once again came back abnormal.[82] It was read a "mild dysplasia with koilocytotic changes" (this refers to specific changes in the nucleus of the cell, usually associated with an active HPV infection). She underwent a colposcopy and biopsies, which confirmed that she still had the abnormal cells in her vagina. Treatment consisted of removing the abnormal cells.

Because of the recurrent nature of Barbara's problem, we knew that there was nowhere for her to go but inward—to explore, if possible, why her body kept giving her the same message. We wanted to work with her to bolster her immune system and stop the process of disease that was resulting in more and more pieces of her vagina being surgically removed, frozen, or cauterized. All the treatments that she'd had so far—surgery, laser, cautery, and various medications—had failed to "cure" her problem.

As we took a deeper history, Barbara told me that her husband had been an alcoholic for the first fifteen years of their marriage. Much later, she found out that he had been having a series of affairs for years. As she put it, "He'd be holding my hand in the morning, and that of another woman in the afternoon. All the lies he told me were finally confirmed a few nights prior to when I asked him to leave, truths I had known in my heart. One affair after another, moments with prostitutes, encounters in large cities. He had previously denied this and more. The truth left me empty and alone." When she originally came to the center, Barbara had started to see a therapist and was in the process of piecing together her family history.

Barbara gradually began to put her life back together. She said, "I embarked on a journey that would eventually lead me to believe that I could make it on my own. Asking my husband to leave was the first well-thought-out decision I had made on my own. I was fully cognizant of the impact it would have on my life, and I had the courage to initiate and pursue a life outside of marriage. I missed the closeness and the union one feels in marriage. I missed the special person next to me and the knowledge that he would come home. He was my rock. He defined me. He owned me. He abused me. He left me. It hurt, and the pain has lightened, yet it will never fully go away." (This series of revelations on Barbara's part nicely illustrates the lifting of denial. As Anne Wilson Schaef once remarked, "It's hard to lose what you never had.")

Barbara kept a journal and told me that its pages revealed a frightened woman—a child, in many ways. She said that she feared tomorrow and that staying positive felt unnatural and uncomfortable to her. Aloneness and learning to live alone seemed insurmountable to her. Her one real joy was caring for her daughter, then eleven, and watching her grow.

Barbara started to do creative visualizations of her tissues as strong and healthy while also undergoing therapeutic touch treatments to help her move the "stuck" energy in her pelvis.[83] This modality helped her learn how to relax and become less stressed. She told me that up until that time, she had never thought about her sexuality, her breasts, or her vagina as free of disease, clear, healthy, and pink. "My body parts had always been dirty and not a part of me. They did not exist," she said.

She described her therapeutic touch sessions as follows: "Therapeutic touch began as I sat in the chair. I was asked to put my hands on my knees and to think about warm water and a clean, healthy body. Trust this woman, I kept saying. Trust! For the first time—ever—my body felt free of anxiety. A true sense of peace prevailed, a high that was truly unexplainable. Empowered. They want me to become empowered. I should change my diet and continue to envision my life as it could be. Trust, I kept saying. This may work. This *will* work."

Barbara attended a conference with Bernie Siegel, M.D., and Louise Hay and went through a guided imagery experience that focused on the highlights of her life. She said that during this experience, pictures and pain surfaced that caused a knot in her stomach that she thought would never go away. She also did some releasing rituals to try to let go of her past. One of these was to bury her wedding ring in a creek that flowed away from her home. She said the affirmation "I'm open to receive myself." She continued working with this theme repeatedly, returning to it over and over.

Despite all of this work, another Pap test returned as abnormal six months after her first treatment. This time Barbara was treated with a chemotherapy cream called 5-FU for ten weeks. (This treatment is reserved for very resistant cases.) She decided at this point to work with her dreams and try to listen more deeply to her cells.

Around this time Barbara's father died, and another part of her past began to surface. A mentally ill woman had lived with Barbara's family from the time Barbara was born. Barbara noted that this woman, Kerry, had great power and controlled the entire family through manipulation. Barbara wondered if Kerry had been having a lesbian relationship with her mother all these years. Was that why Kerry had always come first in the eyes of Barbara's mother—first over her husband and children?

Barbara writes, "My dreams eventually revealed the horror that I had denied. Kerry had sexually abused me as a child. My anger at this was profound. She had violated me, and how I hated her for what she had done! She often told me that I was dirty. I can still feel her hands on my body. And then she would place me in the tub and tell me to wash all the dirt away. She made me scrub my vagina until it was raw. I felt ashamed and feared the loss of those who loved me.

"I'll never know where my parents were and why they did not protect me from the witch that had bound me for so many years. She can no longer hurt me. She is old now and suffering from the pain of her own cancer, a cancer that has bound her for many years now in a home. The family's codependency has been altered. My work with the twelve-step programs has confirmed my thoughts that we all must separate and become individuals and learn to live alone.

"I struggle to forgive her for taking my mother and father from me. She also took my freedom, my dignity, my sexuality. These attributes are returning, and I've begun to love myself. The shame has lessened and the guilt is dwindling. I have begun to recognize other Kerry figures in my life. I am drawn to them; I fear them; I now avoid them.

"In my search for peace and contentment, I continue to take three steps forward and two steps back in all phases of my being. I refuse to give up the fight. I have fulfilled my promise to see my daughter through college and to present her with a model that strives to validate her while validating others and their efforts."

Barbara eventually made peace with her losses—her loss of her mother and father, and her loss of her relationship with a brother who is alcoholic. She says that she is grieving the "loss of the dream that someone special will come into my life and rescue me from my aloneness." She is angry that it has taken her so long to realize that no one can save anyone else, she says.

"Now I know that no one can get under my skin and do for me what I must do for myself. I have let my daughter go. I have released her from being my social support and comfort. The aloneness is a new reality that I no longer deny. I will look to embrace special times with others and special times with myself. For I now see myself as a person who does not have to change. I like me. I like the warm, loving woman who peeks her head out occasionally. I will work on showing her off more. I have some wonderful qualities that can be offered to the universe. I'll be there if you'll be there."

Barbara's body is now healthy. Her six-month checkups and Pap tests all returned to normal. She has become a vibrant, beautiful woman whose entire being radiates health. When she smiles, her smile comes right from her center. Her mask is gone. She is a healed woman.

For Barbara and so many others, the entry points of our bodies have been defiled and denied as part of us for too long. But though we often have pain and shame stored there, we can reclaim the pleasure of these sacred gateways. This journey starts with awareness and compassion.

VAGINAL HEALTH: WHAT IS NORMAL?

Almost all women normally have some kind of vaginal discharge. A yellowish or whitish stain on a woman's underwear at the end of the day, particularly if she has been wearing pantyhose or pants, is almost inevitable. Many women don't know this and often think that they have some kind of infection, but it is quite normal and does not require a visit to a gynecologist. Vaginal discharges can begin the year before a girl gets her first period. Her gradually increasing estrogen levels stimulate the estrogen-sensitive cells of the vagina and cervix, resulting in an increased production of cervical mucus and increasing the cell turnover rate in the vagina.

A normal vaginal discharge comprises vaginal and cervical cells mixed with cervical mucus and also the normal healthy bacteria that are part of what's called the microbiome. When one looks through the microscope at a test on the slide, one sees mostly normal vaginal squamous cells. Normal cell turnover of the lining of the vagina can increase when a woman is under stress, so she will have an increased amount of discharge. But this discharge, too, will comprise normal cells and healthy bacteria.

Vaginal discharges differ at different times in the menstrual cycle. Many women notice an increase during the days surrounding ovulation; some feel that they have "wet" themselves. Ovulatory flow, or fertile flow, sometimes resembles egg white. Some women have premenstrual spotting of brown old blood. This in itself is not an abnormality.

VAGINITIS

Just about every woman is susceptible to a vaginal infection at some point in her life. Both the vagina and the vulva are often involved in this infection. Hence, when I use the term *vaginitis,* understand that the more inclusive term would be *vulvovaginitis.*

Vaginal infections occur when the vaginal ecosystem becomes unbalanced and the microorganisms that normally live peacefully with each other as an ecosystem become imbalanced. Under the right circumstances these infections include chlamydia, *Gardnerella,* trichomonas, and yeast (a type of fungus, of which there are more than twenty species, the most common being *Candida albicans*). The key concept here is "the right circumstances." The vagina, which normally maintains an acidic pH, is colonized by many different types of organisms, all of which work together to form a healthy vaginal ecosystem and functioning immunity. Even yeast and *Gardnerella* usually live in the vagina normally.[84] When a woman is healthy, well rested, and well nourished, these organisms do not cause problems. Only when something in this area becomes imbalanced are these organisms associated with infection.

Almost every type of organism that can cause a vaginal infection when conditions are out of balance can also be found in women who have no symptoms. For instance, some women have trichomonas protozoans, a well-known sexually transmitted cause of vaginitis, present in their vaginas for years with no symptoms whatsoever. Others are incapacitated by the itching and burning the protozoans can cause.

Carolyn Dean, M.D., N.D., says overgrowth of yeast can produce up to 180 different chemical toxins. This can have effects more far-reaching than a vaginal infection, including setting off cravings for sugar and alcohol, slowing your thyroid, causing hormonal imbalance, and even causing dizziness and fatigue. Yeast overgrowth can even be a contributing factor for chronic fatigue syndrome, fibromyalgia, autoimmune disease, irritable bowel syndrome, and even heart disease and cancer.[85]

Symptoms and Common Causes

Most vaginal infections make their presence known by a burning or itching sensation, sometimes accompanied by a change or increase in vaginal discharge.

Anything that disrupts the pH balance or bacterial balance of the normal vagina can result in an infection. The time you're most likely to get a vaginal infection is during or right around your menstrual period, when your mucosal immunity is at its lowest point in the monthly cycle. The pioneering work of Charles Wira, Ph.D., on mucosal immunity has shown that immunoglobulins A and M are affected by the levels of estrogen and progesterone. These hormonal levels decrease just before the onset of a period, making you more vulnerable to infection. The immune system thus mirrors the emotional permeability of this time in the cycle.[86] Some women experience a similar sensitivity to infection after menopause, when both hormone levels and mucus production drop, but this is not inevitable. If women were able to withdraw from their regular daily schedules during these times and rest and reflect more, there would be less chance for imbalances to occur.

Repeated Intercourse over a Short Period of Time. Semen is buffered alkaline fluid, with a pH of about 9. One episode of intercourse with ejaculation can increase the pH of the vagina for eight hours. When vaginal pH is higher than normal for long periods of time, the bacterial balance can be lost. Those organisms that are normally present only in small numbers can begin to grow and cause infection-like symptoms. If a woman makes love with ejaculation of semen into the vagina three times in a twenty-four-hour period, her vagina will not return to its normal pH for that entire twenty-four-hour period. For some women, this is a setup for infection, particularly women who are in long-distance relationships and whose sex lives are sporadic and limited to increased activity over a few days. To prevent problems, you can douche within a few hours of intercourse with a douche containing povidone-iodine, which will lower pH and also effectively kill bacteria. (Trade names include Summer's Eve Medicated Douche and Betadine vaginal douche.) Or use a vinegar douche—one tablespoon per quart of warm water. Douching to reduce vaginal pH after sex is meant as a preventive treatment *only* in those women whose vaginitis is triggered by contact with semen. It's not meant as an endorsement of douching as a standard practice for women.

Chronic Vulvar Dampness. The vulva sweats more than any other place in the body, especially when a woman is emotionally stressed. Thus, wearing restrictive, nonabsorbent, synthetic clothing close to the skin in the vulvar area can be a setup for chafing and subsequent infection. This is especially true if a woman exercises in this type of clothing. Riding a bike or a horse or using a rowing machine in such clothing can also cause vulvar irritation. Instead, switch to looser garments and underwear made from natural fibers like cotton, bamboo, linen, or silk.

Chemical Irritants. Some women develop vulvar irritation through chemical irritants found in scented, softened, and colored toilet paper; bubble baths; and sanitary tampons and pads that contain deodorants. Tampons and pads made from conventionally grown cotton have been shown to have the chemical dioxin in them, which is a by-product of the bleaching process. This is a known toxin that can build up in the body after years of tampon or pad use. In addition, commercially grown cotton is grown using a huge amount of pesticides, the residues of which end up in pads and tampons.

All women should avoid using pads and tampons that contain deodorants. These tampons can produce vaginal ulcers, and the pads can cause vulvar irritation. Ideally, organically grown cotton and all-natural tampons and pads should be used if possible. No tampon should ever be left in for more than eight to twelve hours at a time.

Other irritants can include chemicals in swimming pools and hot tubs, scented douches, and vulvar deodorant.

Emotional Stress. Some women respond to a perceived boundary violation with a vaginal infection. Many yeast infections also occur premenstrually, when a woman's stress is more apt to manifest in symptoms—and when the hormonal milieu is more susceptible as well. They often clear up spontaneously once the period starts.

Antibiotics. After the introduction of broad-spectrum antibiotics in the 1940s and 1950s, the incidence of yeast vaginitis increased dramatically. Many women can date the onset of their vaginitis to their teen years, when they took antibiotics such as tetracycline to treat acne. Unfortunately, every time we take an antibiotic, we disrupt the natural balance of organisms in the vagina and bowel, and a yeast infection, either full-blown or chronic, can result. In the last decade, while the percentage of women over the age of eighteen has increased by only 13 percent, the number of antifungal prescriptions for women has increased by 53 percent.[87]

Birth Control Pills. Some women notice more yeast infections on the pill, which may be related to the type of progestin in the pill. Try switching pills or stopping the pill for three months and see if the yeast infections clear.

Diet. Many books have now been written on the connection between repeated courses of antibiotics, a diet high in sugars and refined foods, and excessive yeast growth in the vagina and bowel. Eating a lot of food made with refined sugar and flour can favor the overgrowth of vaginal yeast. Dairy products can also contribute to yeast vaginitis in some women because of their high lactose (milk sugar) content, which favors the overgrowth of yeast in the bowel and vagina. One of my patients developed recurrent yeast infections when she drank an instant-breakfast-type milk drink every morning. The high sugar content of this so-called healthful meal substitute threw off her body's ability to fight excessive yeast growth.

Many conventionally trained physicians don't look at repeated courses of antibiotics and poor diet as factors in chronic vaginitis. Many women have seen ten or more doctors for their vaginitis and have had every conventional culture and biopsy done without uncovering a definitive cause. Once these women begin to support their bodies' natural healing abilities through emotional work, dietary improvement, and supplements, their vaginitis problems have often gone away.

Diagnosis

The vast majority of common vaginal infections can be diagnosed by looking at a sample of the vaginal secretion under a microscope and testing it for pH. Some infections, such as chlamydia and herpes, require that a culture be sent to a laboratory for further testing.

Women with chronic vaginitis are suspected to have a condition known as intestinal dysbiosis, or an imbalance of bacteria in the bowel that is often accompanied by an overgrowth of yeast. Women with this condition often reintroduce yeast into their vaginas, even after repeated treatment. This is because yeast in the bowel reinfects the nearby vagina.[88] When intestinal dysbiosis is suspected, a special stool culture can be sent to a laboratory that specializes in proper diagnosis of intestinal dysbiosis.[89] Alternatively, simply changing your diet and adding probiotics and digestive enzymes is all that is usually necessary. (See "Nutrition," page 365.)

Treatment

Over-the-Counter Preparations. Many women can treat an occasional episode of vaginal burning or itching with one of the over-the-counter preparations that are widely available, such as Monistat and Gyne-Lotrimin. Essential oils also have antifungal and antibacterial properties. Just put a couple of drops of myrrh, tea tree, or lavender oil into some organic coconut oil and apply to the vulva and vaginal area with your fingers.

Yin-Care Herbal Wash contains a combination of fourteen highly concentrated herbs used in traditional Chinese medicine for their antipathogenic properties. You can use the wash externally as either a douche or compress to treat viral, bacterial, fungal, or yeast infections and to help restore (and then maintain) proper pH balance. (See www.radiantwonder.com/Yin-Care.)

I also recommend She*Pak, an L-shaped gel-filled ice pack for relief of inflamed tissue in both the vagina and the labia. Store it in your freezer until you need it, then apply the lubricating jelly that comes with it (or use your own) before inserting it into your vagina for up to fifteen minutes at a time. You can use it several times a day, but allow for one hour between uses. (See www.femicorp.com.)

If you've tried an over-the-counter preparation or essential oil for a week or so with no improvement of your symptoms, see a healthcare practitioner to be certain that you're not missing something. Once a diagnosis of a vaginal infection is made, the practitioner can prescribe the proper treatment.

Resistant cases of bacterial vaginitis can be treated with vaginal antibiotic creams available by prescription: Cleocin (clindamycin) vaginal cream or MetroGel (metronidazole) vaginal cream. A single-dose oral antibiotic called secnidazole (sold under the brand name Solosec by Symbiomix Therapeutics) has recently received FDA approval for treating bacterial vaginosis. Secnidazole comes in a 2-gram packet of granules that you sprinkle on applesauce, yogurt, or pudding and then eat (without chewing or crunching the granules).

A trichomonas infection can be treated with Flagyl (the oral antibiotic metronidazole), available by prescription. The side effects from this treatment are nausea and an adverse reaction to alcohol. If a woman has trichomonas and has a sexual partner, both partners must be treated. Otherwise, they may reinfect each other. A male has no symptoms but carries the trichomonas in his genital tract.

Evidence also suggests that some women have chronic yeast infection even after treatment because they are continually reinfected by their sexual partners.[90] In these cases, treatment of the partner is helpful.

Preventing Recurrence. Avoiding the chemical irritants involved in vulvovaginal infections can be very helpful for susceptible women. Women with a history of repeated infections may choose to avoid using all tampons for six months. Use an all-natural brand once tampon use is resumed. Avoid panty-hose when possible, or cut out the crotch. Oral sex has also been associated with an increased risk for yeast infection, as has consuming yeasted bread. This is most common in those who have systemic yeast overgrowth, which can manifest in the mouth, skin, nails, and gut.

Douching. I don't recommend douching except for specific symptoms that you are treating or after repeated intercourse to prevent infection. Especially with commercial preparations, douching simply disrupts the normal bacterial flora of the vagina and may actually increase the risk of infection. It is not necessary to "clean" the vagina.

Nutrition. For women with recurrent yeast infections, I recommend the Master Program for Optimal Hormonal Balance and Pelvic Health in chapter 5. I also suggest avoiding all antibiotics. Note that sugar in all forms (including foods that become sugar quickly—including white flour, potatoes, and most processed grains) feeds yeast.

Promising research from Tufts University shows that mice fed coconut oil had less *Candida albicans* than those fed beef fat. The study notes that "these findings suggest that coconut oil could become the first dietary intervention to reduce *C. albicans* GI colonization."[91]

To eliminate yeast in the intestinal tract and rebalance intestinal flora, which will help avoid reintroducing yeast into the vagina, you can use a variety of supplements, such as acidophilus and bifida factor, both intestinal biocultures. Fem-Dophilus, marketed by Jarrow, is a probiotic developed specifically to replenish normal vaginal flora. It is widely available at Whole Foods or drugstores and is also useful for fighting bacterial vaginosis and vaginal yeast infections and for lowering the risk of recurrent UTIs.

PB 8 is a good all-purpose probiotic to replenish gut flora that doesn't require refrigeration. Many other good ones are available as well. Also check the refrigerated section of your natural food store. Finally, decrease stress as a way to enhance your immune system functioning.

Psychological and Emotional Aspects

Some women with chronic vaginal infections fail to respond to any treatment. Some, too, are not open to trying any but the most conventional treatments, convinced that "there's a reason for this that you doctors are simply not finding—so do more tests." These situations present a very difficult dilemma for both the patient and the healthcare practitioner.

For a true cure of the problem, the emotional aspects of chronic vaginitis and vulvovaginitis must be looked at and worked through.[92] This is not to say that the problem is just in those women's heads. What might have begun in the head becomes physical. Studies have shown that many women with these infections have antibodies that work against their own immune and reproductive cells.[93] One of my patients consulted a medical intuitive for her chronic recurrent yeast infections. She was told, "You've got Doberman pinschers in there. You go near there, and you'll lose a limb." As it turned out, this woman had experienced incest as a child. She came to see that one of the decisions she had made in her early teens was that no one was ever going to get near her vagina again. Because she had not made this decision with her intellect, on a conscious level, it manifested through her body. This is nearly always the case. If we were conscious of the conflicts that were driving our diseases, we wouldn't manifest them physically.

Chronic vaginitis is also a socially acceptable way for a woman to say no to sex. For some women, saying "No, I'm not interested in having sex with you tonight or the rest of the week" is not acceptable, given the mate they have chosen and the home in which they grew up. If they believe that sex is one of their duties, regardless of whether they derive pleasure from it, no matter how unconscious this belief may be, chronic vaginitis may well represent an out for them. But the immune system is never fooled.

Another common problem associated with chronic vaginal and vulvar infections is infidelity by the woman's partner. Even when a woman doesn't intellectually "know" that her husband is having an affair, her body may well be aware of it. I've seen several women in whom chronic vaginitis began at about the same time their mate started an affair. Of course, we might explain this by saying that the husband was bringing something home to his wife in the form of germs, and that does happen. But in most of these women, I've been unable to find a physical cause for the vaginitis.

In a woman who has been in a monogamous relationship for years, a sudden onset of primary herpes, fever, general illness, genital sores, warts, or other obvious infections can be classic indicators of infidelity. For reasons already discussed, however, this is not always the case and is almost impossible to prove. Women may also have vaginal problems exacerbated by guilt over affairs that *they* are having.

It's not uncommon for a spouse to lie if he is confronted about having an affair. Several of my patients, especially premenstrually, have had dreams that their husbands were lying to them. After years of questioning their own sanity, they've found out that the dreams were correct—they had in fact been lied to. And guess what? A woman's body knows it, often long before her intellect accepts the information.

Joyce: Vaginitis as a Message

Joyce was fifty-three when she first came to see me. For almost twenty years she had had chronic vaginal infections that always returned after treatment. When I met her, she was bitter and angry over her recent divorce. Her husband of many years, a wealthy and charming alcoholic, had left her for one of her own friends. She felt abandoned and cast aside, even though further questioning revealed that her relationship with her husband hadn't been satisfying for a long time. His drinking and workaholism had been constant problems, and her sex life had been complicated by painful intercourse and frequent infections for almost twenty years.

Joyce's physical exam on this first visit was basically normal, though her vaginal tissues were thin and tender. As long as she wasn't having intercourse, she didn't have any vaginal infections or other discomforts, and no treatment was necessary. Over the next several years, I saw Joyce for her annual exams. Each year she was a little less bitter about her ex-husband and was slowly able to see how much better she felt without him. She then remarried. When she moved in with her new husband, she had a dream in which their house was part hospital and part school. This dream was very meaningful for her because it symbolized this new marriage as one in which both healing and learning would take place. She felt cared for for the first time in her life. She realized that she had never experienced true intimacy before her marriage to this man.

Her sex life with her new husband was wonderful, she reported. In fact, she had never dreamed that it could be so good. She has never had another vaginal infection, and her vaginal tissues are normal and healthy in every way. She has come to see that for years her body, through chronic vaginitis, was sending her a message about her prior relationship, before her intellect "got it." It is entirely possible to heal chronic vaginitis once the stage is set for healing.

Katherine: The Body's Wisdom

Katherine came in for her annual visit complaining that she had had several recurrent vaginal infections in the previous two months. But by the time of her visit, these infections had started to go away by themselves and she was already virtually free of the symptoms. She had recently ended a relationship that she'd been in for only two months. She said, "When he said to me, 'I want to keep you all to myself and keep you away from the world,' I knew I had to get out of there." After leaving this man, Katherine thought she would feel better—but instead she found herself bingeing on food a great deal.

As we talked, I suggested she look back over her life since her last visit a year earlier, when she had just gotten out of a ten-year relationship with a drug addict and was in a group working on incest issues. When I asked her if she'd listened to a recorded lecture on love addiction, something I'd suggested the year before, she replied, "I don't even dare to." We both laughed, and I reminded her how much progress she had made. As we were discussing the fact that the body gives us signals long before the intellect is willing to hear them, she said, "You know, I developed endometriosis in the second month of my relationship with that drug addict, and I knew at that time that it was probably caused by the stress of the relationship. But I didn't let my intuition speak to me." Now, however, she was able to appreciate her body's wisdom, both in her long-term relationship and in the one she had just ended.

A NOTE ON SEXUALLY TRANSMITTED DISEASES

Our current media-driven atmosphere often leads women to believe that it's both desirable and expected to have sex on the first or second date with a person who is almost a complete stranger. Simultaneously, we're all more aware than ever about the risks for contracting sexually transmitted diseases (STDs) of all kinds, including AIDS—a risk that increases with the number of sexual contacts that we (or our partners) have. This double message—sex is expected of you, but make sure you don't catch anything or infect someone else—has resulted in virtual sexual paralysis for some women, and outright risky behavior in others who are fortified mostly with denial. Yet being older does not mean you are immune to the same sexually transmitted diseases and conditions as younger people. For example, the CDC reports that nearly half of those living with diagnosed HIV in the United States are fifty and older. The number of new diagnoses is declining among this age group, yet still around one in six HIV diagnoses in 2016 were in this group.[94] Further, in Americans ages fifty-five to sixty-four, chlamydia cases nearly doubled between 2012 and 2016.[95]

I've seen the unpleasant consequences of behavior at both ends of the spectrum. I've sat with women who reacted to a diagnosis of herpes as though their lives were over. And I've seen many others who've ended up with pelvic inflammatory disease and subsequent infertility—the result of sexually transmitted infections that did their damage before treatment was started. There is a better approach. For a sexually active person, there is no guaranteed way to avoid exposure to sexually transmitted diseases. Despite this, exposure in itself does not make developing a sexually transmitted disease inevitable. Even in the case of AIDS, the overall chance of contracting HIV from one act of intercourse with an infected person is about one in a thousand.[96] And even with repeated exposure to HIV, some people have not become seropositive.[97] Immune function depends in part upon how safe and secure you feel in the world throughout your life in general, or during a particular time. A large individual variation in immune status is common. This information is certainly not meant to suggest that a woman should ever neglect safe sexual practices and condom use. Instead, I present it as evidence that there's a great deal of potential within the human body for resilience and health. A woman's biggest defenses against sexually transmitted diseases are taking commonsense measures, such as using condoms and being discriminating about sex partners, as well as having self-respect, self-esteem, love and acceptance of her sexuality and genitals, and a functional immune system (which goes hand in hand with intact and healthy vaginal mucosa).

You have only two choices when dealing with STDs:

1. Become so paralyzed by fear that you make a vow of celibacy, don't touch anyone—including yourself—"down there," and sterilize everything in sight. (This doesn't work—the world is crawling with germs, and so are we all.)

2. Keep your vaginal mucosa healthy through the power of safe sexual practices as well as your thoughts, diet, and emotions. Practice safe sex as best you can until you've made a monogamous commitment—always follow Frank Pittman, M.D.'s hard-and-fast rule of condom etiquette: "Bring it up before he gets it up."[98] Accept yourself for who you are and what your natural talents are; expand your understanding of what sexuality is and how your views of it affect you; and eat healthfully and take a good multivitamin-mineral supplement.

A Word About AIDS

I am not an authority on AIDS and I don't treat AIDS patients. I *am* often asked questions about it, and have sent many women for testing. Of the estimated 1.1 million people in the United States who are infected with HIV, about one in seven don't know that they are infected, thus jeopardizing their own care and putting others at risk.[99] Though the number of new cases of AIDS increased in the mid-1990s, it declined slightly after 1999 and then leveled off before finally beginning to decrease. From 2010 to 2015, the estimated number of annual HIV infections in the United States declined by 8 percent, and in 2016, there were 39,782 new cases reported.[100] The incidence of HIV infection is greater in certain at-risk populations, including men who have sex with men, African Americans, Hispanics, and women—all of whom are disproportionately represented among people who are HIV positive, have AIDS, or both.[101]

Though it is a much more serious disease, AIDS is related to herpes and warts in that one of the modes of transmission is sexual contact. Because people can have HIV for years before it shows up as AIDS, there are potentially *no* safe sex partners until we have been monogamous with someone for at least eight to twelve months and both have negative HIV tests. (Even a negative HIV test is not a 100 percent guarantee, because you can have the virus when the test is taken but not yet have the antibody in the blood that is the basis for the HIV test.) The concept of the asymptomatic shedder of the herpesvirus (one who potentially sheds the virus and infects someone else without ever knowing that he or she has it) essentially applies, in my opinion, to almost *all* infectious diseases, especially the sexually transmitted ones.

I believe that the AIDS epidemic is a consequence of a large-scale breakdown in human immunity, resulting from such factors as chronic drug and alcohol abuse, relationships in which sex is the central focus, pollution of the environment, soil depletion, poor nutrition, and generations of sexual dysfunction and repression. AIDS has been called a metaphor for the breakdown of planetary immunity as a result of excessive dumping of toxins into the earth's—and thus our own—lymphatic systems.[102]

Fortunately, the number of long-term AIDS survivors is increasing. Since antiretroviral therapies were introduced in 1996, there's been a marked reduction in the rates of illness and death due to HIV infection in the developed world. HIV is now considered a chronic disease, and life expectancy after diagnosis can be decades. In a 2005 article on the subject in the *New England Journal of Medicine,* Scott Hammer, M.D., an HIV researcher, writes, "An otherwise healthy person with asymptomatic HIV infection and no coexisting illnesses . . . should be advised that decades of productive life, which can include intentional pregnancies if desired, are possible with proper care."[103] I am also certain that the fact that HIV is no longer an automatic death sentence is immune-system-enhancing in and of itself.

Several years ago, I met a university professor who has been HIV positive since she was originally infected back in college in the 1980s. Though she has had occasional bouts when she's been really sick, for the most part she remains healthy and functional. She told me that she finds hope and solace in the Buddhist approach of nonviolence and endeavoring to live in peaceful coexistence with the HIV virus instead of seeing it as "the enemy." It's certainly working. And yes, she also takes antiretrovirals.

CHRONIC VULVAR PAIN (VULVODYNIA)

Women with chronic vulvar pain and burning—known as burning vulva syndrome—have a condition known as vulvodynia or vulvar vestibulitis syndrome. Women with this condition experience searing pain at the opening of the vagina during intercourse and sometimes also have unrelenting pain and burning, stinging, or redness. There is acute tenderness to pressure in the ring of vestibular glands that are located just outside the vagina. This may preclude intercourse altogether. Because vulvodynia patients may have seen many doctors without finding a straightforward cause or cure, they often require a good deal of compassion. I've put together the best options I've found for this problem, but I must stress the importance of the mind-body connection for anyone who desires permanent relief from this condition. (The same approach applies to those with interstitial cystitis; see page 377.)

What Causes Vulvodynia?

Numerous studies have failed to isolate a cause for vulvar vestibulitis, but some believe that it could be triggered by vaginal yeast infections, gynecological surgery, or childbirth. It has also been associated with sexual abuse. Research has not been able to demonstrate that allergies, human papilloma virus, or bacterial overgrowth are causes of vulvodynia. Under the microscope, the most frequent finding is a nonspecific inflammation in the vestibular gland.[104] Inflammation is, of course, associated with virtually all disorders, so this isn't particularly helpful. Surgical procedures such as laser vulvectomy or vulvar vestibular gland removal often fail to eradicate the pain, though these procedures have helped some.[105] What is interesting is that scientists have found that the glands in this area have associated nerve structures containing the neurotransmitters serotonin and chromogranin. This explains why treatments that work for nervous system and mood disorders sometimes also work for vulvodynia.[106] Anything that affects neurotransmitter levels in our cells can affect our health. And a wide variety of modalities ranging from biofeedback to antidepressant medication have been shown to alter serotonin levels.

I advise my patients to start with nutritional and mind-body approaches to this problem first, and then resort to the other treatments listed here only if necessary.

Nutritional Aspects of Vulvodynia

Some research has indicated that vulvodynia may be associated in some way with calcium oxalate in the urine.[107] The calcium oxalate is thought to be highly irritating to the skin of the vulva in affected women. Not all research bears this finding out. But whether vulvar irritation is caused by high levels of urinary calcium oxalate or simply abnormally high sensitivity to normal levels of calcium oxalate, the fact remains that many women are helped by following a low-oxalate diet and taking calcium citrate daily. Some doctors claim a 70 percent success rate with this approach. Following a low-oxalate diet can take three to six months to work. Foods rich in oxalate include rhubarb, celery, chocolate, strawberries, and spinach. (See Resources for references on low-oxalate foods and low-oxalate recipes.)

Taking calcium citrate also lowers oxalate levels. Citracal is a widely available brand that contains 200 mg calcium and 750 mg citrate per tablet. Take this or another brand with similar amounts at the rate of two tablets one hour before meals three times per day. Sometimes this alone is all that a woman will need to help relieve her vulvar pain and resume a more normal lifestyle.

I recommend that women with vulvodynia follow the Master Program for Optimal Hormonal Balance and Pelvic Health in chapter 5, page 143. Add proanthocyanidins (antioxidant substances found in grape pips or pine bark, available at health food stores) at an initial dose of 1 mg per pound of body weight, divided into two to four doses daily, for two weeks. Then decrease to a maintenance dose of 20 to 60 mg per day. A comprehensive regimen of vitamins, minerals, and antioxidants has been shown to improve immune system functioning and help support cellular healing and regeneration throughout the body. This is probably why this regimen sometimes works to help women with vulvodynia.[108] A diet that decreases inflammation is also important. (See chapter 17, on nutrition.)

Psychological Aspects of Vulvodynia

Like all other conditions, vulvodynia has physical, emotional, and mental aspects. Failure to address all of these aspects of a problem simultaneously may lead to temporary relief only, while your inner guidance tries to find another way to get your attention. Research on the emotional aspects of vestibulitis has compared vulvodynia patients with a control group of women with other vulvar problems. Compared with the control group, women with vulvodynia were shown to be more psychologically distressed, more likely to have sexual dysfunction, and more likely to have increased awareness of completely normal sensations throughout their bodies. But instead of knowing that these are normal, they are more likely to believe they are symptoms of serious illness. For example, they may sense that their abdomen bloats a great deal after meals and fear that this indicates some major disease process. Small pink spots and other normal discolorations on the skin are believed to be cancerous, or they may think that hearing their heart beating in their ears at night indicates a brain tumor.[109] This is known as somatization.

As already mentioned, vestibulitis patients are more likely to have had a history of sexual or physical abuse than women with other vulvar problems.[110] Since it is well documented that women who've experienced sexual or physical abuse or assault often have difficulty negotiating healthy sexual relationships, it is not surprising that the vulvar area of the body might be where a woman's inner wisdom is trying to get her attention for healing. One approach to changing the nervous system's messages in this area is through biofeedback. Vaginal biofeedback—that is, learning how to progressively relax and rehabilitate the pelvic floor muscles—has been shown to decrease the subjective experience of pain in 83 percent of the women in one study who practiced this technique for sixteen weeks. The majority of these women were also able to resume intercourse by the end of the treatment period.[111] Pelvic floor strengthening and toning (see chapter 8) can work in the same way, so a woman can try this at home. Many physical therapists are trained in pelvic floor rehabilitation. Those who work with stress urinary incontinence may be able to help with this as well.

Other Treatments

NAET. Though vulvodynia has not been shown to be associated with allergy, clearly it is related to some immune response. It may respond well to Nambudripad's Allergy Elimination Techniques (see page 918 or go to NAET's website at www.naet.com).

Interferon. Interferon is an antiviral substance that stimulates the natural killer cells of the immune system. It is often helpful in certain cases of vulvodynia even though we don't understand how it works. However, in women with chronic vulvar symptoms, it is evident that something is "off" with the immune response in the mucosal system. So it makes some sense that a substance that affects mucosal immunity, such as interferon, might help. Some researchers believe that interferon works only in those women with evidence of HPV infection; others don't make that distinction.

Interferon is injected into the vestibular glands three times a week for four to six weeks. Relief has been reported in 40 to 80 percent of the cases, depending upon patient selection. Since studies suggest that HPV is not the cause of the vulvar pain, the success of this treatment is an interesting paradox that can't be easily explained. Interferon doesn't work well in women with no evidence of HPV.[112]

Surgical Treatment. Surgical excision of the vestibular glands is successful in some women, but not all. I would recommend it only as a last resort, because this procedure doesn't address the underlying imbalance and often doesn't work.

Getting to the Heart of the Issue

Like all distressing symptoms, vulvar pain often has an unconscious emotional basis—for example, it may stem from childhood sexual abuse. It exists to quite literally bring someone's attention back to the scene of the crime, as it were. For that reason, I encourage every woman to have the courage to try one of the mind-body therapies that often work so well. These include tapping (Emotional Freedom Technique, or EFT) and eye movement desensitization and reprocessing (EMDR). I also highly recommend working with a physical therapist who specializes in women's health.

The book *Ending Female Pain: A Woman's Manual* (BookSurge Publishing, 2009, and updated in 2014) by women's health physiotherapist Isa Herrera, owner of Renew Physical Therapy in New York City, is a comprehensive manual that shares just about every technique you can imagine to help the pelvic floor and end chronic pelvic and sexual pain. Herrera details the use of yoga, Pilates, visualization, internal massage, scar therapy, and vulva self-care to lessen the pain not only of vulvodynia but also of vaginismus, interstitial cystitis, vestibulitis, endometriosis, pre- and postnatal pain, and more. Isa also offers a powerful online course called the Female Pelvic Alchemy Jump Start Program. The program includes lifetime access to eight modules on healing the pelvic floor, including videos and supplemental materials. (For more information, see her website, www.pelvicpainrelief.com.)

Given all of the scientific evidence and treatment choices, it is clear that the optimal treatment for vulvodynia must address physical, emotional, and psychological aspects simultaneously. A symptom as persistent as chronic vulvar pain requires a great deal of trust in your inner wisdom, and a lot of compassion and patience.

LICHEN SCLEROSUS

Lichen sclerosus is a chronic inflammatory skin condition that affects both women and men at any age, although it's most commonly seen in women at perimenopause and beyond. It is characterized by white patches and thinned skin around the vagina and anus. It can be quite itchy and irritated, resulting in pain, bleeding, and scarring from scratching. This condition can also make intercourse and urination painful.

The cause is unknown, but it's thought to result from some kind of immunologic problem in the skin.

Treatment

Conventional Treatment. Most doctors prescribe anti-inflammatory steroid creams or antihistamine creams to treat this condition. One approach that works well is to have a pharmacist make up an ointment consisting of seven parts steroid cream (such as Valisone) and three parts antihistamine cream (such as Eurax), which is then rubbed into the affected area twice per day. The symptoms generally come back unless the treatment is continued.

Other Treatments. A homeopathic cream known as Emuaid (available in two strengths) has helped many women with lichen sclerosus and other stubborn skin conditions. It is made from a complex blend of homeopathic remedies including 10X, 20X, and 30X HPUS Argentum Metallicum (colloidal silver), emu oil, bacillus ferment, l-lysine hydrochloride, tea tree oil, phytosphingosine, and ceramide 3. There are no toxic ingredients.

Mind-Body Approaches. As with all chronic conditions, it is fruitful to determine whether you have emotional, dietary, or allergy problems that are contributing to the problem. For this reason, I recommend following the plan in chapter 15, "Steps for Flourishing." Also consider trying EFT to see if symptoms can be relieved this way. Heilkunst practitioner Tammie Quick in Alberta, Canada, is a lichen sclerosus expert who herself has dealt with the condition. She uses EFT, among other holistic treatments, in her practice. (See www.quick-health.ca.) Her self-published 2016 book, *How to Live Happily Ever After "Down Under": The How to Thrive with Lichen Sclerosis Guide* is an excellent resource and includes an EFT script to use in treating the condition.

VAGINAL COSMETIC SURGERY

In the past decade or so, plastic surgical procedures to "upgrade" and change labia size and shape and tighten the vagina have become increasingly common. Unfortunately, while there is very rarely any medical necessity for this kind of surgery, many young women who are displeased because their genitals don't look like those of porn stars sometimes seek out this treatment.

In 2016, labiaplasty (plastic surgery performed on the labia) was the fastest-growing cosmetic procedure in the world, increasing 45 percent from the previous year.[113] The trend has been extremely popular in the United States, where the demand increased more than 217 percent from 2012 through 2016, although figures were down almost 11 percent in 2017.[114] "It remains to be seen if this particular procedure is a passing trend or a permanent one," the American Society of Aesthetic Plastic Surgery (ASAPS) noted in a 2017 summary.

Most disturbing is that desire for the surgery is catching on with adolescents. The ASAPS reports that 400 girls age eighteen and younger had labiaplasty in the United States in 2015, an 80 percent increase from 2014.[115] Naomi Crouch, M.D., chair of the British Society for Pediatric and Adolescent Gynecology, told the BBC that girls as young as nine are asking for the operation in the United Kingdom, where more than 150 girls had the procedure from 2015 to 2016.[116] "I find it very hard to believe there are 150 girls with a medical abnormality which means they needed an operation on their labia," she said in the interview. Drawing parallels between labiaplasty and female genital mutilation (FGM), she noted, "The law says we shouldn't perform these operations [FGM] on developing bodies for cultural reasons. Current Western culture is to have very small lips, tucked inside. I see this as the same thing."

While some girls may truly experience chafing or itching in their labia during sports, most teens who ask about the procedure want it for purely cosmetic reasons. Because so many young women (more than 70 percent of females ages twelve to twenty) now routinely wax or shave their pubic area,[117] this part of the female body is literally exposed to an increasing level of scrutiny, leaving many young women feeling insecure and ashamed when their bodies don't look like the airbrushed pictures they see on the Internet. Yet this procedure is not without risks. Surgery on the labia (which are still developing in the teen years) can lead to a lessening of sensation, thanks to the labia's overwhelming number of nerve endings—not to mention the possibility of numbness, pain, and scarring.

So many teenagers are seeking labiaplasty that the American College of Obstetricians and Gynecologists' Committee on Adolescent Health Care issued an opinion in 2017 stressing that the procedure is rarely appropriate for teens and urging doctors to reassure their patients, suggest alternatives to surgery, and screen patients for a psychiatric disorder that causes obsession about perceived physical defects.[118]

Concerned with this trend, Amsterdam illustrator Hilde Atalanta started *The Vulva Gallery* (www.thevulvagallery.com), a series of illustrations of all kinds of vulvas, to serve as an educational platform celebrating vulva diversity. "I aim for *The Vulva Gallery* to contribute in changing the way we look at vulvas, by showing that all vulvas are wonderful just the way they are," Hilde says on her website. She's amassed a community of nearly 250,000 followers since the online gallery launched in 2016.

Another good reality check is the book *Petals* (Crystal River Publishing, 2003) by Nick Karras, D.H.S., a professional photographer with a doctoral degree in sexology from the Institute for Advanced Study of Human Sexuality. The book includes a series of forty-eight unretouched black-and-white photographs of vulvas, showing both their diversity and their beauty. Dr. Karras has also produced a video documentary called *Petals: Journey into Self Discovery*, to dispel the unspoken myths about the appearance and nature of the vulva. (See www.nickkarras.com.)

Here's what I want all women to know: The size and shape of a woman's genitals are quite variable. And all of those sizes and shapes are normal. Though vaginoplasty is certainly an option for those who truly are unhappy with how their genitals look, it would be far more effective for women to spend their time and energy getting in touch with and learning to appreciate both their genitals and their entire pelvic floor area, including optimizing pelvic floor function. Vaginoplasty can lead to scarring and pain with intercourse, while a program of strengthening and toning the pelvic floor carries no risk whatsoever.

Types of Cosmetic Procedures

Vaginal Rejuvenation Treatments. According to the ASAPS, vaginal rejuvenation treatments are the fastest-growing cosmetic procedure in the United States, with the number of procedures increasing almost 22 percent from 2016 to 2017 alone.[119]

Laser or heat treatment of the vaginal mucosa is an option for many women post-childbirth or after menopause. These treatments (also mentioned in chapter 6, page 215) thicken collagen in the vaginal tissues, helping to restore elasticity and function, and they also improve the blood flow to vaginal tissue, restoring vaginal moisture. (These procedures can also help improve urinary incontinence for women with prolapse because in tightening the tissue, the bladder neck can be lifted back into position.) Both procedures involve three initial treatments, spaced about four to six weeks apart, plus an annual maintenance treatment.

The most well-known of these treatments is MonaLisa Touch (www .monalisatouch.com), which administers a carbon dioxide laser through a probe inserted into the vagina. The procedure is painless, it takes only about five minutes, and downtime afterward is minimal.

Another option is ThermIva (www.thermiva.com), a radiofrequency treatment that uses a thin wand to gently administer a thermal current to the vulva and vagina. The procedure is almost painless and there's absolutely no downtime afterward. It takes between thirty and forty-five minutes, and unlike MonaLisa Touch, it can be used to shrink the size of the labia to some extent.

If you are considering undergoing one of these treatments, know that their effects will be greatly enhanced by exercising and toning your pelvic floor regularly. This alone, over the long run, will be well worth your time and effort. Also please note that these procedures are not without risk, and they are not yet approved by the American College of Obstetrics and Gynecologists.

INTERSTITIAL CYSTITIS
(PAINFUL BLADDER SYNDROME)

Interstitial cystitis has more in common with vulvodynia than with urinary tract infection. (See page 370.) Unlike a UTI, the symptoms are not the result of infection. Both vulvodynia and interstitial cystitis are chronic pain syndromes.

Interstitial cystitis is a condition most common in women between the ages of forty and sixty. It is characterized by disabling urinary frequency and urgency, painful urination, needing to get up at night to urinate, and occasional blood in the urine. Pain above the pubic bone is also common, as are pelvic, urethral, vaginal, and perineal pain; this pain is partially relieved by emptying the bladder. Examination of the urine may reveal some blood cells but no bacteria or white cells. It is often present in women who also experience vulvar pain. Though the cause is unknown, many feel that it is, in part, an autoimmune disorder. There is a significant crossover between the population of women who experience vulvodynia and those who experience interstitial cystitis.

Diagnosis is made on the basis of the patient's history and also by a procedure known as cystoscopy, in which a lighted viewing instrument is placed in the bladder under anesthesia. There are some characteristic findings, such as hemorrhage under the bladder lining and cracking of the mucosal lining; a biopsy reveals evidence of inflammation.[120]

Treatment

Behavioral Therapy. Biofeedback and behavioral therapy—both of which have definite benefits, with no side effects—have been reported to help many women with this problem.[121] Behavioral therapy consists of learning deep relaxation, meditation, or other techniques that boost the immune system and calm the nervous system, thus allowing the body to heal itself. (See the section on stress reduction for treatment of PMS, page 153.)

Nutritional Therapy. Stop bladder irritants such as coffee (even decaf), cigarettes, and alcohol. Castor oil packs help immune system functioning: Lie down with a castor oil pack over your lower abdomen three times per week or more, while saying—and really feeling—the affirmations suggested in the section on urinary tract infections, below. The same antioxidant therapy that has worked for vulvodynia patients may also help those with chronic interstitial cystitis. (See the section on vulvodynia.)

NAET. My acupuncturist, Fern Tsao, reports good results with NAET (see page 918), which I would personally recommend to anyone who is open to this approach.

Mind-Body Approaches. Larry Burk, M.D., uses a combination of tapping (Emotional Freedom Technique), hypnosis, breathwork, and dreamwork in coaching sessions (available in person as well as via Skype) to explore and transform the messages your body is sending you through various physical symptoms and conditions, including interstitial cystitis. He helped one woman with the condition who experienced autoimmune bladder flare-ups every day for four years before she began coaching sessions with Dr. Burk. She now has no urgency and very few flare-ups, and she reports profound shifts in every area of her life, not just with her physical health. (For more information, see Dr. Burk's website at www.letmagichappen.com.)

Bladder Distension. This diagnostic procedure is often also used as an initial therapy and involves filling the bladder with water and allowing it to expand while the patient is under general anesthesia. Although it isn't certain exactly why this works, it's possible that it increases capacity and also interferes with pain signals.

Bladder Instillation. This procedure is also called a bladder wash or bladder bath, and it involves filling the bladder with a solution that the patient must then hold for about ten to fifteen minutes before voiding. Generally, women receive treatments once a week or once every other week for six to eight weeks.

Elmiron (Pentosan Polysulfate Sodium). This pill (the first and so far only oral medication that's FDA-approved for treating interstitial cystitis) is taken three times a day. In double-blind placebo-controlled clinical trials, it improved bladder pain in 38 percent of patients and urgency in 61 percent—although it might take as long as four to six months to notice improvement.[122] Elmiron is thought to adhere to the lining of the bladder, acting as a buffer and preventing irritants in the urine from reaching the bladder wall.

RECURRENT URINARY TRACT INFECTIONS

Most women will experience a few UTIs over their lifetimes. The "honeymoon cystitis" our mothers were told about speaks to one of the primary causes of UTIs—the milking action of sexual activity, which, under certain conditions, causes bacteria from the vaginal or anal area to get into the bladder and urethra. The symptoms include burning on urination, blood in the urine, and fever. If a UTI goes untreated, the infection can ascend into the kidneys, which can be dangerous. This is why a woman who feels she may have a UTI should have a urine culture taken, and an antibiotic prescribed if it is positive for bacteria. This will cure the problem in the vast majority of cases without further treatment.

Many women, however, experience recurrent bladder infections, which are treated with repeated courses of antibiotics. This is a different story, and requires a different approach. Chronic use of antibiotics to treat recurrent UTIs doesn't address the underlying imbalance in the body that is leading to the infections, and antibiotics can also kill off helpful vaginal flora, resulting in yeast infections, diarrhea, and—unfortunately—recurrent urinary tract infection.

Treatment

Nutritional Aspects. Start taking a good probiotic. Many are on the market, and most require refrigeration to keep the bacteria alive. PB 8 is a brand that doesn't require refrigeration; it is available at natural food stores. As already mentioned, Fem-Dophilus was developed specifically for the female microbiome.

Another way to help restore your vaginal flora if you've had repeated UTIs and multiple courses of antibiotics is to dip a stiff tampon (for example, OB is a good brand) in plain, organic yogurt and put it in your vagina. Change "yogurt tampons" every three or four hours. This will replenish the vaginal flora and decrease the risk of repeated infections associated with the yeast problem. You can also douche with yogurt or put a probiotic capsule directly in your vagina each night for a few nights.

Coffee, even decaf, can have markedly adverse effects on your urinary tract and act as a bladder irritant, so if you currently drink it, try going without for a week or so and see if your symptoms improve. If they do, you'll have your answer and can plan accordingly. (You might still want to have a cup of coffee now and then—but you will be prepared for the effects.)

Many women with UTIs are also helped by using cranberries, which contain an ingredient that helps keep bacteria from adhering to the walls of the bladder, thus helping prevent infection.[123] Cranberry juice also acidifies the urine, making it harder for bacteria to grow. Long a popular home remedy, drinking cranberry juice has been confirmed by scientific studies to eliminate bladder infections in a majority of the women tested.[124] Sugar-sweetened cranberry juice partially nullifies the benefits, so use the unsweetened variety. You can buy unsweetened cranberry juice concentrate and use 16 ounces of reconstituted juice daily to treat an infection. (Add a small amount of the herb stevia if you want to avoid saccharin or aspartame. Stevia has been used for decades as a noncaloric sweetener in many countries and is widely available in powder or liquid form.) Use 8 ounces per day for prevention. Or you can look for cranberry juice in pill form; CranActin is a popular brand.

The herb uva ursi contains a substance known as arbutin, which is a natural antibiotic that relieves bladder infection.[125] You can take the powdered solid extract (20 percent arbutin) as capsules, two capsules three times per day. Or take the tincture, one dropperful in a cup of water three times per day. Continue this treatment until symptoms disappear. Both capsules and tincture are available in health food stores.

Vitamin C can be very helpful in preventing reinfection. Take at least 1,000 to 2,000 mg every day, and if your infections are associated with sexual activity, take 1,000 mg before and 1,000 mg after sex. Drink plenty of fluids as well, and make sure you get up to urinate within one hour of having sex. Women who do this do not get as many infections after sex as those who wait for an hour or longer, probably because drinking fluid and then urinating prevents bacteria from adhering to the tissues and starting an infection.

Hormones. Menopausal and perimenopausal women often have thinning of the outer urethra from lack of estrogen in that area of the body, which results in burning with urination. This can be mistaken for a UTI. The condition can be treated well by putting an estrogen-based cream in the upper part of the vagina, right along the urethral ridge. I recommend estriol 0.5 mg vaginal cream. The usual dose is 1 gram (one-quarter teaspoon) once daily for one week, then twice or three times per week or as needed thereafter. This will restore your vaginal tissue to its normal thickness and the burning will stop.[126] Other forms of vaginal estrogen also work well, including Estrace and Vagifem. The small amount needed to reestrogenize the urethra does not raise levels in the blood significantly and is considered safe by most doctors.

Nonprescription *Pueraria mirifica* vaginal moisturizer also works very well and has been shown to reestrogenize vaginal tissue (see Resources).

Sexual Activity. UTIs are often associated with frequent or traumatic sex (sex that involves injury to the vaginal and vulvar tissues). For example, in couples who travel separately or live apart during the week, frequent intercourse during a weekend visit can irritate vaginal and urethral tissue. Treatment for this involves making the necessary adjustments in your sex life to decrease trauma. This may mean using a lubricant if you suffer from vaginal dryness. It may also mean rethinking any aspects of the relationship that are less than satisfactory.

Repeated bouts of infection and/or burning on urination can also be related to a woman's contraceptive method. If your diaphragm is too large, it can irritate your urethra during intercourse, causing bacteria to enter the urethral opening and migrate up to the bladder area. Also, the use of condoms or contraceptive creams that contain nonoxynol-9, a spermicide, can cause urethral irritation and burning on urination. It will go away when you stop using the offending agent.

Other Treatments. Don't introduce bacteria into your urethral area. After using the toilet, make sure you wipe yourself from front to back, not the other way around.

Castor oil packs applied to your lower abdomen two or three times a week can work wonders in preventing UTIs, because they appear to improve immune system functioning. Acupuncture can also be very helpful.

Psychological Aspects. As I've already stated, there are some very specific stresses that affect the bladder and urinary system that are often related to unacknowledged anger at someone or blaming someone—often of the opposite sex. So as you're drinking your cranberry juice, taking your uva ursi, or lying down with your castor oil pack, try the following affirmation: "I flow easily with my life. I easily release and let go of old concepts and ideas.

They flow out of me easily and joyously. I am at peace with my thoughts and emotions."

Women's Stories

Chrissa: Recurrent UTIs

Chrissa was thirty-two when she first came to see me for an annual exam. She was in relatively good health but had menstrual cramps, intermittent bouts of pelvic pain, and also recurrent UTIs, for which she'd been on repeated courses of antibiotics. She told me that every time she went on a short trip or vacation she worried that she might get a UTI and be unable to get an antibiotic prescription filled. She was also tired of the yeast infections she developed when taking antibiotics.

When I asked Chrissa what was going on in her life, she told me that her husband had a job that kept him on the road for about two weeks out of every four. His irregular schedule made her life difficult to plan. When I asked about her sex life, she said, "It's full speed ahead when he's home, and I use a diaphragm and vaginal gel alternating with condoms." I asked if she tended to get a UTI after sex with her husband. She thought about it and realized that if she was going to get one, it was usually a day or two following sex.

I checked her diaphragm to make sure that it fit her properly, and it did. I knew that Chrissa needed a strategy to prevent UTIs, so I suggested that she follow the nutritional and supplement program I've already outlined:

- Decrease the refined sugar and flour products in her diet and switch to a whole-food approach.

- Drink cranberry juice regularly or take a cranberry supplement.

- Start taking a good multivitamin-mineral supplement.

- Take 1 to 2 grams (1,000–2,000 mg) of vitamin C as soon after intercourse as possible. Take the same dose the next day.

- Take a good probiotic the day before, the day of, and the day after intercourse.

I also asked her to observe her emotional triggers. Specifically, was she angry with her husband about any unspoken matters between them—such as whether or not to get pregnant or who should be paying the bills?

Chrissa came back for a checkup three months later. She had had the beginning symptoms of a UTI only once, and they had gone away very quickly with the cranberry juice and vitamin C. She told me, "I realized that the key factor in whether or not my body actually got a UTI was my emotions. As soon as I found myself feeling 'pissy' toward my husband, I forced myself to talk over my concerns with him so that my body wouldn't have to do the talking for me. I also made sure that I never had sex with him when I was feeling angry. I realized that was a setup for an infection. I'm thrilled that I finally know that my body is not betraying me with these infections. There's a lot I can do to prevent them, or at least nip them in the bud."

STRESS URINARY INCONTINENCE

Though many women find it difficult to talk about, even to their doctors, fully 30 to 50 percent of us will experience urinary incontinence (the involuntary loss of urine) from time to time. Ten percent of these women are under the age of forty. And many have never had children, evidence that there's more to urinary incontinence than bladder damage from childbirth. In most, it's just an occasional problem that occurs when coughing or sneezing or laughing really hard. But about one in six women between the ages of forty and sixty-five has a significant problem that interferes with her lifestyle. In their comprehensive book *The Bathroom Key* (Demos Health, 2012), physical therapist Kathryn Kassai and Kim Perelli point out that the number one reason women get placed in nursing homes is because of urinary incontinence—which could have been prevented with the proper care of exercise of the pelvic floor.

There are several types of incontinence. Stress urinary incontinence (SUI) is the most common one, and the one I will be addressing here. SUI occurs whenever you increase your intra-abdominal pressure so much (by coughing, sneezing, or laughing) that your urethral sphincter, the muscle that holds the urethra closed, can't hold back the urine that's in the bladder.

Common Causes

Common reasons for weakness of the urethral sphincter are the following:

~ Overall weakness of pelvic floor muscles

~ Pregnancy (the SUI usually ends after delivery)

~ Damage from childbirth (this is much less likely to happen when a woman is encouraged to birth in a relaxed, conscious, and fully supported manner; prevention of SUI is not an indication for a C-section)

~ Genetic factors that result in connective tissue weakness (women with this problem will often have many female relatives with problems related to prolapse of pelvic organs)

~ Persistent, chronic cough, usually from smoking, which results in repeated chronic intra-abdominal pressure that overrides the strength of the urethral sphincter

~ Excessive abdominal fat, which increases intra-abdominal pressure

Treatment

Strengthening Your Pelvic Floor. The first line of treatment for SUI is to strengthen and tone your pelvic floor, as discussed in chapter 8. Pelvic floor strengthening should be part of every woman's healthcare routine, not only for optimal sexual functioning but also if you have a tendency toward SUI. When your pelvic muscles are strong and flexible, they can better support the urethra so that it doesn't give out when you do anything that increases intra-abdominal pressure.

Unfortunately, the vast majority of women who are told to do Kegel exercises find that they don't work. I have already covered the reasons for this and given a program to get you started with pelvic floor training in chapter 8.

To achieve optimal results in strengthening and healing your pelvic floor if you already have urinary incontinence, I strongly recommend working with a physical therapist fully trained in pelvic floor rehabilitation.

Though strengthening the pelvic floor won't cure every type of urinary incontinence, it is always worth a try before resorting to surgery or drugs. Developing a strong pelvic floor not only helps prevent or cure urinary stress incontinence but also increases the blood supply to your pelvis, making you more resistant to diseases such as urinary tract infections. It also enhances the ability to reach orgasm and improves vaginal lubrication during sex. You can do these exercises anytime and anyplace if you're doing them properly, and not a soul will know. You have nothing to lose, and a lot to gain.

Nutritional Aspects. Many women have stress incontinence only when their urine output is increased, especially from drinking coffee or tea. Even decaf coffee is a diuretic—and so is cold weather (I never drink a cup of coffee in the morning if I'm going skiing, otherwise I'll have to go back to the lodge after every other run). Many women also have increased urinary output on the first day of their period, because they're getting rid of all that premenstrual fluid. Under those conditions, urinary stress incontinence will always be worse because your bladder is always fuller. And coffee is also a bladder irritant. I've "cured" several cases of SUI just by telling the patient to stop drinking coffee! It is also helpful to lose excess body fat. (See chapter 17.)

Hormones. Some women begin to experience urinary stress incontinence after menopause for hormonal reasons and for the same reason that they sometimes experience UTIs—thinning of the estrogen-sensitive outer third of the urethra. (See the section on hormones and UTIs.) If this describes your situation, all you need to do to restore the urethral tissue and regain urinary control is to use a small dab of estrogen or *Pueraria mirifica* cream daily for a week and then once or twice per week thereafter. Use estriol 0.5 mg cream, as opposed to other types of estrogen cream such as Premarin, for this purpose because this type of estrogen works very well locally and has a very weak systemic effect. This means that you can safely use estriol vaginal cream to help restore your vaginal and urethral tissues even if you've had breast cancer or another estrogen-sensitive cancer. Estriol vaginal cream is available by prescription from any formulary pharmacy that carries natural hormones. (See Resources for how to locate a formulary pharmacy.) The usual dose is 1 gram (one-quarter teaspoon) once daily for one week, then two or three times a week as needed thereafter. *Pueraria mirifica* vaginal moisturizer is available without a prescription (see Resources).

Pessaries and Urinary Control Inserts. For mild stress incontinence, simply wearing a menstrual tampon is often helpful because they push on the vaginal wall, compressing the urethra. In one study, 86 percent of women with mild SUI stayed dry during exercise when using tampons, although only 29 percent of women with severe incontinence were helped. If you use tampons for this purpose, remember that they must be changed regularly to avoid toxic shock; don't leave the same tampon in all day long.

Pessaries, plastic or rubber devices that are inserted into the vagina to help women with uterine prolapse, can also be used successfully for those with SUI. Unfortunately, many doctors have never been trained in their use and therefore patients may not be offered this option.

Specially designed "incontinence pessaries" lift the bladder neck and restore the proper bladder angle, so continence is restored while it is in place. They work very well for women who aren't candidates for surgery, who have an incontinence problem only intermittently, or who have failed to get help from surgery.[127] Yoni eggs can also work well (see chapter 8).

A prescription product called FemSoft Insert (by Rochester Medical Products) is a silicone tube inserted into the urethra and surrounded by a liquid-filled sleeve. The sleeve creates a seal at the neck of the bladder, preventing leakage. It must be replaced after urination. It's available by prescription.

Surgery. Surgical approaches to SUI are often very successful. Seek out a surgeon specially trained in urogynecology. Another excellent option for some women involves injections of Teflon or collagen into the urethra.

(For more information on incontinence, visit the website for the National Association for Continence at www.nafc.org.)

Regardless of where you currently stand in relationship to this area of your body, know that each of us has inherited the effects of generations of silence or misinformation surrounding the genital and urinary regions. The only way out of this legacy of shame is to talk about our needs, educate ourselves, and reclaim a healthy attitude toward our genitals. As we each begin to listen to and reclaim the wisdom of these areas, we will discover that, like all the other parts of our bodies, this part of our body responds beautifully to our care, compassion, and respect.

10
Breasts

I am . . . struck with how often women *sense* in their bodies, especially in the breast and heart area, when they are giving, loving and responding to the needs of others.

—Jean Shinoda Bolen

The mammary fixation is the most infantile—and most American—of the sex fetishes.

—Molly Haskell

OUR CULTURAL INHERITANCE

Breasts are the physical metaphor for giving and receiving. Many women who have breast-fed their babies in the past feel the same tingling "let-down reflex" in their breasts years later, when they are moved by tenderness and compassion, or even when they hear a baby cry. The instinct to nurture others can be an extremely powerful and desirable source of health and pleasure not only for others but also for ourselves.

How closely breasts are linked with physical nurturing was demonstrated well by the case of a woman whom I saw in the early years of my practice. Jennifer, four years past menopause, had been referred to me with two very large cysts in her right breast that had manifested almost overnight. (They were five and seven centimeters in diameter.) When I asked her if anything was going on in her life in the area of nurturing others, she told me that her last child was leaving home for college and that a beloved cat, a pet for fifteen years, had recently died. Jennifer was grieving the loss both of her daughter and of her pet. The night before the cysts appeared, she dreamed that she was nursing her baby daughter—the same child who was now about to leave home. When I aspirated the fluid from the cysts, I found that they were filled with milk! Jennifer's body had manifested the fluid of maternal nurturing in response to the change in her own nurturing role. This demonstrated to me that the phrase "the milk of human kindness" is more than just a metaphor. (Dixie Mills, M.D., a breast surgeon colleague, saw an increase in nipple discharge and bloody discharge after September 11, 2001, when the country was grieving.)

In addition to being organs of nurturance, breasts are also symbols of sexual desirability. The cultural ideal of the perfect breast size and shape changes depending on the time in history. Whatever the ideal is, most women won't match it—and some feel that something is wrong with them as a result. I wish that every woman could have an opportunity to know how truly diverse breast sizes and shapes are, could see how much they vary among women. They would then realize how skewed women's perceptions normally are about our own breasts and take steps to celebrate what we've got. I was at a women's health conference once when a young woman got up and started complaining about her breasts (which were clearly beautiful). Another woman, who had had a double mastectomy and reconstruction, stood up and said, "Girls, we don't have that kind of time." We all realized in one moment that our task was to love the breasts we still had.

Undeniably, an occasional woman has a size discrepancy or other abnormality related to her breasts that is striking and a source of great psychological or even physical pain. Breasts can be so large that they cause back pain, for example. Plastic surgery can correct such problems and can be a blessing. But most cosmetic breast surgery is undertaken because women feel they don't look as good as models in magazines or as good as their lovers want them to look, or because our current breast-obsessed culture so favors large breasts. This size concern is medicalized in plastic surgery jargon, which writes the indication for breast augmentation as *chronic bilateral micromastia*. That translates as "two small breasts that have been there for a while."

As with their genitals, women often feel that their breasts exist for the pleasure and benefit of someone other than themselves. And this perception is at the root of many problems. I've heard former colleagues of mine discourage women from breast-feeding because it would "ruin their breasts." Some husbands forbid their wives to breast-feed because of their jealousy of the baby! Clearly, the current trend toward breast implants is a symptom of a much deeper, culturally supported discontent. (I discuss implants later in this chapter.)

Overgiving: A Risk Factor for Breast Disease

Our culture has skewed the nurturing metaphor in such a way that women too often give themselves away to others, without nurturing themselves. Women give and give and give without regular replenishment until the well runs dry, or until they are unconsciously seething with resentment. For centuries, women have been taught that being a good woman meant nurturing everyone and everything, leaving themselves for last. I call this the "burnt toast" syndrome. A woman will make toast for everyone in the family—reserving the burnt pieces for herself. Meanwhile, if there is a man around, he will be served the best part of whatever is available—including the best cuts of meat. I've seen this repeatedly.

Much breast cancer is related to our need to appear to be self-contained and self-nurturing, which is impossible. We don't want to bother anyone. Yet everyone needs the support of others to be fully healthy. Caroline Myss notes, "The major emotion behind breast lumps and breast cancer is hurt, sorrow, and unfinished emotional business generally related to nurturance." Breasts are located in the fourth-chakra energetic center, near the heart. Emotions such as regret and the classic "broken heart" are energetically stored in this center of the body. Guilt over not being able to forgive oneself or forgive others blocks the breasts' energy. (The other organs in the fourth chakra, such as the lungs, are also susceptible to this energy pattern.)

An important 1995 study found that the risk of developing breast cancer increased by almost twelve times if a woman had suffered from bereavement, job loss, or divorce in the previous five years.[1] It is important to note that long-term emotional difficulties were not associated with breast cancer. Another researcher also showed that severe life stress (determined before the diagnosis of breast cancer was made) was associated with increased risk for the disease.[2] Similarly, severe losses occurring after the diagnosis of breast cancer have been shown to be associated with increased risk of later recurrence of the cancer.[3]

As far back as the 1800s, the medical literature has noted associations between breast cancer and loneliness, sorrow, and even rage and anger.[4] Women with breast cancer frequently have a tendency toward self-sacrifice, inhibited sexuality, an inability to discharge anger or hostility, a tendency to hide anger and hostility behind a facade of pleasantness, and an unresolved hostile conflict with their mothers. There is evidence that a woman with breast cancer who perceives herself as having high-quality emotional support from a husband or other source will have an enhanced immune response.[5] In one study, breast cancer patients were more likely than women without breast cancer to be committed to maintaining an external appearance of a nice or good person. They were also more likely to suppress or internalize their feelings, particularly anger.[6] In fact, one study found that the suppression of anger over many years is correlated with adverse changes in the immune system.[7] Given our society's tendency to suppress, ignore, or denigrate women and their anger, it is easy to see why so many women have breast problems. A nurse practitioner once told me that several months before one of her friends died of breast cancer, her friend had the following insight: "I finally realized that I didn't have to die of cancer in order to rest." Studies have demonstrated that severe emotional losses such as divorce, death of a loved one, or loss of a job may set the stage for cancer, depending upon how a woman deals with the loss.

It is not the loss itself that causes the problem—it is the inability to express one's grief fully, release it, and respond to the situation in a healthy, adaptive fashion. In the 1995 study noted above, the researchers demonstrated that the coping styles of women influenced whether or not they got breast cancer. Compared with the control group, those with cancer were more apt to have a type of coping strategy characterized by engaging with the problem, confronting it, focusing on it, working on a plan for action, and lobbying for emotional support in this process. What the researchers noted is this: In most severely stressful life events (loss of a loved one, loss of a job, or serious family illness), the person has no control. Therefore, engaging in efforts to change or control the situation and recruiting others to support one in this strategy, as opposed to letting go, ultimately doesn't work and actually increases stress (and risk of cancer). Examples of this would be working tirelessly with organizations that seek to eradicate breast cancer rather than spending time and energy investigating what you need to do in your own life to grieve, let go, and heal. Severe loss is inescapable and part of the process of life for most of us. What helps is grieving fully, making meaning of the situation, and surrendering to something bigger than we are. This is a painful and difficult process that I call radical surrender. (It's beautifully demonstrated in the 2009 movie *Love Happens,* with Jennifer Aniston and Aaron Eckhart.)

The late Ryke Geerd Hamer, M.D., an internist and oncologist, did extensive research on more than 20,000 cancer patients and demonstrated that in every case the development of cancer followed a severe emotional shock or loss within a year or two of the diagnosis. (Dr. Hamer understood the mind-body connection in cancer on a personal level as well. He was diagnosed with cancer following his son's death from a random act of violence.) Most important, his research shows that "the tissue starts to augment from the time of the onset of the actual conflict and will stop growing as soon as the conflict has been resolved." To read more about Dr. Hamer's research, go to www .newmedicine.ca or read *The Cancer Report: The Latest Research in Psychoneuroimmunology (How Thousands Are Achieving Permanent Recoveries)* by John Voell and Cynthia Chatfield (Change Your World Press, 2005).

I also highly recommend the work of Kelly Turner, Ph.D., author of

Radical Remission: Surviving Cancer Against All Odds (HarperOne, 2014) and founder of the Radical Remission Project (www.radicalremission.com). Dr. Turner has researched and documented hundreds of cases of so-called spontaneous remission of cancer and has identified the factors that are common to those who recover and thrive following a cancer diagnosis.

The following story, from Theresa Fincher, beautifully illustrates how important it is to choose doctors and a treatment strategy that you feel fully aligned with instead of going with what the first doctor recommends because you're coming from a place of blind fear. Not all doctors always agree on what approach to take with disease, even specialists in that specific disease, so it's not only possible but important to find doctors you feel totally comfortable with. Having a strong feeling of support and trust in your medical team and your treatment is vitally important to the outcome of the treatment—it can even be more important than the actual treatment itself.

I never considered that I would be diagnosed with breast cancer, let alone die from it. It doesn't run in my family and I had hardly encountered any friends facing it. A gynecologist I had in my twenties told me heart disease was what I should worry about, not breast cancer, so I was certain that wouldn't be part of my journey. I was rarely sick, and I pushed through any cold or flu I had, not letting any ailment get me down. I was dependable, reliable Theresa—the outward picture of health. But on the inside, I was like a teakettle heating up and preparing to screech. I had pushed so many of my feelings down that I didn't notice how much resentment and anger I was harboring inside.

When I found a lump in my left breast, I nursed it for months, sure it was just a cyst. I didn't get it checked because I didn't want to deal with the repercussions of someone telling me anything different. But by the time I quit putting everyone and everything else first and gave myself permission to go to a doctor, I could barely walk. My breast had doubled in size, and my body was engulfed with inflammation. On October 22, 2016, at the age of forty-eight, I was diagnosed with breast cancer.

The cancer had spread to my lymph nodes, so my doctor ordered a PET scan and asked me to meet with a surgeon and a radiologist while we waited for the results. In the meantime, I began making drastic lifestyle changes, overhauling my diet to eliminate sugar and staying as close to a plant-based diet as possible. When I met with the surgeon, I told her that I was not interested in doing the standard treatments for breast cancer. She responded matter-of-factly that if I were her sister, she would advise the standard cancer treatment. She then proceeded to lecture me that what I ate would not help me reverse this advancing disease. I felt confused, terrified, and defeated.

Two and a half weeks later, I was in the radiologist's waiting room, experiencing this overwhelming, almost suffocating feeling that I did not belong there. She was kind and caring but surprised me by telling me she had just received the PET scan results and wanted to review them with me. I was horrified when she showed me the scan. Cancer was peppered all the way down my spine, with the largest mass hovering over the right side of my sacrum, where I was in so much pain. This mass measured off the charts in size. She broke the news to me that I had an aggressive, stage IV breast cancer and recommended I have radiation on my back right away. This would be followed by an aggressive treatment plan that involved chemotherapy, surgery to remove the breast, and then more chemotherapy and radiation.

I knew in my heart that I did not want to do this. I met with the first doctor two additional times to ask numerous questions and request other options, and each time he strongly recommended the standard cancer treatment plan the team had provided. They scheduled a meeting with their board to review my case, and in the meantime, friends reached out to a top oncologist they knew in Germany. Based on my specific type of cancer, the German oncologist recommended a different treatment plan that I was comfortable with and that felt in alignment with how I wanted to help my body instead of assault it. I felt enormous relief that there might be another way to look at my case, using an individualized plan instead of a "one size fits all" approach. I excitedly wrote a letter to my doctor and the board about this insight and rushed it to the office before their meeting. They came back to me after the meeting and said that they all agreed their approach was still best and that I should start immediately. I was deflated. I asked for a referral to one of the top oncology centers in the country for a second opinion. They gave me the referral, but the nurse's parting words were, "Just know that we all start from here," referring to their treatment plan.

I went home in excruciating pain, scared out of my mind, and feeling more and more that I might not pull out of this alive. Every day was getting harder to manage, but I had a haunting feeling that if I followed their plan, I would not survive. I scheduled the second opinion, which was nearly two weeks out. The days crawled by, and I became more and more terrified and confused. A friend encouraged me to reach out to Dr. Northrup, whom I'd met previously when she spoke at a fundraiser for a foundation I ran. When she called, I told her about my confusion and overwhelming resistance to the treatment the doctors were recommending and that I felt I was running out of time. She said a prayer of Divine Love with me and taught me how to express it. "Theresa, it doesn't matter what you choose," she told me. "Just choose it and *be-*

lieve in it." She reminded me that we can all tap into our divine power from within and our power of manifestation through unwavering faith. This was the turning point for me—Dr. Northrup was the catalyst for what became an incredible healing journey.

That evening I went into my bedroom and prayed as Dr. Northrup had taught me, and for the first time in my adult life, I surrendered completely, without any strings attached, asking for God's will to be done and for divine guidance. Four days later, I walked through the doors of the cancer center for my second opinion, and the doctor there recommended almost the exact same treatment the German oncologist suggested, which involved shutting off my estrogen. I began immediately—and instead of being frightened, now my faith was reinforced and restored. Within two weeks my pain subsided. Within three months I was doing basic yoga again. Within six months I was walking normally and could do my advanced yoga postures. Now, although cancer has mostly disappeared from my body, I focus my energy where I am divinely guided to heal and repair emotional wounds, I take the supplements I need to thrive, and I eat a whole-foods diet that supports a clean temple for my inner guidance to be received. I also nurture my soul through reading, meditation, qi gong, tai chi, and helping others.

The cancer had a meaning for me—it is "c-answer," which represents seeing the answer to the messages my body was sending me (based on where the cancer was located) rather than reacting from a place of fear. For instance, seeing cancer in my left breast was a message to focus on family dynamics. Seeing it in my sacrum was a message about not feeling supported. I discovered that for me, cancer was all about pent-up resentment, and it took me getting all the way to this point to really understand the full effect of that resentment.

Cancer can be a death sentence if you choose it to be, but I experienced it as a dance, a flow that I must step into and move within, centered on listening and responding. I have done substantial work in facing my ego and my fears, connecting with my soul thoroughly. It has not been easy, but it has been rewarding. More than two years later, after following a regimen blending various Western medicines with earthbased and Eastern modalities, most of the cancer is completely gone—yet I haven't had any surgery, intravenous chemotherapy, or radiation. Because of my relationship with the divine, I now follow internal guidance and stand in a stronger place of wellness than ever before. The inside and outside of my being are becoming integrated and congruent, and I feel incredibly blessed.

Drawing on her experiences with cancer, Theresa founded the I Love You Project (www.theiloveyouproject.org) to support people on their wellness journey. She's currently developing an equine-guided wellness program called Gia Milagro for children and families facing trauma.

ANATOMY

The female breast is designed to provide optimal nourishment for babies and to provide sexual pleasure for the woman herself. The breasts are glandular organs that are very sensitive to hormonal changes in the body; they undergo cyclic changes in synchrony with the menstrual cycle. They are very intimately connected with the female genital system: Nipple stimulation also stimulates the clitoris and increases prolactin and oxytocin secretion from the pituitary gland. These affect the uterus and can cause contractions there and also in the pelvic floor muscles. Breast tissue extends up into the armpit (axilla), in what is known as the tail of Spence. Lymph nodes that drain the breast tissue are also located in the armpits. After a woman has had a baby and her milk comes in, she may develop striking swellings under her arms from engorgement of the breast tissue in that area. Breasts come in all sizes and shapes, as do nipples. Most women have one breast that is slightly smaller than the other. Some women (and men) have a third nipple.

BREAST SELF-EXAMS

One of the sacred cows of women's health has long been the monthly breast self-examination (BSE). For many years, women have been told to do it as a way to "save their lives." But in November 2009, new guidelines for breast cancer screening from a government-appointed task force recommended that doctors no longer teach BSE, based on findings from two large studies showing the practice not only does not decrease breast cancer mortality rates but also results in more breast biopsies and more frequent diagnosis of benign lesions.[8]

One of those studies, published in 2002 in the *Journal of the National Cancer Institute,* followed 260,000 women in Shanghai, China, for five years. Half of the group was trained in BSE and had that training reinforced at work, while the other half had no BSE training and was not encouraged to practice BSE at all. At the end of the study, the women in the BSE group had found more benign breast lumps than the other group, although the breast cancer mortality rate was the same in both groups. The researchers concluded that "women who choose to practice BSE should be informed that its efficacy is unproven and that it may increase their chances of having a benign breast biopsy."[9] The other study, from St. Petersburg, Russia, followed

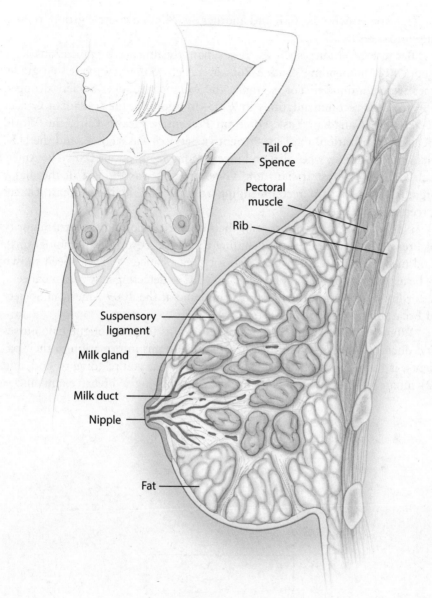

Tail of
Spence

Pectoral
muscle

Rib

Suspensory
ligament

Milk gland

Milk duct

Nipple

Fat

FIGURE 16: BREAST ANATOMY

57,712 women who did BSE and another 64,749 in a control group, reporting similar results.[10]

Because of studies such as these, many healthcare organizations have
stopped recommending routine BSE, even before the new screening guidelines were announced. For example, the American Cancer Society dropped
BSE from its recommendations in 2003. In addition, the Canadian Cancer
Society, the Canadian Task Force on Preventive Health Care, the World
Health Organization, the U.S. Preventive Services Task Force, and the U.K.
National Health Services also no longer recommend routine BSE. The American College of Obstetricians and Gynecologists was the last of the major
organizations to stop recommending routine BSE in their breast cancer
screening guidelines.

Nevertheless, it is women, not their doctors, who find the vast majority
of breast abnormalities (not including those picked up on mammograms).
And in women who are at high risk for breast cancer, BSE has been shown
to be as accurate as mammography and MRI at detecting new breast cancers,
according to the authors of a study presented at the 2009 American Society
of Breast Surgeons annual meeting.

Women's reluctance to do breast self-exams (even among female nurses
and doctors, who are often the ones dispensing this information to their patients) is rooted in two things: (1) fear about what you're going to find, and
(2) innate inner guidance that knows that making a breast exam into a

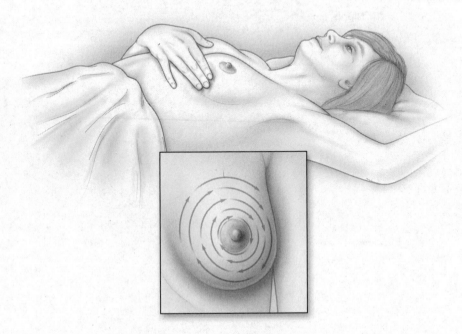

FIGURE 17: BREAST SELF-EXAM

"search-and-destroy" mission not only is counterproductive but may even be harmful. By the law of attraction, that which we focus on tends to expand. So who in their right mind would consciously approach their breasts every month thinking "cancer"? In fact, studies have shown that that's exactly what happens. (See below.)

Transforming the Breast Self-Exam

There is a healthy alternative to approaching a monthly self-exam as though you were conducting a mine sweep. You can get to know your breasts in a healthy, loving way that enhances your health on all levels. And you're not doing this to "find something." A good time to change how you think about and do your breast exams is right after you've had a normal exam with your healthcare practitioner and you know that everything is currently normal. If you don't know what normal feels like, here's what to do. When having your breasts examined by your doctor, ask her (or him) to tell you exactly what she is feeling. Then repeat the exam yourself so you know what normal feels like in your breasts. From then on, whenever you touch your breasts, do so with loving kindness. Rub your hands together until they are warm. Then cover your breasts with them, visualizing your hands transferring love and care to your breasts. You may well feel a tingling in your breasts from increased circulation when you do this.

Approach your breasts with respect. If you are currently afraid of your breasts and find them "too lumpy," start changing your attitude toward them by paying special attention to them during your daily bath or shower. (You can also address the lumps by following the Program to Promote Healthy Breast Tissue in this chapter, page 429.) When you wash this area of your body, pay attention to how the skin feels under your fingers. Imagine that you have healing power in your hands (which you actually do). As you wash your breasts and under your arms, do so in the spirit of blessing this area of your body. As you do so, you will be learning the basic contours and feel of your own breasts. Do this daily as part of your bathing until you have reclaimed some respect for your breasts as an important part of your anatomy. Your breast tissue will respond positively to your intent!

Once you are completely comfortable with this exercise, proceed with learning how your breast tissue feels when you use deeper pressure. You might approach this step in a spirit of curiosity, the same way you might examine your own hand or the sole of your foot. Your breasts are a vital part of your woman's wisdom, and you want to learn to listen to them. Lie on your back with one hand behind your head. This will flatten your breast tissue against your chest wall and make it easier for you to feel and appreciate your breast tissue as it lies on top of the underlying muscles and ribs. With your right hand, using the flat part of your fingers, not your fingertips, explore your left breast. Fingertips are so sensitive that they pick up the little ductules. You may find this frightening until you know what is normal for you, so use your fingertips to explore your breast tissue only after you have become completely comfortable with your breast anatomy and trust yourself. Repeat the exercise, using your left hand to explore your right breast. It is initially helpful to divide your breast into four quadrants and examine each one separately. Then move up to your armpit and back to your nipple so that you can feel the differences in the different breast areas. Breast tissue tends to be the densest in the upper, outer quadrants of the breast. Eventually you will be able to feel the difference between this area and others and to know that these differences are all normal for you.

You can get to know your breasts by understanding their anatomy, feeling your breasts (both from within and without), and looking at them. Your breasts are a normal part of the body and they deserve as much or more loving attention as your hair or complexion. If you approach your breasts in this way, to get to know them, to consciously and lovingly care for them (and *not* just find lumps), you'll be surrounding them with a much more positive energy field than the usual energy engendered by the breast self-exam, in which you examine to find what you don't want to find. Examining your breasts in a spirit of fear simply increases the fear and is the opposite of what you need to create healthy breast tissue. One of my former patients who had had a lumpectomy for breast cancer embodied this healthy way of examining her breasts. She felt her breasts regularly and knew their anatomy well. And every morning, before she got up, she said to them, "Girls, you're safe with me!"

A message I received on Facebook recently said, in part, "Thank you for saying what I felt in my heart was true when it comes to health. I am thirty-nine and have been on a spiritual journey since I was nineteen. I had a troubled childhood and I have always had kind of niggling breast issues. My mother died when she was only forty-eight of cancer, and cancer is a very common theme throughout my family. But I have never identified with it. I refused to have all the genetic testing that my family wanted me to—just because I didn't want that imprinted into my consciousness. In the past few years I have been really trying to send my body love, and I can kind of feel my breasts smiling. My body has given me three wonderful children and I send it gratitude and love."

I have another patient who said she liked to visualize the Divine Mother blessing her and her breasts when she touched them. She told me, "It always helps me feel better and dispels my fear."

Further, if there are any areas of your life in which you are overgiving to others and undernurturing yourself, say to your breasts, "Okay—I see it. I've got this. You don't have to get sick to remind me." This alone can have a very powerful effect on your body.

MONTHLY SELF-NURTURING BREAST MASSAGE RITUAL

Here's a monthly self-care breast massage ritual in which you consciously create breast health. This massage assists the lymph system in removing toxins and impurities from your body tissue because the stroking accelerates the transportation of those impurities to the lymph nodes for processing. (Note: Do not do this ritual if you have been recently diagnosed with breast cancer that hasn't been treated yet, because it may increase tumor spread.)

Before you begin, put on your favorite music (I like anything by Jim Brickman, Wah!, Enya, and Deva Premal) and scent the bath with rose or lavender aromatherapy oil (rose helps dissipate anger, and lavender is very calming). If you don't like baths, use your favorite scented massage oil. Use a light touch, moving the skin instead of massaging the muscles. Enjoy the sensual nature of touch as you do this. The more pleasure you feel, the more healthful the exercise.

1. With the first three fingers of your right hand, find the hollow spot above your left collarbone. Lightly stretch this skin, stroking from your shoulders toward your neck. Repeat five to ten times.

2. With the fingers of your right hand held very flat, cover the hairy part of your left armpit and stretch the skin upward five to ten times.

3. Keeping the fingers of your right hand flat, lightly stroke or pet the skin from the breastbone to the armpit. Do this above the breast, over the breast, and below the breast, repeating each path five to ten times.

4. Finally, with the fingers of your right hand still held flat, lightly stroke your left side from your waist up to your armpit, repeating five to ten times.

Now change hands and massage the right side of your chest. Make this entire process enjoyable.

BENIGN BREAST SYMPTOMS:
BREAST PAIN, LUMPS, CYSTS, AND NIPPLE DISCHARGE

The most common reason women seek medical consultation for breast symptoms is lumps or cysts. Though most of them are benign, these must be closely monitored to make sure that they are not cancerous. (Nipple discharge is a less common symptom but can still be cause for concern.)

Approximately half of all women who go to doctors go because they have some kind of pain in their breasts. Cyclic mastalgia, or breast pain that comes and goes depending on the menstrual cycle, is usually caused by sub-optimal iodine levels, excess hormonal stimulation of the breast from hyper-estrogenism, excessive caffeine intake, or even chronic stress. It is *not* a risk factor for breast cancer.

"Fibrocystic Breast Disease"/Dense Breasts

Currently about 70 percent of women have been told by a healthcare provider that they have "fibrocystic breast disease." In the 1970s and early 1980s a few studies seemed to indicate that women with so-called fibrocystic breast disease had a two to three times higher incidence of breast cancer. A panic ensued, and women were told conflicting stories by different doctors. When the National Cancer Association Consensus Committee investigated the issue in 1985, it discovered that 70 to 80 percent of what is called fibro-cystic breast disease is actually normal changes in breast anatomy and is *not* associated with an increase in breast cancer. Yet many women still believe it is.

Breasts are composed of fat and connective tissue. Over time, the ratio of connective tissue to fat changes. It is therefore normal for some areas of the breast to be denser on examination than others—breast tissue is not homo-geneous. One area may be denser than another simply because there's more connective tissue in that area than another. Most women normally undergo what pathologists call fibrocystic changes in their breasts, so the chance of finding them on a biopsy is very high. Unfortunately, because the term has been used to describe just about any breast thickening, tenderness, or other symptoms, women whose breast tissue is merely dense with connective tissue are sometimes given the diagnosis of fibrocystic breast disease, as are those who simply have variations in tissue density throughout their breasts, all of which are normal. I had a friend who went in for a routine mammogram and the technician made her feel as though her "dense breasts" were an abnor-mality. Why? Simply because they don't show up well on a mammogram—as if her breasts had somehow failed an important health test. She told me it scared her so much she nearly fainted. Such is the power of the words used by medical professionals.

Like the term *cervical erosion*, which simply pathologizes a normal change in the cervix, the terms *fibrocystic breast disease* and *dense breasts* basically don't indicate a disease. I think these terms should be discarded.[11] Misinformation about fibrocystic disease, the constant media exploitation of women's breasts, and our culture's ambivalence toward breasts set up a psy-chological dynamic that is loaded with potential harm for many women. Not only are they made to feel that their breasts are too small, too large, or the wrong shape, but now they are told by someone whom they trust that their breasts have a disease!

Nipple Discharge

Nipple discharge most often happens after nipple stimulation, usually from lovemaking. It is not dangerous. After a woman nurses a baby, it may take a year or more for milk discharge to disappear completely. In cases of persistent nipple discharge that are not associated with nipple stimulation— the discharge can be anything from milky to greenish clear fluid—a blood test to measure the hormone prolactin should be done to be certain that the woman doesn't have a rare pituitary tumor known as a pituitary microadenoma. A bloody discharge should always be investigated to be certain there's no cancer. Sometimes, however, this very rare condition is caused by benign growths in the ductal tissue of the nipple.

Breast Cysts

Breasts are very sensitive to hormonal changes, and nonmalignant lumps or thickenings often go away over time. But it is a standard medical recommendation that you tell your healthcare practitioner immediately about any lump you find. You want to know if the lump is a cyst. Breast cysts are very common in women in their forties when their hormone levels are changing. Breast cysts, which are fluid-filled, are diagnosed by placing a needle in them under local anesthetic and aspirating the contents. Sometimes a physician cannot tell a solid lump from a cyst on examination, so ultrasound is needed to make the distinction. If the lump is a cyst, its contents, usually yellow or greenish brown fluid, can be aspirated. Most experts feel that cyst fluid can be discarded because it is rarely helpful to analyze it. The cyst will disappear following aspiration in most cases and no further treatment is required. If there's any suspicion, however, the aspirated cells should be tested for cancer. If the ultrasound clearly shows a simple cyst and the woman does not want a needle stuck into her breast, the cyst can be watched. Many women track their cycles and stress levels by their cysts. When a cyst gets too painful or too large or sticks out, then she can go in and get it aspirated. Most cysts disappear with menopause.

A friend of mine recently developed a breast lump and was told by her doctor that she needed a mammogram. Because the lump had arisen rather quickly and because she didn't want the radiation exposure of a mammogram, she asked her doctor to do an ultrasound to see if it was a cyst that could be aspirated. Her doctor refused. She said my friend needed a mammogram. My friend called me for a second opinion, and I referred her to a breast surgeon who did the ultrasound in her office, found a cyst, and aspirated it right then and there. Case closed. Of course, my friend also knows that she needs to pay attention to her tendency to overgive to others; the cyst got her attention and she is adjusting her life accordingly.

If a lump is *not* clearly a cyst, the patient should be referred to a surgeon with an interest in breast problems or to a comprehensive breast care center. I feel strongly that women should get the best medical opinions possible about their situation before they embark on any treatment for a breast problem. In women younger than thirty-five (with some exceptions), a breast mass can be watched for several menstrual cycles to see if it goes away.

TREATMENT FOR BENIGN BREAST SYMPTOMS

The vast majority of women have breast pain from time to time. Breast pain (also known as mastalgia or mastodynia) is the number one reason why women visit clinics specializing in breast care and is present in 45 percent of the women who visit these clinics. But it's so common that almost all general physicians see women with this problem. Unfortunately, like so many other women's health issues, breast pain too often has been viewed by the medical profession as a neurotic "all in her head" kind of disease, and so it hasn't received the attention and care that it deserves. But every one of us knows that pain is a sign of imbalance somewhere in our lives. And breast pain is no exception.

The burning question that most women with breast pain want answered right away is this: "Is my pain a sign of cancer?" The answer to this is almost always no. But there are a few cases in which the answer is yes. One study showed that breast pain alone is a symptom in only 7 percent of women who had early-stage breast cancer, and another 8 percent presented with both pain and a lump. Another retrospective study suggested an increased risk for breast cancer in women who have had a history of chronic cyclic breast pain compared with those who did not.[12] I'm going to assume that if you have significant breast pain, you have been to a healthcare practitioner, received a thorough breast exam, and have had a normal mammogram or sonogram if indicated. My own experience with seeing hundreds of women with breast pain over the years is that the link between breast pain and breast cancer is very low. In fact, in one study of women with breast pain in whom no breast cancer was found on routine screening exams, less than 1 percent (0.5 percent, to be exact) actually went on to develop subsequent breast cancer at some point in the future.[13]

What Causes Breast Pain?

To get relief from your breast pain, you first have to understand why it may be there. There is no doubt that the most common type of breast pain occurs premenstrually and is related to the hormonal changes in your body that are part of your menstrual cycle. In the luteal phase of your cycle (the two weeks before your period begins), all women have an increased tendency to retain fluid and to gain a pound or two. But in susceptible women, this slight fluid increase, as well as other hormonal changes associated with the menstrual cycle, can cause pressure or inflammation in the breast tissue, resulting in breast tenderness. The same inflammatory chemicals such as prostaglandins and cytokines that cause menstrual cramps can also cause breast tenderness. Your breast tissue actually goes through cyclic changes each month that mirror those that are happening in your uterus. The difference is that the buildup of fluids and tissue in your uterus passes out of your body in the form of your menstrual flow. But the buildup of fluid and cellular tissue in your breasts simply gets reabsorbed back into your body. So it's not difficult to see how pain might result in many women, particularly if their iodine intake is too low or if they are eating a diet that favors cellular inflammation (see my Program to Promote Healthy Breast Tissue, page 429). These cyclic hormonal changes also explain why women are so often offered a variety of hormonal therapies for their breast complaints—which I'll address in a minute.

Some women experience breast pain that is not related to the menstrual cycle at all. No one knows what causes this. Some sources think it is related to inflammation in the body, whereas others think it is related to neuroendocrine changes resulting from subtle interactions between our environment, our perceptions, and our hormonal and immune systems (breast pain has been linked to alterations in steroid and protein hormones, including estrogen, progesterone, LHRF [luteinizing hormone releasing factor, made by the hypothalamus], and prolactin). The key to pain relief is following an inflammation-reducing diet and supplementation program, including iodine, and at the same time acknowledging and then releasing the various emotional states, including trauma, depression, anxiety, and learned helplessness, that have been shown to alter the body's immune and hormonal systems.[14]

Discovering the Messages Behind the Symptoms

Sometimes a woman's breast pain persists until she addresses a deeper cultural wounding. One of my patients got over her breast pain only after she remembered that at the age of five she had been playing in a barn and some boys forced her to pose nude for them. She remembered that her chest was a major focus of this activity. After her breasts grew at puberty, her emotional and psychological discomfort at this kind of attention became chronic and eventually manifested as physical pain.

A forty-seven-year-old woman told me that when her daughter turned thirteen and became quite independent from her, she became acutely conscious of her breasts for a while. She said that they ached at times, as though they were longing to nourish or cradle a baby. She hadn't given birth to her daughter but had adopted her. She said, "Heading into menopause, I remembered that I never beheld her infant face, nor did she drink from my breast. I experienced an intense desire to hold a baby for as long as I needed to. Several months later, a thickening in my left breast was found during my routine annual exam. It was near my heart. I knew what it was about. I needed to deal with renewed feelings about my infertility and its losses. I felt intense sadness over not giving birth to this wonderful child of mine. Now for the first time, my body was letting me know that it, too, was sorry." Two months after she had this realization, her breast thickening was gone at her follow-up exam. Sometimes the body heals simply when you give yourself permission to listen to its messages and to say to your breasts, "Okay—I've got the message."

Breast Biopsy

Any persistent mass requires further testing for definitive diagnosis, most often (but not always) in the form of a biopsy of some kind. High-resolution ultrasound has decreased the number of biopsies required. Most breast biopsies are done on an outpatient basis under local anesthesia by a general surgeon with a special interest in breast care. A needle biopsy can be done in an office setting under ultrasound or mammographic guidance, thus saving the patient from disfiguring lumpectomy for benign lumps and giving her a diagnosis quickly. In fact, in some breast care centers, diagnosis can be made virtually the same day as the needle biopsy. Sometimes, however, the diagnosis must wait for several days until the pathologist can perform further diagnostic tests on the breast tissue. Many women worry that the needle will spread the cancer. Yet years of experience haven't borne this out. Dixie Mills, M.D., an internationally known breast cancer surgeon with whom I worked for years, has seen only two cases of this in twenty years, and those were of a rare variant of breast cancer.

One of the most unpleasant experiences a woman can have is living with the uncertainty about whether a breast lump is cancerous. Happily, there are better options than waiting and worrying, and I'll cover them later in this chapter.

MAMMOGRAPHY

Mammograms: The Limitations of a Gold Standard

A mammogram is an X-ray study of the breasts used to diagnose breast cancer in its earliest stages, before it can be felt on clinical exam. It has long been considered the gold standard for early detection of breast cancer (and the perception of a greater chance of cure). Fear of breast cancer is many women's number one fear. A 1995 Gallup poll found that 40 percent of women believe they will die of breast cancer, even though the actual risk of death from the disease is less than 3 percent.[15] So women and doctors historically have clung to mammograms and early detection as though they were lifelines.

But in November 2009, the United States Preventive Services Task Force made headlines when it reversed its long-standing advice and released new guidelines recommending that most women start regular breast cancer screening at age fifty (instead of forty, as previously suggested).[16] The guidelines also recommended that women between the ages of fifty and seventy-four have mammograms only every two years. The guidelines did not recommend routine screening for women older than seventy-four at this time because the risks and benefits remain unknown. (These new guidelines did not apply to women at high risk for breast cancer because of a gene mutation that makes breast cancer more likely or because of previous extensive exposure to radiation.)

The task force concluded that the risks associated with mammograms for women in their forties (including a 60 percent greater chance of getting a false-positive result thanks to denser breast tissue, even though they are less likely to have breast cancer) outweigh the benefits (a 15 percent reduction in breast cancer mortality).[17] These risks have long been reported in the literature. For example, as far back as 2000 and 2001, Danish researchers Ole Olsen and Peter Gotzsche published two studies in *The Lancet* of their reviews of seven randomized controlled studies on the benefits of mammography in reducing mortality from breast cancer. They found that five of the seven studies were so flawed they couldn't even be reviewed. In the remaining two, they also found major design flaws and limitations. They concluded that mammograms had no effect on deaths attributed to breast cancer. The studies also showed that mammograms often led to needless treatments and were linked to a 20 percent increase in mastectomies, many of which were unnecessary.[18] Recent research continues to bear this out. A groundbreaking 2012 study in the *New England Journal of Medicine* showed that 1.3 million women over the previous thirty years were overdiagnosed (and, as a result, overtreated), accounting for nearly a third of all newly diagnosed breast cancers.[19] The researchers' conclusion was that "screening is having, at best, only a small effect on the rate of death from breast cancer." A 2013 study concluded that for every 2,000 women receiving mammograms over a ten-year period, only one would avoid dying of breast cancer and ten healthy women would be treated unnecessarily.[20]

The task force's 2009 change in screening guidelines was controversial, however, and consensus has been mixed ever since. For example, the American College of Radiology was so opposed to the change that it went so far as to ask the task force to reverse its recommendation. The college continues to recommend annual screening with mammography starting at age forty and continuing until a woman's life expectancy is less than five to seven years. The American Cancer Society's latest guidelines (released in 2015) suggest women should at least *have the opportunity to begin* annual mammograms at age forty but recommend such screening from age forty-five to fifty-five, at which time women may continue annual mammograms or switch to every other year, with no upper age limit (as long as their overall health is good and they have a life expectancy of ten years or longer). On the other hand, the American College of Obstetricians and Gynecologists' latest guidelines (released in 2017) state that while women should be offered an annual or biennial mammogram starting at age forty, their hard line for starting annual mammograms is at age fifty, with biennial screening beginning at age fifty-five considered "particularly reasonable" until age seventy-five. We have certainly come a long way from the American Cancer Society's awareness campaign from the mid-1980s that admonished women over thirty-five, "If you haven't had a mammogram, you need more than your breasts examined."

Other current research is aimed at improving mammogram technology (which has already progressed to using digital images that can be enlarged and enhanced more easily than the images previously taken using film). Three-dimensional mammography, also known as digital breast tomosynthesis (DBT), takes pictures of thin slices of the breast from different angles. Computer software is then used to construct a comprehensive image. Although DBT uses very low dose X-rays, it is generally performed at the same time as standard two-dimensional digital mammography, so the total radiation dose is higher than with a standard mammogram. Newer strategies are now allowing DBT to be done alone, potentially reducing the radiation dose to a level closer to that of standard mammography. Research hasn't yet shown if this newer 3-D mammography is better than standard, 2-D mammography at detecting early changes or avoiding false-positive test results, but a large-scale randomized breast-screening trial (the Tomosynthesis Mammography Imaging Screening Trial) is currently under way to determine if the method is better at identifying advanced cancers.

Almost all cancer screening modalities (except functional ones such as thermography) identify not just aggressive cancers but also slow-growing lesions that women would die *with,* not *from.* In other words, they would never become life-threatening if left alone. An intriguing and important study published in the November 2008 edition of *Archives of Internal Medicine* suggests that some breast cancers will indeed go into remission without any treatment.[21] This study followed more than 200,000 Norwegian women between the ages of fifty and sixty-four over two consecutive six-year periods. Half of the women received regular, periodic breast exams or regular mammograms; the rest had no regular breast cancer screenings. Researchers found that the women who received regular screenings had 22 percent more discrete occurrences of breast cancer. The researchers concluded that in women who didn't have regular screenings, breast cancer probably developed with the same frequency, but in some of those cases their bodies had somehow naturally resolved those abnormalities without intervention. Other doctors unrelated to the study analyzed the data and concurred that this conclusion makes sense.

People believe that it takes a miracle for cancers to disappear, but this happens more often than you might think. For example, it is estimated that for every hundred women who are told they have breast cancer, as many as thirty have cancers that are so slow-growing that they are unlikely to be life-threatening.[22] Addressing this issue, Barnett S. Kramer, M.D., associate director for disease prevention at the National Institutes of Health, said this: "The health professions have played a role in oversimplifying and creating the stage for confusion. It's important to be clear to the public about what we know and be honest about what we don't know."[23]

The debate about mammograms isn't difficult to understand. Both inside and outside medicine, we as a culture have come to rely on screening to save us. And even though the evidence doesn't support it, individual women and their doctors often feel safer if they perceive that they've "covered all the bases." (By the way, men face a similar experience with PSA screening tests for prostate cancer, long considered to be essential. In one large-scale 2018 study comparing men who had PSA screening to men who received medical exams but no screening, the number of men diagnosed with prostate cancer was the same, as was their survival rate after ten years. Also, PSA testing failed to pick up some aggressive cancers that were potentially deadly, and sometimes it resulted in false-positive results that led to anxiety and unnecessary treatment.)[24]

One helpful way to assess your risk for breast cancer—which in turn can help you decide how often you want to have mammograms—is to use the National Cancer Institute's Breast Cancer Risk Assessment Tool, available online at https://bcrisktool.cancer.gov. After you answer seven simple questions, it calculates both your risk of getting invasive breast cancer in the next five years as well as your lifetime risk, and it compares each to the risk for the average U.S. woman of the same age and race or ethnicity.

A number of other negative studies on mammography have appeared in the medical literature over the years—and these are finally getting the press they deserve. In 2000, the *Journal of the National Cancer Institute* pointed out that the cumulative risk of having false-positive mammograms is quite significant in many women. (Most, though not all, states now have laws requiring women who have had a mammogram to be notified if the radiologist determines their breast tissue to be dense.)[25] And in 2002, a National Cancer Institute advisory panel concluded that the benefits of mammography are uncertain, in part because of the substantial chance of receiving a false-positive result. (There's even research showing that such false-positive diagnoses can cause long-term psychosocial consequences, even three years afterward, that were equivalent to those of women who did indeed have breast cancer.)[26] While this is possible in any age group, it is most common in women in their forties because they tend to have denser and more fibrous breasts that get read as false positives on mammograms and then require biopsy. Andrew Wolf, M.D., an associate professor at the University of Virginia School of Medicine, supports these findings. In an August 2003 review article on breast cancer screening in *Consultant,* Dr. Wolf states, "If a woman begins getting regular mammograms at age 40, there is virtually a 100 percent chance that some kind of abnormality will show up that will warrant at least a follow-up mammogram, an ultrasound scan, or a call from the physician recommending a six-month follow-up examination. It is also likely that over the course of a lifetime, she will undergo an unnecessary breast biopsy."[27] Research from 2011 backs this up, as well, finding that after ten years of annual mammograms, 61 percent of the women had had at least one false-positive result.[28]

Thomas E. Quay, J.D., vice president, secretary, and general counsel for the Athena Institute for Women's Wellness, does not believe this should be taken lightly. "My opinion is that a doctor who fails to advise patients of the pain of mammograms, the downsides of overdiagnosis, false positives, radiation, fear, detriments to the patient's quality of life has not obtained informed consent to a screening mammogram," he says in a statement on the institute's website. "Absent consent," he adds, "the treatment legally is a 'battery,' as in 'assault and battery.'"[29]

For me, the biggest concern about mammography is that it doesn't appear to reduce mortality from breast cancer any better than simple breast exam (which also doesn't decrease mortality). According to a 2000 study from the *Journal of the National Cancer Institute,* after following nearly 40,000 women between the ages of fifty and fifty-nine, researchers found that annual mammograms were no more effective than standard breast exams in reducing breast cancer mortality.[30] A systematic review of nineteen studies including a total of 2.3 million perimenopausal and menopausal women published in 2015 showed that asymptomatic women who received clinical breast exams but no mammograms had a higher cancer-free rate, thanks to the fact that in the women who had mammograms, 30 to 50 percent of those tests yielded false-positive diagnoses.[31] A 2017 study by French researchers evaluating data from a routine screening program in the Netherlands introduced in 1989 for all women ages fifty to seventy-five showed that over a twenty-three-year period, mammograms in fact didn't save any lives in this age group at all, and that more than half of the abnormal results reported were false positives.[32] Yet another study published in the *Journal of the American Medical Association* found that women age seventy and older benefited very little from mammography.[33] The cancers detected at this age never would have killed them.

Then there are those researchers who doubt the safety of mammography because of radiation exposure. A 1994 study published in *The Lancet* addressed another concern that many women have brought up with me—that the breast compression that occurs during a mammogram (the equivalent of about forty pounds of weight on the breast) may cause small, in-situ tumors to rupture, thereby spreading cancer cells into surrounding tissues and potentially leading to more invasive cancers and metastases.[34] Researchers at the UCLA Jonsson Comprehensive Cancer Center found that even when radiation kills half of a patient's cancer cells, the cells it doesn't kill can react to the challenge of that stress by transforming into treatment-resistant breast cancer stem cells. The net result is an increase in the ratio of highly malignant to benign cells within the tumor. Researchers found that the new breast cancer stem cells were up to thirty times more likely to form tumors than the nonirradiated breast cancer cells.[35]

Cornelia Baines, M.D., professor emerita at the University of Toronto and former deputy director of the Canadian National Breast Screening Study, put it succinctly when she said, "I remain convinced that the current enthusiasm for screening is based more on fear, false hope and greed than on evidence."[36] I agree with Dr. Baines completely.

Fortunately, the medical community is waking up to the fact that there is no "one size fits all" approach to breast screening for the average woman. One big step forward is the Women Informed to Screen Depending on Measures of Risk (WISDOM) study, a randomized trial of about 100,000 women that is testing a personalized approach to breast cancer screening.[37] This five-year study began in the fall of 2016 and is being led by Laura J. Esserman, M.D., a University of California, San Francisco, breast surgeon. The study is looking at whether risk-based screening (screening at intervals based on each woman's risk as determined by her genetic makeup, family history, and other risk factors) is more effective than annual screening. While those women at higher risk will receive more frequent mammograms than those deemed to be at lower risk, no one in the trial will receive less than the recommended level of screening in the current U.S. Preventive Services Task Force guidelines.

The bottom line is this: When it comes to mammograms, things are not as cut-and-dried as they seem. There's a lot we simply don't know. After discussing their options with a knowledgeable healthcare practitioner, all women will need to follow their own inner guidance on this issue, taking full responsibility for their choices. Intelligent, informed women can be trusted to do what's right for them, including forgoing mammograms—and I support them wholeheartedly.

The Limits of Conventional Early Detection

Regular screening is not the same as *prevention*. In other words, it is not the same as brushing and flossing the teeth, which actually prevents cavities and periodontal disease. As one of my colleagues said of breast cancer, "We identify the risks, but we don't know what to do until they manifest as disease." Our culture uses mammograms as a fix but doesn't encourage women to change their diets, exercise, stop smoking, and learn how to be in relationships that nurture them. These are preventive changes that favor healthy breasts. But as one researcher has said, it's difficult to put together a constituency for prevention. It is treatment that gets our attention. If your sister or mother dies of breast cancer, you usually give money to programs that do research to produce better treatments; you don't start a whole-food restaurant in your neighborhood or advocate teaching eighth-grade girls how to appreciate their breasts and make sure they have optimal levels of vitamin D. Our culture is crisis-oriented, acting only once the horse is out of the barn.

There is a third option, however. You can use thermography, mammography, and other disease screening as an external guidance system. And if any abnormality appears, you then have the opportunity to ask the abnormal cells what they need that they're not getting. The earlier in the disease process you make adjustments to your diet, beliefs, and lifestyle, the easier it is to transform your cells. (See my Program to Promote Healthy Breast Tissue, page 429.)

Breast Ultrasound: An Adjunct
(and Sometime Alternative) to Mammography

In many women, particularly those with dense breasts, ultrasound screening of breast tissue (reading breast tissue by sending sound waves through it and reading the echoes on a screen) is more appropriate and helpful than mammography. With the advent of high-resolution ultrasound, some authorities feel that this modality may become the method of choice for detecting an invasive breast carcinoma, with mammography reserved for localizing intraductal carcinoma marked by calcifications. One advantage of ultrasound is that it doesn't involve radiation and is also far more comfortable. Routine ultrasound screening of breast tissue with expert interpretation of the scans is not nearly as widely available as mammography, and most women aren't offered this choice.

In the diagnosis of a nonpalpable mass (one that you can't feel but that is discovered on mammography), ultrasound can also be invaluable for guiding fine-needle or core-needle aspiration. High-resolution breast ultrasound has also made it much easier to delineate palpable breast lumps. An ultrasound can easily tell the difference between a cyst and a lump. And if a breast mass is solid, the ultrasound has a 98 percent specificity in terms of being able to distinguish a benign lesion from a malignant one. In fact, some studies have shown that ultrasound is the single most accurate diagnostic test for those women with palpable breast masses, yielding a 99.7 percent positive predictive value if it's used by those who are skilled in this technique.[38] If there's any question about the findings, a needle biopsy can now be done in the office setting to determine whether or not a breast mass is malignant. This has spared many women from disfiguring breast biopsies and the anxiety that comes from not knowing what she's dealing with.

There is another reason why ultrasound is important. Mammography is often not helpful in women who are younger, have dense breasts, have postoperative scarring, suffer from acute or chronic radiation effects, are on hormone replacement, or are less than forty-five to fifty years of age. Sonograms are also more accurate than mammograms for diagnosing breast problems accurately in women who've had breast implants. The highest-risk women are those who've already had radiation to their breasts. Sonography is often a good alternative for these women. Mammography is still the most common screening modality for most asymptomatic women, but ultrasound is helpful as well. Many centers will not do screening ultrasounds because it is very time-consuming and it is difficult to compare pictures from year to year. However, some centers offer screening ultrasounds for high-risk women.

Other Alternatives to Mammography

A few other alternatives to standard mammograms exist, although nothing is currently poised to take their place. For example, magnetic resonance imaging is another tool in the breast cancer detection department. But MRI will most likely never be used as a screening test because it is too expensive (more than $2,000), it's too hard to do (women have to lie still for up to an hour, often medicated), and there are too many false positives. MRI may play a role for high-risk women with dense breasts or suspicious mammograms, though I'd certainly make the decision judiciously. I would recommend having it done only at a breast center whose personnel are highly experienced in their use. (By the way, at least 27 percent of women recently diagnosed with breast cancer have what is called pretreatment MRI in an attempt to gather information for treatment decisions. Yet a 2009 study from a leading U.S. cancer research and treatment center found this practice did more harm than good. The MRI delayed treatment by an average of three weeks and increased mastectomy rates by 80 percent—because of the high rate of false positives—in women who would have been good candidates for lumpectomy.)[39]

A new method of screening called diffuse optical tomography (DOT) that does not involve radiation is currently being studied.[40] DOT uses near-infrared light instead of X-rays to create images that determine blood flow to the tissues and measure changes in the amount of oxygen in them. The method first emerged in the 1990s and is still being perfected, but many researchers believe it has much promise. One 2011 study predicted DOT "will completely change our method of breast cancer screening and therapy monitoring in the future."[41]

True Prevention: Thermography

Thermography—a noninvasive, safe technology that simply records the amount of heat emanating from breast (or other) tissue—is the screening modality of choice. The FDA approved it as an adjunctive breast cancer screening test in 1982, and in my view it could replace the vast number of mammograms women are subjected to. When you get a thermogram, the thermographer uses an infrared thermal-imaging camera to capture the amount of heat on the body's surface. Abnormal heat patterns in breast tissue indicate increased blood circulation to a given area secondary to cellular inflammation, a well-documented precursor for cancer. Thermogram images are scored according to how much inflammation is present. If the image is highly abnormal and there is a high suspicion of cancer, then a mammogram can be ordered to confirm the diagnosis. Standard treatment would follow. In the vast majority of cases, however, a thermogram will indicate a tendency toward breast abnormalities long before these would develop into palpable lumps or mammographic abnormalities.[42] In fact, research suggests thermograms can detect abnormal activity eight to ten years before any other screening test.[43]

This is good news because it means a thermogram allows a woman and her healthcare practitioner to be proactive. If her scan shows inflammation, she can then go on a program (such as the one on page 429 of this chapter) to improve her breast health. Decreased cellular inflammation can easily be documented on a follow-up thermogram. This approach is far more empowering than that of routine mammography, in which a woman simply waits for an abnormality to show up without being given the tools to be proactive about her breast health. And a thermogram can help a woman diagnosed with ductal carcinoma in situ (and her healthcare providers) decide whether or not she requires aggressive or conservative treatment. (See "The DCIS Dilemma" on page 421.) Another valuable bonus is that thermograms don't confuse harmless fibrocystic masses with worrisome lumps as often as mammography.[44]

Routine thermograms could save thousands of women from undergoing unnecessary biopsies and disfigurement. And because breast inflammation is a marker of inflammation in other areas of the body, using thermograms would also help improve overall health at the same time. Unfortunately, thermography is often not covered by insurance (scans cost anywhere from $90 to $250), a fact that has more to do with politics and economics than science.

To find a practitioner in your area who does thermography, visit www.breastthermography.com, www.breastthermography.org, or the websites for the International Academy of Clinical Thermology (www.iact-org.org), the American College of Clinical Thermology (www.thermologyonline.org), or Breast Thermography International (www.btiscan.com).

Philip Getson, D.O., a board-certified thermologist who is both vice president of the American Academy of Thermology and chairman of the committee that formulates the national protocols for breast thermography accepted by the international thermographic community, cautions that not all thermographic equipment is the same. Here are the criteria he suggests for choosing a thermography center:

- The room where the thermograms are taken should be free of outside light, and the temperature should always be at 68–72 degrees Fahrenheit, with a proper cooling system in place.

- The machine's "drift factor" should be less than 0.2 degrees centigrade.

- The thermography center should be backed by qualified, board-certified physicians specifically trained to interpret breast thermograms.

- A physician should be available to explain and discuss all findings.

- The center should retain all images for future comparison.

A BRIEF HISTORY OF THERMOGRAPHY

Back in the 1970s and '80s, a great deal of research showed that thermography was highly effective in screening for abnormalities that included breast cancer.[45] Researchers observed that thermographic scans were highly specific for each woman, providing a unique thermal "signature" that remained remarkably constant from year to year. Like other breast-screening modalities, thermography didn't diagnose anything; it simply pointed out the presence of an abnormality. Here are some highlights of its history:

~ In 1972, a study led by radiologist Harold J. Isard, M.D., of the Albert Einstein Medical Center in Philadelphia analyzed data from 10,000 women, of whom 4,393 were asymptomatic. Dr. Isard concluded that prescreening these women with thermography instead of mammography would have limited the need for mammograms to 1,028 women—a decrease of 77 percent. He also calculated that combining mammograms (when necessary) with thermography would have resulted in a cancer detection rate of 24.1 per 1,000 instead of the expected 7 per 1,000 using mammograms alone.[46] This study was done before the connection between cellular inflammation and cancer was clear, so doctors were not using thermography as a way to address and reverse cellular inflammation. With today's knowledge of how to decrease cellular inflammation proactively, plus knowing that some cancers will regress on their own, thermography is the best modality we have to monitor year-to-year status of breast health.

~ A 1980 study of 1,245 women by Michel Gautherie, Ph.D., and Charles Gros, M.D., at the Louis Pasteur University School of Medicine in Strasbourg, France, concluded that an abnormal thermogram was the *single most important marker* of high risk for developing breast cancer.[47]

~ The next year, Dr. Gautherie spoke at the International Symposium on Biomedical Thermography, reporting on additional research that involved screening more than 600 women over a period of ten years. He and his colleagues found that an abnormal thermogram was *ten times more significant* as a future risk indicator for breast cancer than a first-order family history of the disease.[48]

~ Two other researchers speaking at the Strasbourg symposium (H. Spitalier and D. Giraud) had screened 61,000 women over a

ten-year period with annual thermograms. They found that per-
sistently abnormal thermograms during those ten years were associated with a *twenty-two-fold greater risk* of future breast
cancer (even in patients who showed no other sign of malignancy)
and that of all the patients who were eventually diagnosed with
cancer, thermography alone was the first alarm in 60 percent of
cases.[49]

~ In 1982, the FDA approved breast thermography as an adjunctive
diagnostic breast cancer screening procedure.

~ In 1996, California radiologist Parvis Gamagami, M.D., studied
the use of thermography to detect certain types of blood vessel
formations that often precede breast cancer diagnoses. His research found that 86 percent of nonpalpable breast cancers demonstrated this blood vessel growth, which showed up on
thermograms.[50]

~ In 1998, Montreal oncological surgeon John Keyserlingk, M.D.,
Ph.D., documented that 85 percent of breast cancers could be diagnosed using mammography and clinical breast exams. When
thermography was added, the figure was increased to 98 percent.[51]

~ In 2003, California diagnostic radiologist Yuri Parisky, M.D.,
published a study of 769 women who had suspicious mammograms followed by thermograms. The thermograms were 97 percent correct in detecting breast cancer.[52]

Thermography is the missing link that holds the key to true prevention
of breast cancer, not just early detection—although it also does that very
well. It allows a woman and her healthcare provider to determine the state of
her breast health immediately, and then take steps to improve it long before
a more serious condition develops.

The following account is from Judie Harvey, my former website editor,
about her experience with thermography compared to mammography. She
underwent thermography to experience it herself and to compare and contrast it with the conventional breast care she'd had for years. I believe her
experience has universal implications for all women. Here is her story:

I recently had a thermogram for the first time and found it to be the
most civilized medical test to scan the health of my breasts. Perhaps the
best part was getting the results, because not only were they clear and

conclusive, but they told the tale of *my* unique body! I didn't feel like a statistic or a woman falling into a category who now required another procedure or treatment because "that's the way we handle women with your condition." To truly appreciate the difference between getting a thermogram and getting a mammogram, let me describe each experience.

THE MAMMOGRAM

"Miss Harvey, there's an abnormal image on your mammogram. We'd like you to come back for another mammogram and then possibly a sonogram to confirm our findings." I received this message by phone a couple of days after my routine annual mammogram. *Super!* I thought. *I really enjoyed getting the first mammogram. It's great to be in a room buzzing with radiation with a perfect stranger who's been trained to torture my body.* The Spanish Inquisition would have ended much sooner if there'd been a mammography machine available to squeeze the living daylights out of someone's breasts (or testicles).

But the first exam wasn't that bad. Sure, a perfect stranger touched my breasts, laying them in a tray and squashing them a couple of different ways to see just how flat she could get them. Unpleasant, but the only truly awkward moment was when she asked me the date of my last mammogram. The radiologists in this huge radiology practice in Bethesda, Maryland, where they flatten at least 300 pairs of breasts a day, like to compare the films. I felt just the tiniest hesitation telling the technician it had been twelve years. I knew she'd probably have to sit down to catch her breath. I didn't want her to flinch or twitch uncontrollably when she pushed the button on the X-ray machine. It would only mean more images for me to endure.

"Twelve years? Why have you waited so long?" she asked, trying not to admonish me. *Simple,* I answered her in my head. *Every time I have this test, you find something, because I have lumps and bumps. And every time you find something, I have to have it pushed and pulled like taffy and then stuck with needles and biopsied.* "I just know my breasts are normal and healthy," I responded. I had told my ob-gyn the same thing. He appealed to me, wanting me to know for sure, so I went.

The radiologist looked at me like I had two heads and said, "You know that having an annual mammogram is the best way to prevent breast cancer," leaving off the rest of the sentence: *from killing you.*

After I got the abnormal results of the first mammogram, I scheduled the second exam and then got to wait in the special room with all the other scared women. They looked tense and nervous, and I guessed that theirs were extremely suspicious lumps. I figured mine couldn't be all that bad, since they'd waited three weeks to bring me in for a follow-up. In the radiology practice I go to, which is really quite nice and very professional, you leave the office after your first mammogram without knowing the results. If you get called back, you get to see the radiologist, ask questions, and grin and bear it while another perfect stranger mashes every single sensitive spot on your breasts during a mammogram and sonogram.

Fast-forward. The second mammogram found two lumps and a cyst, likely nothing because cancer doesn't typically present with "friends" (other breast anomalies that are close to each other). But my ob-gyn and the radiologist have to be sure. I've started down the path, and now I'm on the assembly line. Next stop—core needle biopsies.

On the day of the procedure, a nurse assisting the doctor takes me to a very clean room. She explains the procedure: local anesthetic and lots of jabbing with a spring-loaded needle. It's about what I expect, until she tells me about the titanium clip (sometimes called a chip). Apparently, they've just initiated a new procedure in their practice mandating that a small titanium clip be inserted into any mass that's biopsied. The nurse says not to worry, it's the same material they use to make mechanical hips and it almost never goes off when you go through security at the airport. *What a relief!* When I tell her that I don't really want the clip and would prefer to just stick with what God gave me, I feel a little tension from her. *Oh dear, not another patient that won't comply* is written prominently in her eyes. I know I'm probably going to have to break out the "mommy stare"—a look I've perfected that has literally brought grown men to their knees—in order to get out of the clip thing.

"But it's required," she said. "It's part of the procedure. Then, after we place the clips in your breast, we'll take you for another mammogram." *And how painful will that be?* I couldn't help thinking. "We have to make sure the clips are in the right place. This is the best way to track what we've done so you don't have to have any unnecessary biopsies." *Like the ones I'm having now?*

I told her again that I didn't want or need any tracking devices— I'm not an endangered animal in the wild. And because she'd obviously lost sight of the fact, I calmly told her that it *was* my body, so it really should be my choice. She told me they couldn't do the biopsies unless I agreed to the clips. I told the poor woman, who was just following the protocol, that I was happy to leave without having the biopsies.

We agreed to have the doctor come in. And he made a good point: If the tissue being biopsied turns out to be cancer, having the clip will help the breast surgeon zero in on cancerous tissue, which makes the recovery process easier after a lumpectomy.

I looked into his eyes using the mildest version of my mommy stare.

He had a tray full of needles and other sharp objects that he was going to use shortly. One was a needle full of local anesthesia, and I wanted that! I explained that I didn't want the clip and was prepared to leave. (Even though the clip made logical sense, it just felt wrong to me.) He said I was lucky I hadn't scheduled the procedure a few days later (in 2009), when the clips would then be the new standard of care and he wouldn't feel comfortable doing the biopsy without one. He also told me he would "let me slide" because he was pretty sure that my lumps were nothing to worry about. We went ahead with the biopsies. *Darn,* I thought after he was done, *that felt good, having you use my breast for a dartboard!*

Of course, I thanked the radiologist for his work when I left. He was very kind, and I was sure he did a good job. I knew my ob-gyn would be happy I had complied. I put up with pain and extensive bruising for about a week. Everything turned out normal.

THE THERMOGRAM

About eight months later, I scheduled a thermogram because I wanted to experience an approach to my breasts that Dr. Northrup told me was far more proactive. I entered a cozy center near Baltimore called the Cometa Wellness Center, which felt more like a home than a medical office. My thermographer (the thermography technician) met me and took me to a comfortable room. I could tell right away that she was caring and professional, and this helped me relax a little.

Given my history of fibrocystic breasts, a lumpectomy at age seventeen, and multiple biopsies, I was curious to see if there would be heat where these masses were or had been. I, like most women, also have some spots in my breasts that hurt from time to time, and I wondered if those spots would be warmer than the normal tissue.

The thermographer told me I would be having a thermogram of my entire upper body. *What a nice surprise!* I thought. Then a thermologist (an M.D. trained in the science of reading thermograms) would read the digital images taken by the thermographer. The doctor would look at a number of areas, including my sinuses, jaw, and gums; my thyroid and the lymph glands in the neck and armpits; the muscles in my back and neck; and my entire digestive system, including my gallbladder, liver, kidneys, colon, and stomach. Oh—and my breasts!

The thermographer gave me very comprehensive medical history forms. In addition to indicating my previous breast or other surgeries or biopsies, she also had me indicate any area of pain or concern on a chart. There were also extensive questions about the health of my upper body. The information would help the thermologist better interpret the results. *What?* I thought. *No one incites panic in this model? Can this be real medicine?*

Certain things interfere with the test results. I had been told not to bathe, shave, or use deodorants within four hours of the imaging, so I'd showered, etc., the night before. I'd also been asked not to use creams or makeup on the day of the test and not to have bodywork, such as massage or chiropractic manipulation, within a certain number of days before the exam.

I was taken to a dark room where I slipped into a gown, leaving my clothes on from the waist down. When the thermographer returned to the room, she took the images of my head, neck, chest, and back first, while I remained clothed from the breasts down. I stood a few feet from a machine that reminded me of an old-fashioned camera on a tripod. When the thermographer took a picture, the thermal image came up immediately on a computer, with different colors indicating the intensity of the heat. The thermographer told me not to be concerned by what I saw or to try to make sense of it. Still, it did kind of make sense—and it was fascinating.

Next, I dropped my gown for five images of the breast and lymph nodes in the chest and armpits. Because it was dark in the room and she never touched my breasts, I felt that my privacy was being respected. One of the images required my putting one hand behind my head, elbow out. "I feel like a pinup girl, but in a good way," I joked. I was proud and happy to have breasts, not terrified that they were unhealthy.

Finally, she did the abdomen. She didn't like the results at first and asked me to stand with my arms away from my body so I could adjust to the temperature of the room. She explained that it only takes about a minute for that to happen. She stepped out of the room briefly, and this was the only awkward moment for me. I felt a little silly holding my arms up and away from my body, because I was standing there half naked. While waiting, I noticed that the room was the perfect temperature and nothing like the radiology group's setting, which can only be likened to a meat locker. The thermographer said that they intentionally pick a temperature that's comfortable. The entire exam took about fifteen minutes.

A few weeks later, Ariane Cometa, M.D., a practicing internist and the founder of the Cometa Wellness Center, called me to go over the results from the thermologist who read my scan. Normally she just sends a letter outlining the findings; however, I had arranged for a consultation. We talked a little about my thyroid. I had had it tested recently, and it was a little low. Dr. Cometa told me that she saw dysfunction and asked me if I had a history of thyroid disease. I had been taking medication for a while but stopped when it made me jittery. She recommended a different medication and told me something very interesting: Thermography often gives her better information on how the thyroid is functioning than blood work does. So if her patient's blood work for the thyroid is normal but her patient is experiencing symptoms that would indicate thyroid dysfunction, she'll advise a thermogram. Dr. Cometa said that follow-up thermograms of the thyroid taken after the patient has been on thyroid medication for a few months often show positive changes that don't get picked up by blood work. I was so impressed with her knowledge and caring, as well as with the practical, health-promoting solutions she offered. Again, I felt like a unique individual rather than a random widget on a huge medical assembly line, unable to move forward without "their" stamp of approval. The thermogram provided insight into *my* health issues.

Dr. Cometa also explained that asymmetry in the thermogram can be a sign of trouble and that my right armpit showed more heat than the left. Because my right breast had been biopsied less than a year before, this could be explained by the detoxification and restoration process that was still occurring in the lymph nodes in this area.

So what about my breasts? Well, they are perfectly normal. Yahoo! There's no heat or indication of cellular anomalies at all where I have lumps or have had surgeries. In fact, Dr. Cometa told me that she is extremely happy when test results show breasts as healthy as mine. I was so grateful to have had a test that was perfect for a woman with fibrocystic breasts and absolutely no family history of breast cancer. I would return for a follow-up thermogram in three months to check on the right armpit area, and then once every year or so after that. It was such an empowering experience.

RECONCILING THE RESULTS

Ah—but that means the biopsies I'd had in December were unnecessary. So were the mammograms I was told to have in my twenties and all the previous biopsies, with the exception of the lumpectomy I had as a teenager. Yikes. What an awful realization. In an effort to take the best care of me that they could, my doctors put me through a lot of unnecessary pain, expense, and worry. Plus, how can being poked and jabbed and squashed be good for breast tissue?

Then something happened that I never would have expected. I went from being happy that all of my breast tissue was normal to wondering if I could trust the thermogram completely. Maybe I felt like a fool for having put my body through all that. Maybe I was just programmed to think that my breasts weren't healthy until my mammogram said they were.

So I talked to Dr. Cometa. She agreed that because our society places such importance on the mammogram, it might be hard for some women to trust the thermogram at first, even though the technology has been around since the 1950s and more than 800 studies have been published proving its efficacy.[53] Dr. Cometa said that she recommends that these women use the thermogram in conjunction with their mammogram until they can feel completely comfortable. She is sure that once a woman sees the changes that the thermogram picks up from test to test, and how it is completely unique to her, she will be both thankful and trusting of thermography. That's certainly the way I feel.

The DCIS Dilemma

Mammograms, particularly the high-resolution scans, often pick up very early breast abnormalities that may not go on to become actual invasive cancer. These early changes are known as ductal carcinoma in situ (DCIS), or mammary dysplasia or atypia. DCIS refers to cancer cells that are still contained within the microscopic breast ducts and have not broken out or invaded the fatty or fibrous tissue of the breast and formed a lump. DCIS is considered stage 0 breast cancer, and an increasing number of doctors and specialists consider DCIS a precancer. Nevertheless, DCIS is routinely tested to see if it's positive for estrogen receptors (ER positive). And if it's indeed determined to be ER positive, women are given tamoxifen, a drug that has been shown to decrease the recurrence of ER-positive tumors.

However, this is an oversimplification. The multistep progression to breast cancer is not linear. DCIS is an example of a precancer that, in many cases, can be arrestable or even reversible—which means that thousands of women are overtreated for this condition. The Norwegian study mentioned earlier, which suggested that some breast cancers regressed naturally, speaks to this. Nevertheless, some doctors automatically assume that all such abnormalities are fast-growing and potentially lethal. Since these lesions usually occur in many areas of the breast, mastectomy is often recommended.

H. Gilbert Welch, M.D., one of the country's most prominent healthcare policy scholars and formerly a professor at the Dartmouth Institute for Health Policy and Clinical Practice, has researched the problems associated with the ability of technology to overdiagnose diseases such as breast cancer. He cites a study showing that in the breasts of women who died of other causes, 40 percent had microscopic precancerous changes in their breasts. These same types of lesions commonly show up on mammograms, and no one knows which ones will remain dormant and which ones will actually become invasive cancer.[54] In fact, it is now well documented that the majority of women diagnosed with ductal carcinoma in situ of the breast do *not* go on to develop invasive breast cancer. According to a 2015 study done in Toronto that followed 100,000 women for twenty years (the most extensive collection of DCIS data ever analyzed), women with DCIS had nearly the same chance of dying whether they had lumpectomies or mastectomies, indicating that more aggressive treatment isn't needed.[55] Fewer than 1 percent of the women in the study died of breast cancer (the numbers were higher mostly for women under age thirty-five and for African American women), and those who did died despite receiving treatment, not from the lack of it. Interestingly, their chance of dying from breast cancer (about 3.3 percent) is the same as for women in the general population, meaning having DCIS is no death sentence.

Noting this data, Dr. Esserman (the breast surgeon mentioned earlier who is heading up the WISDOM study on breast cancer screening) has called for the word *carcinoma* to be eliminated from the term used to describe this condition and that the diagnosis instead be called "indolent lesions of epithelial origin," or IDLE.[56] Noting that 20 to 25 percent of breast cancer diagnoses today are DCIS, she points out that if this condition were indeed the precursor for a more deadly form of breast cancer, we should be seeing the number of invasive breast cancers drop sharply as more DCIS is detected with screening—yet this has not happened.[57] Therefore, she believes, it's time for DCIS to be seen as a risk factor for invasive cancer, not a precursor, so we can start concentrating on helping women reduce their risk, possibly with hormonal or immunological therapies designed to make breast tissue less hospitable to cancer cells.[58] Finally, an approach that makes sense.

Research has been pointing in this direction for a while now. A 1996 article in the *Journal of the American Medical Association*[59] and a 2005 article in the *Annals of Internal Medicine*[60] both show that the incidence of DCIS has increased dramatically since 1983 due to the fact that mammography screening picks it up. A 2005 study from the Fred Hutchinson Cancer Research Center published in the April 2005 issue of *Cancer Epidemiology, Biomarkers and Prevention* found that the diagnosis of DCIS has increased sixfold since 1980, while the incidence of true invasive breast cancer has remained flat. The researchers also found a fourfold increase in a less common condition called lobular carcinoma in situ (LCIS), which is also noninvasive.[61] While early detection of invasive breast cancer is beneficial, the value of DCIS detection is currently unknown. I am very concerned about the large number of DCIS cases that are being diagnosed as a consequence of screening mammography, most of which are treated by some form of surgery. In addition, the proportion of cases treated by mastectomy is inappropriately high, particularly in some areas of the United States.

Current treatment options for DCIS and LCIS involve varying combinations of lumpectomy (although there is no lump per se), radiation, and tamoxifen, and sometimes even mastectomy. While having a mastectomy for such an early-stage cancer seems extreme, more and more women are opting for this surgery because they're scared to death. In fact, the rate of contralateral prophylactic mastectomy—removing the opposite breast as a preventive measure—more than tripled from 2002 to 2012, despite the fact that studies show removing healthy breasts doesn't improve survival. With celebrities such as actresses Sharon Osbourne and Angelina Jolie having double mastectomies preventively, before any cancer at all is found in either breast, I expect the rate of such "preemptive strikes" against cancer will continue to rise.

While it is very sad for a woman to sacrifice her breast unnecessarily, I can certainly understand why women feel driven to this alternative. It beats the constant worry that stems from the current approach to breast health, which I summarize like this: "We didn't find anything this year. But keep coming back. Eventually we will!" Without being given tools like thermography, which would allow her to make better decisions about her breast health, a woman may feel so powerless over the situation that it just feels like a relief to have her breasts removed and be done with the fear once and for all.

What treatment is recommended often depends on whom you consult. Surgeons tend to recommend surgery for DCIS. Radiation oncologists recommend radiation. Medical oncologists recommend tamoxifen or other anti-estrogen pills. Unfortunately, a 2009 study of more than a thousand women with ER-positive breast cancer (not just DCIS) shows that women who take tamoxifen after lumpectomy or mastectomy for at least five years more than quadruple their risk of developing a rare but more aggressive and more difficult-to-treat cancer (known as ER-negative breast cancer) in their healthy breast.[62] Using tamoxifen for less than five years wasn't linked to the more aggressive cancer, but women don't get the full benefit of the drug until they've taken it for five years. Here's the bottom line: While the majority of women with breast cancer will lower the risk of cancer recurring by taking tamoxifen, one-quarter of them will actually *increase* their risk of getting an even more deadly form of breast cancer—odds I'm not very comfortable with, especially when you consider the fact that this drug also raises the risk of blood clots, stroke, and uterine cancer. Though this study was in women with cancer, not DCIS, women with DCIS are routinely put on tamoxifen. Given that most DCIS isn't going to go on to become invasive cancer in the first place, is tamoxifen worth the risk?

In general, chemotherapy other than tamoxifen is recommended only when there is evidence of invasion. Women should clearly recognize that they have plenty of time to consider all their options. DCIS does not grow rapidly. Some goes away. We know that some untreated DCIS may eventually go on to become invasive cancer, but we do not know which types, when, or why. Shelley Hwang, M.D., chief of breast surgical oncology at the Duke University School of Medicine in Durham, North Carolina, noted in a recent Medscape article that the diagnosis of DCIS didn't even exist before we started doing mammographic screening and that the way it's treated now (as though it was invasive cancer) hasn't changed in forty years.[63] "Because it is a pre-invasive or precancerous lesion," she noted, "it really does not have the ability to spread to any other part of the body. If you catch it at that stage, women are almost 100 percent cured. I think we can make the argument, and many of us do, that many women are cured of a diagnosis that would not have caused them any harm during their lifetime."

Dr. Hwang believes that deescalating treatment for DCIS to active surveillance may well be as successful as a similar approach doctors started to take twenty years ago with low-risk forms of prostate cancer in men. She's part of a team working a new trial called Comparison of Operative to Monitoring and Endocrine Therapy (COMET) for low-risk DCIS, launched in 2017. COMET—the first large phase III randomized clinical trial in the United States to look at different management strategies for DCIS—is following 1,200 women with DCIS at about a hundred cancer centers across the country. Half will receive the current standard treatment, while the other half will be closely monitored with more frequent follow-up exams and tests, progressing to biopsy and surgery only if these tests show changes that require further evaluation. The trial will look not only at cancer outcome but also at quality of life.

Given the new data mentioned here showing that many early breast cancers, including DCIS, disappear without treatment, the angst, fear, and confusion women go through when diagnosed with DCIS create more havoc with their health than the actual disease. The only way out of this dilemma is to realize you have the ability to improve your breast from the inside out, regardless of whether or not you've been diagnosed with DCIS. Here's a better way: Screen with thermography, not mammography; institute lifestyle and nutritional changes; and then do regular follow-ups. (See my Program to Promote Healthy Breast Tissue, page 429.)

BREAST CANCER

Statistics show that one in eight women in the United States will get breast cancer if you distribute the risk over her entire lifetime, up until the age of ninety.[64] Let me put this into perspective. According to BreastCancer.org, at age twenty, the risk of getting breast cancer is 1 in 1,732; at forty, 1 in 69; and at sixty, 1 in 29 . . . far different from 1 in 8![65] Still, breast cancer is the leading cause of cancer death among American women who are forty to fifty-five years of age.[66] On the other hand, lung cancer is by far the leading cause of cancer death in women of all ages. Cardiovascular disease trumps them both—killing six times more women than breast cancer.[67]

When I was in medical school, I was taught that one in twenty-five women would get breast cancer. Experts argue whether the incidence of breast cancer is actually on the increase or whether we are simply diagnosing it earlier these days, with the increase in mammography and public awareness. It's also true that treatments are better than they used to be, so women are surviving longer. Regardless of statistics, however, most of us know at least one person who has had or currently has breast cancer.

For this to be the case, clearly something is out of balance. Evidence is accumulating that certain environmental pollutants contribute to estrogenic activity and may contribute to the incidence of breast problems in the industrialized world.[68] It is well documented that estrogen and estrogen-like chemicals (known as xenoestrogens) stimulate the growth of breast tissue and, in excess, may increase the risk of breast cancer. It is possible that these factors, along with suboptimal levels of vitamin D and iodine, are contributing to earlier signs of puberty in young girls. I'm also concerned about the possible effects on breast tissue of recombinant bovine somatotropin (rBST), which is given to cows to increase milk production.[69] Environmental contaminants such as PCBs, PBBs, and mercury are probably significant as well. A recent study out of the State University of New York at Fredonia revealed evidence of plastic contamination in 93 percent of water sold in plastic bottles worldwide.[70] Unfortunately, there is evidence of plastics in tap water as well.[71] It is well documented that many plastics contain hormone disruptors such as bisphenol A (BPA).

Fifty percent of white girls in the United States now show signs of breast budding before age ten, while 14 percent are showing breast development by age eight. The average age of breast budding for African American girls is just under nine years, with a significant percentage growing pubic and underarm hair before age eight.[72]

Every woman should be proactive about her breast health *now*. Why wait until further studies on environmental toxins come in or the definitive treatment for breast cancer is figured out when you can start, through your thoughts, emotions, and daily choices, to create breast health now—even if you've already got cancer?

The breast is an estrogen-sensitive organ. Many women who have been on birth control pills or estrogen replacement have found that the medication resulted in enlarged and often tender breasts. The effect of these medications, plus the inflammation-causing standard American high-glycemic-index, low-fiber diet, which overstimulates breast tissue, is a setup for breast cancer.

A DIFFERENT TAKE ON ALL THOSE PINK RIBBONS

Every October, during Breast Cancer Awareness Month, a tidal wave of pink hits us. While a campaign in support of preventing breast cancer may seem like a very good thing, there's another side well worth acknowledging. In 2002, Breast Cancer Action, a national grassroots organization founded in 1990 by a group of women who themselves had breast cancer (see www.bcaction.org), started its own campaign called Think Before You Pink to hold corporations selling products that contain chemicals linked to breast cancer accountable for their pink ribbon promotions. BCA's executive director, Karuna Jaggar, notes in a blog post on the campaign's website (www.thinkbeforeyoupink.org), "Few people realize that Breast Cancer Awareness Month (BCAM) was launched by AstraZeneca, a pharmaceutical company that sells cancer treatments on the one hand and carcinogenic pesticides on the other. So BCAM has all along been one big marketing campaign—arguably the most successful marketing campaign of the 20th century. This is why at Breast Cancer Action, we call October 'Breast Cancer Industry Month,' the month when corporations make money professing how much they care about breast cancer by selling pink ribbon products." They point out that the pink ribbon BCAM campaign (and much of the money it generates) is tightly focused on so-called awareness, including getting mammograms, instead of on more helpful and empowering endeavors, such as educating women on how to assess their individual risk, funding research on environmental toxins that can cause breast cancer, and publicizing the many steps women can take to prevent breast cancer. BCA is the only national breast cancer organization that doesn't accept funding from any entities that profit from or contribute to cancer (including the pharmaceutical industry).

Carla Savetsky, a former ob-gyn physician's assistant who founded the holistic healing service Natural Healing for Women (www.naturalhealingforwomen.com), is a BCA proponent. "The pink ribbon extravaganza has nothing to do with empowering or educating women. Rather, it has everything to do with selling a product and promoting fear," she notes in her own blog post on the subject,[73] adding that "the underlying message is that there are no answers to the epidemic of breast cancer, so your *only* hope is to get your yearly mammogram. . . . To me, the pink ribbon is the symbol of this mass unconsciousness, this bait and switch of the *real* issues with the distraction of races and pretty pink ribbons."

The Breast Cancer–Diet–Hormone Link

Breast cancer has often been blamed on high levels of certain types of dietary fat and low levels of some nutrients, such as iodine, vitamin D, and selenium. As far back as 1973, a study at the National Cancer Institute showed that countries with the highest intake of animal fat had the highest mortality rates from breast cancer.[74] But it's not that simple. In 1996 an analysis of 337,000 women in seven prospective studies suggested that there is no association between women's intake of dietary fat and their risk for developing subsequent breast cancer. The researchers found no difference in breast cancer rates between those whose intake of dietary fat ranged from more than 45 percent of their calories to less than 20 percent. It didn't seem to matter whether the fats were from saturated, monounsaturated, or poly-unsaturated sources.[75] More recently, an Italian study showed a decreased risk of breast cancer with increased fat intake but an increased risk of breast cancer when the intake of available carbohydrates in the form of starch (bread, pasta, etc.) was increased.[76]

It didn't surprise me at all to read that a study following data from more than 334,800 European women over eleven and a half years found that those who consumed a diet high in sugars and carbohydrates increased their risk of developing ER-negative breast cancer (the deadliest kind) by up to 41 per-cent.[77] Conversely, a later study following more than 62,000 postmenopausal women in the Netherlands for over twenty years found that eating a Mediter-ranean diet based on fish, fruit, nuts, whole grains, and olive oil (and which traditionally avoids processed foods) reduced the chance of contracting the same form of breast cancer by about the same amount.[78]

Scientific data has long indicated that there's a link between sugar, insu-lin, and breast cancer.[79] Levels of insulin (which regulates blood glucose) tend to be higher in those who eat a diet high in sugar and refined grains—whether or not those individuals are overweight. A 2009 study showed that women with unhealthy insulin levels had a two- to threefold-higher risk for breast cancer.[80]

Although the specifics of this relationship are still being studied, scien-tists do know that insulin is an important growth factor for all body tissues, so it makes sense that it might help breast cancer cells grow and proliferate. A 2015 study of 125 women with metastatic breast cancer found that those who were insulin-resistant (and so had higher levels of insulin) were more likely to have their cancer grow.[81] We now know that estrogen, insulin, and inflammation pathways are associated with early-stage breast cancer, and that having higher insulin levels predicts breast cancer risk even more than being overweight does.[82] All this is why metabolic expert Jason Fung, M.D., believes cancer is, at heart, a metabolic disease. Dr. Fung promotes a regimen of intermittent fasting as well as eating less white flour, sugar, and processed foods, which can help normalize insulin levels. (More about this in the nutrition chapter.)

Breast cancer, like nearly all cancers, is associated with cellular inflammation, which is the final common pathway resulting from a nutrient-poor diet, too much sugar and/or alcohol, or emotional stress. Excessive estrogen (relative to progesterone) over the life cycle that is related to diet and obesity also contributes to cellular inflammation and an increased risk of breast cancer, at least in some individuals.[83] Emotional stress; a nutrient-poor diet full of refined carbohydrates and low in vitamin D, iodine, magnesium, and omega-3 fats; environmental toxins—any and all of these can increase cellular inflammation. And inflammation precedes cancer. (By the way, a 2009 study indicated that chronic cellular inflammation in women who had been diagnosed with breast cancer may also increase the chances of the cancer recurring. Researchers found that elevated levels of C-reactive protein [CRP], a marker for cellular inflammation, measured as long as seven years after the subjects were successfully treated for early-stage breast cancer, were associated with reduced survival rates.)[84]

The latest research shows that a healthier diet can increase your chances of survival after being diagnosed with breast cancer. That's the conclusion researchers came to after performing a secondary analysis of data from more than 161,000 postmenopausal women who were part of the Women's Health Initiative (WHI) observational study conducted in the 1990s.[85] In the new analysis, published in 2018, the researchers set out to compare data from women who didn't change their diets to those who reduced their intake of dietary fat by 20 percent after being diagnosed with breast cancer—although it's worth noting that this change in diet also included eating significantly more fruits and vegetables, which has been proven to reduce risk of breast cancer in general.[86] A decade later, 82 percent of the women who made dietary changes were still alive, compared to 78 percent of the control group.

Some truly exciting mind-body research is adding considerably to this discussion—it appears that not only do activities such as meditation and participating in support groups help cancer survivors emotionally, but these activities have finally been shown to affect their biology. Canadian researchers found that support groups that encouraged cancer patients to meditate, do yoga, and share their feelings instead of suppressing them improved their chance of survival.[87] The focus of the study was the length of telomeres, protein caps on the end of chromosomes that determine how fast a cell ages. While the role telomeres play in our health is not yet completely understood, shorter telomeres are associated with cellular aging and disease, while longer telomeres are thought to be protective.[88] In the study, the researchers followed eighty-eight breast cancer survivors who were experiencing significant levels of emotional distress (thought to shorten telomeres). Those in a mindfulness-based cancer recovery group attended eight weekly ninety-minute group sessions that included instruction in mindfulness meditation and gentle hatha yoga, with the goal of cultivating nonjudgmental awareness of the present moment. These women were also asked to meditate and practice yoga at home for forty-five minutes a day. A second group attended twelve weekly ninety-minute sessions where they were encouraged to talk openly about their concerns and their emotions, with the goal of building mutual support and guiding women in expressing rather than suppressing or repressing their emotions. Those in a third group—the control group—attended a single six-hour stress management seminar. After only three months, the telomere length of those in the two support groups stayed the same, while the telomere length shortened for women in the control group that received no mind-body support.

PROGRAM TO PROMOTE HEALTHY BREAST TISSUE

This program is designed to eliminate breast pain and decrease your risk of breast cancer. Choose from the options in this section on the basis of what appeals to you and what you can easily do without stressing yourself out unduly. You don't have to do everything I've listed here all at once, unless it feels right to you.

First, Consult Your Healthcare Provider. This is to make certain that your breasts are healthy. It is ideal to have a healthcare provider who can also offer you the emotional support you need for dealing with breast pain, a breast lump, or both.

Minimize Estrogen and Inflammation. Follow a low-sugar diet that minimizes excess estrogen and also decreases cellular inflammation in your system (see chapter 17, on nutrition). Breast tissue is exquisitely sensitive to high-refined-carbohydrate (high-sugar) diets, which raise estrogen, insulin, and blood sugar levels, resulting in cellular inflammation. Excessive estrogen production stimulates breast tissue, resulting in breast pain and cyst formation in many women.[89] Many cancerous breast tumors are stimulated by hormones such as estrogen. Tamoxifen, a drug used to treat breast cancer, works by lowering estrogen's effect on breast tissue. The higher the percentage of body fat (because body fat manufactures estrogen) and the higher the insulin levels from too many refined carbohydrates, the higher the estrogen levels and the greater the risk for breast and other gynecological cancer.[90]

Plenty of soluble fiber in your diet from vegetable sources helps increase the excretion of excess estrogen.[91] Lentils and beans are good sources. You can also supplement with psyllium or slippery elm. The cruciferous vegetables (cabbage, broccoli, kale, Brussels sprouts, turnips, and collard greens) all contain the plant chemical indole-3-carbinol, which has been shown to decrease estrogen's ability to bind to breast tissue, thus making the body's own estrogen less apt to promote cancer.[92] This substance is also available as a supplement. About 80 percent of women with cyclic breast pain get relief from dietary change alone because a whole-food, inflammation-reducing diet changes hormonal levels and has been shown to significantly reduce the severity of breast tenderness and swelling.[93]

Get Enough Phytoestrogens in Your Diet. Asian women who consume a traditional diet—including the soy-based products tempeh, tofu, miso, and natto—excrete estrogen at a much higher rate than those who don't. They also have a much lower risk of breast cancer. These soy products, rich in what are known as phytoestrogens, which are plant substances that have biochemical properties similar to weak estrogens, appear to be protective against breast cancer, in part because their weak estrogenic activity tends to block estrogen receptors on the cells from receiving excessive estrogen stimulation from other sources.[94] A Singaporean study showed that diets high in soy products conferred a low risk of breast cancer in premenopausal women.[95] Soy even helps women who have already been diagnosed with breast cancer. The Shanghai Breast Cancer Survival Study, following more than 5,000 female breast cancer survivors in China, showed that the more dietary soy the women ate—either soy protein or soy isoflavones—the lower their risk of death and recurrence of breast cancer.[96] (This was true whether the cancer was estrogen-receptor-positive or estrogen-receptor-negative, and whether or not the women took tamoxifen.) Studies also show that soy exerts a protective effect on breast tissue.[97] And laboratory studies have shown that phytoestrogens inhibit the growth of human breast cancer cells.[98]

Get Enough Lignans. Another study found that vegetarians and women in areas with low breast cancer risk have high urinary lignan levels, whereas those women in areas of high risk have low levels.[99] (Lignans are building blocks for plant cell walls that, when eaten, break down into enterolactones and enterodiol, which have potent anticancer and estrogen-balancing effects.) Flaxseed has one of the highest lignan concentrations of any food. It can be eaten as ground-up seeds (I recommend one-quarter cup three to seven days per week, mixed with soup, yogurt, or other foods) or in capsule form as Brevail, a natural plant extract available at health food stores.

A NOTE ABOUT PHYTOESTROGENS, ISOFLAVONES, AND CANCER RISK

There has been a great deal of misinformation recently about the possibility that phytoestrogens (estrogens from plants) and isoflavones in foods such as soy, flax, and almonds may increase the risk of breast cancer. In fact, many women have been told to avoid these substances. But research has repeatedly shown just the opposite. For example, a study of 502 postmenopausal women who'd had breast cancer and were taking phytoestrogens revealed that phytoestrogen users had lower levels of serum estrogens than those not taking these substances.[100] This is precisely the opposite of what we've been led to believe.

In 2009, an international group of nearly twenty researchers from around the world convened in Milan, Italy, for a meeting on isoflavones and their implication in cancer, sponsored by the Council for Responsible Nutrition. Overall, the information presented in this conference strongly supported the idea that isoflavones are indeed safe both for women with breast cancer and for those who are at high risk for developing breast cancer. This is what Mark Messina, Ph.D., a well-respected soy isoflavone researcher, said at the conclusion of the conference:

> According to the science presented at this meeting, isoflavones do not have an effect on breast cell proliferation or breast tissue density, which are two well-established biomarkers of breast cancer risk. In fact, epidemiologic data presented at the meeting showed that exposure to isoflavone-rich soy foods may improve the prognosis of breast cancer patients. Further, new findings strongly indicated that certain results from some animal studies that have raised concern about the impact of isoflavones on breast cancer are not applicable to humans.[101]

Dozens of research studies on soy isoflavones have demonstrated the same thing: that increasing soy intake decreases risk of breast cancer mortality as well as recurrence, with higher intake related to higher levels of protection. A Japanese study, for example, showed frequent consumption of miso soup and isoflavones reduced risk,[102] while a Chinese study was the first to show that isoflavones from chickpea sprouts may be protective.[103] A 2015 meta-analysis of five studies following women for four to seven years after diagnosis found high soy intake was associated with a 21 percent decrease in recurrence and a 15 percent reduction in mortality.[104] Most recently, a 2018 meta-analysis of a dozen studies showed that women with breast cancer who consumed soy isoflavones reduced their risk of recurrence.[105]

Isoflavones are synonymous with phytoestrogens. The three-dimensional structure of these plant estrogens is what determines how the body uses them. In communicating about this with Margaret Ritchie, Ph.D., a world-renowned expert in phytoestrogens and associated breast cancer research at the University of St. Andrews in Scotland, I received the following explanation from her:

> Interestingly, phyto-oestrogens cannot act in the same way as oestradiol [these are the British spellings of *phytoestrogens* and *estradiol;* estradiol is the most biologically active of all the estrogens] as oestradiol is a three-dimensional molecule, whereas phyto-oestrogens tend to be planar. The geometry in space due to the chemical structure is very different. Another difference is that oestradiol contains a 6-angstrom biophore, found in many carcinogens. Phyto-oestrogens contain a biophore, but it is *not* 6 angstroms and is therefore not able to act as a carcinogen.
>
> In both cases an understanding of the chemistry or shape of the molecules demonstrates the huge differences and hence different actions of phyto-oestrogens compared to natural oestrogens.
>
> Some studies that show a cancer-promoting effect of phyto-oestrogens in rodents have been carried out by Leena Hilakivi-Clarke, Ph.D. The animals were fed neat genistein and exposed to cancer-promoting chemicals. Since no person can eat only one phyto-oestrogen and rodents produce huge amounts of equol [a type of estrogen], these studies are of limited value. Additional studies carried out by the same researchers showed when animals were fed soy with many other phytochemicals present, there was a reduction in tumour size and number.[106]

Eliminate Conventionally Produced Dairy Foods. Stop eating all conventionally produced dairy foods for at least one month as a trial run. Over the years I've seen this relieve the breast pain of many women. If it hasn't helped after one month, then you can add dairy foods again. Though I know of no studies that document this specifically, I have found that conventionally produced dairy foods (pasteurized, produced in factory farms, and from cows who have been given rBST) are associated with breast tenderness and lumps in some women. I believe that the reason for this is that when cows are fed large amounts of antibiotics, genetically modified grains, and hormones to increase their milk supply, these pass into their milk and when consumed by humans can potentially affect human breast tissue. Women who use organically produced dairy foods—especially raw milk dairy—seem to avoid these problems.

Eliminate Caffeine. Stop all caffeinated beverages, colas, and chocolate—even decaf coffee and decaf Pepsi or Coke. The methylxanthines (caffeine and theobromine) in cola, root beer, coffee, and chocolate can cause overstimulation of breast tissue in some women, though not all. Scientific studies show conflicting evidence about this issue, but I've seen women who were so sensitive to these substances that eating one piece of chocolate a month resulted in breast pain. So, as with dairy food, a trial run of elimination (usually for one full menstrual cycle) is worth it.

Decrease Alcohol Consumption. Alcohol consumption is associated with breast cancer risk.[107] The risk increases with the amount of alcohol consumed. In the Nurses' Health Study, for example, researchers found that the risk of breast cancer in women who had one or more drinks per day was 60 percent higher than in women who didn't drink.[108] This link is felt to be due to the fact that alcohol consumption increases hormone levels in the blood. (By the way, a 2009 study found that breast cancer survivors who consumed an average of one drink per week had a 90 percent increased risk of a new cancer developing in their other breast.)[109] In women age fifty and over, the type of alcohol associated with the highest risk was beer.[110] Since many women drink to medicate feelings, unexpressed emotions may enhance the alcohol–breast cancer link.

Take Dietary Supplements. Many different studies have documented the benefit of various nutritional supplements for breast health. While most of the studies done on the various supplements that help breast pain studied a particular supplement individually, all these factors work together. For that reason, it's best to take any supplement along with or as part of a balanced multivitamin formula. Here are some of the more important supplements for breast health:

~ *Omega-3 fats.* There's an ever-increasing body of literature on the anti-inflammatory properties of omega-3 fats, such as those found in hemp oil, macadamia nuts, walnut oil, flaxseed oil, and cold-water fish or fish oil. These oils help with breast pain for the same reason that they help decrease dysmenorrhea. They help decrease inflammation, which stops breast pain. (See the section on dysmenorrhea, page 140, and chapter 17.) There is evidence suggesting that fish oil may also be protective against breast cancer. One recent study of women with breast cancer showed that the composition of breast tissue was altered in a positive direction following the addition of fish oil supplement for three months.[111] I recommend eating plenty of omega-3 fats from foods in addition to taking fish oil supplements (1,000–5,000 mg/day) for optimal breast health.

~ *Antioxidants.* Studies have shown that many women with breast pain are helped by the antioxidant vitamins E and A and the mineral selenium. Research shows that vitamin E actually decreased serum pituitary hormone levels (LH and FSH) in women treated with it for breast pain.[112] (If vitamin E isn't part of your multivitamin-mineral complex, you can add it to your regimen as a separate supplement in the form of d-alpha-tocopherol, 400 to 600 IU per day.) Antioxidants also help reduce the chance of breast cancer, as well as optimize treatment. In one study of women with breast cancer, low serum retinol (a vitamin A by-product) was associated with a decreased response to chemotherapy, while those with higher amounts of vitamin A had a better response.[113] Selenium may help reduce breast cancer risk, too, as suggested by the fact that selenium levels are lower in women with breast cancer.[114] In fact, a double-blind, randomized cancer prevention trial that supplemented selenium at levels of 200 mcg per day for more than six years showed a 50 percent reduction in total cancer mortality.[115] Selenium is a trace mineral that is often lacking in refined-food diets.

~ *Bioflavonoids.* The use of bioflavonoids (found in vitamin C complex) may inhibit estrogen synthesis.[116]

~ *Vitamin D.* Take at least 2,000–5,000 IU of vitamin D_3 per day. (See box on page 435.)

~ *Lactobacillus acidophilus.* Hyperestrogenism and possibly the risk of breast cancer itself may be decreased by including this beneficial bacterium in the diet. *Lactobacillus acidophilus,* the bacterium in yogurt, helps metabolize estrogen properly in the bowel.[117] Most commercially available yogurt does not contain enough of the live bacteria to make a difference, but organic brands do. You can also get lactobacillus in capsules sold in health food stores. Healthcare practitioners can usually suggest a reliable brand; I recommend PB 8, which doesn't require refrigeration.

~ *Coenzyme Q_{10}.* Studies have found that about 20 percent of breast cancer patients have levels of coenzyme Q_{10} that are below the normal range. Coenzyme Q_{10} (also known as ubiquinone) is a natural substance necessary for the production of ATP—the main molecule that powers our cells. It has also been shown to enhance immune functioning. In one recent study from Denmark, thirty-two breast cancer patients were given up to 390 mg per day of CoQ_{10}, together with antioxidants and essential fatty acids. Seven showed partial or complete regression of their tumors.[118] Although these results are preliminary, I recommend CoQ_{10} as part of a supplement program for every woman who has concerns about breast cancer. The usual dose is 30 mg to 90 mg per day. For those women with already diagnosed breast cancer, 300 mg per day is definitely worth a try. Several of my colleagues who treat breast cancer have reported results similar to those found in the Danish study. CoQ_{10} is available in health food stores. Note: Statin drugs greatly reduce CoQ_{10} in the body. Women on these drugs should take supplemental CoQ_{10}.

PROTECT YOUR BREASTS WITH VITAMIN D

There's a paradigm shift going on in medicine as new research reveals a far greater role for vitamin D than merely saving children from rickets. Optimal levels of vitamin D enhance the creation and functioning of healthy cells throughout the body.[119] In addition to protecting the bones and boosting the immune system, studies show that vitamin D helps prevent certain cancers, including breast, ovarian, prostate, renal, pancreatic, colon, and colorectal.[120] Research shows that in the United States alone, if women kept their blood levels of vitamin D at 40–60 ng/ml year-round, it would prevent 58,000 new cases of breast cancer (and 49,000 new cases of colorectal cancer) each year.[121]

Studies by Cedric Garland, Dr.P.H., of the University of California, San Diego, School of Medicine, and other prominent vitamin D researchers show that having vitamin D levels above 52 ng/ml (which you can achieve by taking 5,000 IU of vitamin D_3 per day, plus getting moderate sun exposure when possible) can boost blood levels high enough to cut breast cancer risk in half.[122] A study published in 2018 showed a 78 to 82 percent lower risk of breast cancer for women with vitamin D levels of 60 ng/ml or higher compared to women with less than 20 ng/ml.[123] Getting these levels generally requires an intake of 5,000 IU per day. In addition, an increasing number of studies now link breast cancer survival with this important vitamin. According to a Canadian study presented at the 2008 annual meeting of the American Society of Clinical Oncology, breast cancer patients with very low levels of vitamin D were more likely to have aggressive tumors and were 73 percent more likely to die.[124] In a 2009 study, breast cancer patients with low levels of vitamin D had almost double the risk of their cancer spreading. They were also 1.7 times as likely to die.[125]

A simple blood test is all that's needed to find out your vitamin D level. (See the diagnostic laboratories section in Resources for how to get this done without a prescription.) For quite some time, a range of 20–100 ng/ml was considered normal, but this range has more recently been raised to 32–100 ng/ml. Make sure to ask your healthcare provider what your actual vitamin D level is. Too often women are told that their levels are normal, which is *not* the same as optimal. Optimal serum levels are 40–100 ng/ml, although expert opinion varies somewhat about the higher end of this range. To boost your vitamin D levels into the optimal range, I recommend moderate, safe sunlight exposure (about ten to twenty minutes or so per day—more if your skin is dark) without sunscreen on a regular basis as well as taking supplemental vitamin D. Initially, you may need to take 5,000 IU per day. After you've established a healthful level, I recommend supplementing with at least 2,000 IU per day, because it's hard to get all you need from food. (Some healthful fish, for example, provide 300–700 IU, but milk only provides 100 IU per glass.) According to Dr. Garland's research, for maximum benefit, girls should get enough vitamin D during the entire phase of breast development—which starts at breast budding and continues until the age of twenty-eight. One of my colleagues recently told me that in an in-house study at his company, almost everyone required a full 5,000 IU per day to maintain optimal vitamin D levels without daily sunbathing.

You may be surprised to learn that the sun is actually the best source of vitamin D. The sun's UVB rays enable our bodies to manufacture vitamin D in the fat layer under the skin, as long as we don't use sunscreen. The body can make up to 10,000 IU of vitamin D in thirty minutes of total body exposure, depending on skin pigmentation level. And it will never create toxic levels. Although we are taught to fear the sun, sunbathing in moderation—exposing but never burning the skin—is good for us. Your breasts and your entire body will benefit. This is preventive medicine at its finest. And it may explain why the incidence of breast cancer is higher in northern latitudes than at the equator. (By the way, in the winter, you can even visit a tanning salon that offers UVB tanning rays, to ensure your body is manufacturing enough vitamin D. Just keep your exposure to ten minutes or less.) For more information, go to www.grassrootshealth.net.

Increase Your Intake of Iodine. Every cell in your body needs iodine. As with vitamin D, many women have suboptimal intake of iodine. The average Japanese intake of iodine is about 45 mg/day, mostly from seaweed consumption—and the Japanese have the lowest rate of breast cancer in the world. In the United States, however, average iodine intake is only 240 *micrograms,* which is far too low for optimal health. Iodine intake has fallen over the past fifty years as people have decreased their intake of iodized salt and also because the dough conditioners used in commercial bread making now contain bromate instead of iodate. Furthermore, the dairy industry no longer uses iodine to clean cows' udders. In addition, water fluoridation, fluoride in toothpaste, and the use of chlorine in municipal water systems all interfere with iodine metabolism. That is because bromide, fluoride, and iodine have similar chemical properties (they are all in the category of halogens in the periodic table of elements). But in environments in which iodine is already in short supply, these other halogens actually replace iodine in tissue, with many ill effects. The public health implications of iodine and health are enormous and beyond the scope of this book. For further reading, I recommend the book *Iodine: Why You Need It, Why You Can't Live Without It,* 5th ed. (Medical Alternative Press, 2014) by David Brownstein, M.D.

Please note, however, that if you have Hashimoto's thyroiditis, you may need far less iodine than Dr. Brownstein recommends in his book because iodine can exacerbate Hashimoto's and accelerate thyroid cell destruction. Thyroid expert Izabella Wentz, Pharm.D., feels that for Hashimoto's patients, the risks of high-dose iodine (above 200 mcg/day from food and supplements combined, unless you are breast-feeding or pregnant) outweigh the benefits, although she adds that a low dose of iodine on a daily basis may actually be beneficial.[126] Dr. Wentz adds that Hashimoto's patients who are exposed to high doses of iodine may find it helpful to take a selenium supplement (up to 600 mcg per day) to counter the negative effects of the iodine. Taking selenium without iodine can cause iodine deficiency, and taking iodine without selenium can cause selenium deficiency.

Breast tissue requires iodine to function optimally, just as do the thyroid and the ovaries. In fact, there may be an association between thyroid disease and breast cancer—perhaps because both of these conditions are associated with inadequate iodine intake.[127] Research shows that those who take iodine in doses ranging from 6 mg to 90 mg per day feel healthier and have a greater sense of well-being. That is because iodine acts as an antioxidant (as powerful in that regard as vitamin C, in fact) and also as an immune system booster, protecting cells from environmental and chemical toxins. Low levels of iodine can increase the amount of circulating estrogens in breast tissue, making the breasts a target for toxic estrogens.[128] Taking iodine at these doses eliminates breast pain from fibrocystic changes about 70 percent of the time.[129] In one study of women with breast pain, more than half of those who took

6 mg of iodine daily reported a significant reduction in overall breast pain.[130] Another study of women with fibrocystic disease showed that 3–6 mg of iodine per day led to subjective and objective improvement in 65 percent of the study group.[131] The iodine decreases the ability of estrogen to adhere to estrogen receptors in the breast.[132]

There is fairly compelling evidence that iodine deficiency is a cause of breast cancer. The ductal cells of the breasts, those most likely to become cancerous, actually have an iodine pump in them, indicating that they have the ability to actively absorb iodine. Iodine helps keep the immune system healthy, and it provides antiseptic mucosal defense in the mouth, stomach, and vagina. After all, it is hands down one of the most powerful antiviral and antibacterial substances known to humankind. (It's even been used orally to cure malaria.) Most doctors don't know about all the uses for this vital supplement.

For years I have prescribed iodine supplements for women with breast pain and seen excellent results, usually within only two weeks. In these cases, I recommend dosages in the range of 4–12.5 mg/day, which you can get from kelp supplements, sea vegetables, or Lugol's solution (which is made up of iodine and potassium iodide). A good maintenance dose for breast health is 1–3 mg/day. There are other iodine supplements available as well, including one called Nascent Iodine drops. Nascent Iodine is based on the work of the psychic Edgar Cayce, who channeled a way to make the iodine work better. The advantage to this one is that it's very easy to titrate your dose. To accurately gauge your iodine levels before you begin supplementation, I recommend a twenty-four-hour urinary iodine loading test, such as the one from Hakala Research Laboratory that's available at LifeSpa, the website of John Douillard, D.C. (see www.lifespa.com).

Another way to get iodine safely into your body is to apply tincture of iodine to your skin. You can paint a quarter-size dot right over the painful spot on the breast or on the nipple once a night for two weeks. Very often this will decrease any pain. There have also been anecdotal clinical reports of high doses of iodine resulting in the disappearance of breast tumors.

THE IODINE PATCH TEST

An estimated 80 to 90 percent of the population has suboptimal levels of iodine. A quick and easy way to determine your iodine status is the following: Paint a 3-by-3-inch patch of tincture of iodine on your inner thigh, inner arm, or abdomen. Use the orange kind, not the clear kind. If your body is replete with iodine, you will still see the iodine patch in twenty-four hours. (Try to keep the area dry, but if you do bathe or shower, it's not likely to affect the results.) If you need more, you will find that the patch will fade much more quickly—sometimes within an hour or two. Of course, there are several factors other than iodine deficiency that might contribute to the inaccuracy of this test. But overall, it's a good place to start. An iodine loading test, which must be ordered by a physician, will be more accurate, but this patch test is certainly worth a try.

Sometimes, albeit rarely, a person will get a reaction (usually in the form of a skin rash or bad taste in the mouth) to adding iodine to her diet. The reaction is known as iodism, and it is a result of the iodine releasing excess bromide, fluoride, and other toxins from the system. It's actually a detox reaction and not an iodine reaction per se. Just decrease your dose of iodine and go more slowly.

If you are on thyroid medication, taking higher amounts of iodine will often decrease your need for thyroid medication. But if you don't know this, you can end up with heart palpitations from the effect of too much thyroid hormone. So add iodine to your diet very, very slowly, and discuss this with your healthcare provider. (But please note that most conventional healthcare providers are not up to speed on the benefits of iodine. So please be prepared for this.)

Consider Progesterone. Make sure you have enough progesterone in your system. Because breast pain is often related to estrogen overstimulation, it can be alleviated by increasing your levels of progesterone. Progesterone downregulates estrogen receptors in your breast after you've been on it about a week or so, which means that your breasts will be protected from the effects of too much estrogen. In fact, studies have shown that when a 2 percent progesterone cream is applied directly to the breasts, it decreases the cellular proliferation of breast tissue, whereas applying estradiol (a form of estrogen) to the breast increases cellular proliferation. Uncontrolled proliferation of breast tissue is associated with an increased risk for breast cancer.[133]

Several studies have strongly suggested that premenopausal women who have breast surgery for suspected or already diagnosed breast cancer during the luteal phase of their menstrual cycle (after ovulation and before the onset of menses) have a better prognosis than those who have surgery during another stage of their cycle. In a study of 289 premenopausal women with operable breast cancer who were followed from 1975 to 1992, women with node-positive breast cancer who had serum progesterone levels greater than 4 ng/ml at the time of surgery had a survival rate that was 70 percent higher than those with lower progesterone levels at the time of the surgery. This may be because progesterone decreases blood-clotting effects and also increases the natural killer cells in the immune system. It also decreases breast cell proliferation. Given these three factors, it is possible that progesterone works by decreasing the chances of tumor cells seeding themselves in remote places when breast surgery is done for cancer.[134] I would recommend that any premenopausal woman facing breast cancer surgery make sure that her progesterone levels are optimal before proceeding. This can be done by using 2 percent progesterone cream at the dose recommended on page 156. There is also a substantial body of evidence that women who have adequate progesterone levels during their menstrual and perimenopausal years may be at decreased risk for breast cancer development. (Note: I'm talking about physiologic levels of progesterone, not megadoses. Theoretically, the body can convert high levels of progesterone into estrogen. It's a question of balance.)

Apply one-quarter teaspoon (about 20 mg) once or twice a day for up to three weeks before menstruation. Give progesterone about one month to work; 2 percent progesterone cream may increase breast tenderness initially because it increases estrogen receptors initially, but then they decrease.

Don't Overdose with Estrogen. If your breast pain began when you started taking estrogen replacement therapy (or birth control pills), chances are your dose is too high. Have your dose adjusted accordingly. You can also add progesterone as above. (See chapter 14.)

Apply Castor Oil Packs. Castor oil packs applied to the breasts three times per week for one hour over two or three months often eliminate breast pain, particularly if there is inflammation of breast tissue. A maintenance program of once per week thereafter is recommended.

Change Bras. Stop wearing an underwire bra (or wear it less often). Too often this kind of bra cuts off the circulation of both blood and lymph fluid around the breast, chest wall, and surrounding tissue. Tight bras can also cause chest pain.

Learn About Your Breasts. Understand your breasts' anatomy and keep a calendar, noticing how your breasts change with your menstrual cycle, so that occasional cyclic breast pain doesn't scare you. Talk to your breasts. Ask them, "What are you trying to tell me?" And watch what you say: "My breasts are killing me" is not a useful slogan. Do the breast massage ritual on page 399.

Avoid Certain Drugs. Don't take any of the following drugs for treatment of breast pain unless you feel you have no other choice. All of these have very significant side effects.

- *Danazol (Danocrine).* This drug causes a decrease in levels of estrogen and is also used for the treatment of endometriosis. It often has the following side effects: changes in menstrual cycle regularity, weight gain, acne, flushing, breast reduction, hirsutism, voice change, and depression.

~ *Bromocriptine.* Bromocriptine is also used to suppress lactation after childbirth. It can cause nausea, vomiting, low blood pressure, dizziness, and depression.

~ *Birth control pills.* These are all made from synthetic hormones, with no bioidentical contraceptive available. There are far better options for the treatment of breast pain.

All drugs have the potential to cause side effects, depending on the individual. Some statin drugs (cholesterol-lowering medications), SSRIs (antidepressants), and cardiac pills can cause breast pain, so women should look at what new drugs they have been taking.

Exercise Regularly. It is well documented that women with a lean body mass index (less than 22.8) who exercise regularly have a breast cancer risk that is reduced by a whopping 72 percent.[135] Research from Norway found that women who exercise regularly (four hours per week) had a 37 percent reduction in risk for breast cancer compared with sedentary women.[136] Data from the Nurses' Health Study (covering more than 85,000 women) showed that those who did daily moderate to vigorous exercise were 20 percent less likely to get breast cancer than those who exercised less than one hour a week.[137] This is true even for women who were not regular exercisers in the past.[138] The most likely reason for the reduced risk is that regular exercise is associated with lower levels of body fat and less total circulating estrogen. (Body fat itself manufactures estrone, a type of estrogen, through the conversion of cholesterol to androsterone.) There's no drug that even comes close to the benefits of regular physical activity.

Get Plenty of Sleep. Some of the newest research shows that getting adequate sleep (in a dark room) is more important to breast health than most of us realize. A 2005 Finnish study of more than 12,000 women found that those who consistently sleep nine hours or more a night have less than one-third the risk of breast tumors compared with those who get seven or eight hours of sleep nightly.[139] Several other recent studies have shown that exposure to bright light late at night may increase the risk of breast cancer (and indeed, female night-shift workers have about a 50 percent greater risk of developing breast cancer than other working women).[140] Researchers discovered that bright nighttime light interrupts the production of the hormone melatonin. Inadequate melatonin levels can promote breast tumor growth.[141] Women with above-average melatonin concentrations are less likely to develop breast cancer.[142]

Learn to Pay Attention to Your Dreams. Holistic radiologist and certified energy healthcare practitioner Larry Burk, M.D., conducted a research project culminating in a peer-reviewed study about breast cancer warning dreams.[143] He recruited eighteen women from around the world (including

England, Austria, Colombia, and the United States) who reported having such experiences. Common characteristics of warning dreams the subjects reported included dreams that were more vivid, real-feeling, or intense than usual; a sense of conviction about the importance of the dream; and a feeling of threat, menace, or dread during the dream. Many of the women heard the specific words *breast cancer* or *tumor* during the dream and had a sense of physical contact with their breast. "In more than half of the cases," Dr. Burk reports, "the dreams prompted medical attention, were shared with consulting doctors, provided the location of the tumors, and led directly to diagnosis." Burk, the author (along with Kathleen O'Keefe-Kanavos) of *Dreams That Can Save Your Life: Early Warning Signs of Cancer and Other Diseases* (Findhorn, 2018), suggests keeping a dream diary as part of a breast self-care program, particularly for women in a high-risk category. Of course, this is good advice not only for breast health but also for overall physical and mental health.

Accept Support and Nurture Yourself. Be open to accepting support from others in your life. Breast symptoms are often the body's way of getting us to nurture ourselves more fully and allow others to help. Remember, all human beings deserve and need social support. There's nothing to be gained by suffering in silence! Have compassion for yourself. And learn how to say no to what you don't want.

I can't think of a better way to illustrate this last point than by sharing an inspiring story from my friend Barbara, who was, I'm certain, headed for cancer. She was able to completely turn her situation around, and she did it relatively quickly. Here's her story:

> While on a trip with my husband to celebrate my fiftieth birthday I received a phone call from the clinic where I had recently gone for my comprehensive annual exam, including my first thermogram. The report from my breast thermography was back—and it wasn't good. At first I was shocked. I am physically very active, have good eating habits, and lead a healthful lifestyle. I have no family history of breast cancer—and I have had annual screening mammograms since I was thirty-four. But as I reflected honestly, I knew deep within myself that these abnormal cells were just a warning. Despite the healthy exercise and eating, I had spent the past decade in an unhealthy pattern of overworking, over-caretaking, overgiving, and feeling resentful and angry. In the past year I had made major strides in self-care and releasing resentment. In fact, it was ironic that I found out the news while on a birthday trip with my husband! That trip was the first time we had done something alone for ten years.
>
> My doctor suggested that I immediately get a digital mammogram and an MRI to get more information about the nature of the situation,

but I still had five more days of the trip. So I decided to completely immerse myself in pleasure as a way to jump-start my healing process. I knew instinctively that the more appreciation and pleasure I could feel, the more healing my body would be able to do. I let my husband know what my intentions were so that he could be my partner in healing. As he and I hiked in the Rocky Mountains, I focused on the beauty of the changing aspen leaves, the feel of the crisp breeze, the sound of mountain streams, and the clean, fresh scent of the mountain air. I allowed myself the luxury of long naps in my husband's arms. I enjoyed every bite of food as if I had never tasted it before. I prayed for the ability to release any residual resentments, and I enjoyed sacred intimacy with my husband. Those five days, which could have been frittered away with worry and fear, were magical.

When I returned home, I had a knowing that any abnormalities that had been in my breasts were now gone, but I continued to follow up with more diagnostics. The digital mammography indicated something suspicious, so I also had an MRI. The MRI showed nothing. Nothing at all. My healthcare team told me that no further testing was needed. A follow-up thermogram six months later was completely normal.

I am so grateful for the breast thermography and intend to have one every year. Meanwhile, my new mantra for staying healthy is: "I take care of myself with the same loving care that I give to my husband and son." When I follow my mantra, I can feel every cell in my body glowing with health!

Family History of Breast Cancer and the Breast Cancer Gene

Certain women have been identified as having genetically higher chances of early-onset breast cancer and sometimes ovarian cancer because their families carry mutations in the BRCA1 or BRCA2 genes.[144] The men in these families may have increased rates of not only breast cancer but also testicular, pancreatic, and early-onset prostate cancer.[145] Because 60 percent of women who have inherited the mutated breast cancer gene will develop breast cancer at some point in their lives (compared to 12 percent of women in the general population), those testing positive for the mutation are opting more and more often to have a preventive bilateral mastectomy (the removal of two, usually healthy, breasts).[146] Yet the largest study to date to compare survival rates of breast cancer patients with and without BRCA gene mutations—a 2018 study in the United Kingdom looking at 2,733 women who were forty or younger when first diagnosed with invasive breast cancer—showed that having the mutation didn't influence survival, even after ten years, and that having a bilateral mastectomy did not improve the chances of survival.[147] I'm very concerned that way too many women are having these procedures who don't need them, especially after they read about celebrities who have opted for this, as mentioned earlier.

It's clear that the genes we are born with are only one part of the story. How they get expressed is another matter entirely. Genes don't operate in a vacuum. They're turned on and off by environmental factors.[148] According to one recent study of 2,000 women from different countries headed by Colin Begg, Ph.D., chair of the Department of Epidemiology and Biostatistics at Memorial Sloan-Kettering Cancer Center, several other factors contribute to a woman's risk, including family history, diet, and lifestyle choices.[149] This means that testing positive for the gene mutation doesn't mean you will get breast cancer *and* that testing negative for the mutation doesn't mean you are protected from developing breast cancer.

The first thing I tell women who have a positive family history—usually of a mother with breast cancer—is that they are *not* their mothers and that genetics is only *one* part of whether somebody gets a disease. In fact, the majority of women diagnosed with breast cancer *don't* have a positive family history of the disease, nor do they have the genetic mutation. (In one major study, only 10 percent of young women with breast cancer had the gene.) But women who test positive for the mutation *and* who have more than one close relative (a mother, sister, and/or daughter) with breast cancer have a greater than 60 percent risk, according to the National Cancer Institute.[150]

If you fall into this category, your doctor will most likely recommend vigilant breast cancer screening, including mammography and breast exams (and possibly MRI or sonography), every six to twelve months. Conventional medicine believes in more radical treatments as well, such as:

~ Preventive mastectomy (an option that doesn't increase your chances of survival if you do get breast cancer)

~ Preventive chemotherapy (usually in the form of tamoxifen)

~ Taking estrogen-inhibiting drugs for the rest of your life (presumably to thwart tumor growth)

I'm saddened by these recommendations because they simply don't take into account all the things a woman can do proactively to change the way her genes are expressed. I don't believe any woman should think of her breasts as lumps of tissue that are destined to kill her. And I wouldn't want a woman to think these are her only three options for staying healthy. These protocols can create more problems and diminish a woman's quality of life. And as already mentioned, frequent mammograms have been shown to increase your risk of cancer because of excessive doses of radiation.[151]

A Word About Genomic Profiles

With the completion of the Human Genome Project in 2000, an ever-increasing body of research is showing that certain gene mutations run in families and may predispose them to an increased risk of breast cancer, heart disease, and so on. Genomic profiles typically consist of tests for combinations of gene variants; the specific combinations are considered proprietary and are usually not disclosed in online or printed product information.

Genomic profiling for guiding individualized health promotion and disease prevention is in its infancy but becoming more popular by the day.[152] This type of testing can be a very valuable tool if it is used proactively. For example, the mother of one of my medical colleagues has had two different types of breast cancer. My colleague, a practitioner of functional medicine who understands the link between our genes and our environment, had her mother and herself tested for the type of gene mutations that are associated with some types of breast cancer. Sure enough, she and her mother have exactly the same genomic profile in the area of estrogen metabolism. But rather than feel as though she is a sitting duck for developing cancer, she used the data to spur her on to do what she already knew she should do: exercise more, increase her intake of indole-3-carbinol, decrease her consumption of sugar, and so forth. Increasingly, genomic profiling—and understanding how we can change the way our DNA gets expressed—will be the medicine of the future. If you work with a skilled healthcare practitioner who knows how to interpret a genomic profile and use it to help you improve your lifestyle, then getting one might be worth it. For the vast majority of people, family history is all the genomic profiling they need. The key is to make the changes that the family history—and common sense—tell them they should make. (To find a practitioner who is combining genomic profiles with specific lifestyle suggestions, check out the website of the Institute for Functional Medicine at www.functionalmedicine.org.)

Changing Your Legacy: Prevention from the Inside Out

Here's the story of one woman, a social worker, who has engaged proactively with her family history. (Note the reference to her mother. Breast issues always go back to our mothers—the people from whom we learned our earliest and deepest lessons about self-nurturance.)

Life had been hectic for some time. Working as a social worker in a large Boston teaching hospital, I covered the oncology unit and the two intensive care units and had a beeper that went off nonstop. At home, I felt continuously assaulted by the noise from the street and from the

huge radios that every kid on the block played. I vowed that by the age
of fifty I would retire from the rat race and find someplace quiet where
I could do some teaching and consulting and have a small private practice and a big garden.

I had been working in oncology for a few years. Initially, I felt
somewhat compelled to do so, knowing that it had to do with my own
mother's death, around the age of forty, from breast cancer. It was something of a death-defying act. If I could learn as much as possible about
cancer, it would never "get" me. All I had to do was get past the age
of forty. In my own therapy, as I approached forty, I faced the issue of
"having" to do oncology work. After some struggle, I finally decided
that I did what I did because I was very good at it, and that when the
time came to work in some other sphere, I could do it.

The age of forty came and went. And the angst remained.

In September of my forty-first year, I came to Maine for a vacation.
I was having dinner with an acquaintance and we were talking about
our dreams for the future. When I said that my dream was to retire to a
place like this when I turned fifty, she challenged me with the question
"Why not now?"

My answer was that I made good money for a social worker, I had
a manageable mortgage, and I was vested in the hospital pension plan.
Her observation that I was being held by the "golden handcuffs" irked
me, because I like to think my values are elsewhere. "Besides," she said,
"what makes you think you'll get to fifty?" Not only did my mother die
young, but every day I was working with people younger than I who
were dying.

At that moment I know that my life changed. I felt it in every cell of
my body. And I *knew* there was no reason not to come to Maine. The
next day I told a Realtor what I wanted, and on the following morning
at nine A.M. I walked into the house that I now own. The first house that
I looked at was just what I had dreamed about.

In January I moved to Maine and continued to work in Boston,
never minding the commute, which was made easier by a flexible schedule. In March, Claudia, a young leukemic of whom I had become very
fond, died. I had worked with Claudia and her family for four years.
I dreaded her death. The morning she died, I experienced chest pains.
Knowing that there was no physical problem with me, I paid attention
and tried to figure out what my body was saying to me. By the end of the
day, I had named the pain "collective heartbreak." I realized that I knew
more dead people than live people and decided that I needed a weekend
away to think about things. A few Sundays later, I was sitting out on the
rocks in front of a big resort, looking at the ocean. My thoughts were

of Claudia, of many of the others I had worked with who had died, and eventually of my mother.

For some reason I was curious about exactly how old my mother had been when she died. Surprisingly, I had never done the arithmetic that would give me that information. Simple calculations told me that she had been forty-one and nine months old when she died. On that very day, I was exactly forty-one years and nine months old! And I had been working on the oncology unit for five and one-half years—the same length of time she had been sick with her breast cancer. I had done it! I had survived!

The next day I handed in my resignation. I took the summer off to think about what to do with my life. Those few months turned into a few more, and before I worked again, nine months had passed—an appropriate amount of time to be reborn.

During that time, I had the birthday my mother never had and began to rethink my identity and priorities. Eventually, I began what has turned into a very successful psychotherapy practice. I get to teach now and then, do a bit of consulting, and have that big garden. And I know for sure that although I'm my mother's daughter, I never have to *be* her.

As part of my journey, I have come to believe in the strength of the body and spirit—a helper even in the most impossible situations. In the 1950s, when my mother had breast cancer, I know that there were few options for a Roman Catholic woman stuck in a bad marriage, even fewer if she had been physically disabled in childhood, as was my mother. I now believe that my mother's breast cancer was her only way out of an impossible situation, a bad marriage, a stultifying existence of guilt and self-sacrifice. I regret that her escape cost her her life.

Breast Cancer Treatment

Treatment modalities for breast cancer are beyond the scope of this book and are not my specialty. Though the experts may disagree somewhat on the statistics, the data suggest that the overall mortality rate from breast cancer is going down. Though the National Cancer Institute reports that the mortality rate for U.S. women with breast cancer has been falling an average of 1.8 percent each year from 2006 through 2015,[153] I'm not sure how meaningful this figure really is, given the large number of noninvasive ductal carcinomas in situ that no doubt have been included as part of these statistics. In some areas of the country, mastectomies are still being done, even though lumpectomy to preserve the breast has, in most cases, been proved equally effective. I urge every woman faced with breast cancer treatment decisions to seek a second opinion if mastectomy is the only option she is given.

One major advance in the surgical treatment of breast cancer is the sentinel node biopsy, whereby a surgeon is able to remove a single axillary lymph node, the sentinel node, which is the first to process cancer cells. When this node is negative, no further nodes are removed. This prevents women from experiencing so much pain and subsequent lymphedema from removal of large numbers of lymph nodes.

Chemotherapy is another standard treatment option that deserves more careful consideration. For example, the groundbreaking Trial Assigning Individualized Options for Treatment (known as the TAILORx trial) showed no benefit from chemotherapy for 70 percent of women who have the most common type of breast cancer—HR positive, HER2 negative, axillary lymph node negative—even after nine years.[154] This trial, the results of which were published in 2018, enrolled more than 10,000 women from the United States, Australia, Canada, Ireland, New Zealand, and Peru who were diagnosed with early-stage breast cancer and was one of the first large-scale trials to examine methods for personalizing cancer treatment.

Women now have as much access to information from other people, books, and the Internet as they could want. Some feel overwhelmed by it, while others welcome it. Every woman has her own unique decision-making process and should feel validated in using it. Everyone can read the same statistics and feel differently about them. Some want everything done even if the benefit is statistically very small (less than 5 percent). Others are more concerned about treatment risks and are willing to trust their own intuition. Different doctors can present statistics to patients in different terms. While doctors are rarely malicious, some oncologists (because they deal with so much death) can be quite frightening and full of doom and gloom. A woman should feel she has a support system of healthcare providers whom she can trust and who trust her.

One online resource is Predict (www.predict.nhs.uk/tool), from the University of Cambridge Winton Centre for Risk and Evidence Communication in England. Predict is an evidence-based tool designed for women who have had surgery for early invasive breast cancer to help show how breast cancer treatments after surgery might improve survival rates. After patients answer questions about themselves and their type of cancer in the online form, the tool shows how different treatment options would be expected to improve survival rates up to fifteen years after diagnosis.

Another good online resource is the breast cancer nomograms from Memorial Sloan Kettering Cancer Center (nomograms.mskcc.org/breast). You can choose from three nomograms: one for newly diagnosed patients to assess the likelihood that breast cancer has spread to the sentinel lymph nodes, one for those whose cancer has already spread to the sentinel lymph nodes to assess the likelihood that the cancer has spread to additional lymph nodes under the arm, and one for women diagnosed with DCIS to assess the chance of breast cancer recurring in the same breast after receiving breast-conserving surgery.

CancerMath's online calculators (www.lifemath.net/cancer/index.html) show the relative frequency of a given surgical procedure for a given tumor type. These calculators are based on data for cancer patients from 1987 to 2007, with greater weight given to more recent patients. They're based on data that include surgical treatments used during this time period, so any newer therapies won't be reflected.

Whatever the form of treatment, women all over the world today are transforming their experience of breast cancer and healing at the deepest levels to go on to live full, dynamic, and creative lives. You must choose the treatment option that feels right to you, whether that is surgery, chemo, or radiation, alone or in combination with diet, supplements, and meditation—or even forgoing conventional treatments altogether.

Inner reflective work to change emotional patterns associated with breast cancer, certain types of support groups, and dietary improvement are important parts of treatment, regardless of your treatment choices. Though the vast majority of women with breast cancer choose surgery, chemotherapy, or both for treatment, I've worked with several women whose choice has involved dietary change and inner healing work only—without any aid from conventional medicine besides the initial biopsy to make the diagnosis. After several years, some of these women now have clear mammograms and no evidence of cancer anywhere. One was called at home by her surgeon at the time that she first refused treatment and was told that if she didn't have the recommended surgery she would die. She refused, and twenty years later she is still cancer-free.

Many women choose some, but not all, of the treatment options offered to them. Mildred was forty-three years old when her diagnosis of breast cancer was made. She was married to a university professor and lived in a midwestern college town. She had never worked outside of her home, having chosen instead to marry in her early twenties and raise three children. Shortly after she turned thirty-five, she realized that her husband had been having a series of affairs with students. For financial reasons, she chose to stay with him until their children were older. When her diagnosis of breast cancer was made, however, she left her marriage, went back to school, and got a job. She is now living happily and independently. She had a lumpectomy only. When her daughter asked her why she didn't get a mammogram and exam every six months, Mildred replied, "I know why I got breast cancer. I know I will not get it back again." She knew that she could not maintain her health and stay in a marriage with a man who was sexually unfaithful to her. After more than ten years, she hasn't had a breast cancer recurrence. One of my patients,

Julia, was thirty-eight when she had a lumpectomy. The biopsy showed that not all the tumor had been removed during this procedure. A mastectomy and lymph node dissection were recommended because of the nature of her cancer. Instead, she chose to return to her childhood home in the South and confront her demons—a lifetime of de-selfing herself to please others and a marriage she had outgrown. This process was accompanied by a deep emotional cleansing and a letting go of her past ways, unhealthy behaviors, and habits. Julia also changed her diet to a healthy vegetarian one. Though she is cancer-free at this time, she knows that she must stay in touch with her innermost needs and her bodily wisdom. She recently felt called to move to the Southwest. Though unsure of how she would make a living, she decided to go anyway. Almost immediately she found a job at a bed-and-breakfast. Her circumstances there were very healing and afforded her not only room and board but a great deal of time and space alone and close to nature. Julia is extraordinarily courageous and continues to do well.

Another of my patients, Gretchen, was diagnosed with a type of breast cancer that is known to be very aggressive and fast-growing. She refused conventional treatment and instead changed her diet and left an abusive marriage. She eventually found a job in a publishing house doing work that she loves. Three years later, she has no obvious cancer. But she doesn't think in terms of "being cured." She says, "The essence for me is living my life one day at a time." Gretchen believes that the lifestyle changes she made have been the major factors in her healing.

Women's Stories

Caroline Myss and other healers teach that cancer is the disease of timing. It can result when most of a person's energy is tied up dealing with old hurts and resentments from the past that they can't seem to release. These old hurts need a witness—someone who validates the wounds—before healing can begin.

Our relationship to time can and does make us sick. Feminist and author Sonia Johnson says, "Time is not a river, we all have all the time there ever was or ever will be right now. Linear time, itself, is a workaholic construct."[155] In a materialistic, addictive culture, we learn that time is money and that we should spend each minute of our lives accomplishing or producing more and more. Instead of enjoying each moment we have and living our lives fully, we are instead taught at an early age that there is never enough time. We are always running out of time. Far too many of us suffer from "hurry sickness." We rush around, our hearts beating faster, feeling that there is too much to do and not enough time to do it. The state of our bodies and the cells that constitute them reflect this.

Monica: A Summer of Healing

Monica was forty-eight when she first came to see me. She had recently had a positive biopsy for breast cancer. Her general surgeon wanted to do a mastectomy as well as remove the lymph nodes from underneath her right arm. Monica and her partner had both read extensively on the topic of breast cancer, and she objected to the mastectomy. After full discussion, the surgeon stated that he felt comfortable doing a lumpectomy. However, after the lumpectomy, he found that her tumor margins were not clear on the specimen, leading to a concern that cancer cells still remained. He sent her to see an oncologist who explained that chemotherapy was a standard recommendation for her type of cancer. But she wanted to find out about other things she could do before having the conventional treatment.

I suggested to Monica that she could switch to a diet that would lower her circulating estrogen levels, apply castor oil packs to the affected breast to enhance her immune system functioning, and begin a good supplementation program. I stressed that these measures were not considered "cures" in a conventional sense and that they hadn't been studied nearly as well as surgery and chemotherapy. She understood that. I told her that it was imperative that she spend the next few months learning how to take care of herself and do things that brought her pleasure. She and her family left to consider all her options, and I planned to see them three months later, in September.

When Monica returned three months later, she looked fifteen years younger and was radiant with health. I asked her what she had done. She told me, "When I left here, I knew that I had to change my life. This summer I decided to do whatever felt wonderful and healing. So I rode my bike every day and spent long hours lying in the fields looking up at the sky and the clouds. I took summer into every cell of my body. I haven't had a summer like this one since I was a kid. It seemed to go on forever."

Monica had changed her relationship to time, stopping the clock and bringing her cells into the present. Many of us need to take the time to "take summer into every cell of our bodies." It has been more than ten years since Monica has had any evidence of cancer. Though she eventually decided *not* to have chemotherapy or further surgery to try to eliminate tumor cells, she has remained cancer-free.[156]

Serena: Releasing the Past

Serena was forty-eight when she first came to see me following a mastectomy for a fairly large breast mass that was a poorly differentiated breast cancer—a tissue type associated with faster growth and a poor prognosis. Though she had been involved in alternatives to conventional medicine for years, her inner guidance led her to chemotherapy, which she went through without any problems by using meditation and relaxation. (See "How to Prepare for Surgery (or Chemotherapy) and Heal Faster," page 822.)

When I met her, she had just moved to the East Coast from California. Two years earlier she had broken up with a man with whom she had lived for ten years when he fell in love with and married another woman. This man was the creator and founder of a very popular self-help group, and the group activities, workshops, and trips had not only provided Serena's income but also functioned as a family and support system for her. In addition, Serena had contributed substantial money toward a center where this group met regularly. When her significant other left her for another woman in the group, Serena found herself on the outside and was no longer welcome at group activities in the same way as in the past.

Soon after her relationship breakup, she consulted a lawyer to help her get her money and personal belongings back from the group. This lawyer told her that, given the legalities of her situation, it was highly unlikely that she could get her money back. After talking with members of her support group, she decided to get another lawyer and "take it to the Supreme Court if necessary."

When Serena moved back to the East Coast following the breakup of her "family," she immediately went into therapy (both individual and group) to help her deal with the rage, grief, and abandonment she felt. As a result of this experience, she found herself meeting and taking comfort from many other women who also found themselves in the position of having been taken advantage of financially, sexually, and in other ways. She joined a breast cancer support group, too.

When I first met with Serena, she told me that she was feeling fatigued and listless. She wondered why this was so, given that she had finished her chemotherapy and radiation almost a year before and that she had always eaten a healthy, whole-foods diet, taken supplements, and exercised. When she told me her recent history, I suggested that in the future, she needed to make sure that every relationship she was in was a true partnership, in which she gave and received in equal measure. And I also suggested to her that she take a retreat and make a list of all the aspects of her life that were working and another of all the aspects that needed to change. Then, having meditated on the lists, she could come up with a plan for changing those things she was willing to change right now.

She went off by herself to a meditation center. While there, she had the following dream: She was on a raft and saw a house burning in the distance. Her former friends from her self-help community were in the house. At that point in the dream, she realized that she had a choice: to go to the burning house and rescue them, or to stay on the raft and allow the river to take her where she was supposed to be going. In the dream, she noticed that making the choice to leave the river and go to the house was associated with feeling tired and struggling. Even though her mind was pulling her toward the house, her heart (and body) were drawn to going where the river was taking her.

She woke up abruptly and knew what she had to do. She had to allow herself to float on the river of a new life.

Even though all her thoughts told her that the community owed her financially, she realized at a very deep level that continuing to hang on to that old community was draining her life's energy away from her—and keeping whatever energy she still had stuck in the past, so nothing new or better could come to her. One week after she returned from her retreat and had her dream, she stopped her legal proceedings against the old group and created a ceremony to release her past and let her move on to a new life. In time, she also stopped seeing unsupportive friends from that group, since she realized that these visits simply re-created her past. She also noticed that when she went to the meetings, she always felt more tired when she left than when she went in. She knew that although the group had originally been very helpful, it was now time to leave.

Two months after this healing phase, Serena was offered a job in publishing—something she had always dreamed of doing. She took it, and while there met a new man to whom she is now married. This marriage, unlike her former relationship, is a true partnership of the heart for Serena, and she is able to look back on her breast cancer as her inner guidance coming to her at a critical time. She feels that it gave her the gift of a new, better life. She continues to do well. Most of the time she does not worry about breast cancer. And when she does, she turns it over to her higher power.

Though Monica and Serena chose different healing approaches, both have changed their relationship to time, and both know that they've chosen the right path for themselves. Most important, they are no longer afraid of breast cancer.

COSMETIC BREAST SURGERY
Implants: Are They Safe? Should You Get Them?

In 2017, breast augmentation became the most popular cosmetic procedure performed in the United States, according to the American Society of Plastic Surgeons. Indeed, cosmetic surgery of all kinds is far more acceptable now than ever before, and techniques and results are improving all the time.

Breast augmentation is favored by some women whose breasts have sagged after nursing or weight loss or who simply want bigger, fuller breasts. Some of this, of course, is fueled by the constant bombardment (and perhaps alteration) of our senses by media images of enhanced breasts. In fact, it's rare to see a non-augmented breast on a popular television show, in music videos, or in movies. The new "ideal" models of feminine beauty are seen in the hugely popular Victoria's Secret website. So the bar has been raised artificially high on what our culture considers an ideal breast size and shape. The average implant is a C cup, and many are even bigger. To put the entire area into perspective—and to make sure that women are really informed about it—let's first start with a little history.

The first silicone injections were done into the breasts of Japanese prostitutes in order to satisfy the desire of their American GI clients for larger breasts in the 1940s and '50s. Problems were reported with silicone leaking into other areas of the body because it was never confined to an implant. Little wonder that these women reported health problems! Later, given the "bigger is better" American desire for larger breasts, the first silicone breast implants were developed by two plastic surgeons from Texas, Frank Gerow and Thomas Cronin, in the 1960s. And in 1962, a woman named Timmie Jean Lindsey became the first woman to receive silicone breast implants.[157]

At the time of the first implants, these devices were not regulated by the FDA or any other agency. In the ensuing three decades, it is estimated that anywhere from 800,000 to 1 million women received the devices.[158]

No one questioned the safety of implants until the 1980s when some of the women with implants began to attribute their symptoms to having breast implants. Chronic fatigue, arthritis, immune system disorders, and connective tissue syndromes such as lupus were said to be associated with silicone implants. This resulted in a decade of controversy in which emotion took precedence over science. Though there was never any convincing evidence that implants were, in fact, associated with connective tissue disorders, that didn't stop a series of huge class-action lawsuits against Dow Corning and an enormous amount of fear in women who had had implants. It also resulted in difficulty in obtaining raw material and fear of litigation in manufacturers of other silicone medical devices including vital shunts, catheters, artificial heart valves, and Dacron grafts.[159]

In the end, researchers could find no solid data linking implants, per se, with an increased risk of death. In fact, in June 1999, a panel of experts appointed by Congress to study the issue under the auspices of the Institute of Medicine (part of the National Academy of Sciences) failed to find any scientific evidence connecting silicone breast implants with an increased risk of death. This group released a 400-page report prepared by an independent committee of thirteen scientists that concluded that although silicone breast implants may be responsible for localized problems such as hardening or scarring of breast tissue, implants do not cause any major diseases such as lupus or rheumatoid arthritis. The committee did not conduct any original research; instead they examined past research and other materials and conducted public hearings to hear all sides of the issue. Despite this lack of data on their harm, silicone breast implants were taken off the market in the United States and replaced by saline implants until the newer "gummy bear" type of silicone implant was developed. This type of implant has a more normal feel and virtually no risk of leakage into surrounding tissue.

Interestingly, several studies have been done on long-term mortality among women with silicone implants. A 2001 study by the National Cancer Institute found that women with breast augmentation were more likely to die of brain cancer or lung cancer compared to other plastic surgery patients. In fact, the results showed a doubling of brain cancer and a tripling of lung cancer, emphysema, and pneumonia in women with implants. There was also a fourfold increase in the risk of suicide among implant patients.[160] A 2007 review conducted by the University of Pennsylvania Medical Center of six different studies found that women with cosmetic breast implants had approximately twice the expected rate of suicide.[161] Researchers in one such study from Sweden felt this increased risk was likely not related to any effect of implants; rather, there is a link between the desire for plastic surgery and psychiatric disorders,[162] a risk that is well documented.[163]

It's intriguing that both brain cancer and suicide risk appear to be higher in women with breast implants. Those are both sixth-chakra issues— involving perception, thought, and morality. In other words, it is not the implants themselves that are causing the problem. It is how each woman is thinking about and perceiving herself and her worth that either sets the stage for health or illness concerning implants.

Having seen dozens of women over the years who have done very well with their breast implants (and some who haven't), I'm convinced that the women who are most likely to do well are the ones who generally already feel good about themselves and their worth but are getting the implants to enhance how they look in clothes or because of their professions, such as modeling or acting. (See stories, below.) They are not getting implants to get or keep a man or because they don't feel feminine enough. That said, there are plenty of women who love the look of their implants and who therefore feel sexier and more desirable as a result of having them.

It doesn't take a sociologist to figure out why women would want to look like the images that have been burned into our brains since childhood by everything from Disney movies to music videos. The pressures on girls to match the cultural ideal is far greater now than in the past. This helps to explain why the average person requesting breast augmentation is a twenty-something who doesn't feel good about her breast size and shape.

When I first watched a breast augmentation and saw the amount of tissue damage done by lifting the chest wall off the underlying tissue, I instinctively held my own breasts protectively. I realized that I could never elect to have this procedure, as it is currently performed, done for cosmetic reasons. For one thing, implants can decrease or eliminate nipple sensation, which is part of a woman's sexual pleasure. The implants can become very hard (though that is less common with the materials used now), and they can cause the breast tissue to develop fibrous capsules around them. (To prevent this, take omega-3 fats as supplements, 1,000–5,000 mg/day; see chapter 17, on nutrition.) In some cases they make it difficult (though not impossible) to nurse a child.

There are other risks associated with implants that all women who plan to get them should keep in mind. One concern is the risk, while low, of a condition called breast-implant-associated anaplastic large cell lymphoma (BIA-ALCL), a rare type of lymphoma that can develop around breast implants, both silicone and saline. When caught early, this lymphoma is highly curable. The condition occurs most frequently in women who receive implants with textured as opposed to smooth surfaces and seems to be related to an allergic reaction to the implant. Common symptoms include breast enlargement, pain, asymmetry, a lump in the breast or armpit, skin rash, hardening of the breast, or a large fluid collection typically developing at least one year (and usually eight to ten years) after the implant surgery. Another concern is the risk of having an autoimmune reaction to the silicone. Such reactions are rare, but they are becoming more widely recognized as time goes on.[164] Some researchers are concerned that the silicone in implants may even increase risk of autoimmune diseases and immune deficiencies.[165]

Data show that about 40 percent of augmentation patients and 70 percent of mastectomy reconstruction patients have at least one serious complication within three years after getting their implants. Within the first three to five years after surgery, 12.5 to 25 percent of breast augmentation patients can expect to have additional surgery, and within ten to twelve years, most women will need at least one additional surgery. The reason is that by then, at least one implant is likely to have ruptured. Like most new products, the majority of implants are often fine for the first few years. Then, like with anything (such as a car), problems can happen over time. The older they get, the more likely they are to rupture. After ten years, 10 to 14 percent of implants rupture. These ruptures are not always obvious.

All breast implants have the same basic design. They are made up of a silicone envelope with a filling of some sort, usually saline or silicone gel. Silicone implants have a more normal feel than saline, and a big advantage of the newer ones is that it's impossible for them to leak. The silicone is in a matrix, sort of like a gummy bear candy, so it adheres to the shell that encases it. Even if the implant develops a hole or a tear, called a rupture, the silicone stays put and can't migrate into the body and cause tissue reaction. This is thought to be why the newer silicone implants are less likely to develop hard encapsulations around them.[166] (Before getting breast implants, check out the information at www.breastimplantinfo.org.)

Mammograms can potentially cause an implant to break, especially with older implants or with a technician who is not trained to work with breast implants. (Make sure the mammogram technician knows you have implants and is qualified to do the procedure.)[167] Women who have had implants after a mastectomy do not need mammograms of the reconstructed breast. MRIs are useful for imaging both the breast and the implant when mammograms are not helpful or are intolerable.

At the end of the day, I would never judge women who have had implants or who want them, any more than I would judge women who have had their nose size and shape cosmetically altered. Breast implants and the newer breast reconstruction methods can give women who have lost a breast to cancer a body image that approaches wholeness. This surgery can be key to a woman's healing. Sharon Webb, M.D., Ph.D., a plastic surgeon who specializes in breast reconstruction following breast cancer surgery, says that she often receives letters from her patients and their family members telling her how grateful they are for her work and how much the surgical breast reconstruction has contributed to their overall sense of well-being.

None of us is immune to our cultural inheritance and its impact on how we approach our breasts, and we need to exercise compassion for our own and other women's choices. Each woman has to decide for herself what feels best for her body and why. Here are a few stories concerning cosmetic breast surgery and its consequences.

Women's Stories

Janice: Family Pressure

Janice came to see me ostensibly for a routine annual physical exam. She had been there on two previous occasions for diaphragm fittings. A working woman, she was slim and attractive. When I entered the exam room, she said that she had some other issues she wanted to discuss after her exam, so afterward she came into my office.

Janice told me that she had had a breast enlargement procedure a few years before and that everything seemed fine. (My exam had confirmed that.) In my office, however, her eyes filled with tears, and she said she was afraid she would cry because she had something to ask me that she had never before asked a doctor. I suggested that she stay with her emotions because whenever we're moved in this way, we are onto something very important. She continued, "I first went to see a gynecologist when I was sixteen. I was having terrible menstrual cramps, and I wanted to see if anything was wrong with me. He wouldn't let my mother remain in the room with me when he examined me. His exam was very painful and I asked him to stop, but he wouldn't. Then when he saw my breasts, he laughed and said, 'Maybe if you marry and your husband fondles you enough, they'll grow.'" He prescribed birth control pills for her cramps, and she left the office feeling humiliated.

Janice went on to describe her early breast development. She said that at first her nipples had grown and started to stand out. It felt, she said, as if she had a walnut-size mass under each nipple. The tissue grew to about the size of an avocado pit and stopped. What she was describing was normal breast budding, with normal glandular tissue underneath the nipple. This had happened around the time she got her first period. I told her that it all sounded very normal to me. She cried again. Her breasts were naturally small, but her mother, her brother, and a sister had always referred to her as "deformed."

One day while clothes shopping with her mother, her mother commented on Janice's "deformity" and told her that if she ever wanted anything done about it, she'd be willing to pay for it. (I frequently hear stories of mothers telling their daughters that their breasts are not big enough. Sometimes they suggest that their daughters wear padded bras or stuff their bras with tissue.) Janice surprised her mother and said that she did in fact want something done. Soon after, she had an augmentation mammoplasty, or breast enlargement procedure, with silicone implants.

I asked Janice how she felt about her breasts now. She replied that she had mixed feelings because of the circumstances under which she had had the surgery. Since she was also having acupuncture treatments and was more interested in natural healing than she had been in the past, she was afraid that she'd messed herself up by doing something so "unnatural."

My reply was to share with Janice that many women have elected to have their breasts enlarged and have been very happy with the procedure. The women who are happiest with it are those who have given it a lot of thought beforehand and are doing it to please themselves and not anyone else. These women usually have good results and no complications. When someone feels positive about a decision such as this, I believe that her immune system function is enhanced and that the complication rate is apt to be lower. I wanted Janice to know that I didn't think that having the breast surgery had damaged her health in any unalterable way.

Most important, I affirmed that she was normal, not "deformed," and that she had always been normal. She simply had small breasts, like all the women on her father's side of the family. Unfortunately, she had grown up in a family that was emotionally abusive about her body at a time when she was very vulnerable. Her visit to the gynecologist had reinforced that pathology.

Now, at the age of thirty-three, Janice was finally ready to bring up this history about her body. Before she left, she said to me, "You have no idea how important it is for me to hear this stuff from a doctor." I suggested that she spend the rest of the day staying with her tears and any other emotions that came up. I asked her to express them through sound. All of the tears and all of the emotions that we stifle stay in our physical bodies as unfinished business and are waiting for us to attend to them. Janice now had the opportunity to finish a significant amount of healing. She was ready to heal on all levels her relationship with her breasts.

Sarah: Implants to Please Her Husband

Sarah was about fifty-five when I first saw her. She had raised several children and had been married for twenty-five years to an alcoholic but was now divorced. As is so often the case with people like Sarah, her father had also been an alcoholic. Fifteen years before, Sarah's husband had become impotent. He had blamed her for his condition, telling her that her body just wasn't the way it needed to be for him to be able to get an erection.

Like so many women who are in dominator relationships, Sarah believed him and took on his problem as her own. Her husband said that maybe he wouldn't be impotent if her breasts were bigger. She dutifully went to New York and had breast implants placed. She hated them from the first, and her husband's impotence remained—except that now he told her something must be wrong with her vagina. Their relationship continued to deteriorate, and his drinking worsened.

Several years later Sarah's husband left her. (He is now with a younger woman, for whom we can all feel sorry.) Sarah went into codependence recovery and realized that she was *not* the cause of her husband's impotence and never had been. But now she is stuck with silicone implants that she hates. She said that when it's cold outside, her breasts don't get warm because it takes so long for the implants to warm up. She had apparently looked into having them removed but was told that it would cost her thousands of dollars, which her insurance wouldn't cover. Every day she is reminded of the price she's paid with her body. (Sometimes insurance will cover implant removal. And many plastic surgeons will remove them for a minor fee.)

Kim: Implants to Please Herself

Kim is a vivacious woman in her late thirties. She works in the fashion industry now, but she was a teacher for years. When she was a teenager, she had large hips and very small breasts. She was never able to buy a suit because she could never find a top and a bottom that both fit. For years she was unhappy with her figure, even though she was a multitalented woman. She exercised and followed diets to correct as much of the imbalance as she could, and she elected to have her breasts enlarged after giving it years of thought. The procedure went beautifully and was healing for her because she chose this procedure under optimal circumstances: She did it for herself. She already had high self-esteem, and her expectations for the procedure were appropriate. She has never had a problem. I spoke with her nearly ten years after her surgery, and she said she still loves her implants and is certain she'll have no trouble with them.

Beth: Caught in the Middle

Beth was a patient of mine for years. She had two pregnancies and nursed both children. Her husband left her after her second child was born, and she was raising her children by herself. She was independent and strong. Several years ago, she had a breast augmentation. After childbirth and nursing, her breasts seemed to be flaccid. She couldn't find a bra to fit, and she was uncomfortable with her appearance. She had always had a very attractive body. (I realize that this concept is loaded: Attractive to whom? Why? For what purpose?) In any case, though she had a very low income, she managed to get the money together to have her breasts enlarged. The outcome was excellent, and she was very pleased with the results. An anthropologist might say that her "social" body was improved by this surgery. (She's currently at work on overcoming her uncanny ability to attract men who aren't supportive of her.)

I believe that the circumstances surrounding a woman's breast implantation—why the surgery was done—are as crucial to her freedom from side effects as any potential problems from the silicone. Women with implants should know the following: Thousands of women have *no problems* with implants. And neither do transgender individuals who opt for them. The same holds true, in general, for postmastectomy reconstruction patients and for those who have had implants to equalize the size of their breasts. If you want to breast-feed, you should also know that recent studies have failed to show any increased incidence of immune problems in babies whose mothers had silicone implants. However, though 40 percent of women with implants had no problems with breast-feeding, one study showed that women with implants were three times more likely to experience breast-feeding difficulty than women who haven't had breast surgery. Implants placed through an incision in the nipple were associated with the least success.[168]

If you do decide to have implants, make sure that your diet supports your immune system. Include vegetables rich in beta-carotene, phytoestrogens, and plant lignans. (See the Program to Promote Healthy Breast Tissue, page 429, for more details.) Make sure you get lots of omega-3 fats. I've been very pleased by how well the encapsulation on implants softens when women follow an inflammation-reducing diet that includes enough omega-3 fats.

Breast Surgery to Decrease Breast Size

Sharon's breasts started to develop when she was only eleven years old. By the time she was fifteen, she wore a size 38D bra. She felt embarrassed at school and was self-conscious about sports. Running was uncomfortable for her, and in the summer she developed painful rashes under her breasts from sweating. Buying clothing was difficult because her hips were slim relative to her chest. At about thirty she had a reduction mammoplasty—a breast-reduction procedure. Even though she now has visible scars across each breast, she is thrilled that she had the procedure done.

Erin, a strikingly beautiful woman in her thirties, came to see me for a tubal ligation. During her physical, I noticed that she had the characteristic scars of a breast-reduction procedure and asked her when she had had the surgery. She told me that she'd had it in her mid-twenties, because she had simply been tired of all the attention that she got from being both beautiful and having an ample breast size. Though her size had only been about 38C—not unusually large—she still had elected to have the procedure.

One of my friends has a jogging partner who is about a 38C as well. Men slow down their cars and make comments as she jogs by. Even twelve-year-old boys feel that they have the right to follow her on their bicycles and make comments!

These experiences are typical of women who have chosen to have their breast size reduced. Though this procedure often decreases or eliminates nipple sensation, leaves scars, and may make it difficult for a woman to nurse her baby, most of the women who've had this surgery are very happy with the results. Janette Hurley, M.D., a family physician and breast-feeding advocate in Calgary, Alberta, told me that in her practice, women can often nurse successfully following reduction mammoplasty, as long as they feel good about their choice to breast-feed and have no difficulty appreciating their breasts' normal function.

Women have had a range of experiences with cosmetic breast surgery. Plastic surgery of the breast or any other area of the body is neither right nor wrong—the demand for it merely reflects the values of our culture. The changes it effects can be very rewarding, but as Naomi Wolf so aptly points out in *The Beauty Myth,* they are not a panacea. Surgery will not heal a woman's life or her relationship with her body. The most important factor in a successful outcome, aside from a skilled surgeon, is the context in which the procedure is done and the expectations that the woman has of it.

The Power of the Mind to Affect Your Breasts

Research has shown that it is possible to increase breast size and firmness through hypnosis and creative visualization. This makes complete sense, since it is well known that our subconscious mind has an enormous effect on our physical body. In four separate studies, hypnosis not only increased breast size and firmness in those who completed twelve weeks of treatments but also resulted in decreased waist size and even weight loss in some.[169] In one study, twenty-two volunteers ages nineteen to fifty-four were asked to feel the warmth of a towel on their chests, or to otherwise feel a sensation of warmth in their breasts. Then they were asked to feel a pulsation in their breasts, and to merge that with their heartbeat, allowing heart energy to flow into their breasts. They were instructed to practice this same imagery in their home once per day for twelve weeks. At the end of this time period, 85 percent experienced measurable breast enlargement (the average was 1.37 inches).[170] In this study, those who were good at visual imagery got better results, but even those who weren't good at it got results. It did not matter how small a woman's breasts were to begin with; the technique also worked for women over age fifty.

In another study, the subjects were asked to go back in time, while in a mild trance, to an age between ten and twelve, when breasts normally start to grow. The suggestions for this group included feeling swelling sensations, tightness of the skin over the breast, and slight tenderness. The subjects were asked to put their hands on their breasts during the sessions, and the suggestion was made that they could feel their hands being gently pushed upward as their breasts grew larger. Usually, the subjects' hands could be observed to rise a few inches off the chest during the course of the suggestions. The third component of the treatment consisted of telling the subject that she was at a point in time two to three years later. It was suggested that she imagine herself after a shower, standing nude in front of the bathroom mirror. She was asked to inspect her appearance, noting the larger and more attractive breasts that resulted from the posthypnotic suggestions. The authors of this and other studies suggest that the reason breasts may not have achieved their full growth potential in adolescence is because there was some adverse message the girl was receiving about her femininity or her breasts. In one study, the researchers worked with the study participants to clear this material, but not always successfully. In the first study, more than half of the subjects dropped out "for personal reasons"; obviously, using hypnosis to regress to this vulnerable time may be fraught with emotional peril for some women, though if a woman can work through this safely, the potential for emotional healing (and getting full breast development) exists.

In a third study of eight women, ages twenty-one to thirty-five, who underwent hypnosis, all gained from one to two inches in breast size except one woman who didn't want to be a female at all and instead wished she were a man. The greatest breast size gain in this study was made by the older women in the group who were married.

A recorded self-hypnosis session for breast size enhancement designed by certified clinical hypnotherapist Sarah Dresser is available on YouTube (see https://youtube/Ln7CRb-oA-s). The script is wonderful, and the beautiful voice is quite soothing. Additional MP3s of breast enlargement scripts from hypnotherapist Andrew Dobson, Ph.D., are also available at www.mind fithypnosis.com/downloads/breast-enlargement-hypnosis.

Clearly, if women can use the power of focused intent and visualization to change their breast size and consistency, we also have the power to maintain and create healthy breasts by imagining our breasts as healthy and beautiful. If our bodies are nothing but a field of ideas, let's make sure that those ideas represent our best interests.

One more thing: Breasts can be thought of as "heart pillows." They are very much influenced by the amount of love and touch they receive from a woman herself and from others. In fact, sex and relationship coach Kim Anami says that saggy breasts often become firmer and perk up when massaged and loved regularly. I've actually seen this happen, even though I certainly can't cite any studies on the matter. But it makes sense. Given that breasts are right in the heart chakra area, they certainly are directly influenced by the energy of love and pleasure. It is possible to regain your pre-nursing breast shape to a large extent through pleasurable breast massage, self-love, and hypnosis—which is nothing more than using the power of your mind in a positive way.

If You've Had Breast Cancer

A thirty-eight-year-old midwife whom I met at a conference had had a breast removed at the age of twenty-one. Instead of having reconstruction, she wore a prosthesis that could be removed. She said that in looking back, she realized that she had profoundly rejected her breasts early on in life because she'd been given the message since birth that she should have been a boy. She attributed her breast cancer to her chronic negativity about being female. Now, more than twenty years after her mastectomy, she has decided to discard her prosthesis. She told me that the "fake" breast created a block between her chest, her heart, and the loving energy that this part of her body needed to feel. She said that now when she gets a hug from someone, all of her chest gets in on that loving energy, too.

For many other women, breast reconstruction following mastectomy is a real blessing. If this is your truth, spend some moments regularly appreciating the work of the surgeon, combined with the healing power of your body. And with or without a breast implant, if you've had a mastectomy, touching your scar with respect and reverence is a help—an acknowledgment of your sacrifice and ongoing ability to flourish.

11
Our Fertility

A fertile, sexually active woman using no contraception would face an average of fourteen births or thirty-one abortions during her reproductive lifetime: altogether, a mind-boggling disruption in this period of hoped-for independence and equality for women.

—Luella Klein, M.D.

A broader vision of fertility is one that is not solely determined by whether or not one has a biological child. Fertility is a lifelong relationship with oneself—not a medical condition.

—Joan Borysenko, Ph.D.

*F*ertile. How does that word feel? It feels rich, juicy, yin, abundant—as in fertile fields, fertile minds. It conjures images of dewy youth and infinite possibilities. No wonder all women have a desire to be fertile, to know they could have a child if they wished. It is this feeling of being fertile, this potential within, that so many desire and identify with. Fertility is a form of female power, a power we must work with responsibly and consciously if we are to truly flourish. The number one predictor of a woman's status worldwide is whether or not she has dominion over her fertility. The ability to say when and how many when it comes to having babies is one of the most significant factors leading to the greatly expanded role of women in business, education, and self-development in the last fifty years.[1]

We have now reached a time in our planetary history when we must learn to procreate from our conscious choice, not just to fill up an empty space inside ourselves or to try to keep a man. These latter reasons for getting pregnant are remnants of an unconscious tribal programming that no longer serves us. The late writer and midwife Jeannine Parvati Baker described herself as both pro-choice *and* pro-life: When she was seventeen, she made a decision that she was ready to become sexually active. She also vowed that she would never make love with a man whose child she wouldn't willingly bear, should she become pregnant inadvertently. She says that it took her three years to find such a man. Now that is a powerful example of taking responsibility for what we create! Baker's story, like the stories of birthing women in chapter 12, are beacons for how women might be if they loved and appreciated their bodies and their creative capacities.

Ideally, prenatal life, close to the mother's heart, is bliss for the unborn. Women need to choose to live out their pregnancies wisely, because the way they do so affects both themselves and their offspring for generations to come. Though Sigmund Freud coined the term "infant amnesia" to explain the fact that most people don't consciously recall much that happened to them before the age of three, the truth is that our bodies always remember our life in the womb, birth, and early childhood. Parents have a huge influence on the mental and physical attributes of their children, and this influence starts long before birth and continues throughout life.[2]

All of us retain the imprint of our entire lives within our cells, starting before birth. It is well documented, for example, that we are influenced—for better or for worse—by emotional and genetic patterns handed down to us from those who came before. This has been described in detail by Mark Wolynn in his book *It Didn't Start with You: How Inherited Family Trauma Shapes Who We Are and How to End the Cycle* (Viking, 2016). The key here is how to end the cycle. And that's where each of us has more power than we realize.

Our lives begin in the water of amniotic fluid, our first environment. This period and early childhood are the critical times when most of our expectations and potential are created. Prenatal and birth memories, and their impact on the unborn, are among the many reasons why women must learn to manage their fertility well. We must become conscious vessels.

When a child perceives that she is loved and wanted from the very beginning, her sense of safety, security, and belonging creates an enormously resilient immune system as well as bone and blood health that set the stage for a lifetime of health. On the other hand, many women have told me that they knew their mother didn't want them, and that they had felt it their entire lives. "I know I was conceived during my mother's grief for a son who died nine months before," one woman said. "I remember taking this on in utero. I vowed to try to make it better for her. I've spent sixty-four years trying to do that for her. It has never worked." One menopausal woman, Beverly, said that her mother visited her on her fiftieth birthday with balloons and a rose, then proceeded to tell her, "You are fifty. Your life is downhill from now on.

You're not a kid anymore." She told her daughter how much she had suffered in giving birth to her, and how ugly Beverly had been when she was born. She went on to sing the praises of her son, Beverly's brother, saying that that labor had been virtually painless and that her son had been beautiful ever since birth. Listening to her mother, Beverly felt that in a perverse way she had been given a true gift on her fiftieth birthday. Her mother had confirmed what she had always thought—that she had been rejected since birth.

An existential depression can be felt by people who have been gestated and born under circumstances in which they are not wanted. One woman described feeling ashamed for breathing the air and for taking up space—she had a sense of never belonging, that she was causing someone else pain simply by being here. She told me that she knew she hadn't been wanted and had felt this as far back as she could remember. Another woman, a physician in her fifties, said that she recently had gone through an emotional healing session in which she realized that she had never felt safe in her mother's womb—that she knew she hadn't been wanted. She had been trying to compensate for this her whole life by studying, becoming a doctor, and having a series of relationships. But none of this ever fulfilled a need that had been within her since before she was born—the need to be well loved and desired as a child. As she recalled, "My mother's heartbeat, so close to my own, was *not* a comfort and reassurance to me." Though her mother is now dead, she had gone through the process of forgiving her. In tears she said to me, "Now I finally miss the mother I never had. I realize that she was doing the best she could. She never had a chance for herself."

ABORTION

For many women, abortion is an area of "unfinished business," and as such, it deserves a thorough discussion. If we lived in a culture that valued women's autonomy and in which men and women practiced cooperative birth control, the abortion issue would be moot. If abortion were forced on women in the United States as it has been in places like China, it would hold a different meaning here than it does now.[3]

According to Trudy M. Johnson, a licensed marriage and family therapist with twenty-five years of experience counseling women who are grieving what she calls VPT (voluntary pregnancy termination), 43 percent of women under the age of fifty-five have had voluntary pregnancy terminations. Thirty-eight percent of these are church members. That's 55 million women.

Abortion deliberately ends one potential life. But *not* allowing an abortion potentially murders two lives. The bond between mother and child is the most intimate bond in human experience. In this most primary of human relationships, love, welcome, and receptivity should be present in abundance. Forcing a woman to bear and raise a child against her will is therefore an act of violence. It constricts and degrades the mother-child bond and sows the seeds of hatred rather than love. Can there be any worse entry into the universe than forcing a child to inhabit a body that is hostile to it? Life is too valuable to inhibit its full blossoming and potential by forcing a woman to bear it against her will. Since we know that the early lives of criminals and societal offenders are often filled with poverty and despair, it may even be dangerous to bring a being into the world who isn't wanted. (In their best-selling book *Freakonomics* [William Morrow, 2005], authors Steven Levitt and Stephen Dubner hypothesize that the reduction in crime over the past few decades can be traced to the legalization of abortion.) The specter of more and more women trapped in unwanted pregnancies looms on the horizon as women's reproductive capacity is treated as political barter.

On some level, everyone knows this—even those who publicly would deny women the right to control their own fertility. During my residency in Boston, it was not uncommon for pregnant young Catholic women to be brought to me by their parents, who would say, "We don't believe in abortion, but if our daughter has this child, it could ruin her life. Can you arrange something?"

One thing I've learned over the years is that there is no such thing as sexual freedom. I think that's why I've always been uncomfortable with the phrase "abortion on demand." Having worked in the area of women's reproduction for years, I realize that the current abortion debate is a symptom of the much-deeper problem I described in earlier chapters: As long as women continue to misunderstand how to meet their erotic needs, as long as they continue to sacrifice their bodies for the sexual pleasure of men, we will get nowhere. And as long as abortion is seen solely as a "women's issue," we'll get nowhere.

I performed abortions for years, and I will always be a proponent of reproductive choice for women. But along the way I've come to see how complex the issue of abortion is, and I've learned that there are no easy answers.

Abortion is always a loaded topic because it forces each woman to face her deepest feelings about men's ability to impregnate women and women's power to either retain or reject the result of this impregnation. Abortion hits at the heart of our society's beliefs about the roles and worth of women and men. Is society committed to women's full participation in the economy? What is our appropriate role in the home and in society? "Abortion exemplifies political control of the personal and the physiological," writes historian Carroll Smith-Rosenberg. "It thus bridges the intensely individual and the broadly political. On every level, to talk of abortion is to speak of power."[4]

I always felt as though I were sitting in the middle of a minefield when I performed abortions. Sometimes I got angry when I performed a fourth abortion on a woman who simply didn't use contraception. At other times I'd perform abortions on women who really didn't want them but felt they had no alternative. Of course, many unintended pregnancies happen in women whose method of contraception failed, even though they used it religiously.

Numerous women who have had repeated abortions have told me they later came to realize that their sexual acting-out with men was a form of self-abuse, stemming from their self-loathing and lack of self-esteem. The number of unintended pregnancies in women who have access to birth control is the result of magical thinking that sex can be divorced from its consequences. We should be resisting *any* sexual contact with men who don't respect our souls and our innermost selves.[5] I also realize that in many parts of the world, this is simply not possible yet. But what if a society were willing to hold men accountable for their role in conception and to punish them accordingly for getting a woman pregnant who doesn't want to be? Think about it. Women can get pregnant only a couple of days per month. A healthy man can impregnate a woman 24/7 for his entire life. Talk about inequality! How is it that we continue to think of unwanted pregnancy as only a woman's issue?

At this time in history, many women are rethinking their sexual programming. The first step in this process is to get clear on what that programming is. When a woman chooses to terminate a pregnancy on behalf of herself and her own life, she is swimming against a 5,000-year-old tide of conditioning, of social agendas propounded by churches and other male-dominated institutions, all of which say that a woman's primary purpose is to have children and to serve her children and her husband. Allowing women to choose the course of their own lives goes very deeply against a very old grain.

Ever since the historic *Roe v. Wade* decision legalizing abortion in 1973, the number of women going against this grain has vastly increased. Hence the political and societal forces that want to "keep us in our place" have become more and more vocal—and more destructive. A century and a half of rhetoric designed to make women feel guilt and shame surrounding abortion and the choice of self-development over motherhood (at least for a time) leaves little wonder that abortion is not an easy issue for women to talk about freely. Yet if every woman who ever had an abortion, or even one-third of them, were willing to speak out about her experience—not in shame, but with honesty about where she was then, what she learned, and where she is now—this whole issue would heal a great deal faster. Trudy Johnson wrote *CPR: Choice Processing and Resolution* (Outskirts Press, 2009) to help women who have terminated their pregnancies by choice to process their grief. She points out that decades after abortion was made legal, it's still not okay for women to grieve about this experience without the spotlight of political or religious rhetoric. She writes, "There is no place or public venue to grieve an abortion loss in our culture. This type of grief is called disenfranchised grief. Women sit in silence out of fear of being misunderstood or further shamed. Who are these women? They are your mother, your sister, your girlfriend. Maybe even you."

Since the first edition of *Women's Bodies, Women's Wisdom,* many women have written to me expressing their gratitude that I have addressed this issue. And they have written about how their willingness to tell the truth about their abortion experience has healed them. The late Kris Bercov, who was a therapist offering abortion resolution counseling, wrote a poignant booklet (sad to say, now out of print) entitled *The Good Mother: An Abortion Parable.* When she sent me a copy, Kris wrote, "The abortion experience has tremendous potential to either wound or to heal—depending on how it is handled and interpreted. As you well know, so many women go through the experience unconsciously—leaving their bodies the challenging (and sometimes dangerous) task of communicating the women's unresolved feelings." That was certainly what I observed during the many years I performed abortions. Not having fully grieved a pregnancy termination can be a setup for pregnancy problems in the future.

Now, with the advent of the Internet, we finally have a way for women to end the isolation of grief and shame of abortion. (For resources and community, see Trudy Johnson's website at www.missingpieces.org.)

The cultural climate of any historical era can have profound effects on the overall emotional and physical well-being of that era's people. It is estimated that in the 1840s half of all pregnancies ended in abortion.[6] Currently, as women's power is rising, so is the antiabortion rhetoric. Though no culture at any time in history has been a stranger to abortion, Carroll Smith-Rosenberg's research documents that abortion becomes a political issue only when there are "significant alternations in the balance of power between women and men, and of male heads of household over their traditional dependents."[7] At just such a time, these changes are reflected in laws concerning women's right to manage their own fertility.

Healing Post-abortion Traumas

The technical aspects of the various abortion procedures are very simple and don't usually cause women any physical problems, though it is always somewhat of a shock to the body when the process of gestation is abruptly halted via outside intervention. All the studies done so far on the long-term health consequences of abortion, whether done by D&C, suction, or drugs, have failed to show an increase in infertility or any other problems. The anti-progesterone drug mifepristone (formerly known as RU486) is even safer than D&C or suction abortions. When it is used with misoprostol, a prostaglandin, its efficacy rate is 95.5 percent. This drug works to block the action of progesterone and is usually used within fifty days of a woman's last menstrual period. This medication can be administered confidentially in a healthcare practitioner's office, including at many Planned Parenthood clinics. In some states, it is possible to get a prescription for this pill in a clinic with no doctor present, via telemedicine. Typically with this option, a woman visits a clinic where a healthcare practitioner checks her vital signs and blood pressure and then performs an ultrasound. The information is sent to an off-site doctor, who then talks to the woman via videoconference before prescribing the medication. The woman can fill the prescription at a local pharmacy and take the medication at home, using on-call medical support if needed and following up with the clinic afterward. After the first telemedicine program for abortion was begun in Iowa in 2008, a study of nearly 20,000 patients showed the telemedicine service was just as safe and effective for abortion as meeting with a doctor in person.[8] Another three-year study of 1,000 women in Ireland (where abortion was until recently unavailable through the formal healthcare system) who used an online telemedicine service also showed the telemedicine option was safe and effective.[9] Medication abortions are a big step forward in women's health when you consider that worldwide about 43,000 women die each year as a result of not having access to safe and legal abortions,[10] and millions more suffer complications.[11] (See www.plannedparenthood.org.)

With decades of guilt and shame as an emotional backdrop, however, many women never adequately process the emotional aspects of abortion. Many have never even told another person that they had one. Not infrequently, a woman will tell me not to tell her husband about the abortion she had prior to their relationship because she doesn't want him to know about her sexual history. Through the years, I've heard many women's stories about illegal abortions—some of them painful, and some quite healing. Several older women, for example, have told me that they were raped by the abortionist before he performed the procedure—"just to relax you," he would tell them. Because they were so scared and so dependent upon his services, they simply went through the humiliation and said nothing about it for decades. Another woman who had gone through an illegal abortion said that she would be forever grateful to the wonderful man who did her procedure. She felt that his gentle touch and medical skill were a godsend to the many unfortunate women such as herself, in a time when choice wasn't available. May we never see that time again.

The physical results of a woman's shame and regret about abortion can live on in her cell tissue for years. This is one of the reasons why, when the supposed link between abortion and breast cancer was first reported, it seemed plausible; however, a 1996 study failed to substantiate this link.[12] But unresolved emotional pain does become physical and can set the stage for later gynecological problems such as fibroids and pelvic pain. Remember, it is the *meaning* surrounding an event or procedure that gives it its charge and potential to harm or heal—not necessarily the procedure itself. Despite the safety of abortion, I believe that repeated abortions weaken the *hara,* or body energy center, of the female.

The most difficult abortions I ever did were for those women who had already had one or two children and had homes and resources, but who found themselves pregnant at inconvenient times. I told one of these women, whose husband didn't want the pregnancy, that she might well find herself grieving after this abortion, since she clearly wanted the child and was having the procedure mainly to keep peace with her husband. She assured me that she had made a firm decision—that she was finished with car seats for infants and diapers and that she wanted to get on with her life. So I went ahead. Exactly one week later, this woman was back in the office crying, "Why didn't you tell me how bad I'd feel? Why didn't you talk me out of this procedure?" She decided that she wanted to get pregnant again as soon as possible, to "relieve her sense of loss."

Time and time again, women have abortions that they don't want because the men they are with insist upon it. Under these circumstances abortion is a self-betrayal, even a kind of self-rape. It can poison the relationship unless the issues are dealt with openly and honestly. The first step is for a woman to be totally honest with herself about how she really feels.

A patient of mine in her fifties developed continual spotting and an abnormal condition in her uterus called cystic and adenomatous hyperplasia of the endometrium, accompanied by pelvic pain. (See chapter 5.) This problem, she feels, was triggered by watching her daughter give birth to a girl and experiencing her husband's unconditional support for this birth. This birth experience caused her to feel a great deal of anger at her husband and a sense of deep sorrow—emotions that she couldn't understand intellectually. Later, after letting herself sit with these feelings, she realized that she still had unfinished business about an abortion she'd had years before that she hadn't wanted. Her husband hadn't been supportive of the pregnancy, so she had gone ahead with the abortion. Now, watching the same man fully support the birth of a grandchild, her old unprocessed grief came roaring back, to be felt and released.

In the mid-1980s, I stopped doing abortions. I was tired of mucking around in women's ambivalence about their fertility, and I was tired of performing repeated abortions on women who came back every year for the procedure. I needed to take a break from this arena and preferred to work on other aspects of the problem—like helping women understand their sexuality and their need for self-respect and self-esteem, regardless of whether they had a relationship with a man.

Unintended pregnancies will continue to occur. It's simply the nature of nature. And some women, particularly those whose boundaries have been violated in the past, do not yet have the strength or self-esteem to assume dominion over their own fertility and sexuality. We are still evolving on this point. Voluntary pregnancy termination will always be necessary. I will support its availability. Still, I look forward to the day when abortion is rare, when women and men in cooperation will conceive carefully, thoughtfully, and purposefully, and every child will be wanted and cared for.

Another View of Abortion

I first heard about communication with the unborn from Gladys McGarey, M.D., M.D.(H.), in her book *Born to Live* (Inkwell Productions, 2001). Dr. McGarey writes of her many years of delivering babies both at home and in the hospital. Her deeply spiritual approach to medicine and women's healthcare has been a great comfort and guide to me over the years, particularly as it relates to the abortion issue. She told me the following story: "I can see that abortion is frequently reasonable, understandable, and the 'right' thing to do. The new light dawned with a story one of my patients told me some time ago. This mother had a four-year-old daughter, named Dorothy, whom she would take out to lunch occasionally. They were talking about this and that, and the child would shift from one subject to another, when Dorothy suddenly said, 'The last time I was a little girl, I had a different mommy!' Then she started talking in a different language, which her mother tried to record.

"The magic moment seemed over, but then Dorothy continued, 'But that wasn't the last time. Last time when I was four inches long and in your tummy, Daddy wasn't ready to marry you yet, so I went away. But then, I came back.' Then, the mother reported, the child went back to chatting about four-year-old matters.

"The mother was silent. No one but her husband, the doctor, and she had known this, but she had become pregnant about two years before she and her husband were ready to get married. She decided to have an abortion. She was ready to have the child, but her husband-to-be was not.

"When the two of them did get married and were ready to have their first child, the same entity made its appearance. And the little child was saying, in effect, 'I don't hold any resentments toward you for having the abortion. I understood. I knew why it was done, and that's okay. So here I am again. It was an experience. I learned from it and you learned from it, so now, let's get on with the business of life.' "[13]

My own sister, the mother of three strong-willed and active sons, became pregnant inadvertently when she ovulated during her menstrual cycle—a rare event. She knew that the pregnancy was not right for her—in fact, she felt that it was actively *wrong* on all levels. So she began to work on communicating with the unborn baby, asking its soul to leave. She continued this inner work daily for two weeks. Still she remained pregnant. Finally, she called an abortion clinic to make an appointment, a step she had never dreamed that she would make. No sooner had she hung up the phone than the bleeding started. She miscarried later that day.

Stories such as this one shed a whole new light on the "morality" of abortion, not to mention parenting in general. And such stories reflect my belief that our souls choose our parents and the circumstances of our births. Caroline Myss is very clear that the energy of spirits remains behind after abortion and needs to be fully released. Many ancient traditional cultures acknowledge this as well. (See the story of a patient who went to a Native American shaman for healing around three past abortions that were still emotionally unresolved, in chapter 6.)

Years ago while I was attending an international meeting of the Association for Pre- and Perinatal Psychology and Health, I participated in a healing abortion ritual performed by Jeannine Parvati Baker, coauthor of *Conscious Conception* (North Atlantic Books, 1986). Baker had learned the ritual from a Native American medicine woman. All the women at the meeting who had had abortions and all those who had been deeply affected by them sat in an inner circle. Included in this latter group were a man whose mother had unsuccessfully tried to abort him and a man whose wife had aborted a child he had wanted. In an outer circle surrounding this one sat all of us who had ever seen or done an abortion. We were considered the "eyes" that had witnessed abortion. The outermost circle also included people whose friends and loved ones had had abortions. They were the "ears" that had witnessed abortion. Throughout an entire afternoon and into the evening, both men and women spoke of—and let go of—years of previously unvoiced personal pain surrounding abortion. Baker, representing a conduit between the worlds, helped release the energy of the aborted spirit. For many, it was a powerful healing.

Another powerful story about abortion comes from Sara Avant Stover, the author of *The Way of the Happy Woman* (New World Library, 2011) and *The Book of SHE* (New World Library, 2015). Sara also communicated with her unborn child, as she recounts in her touching and empowering story below:

> In April 2017, while leading a women's retreat in California, I received an email from a stranger named Amanda. She shared with me that she'd been sleeping with my partner, Jack, for the past nine months—beginning one month after we started dating. While Jack had led her to believe that he was single, she found out about me through his Facebook page and a subsequent Google search, where she read an article I'd published the previous week, announcing our pregnancy.
>
> After being bedridden with nausea for three months, I'd just en-

tered my second trimester. Throughout those months, I struggled. I was thirty-nine and my heart's deepest desire was to become a mother. When I found out I was (accidentally) pregnant, it seemed that my prayers had been answered. However, fear and doubt swelled inside me. I was in a brand-new relationship with a man who I wasn't yet certain I could entirely trust. Plus, despite the fact that I had guided countless women to connect with the souls of their children in utero, I couldn't for the life of me connect with the one growing inside of mine.

At eight weeks, I almost had an abortion. I'd gone so far as to schedule one, only to have it cancelled at the last minute when the doctor had her own medical emergency. Taking that as a sign, after much soul-searching, I decided to move forward with the pregnancy. I felt relieved, as abortion had always scared me. If I needed to, I would exclude Jack from the birth certificate and create a simple legal agreement with him stating that if we broke up, he would relinquish full custody to me.

After speaking with Amanda to confirm the truth of her testimony a couple of months later, while leading my retreat in California, I was thrust back into inner turmoil. I knew I had two choices: get full, legal custody and raise the baby on my own or terminate the pregnancy. I told Jack our relationship was over and asked him for custody of the baby. With shock and disgust, he replied: Absolutely not. Paternity rights in Colorado, where I lived at the time, are some of the most progressive in the country. Courts don't care about character disorders or infidelity. Unless there's concrete evidence of physical abuse or drug abuse, a father gets a minimum of 50 percent custody.

Over the next week, I gathered as much information as I could. I consulted with a traditional Chinese medicine doctor who had supported women in becoming pregnant again after second-trimester abortions. I met with a family lawyer who walked me through the challenges I would face—both financially and emotionally—without any guarantee of success, should I try to gain full custody. I met with my ob-gyn, who referred me to a women's health center where I could safely have a second-trimester abortion.

Simultaneously, more truth surfaced about Jack. It turned out that his good looks, his fun-loving nature, and the keen intellect that led him to be highly respected in his career were all a cover. Underneath his flawless external image, not only had he been sleeping with many other women and trying to win his ex-wife back while he was with me, but he also had a recent history of drug abuse and financial exploitation.

I concluded my long list of meetings with my mentor, who confirmed my suspicion. "Be careful, Sara," she warned. "From all you've shared here, it sounds like Jack shows strong sociopathic traits. Sociopaths feel no shame, remorse, or empathy. Literally, no behavior is off-limits for them."

Equipped with all the facts, I needed to make my decision within the next day. The clock was ticking, and waiting any longer would be harmful to both me and my baby. So I headed to bed, knowing it was time to turn inward and strive to make contact with my baby. Only once he told me what he wanted would I move forward. With my head propped up against a mound of pillows and my journal in my lap, I closed my eyes. Then I felt clarity—the clarity I always wait for before making any big decision—and along with it, the rinse of relief I experience when every part of me *harmonizes* and *knows*. A warm, powerful peace surrounded me. It was my son, greeting me for the first time. *My son!*

"Mom, I'm not supposed to be born," he told me. "You're meant to terminate this pregnancy. I came into your life to teach you some big lessons. I love you. It's okay." His voice boomed down into my guts and through my bones. Tears began to roll down my face—as they do now, writing these words just over one year later—tears of relief, tears of gratitude for being in the presence of such a great being, and tears for my and my son's fate. Tears calling me to trust the perfection of it all.

On my nightstand sat the small painting of Mother Mary that I received for my First Communion and have kept close by ever since. From the strength that only a mother's love holds, I knew that it was time to break my own heart and end my son's life. I invited my son to stay with me in spirit and to come back in a way that was best for him—whether that was to his father through another woman, to me at a time when we could have a happy life together, or to another family. As I cried myself to sleep, I set my son free, knowing he didn't need it. He was already Freedom itself.

In the year following my abortion, I learned just how challenging and messy recovering from the initiation of abortion can be. While my mind knew I was doing the right thing, it took time for my heart and body to catch up. What made the healing journey the most complicated, however, is the social stigma—and subsequent silence and invisibility—that surrounds abortion. In response to this, I partnered with the soul of my son to birth Redemption Circle (www.redemptioncircle.org), a nonprofit global movement to heal the stigma of abortion and create a support network to empower women to heal—physically, mentally, emotionally, and spiritually.

Each woman's situation is unique regarding whether to have or keep a pregnancy, and no one but that individual woman can or should decide. Whatever her choice is, however, there will be consequences. What is important is that each woman be clear that she had a choice.

EMERGENCY CONTRACEPTION:
ABORTION PREVENTION

Though emergency contraception has been available in the United States and Europe for more than twenty years as an off-label use of birth control pills, it wasn't until 1998 that the FDA first approved a standardized regimen that was safe and effective for preventing pregnancy. Now, emergency contraception is available in just one pill, which is effective if taken within 72 or 120 hours of unprotected intercourse (depending on which of two forms you take). The first emergency contraception on the market was Plan B, which contains levonorgestrel, a synthetic progestin found in birth control pills. Now several other brands containing levonorgestrel are also available (such as Aftera and Next Choice). These products are available over the counter (or on the Internet) and are safe and effective. It's estimated that they prevent pregnancy in about seven out of eight women who otherwise would have become pregnant and that regular use of emergency contraception could cut the number of unintended pregnancies and abortions in half.[14]

A newer form of emergency contraception called ella (Fibristal in Canada) prevents pregnancy if taken within 120 hours (five days) after having unprotected sex and has a higher effectiveness rate (preventing pregnancy in 98 out of 100 women as opposed to levonorgestrel's 87 to 88 percent). Ella, which contains ulipristal acetate (a selective progesterone receptor modulator, which prevents the effects of progesterone) instead of levonorgestrel, is available only by prescription in the United States but over the counter in Europe. However, if you need emergency contraception because you made an error taking a hormonal method of birth control, ella may be less effective than the pills containing levonorgestrel, and it can also make hormonal forms of birth control less effective, requiring the use of a barrier method of contraception, such as condoms, for the remainder of that cycle.

Emergency contraception prevents pregnancy by inhibiting or delaying ovulation or altering the lining of the uterus, making it inhospitable to implantation of an egg. It also alters sperm and egg transport. It does *not* cause abortion of an established pregnancy. However, if a woman needs emergency contraception, she should take a pregnancy test first. If she does not have an already established pregnancy, she should take the pill within 72 or 120 hours of intercourse (depending on which product you are taking), the sooner the better. Side effects include nausea in some patients. The vast majority of women will menstruate within twenty-one days after treatment. Having an IUD inserted soon after unprotected intercourse will also prevent pregnancy; I recommend this only for those who are at very low risk for sexually transmitted disease, are in a monogamous relationship, and will want to continue this birth control method.

CONSCIOUS CONCEPTION AND CONTRACEPTION

If you are contemplating pregnancy, think of yourself as a vessel for new life. Prepare your vessel with intent. Traditional Tibetan women have always spent time in prayer and meditation before conceiving. I believe that there are thousands of souls waiting to incarnate. Not all of them are highly evolved. When you raise your vibration through conscious prayer and meditation, alone or together with your partner, you make it more likely that you'll conceive a like-minded soul. So many women have told me that they have "felt" their child around them even before they became pregnant. You can conceive consciously even if you're considering single parenthood through donor insemination! The important point is to see your body as a channel for a new spirit and to surrender yourself to the experience—to be open to all that it has to teach you. A high-vibration soul isn't necessarily a physically perfect baby. One of my friends gave birth to the most incredible little boy ever. He was born with all kinds of so-called congenital defects and lived until he was four. But he opened her heart and the hearts of her entire family (who tended to be quite serious and scientific) in ways that were miraculous. (For those women who are considering single motherhood, I recommend the book *Single Mothers by Choice* [Harmony, 1994] by Jane Mattes, C.S.W. Another helpful resource is Emma Johnson's *The Kickass Single Mom: Be Financially Independent, Discover Your Sexiest Self, and Raise Fabulous, Happy Children* [TarcherPerigee, 2017], as well as her website www.wealthysinglemommy .com. A host of other online resources in support of single mothers is available, including www.singlemothers.us and www.singlemom.com.)

Conscious Contraception

All the currently available methods of birth control—pills, IUDs, diaphragms, condoms, and the rest—have their place. (See table 6, page 496.) Unfortunately, many healthcare practitioners do not present birth control methods objectively. Birth control pills have been pushed by the medical profession as the optimal method of contraception for the last fifty years, while the reliability of other methods—such as the diaphragm and/or condoms, as well as fertility awareness—has been downplayed. Given our cultural approach to control of the female body, and the reality that many women still don't have conscious dominion over their fertility, this is not surprising. The pill (and now the patch) is easy to prescribe, easy to use, very reliable, and very convenient. We can use it to manipulate our menstrual cycles, avoiding periods altogether or on weekends. In short, it fits our cultural ideal. The pill is the most-studied medication in history. Unfortunately, because it's made from synthetic non-bioidentical hormones, it has more side effects than it should. Though we have the science and technology to make safer oral contraceptives from bioidentical hormones, there is no profit in doing so—and therefore no support for it. None is currently available.

Most other birth control methods require more education about the body and more active participation than the pill. They are not geared to the average busy doctor's schedule. Many physicians feel that women will not use barrier methods of contraception, such as diaphragms, condoms, or contraceptive foam, because they have seen too many "failures." This is true of some women but not all women. The data show that in the women who are ideal users—who use the method correctly every time—barrier methods and even "fertility awareness" (natural family planning) can be 95 to 98 percent effective.[15]

It is important to distinguish between the failure of a birth control method itself and the failure of a woman to use it properly. Many women are socialized to be available for sexual intercourse without involving their partners in contraceptive responsibility. Many women are involved with men who will not cooperate with contraception and feel that it is the woman's job. Though I'd like to suggest that it is not worth having sex with such men, I know that this is not always an option—especially in the all-too-common situation when domestic violence is an issue. Obviously, it is best for women in this situation to use a contraceptive method that requires no male cooperation. Such methods include birth control pills, the birth control patch, implants, NuvaRing, the IUD, Depo-Provera, tubal ligation, and the female condom known as FC2, which is available online or at Planned Parenthood.

Methods that require conscious partner participation, such as condoms, simply are not appropriate for these women. In fact, in one study, when the Philadelphia Department of Public Health offered a choice of birth control to a group of low-income women, the majority chose the female condom because this method gives more control over their risk of pregnancy and infection than they otherwise would have experienced.

In order to choose the right birth control method for you, you need to decide *honestly* where you are in your own life—and how much responsibility you are willing to assume over your fertility. Some women don't even want to think about getting to know their times of ovulation and checking their cervical mucus, let alone inserting a diaphragm before each intercourse. That's fine—they often do well on the pill or another "automatic" method. Other women prefer barrier methods, such as diaphragms, and I encourage these methods, too—but only in those women who are committed to using them conscientiously. I've worked repeatedly with women who've had three or four abortions because they refuse to use what they call "unnatural" contraceptives. I counsel that there is nothing natural about abortion when a woman fails to use her "natural" method of birth control conscientiously. These women, though conscious about food and the environment, often suffer from the mind/body split we've all inherited—that it is part of being a desirable woman to be available sexually, without asking our partners to share in the responsibility. This is a shame, particularly given that there are so many ways to express oneself sexually without the risk of unintended pregnancy. (See chapter 8.) I recommend that all women make every effort to put their own sexual and fertility needs first in every relationship. Doing so takes courage and support.

Intrauterine Device

The intrauterine device (IUD) is a good choice for some women and is now making a comeback after falling from favor for several decades. It carries an increased risk of pelvic infection for some, but many have done beautifully with it for twenty years or more. The downside is that IUDs are associated with an increased risk of tubal pregnancy. They are also associated with increased cramping and bleeding in some women. They work best for women who've had a child, though that isn't always necessary. Although there used to be some dangerous IUDs on the market (the infamous Dalkon Shield caused pelvic inflammatory disease in so many women that it was taken off the market in 1974), IUDs were redesigned in the 1990s, resulting in far safer products now available (but underutilized, given their safety and effectiveness).

Combined Hormone Methods

Oral Contraceptives (The Pill)

Oral contraceptives have been a boon for many women, though they may contribute to suboptimal nutrition and an increased incidence of yeast infection in many (the pill has been associated with lowered serum levels of B vitamins and other metabolic changes).[16] It is also associated with a slightly increased risk for cervical adenocarcinoma,[17] elevated triglyceride levels,[18] and systemic lupus erythematosus.[19] Women on the pill are also at a higher risk of depression,[20] and while there may be several different reasons for this, recent research shows that the pill interferes with biological pathways that regulate the immune system (which includes mood-altering hormones like serotonin).[21] In fact, a recent review of hundreds of studies found good evidence that the use of hormonal contraceptives (including the pill, implants, and vaginal rings) is associated with an increased risk for several serious autoimmune diseases (such as Crohn's disease, lupus, and interstitial cystitis) as well as other less common autoimmune disorders.[22]

Although the announcement didn't get much press in the United States, the World Health Organization has classified birth control pills with combined estrogen and progestin (as well as combined-hormone HRT) as carcinogenic. (The latest such designation came after the cancer research agency of the World Health Organization convened a group of twenty-one scientists from eight countries in France in June 2005. Reviewing the scientific literature on the pill and cancer, the group pointed to evidence for an increase in cervical cancer, breast cancer, and liver cancer in making its decision, while also stressing that convincing evidence existed for a protective effect against endometrial and ovarian cancers.)[23] Yet other authorities don't think the slightly increased relative risk for breast cancer is significant.[24] In fact, recent research following 1.8 million Danish women for an average of 10.9 years shows only a small increase in risk among women under age fifty taking the pill, a risk amounting to about one extra case of breast cancer annually per 7,700 users.[25] In addition, the pill has been shown to reduce the risk of ovarian and endometrial cancer in postmenopausal women by one-third as well as offer protection against colorectal cancer, for a total effect of modestly reducing the total incidence of cancer.[26]

In my experience, however, the pill is associated with mood swings, weight gain, and decreased sex drive in many women. Going off the pill makes many women feel much better, although not all symptoms always subside. Ironically, some research has shown that oral contraceptives might actually contribute to long-term sexual dysfunction in some women. The January 2006 issue of the *Journal of Sexual Medicine* reported that the pill lowers levels of testosterone, even after the women have stopped taking oral contraceptives. Such problems occur because pill users have elevated levels of a protein called sex hormone binding globulin (SHBG) that binds testosterone, rendering it unavailable for use by the body. Such low values of "unbound" testosterone potentially lead to side effects such as decreased desire, arousal, and lubrication and increased sexual pain. Although the research showed that such problems persisted even after the pill was discontinued (a result of the continued elevation in SHBG), long-term studies are still needed to determine if the problems are permanent.[27] It is very important that physicians whose patients complain of sexual problems related to the pill take these problems seriously and not chalk them up to psychological issues.

Health benefits of the pill include lowered risk of ovarian cancer, endometrial cancer, acne, and pelvic inflammatory disease. In general, the pill's benefits outweigh its risks for the vast majority of women because the health risks from unintended pregnancies far outweigh any risk from the pill. Women who are on the pill should take a good multivitamin-mineral supplement containing B complex. The majority of women who have serious health problems with the pill are smokers. Smokers should not use the pill after the age of thirty-five. Oral contraceptives are now being used for women right up until menopause, at which time these same women may start on estrogen replacement therapy. Such women are on chemical birth control or hormone replacement for most of their adult lives. When a woman uses hormones in this way, she misses out on the messages she'd normally get from her uterus and ovaries (as discussed in chapters 6 and 7).

Note that the antibiotic rifampin, certain psychiatric and anti-seizure drugs, some oral antifungals prescribed for yeast infections, and certain HIV protease inhibitors may interfere with the effectiveness of oral contraceptives.

The Ring (NuvaRing)

The contraceptive ring, approved by the FDA in 2001, is a flexible ring about two inches in diameter that is inserted into the vagina and held in place by the muscles in the vaginal wall. The ring is worn continually for three weeks (including during sex) and then it's removed for seven days to allow a menstrual period. After seven days, a new ring is inserted.

Like the pill, the ring contains low doses of estrogen and progestin, which are absorbed by the walls of the vagina and distributed throughout the bloodstream in a steady supply to suppress ovulation. Because users don't have to remember to take a pill at the same time each day, women who use the ring have fewer hormonal ups and downs. As with the pill, users also experience more regular, lighter, and shorter menstrual periods, and fertility returns quickly after use of the product is stopped. When used as directed, the effectiveness rate is 99 percent.

Initial side effects are similar to those of the birth control pill and include weight gain or loss, nausea, moodiness, and breast tenderness. However, some users have also reported increased vaginal discharge, vaginitis, and irritation. The biggest and most frightening risk is getting blood clots that can result in pulmonary embolism and death. Some studies suggest that the type of progestin used in this product has more risk than the low-dose pills on the market. As with the pill, women over the age of thirty-five who smoke should not use this form of birth control.

As with oral contraceptives, certain medicines—including the antibiotic rifampin, certain drugs used to treat mental illness or to control seizures, certain oral antifungals prescribed for yeast infections, or certain HIV protease inhibitors—may make the ring less effective. (For more information, see www.nuvaring.com.)

The Patch

The birth control patch, also approved by the FDA in 2001, is applied to the upper arm, upper torso, abdomen, or buttocks, and replaced once a week for three consecutive weeks. It's then removed for one week to allow a menstrual period. Like the ring, the patch delivers a steady flow of estrogen and progestin absorbed into the bloodstream to prevent ovulation. It's also 99 percent effective when used correctly.

Most side effects are similar to those of the pill, although trials showed that breast discomfort and dysmenorrhea are significantly more common in women using the patch than in those using the pill. Also, estrogen levels in women who use the patch (both the original patch, Ortho Evra, and the generic version, Xulane, that took Ortho Evra's place in 2014) are 60 percent higher than estrogen levels in women taking standard birth control pills. The increased estrogen may raise the risk of blood clots (some of which are fatal) and may also, after several years of use, cause other side effects as well. Studies are currently looking into the risks of this higher estrogen level.[28] As an answer to the concerns about the effects of this higher level of estrogen, a new low-dose patch called Twirla has been developed by Agile Therapeutics that releases about half the amount of estrogen compared with previous patches. As of 2019, however, this product is still working to receive FDA approval and so is not yet on the market. Some women also report an increase in depression, changes in sexual desire, and a skin reaction at the site where the patch is applied.

The patch may also be less effective for women weighing over 198 pounds, those taking St. John's wort, or those using the same medications listed above that make the contraceptive ring less effective. And as with the ring and birth control pills, women on the patch who smoke are at greater chance for cardiovascular problems.

Progestin-Only Contraceptives

Depo-Provera (an injection that's given every twelve weeks) and Nexplanon (a contraceptive implant, the next generation of the Implanon implant) both have synthetic progestins as their active ingredient. Nexplanon is a thin and flexible plastic implant (about the size of a matchstick) that is inserted under the skin of the upper arm using local anesthesia. It protects against pregnancy for up to three years.

Synthetic progestin of all kinds can result in headache, bloating, and irritability in some women. This last effect is so common that a professor of ob-gyn with an interest in natural hormones once remarked, "It's no wonder Depo-Provera works for birth control. It makes women so ornery, they don't want anyone near them." A 2009 study showed that about one-quarter of Depo-Provera users experienced more than a 5 percent weight increase within the first six months of use. This weight gain was specifically linked to increased abdominal fat, a known marker for metabolic syndrome, which in turn is associated with increased risk for cardiovascular disease, stroke, and diabetes.[29] Irregular spotting and acne are other problems with these methods. On the other hand, they are highly effective and "automatic" compared with other methods, and they work well for some women.

Note: Most IUDs also contain synthetic progestin, which may have some of the same side effects as above. Mirena and Liletta are effective for up to seven years, Kyleena for up to five years, and Skyla for up to three years.

Barrier Methods

A wide range of barrier contraceptive methods is available. Condoms have the distinct advantage of protecting individuals from STDs. Many couples alternate between condoms and diaphragm use, thus sharing responsibility for contraceptives. See table 6 (page 496) for a list of barrier contraceptive options, all of which have their place.

Outercourse

Outercourse is just about any form of sex play that does not involve intercourse, making pregnancy impossible (as long as care is taken that no semen gets onto the vulva or in the vagina). Some of the most common forms include oral sex and manual stimulation, which can be just as satisfying—and sometimes more satisfying—than intercourse. Activities such as erotic massage, fantasy, role-playing, and the use of vibrators or other sex toys also fall into this category. As long as it eliminates exchange of bodily fluids, outercourse also reduces the risk of sexually transmitted diseases. Another big benefit of outercourse is that it can enhance orgasm because, like foreplay, it helps build excitement. (See Steve Bodansky and Vera Bodansky's book *Extended Massive Orgasm* [Hunter House, 2000] for great instructions.)

Fertility Awareness: Natural Birth Control

My colleague Joan Morais taught natural birth control at the University of California, Davis for years. She wrote, "The most common response I have gotten when I tell people I am a fertility awareness instructor is 'Is this the method that Catholics have used that doesn't work?' They presume it is the old and unreliable rhythm method that Catholics used many years ago. They have already made up their minds that it sets women back a hundred years and takes away our reproductive freedom. I can relate, as I also used to think this. I opposed natural family planning and I thought the birth control pill was the best thing ever. I took the birth control pill on and off until my late twenties. I didn't do well on it. I couldn't feel my cycles. I couldn't feel my body! I became depressed and I lost my libido. Somewhere inside me I had an innate wisdom that was telling me that the birth control pill wasn't right for me.

"There is another way besides chemical contraceptives, devices, and sterilization. Fertility awareness is a beautiful way that allows a woman to feel her cycles as she wanes or waxes while also preventing pregnancy. This fundamental knowledge of a woman's fertility and infertility should be taught to every menstruating girl and woman. It is our birthright. These are the operating instructions of our female body that somehow got thrown out along the way. Fertility awareness includes natural birth control, knowing your cyclical body, your menstrual cycle, your reproductive health, and your fertility and infertility. To know how to prevent pregnancy naturally or to consciously know when you can become pregnant is the most profound and empowering knowledge a woman can learn. There are only five days a month a woman may become pregnant, yet we medicate our bodies twenty-four hours a day, three hundred and sixty-five days a year. This is like medicating our body every day to prevent a monthly headache."[30]

Though it's not well known, fertility awareness and natural family planning are well studied and very effective.[31] Joseph Stanford, M.D., a family physician and expert in natural family planning, defines fertility awareness or fertility appreciation as "the use of physiologic signs and symptoms of the menstrual cycle to define the fertile and infertile phases of the menstrual cycle. This information can be used for natural family planning or the diagnosis and treatment of infertility." Fertility awareness involves learning how to determine your time of ovulation. While studies have shown that some symptoms associated with ovulation in some women, such as breast tenderness, mittelschmerz (midcycle pain associated with ovulation), and change in the position of the cervix, may not be accurate indicators of ovulation, there are reliable techniques for assessing the fertile phase. These include cervical mucus checks, observation of vaginal discharge of cervical mucus, or measurement of basal body temperature (BBT).[32] Observation of cervical mucus, combined with monitoring BBT and other symptoms that occur around ovulation, is called the symptothermal method of natural family planning. But in a comparative study of fifteen different methodologies, including variations of the most common methods used to determine ovulation, it was found that the observation of vaginal discharge alone, known as the Ovulation Method, was the most precise and practical way to determine time of fertility.[33] (The addition of basal body temperature graphs did not improve accuracy over the mucus discharge alone.) Commercially available ovulation indicators that test urine pre- and postovulation are also available in most pharmacies, but it is much easier, and cheaper, to learn how to determine your own ovulatory time from changes in cervical mucus.

Fertility awareness techniques (with or without barrier contraceptives during ovulation) can be a highly effective means of birth control. The Ovulation Method has been studied most rigorously at Creighton University in Omaha, Nebraska. Three major studies show that the effectiveness of the method for avoiding pregnancy can be 99.1 to 99.9 percent, while actual user rates ranged from 94.8 to 97.3 percent. The differences in these figures were attributable to teaching- and use-related errors.[34]

Newer methods of determining ovulation have recently been developed that are similarly precise. Most notably, women are increasingly turning to

technology to determine fertility. An app called Natural Cycles (www
.naturalcycles.com), developed in Europe, allows the user to take her temperature (under the tongue) first thing in the morning with the included thermometer and load this data into the app. The app then lets her know what
days are considered "red" (avoid intercourse) and which ones are considered
"green" (unprotected sex won't result in pregnancy). Ideal use achieves
99 percent effectiveness (93 percent with typical use), and this method has no
side effects.[35] Natural Cycles is now an FDA-approved method in the United
States.

Daysy is a similar product that can be used with or without the accompanying app (usa.daysy.me). After using the special thermometer to take
your temperature in the morning, the device lights up red (for fertile), flash-
ing red (for ovulating that day), yellow (for days when Daysy is still learning
your cycle variations, so it's possible you're fertile), or green (for not fertile).
Daysy is 99.4 percent accurate and is based on data from 5 million menstrual
cycles and an algorithm developed from more than thirty years of research,
plus clinical studies.[36]

Another reliable app, OvuSense (www.ovusense.com), provides a sensor
that is worn in the vagina overnight. The user removes it each morning and
then records its data in the app. OvuSense is more accurate than either urine
or basal body temperature taken under the tongue because it takes temperature measurements every five minutes, indicating the subtle temperature elevation from rising progesterone levels that precede ovulation. Because
everyone's fertility imprint is a bit different, it works even for those with irregular cycles or PCOS. OvuSense predicts ovulation up to twenty-four
hours in advance with 99 percent accuracy.

It is important to keep in mind that with all fertility apps such as these,
women counting on them for birth control should know how fertility awareness works instead of relying solely on the app to determine fertile and non-
fertile times.[37] Several factors can affect accuracy, including variation in the
time temperatures are taken, poor sleep, stress, and alcohol. They may not be
as accurate for women with irregular or anovulatory cycles or with endometriosis. Fertility awareness apps are a great step forward and can be an extremely valuable tool, but as with any other tool, knowing the right way to
use it and what its possible limitations are is important.

I also highly recommend the book *Taking Charge of Your Fertility*
(HarperCollins, 2015; originally published in 1995) and the charting apps
developed by world-renowned fertility awareness specialist Toni Weschler.
Her fertility awareness app, OvaGraph, allows for individual preferences
and personally tailored formatting, forecasting, charting, and reporting. Plus
there's a community section that allows women to share information with
one another. (See www.tcoyf.com.)

The advantage of becoming familiar with your fertility cycles—whether through getting to know your own body or using an app to assist with this awareness—is that you will be able to tell beforehand when you are becoming fertile. This is very empowering, and it helps women embrace their fertility when they want to conceive and avoid conceiving when they don't wish to become pregnant. Dr. Stanford told me, "When a couple uses this method, they often develop a deep respect for each other, for their fertility, and for their sexuality. This enhances all aspects of the relationship. It is a spiritual thing."

Fertility awareness techniques that let you know when you ovulate also can enhance chances of conception considerably. It is generally accepted that the probability of conceiving in one cycle for couples with normal fertility is in the range of 22 to 30 percent. But in one study of couples using fertility-focused intercourse, 71.4 percent of the clients who had a previous pregnancy achieved pregnancy in the first cycle. With those clients who had never had a pregnancy, the rate was 80.9 percent. By the fourth cycle, 100 percent of those who had never been pregnant had conceived.[38]

In couples who are having difficulty conceiving, using the Ovulation Method alone without any other testing can considerably enhance the chances of conception. Dr. Stanford notes that "of couples referred to the NFP [natural family planning] center at Omaha for inability to achieve pregnancy [for an average of three years], 20 to 40 percent have achieved pregnancy within six months of use of the Ovulation Method, before any further medical evaluation and treatment is undertaken."[39] The Ovulation Method also works well for those who have irregular periods, are breast-feeding, or are perimenopausal.

I strongly recommend fertility awareness to all women who want to strengthen their relationship with their bodies and truly understand their fertility cycles. Obviously, introducing fertility consciousness into the whole area of sexuality and working with it daily is a pretty new concept for many. Adequate personalized instruction by qualified teachers—or online communities—is essential for the successful use of fertility awareness. It is not learned well from a book, most likely because of the emotional and psychological issues it brings up. The quality of a woman's (or couple's) experience with this method often depends upon the quality of instruction given, the motivation of the individual, and the follow-up care received.

Couples who use fertility awareness effectively throughout their reproductive lives experience no side effects and often find an increased intimacy in their relationships, which includes a shared responsibility for their combined fertility. Though we tend to associate interest in natural family planning with certain religions, many women are drawn to this method because it is, inherently, a holistic approach to fertility. I suspect that if fertility awareness were more widely known and supported by healthcare professionals, it would be more widely used. Whether or not you use fertility awareness for contraceptive or conception purposes, it is empowering to know your fertility cycle. Here's a brief overview of the method.

Defining the Fertile Phase. The egg lives anywhere from six to twenty-four hours after ovulation. But sperm can live for up to five days in fertile mucus, which means that sperm deposited up to five days before ovulation actually occurs can cause a pregnancy. (Without fertile mucus, they die in a few hours.) Therefore, there is about a seven-day time period during every cycle when pregnancy is at least theoretically possible. One study found that among healthy women trying to conceive, nearly all pregnancies could be attributed to intercourse during a six-day period ending on the day of ovulation. Though no one in the study conceived on the day after ovulation, the authors of the study concluded that there was probably a 12 percent chance of conceiving on the day after ovulation and also on the seventh day before ovulation. The study also concluded that for those couples trying to conceive, having intercourse every other day was just as effective as every day. Practically speaking, if you are trying to get pregnant, have intercourse four times during your most fertile week. This is usually more effective, and less stressful, than trying to stick to an every-other-day schedule.[40] It has been my experience, however, that despite the best information science has to offer, sometimes when a soul is meant to come in, it will—no matter what you do or don't do.

Mucus Checks (Natural Birth Control). Studies have shown that almost all women can easily learn to check for the presence or absence of fertile E-type (estrogen-stimulated) mucus by the routine observation of vaginal discharge on the vulva.[41] As menstruation stops, cervical mucus is at a minimum. You feel dry. There is no mucus in the vaginal opening and no discharge on your underwear. This lack of mucus is associated with being infertile. These "dry" days are usually safe for unprotected intercourse. The cervix begins secreting E-type mucus about six days prior to ovulation, so, using this method, you will know when ovulation is apt to occur before it happens. When you see mucus on your underwear or can wipe it off with toilet paper, you know your fertile time is beginning. E-type mucus, when looked at under the microscope, contains channels that help the sperm swim up through the cervix. It also dries into a characteristic ferning pattern. Fertile mucus is similar in feel and quality to uncooked egg white. Some women may even notice that it wets their underwear. You are fertile from the time when fertile mucus first appears until the fourth day after your peak mucus discharge. The last day of any mucus that is clear, stretchy (greater than or equal to one inch of stretch between thumb and index finger), or lubricative is called the peak day of mucus discharge. This peak mucus day is highly correlated with ovulation, which occurs plus or minus two days from this peak day more than 95 percent of the time.[42]

FIGURE 18: FERTILITY AWARENESS:
OVULATION AND BASAL BODY TEMPERATURE

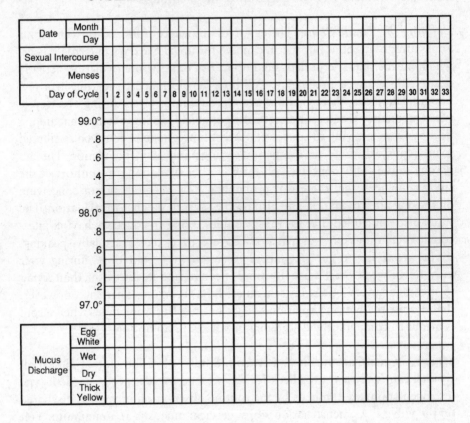

G-type mucus (progesterone-stimulated) appears immediately after ovulation. This type of mucus lacks elasticity. It also has an opaque and adhesive quality. G-type mucus, when looked at under the microscope, lacks the channels that facilitate the swimming of sperm. This type of mucus actually blocks the passage of sperm. Following ovulatory mucus discharge, cervical mucus may cease (you become dry) or become thicker and more dense (G-type mucus). Either way, the change is distinct and noticeable. Your period will start about twelve to fifteen days after the peak ovulatory cervical flow.[43]

As already mentioned, saliva also changes cyclically with your hormonal cycle. As your hormones change during your cycle, your saliva, when dry, develops a special microscopic ferning pattern that matches that of the cervical mucus. Special small microscopes are available and widely used in Europe and Japan as yet another way for women to learn about and therefore make the best use of their fertility cycle, whether the goal is to conceive or avoid pregnancy.

FIGURE 18: FERTILITY AWARENESS:
OVULATION AND BASAL BODY TEMPERATURE

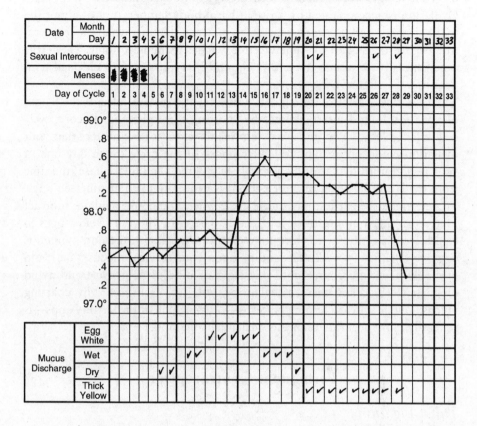

***Keep a Record of Your Basal Body Temperature for Three Months to See if
You Are Ovulating.*** Though learning how to assess your cervical mucus is
also accurate, taking your basal body temperature and recording it for a few
cycles is an empowering way to learn about your body and its internal
rhythms. It also enhances your ability to correlate your cervical mucus and/
or salivary changes with ovulation.

The temperature rise that occurs with ovulation is due to the effect of
progesterone. (You can use any of the apps mentioned above to track this.)
If you become pregnant during the period in which you have been taking
your basal body temperature, you will notice that it stays up and doesn't
drop down again. This elevation of BBT is a very early sign of pregnancy.
(When women are pregnant, they have a great deal of progesterone in their
systems and their temperature is higher than in the nonpregnant state. Pregnancy was the only time I could comfortably swim in the ocean in Maine.)

Take your basal body temperature first thing each morning starting on
the first day of your menstrual period. (This is considered day one of your

cycle.) Do this for three cycles, and chart each cycle separately. You can then use your temperature graph to record cervical mucus and salivary changes. Ovulation is accompanied by a rise in basal body temperature of about 0.6 to 0.8 degrees, and it occurs somewhere between the time when the temperature begins to rise and the time when it reaches its highest point. The fertile time generally is over at the end of the third day in a row of elevated temperature. (See figure 18.)

If your cycles are quite regular, you can get a general idea of the length of your fertile and infertile times by charting the following: Record cycle length for at least six months to determine the earliest possible day that your ovulation could occur. The follicular phase of the cycle (from day one of your period until ovulation) is variable in length. The luteal phase (the time from ovulation to onset of your period) is generally fixed at fourteen days. To determine the earliest day of the cycle when you could ovulate, subtract fourteen from your shortest cycle length. Therefore, if your cycle ranges in length from twenty-six to thirty-one days, the earliest you could ovulate is day twelve (26 − 14 = 12). Depending upon your cervical mucus, you could probably have intercourse until day eight or nine of your cycle and avoid pregnancy. (In doing these calculations, you can easily see why charting mucus flow or salivary ferning patterns—or using one of the fertility apps—is generally more accurate than this "calendar" method.)

Permanent Contraception

Tubal Ligation

Tubal ligation is the most common form of permanent contraception in the United States. Many women are ambivalent about it, however, even when they know intellectually they don't want more children. Most of us value the *ability* to conceive, even if we choose not to use that ability. Permanent contraception closes a door that usually cannot be reopened. For centuries, women were valued solely for their ability to bear children, and bearing children has been the most important socially acceptable outlet for women's creative power. Voluntarily giving up this capacity stirs primitive fears. Yet many women find that being free of the fear of pregnancy is health-enhancing and rejuvenates their sexuality.

Tubal ligation is an excellent choice for some women—but not all. I chose this procedure after waiting until my younger daughter was four. Somehow, though there is no logic to it, this made me feel that she was "safe" and "permanent." At about the age of thirty-seven, my path was split in front of me in terms of childbearing. I knew that having another child would mean at least another five years of energy diverted to the needs of the child and away from my own pursuits. I still went mushy sometimes looking at babies in airports, and I harbored a secret fantasy of having the ideal pregnancy and the ideal labor, in which I would rest and really enjoy the pregnancy *and* the new baby—things I had not done fully with my other two children.

But I had seen far too many women become pregnant "accidentally" in their late thirties and early forties, just as their lives were settling down after a decade or so devoted to the demands of raising children. I was at a point where I had to make a conscious choice one way or the other about having another child. I wouldn't have had an abortion if I became pregnant at this time in my life. (If I had become pregnant during my training years, however, I would have had an abortion without hesitation.) Still, I didn't want a pregnancy just to happen. I wanted to be a conscious decision-maker, not have my life decided by "fate."

My husband and I made our decision together. Though the final choice was mine, we both realized that we didn't really want more children. After that, making the decision to have a tubal ligation was not difficult. Even though vasectomy is technically easier to perform, in the event that I acquired another sexual partner one day through a change of circumstances, I wanted to be sure I would not get pregnant. Besides, I had performed many tubal ligations and felt comfortable with the procedure. (Other couples feel much more comfortable with vasectomy. It is safer and cheaper than tubal ligation.)

A tubal ligation changes the blood supply to the ovaries somewhat. There may even be a slight risk of an earlier menopause following tubal ligation if the blood supply to the ovary becomes severely compromised, but this is rare. Some women develop "post-tubal-ligation syndrome," an ill-defined problem characterized by increased cramping, irregular periods, and heavier bleeding. (Many studies do not show this effect, so its existence is controversial.) This is mostly a problem for women who have been on the pill prior to their tubal surgery and haven't experienced natural periods for years. Indeed, they may have developed bleeding problems anyway when they went off the pill, not necessarily *because* of the tubal ligation. Tubal ligation may even be somewhat protective against ovarian cancer.[44]

Tubal ligation lowers progesterone secretion significantly, and even a year after the ligation, these levels may not recover fully to what they were previously. The menstrual pattern isn't affected, however.[45] These data certainly do explain, in part, why some women develop PMS following a tubal ligation.

ESSURE: FROM GODSEND TO NIGHTMARE

The first permanent method of birth control for women that doesn't involve surgical incisions or general anesthesia, called Essure, was approved by the FDA in 2002—and then taken off the market in January 2019. This office procedure was just as effective as tubal ligation and was performed in the doctor's office in about half an hour. The procedure involved a doctor inserting a small scope through the vagina, cervix, and uterus and using it to place a tightly coiled spring-like device 1 or 2 millimeters long into each fallopian tube. (They are about the size of the springs in a Bic pen.) Most women could return to their normal activity the same day or the next day. The body would then start to develop scar tissue around the coil, which became thick enough to fully block the fallopian tubes in about three months (so an alternative method of birth control was necessary until the physician confirmed that the scarring was sufficient).

In addition to the benefits of not requiring anesthesia and a hospital stay, Essure didn't block the blood supply in the tube or interfere with the blood supply to the ovary at all. Another plus was that it was available to women who weren't good candidates for tubal ligation, such as those who are obese, those with previous multiple abdominal surgeries, and those with heart disease or other contraindications to general anesthesia. I was initially so enthusiastic about this device that I visited a local ob-gyn office to see the procedure myself.

Over time, however, the initial enthusiasm of many of us diminished once the FDA began receiving complaints related to the device, complaints that now number more than 16,000. Reported problems have included chronic pelvic pain, headache, fatigue, allergic reactions, hair loss, and more. In October 2016, the FDA approved a new label for Essure that included a black-box warning, noting risk for implant perforation, device migration, allergic reaction, pain, and other possible adverse effects. In April 2018, the agency restricted Essure's sale and distribution by adding a new requirement that doctors review a checklist of potential risks with patients (and that both doctor and patient sign an acknowledgment that this review had taken place) before the device was implanted. At the same time, Bayer, Essure's manufacturer, was also ordered to begin conducting a three-year post-market study to determine heightened risks for particular women. Sales plummeted, and three months later, once 16,000 lawsuits had been filed against the company, Bayer announced it would no longer sell or distribute Essure after December 31, 2018. The FDA assures women who still have the implant that they do not need to have it removed as long as they are not having problems.

Some of Essure's complications appear to be related to adverse reactions to the nickel the inserts contain, which causes autoimmune problems in susceptible women. Some women have even required a hysterectomy to retrieve the device. More than 35,000 women have detailed their adverse experiences in a Facebook group expressly set up to share such experiences. *The Washington Post* did an investigative report on the device in 2017.[46]

Bottom line: The vast majority of women who underwent the Essure procedure appear to be happy with it and have no issues. However, for those in whom it caused an adverse reaction, it's an entirely different story. If you were one of the women who opted to have Essure implanted, be sure to see your doctor if you develop any adverse symptoms.

Though some ancient Taoist traditions feel that tubal ligation or vasectomy interferes with the energy flow of the body, my medical intuitive consultants say that the life energy around the body simply reroutes itself—that there is no permanent damage to the body after a so-called sterilization procedure. Caroline Myss says that the only problem with a tubal ligation or vasectomy is when the person is ambivalent about it and really doesn't want it done. As with abortion, it's not the procedure itself that can potentially cause problems—it's the *meaning* of it.

I was very clear that the potential problems associated with tubal ligation were *nothing* compared with the disruption that an unplanned pregnancy would cause in my life. So I made an informed choice. Then I called my sister.

Moving into Greater Creativity

My sister, Penny, had her miscarriage a year before I decided to have a tubal ligation. (We're eleven months apart in age—the doctor asked my mother if she had poked holes in her diaphragm.) After the miscarriage, I said to her, "Why don't you have a tubal ligation and be done with the worry?" She said, "I'll do it when you do." So when I finally decided to do it, I called her up and asked her if she wanted to join me for the event and schedule them at the same time. She said she did. I made arrangements for both of us to have our procedures done in the office via a technique known as a mini-laparotomy (small operation). After I made the appointments, I hung up and experienced about thirty seconds of sorrow about what I had just done. I vowed that if this feeling of loss continued, I'd cancel the procedure. But the feeling passed very quickly.

We decided to make this a meaningful event for both of us. Penny has no daughters; I have no sons. Each of us had to make peace with that. We named our operations and the ceremony we had beforehand "Moving into Greater Creativity" because we saw our lives after childbearing as rich with potential to develop ourselves further and to use our fertility in the outer world more fully. (By the way, that is exactly what has happened for both of us.) I've always hated the word *sterile* because of its negative connotations— "barren" women are sterile; a bare, cold room is sterile; hospitals are sterile. I didn't consider myself sterile before the tubal ligation, and I certainly didn't see how having my fallopian tubes cauterized would change how I felt about myself. I had simply chosen to be proactive about avoiding future pregnancy.

Our operations were scheduled at nine and nine-thirty on a Friday morning in May. Springtime—a perfect time to celebrate newfound fertility and also, according to Caroline Myss, a good time to have surgery, as the energies associated with spring bode well for healing and new growth. The night before, Penny and I participated in a beautiful ceremony—one prepared for us by Judith Burwell, a friend who guides people via ritual through significant life changes. Another friend, Gina Orlando, had made us two exquisite spring flower wreaths to wear on our heads during the ceremony. I felt like a bridesmaid—virginal in the true sense of the word, a woman complete unto herself.

Each of us spoke in turn about how she felt taking this step—and about how, when we make a conscious choice, there's always grieving for the choice not taken. Yet we must fearlessly go forth and consciously work with our circumstances to the best of our ability, trying to manifest our dreams. In the ritual Penny and I made space to grieve aloud our unborn children—me for my unborn sons, and Penny for her unborn daughters—knowing full well that Mother Earth doesn't really require more people right now, that that part of the earth's history—the order to go forth and multiply—is over. "For now," I said, "may we go forth and multiply many spiritual children and give birth to ourselves."

The next morning we arrived at the doctor's office, three miles from my house. We had brought a special music tape with us to listen to during our surgery, which was to be performed under local anesthesia with a very light intravenous sedative. My sister went first. I held her hand and checked to see that her tubes were cauterized in just the right way—not so much that the blood supply would be compromised.

Penny walked into the recovery area, and then it was my turn. It was all quite painless. The doctor at one point said, "Do you want to see your tubes? They are very long and perfect." I said, "No, I'd just as soon have a mind/ body split right now." I didn't like the idea of actually burning nice healthy fallopian tubes, something that so many women would love to have. But I had made my choice. If I had changed my mind even *during* the procedure, though, I would have told the doctor to stop.

Afterward, my husband drove us home and fed us lunch and dinner while we rested on the couch, kept ice packs on our lower abdomens, and watched all the episodes of *Anne of Green Gables* on videotape. We developed shoulder pain, which often results when the abdominal cavity is opened and excess gas from room air or carbon dioxide gets trapped under the diaphragm and then is "referred" to the shoulder because the nerves that supply the diaphragm are connected to the nerves that innervate the shoulder. This gas gets reabsorbed after a day or two, and the pain goes away. The intensity of our shoulder pain was unexpected, but we were very happy with our choice.

The following morning we gathered spring flowers from the yard and floated them in the bathtub while we sat on the side, soaked our feet, and talked about our parents, our childhoods, and how happy we were to be celebrating this momentous event together. While listening to the singing of Susan Osborne, we gave each other a foot massage. Then we rested some more.

Later that afternoon, we drove into Portland to a special store called the Plains Indian Gallery. I bought a piece of art called *Tree Momma*, a magical figure of a woman made out of a weathered wooden branch, fur, and some clay. Penny bought a painting that had deep meaning for her of two Sioux warriors riding away from a burial platform. These purchases were personal symbols of our conscious choice to shape our destiny by clarity and intent— not chance.

Neither my sister nor I had any regrets. One chapter of our lives closed, but we each opened an entirely new one. At a family reunion in which we watched our then teenage children have fun together, we remarked on the wisdom of our decision.

TABLE 6

COMPARING CONTRACEPTVE METHODS

Effectiveness figures assume perfect use every time; effectiveness rates of actual use may vary significantly from those shown. Additional information comparing methods of birth control is available on the website for the Office on Women's Health at the U.S. Department of Health and Human Services (www.womenshealth.gov/a-z-topics/birth-control-methods).

Method	Effectiveness	Requirements	Advantages	Disadvantages
FERTILITY AWARENESS	76%–93%*	Conscious understanding of fertility cycle Continual conscious commitment Willingness to use barrier methods of birth control or abstinence during fertile periods	Maintains natural hormonal/ fertility cycle Apps make the entire process far easier than it's been in the past	Requires cooperation and high awareness Medication that affects cervical mucus, body temperature, or menstrual regularity may compromise effectiveness
DIAPHRAGM, WITH CONTRACEPTIVE CREAM OR GEL	94%	Fitting by healthcare professional Faithful use at each intercourse	May protect against pelvic infection and cervical abnormalities Maintains normal hormonal/ fertility cycle Can be inserted hours before sex It holds blood in nicely during menstruation, making sex less messy	Unacceptable to some people May cause genital irritation Failure rate is higher if intercourse frequency is greater than 3×/ week Must be resized after pregnancy, some miscarriages, abortions, or weight change of 20 percent May cause frequent urinary tract infections in some women

*Figure is from research studies, not Planned Parenthood.

Method	Effectiveness	Requirements	Advantages	Disadvantages
CONDOM	98%	Conscientious use for maximal effectiveness	Protects against STDs Decreases risk of cervical dysplasia Does not require a prescription Can help premature ejaculation	Requires male partner to be cooperative Unacceptable to some people Some people are allergic to latex condoms (other kinds are available) Erection must be maintained Loss of sensation
FEMALE CONDOM	95%	Conscientious use for maximal effectiveness Faithful use required at each intercourse Requires a prescription from a healthcare professional	Protects against STDs Protects labia and base of penis during intercourse Can be inserted up to eight hours before intercourse Decreases risk of cervical dysplasia Can be used without partner participation Stronger than latex and less likely to break External ring on condom may stimulate clitoris	One-time use only Unacceptable to some people May be noisy May be difficult to insert May cause genital irritation May slip into vagina during sex

Method	Effectiveness	Requirements	Advantages	Disadvantages
BIRTH CONTROL PILL	99%	Prescription from a healthcare professional Taking a daily pill	Decreases risk of ovarian and uterine cancer Decrease in monthly bleeding and reduces chance for iron deficiency Decrease in menstrual cramps and PMS Decreases risk for benign breast tumors Acne improvement Requires no planning	Blocks natural hormonal/fertility cycle May lower sex drive May increase risk of cervical adenocarcinoma Increases incidence of depression and some autoimmune conditions Increases risk of chlamydia infection Increases risk of thrombophlebitis, pulmonary emboli, stroke—especially in smokers Nausea and vomiting Headaches Certain medications compromise effectiveness May cause spotting, breast tenderness, moodiness, headache, nausea, and weight gain

Method	Effectiveness	Requirements	Advantages	Disadvantages
IUD Copper (ParaGard) Hormonal (Mirena, Kyleena, Liletta, Skyla)	99%	Insertion by healthcare professional	Requires no planning	May increase risk of pelvic infection following insertion or in women exposed to STDs May cause spotting Periods may be longer and heavier May cause cramping after insertion May cause PMS-like symptoms
SPERMICIDAL FOAM, CREAM, JELLY, FILM, OR SUPPOSITORIES	82%	Conscientious use for maximal effectiveness	Free from systemic effects No advance planning required Available with no prescription	Unacceptable to some people May cause genital irritation that can increase your chance of getting an STD or HIV Must reinsert with each act of intercourse May be messy
IMPLANT Nexplanon	99%	Insertion by healthcare professional	Can be used by women who can't take estrogen Fertility returns quickly when removed Can be used while breast-feeding No advance planning required	For most women, periods become fewer and lighter, and after one year, 1 out of 3 women stops having periods completely

Method	Effectiveness	Requirements	Advantages	Disadvantages
IMPLANT Nexplanon (cont.)			Provides continuous protection for up to five years after insertion	May cause irregular bleeding (especially in first 6–12 months), including longer and heavier periods or spotting and breakthrough bleeding
SPONGE Today Sponge	80%–91%	Conscientious use for maximal effectiveness	No prescription necessary Can be inserted hours before sex Can be worn for 30 hours after insertion, and intercourse can be repeated without additional preparation during the first 24 hours	Use during vaginal bleeding, including menstruation, may decrease effectiveness Slight increase for toxic shock syndrome Spermicide used with it may cause genital irritation that can increase your chance of getting an STD or HIV
CERVICAL CAP FemCap	71%–86% (Note: Figure is for typical use; stats for perfect use not available)	Prescription from healthcare professional required Conscientious use for maximal effectiveness	Requires no planning Provides continuous protection for up to 48 hours, no matter how many times intercourse occurs	Current caps come in only three sizes—therefore accurate fit is not always assured Some risk of toxic shock if cap is left in longer than 48 hours May cause odor problems with some women if left in too long

Method	Effectiveness	Requirements	Advantages	Disadvantages
CERVICAL CAP FemCap (cont.)				Not as effective in women who've had children Not as effective after a recent abortion Can be difficult to insert Use during vaginal bleeding, including menstruation, may render it less effective
THE RING NuvaRing	99%	Conscientious use for maximal effectiveness Ring is worn for 21 days, then removed for seven days before being replaced with a new ring	Decreases risk of ovarian and uterine cancer Decrease in monthly bleeding and chance for iron deficiency Decrease in menstrual cramps and PMS Decreases risk for benign breast tumors Acne improvement Requires no planning	May be less effective in women weighing more than 198 lbs. May decrease libido Increases risk of thrombophlebitis, pulmonary emboli, stroke—especially in smokers Nausea and vomiting Headaches Certain medications compromise effectiveness

Method	Effectiveness	Requirements	Advantages	Disadvantages
THE RING NuvaRing (cont.)				May cause spotting, breast tenderness, moodiness, headache, nausea, and weight gain as well as skin irritation at site of application May cause increased vaginal discharge or vaginal infection or irritation
THE PATCH Xulane	99%	Conscientious use for maximal effectiveness Patch is worn for 21 days, then removed for seven days before being replaced with a new patch	Decreases risk of ovarian and uterine cancer Decrease in monthly bleeding and chance for iron deficiency Decrease in menstrual cramps and PMS Decreases risk for benign breast tumors Acne improvement Requires no planning	May be less effective in women weighing more than 198 lbs. May decrease sex drive Increases risk of thrombophlebitis, pulmonary emboli, stroke—especially in smokers Nausea and vomiting Headaches Certain medications compromise effectiveness

Method	Effectiveness	Requirements	Advantages	Disadvantages
THE PATCH Xulane (cont.)				May cause spotting, breast tenderness, irritability, headache, nausea, and weight gain as well as skin irritation at site of application
WITHDRAWAL	96%	Conscientious use at each intercourse Great self-control, experience, and trust of partner	Requires no planning	May decrease sexual pleasure The male pre-ejaculate (fluid at the end of the penis after erection) may contain sperm Less effective in men who ejaculate prematurely
INJECTABLE PROGESTIN Depo-Provera	99%	A shot every three months	Requires no planning Can be used by women who can't take estrogen May help prevent endometrial cancer Fewer and lighter periods	Spotting and headaches, moodiness, irritability, and decreased sex drive Takes an average of nine to ten months to regain fertility after stopping May cause temporary bone thinning
VASECTOMY	Almost 100%	Surgery	Requires no planning	Difficult to reverse
TUBAL LIGATION	Almost 100%	Surgery	Requires no planning	Irreversible

Effectiveness statistics from Planned Parenthood (see www.plannedparenthood.org) except where noted.

TRANSFORMING INFERTILITY

The ability to conceive and bear children can profoundly affect the way a woman feels about herself on a very deep level. So when a woman finds that she is unable to have a child, she's often thrown into great despair and feels a sense of injustice: "Why me?" Seeing teenage mothers having no problems getting pregnant becomes almost impossible to bear, unless the woman can find some meaning in the experience and come to terms with it. The pioneering work of Alice Domar, Ph.D., founder and executive director of the Domar Center for Mind/Body Health in Waltham, Massachusetts, has clearly documented that women who've been diagnosed as infertile are twice as likely to be depressed as a control group, and that this depression peaks about two years after they start trying to get pregnant. And even though infertility is not life-threatening, infertile women have depression scores that are indistinguishable from those of women with cancer, heart disease, or HIV.[47]

Approximately one in every six to ten couples has a problem with infertility. About 40 percent of the problems are related to a male factor and 60 percent to a female factor. Statistics show that sperm counts have been gradually falling over the past century. Decreased sperm counts are associated with cigarette, marijuana, and alcohol use as well as with environmental factors. Humans cannot pollute this planet and their own bodies without consequences, and infertility is one of them. Conditions on the earth may not favor fertility the way they used to. It's as though the collective species brain were generating a great deal of energy toward making many women and men less fertile, due to the stresses of today's families, social environments, and personal addictions, and to stress on the planet itself. Too many stressful childhoods remain unhealed; too many children grow up too fast. We're not allowing nature's rhythms to click into gear naturally. Reproductive problems associated with toxic chemicals and with electromagnetic field disturbances may be part of the reason why fertility rates have been decreasing in industrialized nations for decades.[48] But that doesn't mean that an individual woman's fertility will necessarily be adversely affected.

Fertility is affected by many different factors, such as diet and environment, but in about 20 percent of the cases, the causes are unknown—meaning that medical testing cannot explain the problem. In my experience those couples who are most willing to look at and work with the mind-body connection in addition to the other aspects of fertility are the ones who are most successful either conceiving or healing their relationship with fertility.

The most common (and often interrelated) factors affecting female infertility are the following:

~ Smoking

~ Following a high-glycemic-index diet with inadequate micronutrients

~ Irregular ovulation

~ Endometriosis

~ A history of pelvic infection from an IUD or other source, causing scarring of the fallopian tubes

~ Unresolved emotional stress, sometimes from inherited trauma, that results in subtle hormonal imbalances

~ Immune system problems—some women make antibodies against the sperm of some men and not others, or against the fertilized egg that is created with some partners but not with others[49]

~ Age

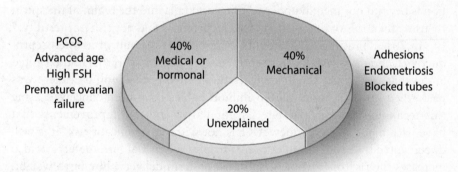

PCOS
Advanced age
High FSH
Premature ovarian
failure

40%
Medical or
hormonal

40%
Mechanical

Adhesions
Endometriosis
Blocked tubes

20%
Unexplained

FIGURE 19: THE CAUSES OF INFERTILITY

A certain percentage of women who've been told that they are infertile for a medical reason get pregnant even without treatment. Infertility is never a completely straightforward affair. Many physical, emotional, and psychological factors are involved in conception, so many that it is ridiculous to try to reduce fertility to a matter of injecting the right hormone at the right time. An infertility specialist I met once said, "I do all the latest high-tech surgery and hormone treatment to try to make someone pregnant. When it is all said and done, I still don't know who will get pregnant and who won't and why. After all my years of training, this area is still a big mystery that I can't control."

The conventional "management" of infertility generally focuses on the body as a hormonal machine and in large part ignores emotional, psychological, and even nutritional factors that have physical and hormonal manifestations.[50] Though the mind-body connection in infertility has been appreciated for decades, only recently has this important link begun to be explored more seriously. As our society has become more technologically focused, the study of the mind-body connection in infertility holds the potential to help many couples, and a thorough psychological interview should be a routine part of every fertility investigation.[51] When we focus only on the extremely expensive (over $4 billion is spent annually on overcoming infertility, and this figure is increasing)[52] and invasive technology currently available for fertility, and forget the hearts and spirits of those going through these procedures, the results are often disappointing and even devastating.

Julie Von, O.M.D., author of *Spiritual Fertility Integrative Practices for the Journey to Motherhood* (Hay House, 2019), has worked with couples from all over the world. She writes, "After working with fertility clients for over a decade, I've learned that fertility depends on much more than age, hormone levels, or ovulation windows. Much of what is happening in conception is beyond our mental understanding and falls into the realm of the spirit. By using the tools of the spiritual, we can promote and nourish our fertility."

In 2016, almost 77,000 infants were born as a result of assisted reproductive technology (ART); this represents 1.9 percent of births in the United States that year. Since the first successful in vitro fertilization treatment was performed in 1978, more than 5 million babies have been conceived using this technology alone.[53] Despite its popularity and the improvements that have been made to techniques, ART is not without significant risk. It is well documented that ART doubles to quadruples the risk of birth defects. It also increases the risk of multiple gestations, preterm delivery, low birth weight, chromosome abnormalities, neurodevelopmental disorders, eclampsia, prenatal mortality, and placenta previa, and it results in an increased rate of C-section delivery.[54] The bottom line here is that Mother Nature has some checks and balances that technology can't bypass entirely.

Psychological Factors

On a personal level, many women do not get pregnant because in their hearts they really do not want to—they are afraid of the demands a child will make on them. In one study, women who were unsuccessful with fertility treatments were found to be more successful in the outer world than those who conceived. The authors of the study interpreted this result as "an exaggerated positive attitude as an attempt to overcome inner fears, doubts, and ambivalence" about having a child.[55] Caroline Myss explains that women have only so much second-chakra energy. If a woman is using her ambition for career success and is already very busy in this area, she may simply not have enough energy circuits available in her body to conceive a child unless she cuts back on other commitments. Many infertile women are working sixty to eighty hours per week and are exhausted; then they pursue having a child as though they were writing a Ph.D. dissertation. A prospective study done in Italy of women going through in vitro fertilization (IVF) or embryo transfer (ET) found that both vulnerability to stress and working outside the home were associated with a poor outcome of IVF or ET treatment, even though the straightforward medical causes of infertility were distributed equally throughout the study group.[56]

Conceiving a child is a receptive act, not a marathon event that can be programmed into your cell phone calendar. Several studies indicated that excessive focus on the goal of having a child may result in premature maturation of the eggs in the ovary and subsequent release of eggs that are not ready for fertilization;[57] while those studies are very dated, there is no doubt that the mind-body-spirit connection plays a major role in fertility. Stress hormones, from whatever cause, have a direct and powerful impact on ovulation and subsequent hormonal balance. I'd also like to emphasize that having a job or career need not affect your fertility. Problems can arise, however, as a result of certain factors that are often associated with work, such as a perceived inability to get your needs met; a sense of lack of control in your life; and not feeling good about the work you're doing, what that job represents in your life, or a career that is not an extension of your inner wisdom.

One fascinating older study of heterosexual women undergoing donor insemination noted that after the first several attempts to produce pregnancy, the women, who were previously ovulatory, actually stopped ovulating. The authors concluded that artificial insemination—and any other mechanized, unnatural technique for "forcing" pregnancy—is on some level a traumatizing procedure that leads to the inhibition of the very process it is trying to accomplish. (This may or may not be true with lesbian couples or single women choosing motherhood because donor insemination is the only method for achieving pregnancy in these situations.) Interestingly, orgasm has been found to enhance a woman's chances of conception. Involuntary vaginal and uterine movements that promote conception accompany orgasm. Failure to achieve orgasm may lead to circulatory changes in the blood flow to the pelvis, which can affect fertility.[58] High-tech conception techniques, by their very design, completely ignore this aspect of fertility.

Whenever a woman feels conflicted over birthing, children, or the restrictions that children may impose once they arrive, infertility may result. Some studies from the 1940s through the 1990s have suggested an association between infertility and ambivalence toward pregnancy and children.

The relationships between husbands and wives who are infertile have also been studied. Many of the women in these studies had an actual aversion to intercourse; they had lower frequency of orgasm when they did have intercourse, and they felt a marked sexual disharmony in their partnership. When these women found more suitable partners, however, they became fertile.[59] I saw this phenomenon repeatedly in my practice, just as I saw countless so-called infertile women conceive shortly after adopting a baby. Psychological testing done on 117 husbands in infertile couples in one study indicated that the men had a pronounced lack of self-confidence, were introverted, and had decreased social assertiveness.[60]

The fertility-stress link remains controversial in conventional science, and it's difficult to document a causal link between psychosocial distress and fertility. Though many studies do show that women with infertility are more apt to have depression and anxiety, most doctors believe that the depression and anxiety are the result of infertility, not the other way around. In any case, studies tend to be conflicting and not well controlled, and there are no prospective studies. In their review of forty years of research on psychological distress and infertility, psychologist Dr. W. A. Fisher and his colleague A. M. Berkovich summarized the viewpoint of most conventional doctors when they wrote: "Much research has been done to try to corroborate the proposition that psychological factors may be causally related to the occurrence of infertility, but no study has been able to confirm a causal relationship to date. In fact the very assumption of a psychological distress–infertility link has become quite controversial because some feel it blames women for their inability to conceive."[61]

Despite this conventional opinion, failing to explore the psychosocial aspects of fertility is a big mistake and robs a woman of all her options. There's no doubt that subconscious fears about having a child can and do exert a powerful influence over the subtle endocrinologic processes that are required for conception. Perceived stress changes the way the hypothalamus of the brain functions, which affects ovulation. It also changes the immunologic functioning of the cells in the reproductive tract as well as elsewhere. When a woman learns how to modulate her stress effectively, her fertility can change. This was demonstrated by Alice Domar, Ph.D., based on her work with a group of women with unexplained infertility in her mind-body program at Beth Israel Deaconess Hospital in Boston. Thirty-four percent of these women became pregnant within six months—which is much higher than the average pregnancy rate for infertile couples at six months. The mean duration of infertility had been 3.3 years.[62] There is enormous potential for healing infertility when a woman is willing to acknowledge the role of her beliefs and commit to bringing them to consciousness and healing them. The first step—and the hardest step—in healing adverse subconscious programming about anything is being willing to accept yourself fully and unconditionally right now. This process involves never beating yourself up for "failing" to conceive because you waited too long, or "failing" at anything else. It's just the opposite of blame.

I've seen many women get pregnant once they committed to healing themselves on the deepest levels. One of the most striking examples of this is the story of my colleague Julia Indichova, who at the age of forty-three was unable to conceive a second child. She was told that her FSH level (the follicle-stimulating hormone from the pituitary gland, levels of which are often used to judge whether a woman is still producing fertile eggs) was too high. But her inner wisdom told her that wasn't true. She changed her diet, began to do some deep soul searching, read everything she could, got her FSH down naturally, and eventually conceived and delivered a healthy daughter. Her book, *Inconceivable: A Woman's Triumph over Despair and Statistics* (Broadway Books, 2001), tells her story. Julia now leads workshops for women diagnosed with infertility and has helped many heal their fertility and their lives. (For more information, see Julia's website, www .fertileheart.com.)

The late Niravi Payne, author of *The Whole Person Fertility Program* (Three Rivers Press, 1997), was a therapist who devoted her professional life to helping couples conceive. Her view of current fertility problems was both enlightening and empowering. She said that it was no accident that so many baby boomers had problems with fertility. A series of complex psychological, sociological, and political factors led to unparalleled changes in our society over the past fifty years that has given rise to the decision of many to delay childbearing, thus altering the reproductive life patterns familiar to their parents and the 30,000 generations before them. Niravi wrote, "In the space of one generation, middle- and upper-class Americans decided to defer childbearing for ten to twenty years. This may be the most radical voluntary alteration of the lifestyle of all of them, and, unquestionably, there have been physiologic consequences."

Millions of boomers rebelled against the circumscribed lives that they saw their mothers living in the 1950s and 1960s. They said no to early marriage and childbearing and yes to defining and developing themselves. And many mothers of baby boomers, recognizing the lack of fulfillment and frustration that characterized their own lives, encouraged their daughters to seek college educations and professional careers. Ironically, many baby boomers had their first abortions around the same time that their mothers had their first children. Acknowledging how factors such as these may be affecting her in the present is often a woman's first step toward healing her relationship with fertility—and what we acknowledge in the present, we transform, thus freeing our daughters from an ongoing familial burden.

Time and again, I have witnessed how unconsciously absorbed beliefs about pregnancy, sexuality, and having children can, in some cases, actually block fertility. For example, some women are actually very unhappy with their current partner but are afraid to say so because they feel they have no alternative but to stay with him. Other women were told by their mothers that having babies could ruin their lives. Many mothers had no choice but to stay home and raise children, even when they had lots of talent and ambition in other areas. Their daughters often picked up on this and blame themselves for their mothers' frustrations. They don't want to risk passing this pain on to the next generation.

We have now passed the torch on to our daughters and granddaughters, who are facing more choices and decisions than ever before. And they are rewriting the script. Currently many thirtysomethings are being convinced they require reproductive technologies to get pregnant the moment they turn thirty-five, and so that age becomes a cultural portal that looms over them—causing the production of more stress hormones than necessary and possibly (adversely) affecting fertility. There is no abrupt drop-off in fertility the moment you have your thirty-fifth birthday, and most women have no problem getting pregnant between thirty-five and forty. There is a huge difference between your chronological age (the age on your driver's license) and your biological age (the age of your cells). We all know women in their early thirties who seem to be going on fifty and women in their forties and even fifties who look like they're no older than thirty.

Regardless of your age, it's crucial that you connect with your cyclic wisdom and your fertility—no technology can match your understanding of your body. In those women who are willing to come to terms with the unconscious beliefs that are really running their fertility, Niravi reported a subsequent pregnancy rate significantly higher than expected.

SHOULD YOU FREEZE (OR DONATE) YOUR EGGS?

A thirty-five-year-old friend of mine recently attended a party where she met and spoke with an infertility specialist who told her that she should freeze her eggs right away. She is not married but wants children. She asked me what I thought. She is very healthy, doesn't smoke, and looks like her biological age isn't much over twenty-five. I told her that chances were very good she'd be able to conceive on her own, and that once she meets the right guy, it won't take very long to have a family. On the other hand, if she were undergoing chemo, I'd definitely suggest storing some eggs for the future. When it comes to donating eggs (which college students sometimes do for the money), I'm hesitant. I sure wouldn't want my daughters to do it—for a couple of reasons. One is that the drugs used to stimulate the ovaries for egg retrieval are designed to produce lots of eggs at one time. This can trigger ovarian hyperstimulation syndrome, the symptoms of which include nausea and vomiting, abdominal discomfort, shortness of breath, labored breathing, clotting disorders, renal failure, and occasionally death.[63] There's also the possible risk that egg harvesting will result in decreased fertility in the future. You might donate your eggs in college to pay tuition, only to have trouble starting your own family in your early thirties. Talk about regretting a decision! These are a few of the reasons why egg harvesting must be thought through very carefully.

Integrative Program to Enhance Fertility

If fertility is an issue that concerns you, I highly recommend that you explore the mind-body connection thoroughly. The steps below will get you started.[64] I'd recommend that you have your journal ready as you read through this so that you can write down any thoughts, feelings, or beliefs that arise as you go through the steps I've outlined. Your responses will be an invaluable guide on your journey toward healing your fertility.

The mind-body approach to fertility is based on the premise that knowledge is power and that a change in perception based on new information is powerful enough to effect subtle changes in your endocrine, immune, and nervous systems. Regardless of what you've been told about your fertility, know that your ability to conceive is profoundly influenced by the complex interaction among psychosocial, psychological, and emotional factors (basically your thoughts and emotions), and that you can consciously change these to enhance your ability to have a baby.

The first thing that's needed in the area of fertility is a new language. Few labels are more damaging to women (or to men) than the label "infertile." It strikes at the very heart of one's self-concept and self-esteem and results in a punishing internal dialogue in women who are going through this experience. Many feel inadequate, guilty, and to blame for their condition, which creates a vicious cycle inside them. The word *infertility* conjures up images of barren, dry, sterile earth that can't bear fruit. If you currently carry this label, try replacing it with the following: "I am a sensual, sexual, fertile being with a great deal of love and nurturing to give to others—and to receive for myself," or "My body is a wide-open channel for new life and new love." Internalizing the feeling that goes along with these words will help you change your self-concept (and physiology). Remember that changing your self-concept is a process, not an event. Give it time.

Denise Wiesner, a licensed acupuncturist and author of *Conceiving with Love: A Whole-Body Approach to Creating Intimacy, Reigniting Passion, and Increasing Fertility* (Shambhala, 2019), points out that babies are made out of love, not desperation. She helps individuals and couples reconnect with their ability to give and receive pleasure, count their blessings, and interrupt the stress caused by the relentless quest to have a baby at all costs. Anyone can make this shift simply by reframing the entire endeavor starting with their approach to love and sex. Wiesner's approach includes the ancient art of tantra, the *tao* of self-pleasuring, the healing of trauma through sexual intimacy combined with love, and a thorough knowledge of one's female erotic anatomy (see chapter 8). This book is a deep dive into transforming your body into a sensual vessel for new life.

~ Look at the big picture. Know that you're not alone—millions of women are charting new territory when it comes to balancing their personal and professional lives. Your fertility situation may, in part, be the result of sweeping psychosocial forces that have unconsciously influenced an entire generation, with very real physiologic effects.

~ If you are over thirty-five and want to become pregnant, examine your programming about your biological clock. The popularity of and widespread publicity surrounding assisted reproductive technologies have made it seem as though every woman over the age of thirty-five is apt to have problems conceiving. But this just isn't true. Here are the statistics: About one-third of women who defer childbearing until their mid- to late thirties will have a problem with fertility. But fully two-thirds won't have any problem. And 50 percent of women in their early forties won't have a problem, either.[65]

Though statistically a woman's fertility decreases with age, it's important to keep in mind that statistics are based on the experience of an entire population. Within a given population there are very big individual differences. For example, the oldest spontaneous pregnancy in modern times recorded in *Guinness World Records* was in a British woman who delivered at the age of fifty-nine. In earlier times, it was reported, a Scottish woman delivered six children after the age of forty-seven—the last one at age sixty-two.[66] Interestingly, Brant Secunda, an American-born shaman trained by the Huichol Indians, who live in a remote region of Mexico, reports that Huichol women routinely get pregnant in their fifties and even in their sixties.[67] (Perhaps because they haven't been told that their eggs are too old, their fertility doesn't suffer much with age.)

This information is evidence of just how miraculous the human female body is when it comes to fertility. Things are not always what they seem. Indeed, research from Jonathan Tilly, Ph.D., and colleagues at Harvard

Medical School found that female mammals are able to create new eggs even into adulthood.[68] This preliminary research has exploded one of the most sacred tenets of reproductive biology.

CDC data show that the birth rate for women ages forty to forty-four is the highest it's been since 1968, and it's been rising since the mid-1980s (even while the overall U.S. birth rate has fallen to a record low). The total number of births in 2017 for women ages forty and up was more than 114,700.[69] A lot of women over forty may not realize how fertile they are. Fifty-one percent of pregnancies that occur among women in their forties are unintended.[70] This may be one of the reasons why women over forty are second only to women between the ages of eighteen and twenty-five in frequency of abortions. So who says your eggs are too old?

~ Make the connection between your emotions, your family, and your fertility. The crux of the mind-body approach to fertility is discovering how the messages you internalized from childhood are currently affecting your ability to conceive. It is very clear that your physiology may well be responding automatically and unconsciously to situations directly related to your early childhood and family conditions. Though most people, especially other family members, may believe that it's easier and healthier to forget painful childhood experiences, and may urge you to avoid emotionally volatile subjects, your willingness to remember and release your emotional ties to past experiences will free up energy that will help you heal your fertility. Please remember that recalling painful childhood experiences is not done at the expense of happier memories. Usually, you'll find that this work will be a mixture of profound joy and sadness that ultimately leads you to a place of greater love and forgiveness for both yourself and your parents.

To get started on this, construct an *ephistogram,* an emotional and physical family health history that diagrams family patterns. It was developed by Niravi Payne as an adaptation of the genogram used by family therapists. It can help you understand what circumstances, over many decades, may have caused you to experience reproductive problems. "Filling it out," wrote Niravi, "is a powerful method for creating new pathways for healing, conceiving and carrying a baby to term." To create an ephistogram, you use the same diagram you would use when drawing a genealogy, or family tree, except that in addition to the names of your grandparents, parents, aunts, uncles, and siblings, you also put in any illnesses or physical symptoms they had, any emotional patterns you remember, and any reproductive difficulties they may have had. This is like detective work. Another fascinating resource is the aptly named book *Wombology: Healing the Primordial Memories and Wounds Your Grandmother's Daughter Gave to You* (iUniverse, 2009) by C. J. Johnson, Psy.D. Remember, for better or for worse, your family served as the model for your current intimate relationships. Ask yourself the following questions about each member of your family tree: "What message did I receive from this person about having children? Was it positive? Was it negative? Did I internalize any of it? What did they lead me to believe about the process of conception, pregnancy, labor, and birth? Were there any family secrets, such as miscarriages or pregnancies that were kept hidden?"

Niravi pointed out something very empowering: "The real freedom from our negative parental conditioning occurs when we stop denying that we are like them. Rather, asking ourselves how we feel, think, act, and react like our parents is the beginning of our separation and healing process. When we look at our lives in this way, it is easier to bring to light multigenerational ambivalence about conception that the ephistogram outlines." And this brings us to the next step.

⁓ Name your ambivalence. It is perfectly normal to be somewhat ambivalent about having a baby. It is possible to very much want a baby and be terrified of the process at the same time. Why wouldn't you be? It changes your life permanently and in ways that you can't really plan for. I certainly was ambivalent . . . so much so, in fact, that when I was pregnant with my first child, I didn't buy a single baby item until after she was born! And I went about my duties in the hospital as though nothing were happening to my body. Ambivalence is a problem only when it isn't acknowledged and worked through. Many women desire pregnancy but are unsure about raising a baby. Others want children but don't want to go through a pregnancy, believing that it will be too painful, too damaging to their figure, or whatever. Others are afraid that they will treat their children as they were treated by their parents. These feelings of ambivalence need to be brought to consciousness so that they won't interfere with conceiving. Ask yourself the following and write the answer in your journal: "Why don't I want a baby?" Be completely honest when you do this exercise.

⁓ I also highly recommend the book *Spiritual Fertility: Integrative Practices for the Journey to Motherhood* (Hay House, 2019) by Julie Von, O.M.D. Dr. Von counsels clients worldwide and helps them understand the principles for becoming receptive to the spiritual energies involved in creating life—whether that be through natural conception, assisted reproductive technologies, or adoption. (See www.drjulievon.com.)

Other Factors to Consider

Stress

Unabated emotional stress results in high adrenaline and cortisol levels. This leads to imbalances in other hormones that are important for optimal fertility, including thyroid hormones, progesterone, and estrogen. One of the most tried-and-true ways to decrease emotional stress and its physiological effects is with guided imagery, meditation, breathing through the nose, and relaxation. A wide range of well-documented modalities is available to help with this.

Mindfulness meditation and techniques such as Herbert Benson's relaxation response[71] (see page 153) have been successfully used by Alice Domar, Ph.D., to help women heal from the stress of infertility while also increasing conception rates substantially.[72] A practical guide to Dr. Domar's program can be found in her books *Conquering Infertility* (Penguin, 2002), *Healing Mind, Healthy Woman* (Henry Holt, 1996), and *Self-Nurture* (Viking, 2000).

Mindfulness and relaxation training are especially important if you're going through any high-tech medical fertility treatments, since it is clear that unresolved and unexpressed emotional and psychological stress has physiologic consequences that may hamper the effectiveness of fertility treatments.[73] But when emotional stress is addressed and resolved, pregnancy rates go up. My colleague Belleruth Naparstek has created helpful guided imagery for enhancing fertility. (See www.healthjourneys.com.) Yoga programs, such as those created by Sue Dumais specifically to enhance fertility, can also be extremely beneficial. Dumais is the author of *Yoga for Fertility Handbook* (Trafford Publishing, 2009). (For more information on her program, see www.yogaforfertility.blogspot.com.)

The Male Factor

When people hear the words *biological clock* we usually think "women." But this simply isn't true. Fully 40 percent of infertility problems lie with the man, not the woman. Because treating female fertility is far more lucrative and well accepted than thoroughly investigating and treating male fertility problems, however, the male factor often remains hidden. According to urologist and male infertility specialist Harry Fisch, M.D., author of *The Male Biological Clock* (Free Press, 2005), roughly 10 percent of men trying to father a child—about 2.5 million men in the United States alone—are either infertile or subfertile. Many don't know they have a problem because they haven't been tested, or tested thoroughly enough. As Dr. Fisch notes in his book, "Men's fertility is often checked only by a simple semen analysis. If a man seems to have enough sperm and those sperm seem healthy, he is presumed fertile. This kind of cursory 'exam' fails to detect a host of problems that could contribute to a fertility problem—most of which can be fixed relatively easily and inexpensively."[74] (For example, taking ibuprofen daily for as short a period as two weeks has recently been shown to reduce male fertility, at least while men continue to take the drug.)[75] So the problem remains undetected and medical attention shifts to the female. This is a tragedy that is completely preventable.

Many of the factors that affect female fertility also affect male fertility. For example, sperm quality is greatly affected by nutrition. I once had the pleasure of having the husband of a former patient come up to me to show me pictures of his children. He said, "I can't thank you enough for recommending vitamin C and zinc to me so many years ago. We got pregnant within three months of my cleaning up my diet and starting those supplements."

Acupuncture can significantly improve both total sperm counts and sperm function in men.[76] Unabated stress and the hormonal imbalance that results are also often a problem. "Over the decades that I have been in this line of work," Dr. Fisch writes, "I have seen firsthand that the male biological clock can be slowed down, or even reversed, and problems with sexuality or fertility that arise at any point in a man's life can usually be fixed."[77]

Though male-factor infertility is beyond the scope of this book, I urge every couple who is undergoing fertility evaluation to read Dr. Fisch's book, which gives a detailed plan to enhance male fertility and overall health.

Artificial and Natural Light

Living in artificial light without going outside into natural sunlight regularly can have adverse consequences on fertility, because light itself is a nutrient. Far too many people not only are stressed at work but don't get outside much. When I was trying to conceive my first child, my basal body temperature rose very slowly at ovulation. (As I've already mentioned, ovulation causes a rise in basal body temperature of about 0.8 degrees. The ovary produces progesterone at ovulation, which in turn produces this rise in body temperature.) I decided to walk outside in the sunlight without glasses or contact lenses for twenty minutes each day. (To be effective, natural light has to hit the retina directly; we shouldn't look at the sun directly, but we must be out in the daytime.) Within one menstrual cycle, my basal body temperature began to rise very sharply at ovulation—a big improvement in the pattern. I got pregnant within two cycles of doing this, having tried for five months before. Though this isn't scientific proof of anything, it is an example of a simple change that had immediate measurable effects. The scientific literature on light and human biocycles is extensive.[78]

Nutritional Factors

Nutrients affect every hormonal interaction in the body, and adequate levels of them are clearly important in human reproduction. The standard American diet, high in processed foods and low in nutrients, is a setup for suboptimal nutrition at the time of conception. Recent research from the University of Adelaide in Australia that analyzed data from more than 5,500 women showed that a woman's diet before conception not only affected her ability to conceive but also affected how quickly she was able to do so.

Women who ate fruit three or more times a day had a lower risk for infertility and also conceived quicker—and the same was true for women who ate the least amount of fast food.[79]

Studies have shown that taking vitamin C (500 mg every twelve hours in one study) and zinc supplements has helped infertile couples.[80] Other studies have shown beneficial effects from folate and B[12] supplementation.[81] Adequate levels of vitamin D have been shown to increase the success rate of assisted reproduction treatment (not to mention the fact that vitamin D deficiency is associated with an increased risk of problems with fertilized eggs implanting properly in the uterus as well as with several obstetric complications).[82]

A double-blind placebo-controlled study on nutritional supplementation done at the Stanford University School of Medicine Department of Obstetrics and Gynecology and published in 2004 documented the benefits of nutritional supplementation in fertility patients. Researchers gave infertile women ages twenty-four to forty-six a nutritional supplement containing vitamins, minerals, green tea extract, and chasteberry. After five months, fifteen women (33 percent) of the nutritionally supplemented group were pregnant. None of the placebo group had conceived. There were no side effects.[83]

If a woman has been on the pill, especially if she is coming off it to conceive, I recommend that she take a good multivitamin if she isn't doing so already. Given the standard diet today and the stress levels of modern life, I suggest that all couples who are trying to conceive begin taking a multivitamin-multimineral supplement. (Nutritional deficiencies can affect sperm quality in males.) It's also important to follow a diet that decreases cellular inflammation. (See chapter 17.)

Eating disorders have also been associated with infertility because they are associated with endocrinologic disturbances. In one study, the investigators determined that 16.7 percent of their infertile subjects had eating disorders ranging from bulimia to anorexia. They recommended that a nutritional and eating disorder history be taken in infertility patients, particularly those with menstrual abnormalities.[84] Once the eating disorder is successfully resolved, endocrine balance is often restored.

Smoking, Drugs, and Alcohol

Smoking, drugs such as marijuana and cocaine, and alcohol intake have been shown in many studies to have adverse effects on all aspects of reproduction, from conception (both women's and men's roles) to labor and delivery. Smoking causes significant increases in miscarriage and prematurity. Women who smoke are less successful with fertility treatments of all kinds than are nonsmokers. If you're serious about becoming pregnant, get help for your addictions. (See "How to Quit Smoking" in chapter 17, page 924.)

Tubal Problems

In order to become pregnant, the fallopian tubes have to be able to pick up an egg and assist its passage to the waiting uterus. This process is dynamic and can be affected by a myriad of factors, one of the most common being scarring of the tubes from previous pelvic infections that are often the result of sexually transmitted diseases. This can be treated with a variety of techniques including deep tissue massage (see information on the Wurn Technique on page 157). In cases where the tubes are open but not fully functional, emotional work may need to be done. Tubal problems, says Caroline Myss, are centered around a woman's "inner child," while the tubes themselves are representative of unhealed childhood energy.

Amazingly, even women who are born without a uterus (a condition called Mayer-Rokitansky-Küster-Hauser syndrome) as well as those whose uterus has been removed because of cancer, other illnesses, or complications of previous childbirth can go on to give birth with the help of a uterine transplant, plus IVF. This happened for the first time in 2015, after a woman in Sweden received a uterus from a living donor, and for the first time in the United States in 2017. The following year, a woman in Brazil gave birth after receiving a uterus from a deceased donor—a significant step forward, since these organs are easier to procure. An estimated 50,000 women in this country might be candidates for this procedure, which is still considered experimental.

Helpful Modalities for Enhancing Fertility

Traditional Chinese Medicine

Though our culture is quick to bring in the big-gun technologies when it comes to fertility enhancement, these are often not necessary. One of the most helpful modalities for enhancing fertility is traditional Chinese medicine. I've been referring patients to practitioners of acupuncture and herbology for years with great success. It's the first place I go for any health problem myself. My colleague Randine Lewis, Ph.D., has dedicated her life to helping women enhance their fertility through the use of TCM. Dr. Lewis, author of *The Infertility Cure* (Little, Brown, 2004), was in medical school when she began to have fertility problems herself. After exhausting the Western medical approach, she discovered the ancient wisdom of traditional Chinese medicine. Not only did TCM resolve the imbalances that were leading to her own fertility problems, but Dr. Lewis realized that it was the perfect solution for many other women as well. She eventually dropped out of medical school to pursue training in traditional Chinese medicine. Following training in China, she returned to the United States, where she opened a clinic that has a 75 percent success rate helping women achieve optimal fertility. Her fertility enhancement work also supports women who are using assisted reproductive technologies, helping them achieve better outcomes. Her fertility enhancement program includes three sections:

1. New Hope: Enhancing Ovarian Response—opening up to Source energies to improve the function of the reproductive system

2. Paradigm Shift: Improving Reproductive Capacity—improving the endocrine system's hormonal status and the energies between all the glands

3. Nurturing the Mother Within: Opening to Implantation—the coming together of ovarian and hormonal responses, and allowing the body to receive

Dr. Lewis points out that in Chinese medicine, *a disturbed ovarian cycle is thought to take a full ninety days to regenerate.* That's why she urges her patients to complete a ninety-day program. TCM, like most holistic methods, is aimed at rebalancing the body from the inside out. It's not a quick fix the way Western medicine claims to be. Dr. Lewis offers two-day personal fertility-enhancing retreats, delivered via prerecorded online video sessions that include multiple exercises and self-inquiry processes. (See www .thefertilesoul.com.)

Treatment of Pelvic Adhesions

Pelvic adhesions from infection, trauma, surgery, or endometriosis can interfere with fallopian tube function and have long been associated with fertility problems as well as chronic pain. It is estimated that approximately 40 percent of female infertility is associated with scarring of the pelvic organs from either prior surgery or infections. A noninvasive, nonsurgical type of deep tissue massage performed by specially trained physical therapists (known as the Wurn Technique after its founders, Larry and Belinda Wurn— both physical therapists) has been shown to do the following:

~ More than 75 percent reversal of fallopian tube occlusion in women with diagnosed tubal occlusion

~ More than 70 percent infertility reversal in women who were physician-diagnosed as infertile

~ Significant improvement in IVF results when therapy was performed prior to IVF transfer

This technique also helps relieve many other conditions, including inability to reach orgasm, severe recurring menstrual pain, irritable bowel, painful intercourse, endometriosis, and pelvic pain. Numerous studies in peer-reviewed medical journals have documented the effectiveness of the Wurns' work. (For more information, read *Miracle Moms, Better Sex, Less Pain* [Med-Art Press, 2009] by Belinda Wurn and Larry Wurn, with Dr. Richard King, or contact Clear Passage Physical Therapy at 352-336-1433 or visit www.clearpassage.com.)

Maya abdominal massage, a technique used for centuries by indigenous healers in Central America, is another form of deep tissue massage that has been used to successfully treat infertility as well as other reproductive and pelvic disorders. (See the dysmenorrhea section of chapter 5, page 140, for a fuller explanation; for a directory of certified practitioners of Maya abdominal massage, visit arvigotherapy.com/arvigo-practitioners.)

Women's Stories

Grace: Childhood Fears

Grace was a successful businesswoman from the Midwest when she first came to see me about her infertility. Married for three years, she had been unable to conceive. Like many of my patients, she preferred to avoid extensive and invasive testing to investigate her problem unless it was absolutely necessary. Her reason for this was that she didn't want anyone "mucking around in there."

Grace ovulated regularly, had a normal pelvic exam, and experienced regular pain-free periods. She had no history of infection, IUD use, or prior pelvic surgery. In short, nothing about her history would lead me to think that there was anything wrong with her reproductive system. Her husband's sperm count was normal.

Over the course of her care, she got in touch with a memory from when she was four years old. At that age, she recalled, she had become so ill that she passed out with a high fever and ultimately had to be taken to the hospital. Though she'd felt sick for several days, she had not said anything to her parents until she was quite ill and had developed urinary retention. In the hospital she had to be held down by several nurses and orderlies while they inserted a urinary catheter into her bladder. Her mother felt that this represented very unseemly behavior on her daughter's part.

After Grace's recovery, her mother took her by the hand and made her apologize for being a "bad girl" to each of the nurses and orderlies who had taken care of her. She remembered acutely how ashamed she had felt. She had always felt that she had had a happy childhood, though she admitted that she couldn't remember much about it. But her hospital experience and her mother's abusive behavior had left a very deep wound. I suspect that her childhood was not nearly as happy as she remembered it.

After Grace told me about that childhood hospitalization, her reluctance to undergo invasive testing became understandable. As of this writing, she is working with a therapist and has decided to put her fertility workup on hold so that she can transform her old fears. She recently told me, "I realize I'm not ready to have a child now. I have too much work to do on myself. I don't want to pass my own unfinished business on to a child."

PREGNANCY LOSS
Miscarriage

Approximately one in six pregnancies ends in miscarriage. I tell women that miscarriage is usually nature's way of getting rid of conceptions that will not result in healthy babies. Generally speaking, healthy babies don't just miscarry, though there are some factors that may cause that to happen. Women who smoke, unfortunately, do have two times the usual rate of miscarriage, and it appears from studies of the miscarried fetuses that a much higher than usual percentage of them were otherwise normal. Smokers also have decreased success in all aspects of fertility treatments. There are also some data on the link between mercury exposure (usually from dental fillings) and subsequent miscarriage. Mercury should never be used for filling teeth in any case and it should *never* be used in pregnancy. Far better, less toxic materials are readily available. A study by Claire Infante-Rivard, M.D., Ph.D., of McGill University in Montreal, found that consuming an amount of caffeine more than that in three cups of coffee a day during pregnancy nearly tripled the rate of miscarriage.[85] However, a later study of 5,144 pregnant women from the State Department of Health Services in Emeryville, California, Kaiser Permanente Division of Research, and the University of California at San Francisco found no significant increased risk for miscarriage: Among heavy users (300 mg caffeine or three cups of coffee per day) the miscarriage rate increased only slightly. Given that caffeine is a well-documented stimulant and neurotoxin, it's advisable for women to decrease or eliminate caffeine consumption before conception and during pregnancy.[86]

A number of more recent studies have reported recurrent miscarriage secondary to blood clotting or platelet disorders.[87] In a recent case report, this syndrome was completely healed in a patient using acupuncture and an allergy elimination technique called Bioenergetic Sensitivity and Enzyme Therapy (BioSET), which is similar to NAET; the woman went on to have a normal pregnancy. Given the intricate and intimate connection between genes and the environment, I consider this a very encouraging collaboration between Eastern and Western medicine and would certainly recommend giving it a try if you've had recurrent miscarriages.[88]

Women who miscarry still must grieve the potential child, though, even if they believe the pregnancy wasn't "meant to be." In some cases, they go through as much grief as women who deliver stillborn babies. After a woman has a miscarriage, her chances of having another one are not increased, but many women nonetheless lose trust in their bodies after miscarrying. Grieving and learning to trust again are major issues for women following miscarriage. Another major issue is guilt: Many women have the mistaken impression that something they did must have caused the miscarriage. If you've had a miscarriage, don't spend a lot of time trying to figure out *why*. Just stay with what you're feeling, and give yourself time to mourn your loss.

Several studies have indicated that in women who have repeated (three or more) miscarriages, there may be an interplay between emotions and the hormonal systems involved in pregnancy. Dr. Robert J. Weil, a researcher on the emotional aspects of infertility, and C. Tupper write, "The pregnant woman functions as a communications system. The fetus is a source of continuous messages to which the mother responds with subtle psychobiological adjustments. Her personality, influenced by her ever-changing life situation, can either (1) act upon the fetus to maintain its constant growth and development or (2) create physiological changes that can result in abortion."[89] The ways in which a woman's body modulates her feelings about her pregnancy are diverse, but all are mediated by the immune and endocrine systems and also by the ways in which our thoughts impact cells directly. Thus, studies have shown that there are endocrinologic imbalances resulting from emotional stress in women who habitually miscarry (known as "habitual aborters" in medical circles) and in those who have what is known as an "incompetent cervix," a cervix that dilates too quickly, so the uterus cannot hold on to a baby. Some studies of women who habitually miscarry or who have an incompetent cervix have suggested that some of them have difficulty accepting motherhood and their feminine role. Femininity, to these women, means being self-sacrificing, passive, and suffering and having to serve and cater to their husbands (yet control them). They became pregnant "because their husbands wanted a child so badly." They also felt that "having a child was a woman's main accomplishment and that not being able to have children meant being inadequate as women."[90] They frequently chose dependent, nonverbal husbands and had restricted social outlets and low adaptability. Due to their aloofness, they were often unable to take part in life around them. The control group of non-miscarrying women in these studies had much healthier images of womanhood.[91] Another study found that "habitual aborters" basically received their pleasure in life through fulfilling the expectations of others. They appeared to react compliantly to the demands of others, despite tension and hostility building in their bodies. Feeling guilty about directly expressing their anger at other people's demands, their frustration built until their body responded with a physical illness. Miscarrying the child (the "psychosomatic" or "autoimmune" illness in this case) relieved the tension that had built up in their bodies. Interestingly, when many of these same women later underwent psychotherapy and learned how to deal directly with their anger rather than storing it in their bodies, their success rate for subsequent pregnancy was 80 percent, while it was only 6 percent for those who did not go through therapy.[92] Though these studies are fairly dated, they certainly support the role of psychological factors in fertility—factors that are very important to address but not beat yourself up with.

Miscarriage is multifactorial, and there's still a great deal we don't know. After his wife had her third miscarriage, science writer Jon Cohen embarked on a thorough investigation of the topic and wrote an incredibly comprehensive book on the subject entitled *Coming to Term: Uncovering the Truth About Miscarriage* (Houghton Mifflin, 2005). Cohen points out the downside of early pregnancy tests—something I've seen repeatedly. Early pregnancy tests have actually increased the rate of so-called miscarriage. By diagnosing pregnancy so early—often before a period is even missed and long before the body has had a chance to say yea or nay to the health of a potential embryo—women with a positive early pregnancy test begin to invest emotionally in the pregnancy. And then when the body says no to this embryo, which was never meant to reach viability, the woman may experience enormous grief and feel like a failure when in fact her body was acting appropriately. I've seen women repeatedly fall into utter despair over something that is really a gift of wisdom from the body—getting rid of a defective fertilized egg.

Back before early pregnancy tests were available, this so-called miscarriage would have been nothing more than a slightly late or heavier than normal period. And this experience wouldn't be perceived as a sign of failure or inadequacy by the woman herself. (Some experts suggest that up to 90 percent of fertilized eggs never make it to term. And most of these don't even get far enough to make sufficient hormone for a positive pregnancy test.) The good news, as Cohen documents, is that a woman's chance of successfully carrying a baby to term actually increases after each subsequent miscarriage. The books mentioned in the approach to fertility resources for this chapter have helped many women heal miscarriage problems.

Ectopic Pregnancy

A fertilized egg normally implants in the lining of the uterus. Implantation anywhere else is called an ectopic pregnancy. Approximately 1.9 percent of all pregnancies are ectopic, with the risk (higher in nonwhite women than in white women) having increased tenfold from 1970 through 2004 before leveling off. These increases have been reported not only for the United States but also for Eastern Europe, Scandinavia, and Great Britain. The most likely causes for this increase in ectopic pregnancy are the following:

~ The prevalence of sexually transmitted diseases, which can lead to tubal scarring

~ The ability of transvaginal ultrasound and early pregnancy tests to pick up the diagnosis in pregnancies that would simply reabsorb on their own

~ The use of tubal sterilization techniques

~ The increase in C-sections, which increases the risk of ectopic pregnancies in subsequent pregnancies

~ The use of tubal surgery to repair damaged tubes

The diagnosis of ectopic pregnancy is made in a woman with a positive pregnancy test when an ultrasound fails to find evidence of pregnancy in the uterus (a small sac of fluid surrounding an embryo and known as a gestational sac). When this happens, a series of blood tests several days apart are drawn to determine whether the amount of the pregnancy hormone beta HCG (human chorionic gonadotropin) is increasing or decreasing. If it is decreasing, then it is safe to watch and wait and simply follow the patient carefully with blood tests every other day or so. But if the beta HCG level continues to increase and there is still no evidence of pregnancy in the uterus itself, then the pregnancy is presumed to be in the wrong location. Often it will show up as a mass in one of the tubes on ultrasound. Sometimes you can even feel it on pelvic exam. Since a ruptured fallopian tube can be life-threatening because of hemorrhaging, ectopic pregnancies that are growing must be treated. This is usually done with the chemotherapy drug methotrexate, which kills rapidly growing cells. This works in the majority of cases, and the tube reabsorbs the ectopic tissue over time. When medical treatment fails, surgery is necessary. A woman who has had an ectopic pregnancy has a 7 to 15 percent chance of having a recurrence because of scarring in the tube.

Though ectopic pregnancy accounts for 10 percent of all pregnancy-related deaths, the actual death rate from this pregnancy complication has decreased tenfold in the past few decades, most likely due to improved diagnosis and management.[93] Whenever a pregnant woman has pain and bleeding in the first trimester, an ectopic pregnancy needs to be ruled out.

I would strongly recommend deep tissue massage such as the Wurn Technique or Maya abdominal massage for any woman who has had a history of tubal infection, tubal surgery, or ectopic pregnancy. (See chapter 5.) That's because this technique might well be able to help prevent or eliminate the tubal adhesions that favor a future ectopic pregnancy.

Ended Beginnings: The Experience of a Stillbirth

While I was in my residency, a lovely young Catholic woman gave birth to two perfect identical twin girls. Unfortunately, these twins had gotten their cords wrapped around each other and died just before labor started (a very unusual event). As I was helping the attending physician deliver these two babies, I asked the mother if she'd like to see them and hold them. I had intended to wrap them in baby blankets and spend some time with her after the delivery, sitting with her while she held her babies. But her doctor scolded me, and he said to her, "Regina, it's better if you don't look. We'll just give you something to put you to sleep so you can get on with your life and get this behind you. It will bother you if you see them." An obedient woman, she complied. As a physician in training, I understood that it wasn't a good idea for me to argue with her doctor.

I knew instinctively that this doctor was wrong and that this mother needed to interact with what she had created, lest she go on to dream for years of babies with no faces. Her babies were in fact beautiful. She needed to see their little hands, their perfect bodies, and their angelic faces—and to know that her body had created them. It is so much easier to deal with what is than with our fantasies about what is.

Most women need to interact with their "creations"—their stillborn babies. Otherwise, unfinished emotional business may result. When a couple has a deformed baby or a stillborn (or suffers the death of any child or loved one, for that matter), they need to look at and touch this being, take pictures, name the child, and perhaps have a ceremony of some kind that acknowledges that this child existed. Thanks to the vision of Kathy Adzich, many hospitals now provide a room where couples can hold their babies who are sick or who have died, bathe them, and take pictures of them—so that parents have something tangible to hold on to. The process of simply holding the baby and interacting with him or her can be extraordinarily healing.

I met Kathy Adzich, a wonderful, light-filled human being who is obviously doing the work she was born to do, in San Diego in the fall of 2005. Kathy lost her son Jakob to sepsis when he was twenty-six days old (as well as two other infant sons before Jakob). Not ready to have Jakob taken away to the hospital morgue, she asked the nurses if she could have a room where she could hold her baby for a while (and for her, "a while" meant two days). To their credit, the hospital staff complied. Though some thought Kathy should move on, she felt that staying with her son was perfectly normal. She needed time to sleep with her son nestled in her arms, keep him close, stroke him, bathe him, and sing to him. She made prints of his hands. She invited friends and family to visit, and together they told stories, laughed, and sang. No one thought it was weird or morbid.

The process helped Kathy transform her grief into a living force to help others. She started a movement to humanize death, convincing an increasing number of hospitals to develop protocols and even offer special resources to help grieving parents. Many others have taken up this work as well, most notably a professional organization called Pregnancy Loss and Infant Death Alliance (www.plida.org), whose mission is education, advocacy, and networking for healthcare providers and parent advocates.

When the work of the late Elisabeth Kübler-Ross, M.D., on grief and dying became better known with the publication of her classic work *On Death and Dying* (Macmillan, 1969), hospitals started to realize that avoiding and denying death didn't help patients' healing process. Far too many women who have lost babies never grieved properly—in fact, they were often told, "You have other children at home" or "You can have more" or "You must be strong." Grief was considered self-indulgent.

But that which isn't fully grieved cannot be released. (This is also a problem with infertility.) Healing from the pain of pregnancy loss or loss of a child is a process. It requires time. It requires that a woman give herself the time and space necessary to grieve and heal.

Barb Frank wrote me the following letter about the unexpected stillbirth of her son, Micah, after a normal and healthy pregnancy. "I was very porous after this experience. It has been a time of intense emotional and spiritual growth for me. Initially it was the opening experience of allowing vulnerability and being willing to openly grieve with my friends . . . to cry in front of and with other people was really healing and a very new experience. (I am usually 'in control' and a real 'planner.') This also has become an emotionally transforming experience for three women friends who came to the birth center and were able to spend time holding Micah with us and being in the midst of that mysterious energy between birth and death present in that room. Subsequently it has made my compassion and understanding so much deeper; it has affected my work as a pediatric occupational therapist with families dealing with their own fear and loss over their children with disabilities. I am no longer afraid of their tears or even anger, because I've been there. The need to create a space and time for grief and reflection in the midst of busy days has brought me closer to a spiritual discipline of regular prayer/meditation time that I always wanted to make time for, but never did until now, when I've had to for emotional survival. So I guess I'm getting the message."

Barb also created an announcement to be able to share the news of her birth. She used it for everything from shower gift thank-yous to enclosures at the memorial service—and even put it into some Christmas cards. It reads:

Facing the mystery of
life and death
we mourn the loss of our son
—Micah—

who accompanied us through a healthy
and hopeful pregnancy . . . but was stillborn
on September 21, 5 lbs. 6 oz., 19 inches.

At the request of her midwives, she also wrote the following list of things that helped her in her recovery process. This is a most helpful and universally applicable list of things to help with grieving a loss of any kind. I am honored to share it with you from Barb.

Having enough time, initially, with the baby and taking photos to have and share later. Some couples have also dressed and bathed the baby. One couple took the child home with them for several hours.

Having friends come and see and hold the baby with us. This validated the whole experience for me, as no one else would get to meet Micah, and in that sense it still isn't "real" for most friends and family.

Crying with people, and seeing others cry, made it easier for us. When people tried to hide their emotions in an effort to be "strong" or "professional," it made things feel worse.

Notes and phone calls from people who have been there and experienced loss themselves, and could articulate this. Also communication from others who had just spent time thinking about what we have experienced and were able to reflect on it beyond "I don't know what to say."

Physical presence of people and physical contact with people, especially in the early days and weeks. I had a need to literally hang on to people to feel grounded and "present" in the world, which is uncharacteristic of me. As time has passed, phone calls still serve that purpose, especially when I need to connect when I'm having a hard time.

Creating a "shrine" of important gifts, notes, photos, remembrances of Micah. This has been a tangible way to remember and honor him, and I never understood the importance of shrines/altars in other cultures and churches until this happened. Lighting a candle (and carrying it around the house) still helps a lot when I feel depressed.

Getting back in shape physically, getting as much exercise as my body could deal with at each stage.

Being involved in purposeful activity. Achieving concrete tasks around the house, in the garden, that gave me a sense of accomplishment but didn't require too much problem-solving (I was easily frustrated, had memory problems, and not much creative energy for a time).

Being outside. For me, getting back into work in the garden puts me in touch with the cycle of life and is grounding and gives me a sense of hope and renewal. Going to the beach is good, but the ocean was almost too emotionally powerful at first . . . so infinite and symbolic as a source of life.

Reading the books and handouts on grief and loss of a baby. We read many out loud together, which also let us talk about our feelings. They always made me cry, but it has been important and positive to cry. Afterward I usually feel better. (I highly recommend *Life Touches Life* [New-Sage, 2004] by Lorraine Ash.)

Barb went on to give birth to a healthy baby girl. She told me that that pregnancy was difficult because she was always worried about the health of the baby. But with the support of her midwives and the staff of the birth center, she made it through and is now enjoying her new daughter.

ADOPTION

Adoption is receiving more attention than ever these days. The CDC reports that nearly 40 percent of American adults have considered adopting a child[94] (and according to the Evan B. Donaldson Adoption Institute, if just one in 500 of them ended up adopting, all the children in foster care waiting for adoption would have permanent families).[95] Currently, a large number of American couples have adopted foreign infants. I can't think of a better way to promote global awareness and intercultural understanding. A patient who adopted two Chinese children told me the following story, which she calls "Listening with the Heart."

Susan and her husband, Bob, went to Taiwan with the intention of adopting a child. One month later, they returned as a family of four with Anio Nicholas, almost six, and Shao-Ma Annie, almost four. "Christmas was a wonderful celebration of the birth of our new family," said Susan. The following Thanksgiving Susan invited her extended family of origin to share the holiday with her "new" family. Near the end of that day of celebration, Annie, sitting on the stairs, asked accusingly, "*Why* did you come to get us in that taxicab in Taiwan, anyway?" Susan wondered what had prompted that question. Then it dawned on her that for the first time since the adoption Annie was sitting in a roomful of people whom Susan dearly loved, to whom she had been paying a great deal of attention—the kind of attention that up until then Annie had seen her give only to Bob, to Nicholas, and to herself.

Focusing on her daughter's question, Susan told her the truth: that she had had a very happy life, full of friends and family, work and play, but that she had still felt filled with a love that wasn't used up. And so she and her husband had gone looking for someone to love and had found her and her brother. Annie tipped her head pensively to one side, then went off to brush her teeth. Susan joined her for their nightly ritual together. As Annie squirted toothpaste onto both their toothbrushes, she said defiantly, "I want to go back to Taiwan to see my *Chinese* mother"—even though she had been told that there was no record of her mother and that it wasn't known who had brought her to the home. Susan realized that her daughter's desire to go back to Taiwan at that moment was symbolic and important. So Susan asked her, "Would you like me to go with you, or would you like to go by yourself?" Annie answered, "By myself." Susan was struck by a sense of loss, emptiness, and despair. She later told me, "Welling up in me was the question, 'But what about me? I love you and have loved you with all my heart! Isn't that good enough? What about me?'"

Then she looked at her daughter and knew that her longing for her Chinese mother was simply a natural part of her birth history and who she was. "Annie was, in her love for a woman whom neither of us would probably ever meet, sharing with me her deepest self. I could join her now, at the core of her being, in her love, or I could bar myself from it. And so finally, I, the verbalizer, just listened—actively, achingly—with my heart."

Several Christmases later, Susan and Bob were walking together with Annie swinging between them, holding their hands. She swung high, and as Bob's and Susan's eyes met over her head, she called out to the sky: "Hello, Chinese mother! How are you? I am happy and I hope you are, too! I love you! Goodbye!"

I once participated in a wonderful adoption ceremony with a couple, long infertile, who had successfully found a child with the help, intent, and prayers of their extended family and community. They brought the baby to a large gathering shortly after the adoption to share their joy with us. I would recommend a similar ceremony to all who are adopting a child. It is a touching and conscious way to bring a child into her or his new community.

In a ceremonial fashion, the woman leading the event had the adoptive parents hold up the baby and carry him around to the members of our community to be welcomed. At the same time, she asked those people who had been adopted to please stand in the center of the circle during this ceremony. As we each welcomed the baby, she addressed the people who had themselves been adopted. "As we welcome this new baby and celebrate his birth and his new parents, may this day symbolize for you that you are deeply wanted, that you were always deeply wanted. And from now on, no matter what has happened to you in the past, may you know how meaningful your birth was and, seeing how deeply wanted and blessed this child is, claim the same thing for yourself." This ceremony was a great healing on many levels for many people and was full of wonder and hope.

Through the years I've worked with birth mothers as well as adoptive mothers, and I appreciate both ends of this relationship. Both terminating parental rights to place a baby for adoption and adopting one have consequences and put all the parties involved on an emotional roller coaster. In the past, adoption agencies operated under the illusions of secrecy and denial. Now, through the efforts of birth mothers and adopted children alike, natural parents and their adopted-out babies are finding one another, sometimes with joyous results but sometimes also with great disappointment. Nevertheless, adoption is an area in which society is learning that secrets don't work. They especially don't work with matters of lineage. Bloodlines are very powerful—they hold ancient memories.

Even more important, every baby is deeply imprinted in the womb by the prenatal environment created by her mother. There is no way around this except to acknowledge the fact that none of us is a tabula rasa when we are born. On the other hand, any untoward prenatal imprint can be greatly ameliorated by how the adopted child is parented. I have always believed that we choose our parents, and that includes those who raise us. The children we raise are our children, pure and simple. I recently heard inspirational speaker Les Brown speak eloquently of being raised by an adoptive mother this way: "I was taken from the womb of my birth mother and nurtured in the heart of my adoptive mother." I have never heard a man speak more lovingly about his mother.

It has now become the norm for adoptive parents to gather as much information as they can about their child's birth parents and circumstances, to share it with their child when the time comes. Most children want to know their heritage. Birth mothers, too, almost always want to know where their children are and if they are all right—even when they know that they themselves are not capable of raising them adequately. In matters of adoption, the only thing that works is honesty.

Another woman I know once told me that when her daughter was a high school freshman, she participated in a women's ceremony in which she had a mystical vision of her future grandchild. The woman and her daughter are white, but the baby in the vision was not. "I could see the baby's face and I could actually feel its little body as I held it in my arms. I was overcome with love," she told me. "I wasn't sure of the sex, but I *knew* the baby was South American. I hadn't expected that, which to me made the experience more believable." She told me she wouldn't be surprised at all if her daughter, who is now in her mid-twenties, ended up adopting once she's ready to start a family.

FERTILITY AS METAPHOR

We must deal with the economic and social problems that are the root causes of high fertility rates: widespread poverty and the oppression of women. . . . When women everywhere have control over their own reproductive choices, fertility rates drop.
—The Union of Concerned Scientists

Motherhood is not simply the organic process of giving birth . . . it is understanding the needs of the world.
—Alexis De Veaux

Increasingly, humans are coming to terms with the idea of sustainability, which Friends of the Earth defines as "the simple principle of taking from the Earth only what it can provide indefinitely, thus leaving future generations no less than we have access to ourselves." We are learning that sustainability involves living within the limits of the resources of the earth while understanding the connections between our economy, our society, and our environment.

We have been clever, producing more and more food from less and less land. The Union of Concerned Scientists writes, "Our species simply cannot survive today's recklessly accelerating population growth, the irresponsible squandering of the Earth's resources, and the continuing destruction of our environment. . . . Every day, there are a quarter of a million more of us than there were the day before. Every week, we must find ways to feed another city the size of Philadelphia. Every month, we must wrest from the Earth additional resources to keep alive another New Jersey. And every year, we are adding another whole Mexico to the burden of this small planet."[96]

The time of endless productivity without replenishing is coming to an end. This is why the world's economic priorities have had to shift, fueled by the global recession that began in earnest in 2008. Women *must* use our inherent creativity—our womb power—to regenerate our planet as well as to produce the next generation. We can no longer have baby after baby with no thought for the consequences. Many of us already feel bad about disposable diapers because of what we know they're doing to our planet's landfills—but we must also look at the fact that the average child in the United States uses fifty times the resources of a child born in a developing nation. Few issues are as controversial as population growth, and I don't intend to go into that controversy here.

In the United States as well as elsewhere, women who have no means of child support bear child after child. These are the mothers who are at risk for developing problems in labor, for having growth-retarded, premature babies. But these women's problems are *symptoms* of the imbalance in our culture—they are *not* the cause. The underlying problem is society's treatment of women and the cycles of poverty, victimization, and abuse in which these young women stay locked.

Sixty percent of teenage mothers are victims of sexual abuse.[97] Almost instinctively, they mate with men who then abandon them. That is all they know—a premature commitment that keeps them trapped. The only role they perceive as open to them is that of baby carrier. They don't know that they have choices. When they think they can do little else, they have babies. Happily, that is changing. Birth rates among adolescents (girls ages ten to fourteen) in the United States have been declining, reaching a record low in 2015, while the birth rate for teen mothers ages fifteen to nineteen declined 57 percent from 2000 through 2016.[98] Rates of sexual activity, especially among African Americans and Hispanics, also decreased significantly between 2005 and 2015.[99]

When we teach young women that they have inherent worth—and that though they may choose to have a baby, there are many other opportunities open to them as well—the world changes. It's happening right now. What if all girls knew that their menstrual cycles are part of their sacred connection with the earth and the moon—and that their sexuality needn't necessarily be shared with men? That they could have it all to themselves if they chose? What if they didn't measure their worth by whose baby they had or whom they were sleeping with? What if they knew that their wombs, whether or not they have children, are their bodies' center for creativity and desire?

We need to expand the meanings of *fertility* and *birth*. We must begin to see female birth power for what it is—the basis of all of creation. When enough women sense this creative female power inherent within each of us—not dependent upon what we produce or don't produce with our bodies—the world will change. When women tap in to this power, the children, the ideas, and the new world to which we give birth will be supportive of all beings, including ourselves.

Whether we ever choose pregnancy, every one of us has encoded in our cells the knowledge of what it is to conceive, gestate, and give birth to something that grows out of our own substance. Conception, gestation, labor, and birth are physical metaphors for how all creation manifests on earth.

On some level we all have miscarriages, abortions, dysfunctional labors, and stillbirths, as well as beautifully formed creations. We don't need to go through these processes physically to understand them and heal from them—they're inherent processes in nature.

Each woman must find her own truth about how to use her fertility if she is to truly flourish. The most important thing to remember is that our creative fertility in the broadest sense is with us for a lifetime—whether or not we have children.

12
Pregnancy and Birthing

For all eternity, God lies on a birthing bed, giving birth. The essence of God is Birthing.

—Meister Eckhart

THE TRANSFORMING POWER OF PREGNANCY

Pregnancy is a time to be savored and celebrated as you take part in gestating the future. It's a miracle, really—and a crucial time in your own and your child's development. During pregnancy you can be in touch with your *hara*—your body's center of creation—in the most direct and powerful way possible. When a woman becomes pregnant, the hormone known as HCG (human chorionic gonadotropin, which is the basis for the pregnancy test) is produced by the placenta in vast quantities. The cells of your body haven't seen this particular hormone since you yourself were in your mother's womb. I believe that this is the physiologic reason why pregnancy awakens primal tribal memories about how our own bodies were formed and how they were nurtured. One of my colleagues experienced a great deal of hip pain during and after her pregnancy. When she delved into the matter, she discovered that when her mother had gone into labor with her, she had been told it wasn't time to deliver, and so she had tried to hold back my friend's delivery by squeezing. A psychic told my colleague that this had hurt her left hip during birth—hence the repetition of this pain during her own labor. Because your body is literally awash in the biochemistry of new beginnings, pregnancy and birth are also times to heal your past.

This is true not only for you, but very often also for your entire extended family. The birth of a grandchild can unite families in profound ways. Adult children sometimes move back to their home turf, realizing how important family really is. Almost all of my daughters' classmates from high school have moved back to our town to raise their children and be near their parents. When my first granddaughter was born, I was astounded by how fierce my love for her was. I hadn't expected this at all. I told my daughter, "I'll do whatever it takes to help you raise this child. And if anything happens to you and her dad, put me down as the one who will take it from there." Talk about a new beginning.

Pregnancy is not an illness or a time for us to be treated with kid gloves. Still, it is a period when we need quiet reflective time to tune in to ourselves and our babies. Positive inner communication between mother and baby long before birth translates into a deeper trust of each other after birth. Pregnancy is also a time to rest, which the body is primed to do. The hormone progesterone, released naturally during pregnancy, has calming and soothing effects. (It also relaxes and slows the bowel, which can lead to constipation in some women.) The body is doing a lot of inner work growing a baby. The tenor of the pregnancy itself contributes to the strength of a child's constitution throughout the rest of his or her life. Forty weeks of gestation is a *very short* amount of time in a woman's life, relatively speaking. Yet it is a time that is crucial for the health of the next generation.

Quality care and education during pregnancy, along with a woman's willingness to shore up her internal blueprint for nurturing through optimal self-care, can prevent an untold number of costly problems for the child later, including many cases of prematurity, growth retardation, mental retardation, physical disability, and learning disabilities—all of which also make the process of parenting much more difficult. And by the way, recent news about the extremely controversial ability to actually edit genes in a human embryo just reinforces this. It's so much safer for all concerned, and ultimately more effective, to set the stage for delivering a healthy baby by doing everything you can to first care for the vessel that baby will be conceived and developed in—your own body—on every level, physically, emotionally, mentally, and spiritually. Optimal care of pregnant women, who are simultaneously very powerful and vulnerable at this time, should be the highest priority in the world. Because women tend to take better care of themselves during pregnancy, it is a fantastic opportunity for them to learn more about themselves and the sources of their own vitality.

For centuries, midwives helped mothers through the pregnancy and birthing processes, standing by them with medical and emotional aid. The very word *obstetrics* is derived from the Latin word *stare,* which means "to stand by." A woman's body knows instinctively how to give birth and will respond in settings in which she is encouraged to move in the ways that feel right and to make the sounds that she needs to make. Modern obstetrics, however, has changed from a natural process of "standing by" and allowing the woman's body to respond naturally into a domineering and often invasive practice. Hence the aptly named book *Pushed: The Painful Truth About Childbirth and Modern Maternity Care,* by Jennifer Block (Da Capo Press, 2007), a volume that accurately documents the current sorry state of maternity care in the United States. Women's cultural conditioning causes us to turn ourselves over to pregnancy experts, so most of us have lost touch with our innate pregnancy and birthing knowledge and power, as have most of these experts, who rely on tests and machines to tell them how to help. I delivered babies for almost a decade and had two of my own before I really came to appreciate the fact that most women's experience of pregnancy, labor, and delivery is nowhere near as empowering as it could be.

Why Have Children?

When I recall the reasons that I had children, I see how emotional and instinctual, unconscious and "tribal" my decision was. The biological pull was so strong. Those of us who've had a child or two have often longed to have another baby, even knowing that another child would tax our emotional and physical resources in an unhealthy way. Some women simply love being pregnant. Others adore little babies and want one around all the time. Some women are even addicted to having babies and giving birth—in part because it's the only thing that is totally theirs in their family structure. I've worked with many women who have become obsessed with having another child in their late thirties or early forties, partly so that they could put off deciding what to do with their lives for another five years.

Some women use pregnancy as a way to try to fill a void in their lives that another human being can never fill. We must know ourselves intimately before we can ever be intimate with another human being. When a baby is brought into being to fill the unmet needs of an adult, the child will carry the unfair and often harmful burden of a parent's impossible expectations. Though having a baby is rarely a strictly rational or logical decision, the decision still can be made consciously and with the wisdom of the heart. My wish for all women is that we gain the courage to understand that having a child cannot in and of itself make us happy and fulfilled. Consider this from Betsey Stevenson, assistant professor of business and public policy at the Wharton School, University of Pennsylvania: "Across the happiness data, the one thing in life that will make you less happy is having children. It's true whether you're wealthy or poor, if you have kids late or kids early. Yet I know very few people who would tell me they wish they hadn't had kids or who would tell me they feel their kids were the destroyer of their happiness."[1]

Probably the biggest factor that contributes to this unhappiness is the fact that a woman's fertility peak also coincides with the time when she is developing her career. And so her feminine nurturing values often are pitted against the masculine traits she must employ to get ahead at work—all of which results in enormous guilt unless she realizes that this problem is far bigger than she is. It's why so many women eventually drop out of corporate America and start their own businesses or work from home. In 2009, women were running more than 10 million businesses with combined sales of $1.9 trillion.[2] And over the past thirty years, the number of women working for themselves has doubled. Today, 35 percent of all self-employed workers are women.[3]

This dilemma was what drove me to start a different kind of practice back in the 1980s. There was simply no way to balance my family and my career in the corporate structure in which I worked. And for many women, this is still the case.

OUR CULTURAL INHERITANCE: PREGNANCY

Pregnancy as a "Condition" to Be Overcome

During my mother's era, pregnant women were not expected to go outside their homes much or travel. Maternity clothes, which included that anathema, a maternity girdle, were ugly and did not enhance women's body image. Many women lost their jobs if they became pregnant. And for women who didn't lose their jobs, there was no formal pregnancy leave, even as late as the early 1980s. That said, pregnancy is a special time. Never again in your life will you be influencing the health of your child in a way that is this profound. You are growing the eyes, the brain, the heart, the liver, and all the major organs of another human being—in your own body. The quality of those organs and that life are directly and powerfully connected to your thoughts and behaviors, for better or for worse. I knew this intellectually, but my behavior when pregnant didn't match what I knew. I also had minimal support.

As the first physician in my former practice to have a pregnancy leave, I experienced some resentment from a few of my colleagues, who felt that pregnancy should not be treated the same way as a broken leg because it was, after all, a "chosen disability" over which I had some control. We've certainly come a long way since then, but pretending that a pregnant woman is just like everyone else and has no special needs is shortsighted and puts her and her baby's health at risk. Our culture can't seem to find a happy medium.

But we need to support women in their pregnancies, for their sake and for the sake of their children. Prenatal influences set the stage of a child's state of health for her entire life. A baby's gene expression is powerfully shaped and guided starting in utero. Thomas Verny, M.D., Psy.D., a psychiatrist and psychologist who founded the Association for Pre- and Perinatal Psychology and Health, writes, "In fact, the great weight of the scientific evidence that has emerged over the last decade demands that we re-evaluate the mental and emotional abilities of unborn children. Awake or asleep, the studies show, they are constantly tuned in to their mother's every action, thought, and feeling. From the moment of conception, the experience in the womb shapes the brain and lays the groundwork for personality, emotional temperament, and the power of higher thought."[4] Studies have shown, for example, that suboptimal conditions in utero set the stage for adult diseases such as high blood pressure, cancer, depression, heart disease, and diabetes.[5] Therefore, pregnancy needs to be treated as a special (and crucial) time that requires a woman to proactively make some arrangements for increased rest and care, or at the very least change any negative thoughts or feelings she has about her pregnancy. Otherwise, she may experience increased fatigue, premature labor, and toxemia.[6] Studies have shown that women who aren't supported or are highly stressed in their pregnancies have a higher incidence of adverse outcomes, and so do their babies. On the other hand, even women who have high-risk pregnancies have been shown to have bigger babies and healthier outcomes if they are optimistic.[7]

An Obstetrician Gets Pregnant

When I became pregnant with my first child, I had recently completed my four-year residency training and by then had worked with hundreds of pregnant women, providing them with prenatal care, labor support, and assistance with delivery of their babies. I had been a proponent of natural, drug-free childbirth throughout my residency, and I was very optimistic about my own. After all, the vast majority of pregnancies end with a normal baby—I had seen the truth of this firsthand.

My attitude toward the pregnancy was one of watching an experiment with the uterus. Wasn't this interesting—to see the changes my body was going through! I realize now that I didn't allow myself what I then considered the luxury of excitement and anticipation, though mine was very much a planned and wanted pregnancy.

I had learned very well how to separate my mind from my body, so I decided that I didn't want to bond much with my baby until after the pregnancy was well along and I knew that the baby was normal—something I would be assured of only *after* he or she was born. Notice the paradox in my thinking here. I felt strongly that everything would be normal, yet I didn't want to make such an investment "just in case." I had watched some women furnish entire nurseries as early as their third month of pregnancy, when the risk of miscarriage is still one in six. I didn't want to go through that kind of grief. I thought that their emotional investment was premature. Years later, I learned that babies know what's going on in utero and hear, feel, and experience emotions long before they're born. When their mothers are detached and not invested emotionally, babies sense this.

Back then I didn't realize for myself, though I taught it to my patients, that a woman's process of bonding with her baby starts when her pregnancy test is positive. At this point, women usually start fantasizing about the baby, thinking about names, and looking at baby clothes and other items. (With the advent of early ultrasound, the bonding process is now earlier and more intense than ever before.) I had never been very interested in babies and could not understand the behavior of women at baby showers—events that I could barely stand. Oohing and ahhing over baby clothes had never appealed to me. (As a grandmother now, I have definitely softened my former left-brained, unemotional stance—and also recovered from a lot of my medical training.)

When the nurses asked me, toward the end of the pregnancy, if I had the baby's room ready, I said, "No, I don't even have a T-shirt." I had no baby stuff at all, not even a diaper. My husband was completing a fellowship in orthopedics and was, as usual, busier than I was. He certainly wasn't up for baby shopping. Although I was clear that I didn't want a baby shower, luckily some nurse friends ignored my adamancy. Though I was mortified at the time, I was grateful later, as I didn't have a clue as to how to go about buying baby things.

At the same time, however, instead of reading parenting guides, I trusted without question my ability to mother. Sentimentality about babies was not, in my opinion, a prerequisite for good mothering. My own mother had been a "lioness" type, with excellent instincts most of the time. She didn't give in much to "experts"—a trait for which I'll always be grateful.

As my baby grew, I watched my body change with interest. I learned a great deal about morning sickness, pain under the rib cage, constipation, excess gas, and heartburn. I'd heard women complain about these things for years, and now I could see why. Although my husband thought my changing body was beautiful, I wasn't convinced. I was concerned about gaining too much weight. How was I supposed to *enjoy* a disappearing waist, puffy cheeks, and increased fat on my hips in a culture that worships quasi-anorexia?

I now regret that I have no pictures of myself while I was pregnant. I was amazed at my patients who showed me entire photo albums of themselves during pregnancy and delivery—they were proud and unashamed of their bodies. At the time, these women seemed like specimens from a different planet—didn't they get it that the culture (and I) didn't think they looked all that great? Two decades have brought about fabulous changes in this area. Now women are justifiably proud of their "bumps." And maternity clothes are fabulous. My own daughter—along with her husband—made a plaster cast of her pregnant belly the week before their second child was born. They plan to decorate it and hang it on the wall at some point. Progress.

During my second pregnancy, I lost my waist almost as soon as I conceived and looked pregnant almost immediately, a common event. This time, I was busier than I had been during my first pregnancy, but I remember taking more time to talk to my baby (although, since she was much more active than my first, I made a sexist assumption and called her William for nine months, an unconsciousness for which I have apologized to Kate repeatedly). Toward the end of this pregnancy, I had difficulty walking because of separation of my pubic bone, which happens so that the baby can fit through the pelvis, but by and large, it was a completely normal pregnancy. Though my belly got a lot bigger, I gained the same amount of weight—twenty-five pounds—in both pregnancies.

I once met a sophisticated professional woman in her late thirties who was in the middle of her first pregnancy. She had finally conceded that she needed to purchase some "ugly clothes" because it had become too hard to "hide" her pregnancy and she had to modify her polished executive look of slim skirts and high heels. Her attitude that pregnancy was something to be endured, ignored, or tolerated used to be all too common—and I was guilty of the same thing myself to a degree. The less pregnant you look, the better everyone tells you you're doing: "Oh, you're so little, you look great—I can hardly tell!" A prenatal-vitamin advertisement in one of the medical journals from the mid-1980s shows a very thin, tall woman who doesn't look at all pregnant, running around taking pictures, working out at the gym, and staying late at the office. The caption reads, "Pregnant, but she won't slow down." The ad reminds me of my own attitude during my pregnancies, when I ran up the hospital stairs to do C-sections or surgery. I didn't want the pregnancies to interfere with my life in any way. How ridiculous.

When I was pregnant with my second child and had to get up at night to go deliver babies, I was so tired that I occasionally walked into walls while I was getting dressed. (My first child, once born, didn't sleep through the night until she was five, so I was up at night for years, whether I was on call or not.) But no one suggested that I slow down. Besides, I was *still* trying to prove myself a worthy professional (think man)—especially now that I'd had children. This is what programming in patriarchy does to most of us to one degree or another.

Unfortunately, studies have shown that not slowing down is sometimes associated with increased health risks. A pilot study of stress and pregnancy in pregnant physicians and nurses showed that certain stress hormones (catecholamines) produced by the adrenals and other tissue under physical or mental stress increased by 58 percent (as measured in the urine) during work periods, compared with nonwork periods. The pregnant physicians' catecholamine levels were also increased by 64 percent over those working non-physicians' control groups of similar gestational age.[8] Higher catecholamine levels increase cellular inflammation, which is a setup for all birth complications. Sylvia Guendelman, Ph.D., a professor of public health at the University of California, Berkeley, has shown that taking maternity leave before delivery can reduce C-section rates fourfold. Again, this is because rest and sleep are the very best ways to metabolize and also reduce secretion of stress hormones, thus decreasing cellular inflammation.[9]

Program for Creating Optimal Pregnancy and Decreased Risk of Complications

Woman literally illustrates the on-going life pattern of how energy becomes matter through pregnancy, labor, and delivery.
—Caroline Myss

The common pathway that leads to nearly all pregnancy complications, including preeclampsia, low birth weight, and prematurity, is cellular inflammation. Happily, cellular inflammation can be curtailed in many different ways, all of which complement one another. The following program will increase your chances of a healthy pregnancy.

~ *Diet.* Eat a low-glycemic-index diet that keeps blood sugar stable and insulin levels low and that also contains adequate protein, essential fats, and micronutrients. Many women cannot tolerate gluten, dairy, corn, or soy very well these days, and pregnancy is a wonderful time to upgrade your nutrition. (See chapter 17.) Such a diet will also help ensure that weight gain remains within healthy limits.

OPTIMAL WEIGHT GAIN IN PREGNANCY

Weight gain in pregnancy is becoming an increasingly important factor, now that 68 percent of adult women are at least overweight, with more than 41 percent of all adult women now meeting the medical definition of obese.[10] Guidelines initially released in 2009 by the Institute of Medicine and the National Research Council recommend a narrower range of weight gain during pregnancy for obese women. These guidelines, based on World Health Organization cut-off points for body mass index (BMI) categories, recommend keeping weight gain within the following ranges for optimal health of both the baby *and* the mother: from 28 to 40 pounds for underweight women, from 25 to 35 pounds for normal-weight women, from 15 to 25 pounds for overweight women, and from 11 to 20 pounds for women who are obese.[11]

~ *Stop smoking (including marijuana) and avoid cigarette smoke.* Smoking deprives the fetus of oxygen, resulting in slower growth and therefore low infant birth weight. According to the Surgeon General, smoking accounts for 20 to 30 percent of low-birth-weight infants, up to 14 percent of preterm deliveries, and about 10 percent of all infant deaths. Even healthy, full-term babies born to women who smoke may have narrowed airways and curtailed lung function. Other studies have shown that smoking during pregnancy is associated with learning disabilities and behavioral problems for the child later in life. Many of the same risks apply when partners of pregnant women or other family members smoke around them during their pregnancy. Even "thirdhand" smoke (the residual nicotine and other chemicals left on clothing, rugs, furniture, and drapes when people have been smoking) can be harmful.

If you think the risks are overstated because you've seen healthy children born to mothers who smoke, consider this story from a nonsmoking colleague: "My mother smoked all during her pregnancy and while I was growing up. I weighed 7 lbs. at birth so I was not small, and I was born after forty weeks so I was not early, and I had no learning disabilities (I graduated from college Phi Beta Kappa with high honors). But when I took up scuba diving, the instructors were amazed at how much oxygen I needed. My tank always ran low well before the others'. They said I must be running underwater to use up that much air, and the joke was that I wore Nike fins!" (For support to quit smoking, inquire if your local hospital has a smoking cessation program; see also chapter 17.)

~ *Don't douche.* Using vaginal douches is not only unnecessary but has also been associated with low infant birth weight and bacterial vaginosis.

~ *Take supplements.* And start before conception, if possible. (One recent study showed, for example, that women who at conception had the lowest levels of vitamin B_{12}—necessary for red blood cell production and a healthy nervous system—had up to five times the risk of having a child with a neural tube defect than women with the highest levels.)[12] For the best results, be sure the potency of the supplements you take is guaranteed and that the supplements are manufactured according to GMP (good manufacturing practices) standards. I recommend a daily supplement with the following vitamins and minerals at the following levels:

Vitamins	Daily Dose	Notes
Beta-carotene	15,000 to 25,000 IU	
Biotin	100 to 500 mcg	
Choline	45 to 100 mg	
Folic acid	800 to 1,000 mcg	
Glutathione	2 to 10 mg	
Inositol	30 to 500 mg	
Niacin (vitamin B_3)	20 to 100 mg	
Pantothenic acid (vitamin B_5)	30 to 400 mcg	
Pyridoxine (vitamin B_6)	10 to 100 mg	
Riboflavin (vitamin B_2)	9 to 50 mg	
Thiamine (vitamin B_1)	9 to 100 mg	
Vitamin B_{12}	30 to 250 mcg	
Vitamin C	500 to 2,000 mg	
Vitamin D	2,000 to 5,000 IU	Aim for optimal blood levels before conception because mothers deficient in vitamin D are almost four times as likely to have a cesarean delivery;[13] see chapter 17
Vitamin E	400 to 600 IU	
Vitamin K	90 mg	

Minerals	Daily Dose	Notes
Boron	1 to 3 mg	
Calcium	500 to 1,500 mg	
Chromium	100 to 400 mcg	
Copper	1 to 2 mg	
Iodine	6 to 12.5 mg	If thyroid is normal
Iron	30 mg	
Magnesium	400 to 1,000 mg	
Manganese	1 to 15 mg	
Molybdenum	20 to 60 mcg	

Minerals	Daily Dose	Notes
Potassium	2,000 to 4,700 mg	
Selenium	80 to 120 mcg	
Trace minerals		From a marine mineral complex or from eating sea vegetables such as hiziki, dulse, wakame, or nori
Vanadium	50 to 100 mcg	
Zinc	12 to 50 mg	

The iodine recommendation may seem high, but a great deal of evidence indicates that the current RDA for iodine in pregnancy is woefully inadequate for optimal fetal health. Given the link between iodine and fetal brain development, I recommend iodine levels beyond the current RDA. (See the iodine discussion in chapter 10.) Folic acid is extremely important in preventing birth defects in the baby's brain and spinal cord (including spina bifida), especially in the first few weeks of pregnancy—so much so that the CDC recommends all women of childbearing age take it daily in case they do get pregnant. In pregnant women who depend on antiepileptic drugs, taking folic acid in early pregnancy may prevent the language delay that is often reported in children of mothers taking such medication.[14] By the way, not only are adequate vitamins important to the baby, but they can be important to the mother. For example, a 2008 study found that vitamin D deficiency is linked to bacterial vaginosis (a common vaginal infection) in the first trimester of pregnancy. As vitamin D levels improved, according to the researchers, the prevalence of bacterial vaginosis decreased.[15]

IMPORTANCE OF VITAMIN D IN PREGNANCY

Up to half of the pregnant women in the United States (and a much higher percentage of African American pregnant women) are deficient in vitamin D—even including those taking prenatal vitamins.[16] Yet this nutrient is vital for the health of both mother and baby. According to research presented at the 2010 annual meeting of the Pediatric Academic Societies, pregnant women who take 4,000 IU of vitamin D (ten times the amount typically found in prenatal vitamins and twice what many health groups previously recommended) cut their rate of pregnancy-related complications—including gestational diabetes and preeclampsia (pregnancy-related high blood pressure)—

in half and were also less likely to deliver prematurely.[17] This research further showed that taking these higher levels of vitamin D caused no harm to either the mothers or their babies, disproving the long-held belief that high doses of the vitamin cause birth defects. A 2017 study confirmed that serum vitamin D levels above 40 ng/ml lower the risk of preterm birth by 60 percent.[18]

~ *Eat enough omega-3 fats, especially DHA.* Essential fatty acids (also called polyunsaturated long-chain fatty acids or PUFAs) help the body fight and ultimately stop cellular inflammation. Eating enough may help prevent prematurity and low birth weight.[19] The main source of omega-3s are fatty fish, eggs, nuts, seeds, sea vegetables, and green leafy vegetables such as spinach, broccoli, cabbage, collards, and kale. Unprocessed vegetable oils (most notably flaxseed, macadamia nut, and hemp seed oils) are also good sources. You can easily find DHA and EPA in supplement form, either from fish oil or from marine algae.

~ *Get regular exercise.* Regular exercise during pregnancy reduces the odds of giving birth to newborns with excessive birth weight by 23–28 percent, according to a study from Norway.[20] A 2017 study from Spain confirms that moderate exercise during pregnancy is safe and beneficial for both mother and baby, not only preventing excessive weight gain but also lowering the mother's risk of preeclampsia, gestational diabetes, cesarean section, lower back pain, pelvic pain, and urinary incontinence.[21] The study further showed that safe exercise during pregnancy does not increase the risk of premature birth, low birth weight, or fetal distress (as long as the mothers had no medical or obstetric contraindication for exercise). For their study, the researchers used the current guidelines of the American College of Obstetricians and Gynecologists, which recommends that women with uncomplicated pregnancies who have approval from their physicians do moderate-intensity exercise for at least twenty to thirty minutes per day on most or all days of the week.[22]

If you're not sure where to start, find out if your local gym offers workout classes specifically for pregnant women. I also recommend Birthfit (www.birthfit.com), which offers support and education through in-person and online programs that focus on fitness, nutrition, chiropractic wellness, and mindset. Their thirty-six-week prenatal program includes four training sessions per week, while their fifteen-week postpartum program offers three sessions per week. In addition, Birthfit offers two different six-week core and pelvic floor courses, one for mothers who have delivered vaginally and another for those who had cesareans. (There's also a six-week preconception program called "Before the Bump.") My daughter Kate did the prenatal program during her entire second pregnancy.

~ *Start a meditation program.* Calm Birth is a form of childbirth preparation that uses proven mind-body and breathing techniques to help create an atmosphere of calmness that decreases fear, pain, and complications for both pregnancy and childbirth. Many medical centers now use this program with good results. The three main methods Calm Birth teaches are the Practice of Opening (allowing the parents-to-be to experience remarkable access to the development of their unborn child), Womb Breathing (where women learn to breathe into their energy bodies to reach full potential in childbirth and also to enrich the child), and the Giving and Receiving Meditation (which teaches how to transform the energy of fear, anxiety, and tension into light in your own body, and breathe it out). The preface to the program states, "When pregnant women practice meditation, an empowering sense of safety and wholeness is generated from the inside. The Calm Birth Methods were developed to give women direct ways to raise the quality of health in childbirth whether or not medical interventions are applied. These methods have been shown to lower the impact of interventions and also lower medical costs and risks." This is a very powerful program, and I highly recommend it. For those who can't find a Calm Birth practitioner in their area (currently, most are on the West Coast), the organization also offers both CDs and downloadable MP3 files of Calm Birth as well as a postnatal program called Calm Healing. (For more information, visit their website at www.calmbirth .org.)

Guided imagery is a particularly useful form of meditation. Psychotherapist, author, and guided imagery innovator Belleruth Naparstek has been a pioneer in the field of guided imagery for decades. She explains that guided imagery is "a gentle but powerful technique that focuses and directs the imagination." Although guided imagery has been called "visualization" and "mental imagery," she explains, it involves not only the visual sense but also all of the senses, all of our emotions, and the whole physical body. "It is precisely this body-based focus that makes for its powerful impact," Belleruth notes, referring to studies showing that guided imagery has a positive impact on health, creativity, and performance. "We now know that in many instances even ten minutes of imagery can reduce blood pressure, lower cholesterol and glucose levels in the blood, and heighten short-term immune cell activity," she says. "And because it results in a kind of natural trance state, it can be considered a form of hypnosis as well." Belleruth makes hands-down the best imagery scripts on the market. Everything is scientifically chosen and recorded, including the fabulous music, and all meditations are available as an MP3 or a CD. Her meditation entitled *The Healthy Pregnancy and Successful Childbirth* is specifically designed to encourage feelings of confidence, support, relaxation, safety, gratitude, and healthy anticipation during pregnancy, as well as labor imagery to ease discomfort, focus breathing, and underline your trust in the divine wisdom of your body. (For more information, visit her website, www.healthjourneys.com.)

~ *Get massage.* Massage has wonderful benefits, including boosting endorphins and decreasing stress hormones. Research by Tiffany Field, Ph.D., founder and director of the Touch Research Institute at the University of Miami School of Medicine, has done extensive research showing that pregnant women who receive massage experience reduced anxiety, improved mood, reduced back pain, and increased sleep. They also have fewer complications in labor, less labor pain, and fewer premature babies.[23] (For more information, see the Touch Research Institute's website at www.miami.edu/touch-research.) A twenty-minute foot rub at the end of a day of work is a good alternative if you can't do a full-body massage.

~ *Expose yourself to natural light.* Morning bright light significantly helps reduce depression in pregnant women, according to a 2002 Yale study. Researchers found that after three weeks of morning bright light therapy, depression ratings improved by 49 percent, and benefits were seen through five weeks of treatment. They also found no evidence of adverse effects of light therapy on pregnancy. Because drugs for depression are best avoided during pregnancy, if possible, and because depression in pregnancy may be a risk factor for preeclampsia, this is significant news.[24]

~ *Enroll in an empowering childbirth preparation program.* I recommend programs that don't merely help women get through childbirth but are specifically designed to help them make it an empowering experience on every level. The practice of hypnobirthing, which involves self-hypnosis, is one excellent option for before, during, and after childbirth. This process helps women retrain their subconscious mind so that they perceive contractions as pressure or squeezing—not pain—leading to a shorter, easier, and more comfortable experience of labor (as well as an easier postpartum period). An excellent resource for learning these techniques is Hypnobabies (www.hypnobabies.com), which offers a six-week childbirth education course that teaches medical-grade hypnosis either in a live class setting (given by certified practitioners across the country) or as a home-study program. Hypnobabies reports that almost three-quarters of the mothers who take their program report feeling nothing but pressure during the birth, with most others able to avoid pain for a significant part of the process.

I also recommend the childbirth preparation taught in the Ecstatic Birth program (www.ecstatic-birth.com), designed by Sheila Kamara Hay, who has done wonderful work bringing the idea of pleasurable childbirth into the collective. Ecstatic Birth covers every aspect of childbirth preparation—body, mind, and soul—in teaching women how to deepen their connection to their sensuality and tap in to it in order to experience physical pleasure during birth. While some women actually reach orgasm in the late stages of labor (more on that in the labor section of this chapter), intense pleasure and ecstasy are possible even without orgasm. Ecstatic Birth training sessions include a series of downloadable audio interviews moderated by Hay and featuring various experts (including myself) in women's health, birthing, and sensuality. The trainings cover both specific preparation for childbirth as well as instruction on accessing power, pleasure, and wisdom from within that you'll be able to integrate into the childbirth experience. Hay also offers one-on-one training with customized sessions and support throughout pregnancy and postpartum.

~ *If you are at risk for premature labor, talk to your doctor about progesterone.* Studies show that this hormone (available in a weekly shot given from weeks sixteen through thirty-six of gestation or as a vaginal suppository) decreases the risk of prematurity.[25] In 2011, the FDA approved the use of progesterone supplementation during pregnancy to reduce the risk of having a premature birth in women who have previously delivered a preterm baby, the first time the FDA has approved a medication for preventing preterm birth.[26] A 2013 meta-analysis of eleven studies showed that progesterone may prevent up to one-third of recurrent preterm births,[27] while an even larger international study published in 2018 showed that progesterone reduced the risk of spontaneous preterm birth at less than thirty-three weeks' gestation by 38 percent. It was also shown to reduce the frequency of infant complications from preterm birth (especially from respiratory distress) and the number of babies born at very low birth weight.[28] If you're carrying twins, however, progesterone may not prevent early preterm birth, probably because the causes of early birth in multiples are different.[29]

Also be sure to get psychological support. Studies have shown such support can decrease the rate of premature birth in those who are at increased risk.[30]

~ *Pay special attention to any prescription and over-the-counter medications you take, including receiving vaccines, particularly in the first trimester.* Nine out of ten pregnant women in the United States take some medication during pregnancy, and two-thirds of them take some form of prescription medication, according to the CDC. Many common medications are considered safe, but others may harm a developing baby or cause miscarriage or preterm birth. (For example, acetaminophen, commonly sold as Tylenol, is considered safe to take during pregnancy, while ibuprofen, found in Motrin and Advil, is not.) With many medications, it's simply not clear. One study noted that more than 90 percent of the medications approved by the FDA between 1980 and 2000 had insufficient data to determine if they were safe to take during pregnancy.[31] Ask your doctor or pharmacist about the safety of any medication before you take it, including prescription medications you were taking before you got pregnant, and avoid taking any prescription or over-the-counter medications that you don't really need. Such caution applies to flu shots as well. In particular, avoid receiving flu shots that include the pH1N1 strain, which has been associated with miscarriage.[32] The CDC has recently been emphasizing its recommendation for all pregnant women to get the flu vaccine during any trimester as well as the TDaP vaccine (designed to prevent tetanus, diphtheria, and acellular pertussis, or whooping cough) early in the third trimester of each pregnancy, even for women who have previously had these vaccines before they became pregnant. The idea is that maternal vaccinations protect the baby before the infant can receive its own vaccinations (which the CDC recommends at two months for TDaP and at six months for influenza). I disagree with the CDC's stance on this because injecting the kinds of toxins vaccines contain into a pregnant woman could possibly compromise fetal neurological development. (For more on the dangers of infant vaccines, see the box called "Vaccines: Helpful or Harmful?" on page 627.)

While most herbal supplements and essential oils are safe for pregnant women, take care with these, too. Avoid the following oral supplements during pregnancy (cooking spices are perfectly safe because they are not as concentrated): arborvitae, beth root, black cohosh, blue cohosh, cascara, chasteberry, Chinese angelica (dong quai), cinchona, cotton root bark, feverfew, ginseng, goldenseal, juniper, kava kava, licorice, meadow saffron, pennyroyal, poke root, rue, sage, St. John's wort, senna, tansy, white peony, wormwood, yarrow, yellow dock, and large doses of vitamin A.[33] Essential oils to avoid during pregnancy include calamus, mugwort, pennyroyal, sage, wintergreen, basil, hyssop, myrrh, marjoram, and thyme.

I also suggest caution about pregnant women taking antiretrovirals for HIV. Some experts believe these antiretrovirals may actually cause the symptoms associated with AIDS instead of preventing the syndrome, as initially expected, meaning the medication itself may be toxic.[34] After all, AIDS is a syndrome of more than twenty separate diseases, not a specific disease in itself. A person determined to have HIV antibodies isn't necessarily sick and may never become so; this has been true for hundreds of thousands of people. And AIDS-like symptoms can surface in people who do not have such antibodies in their blood. In fact, thousands of AIDS victims have never had HIV. HIVNET 012, an NIH-funded trial in Uganda to test the drug nevirapine (designed to prevent transmission of HIV from mother to baby), showed that the drug cut transmission in half.[35] Yet just as with the trials for Gardasil (the supposed HPV vaccine), there was no true placebo group. Instead, the results were compared with those from taking another drug. As with Gardasil, this means that high baseline rates of serious adverse events may surface in the trial that are then simply dismissed because they occur equally in both groups—but again, the comparison is between two drugs, not between the drug and a true placebo. In this case, serious adverse events, including death, were seen in 20 percent of pregnant women taking nevirapine. These are sobering odds.

CELLPHONES: DANGERS REAL OR HYPE?

Cellphones emit an electromagnetic field, using radio-frequency (RF) radiation to transmit signals. They do this not only when you're using them but also anytime they're turned on and searching for a signal. There's been much controversy about whether such radiation can cause cancer, as well as a host of other illnesses and conditions. One study involving researchers from thirteen countries famously found data suggesting regular use of a cellphone increases risk of brain tumors by 40 percent after 1,640 hours or more of use (which equates to half an hour per day over ten years), but they concluded that "bias and error" cast doubt on a causal relationship.[36] In 2011, the World Health Organization classified cellphone radiation as a possible carcinogen.[37] The U.S. National Toxicology Program published data in 2016 that showed possible carcinogenic effects[38] but then reversed that two years later, saying new data shows that typical usage does not result in the levels of exposure that can cause serious harm.[39] Other independent studies, however, have shown reason for concern, keeping the debate open.[40]

Almost everyone, including myself, depends on cellphones on a daily basis not only for communicating but also to stream music, watch videos, and access GPS technology to get directions. Avoiding them is not only impractical but nearly impossible. Various EMF protection chips and stickers on the market purport to protect cellphone users, although studies showing their effectiveness aren't well documented. As long as there's still a question about cellphone safety, it seems prudent to take at least a few easy steps to protect yourself from as much radiation as possible—especially while you're pregnant. A few tips:

⁓ When talking on the phone, keep the device away from your head. Use a headset or the speakerphone setting.

⁓ Don't carry the phone against your body, as in a pocket—and certainly keep it away from your pregnant belly.

> ~ Don't sleep with a cellphone next to your bed. Exposure to elec-
> tromagnetic fields can interrupt sleep cycles (among other poten-
> tial problems) in people who are particularly sensitive to them.
> This is an easy way to cut your exposure time. (I also recommend
> turning off the Wi-Fi in your home or apartment at night while
> you sleep, for similar reasons.)

PREVENTING PREMATURE BIRTH

Despite a great deal of research in this area, the rate of premature birth
has declined only minimally in the past fifty years. It occurs in about 10 percent of pregnancies and contributes to more infant deaths than any other
factor except severe birth defects.[41] Assisted reproductive technologies have
increased the number of multiple gestations—and thus increased the number
of premature babies. The rising popularity of labor inductions has played a
part, too; an increase in late-term prematurity (thirty-seven weeks or so) puts
far too many babies in the intensive care unit because of problems with lung
maturity. As a result, the American College of Obstetricians and Gynecologists recommends that no induction be done before thirty-nine weeks. Quite
frankly, I question all labor inductions that are mostly done for convenience.
These induction-related prematurities would be preventable if women were
encouraged to go into labor normally.[42] I met a German doctor recently who
likened convenience inductions to removing a baby's very first choice—the
choice of when to be born. Thought-provoking.

Though many drugs have been used to try to stop labor, these have only
limited benefit and haven't significantly affected the prematurity rate. Until
the mind-body-lifestyle connection in premature birth is addressed, the rate
is unlikely to change. It is well documented that uterine blood vessels are
exquisitely sensitive to the effects of sympathetic nervous system stimulation
and that the hormones associated with stress of all types can cause changes
in blood flow to the fetus.[43]

In a study of sixty-four women, for instance, Lewis Mehl-Madrona,
M.D., Ph.D., found that a range of the psychological factors (fear, anxiety,
and stress; lack of support from the woman's partner; poor maternal self-
identity; negative beliefs about birth; and lack of support from friends and
family) predicted deliveries that required obstetrical intervention ranging
from cesarean section to oxytocin augmentation or induction. In another
study, hypnotherapy was found to play a statistically significant role in preventing negative emotional factors from leading to C-section or oxytocin
augmentation or induction. Dr. Mehl-Madrona has also used hypnotherapy

to help women avoid giving birth prematurely. Each woman who received hypnotherapy was reassured that she was doing the best she could, asked to state what her stresses were, and then given the suggestion that her body would know what to do to keep her baby safe. As fear and anxiety decreased through supportive hypnotherapy, so did adverse outcomes.[44]

One study followed women with a history of three consecutive miscarriages for which no medical cause could be found. On their subsequent pregnancy, they had a suture placed in their cervix to hold the pregnancy in place. Eighty-nine percent of these women went on to have severe postpartum depression, compared with only 11 percent of the control group who experienced mild to moderate depression. The authors of this study concluded that "these women were forced into motherhood."[45] When severe emotional conflicts about motherhood aren't dealt with consciously, they can be exacerbated postpartum and result in emotional breakdown. It is clear that adverse pregnancy outcomes could be prevented with approaches that help a woman name and work through the particular stresses that can so profoundly affect her pregnant body and her unborn baby.

One of the most underacknowledged but important factors in poor pregnancy outcome is that the pregnancy is unwanted or unplanned or there is some unrecognized ambivalence around it. (Given the lack of support for so many pregnant women and those with young children, this ambivalence is understandable. Who wouldn't be ambivalent about a decision that alters one's entire life and can't be undone?) Current data suggest that about 45 percent of all pregnancies are unplanned.[46] It's much more difficult to ascertain which ones are unwanted because many women adjust well to unplanned pregnancies and end up desiring them. Maternal ambivalence about pregnancy is a setup for complications unless a woman can resolve her feelings during the pregnancy. (See chapter 11.) A woman who feels (usually unconsciously) that she must end her pregnancy as soon as possible to get on with her life, get the pregnancy over with, or "get her body back" may go into premature labor or develop another condition that ends her pregnancy sooner. Numerous studies have documented the profound effects of psychological variables on birth outcome—in other words, prematurity may correlate with poor maternal emotional and physical investment in the pregnancy.[47] Animal studies have indicated that the death of a baby in utero may also be related to marked maternal anxiety. In pregnant monkeys, guinea pigs, and rabbits subjected to emotional stress, the uterine and placental blood flow were constricted from adrenaline released in response to the stress. As a result, the fetuses did not receive enough oxygen, and many died of asphyxia. Marked maternal anxiety and stress also cause uterine blood vessels to constrict via hormonal and neurotransmitter release into the circulation. This reduces oxygen to the baby and may well be related to pregnancy complications, such as placental abruption, placenta previa (a condition in which the placenta covers the cervical opening, which can lead to bleeding and/or prematurity), a prolapsed umbilical cord, a cord around the neck, or breech presentation.[48]

The good news is that mothers can learn to communicate healthful emotions to their babies regardless of their circumstances. After all, the baby is a part of a pregnant woman's own body. When women learn how to get in touch with their inner guidance systems, they can learn how to keep their babies safer and even interrupt premature labor and halt the progression of toxemia. It's really very simple. You just take a deep breath, set an intention to connect with your baby, and tell the child that you are doing everything in your power to keep him or her safe and healthy. Over time, you'll be able to get a feel for your baby's response. And remember that your child knew what he or she was getting into when the baby came to you. Of course, women who develop premature labor and toxemia also have to be willing to stop work, rest more, and change any harmful patterns of behavior and thought. The pioneering work of Dr. Lewis Mehl-Madrona has shown that prenatal intervention consisting of social support, education, and labor support in a group of minority women reduced alcohol intake, smoking, and stress, and also improved birth outcome significantly.[49]

PREVENTING PREECLAMPSIA

Preeclampsia (or toxemia) is a syndrome in which a pregnant woman develops swelling, high blood pressure, and protein in the urine. It's sometimes referred to as pregnancy-induced hypertension (PIH). Women with kidney disease and preexisting high blood pressure are more susceptible than others. Diabetes also increases susceptibility. Toxemia is a leading cause of prematurity and pregnancy disability. If untreated, it can lead to seizures—the condition is then called eclampsia. No one knows exactly what causes preeclampsia, although there are many theories. In one study, electrodes were placed into the nerves adjacent to the blood vessels of four different types of women: pregnant women with high blood pressure, nonpregnant women with high blood pressure, pregnant women with normal blood pressure, and nonpregnant women with normal blood pressure. The women who had preeclampsia were found to have high sympathetic nervous system activity (more adrenaline in their bloodstream), which resulted in narrowing of their blood vessels with a subsequent increase in pressure and inflammatory chemicals at the cellular level. It is well known that the sympathetic nervous system is involved with the fight-or-flight response and perceived stress. One of the researchers in this study suggested that the reason why the preeclamptic women's blood pressure rises is that they have "a defect in the central conflict processing system," which may increase certain hormone levels that not only contribute to an increase in blood pressure but may be associated with feelings of anxiety and hostility.[50] I don't think there's any such "defect." Quite simply, these women don't have the skills or the resources to get their needs met directly. But they can learn them.

Other studies of pregnant women with preeclampsia suggest that they feel less attractive, less loved, and more helpless than do pregnant women without preeclampsia. They may be excessively sensitive to the opinions of others, and orient themselves to what others expect of them. For these women, pregnancy provides an additional crisis that adds stress to their already overstressed lives. Although they view pregnancy as a crisis, they are ill equipped to deal with their emotions about it. They are unable to cope with what they perceive as others' expectations, taking to heart minor criticisms and injustices done to them. I've come to see that these women are highly sensitive people (empaths). Up until very recently, this group hasn't been identified, nor has their sensitivity been acknowledged. These women do not show externally that any of their stresses or inability to get their needs met bothers them. Instead, their body reflects this stress as an increase in blood pressure. In my experience, these highly sensitive women are used to giving but are not good at receiving. Many are in relationships with individuals I refer to as "energy vampires"—people who are self-centered and narcissistic (in psychiatric terms, those with a cluster B personality disorder). Their lack of empathy can create a real crisis if the pregnant woman has been the main person providing this individual with what is called "narcissistic supply," meeting their need for attention, praise, money, and status at the expense of themselves. When a woman is pregnant, she is the one who needs the most care and attention. But chances are good that she has not learned the skills of asking for help or being open to receiving it. And if she is in a relationship with an energy vampire, the vampire's needs will generally take precedence even if she gets up the courage to ask for what she needs. If this strikes a chord, please check out my book *Dodging Energy Vampires: An Empath's Guide to Evading Relationships That Drain You and Restoring Your Health and Power* (Hay House, 2018).

The effect of emotional stress on blood pressure is corroborative of the work of Samuel J. Mann, M.D., a hypertension specialist at New York Presbyterian Hospital/Weill Medical College of Cornell University and author of *Healing Hypertension: A Revolutionary New Approach* (John Wiley & Sons, 1999). Dr. Mann has seen thousands of people with all varieties of high blood pressure. Over time he noticed a pattern that was not in keeping with the common view that stress is linked to this condition. In his book, Dr. Mann writes, "Even patients with severe hypertension did not seem more emotionally distressed than others. If anything, they seemed less distressed. Their high blood pressure appeared to be more related to what they did *not* seem to be feeling than to what they *were* feeling." He began to see that old, unhealed, repressed trauma seemed to be a major culprit in his patients. I certainly agree. Even though pregnancy-induced hypertension is not considered the same as hypertension in the nonpregnant state, I believe that they have much in common. The bottom line is that it is our hidden emotions, the emotions we do not feel, that lead to hypertension (as well as many other physical conditions).

Not surprisingly, women with preeclampsia frequently have conflicts with their employers, and their blood pressure often rises when they try to negotiate their maternity leave. They often attempt to get everything settled before the delivery. Compared with women without preeclampsia, these women's emotions manifest physically through the autonomic (subconscious) nervous system: They frequently blush in the face and neck, talk rapidly, and experience rising blood pressure, dizziness, and heart palpitations.[51] One study showed that women with a set of conditions including excessive weight gain, premature rupture of membranes (one of the leading causes of premature birth), and preeclampsia display high anxiety, social seclusion, and hypochondria compared with controls.[52] These symptoms can all be thought of as bodily cries for help and support. If a woman understands what it's like to have a baby in the intensive care nursery, she can begin the process of seeing her own body as the best intensive care space possible for the baby, not to mention the cheapest. And when she begins to name and put her needs first, this is exactly what often happens. A diet that keeps insulin low is also essential. (See chapter 17.)

TURNING A BREECH PRESENTATION

Nowhere is the mind-body connection more interesting than in the case of breech presentation, in which the baby is oriented feet or buttocks first instead of headfirst. By the time a woman has reached the thirty-seventh week of pregnancy, her baby will usually have settled into her pelvis in a headfirst position. But 3 percent of the time, it will be feet first or buttocks first. Though breech babies can turn at any time, the estimated likelihood that a baby will spontaneously convert from a breech to a vertex (headfirst) position after thirty-seven weeks of gestation is only 12 percent. If a woman enters labor with her baby in the breech position, she is almost always delivered by cesarean section. Some babies are breech for structural reasons, such as a septum or wall in the uterus that can interfere with the baby's position. But in the majority of cases, there is no known medical reason for the breech. It's clear that in some cases the baby is breech because of the tension that the mother holds in the lower area of her body. It has been observed that anxious and fearful women have a higher incidence of breech presentation than do others, attributable to the fact that fear, anxiety, and stress can activate sympathetic mechanisms that result in tightening of the lower uterine segment.[53] My obstetrician colleague Bethany Hays feels that a baby may be in the breech position because it is trying to get closer to its mother's heartbeat—to feel more connected to her.

The key to allowing the baby to turn spontaneously is to help the mother release tension in her lower uterine segment. There are a number of ways to do this. Some women have found that acupressure works. (See figure 20.) I have personally had about a 40 percent success rate teaching mothers a type of bioenergetic breathing, which works to relax the lower abdomen and lower uterine segment, thus allowing the baby to turn. Dr. Hays also reports that if she can get women to relax their lower abdominals, she can often turn the breech with ease. (This manual turning is known as external cephalic version, or ECV.) Dr. Lewis Mehl-Madrona demonstrated that hypnosis can be used to turn breeches, with a success rate of 81 percent—compared with 41 percent for a control group.[54] Dr. Mehl-Madrona has also used hypnosis to decrease C-section rates for those at risk and to decrease use of oxytocin augmentation of labor. (For more information, contact the Association for Pre- and Perinatal Psychology and Health at 720-490-5612 or check the resources on their website, www.birthpsychology.com.)

Our Biggest Challenge:
The Collective Emergency Mindset

Pregnancy is a time when common sense all too often flies out the window, chased by a culture that is out of balance concerning birth. Nowhere is a woman's connection or loss of connection to her inner guidance more evident than during pregnancy. Suddenly, her body is no longer her own. Her entire extended family feels that it is pregnant, and all of them give her advice about what to eat, what to wear, and what to do. I was amazed by how total strangers would approach me when I was pregnant, pat my belly, and offer suggestions. Friends seem to think it their duty to tell pregnant women the worst stories they can think of about cesarean sections, labor pain, and poor outcomes. (This is another example of our dominator culture—glorifying pain and destruction over the life-enhancing qualities potentially available through pregnancy and birth.) I felt blessed to be an obstetrician because I was spared hearing all these horror stories; perhaps people figured that I had been "socialized" by having already learned these horrible stories firsthand. War stories about the rigors of birth are often passed down from generation to generation. Historically, many women have told their daughters "Now you'll see how I suffered with you."

At some very deep level, we are all awed by pregnant women and their power. But instead of emphasizing a woman's awe-inspiring birth power, in

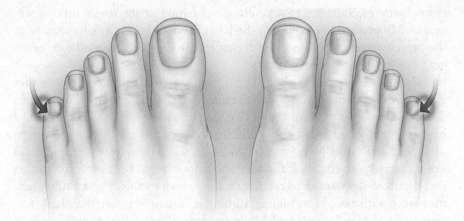

FIGURE 20:
ACUPUNCTURE OR ACUPRESSURE POINTS TO TURN A BREECH

A number of different techniques can be used to stimulate these points, including acupuncture needles or a heat treatment known as moxibustion. If you don't have access to an acupuncturist who is familiar with these techniques, you can try acupressure if your physician approves. Press the point on either toe with your fingernail. Use enough pressure so that the area feels sensitive, but not enough to cause pain. Hold the pressure for one to two minutes once or twice a day. Immediately afterward, get into the knee-chest position for about fifteen minutes. (This position will also help turn the baby.) You can use this technique starting in the seventh month of pregnancy. (Earlier in the pregnancy, the fetus is likely to turn on its own.) Do not attempt this if you have any uterine or pelvic abnormality, a history of habitual miscarriage, or if there have been other problems in the pregnancy. Be sure to consult your doctor before beginning. As an alternative to stimulation of the point with your nail, you can also buy small moxibustion cylinders online. You simply peel off the adhesive backing, stick them to the spot you want stimulated, and light them. Remove them once the heat becomes uncomfortable.

classic patriarchal reversal our culture attends to the fear that that power brings up. Pregnant women are emotionally more porous and more in touch with their intuition than usual, and they are therefore more vulnerable. They pick up on all the collective societal fear of them.

Media images of pregnant women suddenly falling to the ground during pregnancy and shrieking things like, "Oh, John, the baby!" reinforce in our psyches the notion that pregnancy is a time of great danger and unpredictability instead of a normal process. They promote the misconception that pregnancy, like our female body, is a disaster waiting to happen. In every hospital I've ever worked in, pregnant women who come into the emergency room are rushed to the labor and delivery floor as quickly as possible, even if they've come in for some other problem. In Boston, the ER crew once sent up a woman in mid-pregnancy who had a broken leg!

This emergency mindset is especially damaging to women who are having babies in their thirties or forties. Most, if not all, pregnant women over the age of thirty are taught by our culture that they are much more at risk for complications than if they were in their twenties. This perception of increased risk is not necessarily true and depends on the individual woman's health. I remember the first pregnant woman I ever met who was over thirty. It was in the prenatal clinic at the Mary Hitchcock Hospital during my second year of medical school, and I thought that she was very unusual and very brave to be having her first baby at such an advanced age—thirty-two. Looking back, I realize that this woman was at the very beginning of a trend that began in the 1970s and has continued unabated through the present: delaying childbearing until later. Now, decades later, women in their thirties are actually having more babies than women in their twenties. According to CDC data from 2016, women ages thirty to thirty-four had about 103 babies per 1,000 people, while women ages twenty-five to twenty-nine—the group that had the highest birth rate for more than thirty years—had only 102 per 1,000.[55] The same data show that the average age for women to have their first child is now twenty-eight.

Women having their first babies after the age of thirty-five were once referred to as *elderly primigravidas*. Happily, that term has been dropped. Though the term *geriatric obstetrics* is still used occasionally, it should be eliminated, as it sets up all kinds of negativity. Whether or not a woman is more at risk in her thirties must be completely individualized. A forty-year-old in excellent health who has a planned pregnancy is apt to do much better than a twenty-five-year-old who smokes two packs and quaffs a gallon of Diet Coke per day. Too often the medical profession "hexes" women who become pregnant in their thirties and forties by lumping them into statistically high-risk categories that are not necessarily applicable. Older women who are pregnant, as well as infertility patients who become pregnant, have a much higher risk of a C-section. In some places, a woman older than forty will be told that she is very apt to have a cesarean because hers is a "premium pregnancy" (as opposed to a pregnancy in the mother's twenties, whose success doesn't "matter" as much because "you can always have another—you have time"). Because the mother is presumed to be more anxious (or is *made* to be anxious by her culture and her doctor), we should treat her differently. This is a reflection of the healthcare team's own unfinished emotional work. And this is the thinking that has led to a relatively high rate of cesarean birth—now about 32 percent in the United States, down only slightly from the all-time high of nearly 33 percent in 2009[56]—despite the fact that the

World Health Organization says that a 5 to 10 percent rate is optimal and that research shows anything over 15 percent does more harm than good.[57] (By comparison, the cesarean rate is currently 24.5 percent in Western Europe and a whopping 41 percent in South America.)[58] The rate of births by C-section increased by more than 50 percent from about 1975 to 2015. Way back in 1965, the rate was only 4.5 percent.[59] Happily, this trend is starting to reverse as the medical profession wakes up to the dangers of too many C-sections and the fact that a C-section is major surgery with far more complications than a normal vaginal birth. At least in part, these sky-high rates may be linked to doctors' fears of being sued. As of 2017, 85 percent of all American obstetricians had been sued at least once, and 65 percent had been sued two to five times, with 60 percent of plaintiff awards being up to $500,000 and 37 percent being $1 million or more.[60] As a result, many doctors are more likely to opt for performing a C-section at the first sign of a complication.[61] Even so, C-sections are far from benign procedures, and our collective trust in them is mind-boggling.

In fact, age doesn't predict anything when it comes to labor and birth. As noted in chapter 11 in relation to fertility, chronological age (age in years) and biological age (age of one's tissues) aren't necessarily related. One of my friends had her first baby at forty-one. The first stage of her labor lasted only three hours—very short by any standard. And if her hips hadn't been so narrow, she'd have delivered in a total of four hours. Healthy women who are well supported in labor usually do beautifully, regardless of age.

One of the nicest things about women having their first babies in their late thirties and early forties is that by then, these women have established themselves in the outside world of work and career. When they do have babies, they take the time to enjoy them. They already know what it's like "out there." They realize the limitations of the corporate world and are willing to put aside its "benefits" to reassess their lives through the lens of parenting. Many have had time to get in touch with their bodies over the years and are more comfortable with themselves than they were in their twenties. In my mind, such women are actually low risk.

The Magic of Labor and Birth

Having a baby is the true "change of life." Women who go through labor and birth fully supported often emerge from the experience changed forever. One of my patients who had her two children at home told me: "My births were absolute peak experiences of ecstasy and spiritual fulfillment. Nothing I've ever experienced before or since has come anywhere close. As a result of my experiences, I now trust my body implicitly." In order to experience the transformational power of birth, women need to know the following:

~ Labor proceeds on its own schedule. The delicate timing that is a result of the delicate interaction between a baby and her mother needs to be respected. (Despite complications such as increased risk of prematurity, C-section, and maternal death, risky labor inductions for "convenience" nearly doubled from 1990 through 2010. Almost 24 percent of all pregnant women in the United States had induced labors in 2011, although over the next few years that figure finally began a slight decline.)[62]

~ Childbirth is designed by nature to be a peak experience that is joyous, ecstatic, and loving. But if a woman is not supported, her experience may be the exact opposite, plummeting her into depression and despair. A woman's body is designed to labor flawlessly when she is relaxed, well nourished, and well supported. If this weren't the case, the human race never would have survived. During labor, the body is flooded with natural morphine-like substances called endorphins as well as oxytocin, the bonding hormone. This kind of ecstasy is seen in centers such as the Farm Midwifery Center in Summertown, Tennessee, where the legendary midwife Ina May Gaskin practices. Her book *Ina May's Guide to Childbirth* (Bantam Books, 2003) is a must-read for all pregnant women. At a past meeting of the Association for Pre- and Perinatal Psychology and Health, Ina May showed a picture of her niece giving birth naturally with a big smile on her face, something one never sees on television—or in most hospitals!

~ Birth is sexual. This makes sense—after all, the baby is moving down the vaginal canal and stimulating the G-spot and all the nerves connected with sexual feeling. As Ina May says, "The energy that got the baby in is what gets the baby out. Many women experience the most intense orgasm of their lives when they birth in environments in which they are loved, adored, and fully supported." This is probably the best-kept secret in the world.

One woman told me that after her baby was born she said to her doctor, "If I'd known it was going to feel this good, I'd have planned for ten babies!"

Word is, however, getting out. In 2013, French psychologist Thierry Postel published a study that included data from 109 midwives who assisted a collective total of 206,000 births. The midwives reported 668 cases of mothers who said they felt "orgasmic sensations" during childbirth, 868 cases of mothers demonstrating signs of pleasure, and 9 mothers confirming full-blown orgasms.[63] "Pain and pleasure travel along the same neural pathways," explains behavioral neuroscientist Barry Komisaruk, Ph.D., professor of psychology at Rutgers University and coauthor with Carlos Beyer-Flores, Ph.D., and Beverly Whipple of *The Science of Orgasm* (Johns Hopkins University

Press, 2006). "There are many different qualities of sensation that can be elicited from vaginal and cervical stimulation, and that's why some people say giving birth is the worst pain they've ever felt, and others say it feels orgasmic, pleasurable, and even erotic."[64]

My ob-gyn colleague Bethany Hays, M.D., told me that when she was in labor herself with her first child and it was time to push, she recalls being in a place she could only identify as "somewhere I could not stay." At this point she said she wanted to get rid of the baby at all costs. In subsequent births she again found herself in that "terrible, unacceptable place" in which she used all her rational powers to "bypass that terrible transit through the pelvis": "Just get tough." "Get mad and get him out!" "Ignore the pain, just push through it." This resulted, she notes, in "considerable pain and trauma to myself."

Later in her career, Bethany met a woman who taught her—and me—the secret of the second stage of labor, which now seems obvious: Many women don't want to push because we feel disconnected from that part of our bodies and because giving birth is a sexual experience, almost taboo with so many people looking on. Instead of pushing through the second stage of labor as though it were an athletic event, women would do well to let their uterus do the work (as long as there is no fetal distress) while allowing their vaginas to relax into the process.

During my residency training, I was accused of being Dr. Pain by the nurses because I didn't insist on a spinal anesthetic for every delivery. Even then, I knew that pushing the baby out took a relatively small amount of time, and I believed that it was far better for a woman to be alert for her new baby than to have the lower half of her body so paralyzed from a spinal that forceps had to be used to pull the baby out. I witnessed many women who had spinal anesthesia for routine deliveries fall asleep on the delivery table. These women were much less "present" to greet their babies than those who had birthed normally.

Back then, I didn't appreciate the fact that birth is part of the continuum of female sexuality and that by numbing the lower half of the body to feeling anything painful, we were also numbing the possibility for feeling anything ecstatic or sexual.

Though most people don't know this, the art of belly dancing originated for the purpose of getting in touch with birthing power. Grandmothers taught it to granddaughters and daughters. I'm certain that the current resurgence of interest in the arts of belly dancing, pole dancing, and erotic dancing is being fueled by the resurgence of the energy of Aphrodite—the part of the feminine that the baby-boom feminists bypassed trying to be like men. With this luscious energy comes a reclaiming of our essential female birthing power. That's why a young woman friend of mine who had an ecstatic hospital birth after dancing through most of the labor with her husband described the experience as "highly erotic." One more thing: Ample evidence exists that the first drummers were women and that the beat of the drum re-created the beat of the heart, which set up an optimal rhythm for women to bring forth life. (This is laid out in the book *When the Drummers Were Women: A Spiritual History of Rhythm* by Layne Redmond [Three Rivers Press, 1997].)

For more information, see the Orgasmic Birth website (www .orgasmicbirth.com). I also highly recommend the documentary *Birth as We Know It* by Russian-born filmmaker Elena Tonetti-Vladimirova, whose film of natural births, many along the shores of the Black Sea in Russia, is a must-see for all pregnant women. (For more information or to order the DVD or to download the documentary online, see Elena's website, www.birthintobeing .com.)

~ How you do it is what you get. Because of the heightened emotional and neurological receptivity of both mother and baby, the birth experience deeply imprints both mother and baby and impacts their relationship for a lifetime. If you approach labor as a disaster waiting to happen, or turn over your body to experts without consulting your inner wisdom, you will be missing out on a very empowering experience.

~ Natural birth is safe. Studies have repeatedly shown that in healthy mothers with no risk factors, home birth is as safe as hospital birth. One study in the Netherlands looked at almost 530,000 low-risk planned births and found that with the proper services in place (such as a well-trained midwife and good transportation), home births are just as safe as hospital births.[65] In fact, home birth may even be safer. Ina May Gaskin reports that at the Farm Midwifery Center, the C-section rate is only 1.4 percent—a safety rate unparalleled by hospitals. And her experience is clearly not solitary. A landmark study published in the *British Medical Journal* in 2005 found that natural birth at home, under the care of certified practicing midwives, is safe for low-risk mothers and their babies. This study, which tracked more than 5,000 mothers in the United States and Canada, also reported that home births with low-risk mothers resulted in much lower rates of medical interventions when compared with the intervention rates for low-risk mothers giving birth in hospitals. For example, the episiotomy rate was 2.1 percent for the home-birth group, compared with 33 percent for hospital births, and labor was induced in only 9.6 percent of home births, compared with 21 percent of hospital births. The rates of electronic fetal monitoring, C-sections, forceps or vacuum delivery, and epidurals were also much lower with home births.[66] A 2014 study evaluating data from almost 17,000 women over a six-year period (the largest analysis of planned home birth in the

United States ever published) yet again confirmed that for low-risk mothers, planned home births using midwives result in low rates of interventions and no increase in adverse outcomes for mothers and their newborns.[67]

Unfortunately, the American public in general (physicians included) may have a false sense of security about the safety of giving birth today because the statistics on maternal death in the United States are misleading. Unlike most other developed countries, the United States counts in its pregnancy-related death statistics only women who die within a six-week period after a pregnancy ends. Other developed countries include deaths that occur up to one year afterward. According to the Centers for Disease Control, the number of maternal deaths in the United States is probably up to three times as high as the number reported in our national statistics because not all maternal deaths are classified as pregnancy-related on the death certificate.[68] I highly recommend the short video *Reducing Infant Mortality and Improving the Health of Babies* by Debby Takikawa, which you can view for free at https://vimeo.com/6182741. The video shows how using midwives and other means of labor support can help transform the perspective of birth-as-emergency so that laboring mothers and their newborns will not merely survive but truly thrive. (Midwives remain a largely underutilized resource. While the percentage of certified-midwife-attended births has risen nearly every year since 1989, midwives still attend less than 10 percent of births in the United States.)[69] Also, please consult the Birth Survey (www.mothersand babiesfirst.com/the-birth-survey) for feedback and ratings on the doctors, hospitals, and birth resources in your area.

A reader named Katy sent me the following story on Facebook that perfectly illustrates why choosing a home birth attended by a midwife was right for her:

> I wanted to have a home birth because I'd read about the importance of feeling safe during labor, and I had witnessed the overall cultural belief that giving birth is dangerous, an accident waiting to happen, expressed through various people's comments (not to mention through the pressure I felt from friends and family when I was a week overdue). By reading your books and listening to your Hay House Radio show over the years, I was able to tap in to my inner strength and power as a woman. I found an amazing midwife who really supported me. I used hypno-birthing techniques and ended up having a water birth in my home spa pool, in winter under the stars! It was the most profound magical experience of my life, and it has healed me in ways that words cannot describe. We now have a beautiful baby boy, who is so perfect!

Ina May's Safe Motherhood Quilt Project

In the early 1990s, midwifery pioneer Ina May Gaskin began to research maternal death rates in the United States. She was concerned that with escalating hospital birth interventions, such as induced labors and planned C-sections, the rate of maternal deaths would rise dramatically despite the profound medical advances enjoyed by those who live in the United States. Her research shows that forty countries have lower maternal death rates than the United States.[70]

The maternal death rate in any given population is known to be a very good indicator of the overall health status of that population. So it was especially shocking when Ina May found that the maternal death rate in the United States had actually *doubled* in the previous twenty-five years. By now, that rate has more than tripled. In 1982, the rate was 7.5 per 100,000 live births. By 1999, the rate had risen to 13.2, and by 2015, it reached 26.4.[71] Of all developed countries, the United States not only has the highest rate but also has the only rate that is rising.[72] (The second-highest rate for a developed nation is in the United Kingdom, where there are 9.2 maternal deaths per 100,000 women.)

Moreover, Hispanic and African American women continue to have much higher maternal death rates—up to four times that of white women, with even higher rates in some cities.[73] (In New York City, for example, African American mothers are twelve times more likely to die from pregnancy-related causes than white mothers.)[74] This difference in maternal death rates is one of the widest of all the racial disparities in woman's health. The inequalities begin even in the way women of different races are treated by medical professionals, with a national survey of more than 2,000 women published in 2014 reporting that 21 percent of African American mothers say they received poor treatment from hospital staff, compared with 8 percent of white mothers who did.[75] Such differences are not solely a product of socioeconomic class—they persist even for African American women who are college-educated[76]—and they've been well documented in other areas of medicine as well (even down to the amount of pain medication given to patients of different races who have the same symptoms and how often they are referred to specialists).[77] The racial and ethnic disparities in women's health are so great, in fact, that the American College of Obstetricians and Gynecologists issued a strongly worded statement of policy concerning racial bias in 2017. The statement declared that these differences (specifically including higher rates of preterm birth and maternal mortality for African American women) cannot be reversed without addressing racial bias, both implicit and explicit.[78]

This high rate of maternal mortality is particularly shocking in light of the fact that 60 percent of pregnancy-related deaths in this country are preventable, according to a report from a partnership of maternal mortality review committees released in 2018.[79] The project team for the report gathered data from across the country, concluding that nearly half such deaths are caused by hemorrhage, cardiovascular and coronary conditions, cardiomyopathy, or infection, with mental health conditions also representing a leading underlying cause of death.

Ina May found the trend sobering. "When I first became curious about the maternal death rate in the U.S., I wondered why it was so difficult to unearth in the medical library," she recalls. "This was in the early 1990s. I noticed a sharp contrast between how maternal deaths are counted here in the U.S. and the U.K.'s system of confidential enquiries, where four countries cooperate to achieve 100 percent ascertainment of maternal deaths that are directly related to pregnancy and birth. (They claim 97 percent accuracy.) According to the CDC, the actual number may be 1.6 to 3 times the figure that is published annually. I find this shocking, especially since we know that the maternal death rate has been rising in recent years—something that isn't happening in other countries."

To humanize and emphasize this often-hidden problem, Ina May began collecting the names of women who have died from pregnancy-related causes since 1982 (the year when the maternal death rate was the lowest). In 1999, inspired by the AIDS Memorial Quilt, she started the Safe Motherhood Quilt Project. "The purpose is to bring awareness to the rising maternal death rate in the United States and to the substantial degree of underreporting of such deaths," she explains. "Reduction of the maternal death rate depends upon complete ascertainment so that it is possible to learn from past mistakes." The project has since expanded into a non-profit organization headquartered in Sarasota, Florida, whose Facebook page (facebook.com/rememberthemothers) displays the squares collected so far and gives instructions for how to submit additional squares.

I was in San Diego when Ina May unveiled the quilt at the annual meeting for the Association for Pre- and Perinatal Psychology and Health in November 2005. The quilt honors every mother who has died in childbirth or in the postpartum period. As she tells each of their stories, you quickly realize how truly tragic and utterly preventable most of these deaths have been. It raises consciousness because you realize that these women aren't just faceless, nameless statistics. They were mothers, wives, sisters, and lovers—all of whom have left behind motherless families, a mark that will affect their children and families for generations.

When it comes to infant mortality, the news is somewhat better but still not where it should be. Over the past decade, infant mortality rates have declined 14 percent, from 6.86 deaths per 1,000 live births in 2005 (a recent high) to 5.9 deaths in 2016. Currently, the United States has a rate higher than that of any other developed nation. Canada has the second-highest rate, at 4.8 per 1,000, while all the other developed nations have rates under 4 per 1,000.[80] (Japan has the lowest infant mortality rate—2.1 deaths per 1,000 live births.) As with the maternal death rate, infant mortality is a very important measure of public health because it reflects factors such as the quality of prenatal care, maternal health, socioeconomic status, and health insurance coverage. So much for the benefits of high-tech birth.

~ There are many choices for how to have your baby. In fact, there are more childbirth choices now than ever before—everything from high-tech hospital birth to water birth at home. To choose the safest and most mother-friendly option, you must be informed. I recommend that you visit the website of the Improving Birth Coalition, a group of individuals and more than fifty organizations whose mission is to promote a wellness model of childbirth. (For more information, read "Having a Baby? Ten Questions to Ask," on CIMS's website, www.motherfriendly.org.) Other good resources include the Childbirth Connection (www.childbirthconnection.org), Mothers Naturally (www.mothersnaturally.org), and Giving Birth Naturally (www.givingbirthnaturally.com).

OUR CULTURAL INHERITANCE: LABOR AND DELIVERY

Labor and delivery most often go very well. Yet as a society, we continue to treat the normal process of birth with hysteria. The high anxiety about pregnancy and birth in this country is partially the result of our collective unresolved birth trauma—nearly every one of us has unfinished business about her or his own birth that we keep projecting onto pregnant women—and it has also been aided and abetted by the mainstream media. Most baby boomers, for example, were born drugged and were then whisked away from their mothers to the glaring lights and sterility of the hospital nursery. The World War II generation was born at home. Then birth became medicalized and moved into the hospital. Though the maternal mortality rate fell for a while, we also lost a great deal of birthing wisdom with this shift. The tide is starting to turn now—there is a happy medium that isn't either/or. I've been thrilled to see a couple of normal births on mainstream television shows lately (*This Is Us* and *Grace and Frankie*) that depicted normal labors and births that went so smoothly and quickly that the babies were born at home, with no complications. This is huge progress.

It is also true that I have seen cemeteries in New England strewn with the headstones of women who died young, surrounded by the graves of their dead children. Most of these deaths and traumas resulted from poor nutrition, overwork, and lack of maternal support, *not* necessarily from lack of sophisticated medical intervention.[81] Data show, for instance, that women who are unsupported in labor are at greater risk for prolonged labor and poor outcome. Several excellent studies have also shown that the presence of a supportive woman, called a doula, who "mothers the mother" during her labor, decreased the average length of labor from admission to delivery from 19.3 hours to 8.8 hours. The presence of a doula also resulted in the mother being more awake after delivery so that she was more likely to stroke her baby, smile, and talk to her or him.[82]

In so-called primitive hunter-gatherer societies, pregnancies are often spaced two to four years apart by unrestricted breast-feeding, which keeps prolactin levels high and acts as a natural contraceptive. In the course of her lifetime, a woman from one of these societies might have 20 periods, as compared with 500 for Western women.[83] In these societies, provisions are also made to support a pregnant woman and her labor. The birth is celebrated as a community event. Though I don't mean to imply that childbirth is always a completely risk-free, glorious process, even in societies in which women have been well nourished and well supported, we could learn a lot from combining the collective women's wisdom of indigenous, nature-centered people with our current medical technology.

Women Labor as They Live

Having participated in hundreds of cesarean-section deliveries and other forms of medicalized birth over the years, I've learned that our current dilemmas over birthing start long before a woman ends up on the labor and delivery floor. In fact, they originate years before she even gets pregnant. Each of us carries the seeds within ourselves, and we must look at the ways in which we daily participate in less-than-optimal treatment.

A woman's attitudes about pregnancy arrive with her on the labor and delivery floor. One professional woman I know wanted to labor without feeling a thing. She said, "Knock me out—I'm not an Indian." This is the statement of a woman who doesn't understand the power of labor and delivery. It implies that only "primitives" go through labor and that sophisticated intellectuals get babies via technology, keeping their hands clean, their brows uncreased, and their makeup intact.

Too many women approach labor with the wish, stated or unstated, "Take care of this inconvenience, please. I don't want to feel a thing—just hand me the baby when it's over!" Though what women need most in labor is encouragement and loving support for their abilities to birth normally, too often they don't get this because doctors and nurses hold the same attitudes about labor as they do about a crisis or inconvenience—cure it as soon as possible.

I've learned that a woman's entire life leads up to what will happen in labor. Studies have shown that women with prolonged labors have certain personality characteristics. They have inner conflicts about reproduction and motherhood and are unable at the time of the labor to communicate and admit their anxieties. (In our culture, where mothers typically receive so little support, who wouldn't have conflicts?) These psychological factors may result in inefficient uterine action and subsequent prolonged labor.[84] It is also a fact of our culture that violence is common in many women's lives, especially during pregnancy, when the woman's pregnant belly is often the target of abuse. This can certainly increase your chances for pregnancy complications of all kinds. Ask yourself the following questions: Within the last year, or since you have been pregnant, have you been hit, slapped, kicked, or otherwise physically hurt by someone? Are you in a relationship with a person who threatens or physically hurts you? Has anyone forced you to have sexual activity that made you uncomfortable? If you answered yes to any of these questions, you're being abused. To get help, call the National Domestic Violence Hotline at 800-799-SAFE (7233) or your local women's shelter or domestic violence hotline.[85]

Women who have experienced incest or other abuse are prime candidates for dysfunctional labors and subsequent cesarean sections unless they work through this—which is certainly possible. Many of these women have learned at a deep level how to be victims. This plays out in childbirth—a time when, instead of being victims of their bodies, they need to be at one with the process. One of my patients realized that she had gotten stuck in labor because at some unconscious level she was afraid of giving birth to her father's child. Another sexual abuse victim came to realize that she had learned the victim role so well that she could not push her baby out. Like most people living out of a feeling of powerlessness, she simply turned the experience over to the hospital and the staff. On some level she expected them to birth the baby for her. I've worked with countless women who have learned this attitude.

Other survivors of abuse, however, use control as a survival mechanism. During pregnancy these women often come into a doctor's office with a long list of demands: no IVs, no monitor, no medical students, a limit to exams, and no shaving or enemas (despite the fact that shaving and enemas haven't been done for years). Many obstetricians sense that those women who need to control the birth process the most are often the ones who end up with the most interventions. Any birth attendant will tell you that the longer the "laundry list," the greater the chance of an unplanned intervention, such as a C-section. The reason is that the list is often a symptom of the woman's illusion of intellectual control, her attempt to manage a situation about which she feels completely terrorized and out of control. By trying to control all the variables associated with the birthing process, she thinks she can somehow avoid the terror that she associates with her body, with feeling her body in general, and with the birth process. The more a woman operates from this illusion of control, the less likely she will be to surrender to her body's process and the more likely that an intervention will be necessary. And the medical system plays into this seamlessly. There is no question that going through labor is often experienced as a death. As my daughter recently told me after her second child was born, "You can really go to a dark place." That is so true. But deep within, we all have the capacity to move through that dark space beautifully—especially if we feel supported.

Labor also reveals the bare bones of a woman's relationship with her husband or other labor support people. Sometimes women suddenly, when nine centimeters dilated, lash out at their husbands viciously, simply because they are in transition. I was taught that this just "happens," but it never made sense to me. I've since learned that it doesn't just "happen." Any hostility that emerges between people during labor was already there long before labor began. But because of the essential, primitive nature of the process, all pretense at socially acceptable politeness gets dropped, and reality shines through. My father once told me that if I wanted to learn who someone really was, I should go on a camping trip with them. You could say the same thing for the labor and delivery process.

Gayle Peterson, in her book *Birthing Normally*, points out that women labor in the same way they live. Labor is a crisis situation for most women. They approach it the way they approach any crisis: Some believe they are powerless, while others try to assume control. A study of the differences between women who had chosen to induce labor and those who had chosen to let labor come spontaneously showed that those who chose induction lacked trust in their own reproductive systems. They were more likely to complain during their menstrual periods, had more complications in their obstetrical history, and had more anxiety about going into labor.[86] Gayle Peterson and

Lewis Mehl-Madrona did a study of pregnant women in which they were able to predict with 95 percent accuracy which of them would get into trouble during labor based on the criteria in table 7, which is supported by the many studies on individual complications.[87]

THE CERVIX IS A SPHINCTER

Midwife Ina May Gaskin coined the term "Sphincter Law" to explain why so many women's labors stop progressing the minute they get to the hospital and why so many experience "failure to progress" and end up with interventions. The reason is that the cervix is a sphincter—just like the ones that control urination and elimination. It's impossible to let go and relax a sphincter unless you feel totally relaxed and safe. That's why so many people get constipated when they travel.

TABLE 7

POTENTIAL RISK FACTORS IN CHILDBIRTH

High-Risk Childbirth	Low-Risk Childbirth
Passivity	Activity
Dependence	Independence
Reliance on others	Self-reliance
Inability to accept support from others	Ability to accept support from others
Rejection of womanhood	Acceptance of womanhood
Repressed sexuality	Healthy sexuality
Self-view as sexual object	Self-view as sexual being
Childlike	Adultlike
Limiting beliefs about birth	Facilitative beliefs about birth
Nonconducive prior acculturation	Conducive prior acculturation
Dishonest, manipulative communication	Clear and honest communication
Spiritual beliefs that interfere with birth	Spiritual beliefs conducive to birth
Self-image of weakness	Self-image of strength
Split of mind and body	Integration of mind and body
Conflictual relationships	Loving relationships
Departures from birth plan	Adherence to birth plan
Fear not being worked through	Fear being worked through

High-Risk Childbirth	Low-Risk Childbirth
Sedentary	Physically active
Frail body appearance	Robust body appearance
Rigid in resisting change and new ideas	Yielding in accommodating to change
Chaotic home	Comfortable home
Does not want child	Wants child
External control of own life	Internal control of own life
Denial of the reality of birth pain	Acceptance of the reality of birth pain

"Rescuing" Women from Labor

Not uncommonly, a woman in labor will demand that her partner do something to "rescue" her from the situation she's in. How well I remember husbands whose wives sought out their support during their contractions by crying something like "Jer-ry—*do* something!" These men then yelled at me and said, "How much longer is this going to go on? You'd better take care of this soon, or you're going to hear from me." I've been threatened repeatedly by husbands who wanted me to "fix" their wives' labors as soon as possible—or else!

Unable to control their wives' discomfort, and angry at their own feelings of helplessness in a process about which they can do nothing, these men become abusive to the obstetrician—"End this misery!" Their wives, unable to continue their usual roles as male emotional shock absorbers, watch helplessly or expect their husbands to play their Mr. Fix-It roles. These women become even further out of touch with themselves. Labor is *not* an ideal time to educate a couple about transformative experiences. However, if a couple can be encouraged between contractions simply to stay with the process, understanding that it is normal and natural and not life-threatening, then sometimes they can be helped to work *with* the contractions and the process of labor, and not against them. My colleague Bethany Hays, M.D., an obstetrician-gynecologist and former medical director of the now-closed True North Health Center in Falmouth, Maine, always reminded husbands or partners that they couldn't have the baby for their mates, nor could they take away the pain. But what they could do is love their partners. This is a very big gift for most women in labor—simply to feel loved through the entire process. Women who are totally supported in labor emotionally and physically have the opportunity to be transformed forever by the knowledge that they *were* able to go through with it, that they have the inner resources after all. Every woman deserves this loving support—and studies show that such women are more loving with their children as a result. Labor lasts a relatively short time. Yet it's powerful enough to transform a woman's entire relationship with her body and its processes. After having her baby normally, one woman told me, "I have never felt so powerful in my whole life. I was so energized by the process. I was flying. I wanted to call everyone I knew and share my joy with them."

Reversing a lifelong pattern of coping behavior during labor, however, is not always possible. When I was still delivering babies, I found that no amount of cajoling, education, or pleading on my part could reverse many women's inherited belief that they *cannot* give birth normally, that they must have drugs and anesthesia to do it.

The medical system participates fully in treating childbirth as an emergency needing a cure. Because of its patriarchal nature, the medical system too often becomes the symbolic "husband" for all the women crying "Jer-ry, *do* something!" And believe me, doctors are trained in many ways to "do something." Each of our doings has a price. Some studies show, for instance, that epidural anesthesia increases the rate of cesarean section because this anesthetic relaxes the pelvic floor muscles, causing the baby to engage with the head in what's called the occiput posterior position—facing up. It's much harder to push a baby out when he or she is in this position; it also slows down the process and may add to the baby's distress. Epidurals are also a metaphor for our current mind/body split approach to childbirth: "I want to be awake and intellectually aware, but I don't want to feel my body." This was illustrated when a family practitioner friend of mine was attending the delivery of a woman with an epidural who was almost ready to give birth. She was watching a soap opera on TV and completely unaware of anything going on below her waist. At the point when the baby was crowning and actually being born, she asked my friend, the delivering physician, to please move out of the way so that she could see the TV screen. Though the epidural is not the villain here, it clearly made it much easier for this new mother to stay out of touch with her baby and her birth process—and also made the new mother much less aware of her newborn baby than she otherwise would have been. Pain medications also cross the placenta and may affect the baby. Forceps, episiotomies, vacuum extractors, oxytocin augmentation of labor, and unnecessary cesarean sections are other interventions that are not without risk.

A woman has the power within to birth normally and needs to know that drugs and anesthetics have potential adverse side effects. When I was delivering babies, I was frustrated by women who had no intention of delivering normally, and I tried to change them through education. But this was *my* problem, not necessarily theirs. They wanted all the technology that the hospital could offer. I now realize that it was not my job to change them or anyone else. Each woman must look inside and see where she is—and be as honest with herself as possible. My job is to present alternatives in every situation and let each woman choose.

BIRTH TECHNOLOGIES

Fetal Monitors and Cesarean Sections

There is no more striking example of the overuse of technology in childbirth than the high cesarean section rates at many U.S. hospitals, a result of the medicalization of childbirth, fueled by fear of lawsuits if a baby is not perfect. Although as stated previously, the cesarean section rate is now 32 percent, in some cities a white woman with insurance has a 50 percent chance of having a cesarean.[88] This trend, thank goodness, is finally starting to reverse a bit as the medical profession has finally awakened to the risks of too many surgeries.

During my residency training, when fetal monitoring hit the scene and the cesarean section rate began to soar, I remember thinking, "How can it be that such a large percentage of women aren't able to go through a normal physiological event without the aid of anesthesia and major surgery? How could the human race possibly have survived if this many women really need major surgery to give birth? What is going wrong here?"

I was taught that I must treat everyone as though she was going to have a potential complication, as if a normal labor could turn into a crisis at a moment's notice. Whenever a woman arrived in labor, we immediately put in an intravenous line, drew blood, ruptured her membranes (broke the amniotic sac, or "bag of waters" surrounding the baby), screwed a fetal scalp electrode into the baby's head, and threaded a catheter into her uterus to measure intrauterine pressure on the fetal monitor. Then she and her family, the doctors, and the nurses all fixed their gazes on the monitor and pretty much relied on *it* to tell us what to do next. The woman was asked to labor in the position that gave the best monitor tracing—not the one that felt best to her. I recall trying to get these monitoring devices even into women whose babies were about to be delivered when they came through the door. If I didn't have a monitor strip for documentation and there was a bad outcome, I knew that I would be in trouble with my attending physician. So of course I performed all these procedures, including breaking the amniotic sac, even though during my second year of residency, I had gone to a meeting of the International Childbirth Education Association (ICEA) and learned that babies whose mothers' membranes have been artificially ruptured show evidence of more stress in utero—the pH of their scalp blood samples is lower. I also learned at this meeting that the amniotic fluid is the best "packing material" available. It cushions the baby's body during contractions and makes labor much less painful. Why were we so eager to mess with nature's protection? So that we could put in our technological monitors!

Is it any wonder that when you hook up a vulnerable laboring woman to three or four different tubes and wires and then rupture her membranes, she, and subsequently her baby, might get a little scared—resulting in some fetal distress? To make matters worse, there's something about that monitor screen that draws everyone's attention to it—and away from the laboring woman. So despite the data showing that it's not really helping, the hospital staff and the laboring woman herself all pay more attention to the monitor screen than to the mother's own internal experience. Technology designed to help has actually succeeded in cementing a mind/body split in place.

Later, studies would show that electronic fetal monitoring (EFM) does not actually improve perinatal outcome when compared with a nurse listening to the heart rate periodically.[89] What it does do is increase cesarean section rates—a great example of technology catching on before all the data were in. George Macones, M.D., who headed up the development of the latest fetal monitoring guidelines for the American College of Obstetricians and Gynecologists, summarized it quite nicely: "Since 1980, the use of EFM has grown dramatically, from being used on 45% of pregnant women in labor to 85% in 2002. [That figure has now reached 89 percent.[90]] Although EFM is the most common obstetric procedure today, unfortunately it hasn't reduced perinatal mortality or the risk of cerebral palsy." (Back when fetal monitoring was introduced, cerebral palsy was thought to be related to obstetrical trauma. Hence, obstetricians were blamed for it. Subsequent large-scale studies have now proven that cerebral palsy results from in utero neurologic damage that happens long before labor and birth.) "In fact, the rate of cerebral palsy has essentially remained the same since World War II despite fetal monitoring and all of our advancements in treatments and interventions."[91]

A survey of 1,600 women conducted by Harris Interactive for the nonprofit Maternity Center Association showed that 61 percent experienced between six and ten medical interventions during their labor and deliveries, including being hooked up to an IV and being given Pitocin to speed labor—which makes contractions more painful and increases the risk of fetal distress and neonatal jaundice. (In addition, 43 percent had between three and five major interventions—including induction, episiotomy, C-sections, and forceps delivery—and eight out of ten women, including 91 percent of first-time mothers, had pain relief medication during labor.) In this era of so-called evidence-based medicine, why does a practice continue when there is absolutely no evidence to support it? Turns out there are lots of things like that in conventional medicine.

Many cases of fetal distress could potentially have been reversed by soothing the mother and asking her to focus inside on how her baby is and send it messages of reassurance. Biofeedback has documented the profound effects of thoughts on body systems such as blood pressure, pulse, and skin resistance. The baby is *part* of a woman's body. Her thoughts and emotions can and do have large effects on her baby.

Many obstetricians feel inherently that vaginal delivery is just plain dangerous, leading to increased fetal trauma. I've been in discussions with male and female colleagues who believe on some very deep, probably unexamined level that abdominal delivery is the superior mode of arrival. Some strongly advocate elective cesareans as a matter of preference.

Unfortunately, you have to be quite resilient and self-assured to resist the environment of inductions and planned C-sections that is now common in far too many hospitals. The newly pregnant daughter of one of my friends went to a hospital in Texas for her first prenatal visit. The doctor asked, "Would you like to schedule an induction or a C-section?" In some hospital systems in the United States, a woman has to schedule her delivery date in order to fit into the system. The idea of going into spontaneous labor is simply not entertained. Another young woman I know was told that the skin on her vagina was "too thin" to withstand a vaginal delivery and that a vaginal birth might result in tears. The doctor then scheduled a C-section for her. How could one possibly suggest major abdominal surgery (talk about tears!) as a preventive for a possible vaginal laceration that could be easily repaired? And more important, how have we women become so brainwashed about labor that we simply go along with this?

Even women who've had a cesarean section can deliver subsequent babies normally. Approximately 50 to 85 percent of them are candidates for vaginal deliveries. Though obstetricians used to be taught the dictum "Once a cesarean, always a cesarean," by the late 1970s there was a body of scientific literature documenting the safety of subsequent vaginal deliveries. During my medical training, we routinely offered vaginal birth after cesarean section (VBAC) as an option. Yet this option is now withheld from many women who are candidates for it because both doctors and patients are afraid of the rare possibility of a uterine rupture. In an article entitled "When Your Patient Demands a C-section" in one of the ob-gyn magazines, Bruce Flamm, M.D., was right on target when he said, "When someone is scared, it is not an indication for surgery. It is an indication for education."[92]

C-section rates vary tremendously among individual doctors. Some physicians have personal C-section rates of only 6 percent. These tend to be the same doctors who are highly supportive of midwifery.

RISKS OF C-SECTIONS

Although some women elect to have C-sections for convenience or because they fear the birthing process, having a cesarean when there is no medical indication is a controversial practice, and for good reason. A C-section is major surgery that entails some serious risks. The following risks, compiled by the Coalition for Improving Maternity Services (now called the Improving Birth Coalition), are greater in women with C-sections when compared with vaginal births:

~ Maternal death (five to seven times greater)[93]

~ Injury to the bladder, uterus, and blood vessels; hemorrhage; anesthesia accidents, blood clots in the legs, pulmonary embolism, paralyzed bowel; and infection (up to fifty times more common)[94]

~ Difficulties with normal activities two months after birth (one in ten);[95] one in four women who have had C-sections report that pain at the incision site is a major problem, and one in fourteen still report pain six months after delivery[96]

~ Rehospitalization (twice as likely)[97]

~ Internal scar tissue resulting in pelvic pain, pain during sex, and bowel problems[98]

~ Reproductive consequences, such as subsequent infertility,[99] miscarriage, and premature birth[100]

~ Increased risk of unexplained stillbirth in future pregnancies[101]

~ Increased risk of placental problems in subsequent pregnancies, such as placenta accreta, where the placenta grows through the uterine wall, resulting in massive blood loss and possible need for hysterectomy[102]

Risks to a baby born via C-section include:

~ Breathing and breast-feeding problems due to even slight prematurity[103]

~ Being cut accidentally by the surgeon (one to two per hundred)[104]

~ Lower Apgar scores (50 percent more likely) and admission to intermediate or intensive care (five times more likely)[105]

~ Developing persistent pulmonary hypertension, a life-threatening condition (more than four times as likely)[106]

In addition, researchers have found that C-section babies experience certain epigenetic changes connected to higher stress levels during the birth that may be responsible for their increased risk later in life for allergies, asthma, type 1 diabetes, testicular cancer, and childhood leukemia.[107]

For more information, see the CIMS website at www.mother friendly.org.

Episiotomy

Fortunately, episiotomy (the surgical cutting of the tissue between the vagina and rectum, intended to prevent tearing during delivery) is no longer routinely recommended. In 1992, more than 1.6 million such procedures were performed in the United States, yet by 2003, the number had dropped to 716,000.[108] In 2006, the year the American College of Obstetricians and Gynecologists declared that routine episiotomy was no longer recommended, 17 percent of women delivering vaginally had episiotomies, and by 2012, the rate had dropped to less than 12 percent.[109]

Despite what doctors originally thought, women who have an episiotomy are actually fifty times *more* likely to suffer from severe lacerations than those who don't.[110] The reason is that episiotomy cuts frequently extend farther into the vaginal tissues during the delivery. This surgical cut of the perineum can result in excessive blood loss, painful scarring, and unnecessary postpartum pain.[111] The woman's discomfort may affect her bonding with and nursing of the infant. Further research shows that perineal massage with lubricants (done either by the pregnant women themselves or their partners) performed either during pregnancy or during labor itself lessens the need for episiotomy.[112]

During the time that the procedure was still being recommended, whether a woman giving birth had an episiotomy was most dependent upon whether she was attended by a doctor or by a midwife. Midwives are taught how to do normal, noninterventional deliveries. Doctors naturally *do* more—that's what they've been trained to do. Letting a woman push her baby out slowly, gently, and without interference is a rare experience in some hospitals. A retrospective analysis of 2,041 operative vaginal births (meaning that forceps or vacuum extractors were used) in San Francisco showed that the rate of fourth-degree tears (tears extending into the rectum) declined from 12.2 percent to 5.4 percent during a ten-year period as the rate of episiotomy at the hospital fell from 93.4 percent to 35.7 percent.[113] While the rate of vaginal lacerations increased, these are trivial and very easy to repair in comparison with the damage done by episiotomies. They are also far less painful.

A highly publicized review finally laid this matter to rest one year before the change in guidelines. In an exhaustive review of every article published in the medical literature from 1950 to 2004, the authors found that none of the benefits previously ascribed to routine episiotomy did exist. "In fact," the study reported, "outcomes with episiotomy can be considered worse since some proportion of women who would have had lesser injury instead had a surgical incision."[114]

A Word About Pelvic Floor Dysfunction

Ever since the late 1990s, the potential for pelvic floor dysfunction from natural birth has been used to justify cesarean delivery, especially when there is no other indication. In fact, the American College of Obstetricians and Gynecologists released a statement in October 2003 indicating that although physicians are under no obligation to initiate discussions about elective C-section, a physician is justified in performing the surgery if he or she believes that C-section delivery promotes the overall health and well-being of the mother and baby better than vaginal birth. And the potential protection of the pelvic floor through C-section (which I call vaginal bypass surgery) is one of the justifications.

This statement received wide criticism from many organizations, including the International Cesarean Awareness Network, the College of Midwives, Doulas of North America, Attachment Parenting International, and the American College of Nurse-Midwives. The Society of Obstetricians and Gynaecologists of Canada stated in two press releases, in March 2004, that vaginal birth remains the preferred approach and the safest option for most women because it carries fewer of the complications in pregnancy and subsequent pregnancies than C-section.

A thorough review of the medical literature on mode of delivery and pelvic floor dysfunction published in 2006 pointed out the difficulties of comparing modes of delivery because of the varying skill levels of practitioners and also the varying conditions under which birth takes place. For example, vaginal births involving forceps deliveries by unskilled practitioners or vacuum extraction, or the use of episiotomy, are far more apt to be associated with pelvic floor problems than births that don't involve these modalities. The authors state, for example, that "gentle birth in nonlithotomy position [lithotomy position is flat on the back with knees bent and legs spread apart], without urgent directed pushing and without the routine use of episiotomy, will tend to protect the pelvic floor and the perineum and reduce strain on the very structures that we are reviewing, thereby improving outcomes and reducing differences between vaginal birth and C-section where they exist."[115]

Regardless of the statistics, it is clear that the female pelvic floor is designed to give birth without complications in most women and is perfectly capable of doing so in a supportive environment. I was on a panel with the famous midwife Ina May Gaskin at the Annual Meeting of the Association for Pre- and Perinatal Psychology and Health in 2005. Ina May, whose "Sphincter Law" I mentioned earlier, suggested that it's nearly impossible for a woman to birth normally if she is out of touch with her pelvic floor, including her bowel function—a common situation in many women who are terrified of losing control during birth. She jokingly suggested that women might want to follow a horse around so they could see how well the anal sphincter of a horse expands to allow discharge of waste matter and then instantly returns to normal size. The female cervix is also a sphincter that is capable of dilating very nicely under optimal conditions but is heavily influenced by how safe and supported a woman feels in birth. The same thing is true of the pelvic floor. Comprehensive information for helping women prevent pelvic floor problems at birth is available at www.childbirthconnection.org/giving -birth/pelvic-floor/planning-ahead. And if a woman has indeed developed pelvic floor problems from birth, there is still a great deal that can be done to fix the damage—see the information on strengthening the pelvic floor in chapter 8.

Anesthesia

Modern anesthesia is a godsend in many instances, but in labor it is used far too often. This culture believes that if a little is good, more must be better. So there are now obstetrical services in which almost every pregnant woman, long before she goes into labor, is sold on the virtues of epidurals—the "Cadillac" of obstetrical anesthesia. The seed is often planted during hospital-sponsored childbirth classes: "You don't need to feel a thing." Anesthesia is offered as a panacea to many. I've heard women say, "I want that epidural catheter put in during my last two weeks of pregnancy!" One remarked, "I'm making sure I get that 'happy dural'!" But the risks include arrest of the first and second stages of labor, fever, increased forceps use, pelvic floor damage, and fetal distress, with a subsequent increase in cesarean section rates.[116]

In a study of 1,733 women having their first babies, the cesarean rate for those who received epidural analgesia was 17 percent, compared with 4 percent in those who did not receive this type of anesthesia—a fourfold increase.[117] In a study published in 2005, researchers found epidurals were strongly associated with the more problematic fetal occiput posterior position (the baby's head facing up at delivery, instead of the more ideal position of head down, facing the mother's back), which the researchers suggested might explain the higher rate of C-sections in women who have epidurals.[118] The reason for this is that when the epidural numbs the sensory nerves to the pelvic floor, it also affects their motor function. Thus the pelvic floor muscles don't function properly to get the baby in the right position. It's kind of like trying to eat soup after you've had a dental procedure that used novocaine! Despite these studies, there continues to be debate on the pros and cons of epidurals. (How the anesthesia is given, by whom, and when during the course of labor are among the factors that can affect outcome.) But the association of epidurals with C-section accords with my own experience working in a large hospital delivery unit.

In another study of 1,657 women having their first babies, 14.5 percent of those who received epidural anesthesia experienced fever, compared with only 1 percent of the women who did not receive an epidural. Because of these fevers, infants born to the women in the epidural groups were more than four times more likely to be evaluated for infection and about four times more likely to be treated with antibiotics than babies born to women who didn't receive an epidural.[119] Yet of the 356 newborns in the epidural group who were evaluated for sepsis, only 3 actually had it. Epidurals put women at higher risk for fever regardless of the infant's size or the length of labor, two factors also felt to be associated with increased risk of infection. The cascade of adverse consequences of having your baby worked up for an infection include having your baby taken away from you and taken to the neonatal intensive care unit; more pain for the baby, because blood needs to be drawn and IVs started; the risks of antibiotics, which kill all the friendly, normal bacteria in the baby's body, thus increasing the risk of infection from antibiotic-resistant strains of bacteria found in hospitals; increased anxiety for both mother and baby; and possible adverse effects on the establishment of successful breast-feeding. Since this sepsis workup takes place right after you've had your baby, it can significantly affect the important bonding period that nature intended following birth.

Supine Position

Women who deliver in a physiologically normal position, such as standing or squatting, are much less apt to have perineal tears and are more apt to have normal, nonsurgical second stages of labor. Many women also feel most comfortable laboring on their hands and knees. In fact, lying supine while pushing out the baby is a position that is actually unfavorable for birth because this position favors excessive pressure of the delivering baby into the posterior vagina, and it *decreases* the diameter of the pelvic outlet—a setup for vaginal tears. (Ever try to move your bowels while lying flat on your back?) This position, known as the lithotomy position, was apparently popularized by Louis XIV in France, who was a voyeur and wanted to watch the births of women in his court without their knowledge of his presence. In the lithotomy position, with her skirts hiked up, the laboring woman couldn't see who was watching. This position caught on because it was associated with the upper classes and therefore was imitated. It also made things easier for the birth attendant.

Probably another reason it caught on was the popularization of obstetrical forceps. Forceps were originally developed in 1630 by Peter Chamberlen, a male midwife who came from a family of male midwives. These tools remained a Chamberlen "family secret" until they were released to the medical profession in 1728.[120] Training in the use of this instrument was given only to men (usually physicians and surgeons), and they were originally used when all else failed and the woman had been trying to push the baby out for hours. The lithotomy position was the one in which the exhausted woman could rest while forceps were applied. It also allowed the obstetrician maximal control over the process of forceps delivery.

During the second stage of labor, women who squat instead of lie supine increase the size of the vaginal outlet naturally, because this position distributes pressure equally throughout the entire vaginal circumference and helps bring the baby's head down. In the squatting position the anterior/posterior diameter of the bony pelvis (front to back) is increased by a half centimeter or more.[121] The squatting position also keeps the pregnant uterus off the major pelvic blood vessels leading to the heart. The blood supply from the mother to the baby is therefore improved, resulting in increased safety for both. (I've seen countless babies go into fetal distress in the delivery room simply because of the mother's position, flat on her back.) Women who are encouraged to touch their perineum and the baby's head get connected up very quickly with their birthing babies and deliver much more easily. In general, it's not advisable for a mother to overexert herself during the second stage of labor. Pushing the baby out slowly and gently is associated with far less pelvic trauma.

Bottom line: When birth technology is truly needed, it is lifesaving and miraculous. When a physician is in the operating room transfusing a woman whose placenta simply won't separate from the uterus and who is losing blood quickly, she knows that a hundred years ago her patient would have died. In the vast majority of cases, however, more "high-touch" and less "high-tech" would do the job.

MOTHERING THE MOTHER:
A SOLUTION WHOSE TIME HAS COME

Labor support is centuries old, and it is intuitively obvious that those women who feel most supported in labor are apt to do the best. Marshall Klaus, M.D., and John Kennell, M.D., have proved in six controlled clinical trials that the presence of a female labor support person, known as a doula, shortens first-time labor by an average of two hours, decreases the chance of a cesarean section by 50 percent, decreases the need for pain medication and epidural anesthesia, helps the father or co-parent participate with confidence, and increases the success of breast-feeding. Dr. Kennell has shown that if doula labor support were routinely used, this simple step would save the healthcare system at least $2 billion a year in the costs of unnecessary

C-sections, epidurals, and sepsis workups for newborns. He once quipped, "If a drug were to have this same effect, it would be unethical not to use it."

Too often, when we think of labor support, we think of a labor coach—someone who specializes in knowing the right breathing techniques and so on. But a doula embodies women's wisdom. She is a compassionate woman especially trained to give emotional support in labor by tuning in to the needs of the mother and mothering *her*. Doulas create an "emotional holding environment for the mother, encouraging her to allow her own body to tell her what may be best at various times during labor. . . . A successful doula," write the authors of *Mothering the Mother*, "is giving of herself and is not afraid of love."[122] A doula enters the space of a laboring woman and is highly responsive and aware of her needs, moods, changes, and unspoken feelings. She has no need to control or smother. Every pregnant woman should have the benefits of a doula. This person does not detract from the role of the baby's father or co-parent, by the way. A doula enhances it and leaves him (or her) free to do the very important job of loving the mother.

HOW TO DECREASE YOUR RISK
FOR A CESAREAN SECTION

Though cesarean sections are sometimes necessary, many experts in the field feel that a rate of 15 percent plus or minus 5 percent is far more reasonable than the current overall rate of 32 percent.[123] This means, of course, that many women are having cesareans that aren't truly necessary. Because this surgery is so common, however, many women do not realize that cesarean section is major abdominal surgery fraught with potential complications, such as bleeding and infection. This surgery should be avoided unless absolutely necessary. Here's how to decrease your chances of having a C-section.

~ Check out your beliefs and your doctor's. Do you believe vaginal birth is inherently distasteful and too dangerous or frightening for you to get through? Many women and their doctors actually operate under this belief, and it gets played out seamlessly in what happens in labor and delivery. A 1996 study published in *The Lancet* found that of 282 obstetricians surveyed, 31 percent of the women and 8 percent of the men (17 percent overall) said they would want a cesarean section if they or their wives were pregnant. Many said that they would choose the operation even in uncomplicated, low-risk pregnancies.[124] Though I don't know of a similar study from the United States, I've met many physicians who honestly believe that cesarean sections are the superior mode of delivery, and this belief is reflected in their personal C-section rates. Hospitals keep statistics on the C-section rates for individual doctors, so a physician should be able to tell you his or her rate. (Of course, in a practice limited to high-risk obstetrics in a large medical center, the rate will be higher.)

~ If you've had a prior C-section, consider having a normal vaginal delivery for your next birth. Though many women don't know it, both the medical literature and the personal experience of countless obstetricians (including me) who have performed vaginal births after cesarean for years show that the vast majority of women who've had a previous C-section can safely go through a normal labor and delivery. Studies show 60 to 80 percent of women attempting VBAC are successful—even when the mother has previously had two separate C-section births.[125] Only 1 woman out of every 2,000 who undergoes VBAC will have a significant complication from uterine rupture.[126] This makes VBAC far safer than a routine C-section. A 2010 report from the National Institutes of Health says the risks of VBAC are the same as for any other mother giving birth for the first time.[127] Yet many hospitals refuse to offer VBAC because of liability concerns, and nearly half of women who want to attempt VBAC are not given that option by their obstetricians. If your doctor is not comfortable with the VBAC option, find someone who is.

~ Choose your birthing place carefully. Plan to have your baby in a setting in which you know you're most apt to feel safe and secure. More and more, studies are documenting that home births are safe for carefully selected and well-supported women. Family-centered maternity care centers offer many of the comforts of home with the safety net of a hospital. A growing number of hospitals and some freestanding birth centers now offer this kind of care, which is characterized by the following: the laboring woman, with her support person(s), labors and delivers in the same room; the labor and delivery nurse is the same throughout her stay; and the mother's nurse is also the primary nurse for the baby, who rooms in with the mother. In short, in family-centered maternity care, the focus is on keeping mothers, babies, and families together in supportive and healthy ways. This is a vast improvement over the childbirth-as-major-operation approach that has been common since the 1950s; that approach requires a labor room, delivery room, and recovery room, all staffed by different nurses, and the baby is sent to a nursery, where yet another group of nurses takes over. This fragmented care, which was experienced by nearly all of our mothers, can be devastating to a laboring mother and her new baby, and it increases the risk of intervention starting from the time a woman enters the hospital.

~ Hire a doula to mother you during your labor and delivery. (See page 997.) Better yet, work with a doctor or midwife who automatically suggests professional labor support and is comfortable working closely with these individuals. Such doctors and midwives almost always have lower C-section rates than their colleagues.

⁓ Don't go to the hospital too early. It's very common for a woman to go through many hours of "prodromal" mild labor before going into true labor, which is defined as the active dilation and effacement of the cervix. If you're really in labor, you won't want to talk through a contraction, your attention will be focused inward, and you won't want to move around much during the contraction. Consider hiring a midwife who can meet you at your home or at another convenient location to check your progress before you get admitted to the hospital, where the atmosphere may actually slow your labor or cause it to be dysfunctional. (This is not always the case in a good birth center that offers family-centered maternity care.) Remember, your uterus is very sensitive to your environment. It works best whenever and wherever you feel the most relaxed and safe. This will vary from woman to woman.

Recent studies have suggested that labor may take longer than doctors have been led to believe it should and still be completely safe and normal. Many doctors have been trained to follow the now-outmoded Friedman curves—named after a well-known Boston obstetrician whose advice influenced several generations of obstetricians—for determining the progress of labor. If your labor doesn't follow these graphs, it may increase your chances for having a C-section even when everything is normal.

A significant number of C-sections are done for "failure to progress," a condition often attributed to the fact that the baby is "too big." This is usually not the case, since many women who have had C-sections for this indication go on to have even bigger babies in subsequent pregnancies following a normal labor and delivery. Failure to progress, in my experience, simply means that the uterus stops contracting efficiently and the mother becomes exhausted. When this goes on for a number of hours, a C-section is often done to get the whole thing over with. One of my colleagues said that the diagnosis should be changed to "failure to wait."

What you want to do is avoid the chain of events that leads up to this in the first place. Tune in to your body's wisdom. Most women will be able to know when they're really in labor. Don't let the collective emergency mindset of the culture invade your physiology here, because once you get all hooked up to the monitor, you may find that your labor slows—or stops altogether if you are really anxious. And try to avoid letting anyone rupture your membranes to "get things moving."

Unfortunately, all too many women and their mates have been indoctrinated by TV shows and movies showing couples rushing to the hospital at the first sign of a contraction, fearful that the baby will simply drop out if they don't arrive in time. Once they are there, the hospital staff will often be subtly (or not so subtly) pushed to do something because the woman is tired of being pregnant and wants it over with. If, in this state, you get into bed, allow your membranes to be ruptured, and then stay immobile waiting for something to happen, you won't be allowing your body and your baby to find their own timing.

~ Plan to labor without an epidural. When you enter labor with the idea that your body will know how to deal with the sensations, you're more likely to be in the receptive mode necessary for optimal uterine functioning. If, on the other hand, you believe you will need an epidural the minute you enter the hospital, you won't be present with your own labor. The contractions will simply be something to be endured until the anesthesiologist gets there. Although epidurals can be very useful under certain circumstances, they are associated with prolonged labor and with relaxing the lower part of the uterus and pelvis so much that the baby's head engages in the wrong position. And, as I mentioned above, even if an epidural does not increase your cesarean risk, it is still associated with maternal fever and the risk of your baby needing a sepsis workup. It also inhibits the release of the neurotransmitter beta-endorphin, which normally increases during labor and is responsible for the euphoria some women feel. Nature designed that euphoria as the best possible state in which to meet and fall in love with your new baby. If you do find you need an epidural, for whatever reason, wait until your labor is well established and ask for the lowest dose that gives you adequate pain relief.

~ Embrace the process. Labor feels very instinctive and primitive, but because our culture teaches us not to trust our instincts, we usually associate the word *primitive* with *ignorant*. The Random House dictionary defines *primitive* as "unaffected or little-affected by civilizing influences." Believe me, that's exactly how labor feels. We cannot labor with our intellect. We women need to reclaim this animal part of us and embrace ancient and necessary wisdom. Preparing for birth with the Bradley Method (see www.bradleybirth.com) or the Calm Birth method (see www.calmbirth.org) surely helps. Above all, trust that your body knows how to give birth. During labor more than at any other time, women have the opportunity to experience their body's wisdom in a dramatic way. Move into the positions that feel best (usually on your hands and knees). Don't get into bed unless that's the position that feels most comfortable. Don't resist labor—dive in deeply and go with it. I've attended enough labors to know that when women feel comfortable, relaxed, and well supported, their bodies automatically know what to do to keep both themselves and their babies safe.

VAGINAL SEEDING:
GIVING CESAREAN-BORN BABIES "GOOD" BACTERIA

Babies born vaginally come in contact with bacteria living naturally in the mother's vagina during birth, boosting the microbiome of the newborn's digestive system and stimulating the baby's immune system. This reduces the baby's risk for asthma, allergies, and even obesity later in life. But children delivered by C-section (whose gastrointestinal tract is thought to be sterile, without any such healthy microbiome) are at increased risk for immune and metabolic disorders. Similarly, an infant's microbiome is also negatively altered when the child must be given antibiotics for any reason, as well as when a child is formula-fed instead of breast-fed. One option for getting around this is a practice called vaginal seeding (also called microbirthing) that transfers maternal vaginal fluid (and the natural bacteria it contains) to the newborn by soaking cotton gauze or a cotton swab in vaginal fluids and rubbing it on the baby's mouth, nose, and skin. A small pilot study has shown this practice to be effective.[128]

However, the American College of Obstetricians and Gynecologists does not recommend the procedure, citing the risk of spreading potentially harmful bacteria to the baby and the need for more research.[129] Many mothers have taken to making this transfer on their own, a practice ACOG frowns upon because 20 percent of women giving birth are carriers of a common bacteria called group B streptococci, which can cause illness. ACOG suggests mothers who want to do this procedure themselves be informed about the risks and tested for infectious diseases and potentially harmful bacteria before carrying out such a procedure. In my opinion, the practice of vaginal seeding will eventually prove to do much more good than harm and may well become standard within the next decade or so.

MY PERSONAL STORY

As a mother and a women's doctor, I have experienced childbirth from both sides of the bed. Every mother has moments that she cherishes from the birth experience and insights and feelings she'd like to share with other women. I'd like to tell you my story and also some remarkable stories of other women.

The due date for my first child was December 7, 1980. I continued my work supervising the residency clinic at a Boston hospital, and flew or drove to Maine every other week to keep my practice going there. I had watched far too many pregnant women stop work early and then mope around the house eating, waiting for the baby to come, and sometimes begging their obstetrician to induce labor. I didn't want to fall into that category. I had also seen dozens of women go overdue. I certainly wasn't going to get excited about labor—at least, not until my due date.

On Thanksgiving we went to dinner at a friend's house. Later that evening, back home in bed, I started to experience very mild but regular contractions that didn't hurt. Like the good controlled doctor that I was, I went into the bathroom and decided to examine my cervix to see if I was dilating. When I did this, my water broke. I thought, "Damn, now I know this really *is* it."[130] Shortly thereafter, without the natural "padding" that the amniotic fluid provides, my contractions began coming every two minutes and were much more uncomfortable than initially.

I called my mother, who was planning to help me after the birth, and said, "I'm not going to like this." She said that she understood (after six children, she knew) but that it wouldn't last forever. When Mom gave birth in the 1940s, she always had to labor alone, strapped down in bed with no pain relief or personal support. Then for each delivery, she was knocked unconscious by drugs under the mistaken belief that the actual delivery was the worst part and required anesthesia. She was handed the baby later by the obstetrician, as though it was a gift from him and not the fruit of her own labor. Millions of women like her were never given a choice and didn't even know there were other ways to deliver.

The pain of labor was far greater than I thought it would be. (It's always worse after the membranes are ruptured, a point that doesn't seem to stop some obstetricians from doing it prematurely even when there's no need to.) I had seen hundreds of women in labor after five years of OB training. I had always focused on the women who didn't appear to have any discomfort, and I was so sure I would be one of them. But here I was, stuck. I felt as though I were in a box and there was no way out except through. My intellect could not get me out of this—and I was determined to go through the process naturally. I already trusted the natural world more than the artificial man-made one. What I didn't appreciate then was the depth of my own programming into and cooperation with that same man-made world.

We called my obstetrician, a sensitive man with whom I had worked in the hospital for several years. He suggested that my husband and I go into the hospital. The only problem was that all I wanted to do was stay on the floor on my hands and knees. Moving *anywhere* seemed to me the most unnatural thing I could think of. It went against every instinct in my body.

I didn't have a bag packed for the hospital, so my husband ran around and put some underwear, a nightgown, and a toothbrush in a bag. Then he tried to get me dressed, out the door, and into the car. He nearly had to carry me. Left to my own instincts, I would never have left my position on my hands and knees on the floor.

When we got to the hospital, a place where I had worked for half a decade, I had to go through the admitting office as a patient. Admissions had lost the correct papers and would not let me go upstairs to the labor and delivery floor, where my nurse friends and my doctor were waiting. This was my introduction to the bureaucracy of hospitals, something I'd been shielded from for years. (Laboring in a hospital hallway alone is inhumane, but for thousands of women, it is their experience.) I simply walked out of the room, went to the back hall elevator, got in, and went up to labor and delivery by myself.

When my doctor examined me, I was four centimeters dilated. (You have to get to ten to be ready to push.) For the next three hours my contractions came frequently. But I failed to dilate beyond six centimeters, where I remained "stuck" for those three hours. The contraction pattern on the monitor was "dysfunctional." Though the contractions hurt a lot and I never got much of a break between them, they simply were not getting the job done. I had what is known as hypertonic uterine inertia, which means that the contractions, though present, are not efficient—they are erratic, originating all over the uterus at the same time, like the heart when it goes into atrial fibrillation. (Sometimes the "low heart," the uterus in the pelvis, does the same thing as the "high heart," in the chest.) Instead of beginning at the top and moving in a wave to the bottom of the uterus, the contractions originated in many places at the same time. Labor didn't progress well. It was like trying to get toothpaste out of a tube by squeezing it in fifteen places at the same time with a little bit of pressure, instead of squeezing firmly only at the back end of the tube so that the paste comes out uniformly.

When my doctor told me that I had made no progress in three hours, I knew what was next. (Remember, my intellect thought it was in control of my labor.) "Okay," I said, "start the IV, plug in the fetal electrode, and hang the Pit." Pitocin (oxytocin) is a drug that artificially contracts the uterus. After the Pitocin was started, the contractions became almost unbearable, going to full intensity almost as soon as they began.

No amount of Lamaze breathing distracted me from the intensity of the feeling that the lower part of my body was in the grip of a vise.[131] At one point, I looked at the clock and saw that it was 11:15 A.M. What I recall thinking was, "If this goes on for another fifteen minutes, I'm going to need an epidural anesthetic." I didn't know that I was in transition—the part of labor that is most intense, just before the cervix becomes fully dilated. Within the next twelve minutes I suddenly felt the urge to push. It was the most powerful bodily sensation I've ever felt, and I was powerless to resist it. The thought flashed through my mind, "If I ever tell another woman not to push when every fiber in her body tells her to push, may God strike me with lightning!"

In two pushes, Ann almost flew out of my body. My obstetrician quite literally caught her. Though I was laboring in the "birthing room," I wasn't laboring in the "correct" delivery bed, and I barely made it to the delivery bed in time. (Birthing rooms now are equipped with beds that adjust for delivery of the baby, so that moving from one bed to another isn't necessary.)

Ann cried and cried, and though I put her to my breast almost immediately, it still took quite a while to calm her down. I believe this was because the Pitocin made for a far too rapid second stage of labor. It was too intense both for Ann and for me. Neither she nor I had much chance to recover between contractions.

A primiparous patient—one having her first baby—usually takes an hour or more to push the baby out. From the time the cervix is fully dilated to delivery—the second stage of labor—I went from six centimeters to delivery in less than one hour; my uterus was being pushed by a powerful drug, a very intense and distinctly unnatural experience.

During her childhood, my daughter was not particularly "at home" in her body and was afraid to take physical risks, for instance in skiing or hiking. Though there are various reasons for this, I know deep within me that being propelled into the world with so little time to accommodate herself to the process of labor was a terrifying experience for her. She had difficulty nursing, and she was never a good sleeper. Part of the reason is that she was small (5 pounds, 8 ounces) and early (38.5 weeks), and part is her personality—but another part is how she was born. I didn't know then what I know now, and I don't for one minute blame myself about how she was born. I allowed myself to feel sadness about the experience, which would be considered a completely normal labor and delivery by most everyone.

After Ann's birth, the cord got pulled off the placenta, so my placenta had to be manually removed by my doctor. The explosive uncontrolled delivery had left me with some vaginal tears, so removing the placenta was somewhat uncomfortable. But nothing could equal the discomfort of those Pitocin-induced contractions! I was euphoric to have the whole thing over with. I had had a "normal vaginal delivery" and felt lucky to have avoided a cesarean. Most women obstetricians end up being treated like candidates for high-risk pregnancies and deliveries, because women doctors (like other women who have been highly trained out of their instinctual feminine knowing) often split their intellects from their bodies, mistrust their bodies, and unconsciously set themselves up for the possibility of labor problems. We as a group are also at risk for working too many hours during pregnancy to "prove" that we can "handle it" and compete with the men.

When I look back now, I realize that my being stuck at six centimeters was a perfect metaphor for how I felt during my labor and for my ambivalence about having a baby. I had felt "stuck" and trapped by the pain of labor—something my intellect had not prepared me for. My intellect, you recall, thought I was doing an experiment with my uterus. And I wasn't very invested in actually having a *baby*. I had made no room in my life for one. I had spent the previous decade proving to myself and to the world that I was as good as any man—and men don't do babies.

Another factor in creating my dysfunctional labor was the process of moving off my hands and knees in my house, getting to the hospital, going through admitting, and then answering insurance and medical questions for forms that I had already filled out several times. All those things are interruptions of the inner focus required for normal labor. I didn't really know that at the time, though I'd seen countless women come to the hospital in active labor, only to have the process become slowed down or dysfunctional when they were "processed by the system."

Now it was me having a baby—something that I was determined would not change my life. I realized later that what I needed when I got stuck was a midwife or a doctor with good midwifery skills, preferably some wise woman (or wise man—male midwives and male obstetricians with the souls of midwives do exist) who was a parent and who trusted the process of labor and the messages my body was sending. I needed someone who would have said to me, "Go inside and talk to your baby. Let the baby know that it's okay to come out, that she will be fine." Then the midwife would have taken me for a walk in the hall—a very effective way of getting contractions back on track. She might even have helped me work through my ambivalence about having a baby.

With my second labor, I did go to a midwife. I began labor at home and spent some time in the bathtub. (Studies done in Sweden have shown that women who labor in warm water dilate much faster.) I didn't want to go to the hospital until I had to. My husband was asleep, and I didn't wake him until I knew that the labor was moving right along, several hours later. When he examined me, I was already seven centimeters dilated. We called the midwife and then went to the hospital, where my colleague Mary Ellen Fenn, M.D., met me at the front door and parked my car, a gesture of support that I will always treasure.

When I arrived in the birthing room, I was nine centimeters dilated. I spent the rest of the labor rocking from one foot to the other while standing up. This second baby was a lot bigger than the first—8 pounds, 9 ounces. Her head was what is called posterior (she was faceup in my body). I never felt the urge to push, but I pushed her out anyway with a great deal of effort. Even after I was fully dilated, the contractions felt the same as they had at nine centimeters. I didn't have any episiotomy—and I didn't tear. My baby, Kate, and I left the hospital an hour after she was born. Kate was calm and collected, and she has been that way ever since. Her personality and body type are entirely different from her sister's. Part of the reason is that I was a different person during my pregnancy with Kate than with Ann.

Having my midwife in the room with me was heaven. I felt so supported. I had much more trust in myself this time—and I had all the baby things ready. I remember thinking during this second labor that every woman deserved this same amount of support. *Every* woman should be able to labor in whatever position her body wants to take. She should be surrounded by beloved friends of her choice. (Not spectators, but supporters—there's a big difference!) Every woman should be massaged and cared for and cherished during her labor.

In this labor I had pain, to be sure, but I went deep down inside myself with it. In my first labor, I had fought the pain and reached out to my husband in desperation—I wouldn't even let him go to the bathroom. But this second labor felt as though it was between me and my baby. I had plenty of time to rest between contractions and to chat with my midwife, husband, and obstetrics nurse. They gave me backrubs that felt fantastic. No drugs interfered with the labor. I learned to trust my body in a letting-go process that feels like a kind of surrendering to a process that *is* you but that is also *greater* than you. I didn't learn any of this stuff in my residency training— I didn't even learn it from watching women in labor, though I believe that it can be learned that way and that I eventually would have. What you have to do is trust nature, expect the best, and get your intellect's death grip off your flesh.

I now wish I had groaned loudly and let my groans help me expel the baby. But I was far too "professional" (read: out of touch) to do that. I am deeply saddened by all the unnecessarily medicalized births that occur because women in labor don't trust themselves and aren't surrounded by those who could assist them in this process.

TURNING LABOR INTO PERSONAL POWER

Trusting the birth process and knowing how to tune in to the baby are abilities that enhance labor and make it an experience that offers us the opportunity to empower ourselves. Instead of running from these lessons, women could learn a great deal if we were willing to embrace them.

Bethany Hays, M.D., mentioned earlier, is the mother of three sons. She once wrote me the following reflections on the pain of labor and how we can work *with* it: "I used to think that labor was just a matter of dealing with pain and the fear of pain. I knew that with labor the pain was qualitatively different from any other pain experienced in our bodies. I never subscribed to the punishment theory of labor pain. I was looking for a natural and reasonable explanation. I did not believe labor pain was a whim of Mother Nature any more than it was a punishment from God.

"With all other forms of pain, the pain is there to tell us that something is wrong. 'Stop walking on your foot, there's a piece of glass in it.' 'Don't eat any more chili, it's giving you heartburn.' With labor, I knew that the reason for the pain, at least in most cases, is not related to anything being wrong. The physical process of birth is completely normal and exquisitely planned by nature to ensure the safe delivery of an infant with minimal trauma to the mother. Pain was a part of that plan, and I had but to view it in that context to understand its purpose.

"As I observed women through their pregnancies, I began to understand that nature would have to have a signal to get women to stop what they were doing, to find a safe place to give birth, and to gather people around them to help. For some, nothing short of a sledgehammer would do. It needed to be a signal that no one could ignore but that left the mother able to participate in the birth if there were circumstances requiring her to do so."

Certainly, the pain of labor is a strong signal that says, "Stop what you're doing and pay attention." Instead of the "no pain, no gain" cultural mentality that often leads to self-abuse, gaining from the pain of labor is an entirely different way of being with pain. Once a woman has stopped, gathered support people around her, and gotten herself to a safe place to birth, she has reached the point when she must use the pain for something else. Dr. Hays suggests that at this point the pain is something to allow, and she points out that one of the meanings of *to suffer* is "to allow," as when Christ said, "Suffer the little children to come unto me."

Once settled in, women in labor then must *allow* the pain. Thrashing about doesn't help. Going deep within yourself does. Dr. Hays and I were talking recently about the pain of labor and how to help women work with it, and we exchanged a few stories about women who appeared to "go to another place" when they were in labor.

She told me about the wife of a medical student she once worked with who sat quietly in bed with the lights dimmed during her labor and was so focused that her mother and husband figured that she probably wasn't in labor. Not only was she in labor, however, but when she finally opened her eyes and spoke, she said, "I think it's time to push."

"After the birth," Dr. Hays told me, "my curiosity prompted me to ask her where she had gone when I instructed her to go 'somewhere else.' [Early in labor, she had seemed to be very disconnected from her body, and Dr. Hays had told her to get comfortable, relax, and just 'go somewhere else.'] Her answer was totally unexpected. She said, 'Oh, I was concentrating on the pain.' Her answer intrigued me. Could a woman really deal with the pain of labor not, as I had been taught, by distracting herself and concentrating on something else—her 'breathing' or her 'focal point' or her fantasy trip to the Caribbean? Could she, rather, focus on her body—on the work it was doing, on the *pain itself?*"

So Dr. Hays began questioning those women who labored without noise or a lot of activity each time she worked with one. One said, "Well, I was just concentrating on my cervix. You know, letting it open up for my baby's head." The common thread running through all these labors was that the women were *with* the pain. They were going down inside themselves to the place where the pain was and allowing it.

One of Dr. Hays's patients gave her the following beautiful piece of birth imagery in answer to the question "Where do you go during your contractions?" She said, "Well, you know when you are in the ocean, in a heavy surf, if you stay on the surface you will get thrown about against the reefs and the rocks, and you get a lot of water in your nose and mouth and feel like you're drowning. But if you dive down and hold on to something and let the wave pass over you, you can come up in between and feel just fine. Well, that's what I did during labor. When the contractions came, I dived down and let them pass over me." Water imagery is very common when women describe normal birth.

During my own second labor, I realized that I had *allowed* the process quite differently than I had with my first. Labor is a true *process*—with its own rhythm and timing—and it is a process that is bigger than we are. For that reason, learning to go with it—to let it sweep us along—is something that we never forget. And it is great training for the give-and-take of parenting.

ACCESSING THE HEALING POWER OF BIRTH ENERGY

When a woman gives birth, her cervix dilates to allow her baby's body to be born. At the same time, there is also an energy dilation—an aperture of sorts in her energy field—so she can receive the download of the child's birth energy. The birth field is meant to be a sacred and protected energetic space for you and your child; indeed, one of the benefits of resting after giving birth is to preserve its integrity. However, depending on the circumstances of the birth, it may not feel like a safe place. Sometimes this energy process is interrupted or the birth field imprints trauma.

The following two exercises, designed by holistic women's healthcare visionary Tami Lynn Kent and adapted from her book *Mothering from Your Center: Tapping Your Body's Natural Energy for Pregnancy, Birth, and Parenting* (Atria, 2013), can help change the energy of this experience for you. The first exercise is designed to repair the birth field, realigning any aspects that need healing. The second exercise restores the birth energy flow that brings your child into this life. This flow contains all the energy medicine your child needs in their life journey as well as all that you need for mothering them. Tapping in to the potent medicine of this field allows you to receive guidance or healing energy for your child, no matter their age. (For more information about Tami and her work, visit her website at www.wildfeminine.com.)

Realigning the Birth Field

1. In a quiet place appropriate for meditation, reflect upon the experience and the energy of your recent or past birth event. Remember your child's presence in your womb (if your child is adopted, draw on the earliest sense you had of your child) and feel into the mother-child birth space. Remember with your body, and sense the quality of energy from the birth field. How does it feel? What do you notice? Are there any densities or contracted aspects? Remain neutral and simply observe with compassion.

2. Engage the energy by sensing and seeing it with your inner awareness. If you discover aspects of fear or trauma, sweep them away as if sweeping the floor. Let any difficulties dissipate. See these imprints as dust or matter and move them toward the earth with each sweep. If there were any disruptive people or practitioners at the birth, sweep their energy away. Clear any remorse, guilt, or grief as well. Restore the connection with your body, remembering that your body birthed as best it was able. You need this beautiful body to mother your child and reclaim the potential of your creative center. Continue clearing until the birth field is filled with radiant light or a sense of ease.

3. Return to the place where you intended to give birth. Imagine yourself there in a safe and peaceful environment, with the people you desire to be around you. Notice how it feels to be in your desired place; sink into the sensations of ease and comfort. Now let the energy opening expand to allow the birth energy passage. Call upon Mother Earth herself or imagine the earth's energy holding you as a source of support in the expansion of birthing.

4. Begin to bless the birth field. Imagine a golden light moving in the air around you, bringing a divine energy that ignites the life force in all that it touches. See the space around your body responding to this light. Notice how it feels. Breathe toward the sacred energy of your birth field as it realigns. As the field dilates to full expansion, prepare to welcome the soul energy of your child into this life. With your inner vision or senses, witness the pattern that emerges as the spirit door opens and receive its blessing.

5. Continue with the next exercise, Restoring the Birth Energy Flow and Bond.

Restoring the Birth Energy Flow and Bond

1. Begin by sensing your child in the womb; see them in your mind's eye and feel their energy. (If they are adopted, sense them in the same way.) Remember your child's earliest beginning held in the womb space. Also imagine them as their present age, not in the womb but next to you. You will be reconnecting the birth flow energy through your body to your child at their present age. Let the energy between you both connect and align.

2. If your baby was separated from you at birth due to any intervention or trauma, be sure you have swept away all of the trauma or interference energy during the first exercise. If you sense any more of that, sweep it away again and observe it dissipating or moving into the earth. In your mind's eye, bring your baby back to your chest.

3. Begin to visualize the energy moving through the spirit door, from your womb to your child. (If your child is adopted, receive the energy for this child from the birth mother and give thanks for her sharing this thread.) Continue to breathe the energy down through your womb and vagina, toward your child. Sense the soul essence of your child as it moves through the spirit door and then through your center. See the energy moving like a river of light through your body, touching your chest where your baby lay in the first moments after birth and then reaching outward to your child at the age they are now. This river has no end—you are simply opening this current of life and repairing the flow pattern. Sense how as the strong flow of energy moves through your body and the birth field to your child, it fills up your child's energy field in present time. This is the life force that informs their essence and their journey, as well as your journey together. Witness the miracle of this light.

4. As the birth energy continues to flow, notice your own energy field. Are you receiving the blessing of this energy? If you have any hesitations about accepting this path or becoming a mother, let them go. You must step fully through the spirit door with your child's entry to inhabit your full mothering and creative potential. Let the birth energy assist you; it contains infinite resources to make an inspired mothering pattern when you release yourself into the flow. This energy can also assist the family in realigning, so let this birth energy radiate into the whole family's energy field. Imagine talking to your child through this energy current, sharing your original desires for their birth and how the birth energy now contains a blessing for you both.

5. Make an intention for your mothering and set it in this sacred birth space. When it feels complete, let the energy opening of the spirit door close again. Know that you can access this portal and its potent medicine as needed, calling upon this birth flow for inspiration and energy at any point along your journey as a mother.

Women's Stories

Rebecca's Story: Reclaiming Birth Power

The following story is related in the words of Bethany Hays, Rebecca's obstetrician.

"Rebecca was a second-time mother whose first labor had been long, but she did well with the help of her labor support person and a gentle, loving husband. Rebecca arrived at the hospital for her second birth already seven centimeters dilated and feeling great. She walked and talked with her team of supportive people, and she sipped fluids. She tolerated our medical intrusions into her birth with monitor, blood pressure cuff, and thermometer.

"After several hours, Rebecca was still only seven to eight centimeters dilated. She was puzzled and frustrated, wanting to 'get on with it.' We discussed her options, including rupture of the membranes, which might bring the baby's head down against the cervix. The cervix felt ready and soft enough to allow the passage of the head, waiting for some unknown work yet to be done.

"After considering the possible negative effects of it, she chose to rupture the membranes. This was done. Now the contractions got harder, but after some time, the exam showed that she was not quite fully dilated. The head was still high up in the pelvis. She showed some urge to push when squatting, but she was not pushing effectively. Her monitrice [professional labor support person] reminded me that during the first labor, she had also had difficulty pushing—requiring three hours in the second stage and pressure applied to the posterior vaginal wall to encourage her to push.

"Maybe that would help again, someone suggested. So as Rebecca squatted, I knelt on the floor, placed two fingers in her vagina, and pushed firmly on the posterior wall. Her response was an immediate and reflexive withdrawal. I realized that not only was I causing her pain, but I was triggering some much more serious emotional response. My own reaction was equally strong. 'No,' I thought, 'I will not participate in this abuse. This is sexual abuse of another woman's body, and I will not do it.'

"'Rebecca,' I said, 'let's try something else.' Now, I have always been touched at the faith (often undeserved) that patients place in me, and I knew that she trusted me. Whatever the new plan was, she would try it. The joke was that I had no plan. I was flying totally by the seat of my pants. I asked her to get comfortable, and she arranged herself semi-reclining on the bed, with her husband behind her and wrapped around her. 'Now,' I said, 'I just want you to relax and listen to my voice. First, go down inside yourself and find your baby where he is in your body. When you are with him, tell him he is okay, in case he is scared.'

"As we waited, a slow smile came over her face, and I knew that she was with her baby. The fetal monitor no longer disturbed her. It now showed sudden resolution of the small to moderate variable decelerations she'd been having with contractions. [Variable decelerations are heart rate patterns associated with compression of the umbilical cord, which can sometimes produce stress in the baby.]

"'Now,' I said, 'I want you just to listen. Many of us women have not owned all the parts of our bodies. We have not allowed ourselves to feel our vaginas and our perineums. They have seemed separate and are not within our control. They have negative connotations: pornographic or dirty. In many ways these parts of our bodies are problematic for us. But the truth is that they are ours. They belong to us like our hands and our lips and our minds. This part of your body is yours, and you can reclaim it. Right now. Take it back as the sensual, enjoyable part of you that it really is. Since it is yours, you are totally in control. You can allow your baby to move through this part of you as fast or as slowly as you like. It does not have to hurt you, but you will feel very strong signals from this part of your body that you are not used to feeling. Allow those feelings and celebrate them as the return of a long-lost friend.'

"Now we were all watching. Rebecca was totally relaxed, lying in her husband's arms. The room was quiet except for the fetal monitor, which was quietly attesting to the continued well-being of the baby. I was wondering if

I was deluding myself—pretty sure that everyone in the room must think I was nuts.

"Suddenly I realized that with each contraction, Rebecca's perineum was bulging—the head was coming down. It was working. Occasionally, Rebecca lost contact with her body, became frightened, and clutched her husband. Immediately when this happened, the baby's heart rate pattern showed prolonged variable decelerations with slow recovery. At these points, I would say, 'Talk to your baby again, Rebecca. He's scared. Remember, don't go faster than you want to. This is your body. All of it belongs to you.'

"Once again, Rebecca was quiet, and we saw the baby's head begin to crown [to appear, just before delivery]. Soon, with little or no pushing effort, the baby was born into his mother's loving arms."

After hearing this story, I realized that the second stage of my own second labor might have been different if I'd had a doctor like Bethany Hays. I also realized that I have been involved in the unwitting physical abuse of many laboring women by pushing down on their vagina to try to help them push, and by encouraging them, like a football coach, to "push him out." I wouldn't have done that if I had known what I now know.

Amanda's Story: A Home Birth

Bethany also attended a birth in which one of her patients went further into herself than either of us had known it was possible to go. Amanda's first baby had been delivered by Bethany by cesarean section. "I thought we had done everything right," Bethany says. "She had been healthy, confident, and wanted a normal birth, including labor without anesthesia. She had labor support, family, and friends. Though it seemed perfect, the baby simply wouldn't come. We did everything I knew to do, which at that time was not a lot. I finally did a cesarean."

With her second pregnancy Amanda returned to Bethany's care and said, "I want to have a normal birth this time." Bethany agreed and told her that she thought that was entirely possible. The women who are most motivated to give birth normally are those who did not succeed in doing so with their first child but haven't lost the desire to try. Amanda also did not want to have her second baby in the hospital, because she felt that the hospital environment had been part of the problem the first time. Instead, she would have her baby at home.

For years I've had a special place in my heart for those women who choose home birth. The reason for this is that these women trust themselves more than doctors and hospitals. Though they sometimes make mistakes, they have something to teach us. My sister had a home birth, and I wish I had had at least one child at home. Though I left the hospital right after both my children were born and neither one of them went to the nursery, I still would have liked the experience of waking up in labor and not having to get into the car and go someplace. Both times it felt like a very unnatural interruption of my process.

Though Amanda wanted Bethany there, Bethany does not do home births. Finally they reached a compromise. Bethany would be there only as a labor support person, and Amanda herself would hire the best midwife she could find. For an ob-gyn to do a home birth has been politically very unsafe. Many hospitals will not allow physicians who do home births to have hospital privileges, and most malpractice insurance companies won't insure these physicians despite statistics on the safety of such births. But Amanda was determined to have Bethany present, and Bethany was interested in supporting her, as long as she wasn't responsible for being the caregiver.

Long discussions ensued, regarding risks, uterine rupture, fetal compromise, their likelihood, and what Bethany could and could not do if these problems happened at home. Ultimately, Amanda convinced Bethany that she herself was in charge of the safety of her baby and the integrity of her uterus, and that if she felt she could not do this job, she would let Bethany know and they would all go to the hospital.

The day of Amanda's delivery came. Her early labor was long and painful, but she didn't call anyone. When she finally invited her caregivers to join her, they found Amanda in the rocker. "I feel so great," she said in one breath. And with the next she said, "The pain was so bad this afternoon, I thought I would die." Bethany later told me, "I didn't know how to put those two statements together." As the birth neared, Amanda lay in her king-size bed on her side. "As we tried to keep up with her," Bethany told me, "she circled the bed. Her head remained in the center, and her feet made a full circuit around the bed twice, a maneuver that I had not seen before in the hospital. It was very primitive. Though it was not clear to me what it represented, I trusted her need to move in this way as part of her unique birth process.

"There was little talk. Amanda said nothing and made little noise. She pushed her baby out on hands and knees and then kneeled over her. She was somewhere else. We were all commenting on the baby, but she was not looking at her infant. Her body was in a pose of ecstasy. When spoken to, she did not respond. For a moment I was frightened that she might not come back from wherever she was. Then she looked down at her infant and slowly came back into her body—or was it back out of her body?"

Bethany took a picture of Amanda in that ecstatic state, and she showed it at a recent medical meeting in which we both lectured on women's health. From this and reading Vicki Noble's *Shakti Woman* and *Ina May's Guide to Childbirth* (Bantam Books, 2003), I learned that Amanda's experience of ecstasy is potentially available to all women at birth.[132] Since then, I have talked at length with some of my patients who have had home births. One recently told me that during her home birth she "left her body" and became an eagle flying high overhead. She experienced no pain. She had never told anyone about this. From that moment on, however, she trusted her body completely.

Women have learned collectively, though not necessarily consciously, to fear the birth experience, and every obstacle has been put in our collective paths to keep us from experiencing this power. But as Bethany says, "This kind of birth is possible in many environments. It requires a mother who trusts her body and is connected to all of its parts. She must love and want her baby. She must understand that birth is a sexual event and be comfortable with her sexuality. She must feel safe. She needs to know that the people around her accept her body and the sexual nature of what she is doing and are not embarrassed by it and will not interfere with the process. She needs to know that she can go down inside and come back safely. If she has never been there before, she needs the grounding love of family and friends who will, if needed, call her back."

Those women who have already had babies in standard ways should understand that they are not responsible for what they didn't know at the time. I was born drugged, as were all my brothers and sisters. Though we were breast-fed, we were still left in the hospital's nursery for hours while my mother woke up. This isn't the way she had wanted it, but she didn't know she had a choice.

Remember that *being responsible* simply means "being able to respond." No one is guaranteed a perfect birth. In fact, the concept of "a perfect birth" is part of the perfectionism of the addictive system. Sometimes a baby needs to be observed in the nursery right after birth. Sometimes an emergency cesarean is necessary. When this happens, it is not a failure on the woman's part. She is only one part of a complex and mysterious process. The baby herself (or himself) is also an active participant in the labor process. Each baby makes a unique contribution to her mother's pregnancy, labor, and delivery. We can always learn something from it and use the experience for personal growth. But whatever happens, parents should be involved as much as possible, at all stages of pregnancy, labor, and delivery. They need to understand that their input is very important to their baby's health.

Routine Newborn Procedures That Should Be Questioned

Routine Antibiotics in a Baby's Eyes. By law, most states are required to put antibiotic ointment (formerly silver nitrate) in the eyes of all newborns to prevent blindness from gonorrhea. Obviously, this is overkill for those who don't have gonorrhea or any other venereal disease. Giving antibiotics messes up a baby's microbiome—setting up the child for a host of immune problems. When such drops are necessary, that's fine, but the vast majority of the time, the mother will not be infected with anything that can cause problems in the baby. I suggest that you ask your pediatrician or family doctor to write an order avoiding this.

Hepatitis B Vaccination. At this time, almost 99 percent of all babies born in the United States receive a hepatitis B vaccine in the hospital. If the mother does not have hepatitis B at the time of delivery and is not at high risk for contacting it (as IV drug users or sex workers would be), then there is no need to vaccinate the newborn. The vast majority of babies are not at risk at all. The issue with giving the hep B vaccine to newborns is that it contains at least 225 mcg (and sometimes 250 mcg) of aluminum, a known neurotoxin. Why in the world would anyone want to inject a neurotoxin into a newborn, whose brain and nervous system are still developing? The amount in the vaccine is far above the safe threshold the FDA set in 2004 for how much aluminum can be contained in neonatal parenteral nutrition (the IV solution given to those newborns who can't absorb nutrients through their digestive system). That safety threshold is 5 mcg of aluminum per kilogram of body weight per day, which for a 7.5-pound newborn amounts to only 17.5 mcg. Even allowing for the fact that these involve two different pathways— parenteral nutrition is injected into the veins, while the hep B vaccine is injected into muscle tissue—the difference between what's considered safe for one and what newborns receive through the other should be cause for major concern. Of course, these levels can be an even bigger problem for premature babies.

Circumcision. There is no medical justification for the routine circumcision of newborn baby boys, another example of a painful procedure that is unnecessary. While some research shows circumcision reduces the rate of HIV infection and other sexually transmitted diseases,[133] other research challenges this idea.[134] In any case, condoms are the best way of preventing sexually transmitted diseases.

When I was in practice, I did hundreds of circumcisions—and I have publicly apologized to every one of those little boys years after the fact, hoping that this gesture might prevent a mother from unconsciously consenting to this procedure. Though I often used a local anesthetic, even inserting the needle for this caused the baby unnecessary pain and didn't always work very well. Increasingly, doctors and parents alike are appreciating the fact that babies are born with a nervous system that is fully capable of feeling pain and that circumcision without anesthesia is barbaric. Quite frankly, removing a perfectly normal part of the male anatomy without the child's permission—one with at least 10,000 nerve endings—goes against the United Nations Convention on the Rights of the Child.[135]

In the past when I did the procedure, I would ask mothers to come into the nursery to comfort their babies while they were being circumcised, but they wouldn't do it. They couldn't stand the idea. I always made sure I personally took the newly circumcised baby to his mother as soon as I was finished, so that she could comfort her child. I didn't want him wounded and then left alone in the nursery. George Denniston, M.D., sums up the circumcision issue very nicely: "To me the idea of performing 100,000 mutilating procedures on newborns to possibly prevent penile cancer in one elderly man is absurd."[136]

The discussion of circumcision is a perfect example of the strength and influence of first-chakra tribal programming on our thought and emotional responses. This programming is so ingrained that many people cannot even discuss the subject of circumcision without guilt, denial, or other strong emotions. I know that merely addressing the subject of the baby boy's bodily integrity, choices, and pain (if the procedure is done without anesthetic) can cause a "kill the messenger" reaction. But first-chakra programming can be successfully questioned and worked through, if desired. Even many Jewish couples, for whom circumcision is a religious ritual, have rethought the entire circumcision issue and have decided not to have it done to their sons (see www.beyondthebris.com).

Besides the obvious trauma to the genital region, circumcision is known to cause sleep disturbances for at least three days.[137] It can interfere with infant feeding. It also has profound implications for male sexuality and can reduce sexual pleasure as an adult. (See chapter 8.) In fact, I now see the procedure as a form of sexual abuse.

We certainly feel that way about female clitoridectomy and infibulation (what's often called "female circumcision"), but we justify male infant circumcision by pretending that the babies don't feel it because they're too young and it will have no consequences when they are older. I was taught that babies couldn't feel when they were born and therefore wouldn't feel their circumcision. Why was it, then, that when I strapped their little arms and legs down on the board (called a "circumstraint"), they were often perfectly calm; then when I started cutting their foreskins, they screamed loudly, with cries that broke my heart? For years, in some hospitals, surgery on infants was carried out without anesthesia because of this misconception. Women who are going through memories of abuse in childhood know how deeply and painfully early experiences leave marks in the body.

While this view is certainly still controversial in the United States, the decision to keep a male baby's foreskin intact is becoming increasingly popular and the Intactivist movement (see www.intactamerica.org) is growing daily. The CDC reports that while 64 percent of boys born in the United States in 1979 were circumcised, that figure fell to 58 percent in 2010.[138] The fact is that most men around the world (two out of three) have not been circumcised,[139] so this is hardly an unpopular or unacceptable option on the whole. Iceland even introduced a bill in 2018 seeking to make circumcision a crime, punishable by up to six months in prison, although it has yet to be passed. At the very least, make an informed decision before you automatically consent to circumcising your newborn son.

IF INTACT, DON'T RETRACT

One of the biggest issues faced by parents of intact baby boys is the fact that in the United States, many family doctors and pediatricians are ill informed about how to care for a normal penis. They have been led to believe that you need to retract the foreskin to "keep the penis clean." This is just plain wrong. The foreskin is actually an organ known as the prepuce. It is attached to the underlying head of the penis via a cellular layer that gradually goes away as the child grows older. The foreskin is attached to the glans penis in the same way that the eyelids of a kitten are fused shut—we don't forcibly open a kitten's eyelids to keep the area clean, right? Well, the foreskin is exactly the same. Over time, it will retract on its own. Many parents are led to believe that they might as well remove the foreskin now (when the child is a newborn) to prevent later problems. They've all heard of boys and men who have to have the procedure done later in life. Yet many of these later-in-life procedures could have been prevented if the foreskin had simply been left alone. Forcible retraction not only is incredibly painful but also produces scarring and adhesions that can lead to the need for circumcision later on. One of the founders of the organization Doctors Opposing Circumcision told me that they get about four phone calls a day from distraught mothers who took their intact baby boys to doctors or emergency rooms for things like coughs or fevers, and the doctors took down the child's diapers and forcibly retracted the foreskin—leaving the child bleeding and in pain—for no reason other than ignorance of normal male anatomy. This organization actually has stickers that parents can put on their son's diapers before a medical visit that say "I'm intact, don't retract."

There are a couple of YouTube videos that every parent of a son should see before consenting to circumcision. Just type "YouTube, The Prepuce: The Function and Physiology of the Foreskin" into a search engine. You will be amazed at what you didn't know—and what your pediatrician might not know, either. Boys should be allowed to keep the anatomy they were born with. If, for religious or other reasons, they want to get rid of their foreskin later, then it is up to them.

CHIMERISM: DNA FOR TWO

Believe it or not, it's possible for your baby (and even for you!) to have two entirely different sets of DNA, normally thought of as a genetic blueprint that's unique to each one of us. How is that possible? Through a condition called chimerism.

People with chimerism have one set of DNA in certain organs and tissues, and another completely different set of DNA in others, meaning that if they took a DNA test using a blood sample, for example, the result could be different from a DNA test using saliva.

One cause for this benign condition involves something called "vanishing twin syndrome," where a mother actually conceives twins but one embryo dies so early in the pregnancy that it is never detected. (This happens in about 12 percent of pregnancies, or one in eight.) The cells of that embryo can be absorbed by the embryo that eventually becomes a living child, resulting in a person who has both their own DNA as well as some DNA from a twin they never met.

Chimerism is usually not detected until the child becomes an adult and has DNA testing for various reasons, such as to match a child to its parent. It has actually happened that a mother who gave birth to a child she conceived naturally had DNA testing that erroneously reported that her child was not biologically hers. In this case, the baby's DNA matched its mother's unborn twin—an aunt who never existed!

More commonly, however, this shows up when a mother retains a small percentage of cells from her fetus, cells that are naturally exchanged across the placenta. Genetic counselor Kayla Sheets, founder of Vibrant Gene Consulting in Cambridge, Massachusetts, says that between 20 and 90 percent of women harbor cells from previous pregnancies. This might explain why some women suffering from rheumatoid arthritis experience relief from their symptoms during pregnancy, she notes: "The baby's stem cells may be acting to help protect the mother from her own autoimmune condition." Even women who conceive but don't end up giving birth can have DNA from their unborn children. Chimerism can also happen after blood transfusions or organ transplants.

The phenomenon will inevitably become more common as the number of women using assisted reproductive technology rises, since ART tends to result in more twin pregnancies.

Reclaiming Birth Power Collectively

Imagine what might happen if the majority of women emerged from their labor beds with a renewed sense of the strength and power of their bodies, and of their capacity for ecstasy through giving birth. When enough women realize that birth is a time of great opportunity to get in touch with their true power, and when they are willing to assume responsibility for this, we will reclaim the power of birth and help move technology where it belongs—in the service of birthing women, not as their master.

For many women, having a baby is their first experience of being connected with other women and with their vast creativity. It has the potential to transform the ways in which we think about ourselves. As one patient said to me, "I felt at one with every woman who ever gave birth. I felt powerful and in touch with something within me that I never knew was there. I took my place among the lineage of women as mothers."

13

Motherhood:
Bonding with Your Baby

In giving birth to our babies, we may find that we give birth to new possibilities within ourselves.

—Myla and Jon Kabat-Zinn

The process of becoming attached to a new baby begins long before the actual birth and continues long afterward. Still, every effort should be made to optimize the labor, birth, and postpartum environment because this is a particularly sensitive period that deeply imprints both mother and baby, setting the stage for their life together. During this time, the bodies of both mother and baby are flooded with prolactin, oxytocin, and beta-endorphin—neurochemicals that have been called "the molecules of belonging" because they help establish a deep sense of trust and belonging in a baby. Like Cupid's arrow, they help a new mother fall blissfully in love with her baby and also with those who have supported her during labor and birth. These neurochemicals make the mother far more sensitive to her environment as well. That's why the events associated with birth have a very powerful effect on a mother's feelings about herself, her caregivers, and her new baby.

Our understanding of this biologically programmed sensitive period has come light-years in the last few decades. And voluminous research has been done on the biological effects of prolactin and how it engenders trust. In a nutshell, labor, birth, and the postpartum period—and all the experiences the mother and baby have during this time—set down the original wiring between the neurological system, the endocrine system, and the immune system—which in turn sets the stage for one's state of health, and feelings of safety and security, for the rest of one's life.

When I was a medical student, a newborn baby was quickly wrapped in a sterile drape, shown to the mother only briefly, as though the baby's life depended on being somewhere else, and then whisked off to a warmer in the nursery, while the mother looked on with pleading eyes, aching to hold her creation. During my residency, we began to place babies on their mothers' abdomens instead of putting them immediately into the warmer. If a mother holds her baby skin to skin with a blanket over both, the baby doesn't need a warmer, because the mother is the warmer—which is as it should be. At a normal birth, the mother swoops her baby into her arms and holds her full frontal against her skin as soon as the child is born. She knows this baby is hers and needs to be welcomed and comforted immediately. It's also very helpful for the new baby to become colonized with her mother's bacteria by being held skin to skin. This helps establish healthy immunity. When my daughter gave birth to my first grandchild, I was thrilled to see posters in the rooms of the hospital where I used to work stating that "skin to skin" was best. When I spoke to a former colleague there about this incredible leap forward, she said, "It took me twenty years to get this skin-to-skin policy established in the hospital." The wheels of progress can grind very slowly. But progress is progress.

The birth of a baby has great significance not just for the mother but also for the father. The more he is included, the better. Margaret Mead once said that the reason so many cultures banned fathers from births was that if they participated, they would be so hooked by the experience and the new baby that they would never be able to go out, steel themselves, and "do their thing" in quite the same way. I believe that the increased participation of men in childbirth—not as bosses or saviors, but as witnesses to the awe of the moment—holds great potential for balancing our world.

I never wanted my own babies to go to the hospital nursery, because I was aware of how different the atmosphere in the nursery was from what I wanted for them. They had just spent forty weeks listening to my heartbeat, bathed in warm fluid in a darkened space. In the hospital nursery, they would be isolated in small bassinets, alone, under fluorescent lights that were on twenty-four hours per day, cared for by a stranger. (Fortunately, this is now improving somewhat.) I knew that my entire physiology was set up by nature so that my baby and I could become "attached." The breast colostrum (first milk) contains antibodies optimally suited to protect the baby from germs, and the suckling of the child produces hormones that help the uterus contract. Babies are innately most interested in eye contact at a distance of about twelve inches, the distance between a mother's eyes and those of her nursing infant. Looking into my baby's eyes, having her look back at me, having her sleep close to me skin to skin—all of these events have been set up by nature as the "glue" that continues the mother-infant bond that begins in utero. I knew that these experiences were important for both of us.

Too many babies are taken to the nursery to "get cleaned up" after birth (to get rid of all that filthy vagina stuff!). The process of bathing can lower a baby's body temperature to the point that the nurses won't let the baby out of the nursery again to be with the mother until the temperature is back up! I figured, why bathe the baby and make her cold? Why not just nurse her, keep her near me, and hang out together?

When I had my first baby, I went to the postpartum floor, but I kept Ann with me. When I got up to go to the bathroom, I took her with me. A nurse came in and yelled through the door, "Where is the baby?" I replied, "In here with me." She said, "You're going to have to learn to leave her sometime." I replied, "Not on the first day of her life!"

I was afraid of my vulnerability postpartum. So many mothers were undermined by the nurses and their rules, and I didn't want to have to argue with them about when I could and couldn't hold my baby. I wanted my own mother to be able to hold her first female grandchild. In those days, the hospital rule was that only the immediate family could hold the baby, as though the hospital "owned" the child. (Though hospital rules have now changed, even as a doctor I had to fight with the nurses back then to let grandparents hold their new grandchild. Sometimes, depending on the nurse involved, I didn't get very far.)

Expecting a hospital stay to be restful was the stuff of mythology, I knew. My home was where I wanted to be, so I left the hospital on the day of delivery both times. Of course, if you give birth in a supportive setting, leaving your baby in the care of good nurses who will lovingly tend to the child while you get some much-needed sleep can be very helpful. There is no shame in this!

The first few weeks of life are a crucial time of adjustment for both the baby and the parents. I wish now that I had spent even more time with my newborns. The first three months after a baby is born are known as the fourth trimester. During this time, the mother's body serves as a kind of "external" placenta for the baby. And the baby herself is considered an "external fetus" who still requires a great deal of contact with her mother's body for optimal regulation of her breathing, temperature, digestion, and so on.

John Kennell, M.D., is a pioneer in the field of neonatal (newborn) care.[1] He and his colleague Marshall Klaus, M.D., became involved with the treatment of high-risk babies. *High-risk* refers to any baby who requires intensive surveillance at birth and in the first few days, weeks, or months of life. The majority of high-risk babies are born premature. Many premature babies' bodily systems aren't fully developed at birth, and this causes them to have an increased risk of lung problems, developmental and feeding problems, and infection. Back in the 1960s and '70s, Drs. Kennell and Klaus found that there was an unusually high percentage of battering by the mothers of babies who were born prematurely or who were otherwise sick and whose care was taken over by the nursery staff with the mothers not included, and they wanted to understand why. Their research, first on mother-infant bonding and then on parent-infant bonding (adding the father), showed that mothers whose babies stay with them from birth onward bond better and are more attentive to their babies' needs than are those whose babies are whisked away to the nursery to be cared for by "experts."[2] (This is especially true in those mothers who have fewer resources available to them because of poverty, abuse, single parenthood, etc.) These babies are also healthier and more intelligent overall, months and even years later. (The human psyche and soul are very resilient, however. Separation doesn't necessarily cause irreversible damage, but it should be avoided unless absolutely necessary.)

Klaus and Kennell's research verified what should be common sense to everyone—that human touch and concern have a measurable impact on a baby's health. One study on infant touching—known as "tactile stimulation"—indicated that a group of premature infants who were stroked regularly gained weight much faster than those who weren't touched—even when both groups were fed the same diet. And in a study at the University of Miami the touched babies were discharged from the hospital earlier—a cost savings of thousands of dollars per baby.[3] Touch should be thought of as a lifelong nutrient. After all, the skin is derived from the same embryonic layer as the brain and central nervous system. When we stroke a baby's skin (or have our own stroked), it lowers stress hormones, increases the hormones of belonging, lowers blood pressure, and enhances health on all levels. An impressive body of research continues to show these benefits for both mother and baby. (For more information, see the research of Tiffany Field, Ph.D., at the website of the Touch Research Institute at the University of Miami School of Medicine; www.miami.edu/touch-research.)

Touching is so simple, so instinctive. Pregnant mothers automatically stroke their bellies, sending love and energy to the unborn and practicing for when the baby is born. How could we ever have devised a system in which babies were separated from their parents' love and touching in the first minutes of life and sent alone to nurseries run by strangers?[4] No mammal leaves its children unattended and unsuckled the way humans do. A mother bear is at her most dangerous when she's protecting her cubs. She won't let anyone or anything come near them. Many women could use a little more bear energy.

One of the primary ways a baby learns trust and love is through touch. James Prescott, Ph.D., who created and directed the Developmental Behavioral Biology Program at the National Institutes of Health's National Institute of Child Health and Human Development, has done comparative studies of child development in different cultures. His research has found that societies that physically hold and love their children and are not sexually repressive are peaceful. But those societies (like ours) that deprive infants, children, and adolescents of our primal need for touch are far more violent. In fact, children who are touch-deprived often develop a disorder in which they are unable to deal effectively with stress hormone surges, which are a precursor to lashing out in violence. (For more information, visit www.violence.de.) Nature has designed labor, birth, and the postpartum period as a crucial time to maximize touch. This imprints well-being. For more information on healthy attachment (including the benefits of co-sleeping, "wearing" your baby, and more), visit the website of Attachment Parenting International (API), www.attachmentparenting.org. I also recommend the book *Attached at the Heart: 8 Proven Parenting Principles for Raising Connected and Compassionate Children* (Health Communications, 2013) by API cofounders Barbara Nicholson and Lysa Parker.

Culturally, we've all participated in subtle and not-so-subtle abuse of our vulnerable newborns in the name of science, partly out of fear and doubting of our own natural instincts. Putting burning silver nitrate or erythromycin ointment into infants' eyes to prevent gonococcal infection is one example. Why do this to all babies, even those whose mothers don't have gonorrhea or chlamydia? I signed a waiver to forgo putting anything in my baby's eyes. I knew I didn't have gonorrhea or chlamydia, and I couldn't see why my baby should have to undergo treatment for something I didn't have. The waiver absolved the hospital of all responsibility for my choice, which is as it should be. (By the way, laws vary by state on whether or not new parents can refuse such treatment. Check with your local Department of Health for the laws in your area, although be prepared for a bit of a runaround since this isn't a common question and the person you speak with may not immediately know the answer.) I would also recommend avoiding the hepatitis B vaccine, which is now given to 99 percent of all newborns in the United States. As I mentioned in chapter 12, this vaccine contains 225–250 mcg of the neurotoxin aluminum, more than ten times the maximum amount the FDA defined as safe for an IV solution routinely given to infants with certain digestive conditions. (Obviously there will be times when this vaccine is appropriate. But if you don't have hepatitis B at the time of delivery, are not a sex worker, and don't use IV drugs, your baby doesn't need this vaccine.)

Clamping the cord immediately after birth is another example of an overly stressful act against our newborns, which can even be dangerous because it can lead to too little blood volume in the baby—and decreased tissue oxygenation. Nature designed birth so that the baby will receive backup oxygenated blood from her mother via the still-pulsating umbilical cord during the time when her lungs and heart are undergoing the profound changes necessary to switch from a water environment to an air environment. Once the baby is breathing well on her own and her circulation has been established, the umbilical cord vessels naturally close down on their own. And when the cord is allowed to pulsate until it stops, it also helps normalize blood volume in the baby, making sure that the baby's circulation is adequate. Clamping the cord early is not necessary in the vast majority of cases. When babies are sick or premature, the extra oxygenated blood that they can get from a pulsing umbilical cord helps resuscitate them optimally and can make the difference between life and death. (Far too many premature babies who undergo premature cord clamping end up with hypovolemia, not enough blood volume, and then need transfusions once they get to the intensive care nursery.) Clamping the cord immediately after the baby's birth forces the baby to make the switch over to air more quickly than is necessary. Many mothers and doctors feel that this gives the baby a feeling of panic—that there is not enough air. This practice is like shouting a command, "Okay, breathe now—or else!"

After most normal births, the baby can be placed on the mother's abdomen and the cord can be allowed to gradually stop pulsating on its own. Babies often rest very peacefully while this is going on. They breathe gently and don't cry. In fact, mothers and fathers sometimes worry that something is wrong when their babies are calm at birth. They've learned from the culture that a screaming, terrified newborn is *normal*. A nurse friend of Bethany Hays, M.D., recalled that at the first Lamaze birth she ever saw, she thought there was something wrong because the baby didn't cry immediately! (Remember, that which is normal in this culture is not always that which is healthy. A generation ago, a limp, unresponsive baby was considered normal.)

Unfortunately, the collective emergency mindset that permeates high-tech birth makes premature cord clamping the norm, not the exception. Conventional ob-gyn training has argued that delayed cord clamping will increase a baby's risk of hyperbilirubinemia (jaundice). But ob-gyns have no problem using Pitocin for labor induction or augmentation and/or epidural anesthesia—both of which have been conclusively linked with nonphysiologic neonatal jaundice. In fact, any drug given to a mother or baby is likely to compete with bilirubin sites on blood protein, thus causing more free bilirubin, which contributes to jaundice. In healthy full-term infants, and even in sick infants, there are untold advantages to delaying cord clamping until after the placenta has been delivered (or the blood vessels have stopped pulsating), which takes only one to three minutes.[5] For example, a study of more than 1,900 infants published in the *Journal of the American Medical Association* in 2007 showed that delaying cord clamping for a mere two minutes cut the risk of anemia in half because it allows more blood to transfer to the baby from the placenta.[6] According to a review study published in 2009 in the *Journal of Midwifery and Women's Health,* delaying cutting the umbilical cord was shown to have numerous benefits (among them reducing the need for blood transfusions in the first six weeks of life) without additional risk to either the newborn or the mother—and it was found to be especially beneficial for preterm infants.[7] Yet until recently, early cord clamping has remained the norm.

After the World Health Organization, the American Academy of Pediatrics, the Royal College of Obstetricians and Gynaecologists in the United Kingdom, and the American College of Nurse-Midwives all began recommending deferring cord clamping (anywhere between thirty seconds and five minutes after birth), the American College of Obstetricians and Gynecologists followed suit in 2017, issuing a committee opinion recommending delaying clamping for at least thirty to sixty seconds.[8] The opinion cited research confirming that delayed clamping increases newborns' hemoglobin levels and improves their iron stores in the first several months of life, which may have a beneficial effect on the child's development.[9] It is also reasonable and even prudent to clamp the cord after it has stopped pulsating.

FOURTH TRIMESTER

The first three months postpartum are when most women go through enormous physical, emotional, and psychological changes that aren't very well appreciated in this culture. Much of the controversy about sending mother and baby home from the hospital too soon has to do with the fact that for many women, their care and rest end the minute they get home. Though the hospital is often far from an ideal place to rest after your baby is born, it sure beats going home to a sink full of dirty dishes and a load of dirty laundry.

Your body also goes through some unexpected changes. For instance, it is normal to sweat a great deal and have hot flashes during this time—it's part of the readjustment process following the profound adaptations of pregnancy. Also, some women notice that some of their hair falls out from hormonal changes (it grows back). It is also normal to bleed for up to four to six weeks as the placental site heals over in the uterus. The other really common problem many women face is pain during intercourse, especially if they've had an episiotomy. Though many doctors tell women it's okay to have sex after their six-week checkup, this may be far too soon for comfort. Aside from the episiotomy, the hormonal changes necessary for breast-feeding can result in vaginal dryness. This doesn't mean (as some women fear) that you don't love your mate anymore. It just means that you might need vaginal lubricant until postpartum hormonal shifts are completed. You also may find that you're so exhausted from being up at night with the baby that sex is the last thing on your mind.

On the other hand, a fascinating study by Marilyn Moran on do-it-yourself home birthers found that women who gave birth in an environment in which they were totally supported by their husbands and in which they felt safe being sexual actually experienced a marked increase in their sexual activity postpartum. I find this highly plausible and deeply intriguing. It flies in the face of everything we've been taught about sexuality and birth—probably because what we've been taught (and therefore what we experience) has been deeply tainted by our cultural expectations. Modern high-tech birth environments, where more than a third of births are major surgical procedures, certainly do not encourage feelings of sexuality during or after birth. (A full discussion of this topic can be found in my book *Mother-Daughter Wisdom* [Bantam Books, 2005], pages 99–100.)

If I were running the country, I'd make sure that every postpartum woman had full-time help for cooking and cleaning for at least two months after the baby was born and that she had time for a nap or two every single day. In some traditional cultures, women with newborn babies are often cared for by their midwives, mothers, or other women for two to three months after the birth of the baby. It can take babies up to two months to adjust their circadian rhythms so that they sleep at night and are awake during the day. Mothers need a lot of support during this time so that they themselves can be well rested. Their only duties are to nurse, rest, and recover so that they can be fully present for their new babies.

Postpartum Depression

Maternal depression is frequently underdiagnosed. (About 10 to 15 percent of women are clinically depressed during pregnancy itself.)[10] Fully 80 percent of women experience the baby blues for up to two weeks after delivery. Approximately 15 percent of women will go on to experience some form of mood disorder postpartum, ranging from major depression to anxiety disorders such as panic attacks.

If a woman has a history of depression, she is at significant risk postpartum, and many women who suffer one postpartum depression will experience the same thing after each birth.[11] A 2009 study from Norway noted that some new mothers may mistakenly assume their tiredness in the first few months after giving birth is merely a side effect of poor sleep, when in fact it might be a symptom of depression.[12] True psychosis occurs in only about one in a thousand births and is characterized as being out of touch with reality, hallucinating, and hearing voices. It is considered a psychiatric emergency. One of my patients went through this process with minimal medication even though she had to be hospitalized for a time. She said that during that time, she healed a great deal of her past with her mother, father, and, as she put it, "my ancestors before me. It was as though I had to go into this darkness—

that was somehow generations deep—so that I could be present with my baby." Her inner knowing told her that her postpartum reaction was important and loaded with information and energy. By staying with the process and not reducing it to a "chemical imbalance," she was able to heal fully—and, ultimately, so was her family. This is a striking example of staying present with and thus dissolving one's pain body.

Women with any history of depression or psychosis should be sure they discuss this with their healthcare provider before the baby is born, since the right treatment can prevent the problem from becoming severe. My colleague and friend Kelly Brogan, M.D., a psychiatrist, rightly points out that most postpartum depression results from a woman not having the support she requires or from the fact that the postpartum period (like the premenstrual time frame) brings to the surface—in glaring detail—very real issues that are adversely affecting a woman's life. Giving psych meds during this time can greatly delay full recovery. Dr. Brogan points out that the biggest gift you can give your children is a mother who is present and not under the influence of mind-numbing drugs.

Women with moderate to severe PMS may be at increased risk for postpartum depression, especially those who feel their best during pregnancy and who respond well to natural progesterone. In this group of women, taking progesterone as soon after delivery as possible is often very helpful.[13] Estrogen has also been used successfully.[14] Anger, both expressed and suppressed, is emerging as a predictor for postpartum mood disorders. Recent research shows that women who express angry feelings are more likely to report also having baby blues, while those who suppress such feelings may be at risk for full-on postpartum depression.[15] The lesson in this is not that women shouldn't be angry, of course. It's that stuffing unpleasant emotions that arise will usually cause more problems.

In 2019, the FDA approved brexanolone (marketed under the brand name Zulresso) as the first drug specifically for postpartum depression. While the drug must be taken intravenously for sixty continuous hours under medical supervision because in some cases it can cause excessive sedation and sudden loss of consciousness, it takes effect quickly and lasts thirty days. However, the $20,000 to $35,000 price tag will put it out of reach for many women. The manufacturer, Sage Therapeutics, is currently working on a new drug that would be taken as a daily pill.

Fortunately, supplements can help. Consuming adequate amounts of omega-3 fats also decreases the risk of postpartum depression. In fact, omega-3 fats can be used to treat postpartum depression (1,000 to 5,000 mg per day). It's also essential that women keep their blood sugar normal. (Low blood sugar exacerbates depression, and it's very common.) The best way to do this is to be sure to start each day with a breakfast that contains healthy protein and low-glycemic-index carbohydrates. (See chapter 17.) Good choices would be eggs and whole-grain toast or oatmeal with protein powder in it. There is also a wide variety of bars and shakes available for those who don't have the time to cook. A good multivitamin-mineral supplement is essential to help the body manufacture the neurochemicals involved in mood balance, including serotonin, dopamine, and endorphins. Adequate sleep also goes a very long way toward helping maintain mood. (Please see the Program for Creating Optimal Pregnancy and Decreased Risk of Complications in chapter 12, page 540—all of it applies to the postpartum period.) I also highly recommend Dr. Brogan's month-long Vital Mind Reset Program (see www.kellybroganmd.com), offered several times per year, as well as her book *A Mind of Your Own: The Truth About Depression and How Women Can Heal Their Bodies to Reclaim Their Lives* (HarperCollins, 2016), both of which include a nutritional program designed to restore a woman's healthy mood and help her work through her underlying unfinished business. Her breakfast smoothie (described in chapter 17, on nutrition) has made a big difference for many women. The bottom line is to reestablish the hormonal balance that supports emotional stability.

Postpartum depression is made worse by any sense that the birth was not what the woman had hoped for, or that she has somehow failed. A woman from Europe wrote me the following: "I'm the mother of a daughter who is now one and a half years old who was born by cesarean section. This cut changed my relationship with my body a lot. Even now, sixteen months later, I still do have the feeling of being wounded, not so much in the physical body, but in the energetic one. So much physical and emotional pain is connected with such an operation. I know quite a few women who've had the same experience, and there's even a support group in town."

Labor that doesn't turn out the way you planned can be very traumatic to the mind and body, and women can be left with a type of post-traumatic stress disorder (PTSD). A great deal of unfinished business may live in our bodies concerning our labors and deliveries if we weren't fully supported. This is because, on some level, we know that many of these surgeries or procedures may not have been necessary if our circumstances, our thoughts and emotions, and our environments in labor had been different. In these cases, I recommend approaches that help clear the energy body and reprogram the subconscious mind, such as hypnosis, eye movement desensitization and reprocessing (EMDR; for more information, see the EMDR Institute's website at www.emdr.com), and the Emotional Freedom Technique (also known as tapping; see www.thetappingsolution.com as well as the Intuitive Guidance section of the Resources). In addition, I highly recommend getting the C-section scar injected with an anesthetic like procaine—an approach known as neural therapy (an injection treatment that stimulates healing)—as well as having acupuncture to reestablish the energetic meridians that are interrupted by surgical scars (see chapter 15.)

Significant unfinished business with a woman's own mother at the time she gives birth can also increase the risk of postpartum depression. Sharon had her first baby at the age of twenty-nine. About one week postpartum, she became severely depressed and was considering giving up breast-feeding. I helped her stick with it, which enhanced her self-esteem a great deal. She sought help with a psychiatrist for about six months and eventually pulled out of her depression. She later told me that she felt that the depression was directly related to the fact that her mother, an active alcoholic, simply couldn't be present for her during this critical phase of her life. She said, "She wasn't present for me when I was born because of her drinking, and she wasn't present for the birth of my son for the same reason. Nevertheless, something deep within me really wanted her there, and so I invited her to come and help me out after the baby was born. But she wasn't reliable, never could get it together to help me with anything, and ultimately, I ended up mothering her as well as my new baby. It's so painful to have to give up the fantasy that somehow you will one day find the mother you never had."

A woman can have a similar reaction if her relationship with her father is unsatisfactory. What it boils down to is this: When a woman gives birth, the process releases enormous energy for renewal and healing. Something deep within her longs to connect with and heal her own family. If her relationship with them is lacking in some way, this healing feeling will be heightened. The contrast between what could be and what actually is can add to a sense of loss or grief that contributes to depression.

Regardless of your circumstances, every woman needs to realize that having a baby is the real "change of life" and that she may not be fully prepared for this stressful time, especially if she lacks support. In my experience, most women don't have nearly the support that they need during the postpartum time. Many are sleep-deprived and exhausted. I remember that after my first child was born, I left the house to go get groceries when she was about four days old. I closed the front door and walked out onto the porch. Then I remembered, "Oh, God, I can't just leave. I have a baby." In a moment of panic, I realized that I had altered my life forever and that there was no going back. We were preparing to move at the time, and each day my husband would come home from work and ask me how much I had gotten done. I told him that it was all I could do just to keep the baby fed, get some rest myself, and prepare meals. I was too exhausted and stressed out to do anything else. On top of that, I couldn't seem to get motivated to go into overdrive, as I'd done so effectively for so long in my medical training. But I didn't understand this, and neither did my husband, so my "fourth trimester" was not a healing time, to say the least.

When my friend and colleague Donette Morris went through postpartum depression fourteen years ago, she felt called to create something that would help support and educate other women through this period. She became a postpartum doula to change the expectations placed on women in the postpartum period. Donette is devoted to nurturing new mothers to ensure they feel empowered in their femininity, which she believes is the foundation from which a family will truly thrive. (Read more about her at www .donettemorris.com.) Here is her story:

After unexpectedly getting pregnant at the age of forty-four, I became enchanted with the miracle of life and witnessing women fully engaged in the wisdom of their bodies. By immersing myself in books by authors such as Dr. Northrup and Ina May Gaskin, my mind was opened to the idea of what was possible for the birth of my daughter. I was completely focused on my pregnancy, labor, and delivery. I immediately took a leave of absence from my work as an international flight attendant and made self-care my highest priority. Weekly chiropractic visits, massage, and swimming became my new normal. My life felt magical, and it never occurred to me that it would be any different with a newborn.

A beautiful day of nesting resulted in an intimate evening of natural childbirth. I was on the high of my life! The birth of my daughter was the most empowering experience I had ever known. It was as if I was being flooded by a warm, invigorating light. Little did I know that this bliss would be short-lived. Within days the darkness would begin to creep in.

Months went by as I sat stunned and blinded by the wonders of motherhood. I felt confused and bewildered by the tremendous responsibility. The shift in lifestyle seemed overwhelming, and everything felt so complicated. I began to isolate myself and rejected any offers of help. My emotional anguish would soon be compounded by physical symptoms that would affect my ability to hold my daughter. Excruciating pain in my arms (which I now know is reflective of how we give and receive love) kept me practically immobile. I knew I needed help, yet every attempt to reach out was met by the suggestion that I should consider taking antidepressants. Despite studies saying these drugs would have no effect on the baby through my breast milk, I knew different. This realization would change the trajectory of my life.

I started taking yoga classes to get more in alignment with my mind, body, and spirit. I remember moments of lying on my mat sobbing uncontrollably, releasing months of confusion and unprocessed emotions. This was the point at which my postpartum symptoms began to fall away. Yoga therapy combined with dietary changes, supplements, and meditation was the perfect blend to support my healing. In hindsight, I can now see the beauty of my body speaking to me so clearly. By trusting my intuition and embracing an integrative approach, I slowly and joyfully stepped into my role as a mother.

After years of study, I have come to understand the intricacies of the postpartum phase. Our culture places emphasis on "balancing it all" and "losing the baby weight," which often leaves women feeling shamed and desperate. Ultimately, the postpartum period is about so much more. Divine feminine strength comes from a supportive community and the vulnerability in asking for help. My hope is that women will embrace this idea and redefine this time as a sacred bonding experience.

HOW TO ELICIT A CHILD'S NATURAL CALMING REFLEX

Pediatrician Harvey Karp, M.D., author of *The Happiest Baby on the Block* (Bantam Books, 2002), shares several very helpful suggestions both in his book and in his blog that parents can use to help fussy babies calm themselves and get to sleep (see www.thehappiest baby.com). His advice includes:

~ Using a white-noise machine or a *shhh*-ing sound. Either a white-noise CD or a white-noise machine will work well, as does shushing the baby yourself (at a volume as loud as her crying is, and right near her face). This re-creates the noise level in the womb—which is anything but silent—and makes the baby feel more secure. (Dr. Karp offers a CD/MP3 with six specially engineered sounds that work particularly well for this.)

~ Rocking your baby or putting her in a windup or motorized infant swing.

~ Swaddling, or wrapping your baby tightly in a receiving blanket. The feeling of being tightly held re-creates the security of the womb. Dr. Karp recommends wrapping the arms straight at the side while allowing the hips to be loose and flexed.

~ Holding your baby on her side, on her stomach or facing over your shoulder. These positions mimic the baby's position in the womb, making her feel more secure. The classic fetal position—tucking the baby's head down a bit, touching her on her stomach, and then laying her on her side—activates position sensors in the baby's head that trigger a natural calming reflex. (But never put a baby to sleep on her side or stomach, which can increase the risk of sudden infant death syndrome, or SIDS.)

~ Allowing your baby to suck (either by nursing her or by giving her a pacifier).

DEALING WITH DIASTASIS RECTI

As a baby grows inside the womb, it pushes against the mother's rectus abdominal muscles (the ones responsible for "six-pack abs"). While they easily pull apart to accommodate the growing child, the muscles don't always go back after childbirth to the way they were before. Organs and other tissue can bulge out in the gap that's left because there's little or no muscle holding them in place, creating a pooch near the belly button. Even a year after giving birth, one-third of women have diastasis recti—the medical term for a separation of at least one inch between the right and left rectus abdominal muscles.[16] The official diagnosis is made based on an absolute measure of 2.7 mm between the rectus abduminus halves, but as biomechanical expert Katy Bowman points out, you know your own body best. If your linea alba separation (the width of the midline in your abdomen) has expanded, you'll want to do what you can to get your abdominal muscles back to where they should be. This is more than a body issue problem because the resulting weakened core can cause lower back pain. While all sorts of exercises are available on the Internet for fixing this issue, some of them actually exacerbate the condition.

In her book *Diastasis Recti: The Whole-Body Solution to Abdominal Weakness and Separation* (Propriometrics Press, 2016), Katy Bowman goes into great detail about the fact that diastasis recti is the result of not using your core muscles in the way they were designed to be used. This problem is a symptom of a larger problem—not *the* problem itself. You can begin to address it by learning how to move your entire body. A very effective exercise is to get down on the floor and then get up. Do this ten times. Bowman points out that the floor is one of our best exercise options. Once your child is old enough, carry them on one side for a while, then switch. This is far better for both you and the child than a stroller—at least some of the time. Another great exercise is hanging, because you have to use your arms in order to get optimal strength and function in your abdominals. Start just by hanging easily—without removing your feet from the floor. You can use a tree branch, or use the monkey bars at a playground.

I recently installed a pull-up bar in the doorway between my bedroom and bathroom so that I'd use it regularly. I doubt that I'll be able to do a pull-up anytime soon, but I'm noticing that hanging regularly (and also swinging, which increases the load on my ab-

dominals) is getting easier and easier. As a result, my torso and abdominals are getting more and more fit, and better-looking. If you
have diastasis recti after pregnancy—or if you simply want a stronger abdomen and better-looking abdominals—I highly recommend
Katy Bowman's book on this subject. You can also go to her website
(www.nutritiousmovement.com) to learn more. New York City fitness trainer Leah Keller developed an effective pre- and postnatal
fitness system she calls the EMbody Program to realign the rectus
abdominal muscles and flatten the pooch. She teamed up with Geeta
Sharma, M.D., an ob-gyn who was at that time at Weill-Cornell
Medical Center, to put the exercises to the test. After twelve weeks
of doing Keller's exercise ten minutes a day, all the women in Sharma
and Keller's study were successful in fixing the condition.[17]

The key exercise is a very small yet intense core compression
repeated several times for ten minutes a day. Keller teaches the exercise in her subscription-based program, which includes educational
content, the core compression exercise, and workouts. For more information, visit www.every-mother.com.

Testing for Diastasis Recti

Here's how you can test to see if you have diastasis recti:

1. Lie flat on your back with your knees bent and your feet flat.

2. Put your fingers right above your belly button and press down
gently.

3. Lift your head about an inch off the floor while keeping your
shoulders on the ground.

4. If you feel a gap wider than one inch between the muscles right
above your belly button, you have diastasis recti.

FORMULA VERSUS BREAST MILK

Artificial infant feeding is another area that requires rethinking. In the
1940s, infant feeding became very "scientific." Mothers sterilized nipples,
bottles, and everything else, and the medical profession as a group systematically undermined breast-feeding as inferior. Rubber and glass took the
place of a warm human breast. Feedings were timed. Even if a child showed
a need for frequent feedings, the mother was warned not to feed her before

four hours had passed. This information was based on a very early study of dead babies (who had been sick enough to die!) that found that at one, two, and three hours there was still food in the stomach, but that four hours after a feeding the stomach was empty. Like routine episiotomy, the four-hour feeding schedule was accepted into the culture and after a while simply became standard practice. The needs of the individual child were sacrificed on the altar of efficiency and "science"—with all its measuring and weighing. Can you imagine the pain of an infant who cries out to be held or fed, and yet the mother does not do so because the "experts" have told her to ignore all her instincts so she won't "spoil" the baby? (Babies were often weighed before and after a feeding to make sure they "got enough"—a practice that does *not* yield reliable data.)

Even now, women ask their doctors, "How will I know if I have enough milk?" Here's how you know: If the baby is growing, happy, and healthy, she is getting enough. Since women's trust in themselves has been systematically undermined in every area of their lives for centuries, how could we be expected to trust our bodies' ability to feed our babies? (Thank goodness that over the years a few did.) I don't for a minute expect that every woman will want to nurse her babies. For some, it's too anxiety-provoking, while for others bottle-feeding is the only way a woman can get childcare from her husband, because he will be able to help with the feeding. We all have to start from where we are, but we should start from knowledge—not ignorance.

An analysis published in 2007 of more than 500 breast-feeding studies (selected from some 9,000 abstracts) concluded that breast-feeding reduced the risk of ear infections, gastroenteritis, severe respiratory tract infections, eczema, asthma, obesity, type 1 and type 2 diabetes, childhood leukemia, necrotizing enterocolitis (a gastrointestinal disease that mainly affects premature babies), and sudden infant death syndrome.[18] (Breast-feeding cuts the risk of SIDS *in half*, according to a 2009 study done in Germany.)[19] The 2007 analysis further found that breast-feeding is health enhancing for women, too: Mothers who breast-fed were less likely to get type 2 diabetes, breast cancer, and ovarian cancer.

A 2009 study that followed 704 women for twenty years found that breast-feeding reduced the mothers' chances of later developing metabolic syndrome (a cluster of risk factors such as high blood pressure and high triglycerides that are associated with obesity)—especially for mothers who had gestational diabetes. Researchers found that those mothers who did not have gestational diabetes and who breast-fed for more than nine months cut their risk of metabolic syndrome by anywhere from 39 percent to 56 percent. And a similar group of mothers who did have gestational diabetes cut their risk by anywhere from 44 percent to 86 percent.[20] The study reported that risk declined further the longer women breast-fed. It's no wonder that the World Health Organization (WHO), the United Nations Children's Fund (UNI-

CEF), the American Academy of Pediatrics, the American College of Obstetricians and Gynecologists, and the American Academy of Family Physicians all recommend that mothers breast-feed exclusively for six months. WHO and UNICEF recommend that mothers continue nursing (along with giving age-appropriate foods) until age two or longer.

Nature set it up so that when a baby is put to the breast right after delivery, the suckling action causes the hormones oxytocin and prolactin to be secreted by the mother's pituitary gland. Prolactin induces milk production as well as mothering behavior, and oxytocin is the bonding hormone. The longer a mother breast-feeds, the less likely she is to neglect or otherwise mistreat or abuse her child within the child's first fifteen years of life, according to a 2009 study of more than 7,000 mother-child pairs.[21]

Oxytocin and prolactin also set the stage for adequate milk supply. Mothers who nurse right after delivery have fewer problems as well. These hormones help contract the mother's uterus, for example, which helps the placenta separate naturally and thus decreases blood loss. In addition, breast milk is different from cow's milk or formula, and it is unique in that its composition changes over time *depending on the needs of the baby.*

Children who have been breast-fed have one-third fewer hospitalizations than those who are bottle-fed, and they have many fewer allergies. Babies who are breast-fed have a more normal dental arch and palate than those who are bottle-fed. One meticulous study even showed that premature babies fed breast milk had higher intelligence quotients, which is because of breast milk's beneficial effects on neural development.[22] (This study was unusual in that the babies were fed either formula or breast milk by tube, in order to control for the known beneficial effects associated with actually holding a baby close to the mother's body during breast-feeding.) It is a well-known fact that the composition of human breast milk is superior to that found in any formula, including its balance of the essential fatty acids so necessary for brain development. Recent studies have found that breast milk contains stem cells (which play a vital role in healing and regeneration of damaged tissues), and a 2014 study in mice showed that these cells migrate to developing tissues throughout babies' bodies.[23]

Can You Drink Alcohol or Smoke Cannabis if You Breast-feed?

According to the CDC, having up to one drink per day will not harm your baby if you breast-feed, especially if you wait two hours after having a drink to nurse. Although the concentration of alcohol in breast milk is low, levels are usually highest thirty to sixty minutes after having one drink and remain detectable for two to three hours. Of course, the more you drink, the longer alcohol will stay in your milk—after two drinks, alcohol can be detected in breast milk for four to five hours, and after three drinks, alcohol can be detected for six to eight hours—so limiting alcohol makes a lot of sense. There is no need to "pump and dump," because as alcohol clears from your body, it will also clear from your milk.

Similarly, THC—the main psychoactive component of cannabis—also transfers to breast milk in low concentrations. A pilot study notes that although long-term effects on a baby exposed to THC through breast-feeding are not yet clear, mothers who smoke cannabis should be cautious if they breast-feed.[24]

Most women have to go back to work when their babies are six weeks old, making it much more difficult to breast-feed. Our lack of maternity leave is an issue in itself. Of the 193 countries in the United Nations, only New Guinea, Suriname, a few island nations in the South Pacific, and the United States have no national law guaranteeing paid parental leave, making the United States the only high-income country in the world not to offer such protection. Mothers in the United States are guaranteed only twelve weeks of unpaid maternity leave, and even then only if they work for a company with at least fifty employees.[25] This is in striking contrast to Norway, for example, which has the most parent-friendly laws on the planet. There, both mothers and fathers receive paid parental leave, which they take in turn during the child's first year—and sometimes even longer.

Many mothers in the United States who are in the position of needing to return to work have told me that they do not intend to nurse at all. They feel six weeks is so short a time that there's no point. But women who have to go back to work and don't feel that they can pump could still nurse, even if it's just for that first six weeks. Even nursing for only the first few days would be valuable because the antibodies in the colostrum would give the baby's health a head start that no artificial formula can provide. We only kid ourselves when we think that baby formula can do as good a job as nature. No amount of scientific experimentation can come up with food that is more specifically made for a baby than its mother's milk. (Thankfully, however, baby formula is now being manufactured with the all-important fatty acids DHA [docosahexaenoic acid] and AA [arachidonic acid], fats that are crucial for optimal brain, heart, and immune system development. Hydrolyzed baby formulas containing "comfort proteins" that are easier for babies to digest are also available.)

Breast-feeding, in addition to all its other benefits, is also more convenient than carrying around a bunch of bottles, particularly while traveling. Studies have shown that mothers who breast-feed get more sleep (so much for the "convenience" of bottle feeding).[26] I nursed discreetly in restaurants, medical meetings, movies, and theaters. Usually no one noticed. Some, such as Bernie Siegel, M.D., congratulated me and thought it was wonderful. (Some babies are really loud nursers and sound like little piglets, however, so you have to adapt to their behavior and be considerate.) If I had to be away from my babies, I expressed my breast milk into bottles and froze it so that it could be thawed and fed to them in my absence. Both children took both the breast and the bottle, so I had a win-win situation. (So-called nipple confusion resulting from both breast- and bottle-feeding is actually not that common.)

The late renowned anthropologist Ashley Montagu, Ph.D., who advocated breast-feeding for years before it caught on in the modern Western countries, once said, "We learn to be human at our mother's breast." Breast-feeding is one of the most natural, nurturing things that a woman can do for herself and her baby. Yet we live in a culture in which it's perfectly acceptable to walk down the beach in a thong bikini but it is not always acceptable to breast-feed an infant in a public place. That is seen as "obscene." Mothers who nurse toddlers are judged as being somehow "unnatural," fostering unnecessary dependence of the child, though it's been shown that people who feel the most secure in later life are those who had very healthy physical and emotional bonds with their mothers in childhood. The newest research on boys shows how important a solid bond with their mothers is—a bond that we shouldn't be overly quick to sever. Children who feel most secure in their childhoods often are willing to take the most risks later in life. Only in a dominator culture would we get the idea that it "spoils" children to pick them up when they cry and to comfort them when they need it. (An aside: Why should adults get to sleep with someone, while children have to sleep alone?)

Our culture's priorities are completely reversed from what they should be, especially at a time when it has become so hard for mothers to nurture their children adequately and still make a living. I changed my priorities after my own personal wounding with a large breast abscess that developed when I was attempting to work eighty hours per week while trying to prove myself in my group practice—and at the same time provide my firstborn with a diet that was 100 percent breast milk. The abscess, which was invading the muscles of my chest wall, eventually required emergency surgery. The surgeon, who had more than thirty years of experience, told me later that he had never seen an abscess that severe. (I diagnosed it myself at the office—when I stuck a needle into my breast and drew out 10 cc of pus. Such was my immersion in the dominator system. But I knew I was in trouble and finally asked for help.) Fast-forward two and a half years. On the third day after my second daughter's birth, I noticed that milk didn't seem to be coming out of my right nipple. Then the full impact of the damage I had done to myself more than two years earlier hit me fully. I wanted to sob. I remember sitting on my bed, looking down at my beautiful new baby girl, and thinking, "Here you are, and I can't even feed you properly because I screwed up my body two years ago trying to prove I was a man." I *was* able to nurse, but I couldn't maintain an adequate milk supply most of the time and had to supplement with formula, especially whenever I was away from home long enough to miss a feeding.

I came face-to-face with the fact that I had done irrevocable damage to myself. I'd been taught it was normal to feel the "baby blues" on about the third day after a baby was born, but my own depression was exacerbated by the knowledge that I wouldn't be able to nurse Kate completely normally. (I actually felt so depressed I contemplated walking into the river. Kate is now grown up and has two daughters of her own. Life is long. And things that devastated you at the time have a way of healing themselves over the long haul.) On her second day of life I had to supplement her diet with formula. I knew that her stools would immediately start to smell bad. The stools of a breast-fed baby smell like buttermilk because of the bacterial balance. Changing a diaper is a completely different experience with a breast-fed baby. But once you add other food sources, the bacteria change and the smell becomes putrid!

Even though doctors know that exclusive breast-feeding is best for mother and baby, a 2017 study shows that now, compared with ten to twenty years ago, fewer pediatricians—particularly younger doctors—believe that most women are able to nurse successfully and that the benefits of breast-feeding outweigh the difficulties or inconvenience, leaving doctors less likely to actively promote and support it.[27] This is true even though more pediatricians are women now as compared with past decades.

Furthermore, there's been a bit of a backlash to efforts promoting breast-feeding. A nonprofit organization called Fed Is Best sprang up in 2016, not necessarily to steer mothers away from breast-feeding but to warn them of the risks of insufficient breast milk. While it's certainly very important for nursing mothers to be aware of the signs that their babies aren't receiving enough nutrition, it's equally important for mothers to use such knowledge to become more successful at breast-feeding rather than be frightened away from it. Also concerning is a recent article in the journal *Pediatrics* that advises pediatricians to stop referring to breast-feeding as "natural," since this may be "ethically problematic," may promote the belief that natural approaches are healthier, and may influence parents against getting their children vaccinated.[28]

Of course, formula companies exert plenty of pressure of their own. *Mothering* magazine publisher and editor Peggy O'Mara writes in one article on the subject, "It is no coincidence that the formula industry nearly doubled its advertising, to almost $50 million a year, as soon as the Breastfeeding Awareness Campaign [a three-year media campaign to promote breast-feeding initiated by the U.S. Department of Health and Human Services in late 2003] was launched. This aggressive advertising of formula is one of the chief obstacles to breastfeeding success, and the domination of health by profit is a classic feminist issue."[29]

Noting that the global market for infant formula is currently $47 billion (a figure expected to increase by about 50 percent in the next three years, making it one of the world's fastest-growing packaged food markets), the Changing Markets Foundation recently put out two particularly concerning reports. "Busting the Myth of Science-Based Formula" (2018) takes global market leader Nestlé to task for putting effective marketing ahead of science.[30] The report compares the company's marketing claims about the science its formulas are based on with the ingredients of its more than seventy products sold in forty different countries, revealing many examples where formula composition contradicts Nestlé's own scientific advice. The report notes that Nestlé is far from alone in this practice, which is common among other formula manufacturers as well. The organization's 2017 report "Milking It" analyzed more than 400 infant formula products from four industry leaders (Nestlé, Danone, Mead Johnson Nutrition, and Abbott) sold in fourteen countries around the world.[31] The report notes that the differences in the various companies' infant formulas are not science-based, as they claim, but instead are based on sophisticated marketing research into consumer preferences, with so-called premium formulas costing up to two and a half times more than standard formulas without being scientifically proven to be better for infants. Such practices actively discourage mothers from breast-feeding, as they may think formula is better for their baby. This results not only in babies getting less than optimal nutrition but also in economic hardship. For example, the report noted that in Indonesia, formula can cost up to 70 percent of an average parent's salary, while in European countries, even the most expensive formula would cost only between 1 and 3 percent of an average parent's salary. One product analyzed costs the equivalent of $17 per 800 g in the United Kingdom, while the price charged for the same product equates to $24 in Germany and $55 in China.

(By the way, such misleading advertising also extends to toddler drinks in the United States. For example, one product is advertised as being the "number one brand recommended by pediatricians." Yet such products nearly always contain corn syrup and other sweeteners that are not considered nutritious, and they also contain more sodium and less protein than cow's milk. A study from New York University's College of Global Public Health concluded that such marketing practices "undermine the diets of very young children."[32] So don't be fooled.)

While more than 83 percent of all mothers in the United States begin breast-feeding their newborns, CDC statistics show that by the time their babies reach three months, less than 50 percent of mothers are still exclusively breast-feeding, and by the time babies reach six months, the figure drops to about 25 percent.[33] Our culture discourages breast-feeding with the declaration that nursing "ruins" women's breasts. Then there's the issue of women being shamed for nursing in public. I never experienced this, but countless women have. In a culture in which breast implants and pornographic images are everywhere, it is ridiculous to consider breast-feeding anything other than normal.

Some women who've nursed a couple of children do notice that their breasts don't look the same. For a while they can be quite flaccid, and it can take several years after pregnancy and nursing to regain their shape. This usually reverses over time, but that flat appearance, even when it is only temporary, is not what our culture deems attractive.[34] This was illustrated to me once when a friend who had nursed several children told me the following story. She was undressing one night when her four-year-old son walked in. He looked at her chest, looked up at her, and said, "Mom, what happened to your breasts? They died!" Rapid weight loss caused by inadequate food intake while nursing or prolonged nursing with adequate food intake can deplete the fat stores in the breasts and exacerbate this effect. Rapid weight loss also decreases milk supply. Note: Regular loving breast massage—either by yourself or from a loving partner—can help restore breasts to their former firmness. (See the section on breast massage in chapter 10.)

The experience of producing milk, nursing a baby, and feeling the milk "let down" in response to the baby's cries, or even in response to a mother's own thoughts about the baby, is an experience that connects women everywhere. The midwife who delivered Kate used to tell me that she felt her own let-down reflex many times when she heard a baby cry or was aware of a child in need—even after her kids were in college. I, too, can still feel that tingling sensation in my breasts occasionally, especially when I'm feeling a great deal of compassion or appreciation for something or someone. It's my body's way of telling me that I have some love to give to a person or situation. Many women experience this. Our breasts, through this feeling, are reflecting the truth of the concept of "the milk of human kindness." (It has also been demonstrated that levels of the hormone prolactin—which is necessary to produce milk—increase when one is feeling this compassion, love, or appreciation.)

When we trust the makers of baby formula more than we do our own ability to nourish our babies, we lose a chance to claim an aspect of our power as women. Thinking that baby formula is as good as breast milk is believing that sixty years of technology is superior to 3 million years of nature's evolution. Countless women have regained trust in their bodies through nursing their children, even if they weren't sure at first that they could do it. It is an act of female power, and I think of it as feminism in its purest form. One of my friends recently said, "Breast-feeding my son gave me more confidence in myself as a woman than anything I'd ever done before. I felt so powerful."

Newborns who are treated gently are very beautiful. I've seen in their eyes very wise old souls in tiny bodies fresh from God. I heard the following true story at my office. After one couple had their second son, their four-year-old kept wanting time alone with the baby. They were a bit reluctant, feeling that sibling rivalry might be a factor. But the four-year-old kept insisting. Finally they let him have some time alone with the baby. Listening quietly at the door, they heard him ask the baby, "Please tell me what God is like. I'm starting to forget."

VACCINES: HELPFUL OR HARMFUL?

While the idea behind vaccines is certainly a good one—preventing diseases that can be fatal—the truth is that health is *not* a matter of avoiding all infectious diseases. In fact, childhood illnesses are necessary to mature the immune system and render it resilient in the same way that children need to learn to tolerate disappointment to develop into mature adults.

While most parents of baby boomers received only one vaccine (for smallpox), by the early 1980s children were routinely receiving ten vaccinations before they started school—and today they get at least fifty doses in thirty-six separate inoculations by the time they turn six. As I wrote in my book *Mother-Daughter Wisdom,* I am concerned by the sheer number of vaccines very young children receive today. The current CDC schedule calls for sixty-nine doses of vaccine by the age of eighteen years—more than half of which are given before the age of fifteen months. Every one of these vaccines contains neurotoxins and a host of other noxious substances, including formaldehyde. None of the many vaccines given to infants has been tested when given together with other immunizations.

The rate of autism used to be 1 in 2,000. By 2000, it had risen to 1 in 250, and now it is 1 in 36,[35] And we have more chronic illness in children than ever before—the number of children with chronic health conditions increased from 12.8 percent in 1994 to 26.6 percent in 2006.[36] A study published in 2011 in the journal *Academic Pediatrics* put the figure as high as 54 percent.[37] There are many potential reasons for this, including GMO crops, food additives, pesticides, and so on. But read the package insert for a vaccine, see the list of ingredients you're injecting into a vulnerable child, and decide for yourself if there might not be a link.

In 1986, President Ronald Reagan signed into law a bill that exempts vaccine manufacturers from all liability for vaccine injury. Since that time, the number of recommended vaccines has more than doubled, and more are in the pipeline. Why wouldn't there be? It's an incredible business model. No liability, no oversight, no testing—and then make them mandatory to get into school. Though most people don't know this, the U.S. government pays out millions of dollars every year for vaccine-injured children (as of November 2017, the total had reached $3.8 billion), though the government makes it incredibly difficult for parents to prove the vaccine is what caused the problem.[38] I believe that the sheer number of vaccines and the way they are administered in combination are connected not only to an increase in childhood asthma and allergies but also to the increase in diabetes, attention deficit/hyperactivity disorder (ADHD), and autism. By immunizing against so many childhood diseases, we may be unwittingly creating suboptimal immune resilience that is coming out as chronic disease. Although this idea is controversial—vaccines are such a sacred cow that to even question them is considered medical heresy—there is an enormous amount of evidence for it in the medical literature.[39]

The bottom line is that vaccines are neither 100 percent safe nor 100 percent effective. In China's Zhejiang province, for example, where more than 99 percent of children receive required vaccinations for measles, mumps, and rubella, 8.6 percent of children develop measles anyway, and cases of mumps and rubella have been on the rise.[40] Closer to home, Quebec experienced a major measles outbreak in 1989, despite the fact that 99 percent of children there were vaccinated against the disease.[41] There's still a lot we don't know about how vaccines work. The immune responses they cause are not the same as the body's response from a natural infection,[42] and we simply don't yet know what role that may have in inflammation-linked diseases. Immune system response varies and is difficult to predict.[43]

In an astounding TEDxAarhus talk, Danish health researcher Christine Stabell Benn, M.D., points to her studies of children from Guinea Bissau, a small West African country where the mortality rate for newborns is one in fifteen. Her studies show that when a newborn gets a live polio vaccine, it "trains" their newly minted immune system to recognize and fight a host of other diseases—despite the fact that there is no polio in the region. On the other hand, vaccines that contain killed viruses, such as DPT, result in a fivefold increase in mortality from all other diseases (even while protecting against the ones they were meant to protect against). It turns out that all vaccines are not equal, and all of them have unexpected effects. Clearly, we need to rethink the entire field of vaccine science and find out which ones work best and which ones don't—rather than continuing our "one size fits all" and "more is better" policies.

One of the big concerns is that vaccines often contain preservatives that prevent bacterial or fungal contamination, as well as adjuvants—substances that cause inflammation, thus activating the immune system so the vaccine will have the intended effect. Adjuvants often contain mercury or aluminum, which can be toxic to the nervous system as well as to the kidneys. For example, a study in the *Journal of Neurological Sciences* showed that children with severe autism spectrum disorder (ASD) had significantly higher levels of mercury intoxication compared with those with mild ASD.[44] Two studies published in *Alternative Therapies in Health and Medicine* showed a link between vaccines and chronic inflammation of brain tissue, which harms nerve cells and is present in individuals with autism.[45] A growing body of published research from around the world demonstrates a link between aluminum and neuropathology, including both autism and Alzheimer's,[46] as well as various adverse psychiatric events and risk of emotional disturbance.[47] Vaccines contain many other substances as well, any of which can cause an adverse reaction when injected. While clearly not everyone is susceptible to these, children who either have a genetic predisposition or who are exposed to other compromising environmental factors may indeed suffer tragically debilitating effects from vaccines ironically designed to keep them healthy.

Yehuda Shoenfeld, M.D., founder and head of the Zabludowicz Center for Autoimmune Diseases at Tel Aviv University in Israel, has seen so much evidence for the harmful effects of adjuvants in vaccines that he has suggested a new syndrome be recognized, autoimmune (autoinflammatory) syndrome induced by adjuvants, or ASIA.[48] A 2017 paper written by Anthony Mawson, Dr.P.H., of Jackson State University, was the first to compare age-matched vaccinated and unvaccinated children, looking at data from more than 650 homeschooled children (including some from families with both vaccinated and unvaccinated siblings) in four states.[49] The paper reports a dose-response relationship between vaccination and chronic illness, showing that children who were vaccinated were more than three times as likely to have allergies, six times as likely to have pneumonia, about three times as likely to have neurological developmental disorders, five times as likely to have a learning disability, and almost twice as likely to have any chronic illness. A second paper by Dr. Mawson looking at the same group showed that preterm infants vaccinated according to the CDC's recommended schedule had an increased susceptibility to learning disabilities, autism, and chronic health disorders.[50]

It's no secret that drug companies have powerful lobbies in Washington to influence policy on their behalf. They can also pay to fast-track their pharmaceuticals through the FDA's approval process. Not surprisingly, drugs that go through this quicker route have more safety-related label changes, particularly for those with the highest level of warning. One study showed these expedited-pathway drugs have a 48 percent higher rate of changes to black-box warnings and contraindications.[51] So just because a vaccine has FDA approval doesn't mean there's no reason for discernment. Harvard Medical School faculty member Marcia Angell, M.D., wrote in her book *The Truth About the Drug Companies: How They Deceive Us and What to Do About It* (Random House, 2004), "It is simply no longer possible to believe much of the clinical research that is published, or to rely on the judgment of trusted physicians or authoritative medical guidelines. I take no pleasure in this conclusion, which I reached slowly and reluctantly over my two decades as an editor of *The New England Journal of Medicine*."

Again, one of the biggest concerns with the current vaccination recommendations is that there are no studies on the safety of vaccine combinations or the cumulative effect of so many immunizations. British researchers recently published a study documenting what they termed "some of the highest values for aluminum in human brain tissue yet recorded," noting that particularly high levels were discovered in the body of a fifteen-year-old boy who had been diagnosed with autism.[52] The aluminum appeared to have entered the brain by way of immune cells circulating in the blood and lymph. A 2011 study from the University of British Columbia showed that children from countries with the highest prevalence of autism have the highest exposure to aluminum from vaccines—and that children's exposure to aluminum adjuvants in the past twenty years correlates significantly with the increase in autism in this country.[53]

Still other red flags include a study showing a positive correlation between the number of vaccine doses given to infants and the percentage of hospitalizations and deaths reported,[54] as well as recent studies in France on mice showing that low, consistent doses of aluminum adjuvant are actually more neurotoxic than a single large dose.[55] Even the National Institutes of Health committee that assesses studies on vaccines admits straight out that "long-term effects of the cumulative number of vaccines or other aspects of the immunization schedule have not been conducted."[56]

Here's my advice:

- Hold off on vaccinations until babies are at least three months old—especially if you have a family history of ADHD, autism, allergies, type 1 diabetes, eczema, or asthma. Natural health expert Joseph Mercola, D.O., writes on his website (www.mercola .com) about research done in Japan where DPT immunization was delayed until children were two years old. The study reports that these children experienced 85 to 90 percent fewer severe complications than babies who received the vaccine at three to five months.

- Limit the number of vaccinations given at one time and ask to see the vials to ensure that your child is being given individual vaccines instead of a combination shot, which appears to have greater potential for adverse reactions.

- Avoid vaccines containing mercury. Call ahead to ask your doctor to check the package insert to see if the vaccine contains mercury (even trace amounts), and if it does, ask for a different type.

- Don't immunize your child if she's sick or fighting an infection. If the baby's immune system is already working overtime, a vaccine will unnecessarily stress it further.

- Be selective about the vaccines your child receives. I am not a fan of the chicken pox vaccine, for example, because this disease is very benign in the vast majority of children, but more severe for adults who contract it. If all children are vaccinated against chicken pox, they won't get natural lifelong immunity, and then more people will get this disease as adults and when pregnant, when its effects are much more serious. Similarly, I don't recommend the MMR (measles, mumps, and rubella) vaccine until a girl is old enough to get pregnant because those who get it in childhood may well have fewer antibodies against rubella in adulthood, when immunity is important to prevent infection in pregnancy. That said, if you live in a state that requires MMR before a child may enter a public school, I would recommend that you ask your child's pediatrician to separate these three vaccines and space their administration over as long a period of time leading up to school age as possible. I would also hold off on vaccinating a newborn for hepatitis B unless a parent or family member had active hepatitis B when the child was born.

~ If you're breast-feeding, increase your intake of vitamin C to about 3,000 mg both before and after your child's immunization, because the vitamin will pass into the breast milk and help protect the child against tissue damage.

~ Don't make vaccines your primary way of preventing illnesses while ignoring other aspects of immunity and health.

For more information on vaccines, I recommend reading *Saying No to Vaccines: A Resource Guide for All Ages* (NMA Press, 2008) by osteopathic physician Sherri Tenpenny, an expert on the adverse effects of vaccines who substantiates her work with citations directly from CDC documents and respected, peer-reviewed journals, offering irrefutable facts that fly in the face of information generally regarded as truth in traditional medical circles. Dr. Tenpenny's website, Vaxxter (www.drtenpenny.com), has additional valuable information.

I also recommend watching a presentation from Emmy Award–winning producer and investigative medical journalist Del Bigtree, speaking at the Truth About Cancer event held in Orlando in 2017 (youtu.be/RfkkdCg2830) as well as the DVD *Vaxxed: From Coverup to Catastrophe* (see www.vaxxedthemovie.com).

Finally, for solid advice on what positive action parents can take, I recommend the book *The Vaccine-Friendly Plan: Dr. Paul's Safe and Effective Approach to Immunity and Health—from Pregnancy Through Your Child's Teen Years* (Ballantine, 2016) by Paul Thomas, M.D.—a Dartmouth-trained pediatrician who has been practicing medicine for thirty years—and researcher Jennifer Margulis, Ph.D. "We may be overusing a medical intervention so drastically that the cure has, in some cases, become more dangerous than the disease," writes Dr. Thomas. While he describes himself as a pro-vaccine doctor, he's against the current "one size fits all" approach to vaccination, preferring a more discerning individual approach.

The book is designed to help parents partner with their pediatricians to make their own decisions on vaccination, including the best practices for minimizing risk and optimizing immune system health. "I have over 13,000 children in my pediatric practice and I have to say, as unpopular as this observation might be, my unvaccinated children are by far the healthiest," writes Dr. Thomas. "The data is surprising and counterintuitive, perhaps, but it shows very clearly that the incidence of chronic disease and brain abnormalities in the entirely unvaccinated children in my practice, even those with siblings with autism, is much, much lower than in children following the CDC's recommended schedule."

Independent consultants analyzed data from 3,344 patients, born over a ten-year period, in Thomas's pediatric practice. The data included 715 unvaccinated children and 2,629 partially vaccinated children. Analysts found that unvaccinated or partially vaccinated children had a dramatically lowered risk of autism compared with those children who underwent the CDC vaccine schedule.[57]

MOTHERING IN A DOMINATOR CULTURE: THE HARDEST JOB IN THE WORLD

The only thing that seems eternal and natural in motherhood is ambivalence.

—Jane Lazare

Some women say that the most fulfilling time of their mothering was when their babies were small. Others find it exhausting. For me, having young children was—bar none—the most taxing part of my life, a time that I wouldn't care to repeat again unless I had two beloved nannies, sisters, or friends living with me full-time to help with childcare.

The author Lynn Andrews once wrote that there are two kinds of mothers: Earth Mothers and Creative Rainbow Mothers. Earth Mothers thrive on nurturing and feeding. Our society rewards this kind of woman as the "good mother."

Creative Rainbow Mothers, on the other hand, inspire their children without necessarily having meals on the table on time. I know that, beyond a doubt, I'm a Creative Rainbow Mother. I once read the cookbook *Laurel's Kitchen* and fantasized about how wonderful it would be to bake bread daily, relish being what Laurel calls the "Keeper of the Keys," and create that ever-important nurturing home space. But this is not who I am—and to have tried to be something I wasn't ultimately would have done my children and me a great disservice. I love to be alone. I love to read. I love quiet and music and writing. My soul is fed by long hours of unbroken creative time. Young children require a much different type of energy—a type of energy I don't have in abundance.

When my children were little, I became aware of how difficult it is for women to do *anything* for themselves with little children around. Children get and keep our attention through any means possible. They are phenomenal little energy suckers. (I don't blame them for this—it's normal. They're developing healthy egos when they are young. Our culture, however, expects *mothers* alone to meet all their children's attention needs. This is a setup.)

More than one in four children in this country—19.7 million—live without a father in the home, whether biological, step-, or adoptive, according to 2017 Census Bureau data. "Among the children of divorce," writes Ellen Goodman, "half have never visited their father's home. In a typical year, 40 percent of them don't see their father. One out of five haven't seen their father in five years. . . . It is no wonder that the search for a man missing in the action of parenthood is such a recurrent theme in our culture and conversation these days."[58]

Sometimes a woman with young children needs free time, space, and sleep. But for many, there's no one to take over the burden of raising a child. I once said to one of my friends that I thought the optimal adult-child ratio was three adults to one child. "I think your workaholism is showing," she replied. Then she went on to tell me about an Aboriginal culture of Australia she had recently visited where all of the mother's sisters—the child's aunts—are considered the child's mothers. All the father's brothers—the uncles—are considered the fathers. If you ask an Aboriginal child who her mother is, she will point not only to her biological mother but to all her aunts as well. Same with the father. If her biological mother feels the need to go on a "walkabout"—a spiritual initiation—she knows that the child always has a place in the group and is not dependent solely on her, as children so often are in our patriarchal society.

Can you even begin to imagine what life would be like for women if they didn't have the crushing responsibility to provide most of their children's emotional and physical nurturing? What would it be like if we knew that our society would care for our child if we had to work late at the office one night? What would it be like if a woman could still pursue her own interests, even if she had just had a baby? What if we lived in a society in which a woman didn't have to choose between her needs, those of her job, and those of her family? Dream on that for a while.

None of us, male or female, should have to be a prisoner in our own home caring for young children for hours each day without meeting our adult needs for rest, conversation, time alone, and creative pursuits. I remember that the best time I ever had with my children when they were little (three months and two years) was when I went to visit my mother while my sister and her children were visiting. My sister was also nursing a baby at the time, so when I wanted to go out for a while, she simply nursed Kate for me, as women have been doing for centuries. (Kate looked up at her, wide-eyed, the first time, as if to say, "Who is this?" Then she settled right down to her meal.) Our children played together happily, and I was able to enjoy the company of adults *at the same time* that I was enjoying my children. This was my only experience of what a loving tribe must have felt like. On a recent trip to Italy, it was clear to me that everyone in the village cared for the children—not just their mothers.

One widely held misperception about raising children has always upset me. That is the myth that prepubescent and pubescent boys are inherently easier to raise than girls. Even many feminists subscribe to this belief. I'm told by many people, "You just wait—you'll see how difficult girls are when they get to be eleven or so." Well, I've now had two eleven-year-old girls. I've supported them, in every way that I can, to be strong, even opinionated if necessary, and to be powerful. I didn't want them to "dumbify" themselves when they became teenagers. They were *not* difficult then, and they are not difficult now. (In fact, my thirteen-year-old nephew was much moodier on a regular basis than either of my daughters.) That boys are easier to raise than girls might well be the experience of many. But this difference is cultural, a consequence of the differences between the ways boys and girls are treated and reared.

It makes sense to me that girls would get moody around the age of twelve or so. They can see what's coming. In her book *Fire with Fire* (Random House, 1993), Naomi Wolf makes a strong case for the fact that all girls are born with a strong will to power that eventually gets turned inward by what she calls "the dragons of niceness." Thwarting their innate desire to excel and win can make girls very unhappy at this age and can cause them to turn on each other, too. If girls are socialized to be passive and self-sacrificing, their powerful spirits don't like it. (If someone was actively trying to do that to me, I'd be *very* tough to live with.) Instead of attributing this moodiness to the inherent hormonal inferiority of the female, we should be encouraging girls to speak their minds, not to turn their gifts and talents inward. If a teenage girl is taken seriously and encouraged to follow her dreams, she will be no harder to raise than a boy. Young women need to be cherished, honored, encouraged, and praised for their gifts. Otherwise, the world won't benefit from these gifts, and the cycle of oppression will continue. (See my book *Mother-Daughter Wisdom* for a full discussion of this.)

Each of us mothers must also learn to mother ourselves or else we can't possibly be good mothers to our children. When women ask me the best way to mother teenagers, I tell them to do everything in their power to be happy and fulfilled themselves. You also need to know that your girl needs you more than ever when she is being thrown to the wolves of peer culture. My good friend and colleague Sil Reynolds, author with her daughter Eliza of *Mothering and Daughtering* (Sounds True, 2013), points out that peer culture is much like *Lord of the Flies.* Our children need our input and support more than ever at the exact time when peer pressure is at its peak.

Being a woman who cares for herself—and stands up for the integrity of her children—goes further than anything else you could possibly do to nurture daughters who will then know how to do the same. Self-sacrifice and martyrdom are a well-worn path to chronic disease and anger, pure and simple. And though our culture has illuminated this tired old path for centuries—and we've watched our mothers and grandmothers travel along it—it's time to stop. Mothering and nurturing ourselves with the same care that we use to nurture our children takes a great deal of courage. And it's absolutely necessary if you are to truly flourish.

14
Menopause

*Like an electrical charge, menstruation and the ebb and flow of energy
is an "alternating current." During menopause, the flow of energy becomes intensified and steady, like a "direct current." We are charged
with energy to the degree we have opened ourselves to the wisdom of
the Crone.*

—Farida Shaw

The term *perimenopause* refers to the years leading up to the last menstrual period. *Menopause* refers to the final menstrual period—the
term derives from the Greek *meno* (month, menses) and *pauses*
(pause)—which is also known to many women as "the change of life" or
simply "the change." The years surrounding menopause and encompassing
the gradual change in ovarian function constitute an entire stage of a woman's life, lasting from six to thirteen years, called the *climacteric*. When
women say they are "in menopause," what they usually mean is that they are
experiencing the shift from regular monthly cycles to the irregular periods
and symptoms that are so common during the six to thirteen years leading up
to the final period.

Whatever we call it, no other stage of a woman's life has as much potential for allowing a woman to understand and tap in to her own power as this
one—if, that is, she is able to negotiate her way through the general cultural
negativity that has surrounded menopause for centuries. This negativity has
been challenged and changed significantly in the past few decades as the
women of my generation, the baby boomers, have entered menopause by the
millions. This is the generation that changed every stage through which it

passed—from blue jeans and rock concerts to minivans. This is the group that came of age saying "Don't trust anyone over thirty." As a result of the baby boom generation and all who have come after, the perimenopausal experience is now significantly different from how it was for World War II–generation mothers and grandmothers.

By the year 2000, 45.6 million American women had reached menopause, according to the North American Menopause Society, with numbers increasing every year. An estimated 6,000 women in the United States reach menopause every day, which is more than 2 million new menopausal women per year.[1] Worldwide, the number of women over fifty is expected to reach 1.1 billion by the year 2025. At the same time, longevity has increased dramatically. American women now enjoy a mean life expectancy of approximately eighty-one years, up from only forty-eight years for a woman born in 1900. This means that a woman is likely to live thirty to thirty-five years following menopause, making menopause the "springtime" of the second half of life.

Media attention to the subject of menopause has risen accordingly. In the past two decades, more books have been written on menopause than on any other subject in women's health.

Though the advice about menopause ranges from exalting hormone replacement therapy to promoting natural menopause without hormones, the important point is that the silence surrounding this process has now been broken by the women of the baby boom generation. The medical profession stands poised to help women through this life stage, and centers specializing in the health needs of midlife women have sprung up all over the United States. This is a potentially good thing, but every woman must learn to listen carefully to her individual inner guidance to hear her personal truth about how best to deal with this conflicting advice on negotiating this life stage.

When a woman is anywhere from about forty-five to fifty-five, give or take several years on either side, her hormonal shifts will often be in full swing, and she'll want support for these changes. After that, hormonal balance ensues once again for most women, and they are often freer than ever before to pursue creative interests and social action. These are the years when all of a woman's life experience comes together and can be used for a purpose that suits her.

MENOPAUSE: A CROSSROADS

If you want to know where your power really is, you need look no further than the processes of your body that you've been taught to dismiss, deny, or be afraid of. These include the menstrual cycle, labor, and, the mother of all wake-up calls, menopause. The years surrounding menopause are a time when most women find themselves in a crucible, having all the dross of the first half of their lives burned away so that they may emerge reborn and more fully themselves. Menopause can be likened to adolescence in reverse—the same stormy emotions we experienced during puberty often return, urging us to complete the unfinished business of our early years. When we were adolescents, we had neither the power nor the freedom to live according to the dictates of our souls. But by the time we are in our early forties, we have life experience and skills. And now, more than ever before in written human history, we are free to create the life of our dreams. But to do so, we must use this time to question everything we've been taught about what to expect as we grow older.

I've already mentioned that PMS is the wake-up call of the monthly cycle, urging us to clean up everything that isn't working in our lives. Seasonal affective disorder is the wake-up call of the annual cycle. Perimenopause is the wake-up call of the entire life cycle. If we've been pressing the snooze button on any parts of our lives that need attention, like a marriage or a job that isn't working, the years surrounding menopause will bring them to our attention in ways we can no longer avoid if we are to truly flourish in the second half of our lives. Once a woman understands that the true meaning of menopause has been inverted and degraded, like many of the other processes of her body, she can reverse this programming and make her way through the rest of her life fortified with purpose, insight, and pleasure.

Joan Borysenko, Ph.D., refers to the years between the ages of forty-two and forty-nine as the "midlife metamorphosis," when a woman begins in earnest to create her life in such a way that her innermost values are lived out in her everyday activities. During this stage, she is more apt to tell the truth than ever before in her life and less apt to make excuses for others. Many women quest for peace of mind against a background of turmoil and change as they end twenty-year marriages, have affairs, get left by their partners, face the empty nest, start new businesses, and explore new facets of their identity.

At midlife, a woman looks back at her life and ponders where she has been and how far she has come. Now is the time when she grieves the loss of any unrealized dreams she may have had when she was a young woman, and prepares the soil for the next stage of her life. She grapples with many issues that coincide with but are not directly associated with hormonal function, such as caring for aging parents with health problems while also wanting to focus more on herself, perhaps by traveling extensively for the first time or going back to college. Depending upon her degree of success or perceived success in life, she may find herself in a crisis that is not so much physiological as it is developmental. How she negotiates this crisis will affect her health on all levels as she goes through menopause.

During my lectures, I've sometimes shown a slide of Mount Saint Helens erupting to illustrate the stormy emotions that so often characterize these years. This is a time when many women, myself included, begin to manifest some of the fierce need for self-expression that frequently goes underground at adolescence. I like to think of midlife women as dangerous—dangerous to any forces existing in our lives that seek to turn us into silent little old ladies, dangerous to the deadening effects of convention and niceness, and dangerous to any accommodations we have made that are stifling who we are now capable of becoming. By the age of forty-five, I found myself deeply engaged in the process of scrutinizing every aspect of my life and my relationships in an effort to eradicate any deadwood that either held me back or no longer served whom I had become. My tolerance for dead-end relationships of all kinds began to evaporate. This eventually led to the end of my twenty-four-year marriage and was the impetus for writing *The Wisdom of Menopause* (Bantam Books, 2001; revised 2006). Women in midlife are at a turning point: Either we can continue living with relationships, jobs, and situations that we have outgrown—a choice that hastens the aging process and the chance for disease dramatically—or we can do the developmental work that our bodies, and our hormone levels, are calling out for. We must source our lives from our souls now. Nothing less will work. When we dare to do this, we truly prepare for the springtime of the second half of our lives. It all boils down to this: Grow or die.

GRIEVING THE LOSS OF OUR YOUTH: A DEVELOPMENTAL STAGE

Almost no woman I know of gets through the menopausal transition without experiencing loss of some kind. For those with stable and loving marriages or jobs they love, that loss might simply be the loss of their youth. This was beautifully stated by actress Carrie-Anne Moss, who wrote the following poem (published on her blog, "Annapurna Living," at www.annapurnaliving.com) when she began having hot flashes:

The only thing I knew about perimenopause
Came from my mother who told me that it came early for her.
Unlike my mother who had 2 children by the time she was 22,
I give birth to my first baby at 35, then another one at 37, and
    again at 42.

I desired natural birth.
I birthed at home with a midwife.
I nursed for years.

I think, *perhaps this won't happen to me—the whole hormonal deal.
I eat healthy, I exercise . . . I'm different.*

Then I notice the rage coming out of the blue.
My emotions going from zero to 60 in a split second.

I quit coffee.

And one night lying in bed,
Feeling like crap after losing my patience at my youngest over
    brushing teeth,
I face the possibility that hormones may be a part of what I'm
    feeling.

I wrestle with guilt and relief all that night,
waking in the morning as exhausted as a prize fighter who has
    fought a full 10 rounds.

I decide I will get informed.
I'll stop thinking that this "won't happen to me."
My daughter and I have years of
her childhood left, and I don't want to be this version of
    myself.

I cry to a friend about it on my cell phone as I drive back from
    drop-off at school.

I explain what I'm feeling,
and that my 7-year-old deserves more
and that of course I must be dealing with hormones . . .

I'm almost 50.

My friend who doesn't have time for the feelings prescribes
    vitamins for me. (She has a lot of knowledge here and I get
    upset at her for not letting me have my feelings.)
I apologize days later, but rush to the pharmacy for vitamins.
They help.

Oh my god, they help.

My body starts to ache
in ways I'm not familiar with.
I'm a warrior woman . . .
I don't have sore shoulders or feet.
This is not my body, I think.

I go to a chiropractor,
I do a home hormone test,

and go to my natural doctor
(who is also a dear friend) who shares her findings
and gives me supplements.

I don't have hot flashes until one morning in the kitchen
  making breakfast.
I feel a wave of heat
and I end up crying to my husband.
I cry out of the overwhelming sense that I'm old.
Overnight,
in the midst of a hot flash,
I feel my life is ending.
And indeed it is, in some ways.
I am transitioning to a part of life
that I've never really heard about, except in loss.

I decide that morning in the kitchen
with my husband looking at me with total confusion
that I am going to educate and
transform this experience, just like I did with my birth experiences.

I start reading.
I take my supplements (sometimes).
I experience vertigo so badly that I lay on the floor in between
  making French toast
and peanut butter sandwiches.

I keep researching
and I find solutions,
but what I'm mostly interested in is the grief.

The grief of losing the young woman I once was—
the beauty, the skin, the body . . . the superficial things.
I grieve that she never felt worthy or thin enough.
I grieve that time has passed so quickly and that I never really
  took her in.
After fully feeling into this, I decide
that I will feel now
that I will cry now
that I will embrace this time
with honesty and bravery

I'm alive, for god's sake.

In Celtic cultures, the young maiden was seen as the flower; the mother, the fruit; the elder woman, the seed. The seed is the part that contains the knowledge and potential of all the other parts within it. The role of the post-menopausal woman is to go forth and reseed the community with her concentrated kernel of truth and wisdom. (A word sometimes used for the elder woman is *crone*. I don't like it because it has taken on negative connotations and is now usually used to mean a wizened old woman. But what it really refers to is the "crown of age"—when we truly live according to our highest expression.)

In some native cultures, menopausal women were felt to retain their "wise blood," rather than shed it cyclically, and were therefore considered more powerful than menstruating women. A woman could not be a shaman until she was past menopause in these cultures. "Menopause," observes Tamara Slayton, author of *Reclaiming the Menstrual Matrix* (Lantern Books, 2002), "when understood and supported, provides the next level of initiation into personal power for women. With our increased life span, our way of thinking about menopause needs updating from these ancient mythologies. I think of perimenopause and the twenty to thirty years following menopause as a time of ripeness. Instead of rosebuds, we become rose hips—juicy fruit that contains and nurtures the seeds we will sow later."[2] At menopause, we're just getting started. In 1998, I wrote, "What we need is a new Crone archetype—a sort of 'Aquarian Crone'—that reflects these new ways of perceiving this time of life." And that is exactly what is happening. Urban shaman Donna Henes dubs this stage "the Queen" in her book *The Queen of My Self* (Monarch Press, 2005). (See www.donnahenes.com/Queen-of-my-self.) The perimenopausal woman is truly at a stage when she has the tools and experience to become the queen of her own life if she is willing to accept the challenge and not get bogged down in what our culture teaches us about what is "supposed" to happen at a certain age or stage.

The years after menopause are sometimes referred to as the wisdom years. I believe that one of the primary ways this wisdom gets wired in our brains and bodies has to do with the neurotransmitters FSH and LH (see chapter 5, on the menstrual cycle). These levels are high at ovulation, when women are maximally fertile—and also maximally open to new ideas and "cross-pollination" from others. After menopause, these neurotransmitter levels stay permanently elevated in the ovulation range for the rest of our lives—which, in my view, renders us more open to a continual flow of wisdom that heretofore was available only at ovulation.

OUR CULTURAL INHERITANCE

Up until very recently, the conventional medical mindset has been that menopause is a deficiency disease, not a natural process. Jerilynn Prior, M.D., professor of endocrinology and metabolism at the University of British Columbia and coauthor with Susan Baxter, Ph.D., of *The Estrogen Errors* (Praeger, 2009), writes, "Our culture finds it easy to blame women's reproductive systems for disease. Linking the menopause change in reproductive capability with aging, making menopause a point in time rather than a process, and labeling it an estrogen deficiency disease are all reflections of nonscientific, prejudicial thinking by the medical profession."[3] Since menopausal women are no longer using their energy in childbearing, their systems are described in terms of functional failure or decline: Breasts and genital organs are said to gradually "atrophy," "wither," and become "senile."[4] Menopause, viewed through this lens, is the ultimate in "failed production"— a system that is "shut down."

For years the ob-gyn profession has been steeped in lectures and teaching on "managing" menopause and perimenopause. If a woman's healthcare team approaches this life stage with support and respect for a natural process, she will be helped a great deal. But if perimenopause (or any other natural process) is approached from the disease model, with the mindset that it requires management (and its subtext, control), then a woman's ability to flourish during and after menopause will likely be undermined. In our culture, the only ages when female endocrine processes escape potential "management" are the years before menarche and after the age of seventy.

Fear of Growing Older: Symptom of an Ageist Culture

We live in an ageist culture, in which most people believe that it's natural for aging people to become depressed, fatigued, incontinent, asexual, forgetful, and senile. Pharmaceutical companies and gynecologists plant in women seeds of fear that as soon as they go through menopause, their bodies will simply fall apart and waste away unless they are on medication.

An example of this was the cover of a magazine called *Menopause Medicine* from the 1990s. A woman stands by an open window with filmy curtains blowing at her side; only her back is visible. She is looking out on the landscape covered by dead trees and parched earth. The caption under this illustration read, "The Fate of the Untreated Menopause."

It doesn't take a degree in psychology to understand how the pharmaceutical companies influence the sensibilities of the average woman or doctor. For most of my career, we ob-gyns felt enormous pressure to give conventional hormone replacement to everyone, having been led to believe

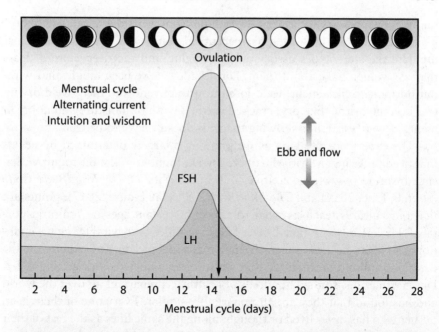

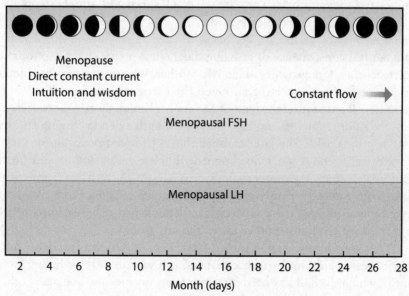

FIGURE 21: CURRENTS OF WISDOM

FSH and LH stimulate ovulation and are realized cyclically each month up until the years surrounding menopause. They then undergo a change during which ovulations gradually cease and FSH and LH levels gradually increase.

that it was necessary to prevent everything from heart disease to osteoporosis. It's easy to see how the pharmaceutical companies and the media manipulate the stereotypes associated with aging and the deep cultural fears that we women have about them. For decades we've been taught that without hormone replacement, we'd lose our attractiveness to men; we'd dry up and become brittle, like dry, cracked earth, devoid of moisture and nourishment. Newer research is showing that this doesn't have to be true.

The experience of aging as we know it is largely determined by beliefs that need updating. Mario Martinez, Psy.D., founder of the Biocognitive Science Institute (www.biocognitive.com) and author of *The MindBody Code* (Sounds True, 2014) and *The MindBody Self* (Hay House, 2017), points out that our cultures teach us what to expect at certain ages or "cultural portals." He has a quote that I love: "Getting older is inevitable, aging is optional." What he means here is that many people do not experience the deterioration and decrepitude that we so often associate with getting older. Dr. Martinez has studied hundreds of healthy centenarians all over the world and has found that they are all remarkably similar. Every one of them is an outlier who has never lived or thought along the same lines as the rest of their families and their cultures. They are the black sheep who simply stepped out of "what was expected at a certain age."

Though many people *do* decline with age in this culture, this decline is not a natural consequence of growing older—it is a consequence of our collective beliefs about growing older. My mother, who is now into her nineties and has never been on estrogen, hiked the entire Appalachian Trail in her late sixties, skied around the base of Mount McKinley shortly thereafter, and spent the summer of 1997 going on a three-month extended hiking and kayaking trip to Alaska. She later climbed the 111 highest peaks in the Northeast with her friend Anne, who chopped all of her own wood for heating her cabin in Vermont. My mother climbed to Mount Everest base camp at the age of eighty-four, probably making her the oldest woman to have accomplished this. Although there is 50 percent less oxygen at base camp on Everest than at sea level, my mother never had any trouble.

Yet as soon as my mother turned sixty, her mailbox was suddenly full of ads for hearing aids, incontinence diapers, and various aids for failing vision, none of which she had any need for. Over time, my mother, like many others, figured out how to ignore the constant barrage of negative messages about getting older. This becomes a spiritual discipline, one that's crucial to your health and well-being. Why? Because as Dr. Martinez confirms, we "co-author" each other's biology. If you are treated as though you are an old woman whose best years are behind you, you may start to believe it and act accordingly. On the other hand, if you stop complaining about your age and focus on what is possible, then you can, quite literally, reverse the aging process. Research has shown beyond a shadow of a doubt that chronological age (the age on your driver's license) can be completely different from your biological age (the age of your cells). Lifestyle and belief changes can, and do, turn back the clock.

Dr. Martinez suggests that we simply stop giving our age. And I agree with him. At this point, I don't want to know anyone's age, because I don't want to start treating them differently as a result of knowing it. I also suggest that you stop celebrating "milestone" birthdays. Celebrate birthdays, of course, but not as milestones that become millstones. Focusing on our chronological age locks us into a way of living in which we feel we are running out of time. This creates stress in our cells and in our bodies. You can learn how to step out of linear time into timelessness.

Harvard professor Ellen Langer, Ph.D., has extensively researched how the context in which we live influences us to feel either younger or older and can have dramatic consequences for our health. For example, she has found that negative stereotypes about aging set the stage for diminished capacity in older adults both directly and indirectly, while the absence of these same cues primes improved health. Dr. Langer and her team looked at women who bear children later in life, curious about whether the youth cues they are given because they are in an environment with mainly younger women would translate into longer lives. That is exactly what they found. Older mothers do, in fact, have longer life expectancies.[5]

The good news is that beliefs about age have shifted dramatically in the last couple of decades. We are finally seeing many more media images of strong, sexy, vital women past the age of forty. Fifty no longer looks old. In fact, it looks downright sexy on an increasing number of women. The same is true of sixty, as we all saw when Helen Mirren went up to claim her Oscar for the movie *The Queen*. We are collectively reversing our cultural negativity about menopause and getting older—one woman at a time. And this change in our beliefs and expectations is showing up in our bodies. For instance, my mother had a health reading from Caroline Myss when she was sixty-eight. Her body read energetically as though she were in her thirties.

The more women ignore ageist stereotypes, the better the chances are that all of us will stay healthy. That's because we are all connected energetically. And when one woman breaks out of a box of limitation, she makes it easier for the rest of us to do the same. Life expectancy is rising steadily as we collectively change our beliefs about what is possible. People live more than 50 percent longer than they did a century ago, and those working in the life extension field believe that there is no absolute limit to the human life span. Our task at midlife is to realize that our most joyful and pleasurable years can be ahead of us. If you want to delve further into the truth of this, check out my book *Goddesses Never Age: The Secret Prescription for Radiance, Vitality, and Well-Being* (Hay House, 2015).

CREATING HEALTH DURING MENOPAUSE

To make the most of the menopausal transition, I encourage a woman to think of it as a period during which she'll be creating the healthy body she needs to last her until the end of life. The menopausal transition is an excellent time to focus on the prevention of problems that, while not necessarily directly associated with menopause, statistically appear to intensify at this stage. At midlife, for example, most women notice that it's no longer possible to just cut back on bread and desserts for a week in order to take off a few pounds and fit into that little black dress. Nor can we stay up all night without feeling the effects the next day. In short, we can no longer continue to ignore our physical, emotional, and spiritual needs and expect our bodies to stay vital and healthy. It's time to make proactive lifestyle improvements. It's not as though our bodies are suddenly "betraying us"—which is what many think. Or that "it's my age." That's not it. What's happening instead is that your body is issuing a big wake-up call: "Stop doing the things that have always been harmful. We gave you a lot of slack. But time's up."

What a woman experiences during this period of her life depends upon a multitude of factors, from her heredity, her expectations, and her cultural background to her self-esteem and her diet. At this time in history, the majority of women in our culture experience some discomfort and some troublesome symptoms at menopause. However, a wide variety of options exist for the treatment of these symptoms, including plant hormones, bioidentical hormones that match those produced in the human female body, homeopathy, and experience. The ideal path through the change is one that uses the best of Western medical knowledge concerning hormone metabolism, bone density, and heart health, combined with the complementary modalities of the East, including meditation, acupuncture, and herbs, to provide optimal individualized care.

Hormone-Producing Body Sites

Though we've been taught to think of menopausal symptoms mostly as an estrogen deficiency state resulting from ovarian failure, this belief is based on incomplete information. It is actually progesterone, another hormone made by the ovaries, that is most likely to be deficient during perimenopause, not estrogen. Total well-being at menopause and beyond depends at least as much on having adequate levels of progesterone—as well as DHEA and testosterone, two androgen hormones also produced in the ovaries—as it does on estrogen. Androgenic hormones are associated with sexual response and libido, as well as general well-being, and they are produced not just by the ovaries but by other organs and body sites, too. These include the adrenal

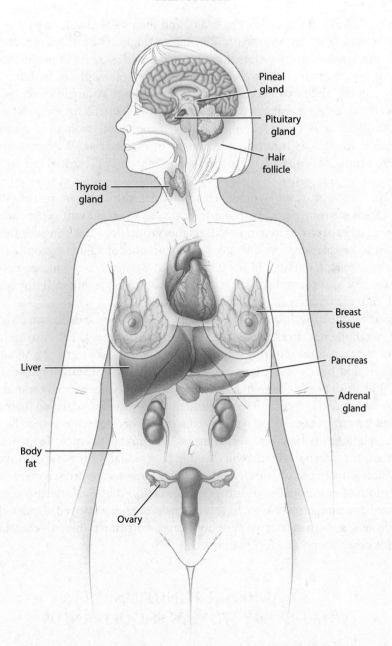

Pineal gland

Pituitary gland

Hair follicle

Thyroid gland

Breast tissue

Liver

Pancreas

Adrenal gland

Body fat

Ovary

FIGURE 22: HORMONE-PRODUCING BODY SITES

Ovarian estrogen and progesterone levels decrease after menopause. Other body sites, however, are capable of making these same hormones, depending upon a woman's lifestyle and diet. The female body, therefore, has the capacity to make healthy adjustments in hormonal balance after menopause.

glands, the skin, the muscles, the brain, and the pineal gland, as well as hair follicles and body fat. (See figure 22.) Interestingly, as hormone production from the ovaries declines at menopause, a twofold increase in production of androgenic hormones from these other sources takes place. In fact, your body has the ability to make hormones throughout your life. Since androgens can act as weak estrogens and can also be precursors for the production of estrogens, it is clear that the healthy menopausal woman is naturally equipped to deal with hormonal changes in her ovaries. Women who are able to produce adequate levels of androgens in their bodies often sail through menopause quite easily.

Nevertheless, some women clearly suffer during menopause. While 15 percent of women are symptom-free, a full 85 percent will experience hot flashes, and approximately one-half of this group does not consider the hot flashes to be tolerable. As time goes on, symptoms of vaginal atrophy (thinning of the vaginal tissue) in postmenopausal women tend to increase; heart disease risk and osteoporosis fracture risk also increase but will not be evident until a woman is in her late sixties or older.

Such menopausal problems are due in part to chronic depletion of women's metabolic resources during the perimenopausal years. The ease and timing of the transition into this stage depends upon the strength of a woman's adrenals and her overall nutrition. For example, an epidemiologic study of 35,000 British women known as the U.K. Women's Cohort Study found that those whose diets were high in oily fish and fresh legumes delayed their final period by an average of 3.3 years.[6] This makes perfect sense given the intimate relationship between nutrition and hormonal balance. In a healthy woman, the adrenal glands will be able to gradually take over hormonal production from the ovaries. Many women, however, approach menopause in a state of emotional and nutritional depletion that has affected optimal adrenal function. And many have had their ovaries removed. Under these conditions, a woman may require hormonal, nutritional, herbal, emotional, and/or other support to feel her best.[7]

ADRENAL FUNCTION:
WHAT EVERY WOMAN SHOULD KNOW

Our adrenal glands provide us with crucial hormonal support that we all need to go through the day with energy, enthusiasm, and efficiency. If your adrenals are depleted from chronic overproduction of the stress hormones norepinephrine (adrenaline) and cortisol, you are much more likely to suffer from fatigue and menopausal symptoms. Here are the signs that your adrenals may need attention: You awaken feeling groggy and have difficulty dragging yourself out of bed. You can't get going without that first cup or two of caffeinated coffee. You rely on sugary snacks and caffeine to get through the day, particularly in the late morning or afternoon. At night, though exhausted, you have difficulty falling asleep as the worries of the day keep replaying in your mind. You wonder what happened to your interest in sex. If this describes you, your adrenals may be running on almost empty, even if all your conventional medical tests are normal.

Functional adrenal testing, which measures the levels of two of the key adrenal hormones, has documented that many women who are tired all the time have adrenal glands that simply aren't functioning at their peak efficiency—usually as a result of chronic emotional, nutritional, or other kinds of stress. Carolyn Dean, M.D., N.D., an expert on the nutritional management of chronic disease, points out that the relationship between adrenal function, thyroid function, and sex steroids is actually a three-legged stool. If one is off, then all of them are off. And by the same token, when you address the health of one of them, the others often get better as well. That's because the function of all three is intertwined. The following symptoms suggest that at least one of the legs of the stool is off-balance: foggy thinking, insomnia, hypoglycemia, feeling cold, recurrent infections, depression, poor memory, headaches, and cravings for sweets.

The adrenal glands are your body's primary "shock absorbers." These two little thumb-size glands that sit on top of your kidneys are designed to produce hormones that allow you to respond to the conditions of your daily life in healthy and flexible ways. But if the intensity and the frequency of the stresses in your life, from either inside yourself (such as your perceptions about your life) or outside yourself (such as having surgery or working the night shift), become too great, then over time your adrenal glands will begin to become exhausted—not unlike a horse that continues to be worked or runs too much without adequate rest, food, and water. And if your adrenals are off, your thyroid and ovaries won't be functioning optimally, either. Eventually your body will produce many different symptoms in an attempt to get you to pay attention and change some aspects of your life—just as a tired horse will sooner or later stop working, no matter how much you whip it.

Here's a list of common stressors that over time can lead to the triad of ovarian, thyroid, and adrenal dysfunction. See how many of these apply to you.

UNRESOLVED EMOTIONAL STRESS

~ Worry

~ Anger

~ Guilt

- Anxiety

- Fear

- Depression

- Lack of pleasurable experiences

- Living with a narcissist or other energy vampire who drains you

ENVIRONMENTAL AND PHYSICAL STRESS

- Excessive exercise

- Exposure to industrial or other environmental toxins

- Chronic or severe allergies

- Suboptimal diet and suboptimal nutrient levels

- Glycemic stress from too many refined carbohydrates

- Overwork, either physical or mental

- Surgery

- Late hours, insufficient sleep

- Trauma, injury

- Temperature extremes

- Chronic illness

- Light-cycle disruption (shift work)

- Chronic pain

- Chronic illness

- Lack of sunlight

Among the key hormones produced by the adrenals are adrenaline, which fuels the body's fight-or-flight response; cortisol, a relative of the drugs prednisone and cortisone; and DHEA. The right balance between cortisol and DHEA is especially important for creating health daily. (So is having adequate amounts of iodine and magnesium in your diet.)

Cortisol in the right amounts enhances your body's natural resistance and endurance. It:

- Stimulates your liver to convert amino acids into glucose, a primary
  fuel for energy production

~ Counters allergies and inflammation

~ Helps regulate mood and maintain emotional stability

~ Stimulates increased production of glycogen in the liver for storage of glucose

~ Maintains resistance to the stress of infections, physical trauma, emotional trauma, temperature extremes, and so on

~ Mobilizes and increases fatty acids in the blood (from fat cells) to be used as fuel for energy production

But, as with most things, too much cortisol can also cause problems. An excess:

~ Leads to diminished glucose utilization by the cells and increases blood sugar and insulin levels

~ Decreases the body's ability to synthesize protein

~ Increases protein breakdown, which can lead to muscle wasting and osteoporosis

~ Suppresses the sex hormones

~ Increases the risk for hypertension, high cholesterol, and heart disease

~ Causes immune system depression, which may lead to increased susceptibility to allergies, infections, and cancer

Under normal circumstances, DHEA reverses many of the unfavorable effects of excessive cortisol, as well as providing important benefits of its own. It:

~ Functions as an androgen to help the body build tissue

~ Is a precursor for testosterone, the hormone associated with sexual desire

~ Reverses immune suppression caused by excessive cortisol levels and therefore increases resistance to viruses, bacteria, *Candida albicans*, parasites, allergies, and cancer

~ Stimulates bone deposition and remodeling, which prevents osteoporosis

~ Improves cardiovascular status by lowering total and LDL (bad) cholesterol

~ Increases muscle mass and decreases percentage of body fat

~ Improves energy and vitality, sleep, mental clarity; reduces PMS symptoms; helps the body recover more quickly from acute stress such as insufficient sleep, excessive exercise, or emotional trauma

So as you can easily see, an imbalance between your cortisol and DHEA levels can leave you susceptible to fatigue and all manner of illnesses, as well as many menopausal symptoms. Levels of DHEA decline in some women with aging, and replenishing this hormone to normal body levels—or using herbal supplements containing phytohormones—may have many benefits. Use of this hormone isn't right for everyone, and once adrenal function is restored, our bodies often have the ability to make enough of this hormone on their own.[8]

To test your current levels of cortisol and DHEA and to see if they are in balance, I recommend that you have your healthcare provider order what is called a DUTCH test (dried urine test for comprehensive hormones), which measures urinary hormones, including cortisol and sex steroids, over a twenty-four-hour period. This test will give you and your healthcare provider an idea of what your circadian rhythms are like, and as a result, you'll be able to track your recovery. The test is available from Precision Analytical, Inc. (www.dutchtest.com). Unfortunately, this test—like many other functional tests—is generally not covered by insurance.

It is not necessary to have your hormone levels tested to benefit from my suggestions for restoring your adrenal, thyroid, and sex steroid glands to optimal capacity, but I find that most women are more motivated to change when they can see their results on paper, especially if the initial results are not optimal. Once you know your starting point with your adrenals or other hormones, there is a great deal you can do to help them recover. If you don't want to have testing done, for whatever reason, just follow as many of the suggestions below as you can without stressing yourself further. In my experience, how you feel is actually a far more accurate barometer of your hormone and adrenal status than any other measure.

Adrenal/Thyroid/Sex Steroid Restoration Program for a Healthier Menopause

Recharge Your Batteries with the Power of Your Thoughts and Emotions

Studies have shown that your natural ability to produce DHEA—the mother hormone that affects all other hormone levels—can be increased by learning to "think with your heart." This is simple: It means choosing thoughts that feel better. So, for example, if you're stressed about something, turn your attention to your heart and think about a puppy, an adorable child, a fabulous meal—anything that feels good and brings you pleasure. Make this a habit. It will change your life! (To get you started, I recommend reading *Ask and It Is Given* [Hay House, 2004] or *The Art of Deliberate Creation* [Hay House, 2006], both by Esther and Jerry Hicks, or visiting their website at www.abraham-hicks.com. A full range of very helpful CDs, DVDs, and digital downloads is available there.) The HeartMath Institute in Boulder Creek, California (call HeartMath at 800-450-9111 or visit Heart-Math's website at www.heartmath.org), has developed a system of heart-focusing techniques that are taught through training programs and books. A study of one HeartMath technique, called Cut-Thru, showed that with sincere practice it could help alter the harmful physiological and emotional responses to emotional stress. The study demonstrated that after one month of using the technique there was a 100 percent increase in the subjects' DHEA levels. Study participants reported significant increases in caring and vigor and significant decreases in burnout and anxiety. The technique helps dissipate emotional static and can help heal emotional patterns of worry, hostility, anxiety, and guilt.[9]

"Thinking with your heart" takes practice, but if you faithfully learn to start thinking with your heart and pay attention to areas of your life that bring you joy and fulfillment, over time you will evoke biochemical changes in your body that will recharge your batteries.

HEART FOCUS EXERCISE TO DECREASE STRESS HORMONES

1. Stop yourself and observe your emotional state.

2. Name what is bothering you—you might even write it down or say it out loud to yourself or a friend.

3. Focus on your heart area (put your hand there if it helps you focus).

4. Shift your attention to a happy, funny, or uplifting event, person, or place in your life that you appreciate, and spend a few moments imagining it.

5. Bring something to mind that allows you to feel unconditional love or appreciation—usually a child or a pet—and hold that feeling for fifteen seconds or more (again, it helps to hold your hand over your heart).

6. Notice how changing your thoughts and your perception has changed how you feel. See that you have the power to shift out of the downward spiral of negativity you may have been caught in.

Make a List of Your Most Important Activities and Commitments

Let everything else go. Before saying yes to a new task or commitment, ask yourself this question: "Will doing this recharge my batteries or deplete them?" If the activity will deplete them, then don't do it.

Get Enough Sleep

Sleep restores adrenal balance more effectively than any other modality. Many women, including me, require eight to ten hours of sleep to function optimally. Get to bed by 10:00 P.M. Getting to sleep on the earlier side of midnight is much more restorative to your adrenals than sleep that begins later in the night, even if you sleep late the next morning to get in your full amount of sleep.

Allow Yourself to Accept Nurturing and Affection

If you didn't learn how to do this as a child, you may need to practice it. Every morning before you get up, spend a minute or two reveling in a memory of a time you felt loved. Do the same at night. Imagine your heart being filled with this love. Dwell on the things you really like about yourself.

Concentrate on activities and people that are fun and make you laugh. This stimulates healthy immune function. Make pleasurable activities a priority—every day. Don't wait until later. "Later" rarely comes.

Get regular massages as well. Way more than merely an indulgent way to relax, massage is just plain healthy. It actually decreases cortisol and increases serotonin (the feel-good hormone), dopamine (a neurotransmitter that increases energy levels), and the natural killer cells that boost immunity, according to research by Tiffany Field, Ph.D., director of the Touch Research Institute at the University of Miami School of Medicine. (By the way, don't think you need a professional massage to get these benefits. Dr. Field's studies are largely based on twice-weekly, twenty-minute massages given for one month by significant others.) Massage therapy helps a host of midlife issues, including endometriosis, fibroids, cramps and heavy periods, arthritis, chronic fatigue, and insomnia, just to name a few.

It also helps with mood swings because touch aids in releasing the stress we all store in our fascia and muscles and gets the parasympathetic nervous system back in line. I know women who have gone from breakdown to breakthrough on the massage table, crying and getting rid of pain that's been stored up for years.

I also have a theory that massage can help normalize weight, in part because it helps bring pleasure into your life. When you don't experience pleasure on a regular basis, you're more likely to turn to sugar and alcohol to feel good.

Support Yourself Nutritionally

Follow the guidelines in chapter 17. Eat a whole-food diet with minimal sugar. Avoid devitalized food as much as possible. Check your vitamin-mineral intake, too. Vitamin C is essential for the blood vessels supporting your adrenal glands: Take 500 to 2,000 mg in divided doses over the day. Vitamin B_5 (pantothenic acid) is involved in energy production via ATP in the adrenals and elsewhere; take the rest of the B complex along with it in a good-quality 25 to 50 mg supplement that includes at least 800 mcg of folic acid per day.

Get Your Minerals

The extensive research of Carolyn Dean, M.D., N.D., author of *The Magnesium Miracle* (Ballantine Books, 2003; most recently updated in 2017), has shown that there are nine minerals essential in supporting the structure and function of the thyroid. Remember the three-legged stool I brought up earlier in this chapter—when thyroid function is optimal, this positively influences the health of the adrenals and thus the production of sex steroids. Here's a rundown of what you need.

Magnesium. This mineral is crucial to the regulation of between 700 and 800 enzyme systems in the body, the most important of which are involved with the body's ability to create, store, transport, and utilize energy. In short, to experience optimal energy, you need optimal levels of magnesium. It is estimated that the majority of people in the United States, if not most people on the planet, have suboptimal levels of magnesium, in part because of depleted soils and the refining of foods.[10] Excretion of magnesium in the urine increases when cortisol is too high, so it's easy to see why chronic stress also leads to magnesium depletion. Magnesium supplementation has been found to increase the adrenals' ability to make DHEA (see below). Note that calcium and magnesium must be balanced in the body to ensure proper bone metabolism as well as optimal thyroid and adrenal function. If there is too much calcium, thyroid hormone function can suffer. Magnesium regulates both calcium absorption and regulation. The focus on calcium as an important nutrient for bones has overshadowed the role of magnesium and led to a host of other problems, including calcification of tissues and increased muscle cramping.

Two good ways to make sure you're getting enough magnesium include taking an Epsom salts bath (pour one cup of magnesium sulfate, commonly called Epsom salts, in a warm bath and soak for twenty minutes) and using transdermal magnesium (apply magnesium lotion—such as Dr. Dean's ReMag lotion; see www.rnareset.com—liberally at night before bed or after exercise).

Iodine. The thyroid hormone known as T4 (thyroxine) has four iodine molecules, while the hormone known as T3 (triiodothyronine), which is T4's more active form, has three iodine molecules. T4 is 68 percent iodine by weight, and T3 is 58 percent. As already mentioned in chapter 10, while iodine is absolutely essential for optimal health, many people have suboptimal levels.

Selenium. This mineral is a co-factor necessary for the production of T4, while it also helps convert T4 to T3. A total of eleven selenium-dependent enzymes have been identified as necessary for optimal thyroid function and hormone production. Everyone who takes iodine also needs to take selenium, because selenium without iodine can cause iodine deficiency (and vice versa). Selenium and iodine go hand in hand.

Zinc. Zinc is also required for the synthesis of thyroid and other hormones. In fact, in many people, zinc deficiency can cause hypothyroidism (too little thyroid hormone). Conversely, you won't be able to absorb zinc without thyroid hormones. Dr. Dean accurately points out that the hair loss we blame on hypothyroidism sometimes doesn't improve until you supplement with zinc. The usual dose is 15 to 30 mg/day.

Molybdenum. This is another mineral upon which thyroid function depends. It works in the oxidative system of thyroid epithelial cells (thyrocytes), and also plays a role in the release of T3 from the thyroid gland. Interestingly, molybdenum also helps break down yeast toxins. Many people with hypothyroidism have problems with yeast overgrowth in part because their body temperature is suboptimal.

Boron. This mineral is essential for the conversion of the storage form of thyroid hormone (T4) into the active form (T3).

Copper. This mineral plays an essential role in the metabolism of an amino acid known as tyrosine, a precursor for the production of T4.

Chromium. This mineral is well known for its ability to enhance insulin sensitivity and for the regulation of insulin release as well as its effect on blood sugar and glucose storage. Chromium also influences the conversion of T4 to T3.

Manganese. Maganese is required to transport T4 into our cells.

Your regular multivitamin-mineral supplement may have all of the nutrients I've listed here, but you will probably need to add more magnesium and iodine than will be included in a standard multi.

Another option is Dr. Dean's ReMag and ReMyte formulations (see www.rnareset.com), which contain all these minerals in a 100 percent absorbable form known as picometer minerals.

Try Herbal Support

Pueraria mirifica has helped countless women recover their hormone and adrenal balance naturally. Its potent phytoestrogen, miroestrol, is related to DHEA and pregnenolone, both precursors for DHEA and cortisol. The usual dose is 80 mg twice per day. (See Resources.)

Licorice root contains plant hormones that have effects similar to cortisol. For low-cortisol states, take up to one-quarter teaspoon of 5:1 solid extract three times a day. Or simply drink licorice tea. Traditional Medicinals is a good brand.

Consider Hormonal Support

If your lab report comes back showing that you have decreased DHEA levels, try the steps listed above first. It's always ideal to restore adrenal function naturally. If you are not successful, you may consider supplementing your program with DHEA until your adrenals have recovered. High doses of DHEA over long periods of time can change the normal daily variation in cortisol levels, and I don't recommend them for most healthy women. However, physiologic replacement doses of DHEA (enough to bring levels up to normal) can help your own adrenals get a rest and start to recover faster.

DHEA is available as a skin cream, a pill, or a tincture. The best brands are pharmaceutical grade (look for "GMP" on the label). (The tincture needs to be made up by a formulary pharmacist.) Each form has a somewhat different effect, but whatever the form, you should start with the lowest dose possible and build up gradually until you notice a difference in your energy. Most women need no more than 5 to 10 mg twice a day; some will need up to 25 mg once or twice a day. Your DHEA levels should be tested again three months later, and if they have been restored to normal, you can begin to taper off the supplementary DHEA.

Progesterone also helps balance the effects of too much cortisol. Use one-quarter to one-half teaspoon of 2 percent progesterone cream once or twice a day on the skin. It also raises DHEA levels.

An occasional individual may also need cortisol supplementation, which can be prescribed for a limited amount of time by your healthcare provider.

Exercise

Light to moderate exercise is very helpful. But if you feel depleted afterward, you are doing too much. Make sure you can breathe comfortably through your nose when exercising. Mouth breathing, discussed in chapter 18, is a stress response. Exercising to the point where you must breathe through your mouth will simply create more adrenal stress and fatigue. Don't do it. Pushing yourself beyond where you can comfortably breathe through your nose weakens your adrenals even further, so start slowly—even if it's only walking down your street and back. Then build up slowly.

Vitamin D and Sunlight

Vitamin D, which is both a vitamin and a hormone, affects every cell in the body. Optimal vitamin D levels (40–100 ng/ml) are essential for optimal adrenal, thyroid, and hormone function as well as bone and breast health. (For a discussion of vitamin D, see chapter 10, on breast health, as well as chapter 17, on nutrition.) Take 2,000 to 5,000 IU per day. (You may need far more initially to get your levels in the optimal range. The protocol of world-renowned vitamin D researcher Michael Holick, Ph.D., M.D., recommends 50,000 IU weekly for eight weeks. This should be done only when under the care of a knowledgeable physician.)

Natural sunlight can also be very helpful for restoring adrenal function, as long as you don't overdo it. I recommend at least ten to twenty minutes of exposure over as much of your body as possible during morning or afternoon hours, avoiding midday sun. (Note: In northern climates—those having a latitude around the mid-30 degrees or higher—you cannot get enough UVB radiation to make vitamin D under the skin between mid-October and mid-March.) We've been made to fear sun exposure, but research shows that getting either too much *or* too little sun is harmful to our health. After doing an epidemiological review of 115 studies, researchers from the Netherlands concluded that regular time in the sun is related to a reduced chance of getting several types of cancers, including colon and breast cancers, as well as a reduced chance of getting multiple sclerosis and metabolic syndrome.[11]

Try a sunbath at least three to four times per week in the appropriate season. This type of exposure, if you are sure not to burn your skin, will not increase your risk of skin cancer. It's also an excellent way to help boost levels of vitamin D. Getting thirty minutes of sun exposure on light skin results in 10,000 IU of vitamin D made in your own body (less if you have dark skin). You can't overdose when you get vitamin D from the sun—your body will stop making it once you get to an optimal level. In the winter, you can use a tanning booth for less than ten minutes once per week, or simply take supplements.

HYPOTHYROID DISEASE

The thyroid—a butterfly-shaped gland located in the area of your neck just below the Adam's apple—is part of the endocrine system and regulates your metabolic rate, although it exerts a profound effect on the function of nearly every organ in the body. Women with hyperthyroidism make too much thyroid hormone, while the far more common condition is hypothyroidism, which occurs when the body doesn't make enough thyroid hormone. About 26 percent of women in or near perimenopause have this problem.[12]

There is a wide variety of symptoms of hypothyroidism. The most common include mood disturbances (such as depression and irritability) as well as low energy level, weight gain, mental confusion, and sleep disturbances. Some women have hypothyroidism without any of these symptoms, while others reporting symptoms have normal (or only slightly abnormal) thyroid function tests—in which case subclinical hypothyroidism is often the cause. (By the way, many symptoms of hypothyroidism are the same as those commonly associated with the hormonal fluctuations of perimenopause. So it's entirely possible to have many of the symptoms of hypothyroidism yet have completely normal thyroid function.)

Low thyroid function can deplete your body of serotonin and other mood-stabilizing neurotransmitters, which is why low thyroid levels are often associated with depression. I suspect these two conditions (hypothyroidism and depression) occur simultaneously. While one does not necessarily cause the other, similar emotional or behavioral patterns—such as learned helplessness or not believing you can have your say—may predispose you to both low thyroid and depression. For this reason, many women do best when their depression and their hypothyroidism are treated simultaneously.

If you suspect you may have thyroid issues, have your TSH (thyroid-stimulating hormone) level checked, along with your free triiodothyronine (T3) and free thyroxine (T4) levels. The TSH should definitely be no higher than 3.0 mIU/L, although many experts, including myself, are more comfortable setting the limit at 2.5. If your levels are higher than that, you have subclinical hypothyroidism. (For information about how to check these levels without a doctor's visit, see My Med Lab in the Diagnostic Laboratories section of the Resources.)

Please make sure you are replete with the nine minerals mentioned earlier. In many women, this is all that is necessary to restore thyroid function. My colleague Kelly Brogan, M.D., who is board certified in both integrative holistic medicine and psychiatry—and who also has recovered from thyroid problems herself—has found that a supplement from Allergy Research Group known as TG 100 Natural Glandulars works beautifully for the vast majority of her patients (see www.allergyresearchgroup.com or order it on Amazon). Also refer to the section on iodine in chapter 10.

If you are already on thyroid medication, it is best to add this nutritional support under the care of your healthcare provider. It's extremely common for these nutritional treatments to restore thyroid function, and as a result, taking the usual dosage of thyroid meds can cause a person to think she is hyperthyroid. She isn't; she will just need to adjust or stop her thyroid meds and get retested.

If you require thyroid medication, note that supplementing with only T4 (which is the hormone found in Synthroid, one of the most commonly prescribed thyroid medications) is not enough. You also need T3. To get that, you need to take natural thyroid replacement, such as Nature-Throid (www.naturethroid.com), Armour Thyroid, or a mixture of T3 and T4 made up by a formulary pharmacist (or simply try the Allergy Research Group TG 100 Natural Glandulars I mentioned earlier—no prescription required).

KINDS OF MENOPAUSE

Natural Menopause and Perimenopause

The average age of menopause is currently about fifty-one, with a range from forty-five to fifty-five. It is possible for some women to experience menopause as early as age thirty-nine. Most women go through menopause at approximately the same age as their mothers, although this is not always the case, especially given the new research on how good nutrition can delay menopause for several years.

The climacteric is a biochemical process lasting six to thirteen years. (New studies show that women who enter menopause at an earlier age generally have a longer menopausal transition, for reasons that aren't clear.)[13] During this process, periods may stop for several months and then return; they may increase or decrease in duration and flow. Some women may experience as much as a year-long interruption in periods only to have them resume once again.

When irregularity in the menstrual cycle begins during perimenopause, a woman's symptoms, such as headaches and irritability, will often be due to increased levels of estrogen relative to progesterone, caused by decreased ovulation. This is known as estrogen dominance. Women who have experienced a difficult puberty, PMS, or postpartum depression are more likely to experience mood swings and other related symptoms during menopause than those who have gone through earlier hormonal changes comfortably. Women in perimenopause can often be helped dramatically by taking the herb *Pueraria mirifica* daily. This adaptogenic herb acts on the beta estrogen receptor and prevents the overstimulation of the alpha estrogen receptor that so often causes symptoms of estrogen dominance. There are two ways to take it, depending upon whether or not your periods are still regular. If they are regular, then take 80 mg twice per day on days seven through twenty-one of your cycle. If your periods are irregular, then simply take 80 mg twice per day, stopping for seven days starting on the first day of your bleeding.

Another option is to take small amounts of progesterone administered in the luteal phase (second half) of the cycle. The usual dose is 50 to 100 mg of micronized progesterone administered orally one to three times a day from the sixteenth through twenty-seventh days of the cycle.[14] A 2 percent progesterone cream can also be used. (The brand I have recommended for years is Pro-Gest, by Emerita, available on Amazon.) Some women will fare better if progesterone or *Pueraria mirifica* is used continuously through the cycle, regardless of whether or not periods are regular. This can be particularly beneficial for women with premenstrual migraine headaches.

Many women who begin to skip periods or experience changes in the menstrual flow believe that they are entering menopause. The final menstrual period is probably at least five years away, making this an ideal time to reassess every aspect of your lifestyle, nutritional levels, relationships, and so on.

While menopause is often heralded by the onset of a change in menstrual flow or skipped menstrual periods, some women simply stop having periods and have no symptoms whatsoever. Others experience hot flashes, vaginal dryness, decreased libido, and "fuzzy thinking." A blood or urine test is often done at this time to "diagnose" menopause. This consists of measuring the levels of the pituitary gonadotropins FSH (follicle-stimulating hormone) and LH (luteinizing hormone), hormones produced by the pituitary gland to stimulate the ovary to produce eggs. During the years of menstruation, FSH and LH peak with ovulation at midcycle each month, producing the emotional and physiological changes discussed in chapter 5. During the climacteric, however, the pituitary gland and the ovaries undergo a gradual change, during which ovulations decrease and FSH and LH levels gradually increase. (The pituitary gland continues to send out LH and FSH because it is not getting the usual hormonal messages from the developing egg to tell it to slow down.) When FSH and LH reach a certain level in the blood, they are said to be in the menopausal range.

I was taught that once a woman's FSH and LH are in the menopausal range, she was indeed menopausal and would stay that way, but this is not always the case. One forty-year-old woman, for example, who had no periods for six months and had menopausal levels of FSH and LH, later went back to having normal periods for years. A recheck of her hormone levels showed that they also had gone back to premenopausal levels. At this point, I don't consider FSH and LH levels very reliable diagnostic indicators of menopause, but they can be useful to confirm that a woman is heading in that direction. (It's also enlightening to watch this trend reverse sometimes when the ovaries and adrenals get the support they need.)

It's important for perimenopausal women to know that even though they may be skipping ovulations, they can theoretically still become pregnant up until one year after their last period. For that reason, I recommend that a woman continue to use some form of contraception throughout this time.

Premature Menopause

A small percentage of women—approximately one in a hundred—experience natural premature menopause at age forty or younger. In some cases, this is due to an autoimmune disorder related to poor diet or chronic stress and resulting in the production of antiovarian antibodies.[15] Rather than thinking that the body is attacking the ovaries via immunity (the autoimmune hypothesis), it is far more accurate (and comforting) to realize that these antibodies are simply the result of cellular inflammation at a deep level—just as in Hashimoto's thyroiditis, another so-called autoimmune disease. Women who undergo premature menopause from any cause and loss of ovarian estrogen supply have been shown to have increased susceptibility to dementia.[16] It is important for a woman with this history to pay special attention to those things that promote healthy brain function. (See the discussion of Alzheimer's later in this chapter.)

Artificial Menopause

Currently, one in every four American women will enter menopause as a result of surgery. Hysterectomy with ovarian removal or bilateral salpingo-oophorectomy (removal of both tubes and ovaries) results in instant menopause in the premenopausal woman, which is very different from natural physiological menopause and should be treated differently. Removal of the ovaries is associated with a dramatic decrease in the production of testosterone and other androgens. Surgical menopause can also result in a major decrease in estrogen production. Symptoms can be severe and debilitating without proper readjustment of hormonal levels.[17]

A startling 2009 study also shows that premature menopause, whether natural or because of bilateral oophorectomy, nearly doubles the risk of lung cancer—even if you don't smoke.[18] Bilateral oophorectomy also increases your chances of coronary heart disease, stroke, and dying from any form of cancer—although it decreases the risk for breast and of course ovarian cancer.[19] In addition to the risks cited above, the Mayo Clinic Cohort Study of Oophorectomy and Aging found that women who'd had their ovaries removed before menopause had a fivefold increase in risk of mortality from neurological or mental diseases. Data from this same study also indicated that women with bilateral oophorectomy before age forty-five experience an almost twofold increase in mortality from cardiovascular disease; an increased risk for Parkinsonism, cognitive impairment, and dementia; and an increase in depressive and anxiety symptoms later in life.[20] Taking hormone therapy after ovarian removal certainly helps to prevent these outcomes, but studies also show that long-term compliance is not sufficient to make up for the impact of hormone deficiency following the surgery.[21]

Because normal menopause occurs at around fifty-one years of age, some kind of supportive therapy—either with mammalian hormones or with phytohormones—should continue at least until this age but can be continued longer depending on individual circumstances.

Hysterectomy without removal of the ovaries may still result in accelerated menopause, as mentioned earlier. In some cases, the ovaries temporarily decrease hormone production, causing menopausal symptoms that disappear when normal ovarian function resumes. It has also been shown that progesterone levels decrease significantly for at least six months following tubal ligation.[22] Obviously this depends upon how much of the tube and underlying blood supply gets interrupted by the ligation method.

Women who have had chemotherapy for any cancer or who have undergone radiation to the pelvis are also apt to undergo premature menopause. For women facing chemotherapy or radiation, it has been my experience that undergoing a course of acupuncture and Chinese herbs at the same time as the chemo or radiation often can prevent premature menopause and also will alleviate many side effects of the treatment. The same is true of a healthy diet. Adding together the women who undergo natural premature menopause and those who undergo artificial menopause through drugs or surgery means that approximately one in twelve women today faces menopause before the age of forty.

THE HORMONE THERAPY QUESTION

A Brief History of Conventional Hormone Replacement

Premarin, the first and most well-known form of estrogen therapy, was introduced in 1949. It consists of a collection of more than twenty different conjugated equine estrogens mostly made from the urine of pregnant horses. (Premarin is an acronym derived from the phrase "pregnant mares' urine." If you doubt this, just put a drop of water on a tablet of Premarin and smell it.) There is no generic form of Premarin because no one has been able to identify and synthesize the same hormones that occur in horse urine.

For historical and economic reasons, Premarin (taken by itself, along with a synthetic progestin called Provera, or in a pill called Prempro, which is a combination of Premarin and Provera) has been the gold standard against which all other menopausal hormone treatments are measured. In the late 1980s through the 1990s, millions of women were put on this drug because studies strongly suggested that it decreased the risk of heart attack and stroke (the leading cause of premature death in women), increased bone density, and decreased the risk of dementia. Although it was associated with a slightly increased risk of breast and endometrial cancer, these risks paled in comparison to the possibility of saving lives lost to heart disease.

In the early 1990s, the Wyeth-Ayerst company, makers of Premarin, helped fund the huge Women's Health Initiative, which was designed to prove that Prempro would save lives by decreasing heart attacks, etc. The study was stopped in July 2002 when researchers found that Prempro actually increased the risk of heart attack and stroke as well as breast cancer, Alzheimer's, and dementia. Overall, it was felt that the risks outweighed the benefits.

The news about Prempro panicked thousands of women, many of whom stopped taking hormones cold turkey and ended up with insomnia, intolerable hot flashes, and a greatly decreased quality of life.

Then in early 2006, a reanalysis of the data from both the WHI and the Nurses' Health Study found that women who started hormone therapy within ten years after menopause did indeed have an 11 to 30 percent decreased risk of heart disease compared with those who didn't use any hormones. But those who started it ten years or more after menopause had an increased risk for stroke, heart attack, and so on.[23] This added a new wrinkle to the entire HT discussion.

Ten years later, in 2016, the International Menopause Society released new recommendations that assuaged those fears and urged a more individual approach, noting that new data as well as reanalysis of older studies show that for most women with menopausal symptoms, hormone therapy has more potential benefits than risks if the therapy begins soon after menopause starts.[24] The guidelines note that the increased risk for breast cancer from using hormones is rare—less than 1 additional case of breast cancer per 1,000 women per year of use—and that this level of risk is similar to or lower than the risk women face from common factors such as a sedentary lifestyle, obesity, and alcohol consumption.

Another closer look at the evidence has shown that hormones that match those found in the female body (known as bioidentical hormones) may not raise the risk of breast cancer the way synthetic or horse hormones do. One of the most recent studies on this is a 2017 review study that found that hormone therapy containing micronized (natural) progesterone has a significantly lower breast cancer risk than therapy with progestins (synthetic hormones).[25] One of the largest studies to date comparing the risk of breast cancer with the use of natural bioidentical hormones to the risk when using synthetic hormone therapy followed more than 80,000 postmenopausal women in France for more than eight years. Data showed that the natural hormones (including progesterone) had significantly less associated risk of breast cancer.[26] The following year, a comprehensive analysis was published in the medical literature by the Holtorf Medical Group in Torrance, California, that examined 200 physiological and clinical studies on both synthetic and bioidentical hormones. The analysis showed that bioidentical hormones were associated with lower risk for breast cancer and cardiovascular disease than were synthetic hormones. In addition, the study showed that bioidentical hormones were better than their synthetic counterparts at alleviating symptoms such as insomnia, cognitive problems, depression, anxiety, and more.[27]

Further, Rowan Chlebowski, M.D., Ph.D., a medical oncologist at Los Angeles Biomedical Research Institute at Harbor–UCLA Medical Center, assembled a team of researchers to determine if the significant drop in breast cancer cases seen after 2003 was due to women halting their hormone therapy or to more vigilant mammography practices.[28] Their research, published in 2009, showed that getting regular mammograms didn't affect the drop in breast cancer cases. But it also showed that the decline in breast cancer wasn't related to all types of hormone therapy. The women who took only estrogen (mainly Premarin) without the progestin were no more likely to develop breast cancer than women who took no hormones at all, which points to synthetic progestin as the likely culprit. This has been borne out in the more recent studies above.

The medical literature on hormone therapy mentioned is very confusing and often contradictory. Here is what is clear. The science supporting hormone therapy is still evolving. There is no "one size fits all" approach for all women. The huge Women's Health Initiative laid that notion to rest once and for all. Hormone therapy decisions need to be individualized. Fortunately, many options exist.

The Case for Bioidentical Hormones

Despite data suggesting a decrease in heart disease if Premarin is started early, and also despite the data indicating that Premarin probably doesn't cause an increase in the risk of breast cancer, I'm still concerned that Premarin just isn't the best choice of estrogen. And synthetic progestin clearly isn't the best choice, either. Back in 1994, concerned about the type of hormone therapy used in the WHI study, I wrote, "In view of the concerns regarding breast cancer associated with estrogen replacement therapy (ERT), the use of synthetic sex compounds with which the human body is not designed to cope would appear to be the equivalent of conducting a vast experiment on the human female population. It is ironic, in this light, that treatment using natural hormones bioidentical to those in a woman's body is designated as 'alternative' medicine."

Now here we are, decades later, and most people, including healthcare practitioners, still don't comprehend the difference between a hormone that is identical to one that is native to the female human body and one that isn't. It's crucial to understand that it is the three-dimensional structure of a hormone that determines how it acts in the body. You can't possibly get an optimal physiologic response from a hormone if its structure is foreign to the human body. And this alteration from what occurs naturally is the main form of hormonal support available today in nearly all conventional medicine approaches. The reason for the continued use of synthetic hormones is that naturally occurring compounds cannot be patented. Therefore, using them has not been in the financial interest of drug companies. Instead, they have altered the compounds (or the delivery systems) so that they can obtain patents on them. (This is also why substances such as iodine, magnesium, vitamin D, and omega-3 fats, for example, have been so slow to catch on as the therapeutic powerhouses that they are. There's little financial profit in producing them.)

Because the hormones in Premarin are derived from horses, they clearly don't match those found in women's bodies.[29] As the late Joel Hargrove, M.D., a pioneer in the use of natural hormones and former medical director of the Menopause Center at Vanderbilt University Medical Center, used to say, "Premarin is a natural hormone if your native food is hay."

Finding Middle Ground:
The Individualized Hormone Solution

Though many of my colleagues and I were disturbed by the way in which the Women's Health Initiative study was stopped and the distress it caused for so many women, the good news is that it changed the hormone therapy paradigm completely. Almost overnight, we went from a "one size fits all," "magic bullet" approach to understanding the need to individualize our approach to hormone therapy. And that is the new standard of care—regardless of what new studies are done in the future. This updated thinking about hormones also led to new terminology. Taking hormones is now called hormone therapy (HT), not hormone replacement therapy (HRT). This change reflects the fact that menopause is now finally viewed as a normal life stage, not as a deficiency state. Hallelujah!

For those women who require hormone therapy by virtue of their symptoms, this is very good news. The field of individualized natural hormone support has positively blossomed since the first edition of this book was published. And instead of reducing the entire hormone question simply to estrogen, it is now clear that HT sometimes includes other classes of hormones that the ovaries also produce: progesterone and androgens.

First, a word about that confusing and much-debated word *natural*. The hormone components of Premarin are indeed natural for horses, but the word is more commonly applied to plant hormones (phytohormones) found in foods such as soybeans and wild yams. The human body utilizes plant hormones very well, because we have been ingesting them for millions of years. But plant hormones are sterols, not steroids. And though they have hormonal effects, they are simply not the same thing as bioidentical human hormones. (See also the phytoestrogen discussion in chapter 10, page 430.)

I use the word *natural* to refer to a hormone that, while derived originally from the plant sterols found in soybeans and yams, has a molecular structure that is modified in the laboratory to be an exact match for those found in the human body. That is why they are also referred to as bioidentical hormones. The issue is not whether or not a hormone is produced in a laboratory; if it matches the hormones found in the human body, then it's a bioidentical hormone. The bioidentical estrogens, progesterone, and testosterone that are used for hormone therapy have been available for years and are listed in the United States Pharmacopeia. Any licensed pharmacist or physician can use them, and they can be produced at strengths that can be standardized, so their effects are measurable and predictable. They do not require FDA approval because, as naturally occurring substances, they do not fall under the jurisdiction of the FDA.

Natural hormone therapy using bioidentical hormones provides no single, uniform program. Prescriptions must be tailored to the individual patient, with adjustments made regularly for the first year or so until an optimal dose is reached. This dose may continue to require readjustment as a woman moves through perimenopause and menopause and her body, lifestyle, and diet undergo changes.

The goal of natural hormone therapy is to provide symptomatic relief of a woman's menopausal symptoms. How much of what hormone is needed to do this varies widely depending on the woman. In general, symptom relief is reached when hormones are at about the same level a woman had in her late thirties or early forties.

An integrated approach to hormone therapy might include estrogen, testosterone, and/or progesterone—all three or just one. Remember that DHEA is the "mother hormone" that can be converted to all the others in a woman whose nutrient levels support the necessary conversions. The female body can also convert progesterone into both estrogen and testosterone. Currently, most women who have had hysterectomies are offered only estrogen, without any consideration for the role of progesterone or androgens. In some, that is all that is necessary. In other cases, a formulation containing all three is needed.

Virtually hundreds of combinations of hormones, including estrogen, progesterone, DHEA, and testosterone, are possible and may be administered by various routes, including orally, transdermally, or vaginally. (Transdermal and vaginal routes are the physiologically best way to take hormones because they don't have to go through the gastrointestinal system and then be processed by the liver. This allows the body to get maximal benefit from a minimal dose.) Because the choices are so numerous and often confusing, I recommend beginning with a hormone profile for every woman who expresses concern about menopause or who is exhibiting menopausal symptoms. Ideally this baseline hormone profile should be done in one's early to mid-forties, when a woman is symptom-free. Then her own normal levels will be known beforehand, making it much easier to create a hormone therapy regimen that is tailor-made for her should she require it. That said, there is still a great deal we don't know about how hormones are metabolized in the body. So much depends upon a woman's mood, thoughts, stress levels, and so on. Having been involved in all kinds of hormone testing over many years, I've found that how a woman actually feels is the best possible indicator of what dose of hormone to take—not a lab test.

Ultimately, relief of symptoms and an overall sense of well-being, not necessarily hormone levels, are the best ways to assess the success of hormone therapy. Since the climacteric can last as long as thirteen years, it may be necessary to vary regimens or to reevaluate the need for continued hormone replacement over the course of the menopausal transition. Happily, a growing number of healthcare practitioners are offering women the kind of individualized hormone replacement regimens that I consider ideal. A number of laboratories and independent formulary pharmacies located throughout the United States and Canada specialize in customized care. (See Resources.)

No one knows the ideal length of time to stay on hormone therapy. Short-term is considered five years or less. I suggest annually remaking the decision about whether to stay on hormones if you are already on them. Many women are finding that individualized nutritional and herbal regimens are working so well that they don't require any hormone therapy at all. (See below.)

Research on the potential long-term benefits of hormone therapy is ongoing. For example, the Kronos Longevity Research Institute, a nonprofit organization in Phoenix that does research on aging, conducted a multicenter prospective trial known as the Kronos Early Estrogen Prevention Study (KEEPS) that compared the use of bioidentical hormone therapy (a natural estrogen patch) to conjugated estrogen therapy (Premarin) in newly menopausal women. Those women who still had a uterus were also given oral natural progesterone (Prometrium). The placebo-controlled study followed 727 healthy women ages forty-two to fifty-eight for four years, starting in 2005. KEEPS was designed to address the issue of whether either of these types of estrogen therapy, if begun within three years of menopause, decreases the risk of heart disease (specifically, it prevents the buildup of plaque in the blood vessels near the heart) and prevents cognitive decline. The KEEPS researchers presented their results at the annual meeting of the North American Menopause Society in October 2012.[30] Hormone therapy had no effect on hardening of the arteries or blood pressure, they reported, although there was some limited evidence that hormone therapy might be cardioprotective.[31] Women taking Premarin lowered their LDL cholesterol (the so-called bad cholesterol) and increased their HDL cholesterol (the "good" cholesterol), but they also increased their levels of harmful triglycerides. Women on the natural estrogen patch didn't experience a change in their blood lipid levels, but their insulin resistance improved. Both groups substantially reduced hot flashes and night sweats, had small gains in bone mineral density, and improved their sexual function (with those on natural hormones also seeing improvements in libido). The researchers further reported no adverse effects on cognitive function (as the earlier WHI study on older women showed). Because the KEEPS study followed only younger women and only for four years, a follow-up study called the Kronos Early Estrogen Prevention Study (KEEPS) Continuation has been launched thirteen years after the original KEEPS research began to follow the effects of hormone therapy and normal aging on brain structure, cognitive performance, and markers for Alzheimer's disease in those women who participated in the original KEEPS trial.

Similarly, the National Institute on Aging sponsored a double-blind, placebo-controlled study on estrogen and heart disease called the Early Versus Late Intervention Trial with Estradiol (ELITE) study, conducted by researchers at the Keck School of Medicine at the University of Southern California. The study followed 643 healthy women divided into two groups—those who had started menopause less than six years earlier and those who had started menopause ten or more years earlier. The study tested natural hormones (an estradiol pill and, if the women still had a uterus, progesterone gel applied vaginally) against placebo. The data showed that natural estrogen therapy reduced the progression of early atherosclerosis if started soon after menopause but had no effect when administered ten or more years after menopause.[32] The same team conducted a second study on the same group of women, examining the cognitive effects of natural hormone treatment, and found no difference—estradiol neither benefited nor harmed cognitive abilities, regardless of time since menopause.[33] Many other aspects of HT continue to be studied. Stay tuned.

Remember, hormone therapy is as much an art as it is a science. Most formulary pharmacists have a great deal of experience working with healthcare providers to individualize optimal hormone solutions. For additional information and guidance that will help you make the right decisions about bioidentical hormones for you, visit the website of the Bioidentical Hormone Initiative at www.bioidenticalhormoneinitiative.org.

Are Bioidentical Hormones the Secret of Youth?

Some doctors who practice antiaging medicine feel that lifelong hormone therapy with levels matching those of a twenty-year-old is the secret of youth. This school of thought also recommends that a woman's hormones be cycled in such a way that she gets her period every month. This is the approach that has been widely publicized by actress and breast cancer survivor Suzanne Somers in her book *The Sexy Years* (Crown, 2004). Though I love the idea of all of us looking as sexy and young as possible for our entire lifetimes, there are other ways to do this that don't involve artificially keeping hormone levels at the level of a twenty-year-old. The jury is still out on the wisdom of taking high-dose hormones for life in order to stay young forever. Besides, I know precious few women past the age of fifty who want to continue having periods. That said, I applaud Somers for her work in letting women know about the many benefits of bioidentical hormones as opposed to synthetic ones and also for being a role model for looking gorgeous and fit after the age of fifty. Many, many women are following in her footsteps, realizing that staying fit and healthy into their fifties and sixties is about far more than taking hormones. In 2015, I wrote *Goddesses Never Age: The Secret Prescription for Radiance, Vitality, and Well-Being* because it is clear to me that our cultural view of what it means to be a woman over fifty truly needs updating. We are not designed to deteriorate and get chronic disease after fifty. But to stay healthy, vital, and sexy, we must continue to move regularly, think differently, and question everything our culture has taught us about what to expect after a certain age. We all need to know that what happens to us as we grow older is largely determined by our lifestyle. We can be fifty going on thirty-five or fifty going on eighty-five. The power to remain vital and healthy is within each of us.

A HORMONE PRIMER

Estrogen

There are three types of estrogen that occur naturally in the female body: estrone (E1), estradiol (E2), and estriol (E3). Estrone is produced in significant amounts in body fat, which is one reason why anorexic women cease menstruating and get premature osteoporosis. They simply don't have enough body fat to sustain normal hormone function. Estrogen acts as a growth hormone for breast, uterine, and ovarian tissue. Overstimulation of these organs by estrogen is associated with excessive cell growth that may lead to cancer. On the positive side, estrogen elevates HDL (the good cholesterol) and has a beneficial effect on blood vessel walls; these were the main reasons why a large number of studies, but not the Women's Health Initiative, have shown a decreased risk for heart disease for those taking estrogen soon after menopause. Estrogen also helps to prevent osteoporosis by inhibiting the activity of bone cells known as osteoclasts, which are involved in the recycling and breakdown of old bone. It also ameliorates hot flashes, prevents vaginal thinning and dryness, and enhances the collagen layer of the skin, which improves elasticity and helps to prevent wrinkles.

The most effective and most commonly used estrogens are estradiol and estrone. These are available in a wide variety of preparations, including transdermal patches and creams, vaginal rings, or oral preparations. (Note: Bioidentical hormones can now be found in conventional pharmacies—because pharmaceutical companies have figured out a way to patent the technologies used to deliver these hormones into the body. The Climara patch, which has bioidentical 17-beta estradiol, is a good example.)

With the exception of estriol, estrogen from any source, natural or otherwise, can be potentially dangerous if the dose used is too high or if it's not balanced by progesterone. The rule for estrogens is this: Use the lowest possible dose that gives symptom relief.

The ideal preparations match the hormones found naturally in the female body. These would include any combination of estrone and estradiol from a formulary pharmacy; Estrace, the Estraderm or Climara patch, or any other type of estradiol; or Ortho-Est, a type of estrone.

Note that estrogen given through the skin by patch or cream often results in much higher levels than oral preparations. In some cases, a woman will need only a tenth of the estrogen on her skin that she was taking as a pill. This is one of the reasons why monitoring hormone levels can be prudent.

Estriol

Women who have had breast cancer or an estrogen-associated neoplasia of any kind, as well as any women with concerns about breast cancer, are usually not considered suitable candidates for HT, although studies are contradictory in this regard. Some have found that taking low-dose estrogen doesn't increase their risk for breast cancer.[34] Suzanne Somers, a breast cancer survivor, has described her very positive experience with bioidentical hormones and has been vocal about their safety. An alternative bioidentical hormone for these women may be estriol, a somewhat weaker estrogen that seems to have a protective effect against breast cancer.[35] Henry Lemon, M.D., demonstrated this in a study of women with metastatic breast cancer. In a test group receiving estriol in dosages ranging from 2.5 to 15 mg per day, 37 percent experienced either remission or arrest of the cancer. A later study from Hebrew University of Jerusalem showed that in sufficient dosages, estriol actually has an antiestrogenic effect, preventing estradiol from binding to estrogen-sensitive tissue (such as breast and endometrium), which then doesn't form tumors.[36] In another study from Berkeley, researchers found that rats receiving a three-week treatment of estriol with progesterone had a significantly reduced incidence of breast cancer.[37] Clearly, more research is required in this area.

The bottom line is that estriol seems very promising as an estrogen for those women who are worried about breast cancer. The same is true for phytoestrogens (see below). Not only does estriol not cause excessive cell growth in the uterine lining[38] or breast tissue, but it's good at helping hot flashes[39] and preventing vaginal dryness, and it has an equal benefit on the skin collagen layer as the other estrogens.[40] But very high doses (12 mg or more per day) are required to affect bone density. Such doses generally cause nausea and are therefore not clinically appropriate. It is also worth noting that estriol has been linked with otosclerosis in some women, a genetically linked condition in which the three small bones in the middle ear fuse together and thus fail to transmit sound to the brain. The usual oral dose is 2 mg per day.

Progesterone

During perimenopause, estrogen levels often rise, while progesterone is the first hormone to fall. This situation is known as "estrogen dominance" and it is largely responsible for many of the PMS-like symptoms so common in perimenopause. Giving estrogen to a woman with estrogen dominance is like putting a match to gasoline. What she really needs is progesterone and/

or a good nutritional program including enough magnesium—and also some good adaptogenic herbs like maca or *Pueraria mirifica* (see below).

The voluminous research of Jerilynn Prior, M.D., coauthor of *The Estrogen Errors* (Praeger, 2009), clearly shows that progesterone therapy, not estrogen, should be given first to symptomatic perimenopausal women. Progesterone is a precursor molecule that the body can use to produce both estrogens and androgens. For example, the body may be able to make adequate DHEA from natural progesterone, which is why a common finding with natural progesterone supplementation is increased sex drive. (Alas, this doesn't work for everyone.)

As already mentioned, bioidentical progesterone is very different from the synthetic progestins, such as medroxyprogesterone acetate (Provera). Unlike Provera—which increases the risk of fatal coronary artery spasm (see the section later in this chapter on heart disease) and is also known to cause bloating, headaches, depression, and weight gain—bioidentical progesterone has no serious side effects at the usual doses and has no adverse effects on blood lipids.[41] Although there are circumstances in which a woman may need the strong pharmacologic effect of Provera, as in cases of heavy bleeding, for most purposes of symptom relief, bioidentical progesterone is far superior, with the additional advantage of a lack of side effects.

For clinical purposes, the usual conversion is 5 mg of Provera equals 100 mg of natural progesterone if a woman is using oral doses. In general, a significant amount of progesterone must be given to downregulate estrogen receptors in breast tissue and the uterine lining in order to inhibit the growth-hormone effect of estrogen replacement.[42] Transdermal 2 percent progesterone cream at a dose of one-quarter teaspoon (about 20 mg) has also been shown to result in physiologic levels of progesterone, and this is often all that a woman needs to counteract the effects of estrogen, though this must be individualized.

Many doctors believe that 2 percent progesterone creams such as Pro-Gest don't work because they don't result in increased blood levels. But research shows that small amounts of progesterone skin cream do indeed get absorbed into the bloodstream.[43] Serum levels of progesterone are often low when a woman is on progesterone creams because when progesterone is absorbed into the bloodstream, 80 percent of it will be bound to the plasma membranes of the red blood cells—the part that is thrown out when serum levels are checked. This is also the reason why salivary levels of hormones often measure higher than serum levels. Ideally, hormone levels will be monitored by a physician in a clinical setting. Most clinicians agree that how a patient feels on hormones is, ultimately, a far better measure of effectiveness than a blood or salivary hormone level. This has certainly been my experience.

For effectiveness, transdermal cream should contain a minimum of 375 mg progesterone per ounce. The following creams meet or surpass the standard: Pro-Gest, PhytoGest, OstaDerm, Progonol, ProBalance, and Serenity. The usual dose of these standardized progesterone creams is one-quarter to one-half teaspoon on the skin one or two times per day. There is virtually no danger of overdose, and many women use 375 to 400 mg, or the equivalent of an entire tube or jar, per week with no ill effects.

Bioidentical progesterone is also available in regular pharmacies in two forms: oral micronized progesterone under the brand name Prometrium and vaginal progesterone under the brand names Crinone 4% and 8% and Prochieve 4% and 8%.

Many preparations sold as wild yam (*Dioscorea*) creams may contain little or no progesterone. Although wild yams are one ingredient used in laboratory manufacture of progesterone and other sex hormones, there are no data to indicate that a yam cream will help a woman in the same manner as standardized formulas. Wild yam may have benefits as a phytohormone (plant hormone); it's just that it doesn't have the same measurable effects.

Androgens

As I pointed out in the section on adrenal function, the androgenic hormones DHEA and testosterone are associated with energy, vitality, and sex drive. However, it's also true that the female brain is the biggest sex organ in the body and optimal libido is critically linked with one's thoughts and emotions. Hence some women with low androgen levels have good libido and some with normal androgen levels have low libido. Androgen levels may drop following hysterectomy even when the ovaries are spared; they may also drop following tubal ligation because of the change in blood supply to the ovary. Many women who don't feel their best even on estrogen and progesterone find that taking a small amount of DHEA or testosterone is all they need to feel like their old selves. DHEA is a precursor for testosterone, so I prefer trying this first. The herb *Pueraria mirifica* has also helped many, many women regain their sex drive (see below).

If you think you might benefit from increased androgen levels, first try transdermal magnesium and/or transdermal progesterone, or try *Pueraria mirifica*. As I've noted, these can help the body produce its own DHEA or the equivalent effect from a plant sterol. If symptoms persist, try oral or transdermal DHEA at a starting dose of 5 mg twice per day. It's rare that a woman will need to increase this much beyond 10 mg twice per day. A study in the journal *Menopause* reported that daily doses of DHEA taken intravaginally improved sexual functioning, including desire, arousal, orgasm, and lubrication.[44] Some women, however, will need testosterone supplementation directly, which can be given in pill form or as a cream. Many women find that natural testosterone at 1 or 2 mg every other day given as a vaginal cream clears up both vaginal dryness and libido problems. A formulary pharmacist can compound either testosterone or DHEA cream for either transdermal or oral use with a prescription. *Pueraria mirifica* as a vaginal gel is also very effective (see Resources).

SYMPTOMS OF MENOPAUSE

What you're likely to experience in menopause has a lot to do with your beliefs, your culture, and your expectations. Given the culture of medicine, it's no surprise that the vast majority of studies through the years have been on women who were experiencing health problems during menopause. The medical system (which is simply a reflection of the larger culture) has only very recently begun to study the menopausal experience of healthy women who exercise regularly, don't smoke, eat a good diet, and lead a healthy lifestyle. And just as one might suspect, these studies are showing that many healthy women have no problems with bone loss, sex drive, cardiovascular disease, or depression.

The research on traditional cultures in which women's experiences are quite different is fascinating. For example, medical anthropologist Anne Wright, Ph.D., studied menopausal symptoms in both traditional and acculturated Navajo women. She found that traditional Navajos exhibited fewer menopausal symptoms than acculturated Navajos, and that economic ranking and social status were clearly related to women's experience of symptoms. Her study suggested that menopausal symptoms are caused by psychological stress rather than physical stress.[45]

A study of !Kung women in southern Africa showed that their social status increased after menopause. Moreover, there is no word for "hot flash" in the !Kung language. This points to the possibility that !Kung women either do not experience this symptom or experience it in a manner different from Western women and do not view it in a negative light.[46] By contrast, 80 to 90 percent of women in our culture experience hot flashes, and a significant number have vaginal dryness and loss of libido.

HOT FLASHES

Hot flashes, or vasomotor flushes, are characterized by a feeling of heat and sweating, particularly around the head and neck. They affect anywhere from 50 to 85 percent of women at some time during their climacteric years. For most women, hot flashes are simply an occasional sensation of warmth and slight sweating, but about 10 to 15 percent of women experience hourly waves of heat and drenching sweats that disrupt daily activities and can result in sleep disturbance and subsequent depression. Hot flashes usually subside in a year or so, but some women have them for anywhere from ten to forty years.[47] The actual cause of hot flashes is not known; it is thought to be related to neurotransmitter changes that are poorly understood. Women may experience hot flashes during their adolescence and reproductive years, after having a baby, and premenstrually for reasons other than estrogen deficiency. Hot flashes have also been shown to increase when a woman is anxious or tense. This is because the stress hormones, adrenaline and cortisol, adversely affect the way other hormones are metabolized. Excess stress hormones from worry, depression, sleep deprivation, and nutritional deficiency are often the root cause of hot flashes that go on for years or that do not respond well to standard treatments.

Treatment

Nutritional Treatments. Many, many women notice vast improvements in sleep and hot flashes when they reduce their glycemic stress. (See chapter 17.) Hot flashes almost always improve when you stop wine, sugar, white flour products, and coffee. (Sorry.) The reason for this is that these substances can raise blood sugar and adrenaline levels, thus resulting in imbalances of neurotransmitters. Take vitamin E (d-alpha-tocopherol), 100 to 400 IU two times per day,[48] and citrus bioflavonoids with ascorbic acid, 200 mg four to six times daily.[49] Omega-3 fats such as those found in flaxseed and fish oil are also very helpful.

Phytoestrogens. Phytoestrogens (also known as isoflavones) are naturally occurring estrogen-like substances found in more than 300 plants, including soybeans and flaxseed (two particularly rich sources). Significant amounts of phytoestrogens are also found in cashews, peanuts, oats, corn, wheat, apples, and almonds.[50] Phytoestrogens contain isoflavonoids, which are chemically similar to the estrogens found in the human body (although not identical). These substances prevent free-radical damage (the number one cause of premature tissue aging) and appear to block the effects of excess estrogen stimulation of the breast and uterus. (The genistein in soy products shows promise for decreasing cancer risk as well.) Phytoestrogens also decrease menopausal symptoms and modulate estrogen levels. It is hypothesized that Japanese women have a lower incidence of hot flashes and other symptoms in part because of their high intake of soy-based products.[51]

Soy protein, when taken in high enough dosages, has been shown to improve hair, skin, and nails; cool hot flashes; increase vaginal moisture; help with weight loss; and also improve quality of life. A double-blind, randomized, placebo-controlled study of ninety-three postmenopausal women done at Johns Hopkins University School of Medicine in Baltimore showed that daily consumption of soy protein (in the form of Revival products) reduced hot flashes and night sweats as well as improved the quality of life for the women in the study.[52] Many women have personally told me how much this high-dose soy product has helped them. One wrote, "Revival has transformed my life! This last summer, my days were plagued by hot sweats, broken nails, and limp hair, plus I was overweight. Now, after four months of using Revival daily, I am twenty-four pounds lighter, my hair and nails are not brittle, and my sweats are completely gone. I am now in a new relationship. I feel like a new woman, young and vital, and without the symptoms of menopause I look and feel wonderful. I know I do not look fifty-two years old." (For more information on Revival, see their website at www.soy.com.)

Botanicals. A wide variety of herbs have been used to alleviate menopausal symptoms since antiquity. One of the most studied is an extract of black cohosh (*Cimicifuga racemosa*), sold under the name Remifemin, and available in pharmacies and natural food stores. It has been shown to improve vaginal lubrication and to reduce depression, headache, and hot flashes. The usual dose is two tablets twice daily.[53] A form of black cohosh known as BNO 1055, contained in the preparations Menopret (formerly Klimadynon) and MenoFem, was shown to calm hot flashes in breast cancer survivors as well as conjugated estrogens did, completely eliminating hot flashes in 47 percent of the women in the study.[54]

Other herbs shown to be helpful are *Vitex agnus-castus,* Siberian ginseng, dong quai, fo-ti, red clover, and wild yam.[55] Tinctures and oral combinations of these are widely available in natural food stores. They must be used for four to six weeks before improvement in symptoms is noted. Chinese herbal remedies have also been shown to reduce menopausal symptoms. Several excellent formulations are available; consult an individual practitioner. Note that botanicals and all other natural treatments for hot flashes tend to take longer to work than estrogen. Recent studies show that while all women improved on black cohosh and red clover, both of which were found to be safe, they didn't improve significantly more than the placebo group.[56] Even so, the botanicals didn't have an adverse effect on cognitive function the way synthetic estrogen did.[57] Moreover, many individual women do very well on these herbs.

Nutrafem is a phytoestrogen combination that has been found to reduce hot flashes by 46 percent in one study.[58] The researchers further reported that 43 percent of women taking Nutrafem (a formulation of two botanical extracts—*Eucommia ulmoides* bark and *Vigna radiata,* or mung beans) experienced a 50 percent reduction in menopausal symptoms. Women reported relief after seven days of taking this supplement. Nutrafem is available online at www.nutrafem.com.

Pueraria mirifica. Also known as Thai kudzu, *Pueraria mirifica* (PM) has been shown to be very effective at relieving menopausal symptoms, including vaginal dryness, hot flashes, insomnia, and irritability. Thirteen different species are native to Thailand, but only one has been used for seven millennia by both men and women for its hormone-like effects. The standardized form of PM contains a potent plant sterol known as miroestrol, which is particularly effective for relieving menopause symptoms safely and effectively. Miroestrol has estrogen-like effects on bone and vaginal tissue, while also protecting the breasts and endometrium from the adverse effects of excess estrogen.[59] In one study that compared PM with conjugated equine estrogens (Premarin), PM had an estrogenic effect that was similar to Premarin but without the side effects.[60] Thai researchers showed that over a period of six months, PM decreased all menopausal symptoms, including hot flashes and night sweats, from moderately severe to mild (with the most significant drop occurring during the first thirty days of taking the herb).[61] More recent research on PM shows it is effective on twenty different menopausal symptoms, including headache and mood instability.[62] Several studies show it benefits bone health[63] and can help prevent osteoporosis if taken early in menopause, before bone loss begins.[64] Aside from menopausal issues, a 2009 study shows PM can halt the growth of breast cancer cells in vitro (in the lab),[65] while a 2017 study on humans shows PM halts abnormal cell growth in the uterus.[66] (Interestingly enough, Thailand has one of the lowest incidences of breast cancer in the world, particularly in the areas where the most potent forms of PM are grown.)

To obtain the benefits of PM, you need a product that contains standardized miroestrol (approximately 20 mg of miroestrol per 100 grams). I have been so impressed with the effects of this herb—both for women and for men (to promote prostate health)—that I started my own company, Amata Life, which manufactures *Pueraria mirifica* products according to the highest standards (see www.amatalife.com).

Maca. Species of maca grow all over many South American countries, but only the maca from Peru has been studied in any significant way. Maca is a dietary staple in Peru and has high nutritional content. It is an adaptogenic plant, which means that it helps modulate the body's response to stress of all kinds. The herb has been traditionally used to benefit the endocrine and reproductive systems of both men and women. Research shows that maca increases the production of sex hormones, enhances sex drive, increases energy, and also results in mental improvement in many. Its properties make it a particularly useful herb for perimenopausal and menopausal women.[67] Femmenessence MacaPause, a formulation of maca that has guaranteed potency and excellent bioavailability, is made by Symphony Natural Health (www.symphonynaturalhealth.com).

Natural Progesterone. Natural progesterone has been shown to help hot flashes in some women.[68] This effect is most likely ascribable to the fact that it is a precursor hormone and also because it downregulates estrogen receptors.

Hormone Therapy. The gold standard treatment for relief of hot flashes is estrogen therapy, but many, many women have quelled their hot flashes with other methods. Note that *not* all hot flashes are related to decreases in estrogen. Hyperthyroidism can cause them, as can alcohol intake and out-of-control diabetes. I had hot flashes during my pregnancies and sometimes premenstrually. Many women report similar patterns.

Energy Medicine. Meditation, relaxation, and slow, deep abdominal breathing can help to relieve hot flashes.[69] The relaxation response (see PMS section in chapter 5) has been successfully used by many women to decrease hot flashes by as much as 90 percent.[70] Traditional Chinese medicine and herbs are also very effective. The reason these work is that they all reduce levels of stress hormones that trigger hot flashes. The adrenal restoration program (see page 654) will also reduce hot flashes.

VAGINAL DRYNESS, IRRITATION, AND THINNING

Thinning of vaginal tissue in menopause is associated with decreased estrogen levels. Vaginal tissue is made of many cell layers. When the vaginal mucosa is well estrogenized, it is called "cornified epithelium." *Cornified* refers to cells that are tough and resilient. After menopause, some women lose the outer cornified layers of their vaginal tissue. This can lead to complaints of vaginal dryness and irritation. Such complaints are highly individual and subjective; a woman who has been diagnosed with atrophic vaginitis may not have any symptoms at all. In some women, thinning and irritation are accompanied by an increase in the vagina's alkalinity. At these higher pH levels, bacterial vaginitis sometimes results.

The phytohormones mentioned above often work well to restore vaginal tissue, particularly *Pueraria mirifica* and high-dose soy (such as Revival). For some women, an application of estrogen cream or *Pueraria mirifica* cream directly to the vagina may be all that's required. Studies show *Pueraria mirifica* to be safe and effective.[71] Transdermal estrogen or the vaginal ring (Estring) are also very effective. In fact, research shows that using 0.1 percent estradiol gel for twelve weeks not only improved hot flashes but also increased the estradiol/estrone ratio in postmenopausal women to premenopausal levels.[72] A low-dose synthetic conjugated estrogen cream (made with Premarin) used twice per week has also recently been shown to be helpful, with no endometrial problems.[73]

Urinary frequency and symptoms of urinary tract infection are sometimes also associated with thinning of the vaginal mucosa and urethral tissues. (See the section on UTIs and hormones in chapter 9.) This problem is easily alleviated by applying a small amount of estrogen or *Pueraria mirifica* cream directly to the vaginal tissue covering the outer third of the urethra, which you can feel running just beneath the top of the vaginal opening.

Treatment

Botanicals. *Pueraria mirifica* (see above) and high-dose soy (such as Revival) have been found to relieve vaginal dryness in many women. Remifemin (black cohosh) works similarly to estriol to effect a thickening of the vaginal mucosa. Herbs such as dandelion leaves and oatstraw have also been used to restore vaginal lubrication.[74] These herbs should be taken orally.

Lubricants. There is a wide range of effective lubricants that have been shown to work well, ensuring that there's a lubricant available to suit just about every taste.[75] Over-the-counter options include K-Y Jelly, Sylk, Probe, and Good Clean Love, to name a few. Organic coconut oil works very well, too. A vaginal gel containing *Pueraria mirifica* is also available.

Testosterone. One-half mg to 1 mg transdermally or as vaginal cream, daily or every third day, will restore vaginal mucosa function without the risk of creating excessively high systemic estrogen levels.[76]

Estriol. Estriol vaginal cream is applied in a dosage of 0.5 mg twice a day for one week, then once a day for one week, and two or three times weekly thereafter. Concerns surrounding the effect of estrogens on breast cancer are mitigated by the use of estriol, which exerts a very powerful local action but is weak systemically.[77]

Estradiol Vaginal Ring. Estring is a vaginal ring made of silicone and impregnated with estradiol. It is placed in the vagina like a diaphragm and continually releases small doses of estradiol for three months. It is a convenient choice for many women. A small percentage of women will experience side effects such as recurrent vaginal infections, headache, and vaginal irritation.

Conventional Vaginal Creams. Estrace (estradiol) is a bioidentical estrogen cream that works well for treatment of vaginal dryness, thinning, and other symptoms.

Use It or Lose It. The very act of regular vaginal stimulation, whether through intercourse or through use of a jade egg, vibrator, or dildo, helps keep vaginal tissue healthy and well vascularized. Many women notice that their initial vaginal dryness goes away with this practice.

OSTEOPOROSIS

Postmenopausal osteoporosis is one of the most common and disabling diseases affecting women in North America today. Studies have shown a 2 to 5 percent loss in bone mass per year in women over a five-year period during and after menopause. A loss of bone in and of itself does not necessarily increase a woman's risk for fractures. It is, instead, the decrease in quality of bone that is the issue. Osteoporosis has been called "scurvy of the bone" and I tend to agree. Treating all women with low bone density as though it were a disease puts far too many women at risk for the side effects resulting from drugs such as alendronate (sold as Fosamax) that interrupt the natural remodeling of bone. So instead of convincing all women with low bone density that their bones are at risk, let's instead focus on what builds healthy bone and what doesn't.

Risk factors for poor bone quality (what we call osteoporosis or osteopenia) include the following: lack of exercise; a diet high in refined carbohydrates; deficiencies in calcium, magnesium, boron, trace minerals, and vitamin D; and never having borne a child. Depression has also been shown to be a significant risk factor for osteoporosis, most likely due to the increased levels of cortisol usually associated with this condition.[78]

As much as 50 percent of a woman's bone loss over a life span is lost before the onset of menopause, which is why it's important to begin following a healthy lifestyle as soon as possible—starting in childhood!

A history of ovulatory disturbances and subsequent progesterone deficiency can predispose women to osteoporosis. Women with a history of amenorrhea due to a low percentage of body fat, as is often found in athletes and dancers, are at greater risk for osteoporosis than the general population.[79] Statistics show that 6 to 18 percent of women between the ages of twenty-five and thirty-four exhibit abnormally low bone density. Although low bone density is responsible for many hip fractures, two studies have shown that a predisposition to falling created by "senile gait" (a shuffling, tentative walking style caused by muscle weakness and general lack of fitness) and poor eyesight is equal to low bone density as a significant factor for hip fracture risk.[80] Hip fracture rates for white women in the United States begin to rise abruptly between the ages of forty and forty-four, before the normal advent of menopause.[81] This is the time when your body will no longer let you get away with the unhealthy lifestyle you've been living up to that point.

Bone density screening is recommended in general for women who are sixty-five and older, or for younger postmenopausal women with certain risk factors (including those who smoke, have a history of excessive alcohol intake, suffer from rheumatoid arthritis, have a history of taking steroid drugs, or have a mother diagnosed with severe osteoporosis).

The best way to determine your current bone density is through a screening test called dual-energy X-ray absorptiometry (DEXA). It can be used on the hips, spine, forearm, or entire body. It is brief (under ten minutes) and safe, because it uses a very low dose of radiation. Make sure that the technician doing the test is thoroughly trained in densitometry. If they are not, your test results could be skewed. You also want to be tested on the same machine for subsequent testing because there can be significant variations between machines.

The biggest problem with the test is that if you are small-boned, it may suggest that you have osteoporosis or are at significant risk for it even if your bone quality is good. In other words, your bones may register in the lower range compared with an entire population, even though they may well have been in this range for your entire life. So do not allow one test result to cause undue stress. But do let it spur you on to a more bone-healthy lifestyle. In general, women going through perimenopause can lose 1 to 3 percent of their bone mass per year for a period of five to ten years. This need not be a problem if you enter perimenopause with peak bone mass. But many women already have suboptimal bone mass in their thirties and forties because of risk factors like smoking, anorexia (even years earlier), steroid drug use, antidepressants, clinical depression, excess alcohol intake, being on diuretics, or a host of other factors. If you are at risk for osteoporosis, it's very important that you seek the care of a professional who understands bone quality and bone health. I also highly recommend urine tests that determine your rate of bone loss. These are the NTx test and Pyrilinks test, which measure collagen breakdown products. The matrix of bone is made from collagen. Minerals attach to it. Testing for bone breakdown products is a very useful way to monitor any bone-building program because it will show improvement long before you are likely to see it on a DEXA test. You also need to be tested for parathyroid abnormalities. Small tumors of the parathyroid gland that cause people to lose bone too quickly require surgery, and the very best place to go for that is the Norman Parathyroid Center in Tampa, Florida (see www.parathyroid.com). Parathyroid surgery is their specialty and they see people from all over the world. If you are at risk for osteoporosis and have had a low DEXA test reading, please read *Dr. Lani's No-Nonsense Bone Health Guide: The Truth About Density Testing, Osteoporosis Drugs, and Building Bone Quality at Any Age* (Turner House Publishing, 2014) by Lani Simpson, D.C.

Bone Health Program

Although estrogen replacement is very effective for decreasing osteoporosis risk, preventing progressive bone loss in women requires dealing with far more complex factors. A program of dietary adjustments; exercise with just the right amount and type of stress on the bones and joints; and supplementation with vitamin D, calcium, and magnesium can also be very effective in preventing, halting, or even reversing bone loss. In fact, suboptimal vitamin D levels are increasingly implicated in osteoporosis. Research presented at the 2009 meeting of the American Society for Bone and Mineral Research showed that combining a home-based physiotherapy program with high-dose supplementation of vitamin D significantly reduced the rate of falls and hospital readmissions in the elderly.[82] And while dairy products are pushed as a panacea to prevent osteoporosis, it's entirely possible to create and maintain healthy bones without eating dairy. (See box below.) In fact, studies in both pre- and postmenopausal women report that consuming soy and soy isoflavones help to support better bone structure.[83] Miroestrol, a potent phytoestrogen found in the Thai herb *Pueraria mirifica* (see above), increases bone density in rats who've had their ovaries removed—a sign that this same herb might work well in humans.[84]

One of my patients went in for a bone density test when she went through menopause at the age of fifty-three. It showed that her bone density was low normal. Her mother had died of breast cancer when my patient was thirteen, so she had no intention of going on estrogen. Instead, she was immediately advised to start taking Fosamax, a drug that prevents bone breakdown, and get the scan repeated in six months. She called me, deeply concerned that her bones were melting away. I reassured her that this wasn't the case and suggested a program of weight training, *Pueraria mirifica,* and supplementation with boron, calcium, magnesium, vitamin D, vitamin C, and trace minerals (see below). Within six months, her bones had shown a significant increase in density. The doctor at the osteoporosis center told her that he was very surprised at her results, and said that she should keep on doing whatever she was doing. She has had a scan every two years since then and her density has remained excellent.

LOW-ACID DIET:
BETTER THAN CALCIUM FOR PREVENTING OSTEOPOROSIS

While for years doctors have been recommending dietary calcium as the best way to ward off osteoporosis, many studies cast doubt on this idea. For example, a 2003 Harvard study looked at diet and hip fractures among 72,337 older women for eighteen years and concluded that "neither milk nor a high-calcium diet appears to reduce [fracture] risk."[85] A more recent Harvard study, this one from 2007, analyzed seven trials that followed a total of 170,991 women for several years and found no association between total calcium intake and hip fracture risk.[86]

The truth is that calcium isn't all it's cracked up to be when it comes to bone health. After all, in Africa and Asia, where people generally don't take calcium supplements and after infancy consume little or no dairy, fracture rates are 50 to 70 percent lower than they are in the United States. Statistics show that most industrially advanced countries have the highest fracture rates, although they consume more dairy products than other countries.

Amy Lanou, Ph.D., an assistant professor of health and wellness at the University of North Carolina, Asheville, and medical writer Michael Castleman came to a remarkable conclusion after reviewing 1,200 studies on the dietary risk factors for osteoporosis in researching their book, *Building Bone Vitality: A Revolutionary Diet Plan to Prevent Bone Loss and Reverse Osteoporosis* (McGraw-Hill, 2009). Of the 136 trials they found that examined the effects of dietary calcium on osteoporotic fracture risk, two-thirds of them showed that a high calcium intake does *not* reduce the number of fractures— even in those who took calcium (with vitamin D) during childhood. They also found that eating fruits and vegetables improved bone density in a whopping 85 percent of studies that looked at the effects of such foods.

It's not that calcium isn't valuable; it's just that it's not the holy grail it's been made out to be. "Think of calcium as the bricks in a brick wall of bones," Castleman writes in an article in *Natural Solutions*. "Bricks are essential, for sure, but without enough mortar— which comes in the form of about 16 other nutrients—the wall can't hold itself up."[87]

The key to preventing osteoporosis, they determined, is eating a low-acid diet. The basic idea is that a diet high in animal protein (including meat, poultry, fish, milk, and dairy), grain, and high-glycemic-index foods (refined carbs) makes blood slightly more acidic. When blood is more acidic, the body tries to balance or neutralize it by adding alkaline material the only way it can—by leaching some of the calcium compounds stored in bone. Eventually, osteoporosis results.

Whether a food is considered alkaline or acidic depends on the effect it has on the body after it's digested. Generally fruits and vegetables are considered alkaline, while meats and dairy products are considered acidic. It's important to note that while some foods (such as tomatoes, citrus fruits, and apples) may *taste* acidic, the effect they have on the body when they're metabolized is actually alkaline. Also, just as the proteins from animal sources are responsible for meat and dairy having an acidic effect, so are the proteins found in soy and most lentils and beans—although vegetable proteins do not generally have as strong an acidic effect as those from animal sources. (See *Building Bone Vitality* for charts showing the relative acidity and alkalinity of several different types of foods.)

In general, it takes three servings of fruits and vegetables to neutralize the acid in just one serving of animal food, and two servings of fruits and veggies to neutralize the acid in one serving of grain. (By the way, consuming dairy foods does add back calcium, but calcium from animal sources such as dairy is highly acidic, so it's like taking one step forward and two steps back.)

The bottom line: For healthy bones, your blood needs to maintain a slightly alkaline pH level (a measure of relative acidity or alkalinity), which you can achieve by eating at least five servings of fruits and vegetables for every one serving of red meat, chicken, or fish. (Another good idea is to eat vegan—no meat or dairy—one day a week, which is very easy given the wide availability of beans, tofu, and other plant-based proteins these days.)

Diet. Bones are dynamic organs that thrive in a mineral-rich environment. A refined-food diet is everywhere associated with weak bones and poor teeth. Follow the dietary program in chapter 17.

Exercise. Two forty-minute sessions per week of weight training have been shown to increase bone density as much as estrogen, according to research by Miriam Nelson, Ph.D., director of the Center for Physical Activity and Nutrition at Tufts University and author of *Strong Women, Strong Bones* (Perigee, 2006). Dr. Nelson further reports that higher-impact activities (including vertical jumping and stair climbing), when done safely, can also help build bone. She recommends a comprehensive exercise program that includes weight-bearing aerobic exercise, strength training, vertical jumping (when appropriate and for women under fifty), balance exercises, and stretching. Walking, bicycling, and climbing all keep bones well mineralized by putting stress on them, which creates a mini-electrical current that draws minerals into the bone.

Several studies have shown Pilates to be helpful in increasing bone mineral density.[88] However, it's important if you already have osteoporosis or osteopenia to avoid exercises that involve forward bending (especially when twisting), including lifting your head while lying on your back (moves that a Mayo Clinic study showed could induce vertebral fractures in those who are susceptible).[89] If this applies to you, just tell your instructor you need to avoid those moves in class, or even better, have a private session. Almost all Pilates exercises can be modified, so that need not be a deterrent. Research also shows yoga to be helpful for building bone. One study with 227 people (202 of them women) assessed the effectiveness of doing a specific twelve-minute yoga routine (with twelve different poses) at least every other day for two years.[90] The average age of the participants at the start of the study was sixty-eight, with 83 percent reporting low bone density at that time. Ten years later, DEXA scan reports showed significant increases in bone density in the spine and femur with lower gains in the hip.

Proper alignment of the skeleton is also crucial for maintaining healthy bones and hips throughout life (see chapter 18, on exercise). Pilates and yoga are also excellent for alignment, as is Esther Gokhale's Primal Posture training (see www.gokhalemethod.com).

Reduce Phosphorus Consumption. Phosphorus directly interferes with calcium absorption. Eliminate cola and root beer drinks (as well as any other dark-colored soft drinks), which are too high in phosphorus and which also contain coloring agents that interfere with calcium absorption.

Quit Smoking and Cut Back on Alcohol. Since smokers, along with women who consume two or more alcoholic drinks daily, are at highest risk for osteoporosis, women should refrain from smoking and limit alcohol intake.[91]

Limit Caffeine. Caffeine increases the rate at which calcium is lost in the urine. Daily intake should be limited to no more than the equivalent of the caffeine in one to two cups of coffee.[92]

Decrease Stress Hormones. If you are depressed or under chronic stress, get help. Depression increases the risk for osteoporosis. The stress hormone known as cortisol is higher in depressed or chronically stressed individuals, and over time, this hormone results in bone (and skin) breakdown.

Vitamin D. As you will recall from the breast chapter, an optimal level of vitamin D is 40–100 ng/ml. According to Michael Holick, M.D., Ph.D., chief of Endocrinology, Metabolism, and Nutrition at Boston University School of Medicine, blood levels less than 20 ng/ml can cause osteoporosis,[93] while the lowest average blood concentration for vitamin D that demonstrates fracture reductions is equivalent to 30 ng/ml.[94] Consuming adequate levels of vitamin D is associated with lower risk of hip fractures in postmenopausal women, according to research from Brigham and Women's Hospital and Harvard Medical School.[95] Take at least 2,000 IU of vitamin D per day.[96] (For a more detailed discussion of the importance of vitamin D, see chapter 17.)

Beta-Carotene. Take 25,000 IU per day (15 mg). Beta-carotene is converted into vitamin A in the body. Vitamin A promotes a healthy intestinal epithelium, which is important for optimal absorption of nutrients, and it also promotes strong joints. It is found in abundance in yellow and orange vegetables such as acorn squash and carrots and also in dark green leafy vegetables.

Natural Progesterone. Progesterone's role in bone metabolism is well documented but frequently overlooked.[97] I recommend one-quarter to one-half teaspoon of 2 percent cream daily on the skin.

Vitamin C. This nutrient assists in collagen synthesis and repair. The recommended dose is 2,000 mg per day.[98] The work of Linus Pauling, Ph.D., suggests that optimal vitamin C intake should be much higher than we've been taught. An orange provides only 60 mg per day, but Dr. Pauling's evidence is quite convincing that vitamin C is beneficial and has no side effects at levels around 2,000 mg per day or even more.

Magnesium. Though calcium gets all the credit when it comes to bone health, magnesium is equally important. Magnesium is a constituent of bone and is essential for several biochemical reactions involved in bone building. As already mentioned in the discussion of adrenal health, the standard American diet is low in magnesium. A diet low in magnesium and relatively high in calcium actually contributes to osteoporosis. Though blood levels of magnesium may be normal, this is misleading. A more accurate test is red blood cell magnesium, which is often low in cases of depression and fatigue. (See the section on magnesium in chapter 17.) Overconsumption of processed food is usually the culprit in magnesium deficiency. This nutrient is found in organically grown vegetables, whole grains, sea vegetables, and meats such as turkey. I recommend a magnesium supplement daily at a dose of 400 to 800 mg per day, depending upon the quality of your diet.[99]

Manganese. This nutrient should be supplemented in the form of manganese picolinate. The recommended dose is 15 mg per day.

Calcium. Taking calcium without vitamin D is almost useless. That said, calcium supplementation is valuable. Take 500 to 1,500 mg per day in the form of aspartate, citrate, or lactate. You can take less if you obtain significant amounts from your food. Despite widespread promotion of the antacid Tums as a way to obtain needed calcium, better supplements are available. Although the calcium carbonate found in Tums has been shown to increase bone density, it also reduces stomach acid, thereby inhibiting calcium absorption and increasing the risk of kidney stones.[100]

Boron. Boron is a trace element found in fruits, nuts, and vegetables. It has been found to reduce urinary calcium loss and to increase serum levels of 17-beta estradiol (the most biologically active estrogen); both of these effects help bone health. The minimum daily dose of boron needed (2 mg per day) is easily met with a diet rich in fruits, nuts, and vegetables; supplements can be taken up to 12 mg per day.[101]

A WARNING ABOUT BISPHOSPHONATES
(FOSAMAX, ACTONEL, AND BONIVA)

I'm very concerned about the long-term safety of bisphosphonates, drugs including alendronate (Fosamax), ibandronate (Boniva), and risedronate (Actonel) that are heavily marketed to women to prevent osteoporosis fractures. They are not the panacea for bone health that they appear to be. In fact, they can be downright dangerous. They inhibit bone resorption by cells known as osteoclasts, which are necessary for the continual remodeling of bone that occurs throughout life. Here's the problem with that. Suppressing bone turnover creates excessive mineralization of bone, which makes it more brittle. When bone gets too thick, blood vessels can't get in to nourish it, either. Animal studies indicate that alendronate also inhibits normal repair of microdamage to bone, resulting in eventual accumulation of microdamage and loss of bone strength. For these reasons, studies have shown spontaneous nontraumatic spinal and also atypical femur fractures in individuals taking this drug. In one study, severe reduction in bone formation was found in all the patients studied.[102] Orthopedic surgeons have increasingly been reporting atypical femur fractures that don't heal in women on alendronate.[103]

Though drug companies quote the widely publicized study showing a 50 percent reduction in risk of fracture with alendronate, what they don't tell you is that this result is seen only in those who already have osteoporosis, not healthy women who are taking the drug to prevent the problem. It is estimated that you'd have to treat a hundred women with the drug to benefit just one woman.[104]

More confusion resulted when two studies reported in 2009 appeared to link taking oral bisphosphonates (including alendronate) with a decreased risk for breast cancer—one study by 32 percent and the other by 34 percent.[105] Yet even top cancer doctors were hesitant to get too excited about this association for some very good reasons. First of all, neither of these studies was a randomized clinical trial—both were observational studies of data that already existed. Also, women taking these drugs for low bone density often have lower estrogen levels, which may give them a lower breast cancer risk to begin with, because a woman's risk for breast cancer increases with higher exposure to estrogen over her lifetime.

Here's another potential side effect that is truly frightening: death of the bone tissue (osteonecrosis) of the jaw—a condition that is not treatable.[106] Many individuals have also found that they require root canals soon after beginning alendronate. The reason for both these conditions is most likely inadequate circulation to the root of the teeth through the jaw and to the jaw itself. Atypical femur fractures (right in the middle of the thigh bone) have also been reported in women who have been using the drug for more than five years.[107] These fractures don't heal.

To make matters worse, bisphosphonates stay in the circulation for decades, even after women stop taking them, because they bind tightly to bone. Therefore, alendronate, if used at all, should be reserved for much older postmenopausal women (age seventy or older) with major risk factors for osteoporosis. And even then, treatment should be limited to five years or less.[108]

SEXUALITY IN MENOPAUSE

What we believe about sexuality and menopause has a lot to do with our sexual expectations and experience. A very common misconception about menopause is that sexual desire and activity significantly decline during this period. Yet research fails to show any significant link between menopause and decreased sexual functioning.[109] Because our society has viewed menopause as "failed productivity" and associates reproductive capacity with sexual capacity, many women have bought the belief that their sex drive is supposed to go away. But in humans, the capacity for sexual pleasure and the capacity for reproduction are two distinct functions. We can always have one without the other.

Research shows that in healthy, happy women, there's no significant decline in libido, let alone in sexual satisfaction, frequency of sexual intercourse, genital responsiveness, and ease or difficulty reaching orgasm after menopause. In fact, a woman's relationship satisfaction, attitudes toward sex and aging, vaginal dryness, cultural background, and overall mental and physical health have a much greater impact on sexual functioning than does being in menopause. That's why many of my menopausal patients who left unsatisfying marriages and found more compatible mates ended up having better sex lives than ever. Since that time, I've been astounded by the number of women who are enjoying great sex in their sixties, seventies, and eighties.

The number one predictor of good sex during and after menopause is a new partner! Instead of trading in your old partner, however, my advice to most women is to become a new partner yourself. In other words, when you begin the work of reinventing yourself instead of being stuck in outmoded patterns of anger and resentment, you will find that your sex life is bound to improve. This is partly why the research of Gina Ogden, Ph.D., shows that women in their sixties and seventies are having the best sex of their lives.[110]

I remember one very proper seventy-five-year-old woman who always came in dressed formally in blouses with high lace collars. She was having a problem with some vaginal dryness and was worried that she'd have to stop her sexual activity. Newly married, she was regularly having seven orgasms per lovemaking session with her husband, after being anorgasmic for her entire forty years of marriage with her first husband. She told me that she had had no idea how wonderful sexual activity could be. All she needed was a bit of estrogen cream and some reassurance that she was normal.

Another woman, age fifty-five, was at her most sexually fulfilled when she began a relationship with a man fifteen years younger than she. The combination of an older woman and younger man in this regard makes perfect sense—though up until very recently, this has gone against everything that our culture has taught us. Sexual preference may also change at midlife. Several of my patients have found themselves sexually attracted to women after menopause, although they had defined themselves as heterosexual beforehand. Research shows that women's sexuality is far more fluid than we've been led to believe, so this makes sense.[111]

Some women truly do notice a decline in libido at menopause. One of them told me that her lack of libido is not a problem for her personally, but she does worry about her husband getting enough sex. I suspect that this concern is shared by many. One of the reasons that libido falls during perimenopause for some women is that their life force, or *chi,* is simply exhausted from years of stress and they have nothing left over for sexual desire. Many women find their energy turned inward for a time as they reinvent themselves at midlife. It is also clear that levels of testosterone, which play a role in sexual desire, decrease in many older women for a wide variety of reasons.[112] If this is the case, these androgenic hormones can be restored to normal levels.[113] (See the section on adrenal restoration in this chapter.) I've also received hundreds of testimonials from women all over the world about the fact that *Pueraria mirifica* has had a significantly positive effect on their sex lives, contributing to enhanced lubrication and libido.

For other women, however, the climacteric and postmenopausal periods are associated with heightened sexual drive and activity. For many, it is the first time that they are truly free from the fear of unwanted pregnancy. Many physicians mistakenly believe older women who are not sexually active lack sexual drive. But studies have shown that the reason they are not sexually active is usually that they have no available suitable partner, or their partner is ill, or they have vaginal thinning leading to pain with intercourse (a condition that is easily remedied with one of the suggestions on page 681). Of greatest importance to continued sexual desire and interest is marital happiness or happiness with your partner.[114]

Another problem for many heterosexual women is that their male partner's ability to get and maintain an erection may change as he ages. (This is not inevitable at all. Many men are sexually capable for life, regardless of age. As a seventy-five-year-old male friend points out, "It's all about the person you are with. This makes a huge difference in strength of erections.") If the male perceives erectile problems as "impotence," however, he may avoid sexual activity altogether. Many women have told me that they would like to enjoy regular sexual activity, but their husbands won't participate anymore because of their fears of impotence. Because these women are afraid of offending their husbands' egos, however, they keep quiet instead of getting help. The most important way they can help is to let their husbands know that they don't require an erect penis to be fulfilled. This is the time to get creative with hands, tongue, and so on. (See chapter 8.) Intercourse is such a limited way of expressing sexuality. And it's time that all couples begin to explore the range of other options.

A word about erectile dysfunction drugs. Pharmaceuticals such as Viagra, Levitra, and Cialis have helped many men achieve erections, but they haven't always helped with true intimacy. Besides, these drugs have been shown to have risks. The Health Research Group of the consumer advocacy organization Public Citizen has asked the FDA for a black-box warning on these drugs because reports of unilateral vision loss (loss of sight in one eye) have been linked to them. Men should also know, however, that the same diet and supplement programs that help support menopausal hormone balance in women also help men maintain optimal sexual function without drugs.[115] Usually all the help most men need is a bit of education. Still, antihypertensive and other medications can interfere with erection and even orgasmic capacity in some men. Lifestyle changes such as weight loss, improved diet, supplementation, and increased physical activity can reverse hypertension in those who are motivated enough to make them.

Recall, too, what I said in chapter 8—that a turned-on woman is what turns on a man. This concept is so important to health and well-being that I wrote a small book about it entitled *The Secret Pleasures of Menopause* (Hay House, 2008), which is really all about the health-enhancing properties of nitric oxide—the circulation-enhancing chemical produced by the lining of all blood vessels and which is the mechanism by which drugs such as Viagra work.

Treatment

Treatment for lack of sex drive must be highly individualized, keeping in mind that a woman's sexual response is strongly related to the quality of her relationship. At midlife, many women wake up to the fact that they've been living with narcissistic or abusive men. And their bodies just won't respond anymore.

Sexual response is also related to a woman's overall health. That said, all women with this problem should first consider the quality of their relationship. If they're in a high-quality relationship and are still having problems, they might consider having their testosterone and DHEA levels measured. If levels are low, the first line of treatment is to follow the program for adrenal restoration on page 654. If there is still a problem, some women report feeling more like their former selves on either phytoestrogens or mammalian estrogens. Others note an increase in libido following the use of a transdermal 2 percent progesterone cream, which may work, in part, because natural progesterone is a precursor molecule and can be turned into androgens and even estrogen when the body needs more of these hormones. Testosterone is the major androgen associated with libido. In those women who don't seem to be able to produce enough of their own androgens, DHEA or testosterone in the form of a cream, a gel, or a capsule can be given.

If both DHEA and testosterone levels are low, I prefer replenishing DHEA first, because it is a precursor of testosterone, and when women take it in the usual doses (10 to 20 mg per day), their testosterone levels increase by one and a half to two times.[116] When given with progesterone, DHEA can enhance well-being in those who don't respond to progesterone alone. Some older women have naturally high levels of DHEA, so not everyone needs it. The side effect of too much testosterone or DHEA is a slight increase in hair growth on arms and legs and sometimes the face.

The dose of testosterone for those who don't respond to DHEA is 1 to 2 mg every other day, depending upon the individual. Transdermal magnesium can also help increase DHEA (see page 676).

Other women have done well with homeopathic remedies, acupuncture, or herbs, especially *Pueraria mirifica*. You might also consider yoni egg practices (see chapter 8). This approach is perfect for women who want to retain their youthful appearance and sexual potency long after menopause. First championed by Grand Master Mantak Chia, it uses the mind to flow life force energy—especially potent ovarian energy—throughout the body.[117]

However, you don't need to get into ancient Taoist techniques to keep your sex drive strong. What you have to do is actually train your body to be able to receive more pleasure. This takes care of the life force all by itself. (See chapter 8.) Regularly experiencing pleasure magnetizes you to attract more of the same.

Whatever therapy you choose, there is likely to be a placebo effect on the libido simply because you are doing something to help yourself. Remember, sometimes it's your *life* that needs "medicine." When you make positive changes (including adding more pleasurable activities), your hormones will balance themselves. Because sexual function and libido are so intimately connected to our thoughts and emotions, it's also important for women who want to enhance libido to actually take the time to think about sex more often. Reading erotic material, watching erotic movies, and spending time self-pleasuring can often jump-start a flagging libido.

Note: Often Estratest, a combination of equine estrogens and synthetic methyltestosterone, is the only solution offered to women with libido problems. However, the dose is too high for many women and it is difficult to make adjustments. The hormones in it are also in forms that are foreign to the female body. I do not recommend it. Instead I recommend that you start with nutritional and herbal solutions, which are safer and don't require a prescription.

THINNING HAIR

Up to one-third of menopausal and postmenopausal women in this culture have problems with thinning hair. Confusingly, hair loss on the head may be accompanied by excess hair growth on the face. This is because all hair follicles are not created equal in their response to hormones. Much of this problem is related to subtle imbalances of hormones, at the level of the androgen-sensitive hair follicle, that do not show up on standard testing. These imbalances are associated with insulin resistance and overconsumption of refined carbohydrates. Here's a typical letter from a member of my online community:

> Dear Dr. Northrup,
> I am currently going through menopause. My hair has always been thick and healthy. I am starting to lose a great deal of hair. I had blood work done by my primary care provider and everything came back fine except for my hormone levels. My estrogen level is low and my testosterone level is at 77. He mentioned that high testosterone levels can cause hair loss. He recommended hormone replacement, which I choose not to do, or spironolactone. My concern is that he mentioned I would have to stay on this for life if I do not wish my hair to fall out. Is this true? I have changed my diet and am working out with weights and cardio. I would greatly appreciate your help. This is truly stressing me out.

The conventional approach to hair loss is drugs such as spironolactone. I do not have experience with them and prefer that women try a natural approach first.

Hair Restoration Plan

Try one or more of these approaches in the following order:

~ Check your thyroid. Hair loss is very often a sign of hypothyroidism. Your TSH should definitely be no higher than 3.0, although I recommend an upper limit of 2.5. If your levels are higher than that, try iodine supplementation or natural thyroid replacement, such as Nature-Throid (www .naturethroid.com), Allergy Research Group's TG 100 Natural Glandulars (www.allergyresearchgroup.com), Armour thyroid, or a mixture of T3 and T4 made up by a formulary pharmacist. (See page 660 for a fuller discussion of thyroid issues.)

~ Follow a diet that normalizes blood sugar and insulin and also decreases inflammation. (See chapter 17.) High blood sugar and high insulin levels skew hormone metabolism toward too many androgens. Also take a good multivitamin-mineral supplement.

~ Lose excess body fat.

~ Decrease stress. Stress hormones make *everything* worse and may even be the reason for the hair loss in the first place. As already stated, hormones produced by excess stress skew hormone metabolism into the androgen range. And if your diet is high in sugar and refined foods (alcohol, white bread, chips, and so on), then you have a double whammy. Massage and foot reflexology can help with stress.

~ Take supplemental iodine. (See chapter 17.)

If these approaches don't work within three months, try laser acupuncture or traditional needle acupuncture.

MOOD SWINGS AND DEPRESSION

Research shows that menopause itself does not contribute to poor psychological or physical health. In fact, menopausal women age forty-five to sixty-four actually have a significantly lower incidence of depression than younger women. Moreover, the major stress in the lives of menopausal women is most often caused by family or by factors other than menopause.[118] For example, approximately 25 percent of women in the menopausal years are caring for an elderly relative, according to some studies, which certainly can be stressful.[119] Sonja McKinlay, Ph.D., formerly an associate professor of community health at Brown University and currently CEO of New England

Research Institutes, who researched a group of healthy menopausal women who were not seeking medical advice, says, "For the majority of women, menopause is not the major negative event it has been typified as. That is basic mythology." She noted that only 2 to 3 percent of the women in her study expressed any regret at moving out of their reproductive years. One unique feature of this study is that it was done on healthy women who were not seeking medical advice. Clearly, many physicians have a negative view of menopause in part because they see only women who have menopause-related complaints.

As I pointed out earlier, however, menopause is a time when we may come up against the unfinished business that we have accumulated over the first half of our lives. We may find ourselves grieving for losses never fully grieved, wanting to get a college degree that we never completed, or longing for another child or a first child. It is as if we have gone down into our basement and found boxes and boxes of stuff to be sorted through and weeded out. If a woman is willing to deal with her own unfinished business, she will have fewer menopausal symptoms. She will find that her symptoms are messages from her inner guidance system that parts of her life need attention. And her changing hormones will provide the impetus to make long-needed changes.

Treatment

When a woman is willing to resolve the unfinished emotional business of her life, often no treatment of her mood swings is necessary. The inner work discussed in part three of this book is a good place to start. (There is a full treatment of this in the *Wisdom of Menopause* [Bantam, 2012].) Dietary improvement and exercise can often work wonders. Many women with depression have been following a diet that is so low in fat, they can't make the proper brain chemicals to lift depression. (See chapter 17.)

Most women require the physical support of their endocrine, energy, and emotional systems through hormone therapy, homeopathy, acupuncture, and/or other approaches. I highly recommend the book *A Mind of Your Own* (HarperCollins, 2016), by Kelly Brogan, M.D. Dr. Brogan's Vital Mind Reset Program (see www.kellybroganmd.com) has helped thousands of women recover from depression naturally. St. John's wort (*Hypericum perforatum*) has been shown to be very helpful in mild to moderate depression, allowing many women to get off their other antidepressant medication. Look for a standardized 0.3 percent formulation. The dose of St. John's wort is 300 mg three times per day with meals.[120] The herb *Pueraria mirifica* has also been shown to help with mood problems (see page 149).

Hormone therapy lifts depression in some women but has no effect on others. Each case has to be examined holistically to determine optimal treatment.

FUZZY THINKING

Many women talk about a perimenopausal change in their thought process. This "fuzzy thinking" is most commonly described as an inability to think straight, and is a normal development that is self-limiting. Marian Van Eyk McCain, in her book *Transformation Through Menopause* (Bergin & Garvey, 1991), calls this "cottonhead," or feeling unable to use the left brain or intellect for such tasks as balancing the checkbook or getting organized.[121] I have asked many women about this and have found it to be common. Many are very relieved to find that it is normal, because they are afraid they are getting Alzheimer's disease. There is no evidence to support the commonly held myth that women (or men) normally lose their memory or get "senile" as they age.[122] In fact, a very reassuring 2009 study of more than 2,000 women, headed by Gail A. Greendale, M.D., from the David Geffen School of Medicine at the University of California, Los Angeles, shows that while learning abilities may decrease during perimenopause, they rebound to premenopausal levels afterward.[123]

After I read about "cottonhead," I realized that I had felt this same way after having my children. I seemed virtually unable to concentrate on linear tasks. My brain felt fuzzy. I wanted to watch movies, be with my baby, and not have to think, at least in the limited way that our culture defines thinking. The way I understand this "cottonhead" state is that it may disconnect us temporarily from our frontal lobes, the part of the brain that is involved with rational, linear, planning-for-the-future thought. We now have a chance to think with our hearts. If we allow this process to unfold, if we don't fight it or see it as a dysfunction, it can be an initiation into a whole new way of experiencing the world, a far more intuitive way. For many women the ability to express themselves in art, writing, or sculpting comes from allowing their "cottonheadedness" to center them and help them withdraw from the world ruled by the steely organized intellect. Neuropsychiatrist Mona Lisa Schulz, M.D., Ph.D., author of *The New Feminine Brain* (Free Press, 2005), points out that temporarily forgetting names or where you put the phone is not caused by memory loss per se. These lapses are related, instead, to attention. Many perimenopausal women turn their attention deeply inward—a natural way to do healing work.

When Peggy, a fifty-eight-year-old kindergarten teacher, went through menopause, she began to experience an inability to concentrate in her classroom. "After thirty years as a teacher," she said, "I couldn't remember the names of the kids in my classes, and sometimes I couldn't even remember how to spell words." Every fiber of her being told her to take a sabbatical from teaching to give her inner life some attention. Her "thinking" problem became so bad that she eventually started crying in front of her classes. She realized that she needed a change. She left her job, traveled to California, and lived in a small cottage near the beach for a year. During that time, she began to knit. She found that knitting was exactly what her brain needed for meditative activity.

On a hunch, Peggy began to teach senior citizens the knitting techniques she was learning. She found that her skills were in great demand. She mailed a beach chair to me. She had hand-knitted the seat and the back in beautiful and unusual designs. In addition to her knitting, she allowed herself to grieve fully for the end of her marriage ten years before. She forgave herself for the impact that it had had on her son. By the time I saw her a year later, she was a healed woman with a great deal of trust in life. She had accepted the challenge of menopause, moved into her intuitive side, and begun a whole new life. She now spends half the year in California and half the year in Maine. She is back to a small amount of teaching, on her own terms. She no longer forgets names or class plans.

LONG-TERM HEALTH CONCERNS

Breast Cancer

The most common concern women have about taking hormones is the fear of breast cancer, and it's the main reason many women don't want anything to do with hormone therapy, even when it could help them. I believe that if the estrogen and progesterone used in HT were bioidentical, as previously described, and if they were used at dosages tailored to an individual woman, we would not find an increase in breast cancer risk.

Jerilynn Prior, M.D., founder and scientific director of the Centre for Menstrual Cycle and Ovulation Research (CeMCOR) in Vancouver, British Columbia, believes that progesterone might actually decrease the risk for invasive breast cancer because studies show it opposes the effects of estrogen.[124] Her research shows that estrogen levels are significantly higher than normal during perimenopause.[125] To counterbalance these high levels of estrogen, Dr. Prior, coauthor of *The Estrogen Errors* (Praeger, 2009), prescribes progesterone to successfully treat hot flashes, low bone density, and menstrual problems. I agree with her practice.

Isaac Schiff, M.D, chief of Vincent Memorial Obstetrics and Gynecology Service at Massachusetts General Hospital in Boston, keeps a breast cancer risk chart on his desk to help his patients see clearly what the estrogen–breast cancer statistics really mean for them personally. I have found this approach so helpful that I have reproduced the chart here. Risk of breast cancer must be kept in perspective.

TABLE 8

THE EFFECTS OF HORMONE THERAPY ON BREAST CANCER RISK

Your Current Age	Probability of Breast Cancer Diagnosis This Year	
	With 5 Years HT	Without HT
50–54	1 in 320	1 in 450
55–59	1 in 275	1 in 386
60–64	1 in 209	1 in 292
65–69	1 in 144	1 in 244

Source: Cancer Statistics Review 1973–1989, excerpted from the August 1995 issue of the *Harvard Women's Health Watch,* ©1995, President and Fellows of Harvard College.

As already mentioned, there is an association between excessive amounts of carbohydrates in the diet, high insulin levels, and breast cancer, so keep the amount of refined carbohydrates in your diet moderate.[126] Also, in a controlled trial of alcohol intake, women receiving oral Premarin and those on estrogen had an average 300 percent increase in estradiol levels for five hours following ingestion of alcohol. Those not receiving hormone therapy showed no comparable increase. Women should consequently be counseled to limit alcohol intake when on oral hormone therapy.[127]

Optimal approaches for a woman with breast cancer concerns include avoiding estrogen; using estriol, small amounts of progesterone, and botanicals; or using the minimum effective dose of estradiol or estrone. (See Program to Promote Healthy Breast Tissue in chapter 10.) Remember, too, that regular exercise dramatically decreases the risk of breast cancer.

Heart Disease

Heart disease is the leading killer of postmenopausal women. If you have any personal or family history of heart disease, understand that diet and lifestyle changes can reverse or greatly alleviate your risk of getting it, with or without estrogen. Chief among the risk factors for heart disease is increased insulin resistance, which is present to some degree in 50 to 75 percent of women in this country. Problems with insulin and overconsumption of refined carbohydrates result in increased body fat and aberrations in lipid profile.[128] (See chapter 17.) An enormous amount of data exists on the link between nutrition and heart disease, particularly with regard to the ill effects of excess insulin and the benefits of antioxidants. A study reported in the *American Journal of Clinical Nutrition* demonstrated that a diet too high in carbohydrates and low in fat increased the risk of heart disease because of its adverse effects on lipids and insulin. The authors concluded that given their results, "it seems reasonable to question the wisdom of recommending that postmenopausal women consume low-fat, high-carbohydrate diets."[129] I couldn't agree more. It has also been demonstrated that in individuals with stable angina (chest pain), a high-carbohydrate meal will induce a reduction in blood flow to the heart during a treadmill test much more quickly than a high-fat meal.[130] This is because the surge in high blood sugar following a refined carbohydrate meal creates free-radical damage in the lining of blood vessels that causes them to go into spasm. Over time, high blood sugar also hastens atherosclerosis.

A lifestyle characterized by overconsumption of trans fatty acids and refined carbohydrates, combined with inadequate amounts of protein and micronutrients and a lack of exercise, sets the stage for cellular inflammation, which in turn creates a predisposition to hypertension, diabetes, and heart disease.[131] By contrast, a diet that contains fish oil has been found to reduce the incidence of heart disease better than statin drugs in a number of studies. As a matter of fact, the regular consumption of fish oil reduces all causes of mortality, not just heart disease.[132] I'd recommend two servings per week of sardines, mackerel, salmon, or swordfish that is virtually mercury free[133] (such as products from Vital Choice Seafood; for more information, call Vital Choice at 800-608-4825 or visit www.vitalchoice.com). If you are a vegetarian, high-quality flaxseed oil, ground flaxseed, hemp seed oil, or macadamia nuts or oil can be beneficial. (See Resources.) Also follow the dietary guidelines in chapter 17.

Weight-bearing exercise can also be very helpful because it lowers insulin resistance dramatically. (See chapter 18.) It will help increase lean muscle, and because lean muscle mass has a higher metabolic rate than fat, it helps to burn excess body fat and thus lower the risk of heart disease. Women who perform such exercise live an average of six years longer than those who do not.

Recent studies have shown that natural progesterone has a protective effect on coronary arteries in women. In addition, low levels of progesterone (common during perimenopause) or consumption of synthetic progestins increase the risk of coronary artery spasm and subsequent chest pain in women. Natural progesterone has been shown to be very helpful in this regard—and at very low doses (one-quarter teaspoon of 2 percent progesterone cream applied to the skin).[134] For those women who are already on synthetic progestin in the form of Provera, Amen, Cycrin, or Prempro, I recommend switching to natural progesterone. A study at the Oregon Regional Primate Center induced heart attacks by injecting chemicals into several groups of monkeys whose ovaries had been removed to simulate menopause. One group was on Provera, one was on estrogen, one was on estrogen plus natural progesterone, and one was not on any hormones. They found that the monkeys on Provera had an unrelenting constriction of their coronary arteries, cutting off blood flow. These monkeys would have died had treatment not been initiated. The chemicals produced the same effect in those monkeys not on any hormones at all. But in the monkeys on estrogen alone, and those on estrogen plus natural progesterone, blood flow was quickly restored with no treatment necessary.

Clearly, the take-home message is this: Get off Provera or Prempro if you are using it for hormone therapy and substitute bioidentical progesterone. (In all fairness, the 2006 reanalysis of the data from the Women's Health Initiative study and Nurses' Health Study showed a decreased risk of heart disease in women who started HT within ten years of menopause, and the risk of heart disease was decreased by 11 percent even in those using estrogen plus synthetic progesterone. But the risk reduction was even better [44 percent] in women on estrogen alone—which may point to the adverse effect of the synthetic progestin.)

Some women experience heart palpitations in menopause, often related to emotions such as panic, fear, and depression, all of which raise adrenaline levels, which causes blood pressure and heart rate to increase. Biofeedback such as the HeartMath technique described earlier (see the section on adrenals in this chapter) can help dramatically with this symptom. St. John's wort may also be helpful (see the section on mood swings and depression in this chapter). Regular expressions of joy and creativity are important for a healthy and functioning cardiovascular system and, in the end, are likely to be the best prevention. These emotions reduce levels of stress hormones. The late Louise Hay likens blood flow to the flow of joy throughout the body. The more pleasure and joy you take in life, the more freely the blood flows!

ALZHEIMER'S DISEASE

The fuzzy thinking many women experience perimenopausally is not a symptom of Alzheimer's disease, but it is important to understand what factors are associated with Alzheimer's, the most common cause of dementia—accounting for more than half of all cases. (Other forms of dementia are caused by chronic drug use, hardening of the arteries in the brain, and the effects of chronic alcohol use and a nutrient-poor diet.) Currently, 5.7 million Americans have Alzheimer's disease, including 5.5 million people (one in ten) age sixty-five and older. Every sixty-five seconds, someone in America develops this debilitating disease. Experts estimate that by the year 2050, there will be 13.8 million Americans over age sixty-five with Alzheimer's.[135] Presently there are 3.4 million Americans over age sixty-five with Alzheimer's, and two-thirds of those are women, according to the Alzheimer's Association.

Though it's hard to predict exactly who will eventually be diagnosed with dementia, a long-term study of nuns showed that those with the highest cognitive function in early life were the least likely to develop Alzheimer's disease decades later.[136] Women who maintain normal memory and brain function throughout life tend to share a set of characteristics, which include:

~ Good health

~ Financial security

~ Above-average intelligence and education

~ Active personal interests

~ Sense of satisfaction and accomplishment in life

~ Physical fitness

Dementia is not inevitable. Most women have a very good chance of preserving our memories as we grow older—and in fact may even improve them. Neuropsychological testing has shown that brain function in healthy older people remains normal at least throughout the eighth decade, with the most recent studies showing there are indeed centenarians with absolutely no evidence of neurodegenerative disease (and some with substantial markers for Alzheimer's who show no clinical criteria for dementia).[137] The National Institute on Aging reports that there's growing evidence that as we grow older, our brains remain able to adapt to new challenges and tasks throughout our lives—if we stay healthy by eating a good diet, drinking no more than moderate amounts of alcohol, and getting regular exercise. Our brain's biological age is not tied absolutely to its chronological age.[138]

There is no question, however, that hormones have an effect on brain function, which is why those who've had their ovaries removed before the age of forty have a much higher risk of neurologic problems later in life, including dementia. Millions of women have taken hormone therapy in part to ward off dementia because estrogen was originally thought to be protective, yet data from the Women's Health Initiative Memory Study showed that the risk of dementia in the estrogen-only HT group, which was taking Premarin, was 49 percent higher than in women not taking hormones.[139] While the individual risk is small (among 10,000 women using hormones, 37 could be expected to develop dementia, compared with 25 in the no-hormone group—a mere 12 extra cases) and the risk was not deemed statistically significant, the data are still cause for some concern. As I've already said, I believe Premarin to be the most problematic of all the choices out there. (In contrast, a study done at Emory University School of Medicine in Atlanta showed that transdermal estradiol may confer at least modest protection against Alzheimer's, especially if it's begun soon after menopause.)[140] In contrast to Premarin, bioidentical estrogen has been shown to encourage dendritic and axonal branching between brain cells—a process associated with enhanced memory.[141] This is one of the reasons why some women on estrogen report better mood and even memory. (DHEA and pregnenolone—a steroid hormone related to progesterone—also aid the proliferation of connections between brain cells.)[142]

To date, there have been a few studies of women with mild to moderate Alzheimer's whose memory has improved initially on estrogen. And, in fact, estradiol (one type of natural estrogen) binds to the areas in the brain that are associated with memory and are affected by Alzheimer's disease: the cortex, the hippocampus, and the basal forebrain.

Brain function and memory preservation—and the acetylcholine levels associated with these functions—are also affected by a wide variety of factors other than hormones, including nutrition and aerobic exercise.

ALZHEIMER'S IS TYPE 3 DIABETES

The most important current understanding about Alzheimer's dementia is that it is associated with chronic high blood sugar and insulin resistance[143]—the end result of which is chronic inflammation and free radical damage in the brain. This is not unlike the adverse effects of type 2 diabetes elsewhere in the body, such as kidney damage, loss of eyesight, and increased risk for heart disease.[144]

Well-known holistic neurologist David Perlmutter, M.D., wrote the classic book *Grain Brain* (Little, Brown, 2013; revised 2018) to highlight the link between a diet high in grain and carbohydrates and the adverse effect that both sugar and gluten can have on neurologic function. It is now abundantly clear that lifestyle and dietary choices are more important than any other factor in preserving brain function throughout life.

A Brain Preservation Program

Update Your Knowledge and Attitude About Memory and Age. Our society currently operates under the mistaken notion that it is normal to become senile, lose memory, and have a change of personality with age—and all of us have been around relatives and friends with Alzheimer's or other dementias and know what a toll this illness can take on everyone concerned. But no one loses neurologic function simply because of age. There are always other factors such as cellular inflammation, suboptimal nutrition, and so on. So the first thing you must do to enhance your brain function is to stop buying in to the self-fulfilling prophecy about memory decline with age. Start by banishing the phrase "senior moment" from your vocabulary.

Here are the facts: We used to believe that we reached peak brain function and size around twenty-five and that it was all downhill from there. Newer research shows that our brains are capable of continuing to reshape and add new cells in the hippocampal memory area throughout life.[145]

In fact, studies have shown that throughout our lifetime, as we move from naïveté to wisdom, our brain function becomes molded along the lines of wisdom. Think of your brain as a tree that requires regular pruning if it is to acquire its optimal shape and function. Neural plasticity—the ability of the brain to upgrade and change—is akin to pruning the nonessential branches of a tree that may actually be interfering with optimal function by clouding consciousness and mental clarity. Complementing this process, the dendritic and axonal branching among brain cells actually increases with age as our capacity to make complex associations increases. What this means is that the older and more experienced you become, the more likely you are to develop new connections that help you synthesize your experiences. This is how wisdom gets wired![146] This is why Mario Martinez, Psy.D., founder of the Biocognitive Science Institute, reminds us that "growing older is the opportunity to increase your value and competence."

Protect Yourself with Antioxidants. Adequate antioxidant and vitamin intake helps prevent Alzheimer's since it reduces the amount of free-radical damage to brain tissue.[147] Free radicals are unstable molecules that are formed in our cell tissue by culprits such as radiation, trans fatty acids, and even oxygen. These free radicals combine with normal, healthy tissue and cause microscopic scarring and damage, which over time sets the stage for loss of tissue function and disease. Antioxidant vitamins, such as vitamin E, help quench these free radicals as soon as they are produced, thus helping to spare our brains, hearts, blood vessels, and other tissues from their ill effects.

Make sure your diet is rich in vitamins C and E, selenium, and the B vitamins, including folic acid. In fact, vitamin E has been shown to slow the progression of already-diagnosed Alzheimer's, but why wait? Another class of powerful antioxidants are the proanthocyanidins found in pine bark and grape pips. Since a great deal of brain health depends on minimizing free-radical damage, women should include a good antioxidant formula in their daily supplementation program.

Avoid Smoking and Excessive Alcohol Intake. Alcohol affects the basal forebrain—an area associated with memory. And cigarettes are well-known factors in causing cardiovascular disease and small blood vessel changes that decrease oxygen to your brain tissue.

Protect Your Brain Acetylcholine Levels. Avoid drugs that are known to decrease acetylcholine levels. Decreased acetylcholine is associated with memory loss and confusion. You'd be amazed at how many of these there are and how few doctors realize their adverse effect on brain function. Check the label of any medication used for sleep, colds, or allergies to see if it contains diphenhydramine (which is commonly sold under the name Benadryl). Examples are Tylenol PM and Excedrin PM.

Consume Omega-3 Fats. All of the cells of the central nervous system (the brain and spinal cord) are made from specific types of fat. The omega-3 class of fats is particularly important for healthy brain function. I recommend 1,000 to 5,000 mg of omega-3 fats daily. (See chapter 17.)

Engage in Regular Exercise. Studies have shown that exercise improves memory even in those who are already showing signs of dementia. Imagine what it does to prevent the problem! A recent study on individuals with early Alzheimer's showed marked improvement in memory and other cognitive functioning from engaging in 150 minutes per week of aerobic exercise.[148]

Remain a Lifelong Learner. I can't stress enough how important this is. In fact, I feel that it's the most important factor of all for optimal brain function. To maintain and enhance your brain function and wisdom, you must remain interested in the ongoing process of life. You must be actively engaged in some form of pleasurable activity involving growth, development, and learning. Take classes, get together with friends, learn a new sport or activity, start a new career or business, or engage in volunteer work. Tone your brain cells and neural pathways with new ideas, new connections, and new thoughts every day. Make sure you're on the path toward becoming a fun-loving wise woman of power—not a "little old lady." I was reminded of this a few years ago when my colleague Gladys McGarey, M.D., and I were having a conversation about a white paper she had just written on healthcare reform. She said, "I love being eighty-nine. I can say whatever I want. It's delightful!" That same joyful spirit showed itself later on when she was ninety-three. She bragged: "Ninety-three and prescription free." That same year she was a flower girl in one of her granddaughter's weddings. This is the spirit associated with agelessness.

DECIDING ON MENOPAUSAL TREATMENT

The Woman's Health Initiative data on Prempro changed the entire field of menopausal treatment overnight. Suddenly all the presumed benefits of HT were replaced with doubt and fear. We moved from black and white to shades of gray. And at the end of the day this is a good thing, though perhaps not as reassuring as the old "magic bullet" approach of the past.

Know this: When it comes to treatment for your menopausal symptoms, even though you may want to consult with your doctor for recommendations and of course prescriptions, the person who is most familiar with your body and in touch with its responses is you, and you need to heed your inner wisdom in deciding upon appropriate treatment.

My own recommendation is that if a woman has tried dietary changes, supplementation, herbs, and exercise and is still experiencing many menopausal symptoms, then she should try bioidentical hormones. After a three-month period on a starting dose your progress should be reevaluated. Remember, a woman's decision to begin hormones is not irreversible. Our bodies are constantly changing and evolving; therefore, prescriptions should be reviewed and updated regularly as hormone levels and life circumstances change. I recommend that women revisit the decision about hormone therapy on an annual basis depending upon how they feel. You have nothing to lose with this approach and a great deal to gain.

Getting Off HT or Changing Types

Many women find that when one type of HT doesn't work for them, another type will. In general, it is fine to switch from one type to another without any time lag in between. For example, you can take your Premarin one day and switch to bioidentical estradiol the next. If you are currently on hormones and want to switch to a phytoestrogen preparation, the best way to do so is to add the herbal supplement while still on hormones—and then, after a month on the herbs plus hormones, gradually taper off the hormones over a month's time.

If you want to *stop* hormones (even if you've added an herbal supplement), do it very gradually. Usually this means taking one less tablet per week until you are off your estrogen completely. When you taper off slowly in this way, there is much less chance of having rebound hot flashes. Some women begin to use 2 percent progesterone cream or *Pueraria mirifica* and after one month or so gradually taper their estrogen so that they are just on the progesterone cream or herbal combination. This gives your body time to feel the benefits of the new regimen while slowly weaning it away from the old.

SELF-CARE DURING MENOPAUSE

When making your self-care choices during the menopausal transition, please keep the following principles in mind:

~ Your body was designed to be healthy for at least a hundred years and probably longer. Menopause is nothing more than a halfway point.

~ Dementia, osteoporosis, heart disease, and cancer are not inevitable—no matter what your mother or grandmother experienced.

~ The menopausal transition is a powerful, biologically driven opportunity to reevaluate all aspects of your life and your health.

~ There is a wide variety of treatments available to support you hormonally and otherwise as you go through the menopausal transition. You have the inner guidance you need to choose the ones that are best for you. This may include hormones, herbs, a complete change of diet, or nutritional supplements.

~ Women are designed to enjoy sexual pleasure for a lifetime. Sexual pleasure can be greatly enhanced after menopause.

~ Menopause is the springtime of the second half of your life.

~ The time and energy you are willing to invest in yourself now will pay off in spades for years to come.

MENOPAUSE AS A NEW BEGINNING

Many menopausal women have dreams of giving birth. These birth dreams are important—they signify that there is much within us that needs to come forth. In this culture, women who are about to go through menopause or who are already in it need more than ever to reach deep within themselves and give birth to what is waiting there to be expressed. We can no longer afford to let our culture silence the wisdom of the wise woman—the woman who contains her sacred blood.

Susun Weed writes, "The process of menopause—not the last menses, the last drop of blood, but the entire thirteen-year menopausal process—sets the stage for initiatory ritual the world 'round, just as menstruating women's natural needs/abilities became the basis for all other initiations.

"During the process of menopause each woman finds herself immersed in and creating the three classic stages of initiation: isolation, death, and re-birth . . . our female bodies insist on completeness, wholeness, truth, change. Much as any woman would like to deny her shadow-self, her body will not let her. Menopause brings the individual woman and thus the entire community face-to-face with the dark, the unknown."[149]

With or without the help of hormones or herbs, every woman will benefit if she enters menopause consciously, ready to gather the gifts available at this stage of life. What we have to lose is not nearly so valuable as what we have to gain: finding our own voices and the courage to speak our own truths. When women do this, they are truly irresistible in their power and beauty. I have noticed everywhere I go that more and more women over the age of fifty look better than ever before. As a culture, we are redefining what it means to truly ripen with wisdom.

When she was in her seventies, my mother began expressing her creativity and connection with animals through learning the art of carving them in stone. Up until then, she never considered herself creative or artistic at all . . . and she was too busy raising five children to discover her gifts in this area. Her work is beautiful and inspiring—and she, like so many others past menopause, has discovered aspects of herself that she didn't know existed. She also speaks up a great deal at town meetings and other forums that concern her. She is no longer afraid to tell the truth in a group or in her own family. She says, "I have nothing to lose, and I've come to see that people can often benefit by what I have to say."

Several years ago, I led a Blessing Way ritual for my brother's fiancée to celebrate her upcoming wedding and to welcome her into our family. Seated in a circle around her were my daughters, my niece, my sister, the mother of the bride, my sister-in-law, the bride's sister, and two of my mother's friends. The age range in that circle of women was sixteen to eighty-three. I felt blessed to have the wisdom of three strong, powerful, and capable older women available for all of us in this circle, but especially for my daughters. What a gift it is to have honest, straightforward, physically healthy women over the age of eighty in our lives. They give us hope, courage, and guidance for the path ahead.

As a culture, we've been too long without those powerful, honest wise women of old—too long without the images of their beauty, power, and strength. Welcome them back. Whether or not you know any of them now, remember that they are inside each of us, waiting to be born through the initiation of menopause.

Part Three

Women's Wisdom Program for Flourishing and Healing

15
Steps for Flourishing

It's up to us each to think like leaders of our own "countries," to be sovereign in our own lives, and to steer our own personal lives on the best course. Ultimately, we *are* the government. Exercise the power you have. Do what you can.

—Anne Ortelee

It is in troubled times that it becomes most important to remember that the wonder of life places the medicine of the self near where the poison dwells. The gifts always lie near the wounds, the remedies are often made from poisonous substances and love often appears when deep losses become acknowledged. Along the arc of healing the wounds and the poisons of life are created the exact opportunities for bringing out all the medicines and making things whole again.

—Michael Meade

The steps in this chapter will help you tune in to the inner guidance of your body, mind, and spirit. By going through this chapter mindfully, you will be practicing preventive medicine at its best, whether or not you are currently being treated for anything. Use a journal or computer to write down your responses to these steps and record whatever material comes up for you. This will give you an accurate record of where you are right now. I'd also recommend that you repeat this process every few months as a way to see how far you've come. Recording your progress will be an affirmation of your own inner wisdom. I have kept journals for many years. When I go back and see how far I've come in so many areas of my life, it provides motivation, hope, and a profound sense of trust in my body, my health, and the fact that I'm connected to wisdom that is far greater than my intellect could ever appreciate on its own. Read your journal a year from now—or even six months from now—and you'll see that you're not the same person!

IMAGINE YOUR FUTURE:
CHANGE YOUR CONSCIOUSNESS,
CHANGE YOUR CELLS

Healing always involves releasing the past as we move into the future. If we don't release the past, we keep re-creating it—and it becomes the future. As we release, it's also crucial to have a powerful vision of a hopeful and exciting future that draws us forward. For years, I had my patients begin their health journeys by exploring their pasts to find clues to how they were creating their present conditions.

Our cells keep replacing themselves daily, and through this process we create whole new bodies every seven years. So it is not really accurate to say that our pasts are locked in our bodies, though sometimes it seems that way. What is really going on is that the consciousness that is creating our cells is often locked in the past—usually stuck somewhere in childhood—and that child's consciousness keeps re-creating the same old patterns via old subconscious nervous system programming. If, however, we change the consciousness and beliefs that create our cells, then our cells and lives improve automatically, because health and joy are our natural state. The easiest and fastest way to do this is to imagine your future self in as much detail as you possibly can. Doing this will assist you through any healing process you're currently involved in. So before you dive into the steps listed here, invite your future vision to accompany you on your journey.

World-renowned medical anthropologist and shaman Alberto Villoldo, Ph.D., calls this "future causation." You literally go into your future and invite it back to guide you in the present. He tells the story of a colleague he visited whom he hadn't seen for a long time. The colleague, who had been diagnosed with cancer and given six months to live, had just met the love of his life. And now here he was with a terminal diagnosis. Knowing that shamanism doesn't view time in a linear fashion, Alberto focused on the 10 percent chance that this man would be alive in ten years. Then he had him visualize himself in that future. It worked. Instead of dying, this man went on to marry and live another twenty years in good health. Alberto took him on a shamanic journey to a future self that was healthy. All of us can take a similar journey, because the subconscious mind doesn't make any distinction between what we can imagine in vivid detail and what actually happens to us in real time. So let's begin.

If you were in optimal health and truly flourishing, what would your life look like?

This question may be answered in the form of an exercise, with a friend who fully supports you; in writing, without worrying about revising or spelling; or out loud to yourself as you look in a mirror.

Answer the following questions (have your friend ask you the questions one by one, or write for three to five minutes without stopping, or talk to your image in the mirror): If anything at all were possible, quickly, easily, and now, what would your life look like? Who would be in it? What would you be doing? Where would you be living? What would you feel like? What would you look like? How much money would you be making?

Don't think about these questions before you answer. Pretend you're a child, creating your life exactly as you want it, no holds barred. How would your life be? Your inner guidance knows exactly what your heart's desire is. When you open your mouth and remove the brakes—and get the judge out of your head for a minute—your inner guidance will come up with the right answers.

If you need help getting going, imagine back to when you were eleven. What did you love to do? Who were you? Who did you think you would be? Imagine yourself now, telling the world who you are—and who you are going to become. Speak it to your image in the mirror; tell it to a friend or to the wind. Call that eleven-year-old back now. She's got something to tell you. Take her into the future with you and let her become everything she ever dreamed she would be.

After you have completed the first part of this exercise, imagine that it is one year from today. You have been able to create everything that you wanted, plus more. Everything that you dreamed could come true is now true. You are celebrating and looking back over this phenomenal year. You've created all of it almost magically, through the power of connecting with your inner guidance and wisdom. After you feel this scene fully, tell your partner (or your journal, or your image in the mirror) in detail about everything that you've created; share how excited you are, and invite her or him to celebrate with you. Keep talking for two to three minutes without censoring yourself. Just let it flow, like a child playing make-believe.[1] If you can't dream up any circumstances for the future, just imagine feeling joyous, light, and happy. Now take it a step further. Imagine that it's five years in the future and you're looking back. Record or say out loud what you see or feel.

I first did this exercise twenty years ago. At the time, I remember visualizing water and wells—and getting the distinct impression that water was the Goddess incarnate and that pure water was absolutely essential for optimal health. Our bodies are, after all, 60 to 70 percent water. I "saw" myself working with water as a healing modality. As I write this now, I'm in the process of creating a campaign for Charity: Water (www.charitywater.org), which provides wells and clean water all over the planet. I have also done some projects with the Hydration Foundation (www.thehydrationfoundation .org), which is dedicated to researching and educating about the profound connection between our hydration levels, the health of our connective tissue, and the fact that our consciousness and beliefs imprint not only the water in our bodies and tissues but also the water in our streams, lakes, and waterways. Gina Bria, founder of the Hydration Foundation, is also the coauthor with Dana Cohen, M.D., of a fantastic book on hydration called *Quench* (Hachette, 2018).

Anyway, know that there is no time in the unconscious. So what I "saw" twenty years ago is only now starting to take form in the three-dimensional world we call reality. We all want to know when something is going to happen. But I've learned that no one can give you this exact answer when it comes to working with energy and the potential future selves that are available to you.

This exercise is extraordinarily simple but very powerful. Part of the reason is that focused thought is what creates the reality around us. It has been said that if you can hold a thought or feeling for at least seventeen seconds without introducing a contradicting thought or emotion, then you'll see evidence of this thought manifest around you in the physical world. For example, start thinking about and talking about blue glass, white lilies, or something else that holds no particular "charge," and watch what happens. I have experienced this repeatedly. This exercise is so playful and fun that it's easy to reach and exceed the seventeen-second mark.[2]

You can change the time intervals by dreaming up your future self one week from now, one year from now, or even at the end of your life. In each case, have your future self look back and take in everything that you've accomplished and healed. It's exhilarating, and it will get you in touch with who you really are. I recommend repeating this experience at least four times per year.

Now, take this a step further. Pretend you are your future ideal self now. That's right. Envision yourself as a confident, fit, prosperous, magnetic, attractive woman right now. Lighten up. Play with this energy now. Call this future self to you now. As you go through the rest of this section, bring your future self along with you. Call her in and let her wisdom and joy help you as you explore your past. She—and your inner wisdom—will always be there for you. You don't have to do this alone.

IMPORTANT SPIRITUAL WISDOM TO KEEP YOU ON TRACK

This exercise seems simple, and it is. But things are not always what they seem. Yes, our habitual thoughts and beliefs impact our reality profoundly. But that doesn't mean that you have "created" your current reality on purpose from the perspective of your intellectual self or from the point of view of your inner child. There are far bigger forces at work in your life. Spiritual teacher Tosha Silver (www .toshasilver.com), author of *Outrageous Openness: Letting the Divine Take the Lead* (Atria Books, 2014), reminds us of three ancient spiritual principles (and their Sanskrit names) that must be taken into consideration whenever we decide to consciously work with the power of our thoughts and beliefs to improve our health and our life. They are as follows: *aparigraha* (nongrasping), *vairagya* (detachment), and *ishvara pranidhana* (surrender). Tosha, like many wisdom teachers, points out that the soul has an agenda of freedom—to not be imprisoned by or addicted to desires. This doesn't mean that desires are bad. They are absolutely essential. Many spiritual teachings make desires and needs "wrong" or "bad" and teach that these desires must be transcended. The usual way is to meditate, fast, or exercise until those needs go away. But they don't. Why? Because they are the cry of our inner child, who won't stop crying out (through sickness, pain, fatigue, loneliness, and so on) until we finally put her needs on the front burner and commit to getting them met. But we can't accomplish this by making someone else wrong or to blame for not meeting our needs (even though we can always make the case in so many different situations in our lives that our doctors, mothers, governments, and partners could and should have done better).

Still, to truly be healthy, happy, and free, you must connect with your own inner wisdom and Higher Power. The needs of your inner child—for safety, connection, being held, being seen, being cherished, and being loved—are nonnegotiable. And they won't go away until you've addressed them and loved yourself for having them. It is our mission and our job to take care of that vulnerable part of ourselves. Loneliness is always our inner child crying out to be taken care of. So when we long for someone to "complete" us, let us start first with the vulnerable little child within who never got the love she needed. Embrace your vulnerability, your needs, and your humanity. Love yourself right there—and at the same time, know that your soul also has its own curriculum, an agenda that I believe you chose before you were born. Regardless of how much you want something (more money, a life partner, a better job, a new living situation) or how well you visualize it, there are likely to be some karmic aspects in your life that you won't be able to override with visualization, vision boards, or exercises alone.

Instead of beating yourself up for this—believing you're not doing something right, you're blocked, you're somehow flawed, or you're not doing enough or working hard enough—it is far more effective to just do the exercises I've presented here and then turn the timing and the results over to the divine part of yourself (your Higher Self) that knows exactly what you need and when. This approach may well drive your small self nuts for a while: "Where is my soul mate? Why am I still tired? Or sick? Or bleeding?" But fear not. Every single one of us has a force of love guiding us every step of the way, if we just allow it to lead us.

Say the following affirmation from Tosha Silver out loud in the mirror: "I *am* the divine nurturing force that loves and nurtures my inner child." This inner divine child in each of us is the ultimate path to fulfillment and divine guidance. It is the path of the heart that far surpasses our intellect's ability to figure things out. Over time you will learn to trust it and know that it is always leading you toward greater and greater fulfillment.

STEP ONE: UNCOVER AND UPDATE YOUR LEGACY

You need only claim the events of your life to make yourself yours. When you truly possess all you have been and done, which takes some time, you are fierce with reality.

—Florida Scott-Maxwell

Every one of us inherits a specific legacy from our families that must be claimed and changed as needed. This legacy, from our own past and our family's past, affects our energy, our health, and our potential for change in each generation. If it is not acknowledged, it will be unconsciously passed on in repeated behaviors, and consciously passed on in the form of advice. Our legacies often nail into place the upper limits of what we believe is possible in life.

Regardless of what happened to our parents or grandparents, it is our job to break through these upper limits with our intent and consciousness. One way to do this is to write down your family history (the medical aspects as well as the emotional ones), thus bringing them to the surface, where they can be examined.

If, for example, all the women in your extended family have had a hysterectomy before the age of fifty, you may be influenced by a self-fulfilling medical family prophecy around the uterus that has nothing to do with genetics and everything to do with belief. The same is true for breast cancer or any other disease that "runs in the family." Putting that fact in writing helps free you from the necessity of repeating the experience. Because conditions such as alcoholism and depression often go unacknowledged within a family system, it's important to address these areas directly by shining a light on subjects we tend to keep in the darkness ("I'm not really an alcoholic, I'm just a heavy social drinker," or "My uncle was just being playful. He didn't really molest me"). Also, the emotional impact of a history that includes the premature death of a parent, the loss of a beloved pet, a secret out-of-wedlock pregnancy, or secretly giving up a baby for adoption—all of these are frequently denied. These issues are often revealed in writing down the family history.

In the past, scientists believed that our genes had a huge role to play in determining our health. This is known as "genetic determinism," or "I'm destined to get cancer because it runs in my family." But newer data have modified this approach considerably. Cell biologist Bruce Lipton, Ph.D., author of *The Biology of Belief* (Hay House, 2008), explains that our genes are a blueprint. But a blueprint sitting in an architect's office can't do anything until it's acted upon by a contractor who takes the plans and builds something from them.[3] The same is true of our genes—ultimately, it's the mind and the environment that together act as the general contractor. The neurotransmitters that the brain makes when it thinks, and that the gut makes when it digests, play a huge role in how a gene gets expressed. This is the science of epigenetics. In his book *It Didn't Start with You* (Viking, 2016), Mark Wolynn, an expert on inherited family trauma, points out that the grandchildren of Holocaust survivors often have anxiety, fears, and nightmares even when they have no knowledge of their grandparent's trauma.[4] The children of women with PTSD are more likely than others to use addictions like smoking and overeating to deal with stress.[5] It's important to acknowledge the impact our family histories have had on us—but not to get stuck there.

I once spoke to a woman on my radio show, *Flourish!*, whose son has cystic fibrosis—a well-known genetic disorder associated with severe respiratory illness and premature death. Early on she decided that she wasn't going to "activate" her son's disease any more than was necessary. She never restricted his activity nor tried to protect him from germs brought home from school by his siblings. At the age of twelve, he had never been hospitalized for respiratory problems—almost unheard of in those with cystic fibrosis.

This woman was not pretending that her son didn't have a chronic inherited disease. She was just setting up his environment for optimal expression of factors other than his disease. This is a wonderful example of how environment plays a huge role in the expression of disease—even diseases such as cystic fibrosis, which are without a doubt genetic. (Most diseases that run in families, such as diabetes, osteoporosis, and breast cancer, are actually multifactorial and, unlike cystic fibrosis, are not inherited in a straightforward way.) The bottom line: Use your power to influence your genes, instead of being a victim of them.

Lois, a forty-three-year-old woman with a history of early cervical cancer and pelvic endometriosis, once told me, "I was a battered wife five years ago and finally got out of that marriage. Then my daughter was in a car accident and I had to take care of her for months. Then this summer I was in another accident and sustained a whiplash injury. I want to cry, but I keep pushing it down. It gets harder to do, though. Is this from early menopause?"

When I went over Lois's history with her, it was easy to see that she had been through a very significant amount of change and loss in the past decade, which she'd tried to deal with by keeping everything in order, going to work daily, and appearing cheerful. She admitted that it seemed to be harder to keep her house in order these days, and that even though there was no current crisis, she still felt inefficient and emotional. In fact, her back pain from the whiplash was gone, her daughter was now in college, and her job was going quite well. What she realized she needed to do was acknowledge the losses she hadn't grieved and give herself the necessary time and space for this.

What Lois was experiencing was what I call "breakdown to breakthrough." She needed to feel what she was feeling. She took a week off from work and family, went to a small country inn, and spent the next week mostly in a robe and slippers, reading, crying, drinking tea with the woman who ran the inn, and gradually getting back in touch with parts of herself and feelings that were long denied. When I next saw her, she looked fifteen years younger. "Now I know that those feelings you mentioned don't come up when you want them to," she said. "They come when they come. It took me three or four days of being quiet and by myself before I could really cry. But I also learned that I can go off by myself when I need to in order to do this for myself. My relationship with my husband [she had remarried] and daughter is better than ever. I learned that *when I take care of myself, everything else takes care of itself.*"

Family History

For each family member, note age (if still living), any important conditions—such as alcoholism, high blood pressure, cancer, diabetes, heart disease, osteoporosis, mental illness, personality disorder (narcissism, borderline personality disorder, psychopathy, sociopathy, antisocial behavior), addictions, other illnesses—and cause of death and age at death (if applicable). Include any additional details that feel relevant.

Mother: _____

Father: _____

Sister(s): _____

Brother(s): _____

Maternal grandmother: _____

Paternal grandmother: _____

Maternal grandfather: _____

Paternal grandfather: _____

Maternal aunt(s): _____

Paternal aunt(s): _____

Maternal uncle(s): _____

Paternal uncle(s): _____

THE PROFOUND ADVERSE HEALTH EFFECTS OF CLUSTER B (PERSONALITY DISORDERED) INDIVIDUALS ON THOSE IN RELATIONSHIP WITH THEM

In the past twenty-five years or so, the mental health field has identified a group of personality disorders that is designated as "cluster B": narcissism, borderline personality disorder, histrionic personality disorder, antisocial personality disorder, psychopathy, and sociopathy. These disorders exist on a spectrum, much like autism. That means that some people just have narcissistic traits, while others are full-blown psychopaths with no conscience whatsoever.

When we hear the word *psychopath*, what springs to mind is a mass murderer like Charles Manson or Jeffrey Dahmer. But most psychopaths operate under the radar and are not involved with the criminal justice system. In her book *The Sociopath Next Door* (Broadway Books, 2005), Harvard psychologist Martha Stout,

Ph.D., points out that one in twenty-five people is a psychopath—meaning they have no conscience and no moral compass (also see the discussion on this in chapter 4). Because the legal, mental health, and justice systems have not understood the true nature of these individuals until fairly recently, many have quite literally gotten away with murder. Psychopaths target openhearted and empathic individuals to get what they want—and what they want is money, sex, status, and power. In her book *Women Who Love Psychopaths: Inside the Relationships of Inevitable Harm with Psychopaths, Sociopaths, and Narcissists* (Mask Publishing, 2009), therapist Sandra L. Brown says, "They are sicker than we are smart." What she means by that is that these individuals can be so charming, seductive, and convincing that almost anyone can be duped by them. The documentary films of Alex Gibney (*Enron: The Smartest Guys in the Room, Going Clear: Scientology and the Prison of Belief,* and *Mea Maxima Culpa: Silence in the House of God,* about the sexual abuse of more than 200 deaf boys by Catholic priest Lawrence Murphy) explore this brilliantly.

About 20 percent of people are considered to have a cluster B disorder—that's one in five people. (I refer to them as energy vampires because they drain the life energy of others to meet their needs.) In normal day-to-day life, they are the individuals who suck all the air out of the room. Very often they are charismatic, fun, and talented. You can't take your eyes off them. But the moment you stop providing them with what they want, they deflate like a balloon with a hole in it. They don't know how to source their life from inside themselves. They require other people's energy to thrive, leaving everyone around them drained.

Every family has at least one such person. They fuel their lives from what is called "narcissistic supply"—the attention, energy, money, sex, and adulation of others. They rarely, if ever, change. Once you wake up to what's going on and set a boundary, they are on to the next person (which feels like a huge betrayal if you've been married to one and realize that they never really loved you).

In any given primary care medical practice, it is estimated that anywhere from 25 to 30 percent of the patients have a personality disorder.[6] They use the medical system for attention but almost never get well. They are one reason (of many) why so many healthcare professionals suffer from burnout.

Conversely, those with whom they live too often find themselves burnt out from constantly trying to meet these individuals' endless demands and cope with their clever manipulation. Empathic, caring individuals may even end up with brain changes associated with executive function disorder (confusion and fuzzy thinking) because of the cognitive dissonance caused by living with such an individual. Cognitive dissonance results when you are living with two conflicting realities at the same time (for example, "If I'm a good person, my love should be enough to heal this person. All people are good at heart, aren't they? He's like this because he suffered as a child. I can heal him" versus "But why does he keep shaming me and making me feel like crap no matter what I do? When do my needs get met?"). I wrote the book *Dodging Energy Vampires: An Empath's Guide to Evading Relationships That Drain You and Restoring Your Health and Power* (Hay House, 2018) to bring attention to this phenomenon because I realized that there is a subgroup of women (and men, for that matter)—empathic, openhearted, practical, and successful—who are targeted by this kind of individual. I include myself in this group. Energy vampires hook us with a sob story, and because we're very skilled in most every other area of our lives, we believe we can help them. We take them on as a project. As a result, we can spend months and even years pouring our life energy into bottomless pits who never change. The end result for too many women is that their immune, endocrine, and central nervous systems begin to suffer from overgiving to the energy vampire and not getting their own needs met. They develop so-called mystery illnesses like adrenal fatigue, chronic Epstein-Barr infection, chronic fatigue, fibromyalgia, and autoimmune diseases such as lupus. Many who suffer from these conditions eat a perfect diet, meditate, and do everything else they can think of to get better. But the real problem is the energy vampire who is constantly draining them.

Since *Dodging Energy Vampires* was published in 2018, I have received hundreds of responses from women (and men) all over the world thanking me for pointing out this pattern and giving them the tools to free themselves from the chains binding them to energy vampires.

HEALTH INVENTORY: WHERE I AM NOW

It's helpful to fill out this form to get an idea of exactly what your health and life look like now. (By the way, research has shown that perceiving that your health is good or excellent is, in and of itself, a very accurate assessment of your state of health—with no further testing needed. Please keep that in mind.)

Medical Status

General health (circle one):   excellent   good   fair   poor

Medications (prescription or otherwise): _____
_____
_____

Supplements (vitamins, herbs, minerals): _____
_____
_____

Health-enhancing activities:

Exercise	Music/artistic endeavors
Meditation	(including dancing and
Hobbies	singing)
Participatory sports	Participation in religious/
Social groups and clubs	spiritual practice
Volunteer activities	Other things you do for fun

Hospitalizations and Operations

Dates   Diagnosis/Operation

Pregnancies (including miscarriages and abortions)

Dates   How far along   Gender   Weight   Medical problems in pregnancy
_____
_____
_____

Past or Current Medical Conditions (circle those that apply)

Vaccines: When and how many?	Heart trouble
Chicken pox	High blood pressure
Hepatitis B	
Hepatitis A	High cholesterol
Meningitis	Stroke
Rubella	
Flu	Varicose veins
Shingles	Phlebitis
Pneumonia	
Childhood chronic conditions,	Clotting defects
such as asthma and	Bleeding tendencies
allergies	Blood transfusion

Diabetes

Kidney trouble

Rheumatic fever

Jaundice/hepatitis

Epilepsy

Arthritis

Colitis

Fractures

Cancer

Asthma

Chronic fatigue/Epstein-Barr

Eating disorder

Other

Habits

Dietary preferences/restrictions: _____

Sample of day's menu:

    Breakfast: _____

    Lunch: _____

    Dinner: _____

    Snacks: _____

Tobacco use (how much currently, previous history): _____

_____

Alcohol use (how much, how often): _____

Caffeine use (how much): _____

Mood-altering substance use (i.e., marijuana, cocaine, etc.), past and present:

_____

Work stresses: _____

Personal stresses: _____

Gynecological History

Age at first period: _____

Any abnormal Pap tests: _____

    If yes, how were they treated? _____

Are you sexually active? _____

Do you have intercourse? _____

Do you have regular orgasms? _____

Do you know your female erotic anatomy? Where your clitoris and G-spot are? _____

Do you practice safe sex? _____

Are you trying to get pregnant? _____

Current birth control method (and how long): _____

    Any problems with it? _____

    Past birth control methods: _____

Normally (when not on hormonal methods of birth control), number of days from the start of one period to the start of the next: _____

Number of days of flow: _____

Amount of bleeding: _____

Amount of cramping: _____

Premenstrual symptoms (and when they start): _____

Any current changes in your normal pattern? _____

Any bleeding between periods? _____

Any unusual pelvic pain, pressure, or fullness? _____

Any unusual vaginal discharge or itching? _____

Any sexual concerns? _____

Any past history of tubal infection? _____

Any past history of sexually transmitted disease? _____

Did your mother take DES when she was pregnant with you? _____

Other: _____

Present Symptoms

General Physical
Fever or chills
Hot flashes
Unusual hair growth
Skin eruptions
Weight change

Abdomen
Bloating
Heartburn, indigestion
Cramps or pain
Nausea or vomiting
Change in bowel habits
Bloody or tarry stools
Diarrhea
Constipation
Hemorrhoids
Flatulence

Head
Headaches
Dizziness
Visual defects
Hearing defects
Sinus trouble
Fainting spells

Bladder
Frequent urination
Painful urination
Blood in urine
Inability to hold urine
Inability to empty bladder
Need to get up at night to urinate

Chest
Chest pain
Shortness of breath
Heart murmur
Mitral valve prolapse
Palpitations
Chronic cough
Coughing up blood
Wheezing

Breasts
Lumps
Bleeding
Discharge
Tenderness
Other concerns

Once you have expressed your desire to make the changes that will help you flourish, be aware that you and your Higher Power (or broader perspective) have what it takes to do just that.

THE CAUSES OF HEALTH

Our entire healthcare system is set up to look for disease. We are taught that disease screening and receiving an ever-growing number of vaccines is healthcare. I have often quipped that women's health has largely been reduced to "We didn't find it yet. But keep coming back. We will." Though there is a place for disease screening, it is no substitute for living your life in a way that actually creates health, a way of living that is also associated with robust immunity, a prolonged health span (not just life span), and vitality.

Mario Martinez, Psy.D., founder of the Biocognitive Science Institute, has researched hundreds of healthy centenarians in countless countries worldwide. Regardless of what country they are from, they all have a number of things in common—they practice what Dr. Martinez calls "the causes of health." These people are outliers whose beliefs and behaviors fall outside their cultural norms of "what to expect at a certain age." The three major causes of health that Dr. Martinez has identified are listed below. As you go through them, notice how many of them you currently practice—and then commit to practicing them more often.

1. *Elevated cognition.* Thinking positive and uplifting thoughts (the glass is half full instead of half empty). Looking for the silver lining in every cloud.

2. *Exalted emotions.* Focusing on feeling joyful and good. Participating in activities and endeavors that bring joy, laughter, deep feelings of compassion, and delight (such as reading poetry, watching the sunset, appreciating moonlight, listening to or playing music, and smelling fragrant flowers).

3. *Righteous anger.* Allowing yourself to feel anger when your own innocence or someone else's has been threatened. An example of this would be stepping up and saying something when you see someone abusing their child. Here's another example: You're in labor, and the doctor comes in with a medical student who begins to examine you without your permission. It hurts. You need to say, "Hey—this is not okay with me." Most of us become a deer in the headlights around medical procedures. That's why it can be important to take someone with you when you go in for medical procedures. Dr. Martinez points out that Tibetan Buddhist monks have unusually high rates of type 2 diabetes. He posits that this is because they've spent

years training themselves to bypass their anger and go right to loving-kindness. Feeling loving-kindness produces a neurochemical called beta-endorphin. It blocks pain and feels good. The problem is that too much beta-endorphin can interfere with the metabolism of blood sugar. Loving-kindness literally sugarcoats righteous anger. Dr. Martinez points out that the Tibetan monks need to feel anger first, if only for a few moments; then they can release it and move on. The Chinese destroyed their monasteries and killed many of them. The spiritual training of the monks is to forgive this and move on, something we all have to do when we've been wronged. But first we have to feel how bad we feel and how angry we are. Only then can we transcend into forgiveness. Please know this. Although it's a health risk to marinate in anger and resentment overly long, it's also true that we have to feel these emotions fully. Only then is it safe to move on.

STEP TWO: SORT THROUGH YOUR BELIEFS

Commit yourself to setting aside some time to answer the following series of questions. You might want to do this with a friend or in a group. Your answers would make an excellent starting place for a personal journal that you can update regularly as new insights come to you. Writing your answers down is, in itself, a significant commitment of your time and energy toward creating health. You learn a great deal about yourself and your relationship with your body. This is healthcare that won't cost you a penny.

Do you understand how inherited cultural attitudes toward our female physiological processes such as menstruation and menopause have contributed to the illnesses suffered by our female bodies? What are the thoughts that arise when you hear the words breast, menstruation, childbirth, vagina, vulva, menopause, *and so on?*

If you've grown up believing that your menstrual period is "the curse," for example, it's quite likely that your attitude toward your female physiology is less than optimal.

To what extent have you internalized negative cultural programming about the female body?

One of my patients became menopausal following chemotherapy for Hodgkin's disease at the age of twenty-seven. Though she had gone on estrogen replacement therapy for a few years, she eventually stopped it because "the thought of getting my periods back was chilling and repugnant to me," she said. I found her statement of disgust and its implications about her attitude toward her body equally chilling, but such attitudes have been common for centuries. Luckily, this is all changing.

Do you believe you can be healthy?

Women who have grown up in a household where the norm is to go to the doctor for insomnia, anxiety, headaches, and the common cold often internalize the belief that the human body is meant to suffer from all manner of ills and that there's a pill for every ill. Enjoying ill health is the norm for some people. The possibility of a sound body that isn't susceptible to every germ in the environment is inconceivable to them. A study at Carnegie Mellon University in Pittsburgh famously showed that people who think of themselves as healthy developed fewer cold symptoms, even when they were infected with cold viruses and their immune system reactions verified the infection.[7]

What challenges were part of your childhood?

Challenges are part of every childhood. They're what build resilience. When it comes to the physical body, for example, childhood illnesses and germs are actually necessary to mature the immune system. Childhood challenges, then, are necessary. What's important in adulthood is to update any outmoded beliefs and behaviors that are still lingering from childhood. Consider how your childhood experiences contributed to your current perceptions and experiences. A childhood history of incest, chronic illness in a parent, divorce in the family, and having a parent abandon the family are common occurrences that, if unresolved, can set the stage for later problems that have similar dynamics. Many women's fathers left them when they were children and never returned. Other women have never talked openly about a parent's death. Though the impact of these events is as variable as our fingerprints, there is always an impact. How we name, express, and fully release emotions surrounding such losses can be a factor in our physical health. Recall that this information is directly related to the health of our first three chakras and the organs they comprise.

An eighteen-year longitudinal study of 413 African American children published in the journal *Development and Psychopathology* shows just how important this idea is. The researchers found that supportive parenting, which encouraged children to feel not only that they were loved but also that they could trust their bodies, seemed to protect against inflammation-induced depression later in life.[8]

Physical therapist Tami Lynn Kent, who specializes in the pelvic floor and how the events of our lives impact our bodies, points out that many women of color have especially deep imprints in their root chakras (sense of safety and security and belonging) from their legacies of subservience, slavery, disrespect, and abuse. White women can begin to appreciate the experience of most women of color by taking every adverse thing that has ever happened to them and multiplying it a hundredfold—a start toward understanding the degree to which they have been privileged and protected simply because of the color of their skin. But the work is the same for every woman—to name and claim our legacies and then use our inner power and connection to Source to heal. This is possible regardless of your background, race, or history.

One of my former patients developed panic attacks and severe PMS around her fortieth birthday, several months after her father was diagnosed with bowel cancer. Her mother had died suddenly from a reaction to penicillin when my patient was four years old. She was sent to live with an aunt with no explanation, no one ever cried in her presence, and she herself was never given permission to speak about or grieve her loss. Now with the possible loss of her father, all the emotions she had buried were working their way to the surface. But once she became aware of what was happening and why, she was able to express them in a healthy manner and release them over time.

What purpose does your illness serve? What does it mean to you?

A forty-two-year-old woman recovering from a car accident told me that there was no question that before the accident, the pace of her life was moving way too fast. To pay attention to her needs, she literally had to be forced to lie in bed and stare up at the ceiling for several months, as she was now. She regards this accident as a very positive turning point in her life. Leslie Kussman, a filmmaker who has multiple sclerosis, said that during one of her morning meditations it occurred to her that perhaps we need to rephrase the question from "What purpose does your illness serve?" to "What is the illness that will serve your purpose?"[9] *Illness is often the only socially acceptable form of Western meditation.* Our society is set up such that taking a nap or meditating in the middle of the day to recharge and renew ourselves is frowned upon as hedonistic or irresponsible, but getting the flu is a socially accepted way to rest.

Without slipping into self-blame, think back on the last time you had to miss work because of illness. Was the illness a satisfying break from your routine? What did you get out of it? What did you learn from it? Do you see any way that you could get the same rest without being sick? A young female doctor developed breast cancer while she was pregnant with her third child. As a result, she changed her diet, her work schedule, and her life. Two years later she told me, "My life has never been better. Every day is a joy. I'm glad I had cancer. It saved my life."

If you had only six months to live, would you stay at your current job?

Would you stay with your current partner? Would it take a serious illness for you to begin making beneficial changes now?

Are you willing to be open to any messages that your symptoms or illness may have for you?

Before you begin working with this question, please note that a willingness to be open to the message is entirely different from a need to control and figure out the exact meaning of an illness, especially while it is happening. The former is associated with vibrant health. The latter is just manipulating yourself and is part of our illusion of control. Being open to meaning means that you allow the illness to speak to you, often through the language of emotion, imagery, and pain. Your intellectual understanding of your situation may well come only after an illness is over with.

Back in the 1980s, when our culture was learning about the mind-body connection, people would actually ask questions like "Why are you needing to create cancer?" as though the intellect could figure that out through cause-and-effect thinking. These sorts of questions keep the intellect running in circles and take us away from our hearts—the place in the body that really heals us. Being open to meaning is an attitude, a process. It's "waiting with," not "waiting for." And it connects us with our soul's voice. Glenda Green, author of *Love Without End* (Spiritis, 2002), puts it beautifully: "The mind will seek to compensate for the discomforts of the heart. But the mind will never seek to cure or remove those discomforts."

When faced with an illness, what is your usual reaction?

Learning the meaning behind the illness is a process that doesn't lend itself to questions like "Why me, why now?" Evy McDonald writes, "Don't get caught in the tangling web of why. The search for the explanation and meaning of your illness can lead to frustration and depression and can paralyze your ability to make decisions and take action." As they say in twelve-step programs, "Whying is dying."

In the days of the ancient Greeks, a messenger would be sent to the leader with news of the current battle. If the news was bad, the messenger would be killed. Your task is not to kill the messenger of illness by ignoring it, complaining about it, or simply suppressing the symptoms. Your task is to examine your life with compassion and honesty while cultivating detachment—which simply means caring deeply from an objective place. From this place, identify those areas of your life that require harmony, fulfillment, and love.

What is preventing you from flourishing?

"Waiting with" this question is a good meditation. Don't expect an answer to spring forth immediately, though it sometimes does. Back in the days when I had two small children and a busy practice, I repeatedly asked myself what changes I needed in my life and what I needed to do next. The answer that kept coming was simple: *Rest. You're burned out.* Taking action on that insight took more than a year. Why? Because at the time, I honestly believed that adequate rest was incompatible with my chosen life's work. It was, and always is, a process.

Some people never heal because they believe that if they were healed, they would be alone and abandoned. Being sick in this culture can be a very powerful way to get our needs met legitimately. Saying to someone, "Please hold me—I feel ill," is quite different from saying, "Please hold me—I want to be held because it feels good and it is a basic human need." The first sentence uses illness to justify the universal human need for closeness. The second sentence simply states the need clearly. Many people don't know that intimacy is possible without using our wounds to get it. We are brought up to be ashamed of our needs for touch, love, and companionship, so we learn very early to bond with each other via our wounds.

During my residency training, I was very proud of the way I had handled a certain woman's care, and I decided to tell one of my nurse colleagues who also knew this patient well and who could celebrate with me. When I told her, she said, "Don't break your arm patting yourself on the back." I was stunned. I had simply been expressing a natural human need to share my success with a colleague who would understand its implications. When I was growing up, my parents had always believed that each of us children needed his or her place in the sun. We were routinely recognized for our gifts and achievements, and we felt good about ourselves and each other when these were shared. (We still do this.) But my nurse colleague had obviously learned that it was not okay to "blow your own horn." Often, the only time good things are said about the life of another person is at their funeral. This is tragic. Each of us needs to accept that no matter how strong, independent, and healthy we become, we will always need others for companionship, celebration, and joyful living. And we need others who will reflect our worth back to us!

Do you take on everyone else's problems and put yourself last?

This is the classic dilemma for women. Feeling the need to be the healer and peacemaker for our entire family or place of work is a pattern that many of us learned in childhood as a way to get recognition. To truly flourish, a woman must face this tendency squarely and commit to changing it. In her book *The Art of Extreme Self-Care* (Hay House, 2009), my friend Cheryl Richardson included a chapter entitled "Let Me Disappoint You." I have never forgotten that title—and its message. Many times, if we are to be true to ourselves, we risk disappointing others or not meeting their needs. Obviously there are times in life when we absolutely must meet the needs of others. It's a sacred obligation to care for and feed any young children you have in your life, or if you work in healthcare, you must meet the needs of your patients. But far too often, we override our own needs until it becomes a habit—a habit that, over time, can be life-threatening, a setup for chronic illness.

Here's an example: One of my good friends got a letter from her nine-year-old daughter, who was away at summer camp. The letter read, "Dear Mom, I wrote you a letter but it didn't get to you. I just wanted to check in. What I mean is I miss you, but I don't." The letter summarized a truth we all need to pay attention to. When we are in the flow of our lives and pursuing those things that bring us joy and fulfillment, we are very much in the moment. We are whole and complete. We are free. Given our culture, most men have no trouble reaching this state of being because they've been supported for it since birth. How many men do you know who routinely make time to play hockey, basketball, tennis, or golf with their friends—even when their wives are at home taking care of the children? They don't feel guilty about it at all.

Notice how your children or friends ignore you when their lives are going along well but reach out to you only when they need your energy for something. Notice how you may be sacrificing your own desire for play and recreation because of your obligations to meet the needs of others. Imagine what would happen if you put your own needs first, just as a privileged white male would, and never gave it another thought. The first thing that would happen is that you would feel guilty, and that guilt would drive you back into self-sacrifice, which would initially feel better than the guilt. But this is all cultural programming, and you can change it.

It is a revelation to many of us that we, too, have needs for friendship, laughter, and companionship separate from our children. When I realized this, around the time my kids were ten and twelve, I let them know that I, too, had needs—individual needs that were as important as theirs (not *more* important—*as* important). I came to see that I had to take a stand for my own needs as well as the needs of my children. Together, we began working on becoming conscious of the ways in which they assumed that I had no life separate from them, and the ways in which I assumed because of my cultural imprinting that I should sacrifice my life for their needs.

When I became clear about this situation and what needed to happen, I had a dream about being given a red 1950s-style gas pump that pumped milk. The name painted on the pump was "The Mother." I had to keep the pump refrigerated so that the milk wouldn't spoil. I kept trying to think of whom I was going to give the milk to. My family didn't need it—we don't drink milk. When I woke up, I realized that the pump represented me and that it was now time to let go of an obsolete kind of mothering.

Do you fully understand the workings of your female body and how intimately your thoughts and feelings are connected to your physical health?

Your body experiences every thought and sensation as a "physiological reality." By thinking of the taste and smell of chocolate, you trigger many of the same physical reactions as when you actually eat a piece. Our bodies are not static structures. The amount of sunlight shining on us in a day affects our physiology. The quality of the sounds we hear affects our physiology. The quality of the relationships we have with others affects our physiology. One woman said to me, "Oh, my breasts are being taken care of by the Lahey Clinic!" Instead of believing that the Lahey Clinic is responsible for her breasts, she would be much better served by assuming responsibility for her breasts herself.

Many women don't understand not only how intimately our bodies are affected by our environments but also the basic anatomy of our bodies. Many who have had surgery don't know exactly what was taken out and what was left in. Yet knowing precisely where the organs in our bodies are is very reassuring. During my residency I once did an emergency appendectomy on a woman. She also required removal of her uterus and ovaries because of a life-threatening infection. Several days later, I learned that she thought her appendix was as big as a large melon and that now her entire lower abdomen was completely empty because we had removed it. I explained to her that her large and small intestine completely filled her lower abdomen despite the loss of her pelvic organs, which was very useful information for her in her recovery because it helped her feel that the loss was less overwhelming. Showing her drawings of her anatomy was also helpful—she learned that her appendix was smaller than her little finger.

I encourage women to get personal copies of all their records and go over them with a healthcare provider who can answer questions, particularly reports of any surgeries they have had, so that they know exactly what is going on inside their bodies, how things look, and what is left. When you go to the doctor, take a friend or use your cell phone's voice recorder. Ask questions. Be proactive. Keeping copies of your own records can also expedite your healthcare if you are traveling or have to make an emergency-room visit.

Do you know where your organs are? If not, consider looking through an encyclopedia or standard anatomy guide. Get to know your body in health, not just in sickness. You also need to own all of it—even the parts that aren't considered socially acceptable.

What do you call your genitals? What was the name given to the female genitals in your family? Too many women were raised in families in which all the functions below the waist were considered shameful and not talked about. One friend said, "In my family, the area below the waist was referred to as 'down there.' It was kind of foggy. I didn't know what to call it. Likewise, women weren't supposed to pass gas!" At a meeting of the Association for Prenatal and Perinatal Psychology and Health several years ago, renowned midwife Ina May Gaskin commented that women would be far better prepared for birth if they allowed themselves more humor and relaxation about bodily functions such as bowel movements and passing gas. I agree.

The first step in reclaiming your women's wisdom is naming and reclaiming all of you. In the book *The Sexual Teachings of the White Tigress: Secrets of the Female Taoist Masters,* Madame Hsi Lai, the matriarch of the White Tigress Taoist lineage, speaks of the genitals as the "Jade Gate Opening." This terminology feels spiritually enlightened to me and brings much-needed healing energy to the area.

This type of language may not work for you. In that case, check out the work of Regena Thomashauer, the author of *Pussy: A Reclamation* (Hay House, 2016). Regena has dedicated her life to helping women achieve their full potential through connecting with the power in their wombs and genitals. She uses the rather shocking but inclusive word *pussy* to refer to all of the genital area—the vulva, the perineum, the clitoris, and the vagina. (Referring to the area as just the vagina is inaccurate.) Many women find this offensive at first because of our cultural programming. However, this friendly word can be used as a term of endearment that aptly describes a warm, fuzzy, and pleasurable area of the body. Plus, it sure beats the other slang terms! Reading Regena Thomashauer's books will help you embrace not only this word but also the power of your genital area. As already mentioned in chapter 9, the Sanskrit word *yoni* is another good, and accurate, choice. Or you can just use the correct anatomical terms, like *vulva.*

Are you following your life's purpose?
Our bodies are designed to function best when we're involved in activities and work that feel exactly right to us and that bring us pleasure . . . at least more than 50 percent of the time. Our health is enhanced when we engage in deeply creative work that is satisfying to us, and not just because it pleases our bosses, husbands, or mothers. This work can range from gardening to computer programming to welding. My friend and colleague Gay Hendricks, Ph.D., calls this our Zone of Genius. When we commit to spending most of our time in our Zone of Genius, as opposed to our Zone of Excellence (doing things we're good at but which don't really fulfill us), then we really start flourishing.

Though all of us will occasionally have to engage in work we don't really want to do in order to get where we want to be, we flourish only when we make a living in our Zone of Genius. (I encourage you to run out and get Dr. Hendricks's brilliant book *The Big Leap* [HarperCollins, 2009] for further reading on this life-changing subject.) For most people, unfortunately, going to work is more like "making a dying" than "making a living." People often put up with very unsatisfactory work environments because of the financial benefits. I call this "dying for our benefits." Financial and gynecological health are intimately connected. The second-chakra area of the body (uterus, tubes, ovaries, lower back) is affected by financial stresses. Health in this area is created when we tap in to our ability to be creative and prosperous at the same time. This is not simply a metaphor. Have you heard the term "shake your moneymaker" as it applies to women? Well, there's a great deal of truth in that statement. Sexuality teacher Kim Anami (www.kimanami .com) teaches that when you increase your orgasmic potential, you often increase your financial potential as well. This is because the genitals reside in the second chakra—the center in the body that is influenced by our relationship with sex, power, and money. When one area is flowing nicely, the others are often positively affected as well.

Living in our Zone of Genius and becoming prosperous often involves as a first step a change in our attitudes toward money, self-worth, and work. We must be very clear on how our culture's belief in the zero-sum model affects us. For instance, many people believe, "If I am doing well, someone else has to suffer. There is only so much money to go around." Or vice versa: "If someone else is doing well, then there is no chance for me to do well also. There is no way to get ahead." Our personal finances are powerfully and directly affected by our beliefs about money. Poverty consciousness pervades our culture on every level. When we change our beliefs, we can change our income!

In their book *Your Money or Your Life* (Viking, 1992), the late Joe Dominguez, a former Wall Street analyst, and coauthor Vicki Robin point out that for most people, money is the substance for which we exchange our life energy.[10] Dominguez and Robin suggest that you figure out how many hours you have left in your life—your total life energy. Then calculate how much your work actually costs you in terms of your life energy. If you work so many hours that you require expensive vacations and frequent illnesses to get enough rest to balance the energy drain of work, you may well find that once you factor in the hidden costs of vacation and illness, your work is netting you much less per hour than you are actually being paid. Their program then helps you balance your relationship with money by determining how much fulfillment you get out of every purchase, compared with how much it has cost you in terms of your life energy. There are many good books on this subject, including two written by my daughter Kate Northrup: *Money, A Love Story: Untangle Your Financial Woes and Create the Life You Really Want* (Hay House, 2013) and *Do Less: A Revolutionary Approach to Time and Energy Management for Busy Moms* (Hay House, 2019). Another book I've found very useful is *It's Not Your Money: How to Live Fully from Divine Abundance* (Hay House, 2019) by spiritual teacher Tosha Silver. It teaches readers how to tap in to true abundance, regardless of their net worth.

Your next step is to consciously make a decision to spend more money on the things or activities that bring you the most fulfillment and less money on the stuff that ultimately has no meaning. What happens is that eventually your expenditures decrease and the fulfillment that you derive from them increases. When you begin to look at money in this way, your entire relationship with it changes. You begin to see that it is not necessary to put off doing what you've always wanted to do until "later." Some of my greatest pleasures, such as walking on the beach, reading, dancing tango, and going to the movies, cost little or nothing. It need not cost you much money to begin living your life in a more fulfilling manner. By going through the Dominguez-Robin program myself back in the late 1980s, I realized that my free time was priceless to me and that I would never again be able to work in any job, regardless of high pay and good benefits, if the job didn't also fulfill my soul and give me ample time to create my life on my own terms. And that is why, to this day, I turn down the vast majority of invitations to speak that come my way.

At midlife when I went through an unexpected divorce, I was once again forced to come to terms with what I really valued. I had had a large fibroid removed from my uterus a couple of years prior to the divorce—a sure sign that I had second-chakra lessons to learn in the area of money, sex, and power. The body never lies! After the divorce, overnight my income was cut in half and my expenses rose significantly. I was also faced with paying the vast majority of two private-college tuitions for my daughters. There's nothing like a financial (or health) crisis to get our attention! Knowing about the connection between prosperity and thought, I read the classic *Think and Grow Rich* (Hawthorn Books, 1996; Aventine Press, 2004) by Napoleon Hill, all of Suze Orman's work, and all of the financial advice from Robert Kiyosaki, author of *Rich Dad, Poor Dad* (Warner Business Books, 2000). (For more information, visit www.richdad.com.) I also played Kiyosaki's ingenious board game CashFlow 101 until I could regularly get out of the rat race (living from paycheck to paycheck) and onto the fast track (creating residual income from business or investments). This game eerily re-creates one's relationship with money—it's a real eye-opener.

Finally, I learned that financial literacy is crucial for all women. I got up to speed on the necessity of creating residual income (the kind that comes in regardless of whether you work or not). Residual income is the biggest difference between those who are prosperous and those who are struggling financially. I also learned how to reprogram my thinking about prosperity through the work of Catherine Ponder, author of *The Dynamic Laws of Prosperity* (Prentice-Hall, 1962). As I was going through my divorce, I happened to meet Suze Orman at the *Today* show. She told me that you can always see health problems start in someone's money situation first, because a balance sheet has no place to hide energy. Sooner or later that energy drain hits the body as a health problem. She also said that the only thing that keeps money away from you is anger or fear. Though I wasn't fully aware of it at the time, I found out that Suze was correct. I had a load of each at the time, which I worked through. By applying the laws of prosperity in my own life (e.g., the Law of Circulation—if you want to receive, you have to learn to give, etc.), I eventually was able to create true financial abundance and also greatly improved health. This process was so empowering that I passed it on to my daughters so that they would not have to be dependent upon a man for financial security.

EINSTEIN TIME

Changing our relationship with time is equally vital to our ability to flourish. Several years ago I had a wonderful conversation with Gay Hendricks, Ph.D., about what he calls Einstein Time. (He has since written about this in his aforementioned book, *The Big Leap.*) He pointed out that everyone is allotted the same amount of time in every day. But in this ever-busier world, people increasingly feel more time pressure and operate under the stressful perception that they are running out of time. Using insights from quantum physics and Einstein's space-time continuum, Dr. Hendricks explained that our perception of time is highly influenced by our feelings about what we are doing with our time. When something is painful or un-fulfilling, our energy field contracts and time drags on endlessly. We feel miserable. On the other hand, when we're engaged in something that lights us up, such as making love with our beloved, our energy field expands and time stands still. One hour of being passionately present passes in a minute, but a few seconds of touching a hot stove feels like an eternity. It's all relative.

Dr. Hendricks notes that we never have enough time to do what we really don't need to be doing in the first place. On the other hand, when we are operating in our Zone of Genius—doing things we love and were born to do—then we are far more efficient and our perception of time changes completely. We get more done in far less time.

We can become masters of time by being fully present in each moment with the understanding that our perception bends time and shapes our experience of it. Dr. Hendricks posits the liberating thought that "I am where time comes from." After being introduced to this most health-enhancing and liberating concept of time, I wrote the following affirmation:

Time is on my side. Time is standing lusciously still for me. I am creating timeless time. I have enough time. I'm having the time of my life!!! I am where time comes from—in slow, sexy, sensual rhythms of joy and pleasure that stretch out into eternity. Ahhhhhhhhhh!

I keep this posted on my bathroom mirror so that I can look at it regularly and feel the truth of it every time I'm tempted to succumb to the health-destroying effects of doing too much or rushing. I suggest that you do the same!

Have you designed your life in a way that fulfills both your innermost needs and your desire to be of service to others?

It is entirely possible to develop yourself fully, meet your innermost emotional needs, and at the same time work with others for the common good. Our culture has taught women just the opposite: that they must sacrifice themselves and their needs for the good of others. But you cannot quench the thirst of others when your own cup is always empty. Many studies have shown, for example, that women who sacrifice work they love and optimal self-development in order to nurture others are at high risk for breast cancer. It is not the sacrifice that creates the health problem—it is the unexpressed resentment that results from it. When a woman doesn't believe that she has a right to self-development, she won't even allow herself to acknowledge her resentment. Her body wisdom must then bring it to her attention so that she can create balance. The most prosperous people I know are also the most generous. They make the world a better place and also enjoy abundance themselves.

A Boston College study showed that patients suffering from chronic pain and depression felt less pain, reported less disability, and reduced their depression after volunteering to help others suffering in a similar way.[11] In talking to the researchers, the subjects repeatedly mentioned making a connection with others and having a sense of purpose. "Despite encountering challenges," the study concludes, "the rewards of this altruistic endeavor outweighed any frustrations experienced by volunteers with chronic pain."

A fascinating study done at the University of North Carolina at Chapel Hill compared the gene expression of two groups of eighty healthy, happy volunteers—one group mainly striving to live a life of purpose and meaning and the other generally seeking a good life filled with pleasure. The group who lived purposeful lives were not as financially well-off or as stress-free as the pleasure-seeking group, but they had low markers for inflammation (which is associated with degenerative illnesses) and tended to downregulate (essentially turn off) genes related to physiological stress. The pleasure-seekers, on the other hand, had surprisingly high levels of inflammation and tended to upregulate (turn on) genes related to physiological stress.[12]

Do you regularly appreciate your strengths, gifts, talents, and accomplishments? Are you a good receiver?

A large part of creating vibrant health—or anything else, including wealth—is giving ourselves credit for where we are now. Learning how to take in praise—to let ourselves really feel success and completion physically—is a skill that can be learned. Amanda Owen, author of *The Power of Receiving: A Revolutionary Approach to Giving Yourself the Life You Want and Deserve* (Tarcher/Penguin, 2010), says, "Those who have trouble receiving attract those who have trouble giving."

A big reason why people get stuck and can't create better lives is that they don't give themselves credit for what they *have* created. This usually comes from the subconscious programming we received in childhood, e.g., "Money doesn't grow on trees," or "You'll never amount to anything." If you chronically skip this step of acknowledging your creations and continue to focus only on what you have *yet* to accomplish, then your subconscious hears only "You are not enough. You haven't done enough. There is so much more to do. You will never be enough," instead of "Good job. Look how far you've come."

One of my medical colleagues learned this lesson well when she developed an ovarian cyst while working on the faculty of a major medical center. Florence had originally gone to work in this center because she didn't believe that she had what it took to start her own practice, where she could use her creativity to the fullest. Following her ovarian removal, however, Florence knew intuitively that she needed to leave her workplace, that it was somehow dangerous for her to stay. In this work environment, others did not value her innate feminine creativity, and as a result, she didn't value it herself when she was there. Florence knew that she was not yet strong enough to hold her own feminine viewpoint without at least some support from others, but the ovarian "sacrifice" really got her attention and mobilized her to make a change. She left the medical center and started her own highly successful practice. Only years later, after learning about ovarian wisdom and releasing her need to blame others, was she able to appreciate how profoundly she had put her creativity at risk in her original work setting.

Many women live with the following beliefs: *There is too much work to do, I will never get it done, but I can't rest or have fun until it's done.* The classic double bind. This belief comes directly out of our cultural obsession with productivity and the belief that our worth depends upon what we can produce for others, whether this be children or goods and services. Operating under this belief system, we create more and more work that doesn't feel complete or fulfilling. Here's the truth: You'll never get it done. There will always be something still to be accomplished in the future, something you could have done better in the past. This is true for all of us. The answer is to build regular pleasure and appreciation into your schedule so you learn to feel good about yourself and your life right now! And do regular "completions." For example, every year on my birthday and again at the new year, I write down both my goals for the new year and the things I've completed and accomplished in the past year. The completion list always amazes me as I look back in wonder at how much I've actually accomplished. It's very satisfying. Regena Thomashauer puts this another way: "Undigested good turns to shit." This observation is absolutely true, which is why you simply must acknowledge and appreciate yourself and others regularly.

Think of one thing that you're proud of that you've accomplished today, this week, or this year. Feel your accomplishment fully. Take it in, until it's more than just intellectual knowledge. Take yourself right into your heart. If we can't feel good about our skills and accomplishments, no one else can, either. Find a few friends you can brag with. (I have several groups of women, including my daughters, with whom I regularly do this. It's one of the most uplifting and useful endeavors I've ever participated in.) Send each other emails or texts regularly, bragging about how wonderful and skillful you are—and what you're most proud of. Recognizing that you are exhausted and choosing to spend a day resting is something to be proud of, too. My friend Melanie Ericksen, a skilled healer (www.soulplay.us), often calls me with what she calls a "celebrag"—a term that combines celebration and bragging. We uplift each other this way on a regular basis. And when we look back, we're always amazed at how far we have come.

Remember, optimal pelvic health requires that we acknowledge our accomplishments as an outward manifestation of our deepest inner need for self-expression. These need not be measured in dollars or productivity to be a valuable contribution to our health and that of others. One of the accomplishments I was most proud of several years ago was the ability to spend a weekend alone at home by myself and be really, really happy and fulfilled with my own company! This took decades, but I finally made it.

That said, it's also time that we properly recognize and celebrate the full value of the financial contribution women make to their family's income. According to a 2018 NBC News/*Wall Street Journal* poll, 49 percent of working women say they work because they are their household's primary wage earner, up from 37 percent in 2000.[13] We are nearly half the workforce today (almost 47 percent),[14] as opposed to a third fifty years ago, which means that our voices and skills are impacting all areas of society—industry, education, medicine, and other professions. That's quite impressive! Even so, there's certainly room for improvement. The same poll reports that 61 percent of women say they are not treated as equals in the workplace, with 44 percent reporting gender discrimination and 49 percent saying they've received unwelcome sexual advances or experienced other kinds of sexual harassment at work. One way we can support ourselves as we navigate this changing landscape is to learn to listen deeply to the wisdom within ourselves and within each other so that we develop strong, self-assured voices that are grounded in innately feminine values.

STEP THREE: RESPECT AND RELEASE YOUR EMOTIONS

Pain is the result of resistance to our natural state of well-being and the more we pay attention to it, the more of it we attract.
—Abraham, via Esther Hicks

Emotions are a vital part of our inner guidance. As I've stressed before, our emotions are part of our aliveness. They let us know whether we're traveling in the direction of our dreams or in the opposite direction. And they always point to unmet needs that we didn't know we had. Many of us have been shamed for having needs. But all humans have needs. The needs to be heard, touched, held, appreciated, seen, and protected—all are sacred. All are natural. All are human. And when we have the courage to be vulnerable and loving enough to ask our friends or family to assist us in meeting these needs, we become far healthier. An example of this is a colleague who recently led a weeklong retreat at a conference center. An introvert, she was afraid of being overwhelmed by the participants when the regularly scheduled sessions were finished each day. So after a lot of praying for guidance, she simply told the workshop participants at the very beginning of the week that she needed quiet time between sessions. She requested that no one come up to her to ask questions during that time. To her great joy and amazement, everyone understood and respected her needs. And the conference was a huge success.

We all must learn emotional literacy instead of trying to override our emotions with our intellect. We must release our judgments about emotions, and be grateful for their guidance. They never lie. If we attend to them and listen deeply, we find that they offer profound wisdom and healing. And no matter how difficult they are to bear or feel, we must give them space, acceptance, and a voice. We must love ourselves "right there" without shame or blame.

Chronic anger or sadness, by the law of attraction, tends to attract to us situations that are filled with anger or sadness. For example, you find yourself stuck in anger, and then you fall on the ice or get pulled over for speeding. Daily doses of joy and appreciation of ourselves and others, on the other hand, tend to attract joy and appreciation into our lives. In his book *When the Body Says No* (John Wiley & Sons, 2003), Gabor Maté, M.D., explains how illness is in large part an emotional expression of maladaptive stress-response habits. For example, suppressing one's own emotional needs in service to others (in other words, classic people-pleasing behavior) can put you at risk for developing an immune-related illness. This is because by suppressing your emotions, you are essentially ceding control to those you are serving, which is disempowering and essentially self-violating. The chronic stress this causes is what then can trigger disease. Dr. Maté notes that every one of his patients has struggled with using this sort of emotional repression as a coping mechanism.

This can start in childhood, he explains, if you believed that in order to survive some sort of acute or chronic trauma, you had to stuff your emotions, usually conforming to an authority figure's or even society's expectations. What can happen is that these emotions go unconscious, confusing our physiological defenses. Those defenses can then go awry, destroying our health instead of protecting it, the way they are designed to do. Dr. Maté describes a Yugoslavian study concluding that the single greatest risk factor for death (particularly from cancer) was "rationality and anti-emotionality." When anger wasn't repressed, the researchers noted, even those who smoked didn't have a greater risk of lung cancer compared with nonsmokers.[15] Similarly, a study from New Zealand shows that unexpressed grief can result in congestion, sneezing, and allergy symptoms, even when there is no allergy or cold virus present; the body essentially cries for the person when the person can't cry on their own.[16]

Yet Dr. Maté also makes the very important point that positive thinking and positive emotions aren't the same thing as genuinely experiencing joy—especially when they are used to distract us from negative emotions. "Negative thinking allows us to gaze unflinchingly on our own behalf at what does not work," he writes. "We have seen in study after study that compulsive positive thinkers are more likely to develop disease and less likely to survive. Genuine positive thinking—or more deeply, positive being—empowers us to know that we have nothing to fear from truth."[17] In other words, we must truly do the work of expressing and releasing our emotions to experience vibrant health.

Children automatically know how to feel their emotions and then let go. When they're hurt, they stop and cry. Within minutes, they are back to playing again. Animals who have just been chased will often get the fight-or-flight reaction out of their bodies by shaking; then, after just a short time, they go back to grazing peacefully. We are animals, too. And if we are supported, our bodies know how to heal and recover from the stresses of life. The late

Elisabeth Kübler-Ross pointed out that a child's natural anger and emotional outbursts last about fifteen seconds. Shaming or blaming the child for that anger, however, often blocks its natural release. The child's natural emotion may get stuck and become a form of self-pity that remains with the person for years. Kübler-Ross noted that people who weren't allowed a natural expression of anger in childhood are often "marinated in self-pity" as adults and are difficult to be around.

Emotional suppression is a pattern that gets passed down from generation to generation. Many women have rage that's been held in check for decades. They hold in oceans of tears that are yet to be shed. One very overweight woman in my practice told me that her mother and grandmother had taught her how to gorge on chocolate whenever their husbands were out of town and they were feeling lonely. The fat on her hips, she told me, represented three generations of stagnated emotional energy held down with chocolate.

Emotional release, or what I've already called emotional incision and drainage, is an organic healing process that is completely natural and safe.[18] When I first went to an intensive workshop and sat with people who were doing deep process work, I felt as if I were on the labor and delivery floor at the hospital—standing by, allowing people to give birth to themselves. All of us have this ability within us. Dorothy's ruby slippers could get her home to Kansas all by herself—she just didn't know it. She thought she needed the wizard. Likewise, we all have the power to choose thoughts of appreciation and gratitude—and release old resentment and tears.

Making sounds is an important part of emotional release. Women naturally make deep primal sounds in labor. They help open the cervix and get the baby through the birth canal. Primal sounds are also part of lovemaking, which is the basis for the multiple orgasm work of Jack Johnston (www .multiples.com). Women naturally vocalize during sex unless taught to suppress these primal sounds. Myron McClellan, a musician specializing in the healing power of sound, says that "singing is part of the emotional body's digestive system." Singing is one form of healing sound. Wailing or deep sobbing is another. These sounds are like grappling hooks that go through the body, cleaning out toxins and old debris. A woman recently wrote me, "I have taken several months of training in the martial arts simply to help release some of the tensions and muscular inabilities that I have felt in my body. An interesting by-product is that I have found my voice. In the process of learning tae kwon do, I had to be able to give a huge yell with the punches and the kicks that are part of the practice. I had never before in my life been able to make a noise with that much authority. As a child, I learned that if one didn't make noise, then one could possibly avoid aggravating or irritating one's abusers and, possibly, avoid abuse. I have carried that legacy with me for many years, even silencing my grief when my husband was killed. In other cultures women are traditionally taught to keen loudly to express grief, sorrow, and rage at death. I had never made that kind of sound, though I certainly have wanted and needed to do so. Not until now, six years after my husband's death, have I been able to make those sounds. They came, not only because of the karate, but as a result of the deep healings to my respiratory tract that I have been able to accomplish through macrobiotics and Oriental medicine."

In many ways, the year or two *after* a traumatic experience are more difficult than the experience itself—possibly because in this culture we have support for crises but are then expected, both from within ourselves and from outside, to get on with it when it's over. A young woman who had recovered from Hodgkin's disease with the help of a bone marrow transplant a year before came to see me once. The chemotherapy had caused an early menopause, and we were working with estrogen replacement therapy to help her hot flashes. She was having problems with fatigue and weakness, but there was no sign that the cancer had returned. In going back over her history, she burst into tears in my office and told me that she had never cried even once during the year in which her diagnosis was made or during her entire chemotherapy experience. She had not allowed herself to experience her fear. She had simply gone through it as best she could. A year later, there was no crisis in this woman's life. Her body was well, but she still didn't feel better. She didn't have the energy to exercise, and she didn't want to cook nourishing meals for herself. After sitting with this for a while, she realized that she needed time to process her recent experience emotionally.

When I first visited an acupuncturist, she told me that in Chinese medicine, emotions such as anger are viewed simply as *energy*. Many women have a problem with the direct expression of their anger and use it to manipulate others instead. But anger can be a powerful ally. When we feel angry, the anger is always related to something we need to acknowledge for ourselves. It is not necessarily about the situation or person that evoked it. It is always a sign that on some level we're not meeting a personal need that we may have. That's one of the reasons why anger is so often part of PMS.

All women must learn that no one can *make* us angry. Our anger is ours, and it is telling us something we need to know. Anger is energy—our personal jet fuel. It is telling us that something needs adjustment in our lives. It is telling us that there is something we want that we don't yet know how to get, and it is dangerous only if we deny it and stuff it in our bodies or lash out at someone else with it. The next time you discover that you're angry (which might manifest as feeling jittery, having shaking hands, or being irritable), go off by yourself. Move around. Breathe. Yell.

Try this: Arrange two chairs facing each other. Sit in one and imagine that the person with whom you are angry is sitting opposite you. Now tell the person everything you really want to say—no matter how loud, off-color, or nasty it is. Truly get your anger up and out. Get into it fully. And when you're spent, love yourself for your courage. Then ask yourself, "What do I need?" Wait for an answer. If the anger arises again, repeat the exercise until the charge is dissipated.

Your anger at another may well be justified. And it must be expressed safely. But if you hang on to it overly long, the one who will be hurt the most is you. At the end of the day, you have to decide whether you want to be justified or healthy and happy! Ask for what you need with kindness. When you get it, say, "Thank you."

SHAMANIC IMPRINT REMOVAL

I learned this particular approach to getting difficult emotions out of the body from the late Peter Calhoun, an Episcopal priest who became a shaman after realizing that the old rituals in his religion weren't particularly helpful for many people. (For Peter's full story, read his book *Soul on Fire: A Transformational Journey from Priest to Shaman* [Hay House, 2006].) I have found Peter's process to be profoundly helpful for those who are open to this kind of divine help. No special skills or training is required. This practice is done as a partnership, with one person doing the imprint removal and the other having the imprint removed. Here are the steps:

1. The person having the emotional imprint removed sits in a chair, as in the anger-clearing exercise above. We'll call this person the "subject." They imagine that the person who has wronged them—the one at whom they directed their anger in the exercise above—is sitting in front of them.

2. The person who is assisting now asks the subject where in her body she feels the stuckness. It's usually in the abdomen, chest, or throat.

3. The assistant now says the following, or something similar in their own words: "With Archangel Michael's cobalt blue sword of light, I cut any energy cords that are binding you. I release any dark or wandering spirits and send them on their path of healing, and I bar them from ever returning." (It's helpful to literally make the same motions with your hands that you would do if you had a sword and were using it to sever actual cords. Those who are clairvoyant can actually see and sense these cords. Clairvoyance is only one type of intuition, of course.)

4. Now encourage the subject to address the person in front of them who is associated with their anger, sadness, or pain, using the following words: "[Name of person subject is addressing], I forgive you for [fill in the blank], and I send you on your path of healing." An example would be: "Mom, I forgive you for never allowing me to express myself or get my needs met because of your extreme jealousy and control. This really hurt me. And I send you on your path of healing."

Or this: "Dad, I forgive you for molesting me when I was three, and for never being a real father. *WTF!* And I send you on your path of healing."

Now comes the most important part: You really, truly let them have it—even though they are not physically sitting there in front of you (and even if they are dead; it's never too late). Let out the angst of the unhealed child within you. This is *not* an intellectual exercise. You must *feel* your feelings here or the process will not work. Really feel and express them.

Here's another example: "John, I forgive you for abandoning me when I needed you most. What kind of asshole does this? You left me so devastated! And I send you on your path of healing."

Note: This is *not* a therapy session. The person assisting the imprint removal encourages the subject to just get it all out. Many people who have been abused have overly intellectualized their pain, so it might take a bit of encouragement. It should take only a few minutes to hit the pain core.

5. Now the subject says, "And I forgive myself for [fill in the blank]." This is a very poignant moment. This is when the subject realizes the degree to which they have adversely affected their own life as a result of the trauma and subsequent beliefs about themselves that resulted from the wound.

6. The assistant says to the subject: "Are you ready to heal this imprint?" If the subject says no, then return to the previous step until the answer here is yes, meaning the subject has nothing further to "say" to the perpetrator.

7. The subject says, "I now release this imprint into the Violet Flame." (The Violet Flame, which is associated with St. Germain, is a potent healing energy that assists in removing all doubt and limitation; see www.saintgermainfoundation.org.) Imagine literally sitting in a violet flame. The subject should feel the release of what they felt in their chest, abdomen, or throat while in the Violet Flame. It often happens immediately. If it doesn't, repeat the steps until the feeling is released.

When I am doing an imprint removal, I always "see" one of three things. Most of the time, the abuser runs away—just literally runs for the hills. Other times, the abuser kneels before the subject in the flame, in contrition, asking forgiveness. Every once in a while, the abuser will jump into the flame with the subject in celebration of the completion of a karmic contract.

8. As soon as the feeling in the body has released, the assistant then "packs" the place where the imprint was removed with golden and midnight-blue light. You literally take your hands and pretend you are packing an open space in and around the body with this light. As someone trained in surgery who has packed wounds with gauze, I know what packing a wound actually is. Removing an imprint is psychic surgery, and packing the resulting wound is just as real as packing a physical wound—except that it's in the energy field.

Note: You don't have to be present with someone to assist with an imprint removal. I sometimes do them on my radio show if I feel it's appropriate and the caller is open to this approach. There is no time or space in the unconsciousness. And in the quantum energy field that surrounds all of us, we are all connected. This means I can assist with an imprint removal sitting at my desk in Maine while the subject is in British Columbia.

9. Make sure the subject can rest. I suggest that people who've had an imprint removal go to sleep or at least lie down afterward. As previously mentioned, this is psychic surgery. It is real, potent, and very effective.

Healing is like peeling the layers of an onion. When one imprint is removed, another might come up. If this happens, just repeat the process. For example, if the imprint removal was with your mother, you may then find that you have unfinished business with your father. And so on.

STEP FOUR: LEARN TO LISTEN TO YOUR BODY

Learning to listen to and respect your body is a process that requires patience and compassion. The following list of suggestions can help you with that process:

⁓ Make note of those things in your life that are difficult, painful, joyful, and the like. As these things come up, notice your breathing, your heart rate, and your bodily sensations. What are they? Where are they?

⁓ Pay attention to what your body feels. Do certain parts of you feel numb? Tired? Do you feel like crying? Do parts of you feel like crying? These feelings are your body's wisdom. They are part of your inner guidance system. You can always enroll a friend to help you process them using the imprint removal process above or just talking things through.

⁓ Ask yourself what your self-image is. Through years of chronic dissatisfaction with their bodies and chronic dieting, many women develop an unrealistic image of themselves. Some feel much heavier than they actually are, a fact that was beautifully documented in the television reality show *How to Look Good Naked,* in which women, wearing nothing but bras and panties, were asked to look at a line of other women dressed the same way and choose the size that most closely matched their own. Invariably women overestimated their size, thinking they looked much bigger than they really were. On the other hand, women who are in touch with their inner guidance will often appear taller and more imposing physically than they are. The way you feel about yourself creates an electromagnetic field of energy around you that broadcasts these feelings to the world and attracts your reality to you. Choose your signal consciously.

⁓ Notice how you routinely talk to and about your body. What happens when you look in the mirror each morning? Do you criticize your face, your legs, your hair? Do you routinely apologize to others for how you look? Now write the following sentence down on a piece of paper and tape it to the mirror: *I accept myself unconditionally right now.* I've often written it on a prescription blank and handed it to my patient with the following instructions: "Say this sentence out loud to yourself in the mirror while gazing into your eyes. Do this twice per day for thirty days." When you do this exercise, you will learn a great deal about the inner critics that live within you. Give them a name, such as Esmeralda or George, so that you won't take them so personally next time they put you or your body down. (Remember—they are just old subconscious and incorrect programs that got downloaded earlier in life. You can change them.) When you don't take their criticisms personally, you can tell them to be quiet. Or you can even choose to laugh at them. And guess what? They eventually lose their power over you and go away! Then you are free to proclaim each morning, "You are gorgeous, adorable, and sexy," every time you look in the mirror.

⁓ Tune in to what your body needs on a daily basis. Are you hungry? Do you have to go to the bathroom? Are you tired? Do you routinely ignore your body?

~ Understand that your health is at risk if you are constantly undermining certain parts or functions of your body. Barbara Hoberman Levine, in her book *Your Body Believes Every Word* (WordsWork Press, 2000), tells the story of a friend who always developed rectal pain during her period. Levine asked her if she thought of her period as a "pain in the ass." The woman gasped and admitted that that was exactly how she felt about it.

~ Identify the fears you hold about your body. For example, do you avoid touching your breasts because you are afraid of finding lumps? Instead, learn about breast anatomy and learn to touch your own with respect and love. You can transform and heal your entire relationship with them. The same goes for your genitals.

~ Notice whether there are parts of your body that you have disowned. What are they? Do you consider parts of yourself "unacceptable"? A patient of mine had frequent abdominal pain until she was thirty-five. In her family, she had learned that it was completely unacceptable for a woman to pass gas, even though it was okay for her father and her brothers. Thus, instead of allowing routine intestinal gas to leave her body as necessary, she literally held on to it, with resulting abdominal pain. Once she realized that she had disowned an entire natural body function, she learned how to allow this function and became free of abdominal pain. Farts are funny. Little children know that. Even Shakespeare knew it. Accept them and learn to laugh and let go!

~ When you experience a bodily sensation such as back pain, "a gut reaction," a headache, or abdominal pain, pay attention to it and see if you can pinpoint the emotional situation that may have triggered it. The late Niravi Payne taught her clients a vocabulary of symptom empowerment. For example, instead of "My stomach is hurting," say, "What is it I'm having trouble stomaching?" Emotions such as anger, or any other emotion that you may consider unacceptable or that you may find difficult to experience directly, will often affect your body instead. When a sensation arises in your body, stop what you are doing, lie down, breathe, and wait with your symptom, emotion, or feeling. You may be surprised at what other feelings or insights come up. The late John Sarno, M.D., who was a physical medicine and rehabilitation specialist at the Rusk Institute in New York, and author of *Mind Over Back Pain* (Berkley Books, 1999) and *Healing Back Pain* (Warner Books, 1991), had a 75 to 85 percent success rate with treating back pain and other related conditions such as neck pain and fibromyalgia, all of which he referred to as TMS—tension myositis syndrome. He noted that the personalities of those who tend to get this syndrome are characterized by being highly conscientious, responsible, and perfectionistic. (This is not the same as the type A personality, which is associated with hostility.) He taught his patients how to make the pain go away by making the link between their emotions and their symptoms and by telling their brains that they've got the message and it's okay for the pain to go. The results were often astonishing. I had a friend who limped into one of Dr. Sarno's meetings with crippling sciatica, which she'd had for weeks. She walked out pain free. (Posture is also a major issue in back pain. See the section on the psoas muscle in chapter 18.)

~ Stand in front of a mirror regularly and thank your body for all it has done for you. Cultivate the link between your mouth and your ear—and the rest of you—so that you get used to hearing yourself say positive things about your body. Remember always that 90 percent of your bodily functions take place without your conscious input. Who keeps your heart beating? Who metabolizes your food? Who tells you when you need to replenish your fluid intake by drinking water? Who heals your skin when you cut yourself? Who tells your ears to listen to beautiful music? Who tells your eyes to see beautiful sunsets? Acknowledge that your body is a miracle and that its natural state is health and joy.

STEP FIVE: LEARN TO RESPECT YOUR BODY

Almost all women in the United States have a body image distortion because of the millions of images of "perfect" airbrushed women that the media flash at us continually. We begin comparing ourselves with these icons of unattainable perfection even before puberty. Thus, we often relate to our bodies via negative comparisons: "My hips are too fat, my breasts are too small, my knees are ugly, my hair is too thin."

Instead of bowing to these cultural dictates and feeling bad about yourself:

~ Understand that your wish to have what society believes is the "perfect body" is completely natural. Know that you may be powerless over it. (By this, I mean that the desire rises up unbidden. You have no control over it.) But you *do* have control and power over what you choose to do with a thought or desire. This is why it is so important to begin to hear ourselves and our thoughts.

~ Love the body you have. If you don't respect, care for, and love your body, no one else will or even *can*. Vow to treat yourself and your body with kindness, especially when put-downs and comparisons come up from deep inside.

~ Be aware that your thoughts and beliefs about yourself send a powerful signal out into the universe that others can sense. In her book *Life Magic*

(Miramax Books, 2005), Laura Bushnell suggests that you imagine a huge mirror in the sky above you. In red lipstick, write the following phrase on that mirror: "I am beautiful and irresistible." Over time, your body will respond to your thoughts. You will become what you affirm.

Most media personalities have had or will have plastic surgery at some point in their careers. The models of perfection who beam into our global living rooms every day set up a standard that is impossible for most to aspire to without resorting to measures such as surgery.[19] And there's nothing wrong with using surgery to look your best. But even with surgery, the models on magazine covers routinely have several inches airbrushed from their thighs and buttocks and duct tape applied to various areas to pull them tight. They are human, after all—subject to the same wrinkles and sags as the rest of us. But their industry standards demand a certain image, and so they meet it, first by having the good fortune to have the right genes, and then by using surgery and often following a rigorous and disciplined lifestyle to maintain their looks. On a TV or movie set, someone follows them around all day with a blow dryer and makeup brush. On some level, almost all women would look their very best (or at least their culturally determined best) if they devoted the same amount of time, energy, and money to their appearance as our cultural media icons do and had all their photo images professionally manipulated—we've all seen evidence of this on the popular makeover shows on television. The enduring appeal of makeovers is that they help us manifest on the outside how we feel inside. The ancient arts of adornment are part of caring for ourselves. Nail polish, eyeliner, and lip colorings were used by the ancient Greeks and Romans. It seems that the human race has always been interested in style and makeup. I applaud the increasing trend toward better self-care through regular massage, pedicures, manicures, and pampering. It's a step in the right direction!

Our approach to dressing, makeup, hair, and personal care can be well served by the wisdom of Dolly Parton, who said, "Find out who you are, then do it on purpose." If we can find out who we are on the inside, we can then express it on the outside. As Coco Chanel once said, "Adornment is never anything except a reflection of the heart." The best source I've ever found for exactly how to do this is the work of Carol Tuttle, who wrote *Dressing Your Truth: Discover Your Type of Beauty* (Live Your Truth Press, 2010). Carol has found that all of us fall into one of four energy "types"— the Bright, Animated Woman; the Subtle, Soft Woman; the Rich, Dynamic Woman; and the Bold, Striking Woman. When you know what your energy type is—and know exactly what colors, fabrics, and styles work best for you—you will find that dressing is a pleasure. Carol's approach to knowing your inherent energy type and dressing according to this is liberating—it's truly life-changing. (See https://my.liveyourtruth.com/dyt/home.)

STEP SIX: ACKNOWLEDGE A HIGHER POWER OR INNER WISDOM

There is an unseen force, a spiritual dimension, guiding our lives like a loving parent guiding its child.

—Pythia Peay

Our bodies are permeated and nourished by spiritual energy and guidance. Having faith and trust in this reality is crucial for lasting health and happiness. When a woman has faith in something greater than her intellect or her present circumstances, she is in touch with her inner source of power. Each of us has within us a divine spark. We are inherently a part of God/Goddess/Source. Jesus said that the kingdom of heaven is within, and we can make this spiritual connection through our inner guidance. We need go no further than ourselves to find it.

Learning to connect with our inner wisdom, our spirituality, is not difficult, but neither our intellect nor our ego can control either the connection or the results. The first step is to hold the intent to connect with divine guidance. The second step is to release our expectations of what will happen as a result. The third step is to wait for a response by being open to noticing the changes in the patterns of our lives that relate to the original intent.

Each of us has a guardian angel available for guidance. But we have to ask for guidance and be open to receiving it. Seeing the patterns, how all the parts connect, is a way of looking at life. This is the paradigm shift I mentioned at the beginning of this chapter. Understanding the big picture doesn't mean getting stuck in the particular moment. Gaining access to spiritual guidance means looking at the pattern of our lives over time. As David Spangler said, "Dreams, events, a book, the words of a friend: All of this might be one word from an angelic being."

About two years before I wrote the first edition of this, my first book, I was standing by my bed on a sunny Friday morning, getting ready for the day. I read through my favorite meditations, which I've written down in a small book made of handcrafted paper. I decided to say aloud a statement taken from Florence Scovel Shinn's book *The Game of Life and How to Play It.*[20] I spoke it out loud clearly with sincere intent: "Infinite spirit, give me a definite lead, reveal to me my perfect self-expression. Show me which talent I am to make use of now." That very afternoon I received a call from an acquaintance who is a literary agent. "I think it is time you wrote a book," he said. It wasn't until much later that day that I put those two events together. Sometimes the guidance comes easily and quickly. When it does, though, you may have to go through the part of your intellect that tells you you're making it up and are crazy for believing this stuff.

Though each of us is part of a greater whole, we are also individuals. The unique part of this whole that we each embody must be expressed fully in order to create health, happiness, and spiritual growth for ourselves and others. The way to best express this divine part of ourselves is by becoming all of who we are. Our bodies direct us toward full personal expression by letting us know what feels good and "right" and what doesn't. Illness is often a sign that we are somehow off track from our life's purpose. That is why Bernie Siegel, M.D., says, "Illness is God's reset button."

Many doctors are open to this realm of mystery, too, but they don't dare to say anything. A highly skilled intuitive here in southern Maine once said to me, "Someday I'm going to have a cocktail party at my house and invite all the doctors in this area who've come to have readings. You will all stand around and be amazed at how many of you there are—and also at who is here."

When we invite the sacred into our lives by sincerely asking our inner wisdom, or higher power, or God for guidance in our lives, we're invoking great power. This can't be taken lightly. The reason people are cynical about this and make fun of it is that they are afraid. When you sincerely invite in the sacred (your inner guidance or spirit) to assist you with your life, you are granting permission for your life to change. Those areas of your life that no longer serve your highest purpose may start to disintegrate—and this can be frightening. Caroline Myss says, "Wiping out a marriage or a job is a day at the beach for an angel." Having been in both situations, I can attest to both the fear and the power inherent in this approach. The key to getting through it is being open to the greatness of your spirit.

Believing in angels, having your astrological chart done, or getting an intuitive reading doesn't excuse anyone from the work of healing and becoming whole. Remember that anything can be used addictively—even so-called spiritual pursuits. Too many people use their "spiritual practices" to avoid addressing the difficult areas of their lives. Using crystals, New Age music, and astrology or going to church twice a week while drinking a bottle of wine every night or being abusive to your children will not help you heal. Doing meditation faithfully twice a day and being beaten up by your husband every night will not keep you healthy. All the "spirituality" in the world won't do your human homework for you. Only you can take the action necessary to compose a vibrant life. As one of my twelve-step friends told me, "God moves mountains—bring a shovel."

To reconnect with their innate spirituality, many women have to get past years of religious abuse, particularly if they've been victimized by organized cults or patriarchal religions. God has too often been portrayed as a vengeful, righteous being, outside of human ability to understand or know, and so it's no wonder that being angry with God and struggling with the concept of a "higher power" or "inner wisdom" is a reality for so many. Some women are stuck at a very childlike stage in which they feel, "If there was a God, he would never have let this happen to me." One of my colleagues says, "If I make God something separate from me and outside of myself, then I get to accuse God of punishing me whenever my life doesn't go well."

We are all spiritual beings with all-knowing souls or higher powers. Connection with spirit is inherently part of being human. For centuries our culture has tried to control our inherent spirituality via religion. Though some women may gain access to their spirituality through organized religions, too many religions rely on static dogma and rules that serve to split us from our daily spirituality. Spirituality is free-flowing and ever-changing. Though it is clear that most religions were originally based on the immediate and profound spiritual insights of their founders, most organized religions today lack the flexibility and ongoing evolution necessary to truly be spiritually connected.

Partly in response to so many years of male-based religions, many women today are drawn to different aspects of the Great Goddess. As women, we need "a sexually affirming image of power and beauty as a focus for prayer and meditation," says Patricia Reis.[21] Having internalized God as male, we can find much-needed balance in the Goddess images that are now rising.

My mother is a dowser and frequently uses a pendulum for intuitive guidance. Others use runes, tarot cards, or Bible phrases. Spiritual guidance comes in all forms, so use the form that works best for you.

Regardless of what you believe about spirituality, it is important to bring a sense of the sacred into your everyday life. Spirituality pervades all that I do. My spirituality is not set aside for special days such as Christmas, nor do I practice it only in special buildings called churches, synagogues, or temples. My spirituality is every part of me. On some level I feel part of God/Goddess/All That Is—not separate from it. When I'm exercising, I'm in touch with my spirituality. When I'm writing, I'm very much in touch with my spirituality. I'm especially in touch with my spirituality when I'm assisting women in opening to their inner guidance system. This is because reaching out to another to help her heal and connect with her spirituality also helps me heal and connect with mine.

Like many women, I feel a deep spiritual connection with nature. Many people find peace and comfort in a special place, a place that they may have gone to as children to feel held close by the nurturing qualities of nature. Women often tell me about special trees, rocks, hills, or other places that connect them very strongly with their own spirituality. Time spent alone in a natural setting is often a catalyst for connection with your spirituality.

A powerful way to tune in to the natural world is to notice what phase the moon is in and see if this natural waxing and waning has any effect on your body, emotions, or perceptions.[22] Notice what effect the seasons have on you. Does the coming of autumn wake up your senses and find you braced for new beginnings—or does this happen for you in the spring? Find out when the equinoxes and solstices are. For centuries, people felt that more spiritual power was available to them at these times. All major religious holidays are held around these times. You don't have to study anything—just be aware of the moon and the rhythms of nature. I live on a tidal river and enjoy the changing water levels outside my window, knowing that, like my body, they're connected with the phases of the moon.

When I was growing up, my father used to go to church on Sundays because he liked the church and his family had always gone there. My mother, on the other hand, often went for a walk in the woods. "He has his church, I have mine," she said. Each woman must find her own spiritual center and her own inner guidance. And for each woman it will be different.

Regardless of whether we believe in angels, God, Jesus Christ, the human spirit, Buddha, the Blessed Mother, the Great Spirit, or the Goddess Gaia, being in tune with our spiritual resources is a vital healing force. Committing ourselves to remembering our spiritual selves and receiving guidance for our lives is part of creating vibrant health.

One of the most powerful things you can do with any dilemma is to turn it over to the divine. What that means is acknowledging that you have done everything you know to do intellectually to figure out how to heal your problem. You then sincerely turn it over to the divine, which can be thought of as a part of yourself outside of time and space that knows far more than you do. You can call it God, your inner wisdom, or your Higher Power. You get to choose.

I have a box I call a God box. When I have an issue that I've pretty much worried to death with no resolution, I put it in the God box and then expect to be shown what to do about it. I literally turn it over to divine Source— sometimes again and again if it's something I've been obsessing over (like belly fat or a relationship). And guess what? Over time, I'm always shown. One of my most persistent areas of unfulfillment in life has been romantic relationships, and so over the years I have put many, many desires, prayers, wishes, and names in my God box. It has taken many years of faithful work on myself and my unhealed inner child, but every year, when I empty out the God box and read the contents, I have found myself closer and closer to true soul mate love—but it had to start with me. I know you've heard this before, but it happens to be true. I finally had to surrender the entire issue of relationship to God and pray to be happy with or without a man. I put the following in my God box: "I surrender my love life to the divine. Help me to let go and allow. If I'm meant to be with someone, please send him." This was not easy work. But it worked—especially after I stopped all the "trying" and just got happy with my life.

Those answers can even come immediately sometimes. A reader and radio show listener named Lori Robin recently shared the following amazing story with me:

> I was sitting in the bath listening to a recorded weekly group call with Tosha Silver. After it was done, I did the Five Breaths exercise, and then I relaxed and affirmed that I embrace fully whatever new beginning was coming for me. I completely surrendered to the divine, offering myself up, releasing all expectations. Within seconds, I felt this sharp painful movement under my right rib cage, an area where I've felt pain for more than a decade and which no gastroenterologist has been able to help me with (even after needlessly removing my gallbladder). The pain began to move, and I could actually see this on the outside of my body, the way when you're pregnant you can see the baby's heel moving against your belly. The pain was intense, but I said out loud, "I don't know what this is, but I give thanks (ouch!) for this and embrace it (ouch!)." It twisted, feeling like a snake uncoiling, which didn't startle me, because I love snakes. I just relaxed and continued giving thanks. And just as suddenly as it began, it was over. After sixteen years of having pain in that area— and after seeking treatments of all kinds in the last seven years—the pain was just over. *How bizarre, how wonderful,* I thought, *and how timely,* because I had been contemplating having an ultrasound. Now there was no need to do that. In the year since this happened, I have experienced only very mild twinges of discomfort now and then. I am still amazed that the almost intolerable pain vanished in this way.

DIVINE LOVE: THE MOST POTENT ENERGY IN THE WORLD

Several years ago, I received a flyer about the work of the late Bruno Groening (www.bruno-groening.org/en), a German healer. I went to the meeting, which was led by doctors from Germany, and learned that many healings from so-called incurable illnesses were well documented by the medical scientific group of the Bruno Groening Circle of Friends. The Circle of Friends teaches a way to tune in to the divine through a process called *Einstellen,* which is a way of sitting with the hands on the thighs in a palms-up position with arms and legs uncrossed. While tuned in this way, one can feel what Groening called *Heilstrom,* German for "the healing stream." Beautiful music has been written to accompany this practice. I went to many meetings of the Circle of Friends and personally witnessed a number of remarkable healings, including a woman with multiple sclerosis and a man with insulin-dependent diabetes. I was also impressed with the scientific rigor with which the healings were documented.

Then I learned about the work of engineer Robert Fritchie, author of many books, including *Being at One with the Divine: Self-Healing with Divine Love* (World Service Institute, 2016). Fritchie worked with the late Marcel Vogel, a scientist who held more than a hundred patents in crystal technology with IBM. Fritchie and Vogel worked on the documentation of energy healing for many years. This healing force, which Fritchie calls Divine Love, is, in my experience, exactly the same thing as the *Heilstrom* that Bruno Groening referred to. Fritchie calls it the most powerful healing force in the world. And he, too, has used it to help heal everything from environmental pollution to cancer.

Vogel developed special crystals to amplify energy, but crystals aren't necessary. Fritchie points out that we are all crystals, able to both send and receive healing energy transmitted through intent. (As I've noted, our connective tissue, teeth, and bones are all crystalline matrixes in which information in one area is instantly transmitted throughout the whole.) Gary Schwartz, Ph.D., director of the Laboratory for Advances in Consciousness and Health at the University of Arizona in Tucson, has documented this, showing also that the human heart emits light.

Divine Love is available to everyone, regardless of religious background. It is God's love, pure and simple. It is not the same as personal love. Using personal love (your own personal compassion and care) to heal someone can be very dangerous for those who are empathic and drawn to the healing professions. That's because we often want an outcome for someone that is not in alignment with what that person's soul and spirit have chosen. Divine Love bypasses all this. It's why we end each petition with "According to the Creator's Will." Divine Love works through the high vibration of your Spirit and your intention. It is a higher vibration than your thoughts, your soul, and your body.

I personally work with Divine Love every day. As Fritchie notes, one must believe in a loving Creator in order for Divine Love to work well. I have come to see that nothing is incurable and that the healing power of Divine Love is essential knowledge for everyone as we move through this time of change on the planet. The following two healing statements (used with permission of Bob Fritchie) are the most current petitions Fritchie has created to help people heal.

First, use the one-symptom healing statement for one symptom and one symptom only. That symptom might be a headache, a sore toe, fear of flying, or grief over the death of a loved one. Pick one, and know that Divine Love works to complete the petition as long as you do the four-cycle breathing exercise associated with clearing your energy field, which is also explained below.

Pop-ups are (usually emotional) symptoms that may arise while you are clearing the original symptom. Use the second healing statement right after using the first healing statement to remove pop-ups before they begin.

Divine Love Healing Statement for One Symptom

Clasp your palms together and say: "I release to the Creator from my entire being all of my [specify symptom] and ask that the Creator heal all damage from my [specify symptom] automatically according to my Spirit's intent and according to the Creator's will."

Draw in your breath with your mouth closed and pulse your breath once through your nose, as if you were clearing your nostrils. Unclasp your hands.

Divine Love Healing Statement to Remove All Symptom Pop-Ups

Clasp your palms together and say: "I release to the Creator from my entire being all of my pop-ups associated with [specify symptom] and ask that the Creator heal all damage from my pop-ups associated with [specify symptom] automatically according to my Spirit's intent and according to the Creator's will." Draw in your breath with your mouth closed and pulse your breath once through your nose as if you were clearing your nostrils. Unclasp your hands.

Four-Cycle Breathing

In addition to these two healing statements, you also need to add four-cycle breathing to your daily activities. Here's how:

1. Breathe in slowly through your nose for a count of five.

2. Hold your breath for a count of five.

3. Slowly release your breath through your nose for a count of five.

4. Hold your breath for a count of five.

This is one cycle. Repeat at least four times for one deep breathing session.

Do at least four sessions of deep breathing per day. Over time you will find this very, very soothing and effective, and it will speed your healing dramatically.

Do not change the symptom you are working with until you know it has cleared. Here's how you know. Look deeply into your eyes in a mirror and say, "With my Spirit's and the angels' help, I send Divine Love throughout my body and ask the Creator if my [specify symptom] is completely healed in my soul, mind, and physical body." If the answer from the Creator is yes, you can move on to another symptom. If the answer is no, do some deep breathing and continue to check once a day.

The two healing statements are part of Fritchie's At Oneness Healing System Advanced Protocol. The benefits of the advanced protocol are that it keeps you connected to the energy of Divine Love, it purges all the emotions you've stored over time as you do the deep breathing, and it stabilizes any life-threatening health issues first, before addressing your petition symptom. To understand how to get the best results with these two powerful healing statements, I suggest studying the Advanced Protocol and Healing Statement training video on the World Service Institute's website (www .worldserviceinstitute.org).

By the way, you can also facilitate a healing for a loved one using Divine Love by proxy. To do this, all you have to do is follow the same protocol outlined above. Say the two healing statements daily, naming the person you want to help, until the person's symptoms have cleared. Simply replace the word *my* wherever it appears in the two healing statements with the person's name. Divine Love by proxy works no matter what the physical distance may be between you and the other person. This can be a powerful and loving act of service, but remember that it isn't possible to force a healing on someone else based on your own personal desires. The healing statements simply won't work unless your intention is in line with the will of the Creator.

Another important point to keep in mind is that you can't use the healing statements to justify making choices that you know are not healthy (like eating junk food). Whenever you use the healing statements, you are protected in your innocence (or ignorance) from whatever you may not be aware of, but you are responsible for your wellness once you are presented with the truth. If a person does not have access to good food or is unable to afford it, however, the protection remains.

For more information (including specific programs that use Divine Love by proxy to assist in healing addiction and Alzheimer's), see the World Service Institute's website (www.worldserviceinstitute .org).

STEP SEVEN: RECLAIM THE FULLNESS OF YOUR MIND

Women need to know that they are capable of intelligent thought, and they need to know it right now.

—Adrienne Rich

The positive thing about writing is that you connect with yourself in the deepest way, and that's heaven. You get a chance to know who you are, to know what you think. You begin to have a relationship with your mind.

—Natalie Goldberg

If we are to reclaim the wisdom of our bodies, we must also reclaim our intellects, our minds, and our ability to think. Once we have experienced how intimately our thoughts and bodily symptoms are related and how intelligent we are, our thinking is less distracted by cultural hypnosis. We come to trust our inner voice. We question our assumptions more critically, thus freeing ourselves from the mental habits of a lifetime.

Journal writing, writing practice, and meditation are methods that many have used to successfully get in touch with their inner voices and get to know their minds. Proprioceptive writing (PW) taught me to trust my mind and inner wisdom. Originally developed by Linda Trichter Metcalf, Ph.D., coauthor of *Writing the Mind Alive* (Ballantine Books, 2002), this writing process engages the intellect, the intuition, and the imagination simultaneously. It is done to Baroque music, which has been found to synchronize brain waves at about sixty cycles per second, a frequency associated with increased alpha brain waves and enhanced creativity.[23] (For more information on proprioceptive writing, see the website for the Proprioceptive Writing Center at www.pwriting.org.)

In doing proprioceptive writing, I noticed that if I simply wrote down my thoughts as I listened to them, at first they seemed random and without order. When I wrote or thought of a word or concept, my mind immediately went in several directions at once—all of them rich with emotional content, and all of them related to one another equally, nonhierarchically, and non-linearly. Thus, my natural thinking process is circular and multimodal, as it is for many women. But as I continued the process, I could see that my thoughts were weaving a web of interconnected meaning that was going in a certain direction. My job was simply to go along for the ride and record what I heard or felt. I would always come back to my initial point of departure, but with a deeper understanding of my beliefs and wisdom.

Through writing I have come to see that every word that comes into my mind has meaning and that this meaning is connected to my entire being. If I write the word *bra,* for example, my mind goes off in all the following direc-tions almost simultaneously: I think of a woman's relationship with her bra, how she purchased her first bra, what it was like for her, what that means about her relationship with her breasts, whether she's ever used an under-wire bra, what her breasts mean in this culture, whether she was breast-fed, and so on. I've come to appreciate that my ideas, thoughts, and wisdom come from all of me—my brain, my uterus, and my higher power—and that they may originate in any one of the numerous interconnected aspects of me. I have learned to trust my thoughts. Women's (and some men's) ways of knowing are not the logocentric left-brain approaches taught in our schools and universities. It's staggering to realize how many highly intelligent women feel that they are stupid and not good enough because of this training.

Writing practice is a profound tool for learning how to hear ourselves. For years, for example, the word *worthy* kept coming up in my writing be-cause on some deep level I didn't feel worthy. I spent hours asking myself what I meant by this word. Images of school, authorities, tests, and church always arose around this word. Eventually, my meditation on the word *wor-thy* led me to a breakthrough understanding of the original sin of being fe-male. How could I have felt worthy, given my cultural programming?

If a word or phrase continually comes into your mind, it is important—it has meaning for you. Explore it. Write about it. Meditate on it. If a thought comes into your mind, learn to accept it without judgment. It will have mean-ing for you, no matter what it is. It is there for a reason. Linda Metcalf says, "There are no tourists in the mind."

To change the conditions of our lives outside, we must make a change in-side. Proprioceptive writing is a tool to explore what is inside. After all, if we don't know where we are, how can we ever expect to get anywhere else? What I discovered within me were layers and layers of *shoulds, oughts,* and other impedimenta of my education and cultural indoctrination. Metcalf describes these as a "mangrove swamp, with all the roots twisted around each other."

Through weeks, months, and years of writing, I gained direct experi-ence of my own indoctrination, and eventually came to hear my true self emerging—my own voice. But I also ran smack up against my guilt about almost everything—not being a good enough mother, not being a good enough doctor, not having a perfect body, and not being able to fulfill everyone's needs! Mine was the guilt stemming from what Anne Wilson Schaef, Ph.D., called "the ongoing sin of being born female." This guilt seemed to be a part of who I was, neatly installed years before. Guilt for not being "enough" is a fantastic tool for keeping women in their place. It is a form of internalized oppression and fear that serves to maintain the status quo. Guilt immobilizes us with "What will they think if . . ." messages. I realized that if I continued to wallow in my own guilt instead of examining its voice within me, I would forever be ineffective at doing the work I am best at—and which I love the most. How could this possibly help me or anyone else? When I reclaimed my right to do my work and let go of guilt (mostly), I broke free from a set of health-destroying beliefs. It's an ongoing process.

My writing was vital in helping me break free from those parts of my life that no longer served me. However you do it, you, too, can learn to respect your intellect, your mind, and the fullness of your intelligence.

Dialogues with the Body: Listening to the Mind That Creates the Cells

I often ask women to carry out a dialogue with their bodily symptoms or with the organ that is giving them problems, through writing, meditation, or drawing. Sitting with your journal open while being receptive to your thoughts, ask your body what it needs or what it is trying to tell you.

One of my former patients, who was experiencing heavy menstrual bleeding and a fibroid, asked her pelvis to speak to her. In her journal she wrote, "What is the wisdom you are trying to convey to me through my bleeding and my fibroid?" Over the next several days, she "waited with" this question for about ten minutes per day.

The answer that eventually came was, "Your periods are symbolic of the way you give yourself away too freely. The heavy bleeding represents your own life's blood draining away. You do the same thing in your relationship with your boyfriend. This is related to your relationship with your father."

Another former patient told me, "You asked me to have a dialogue with my cervix. [She had had an abnormal Pap test.] It's all about shame, it's all about deprivation, it's all about not being good enough. I think I need to listen some more."

Many fine publications have been written, and workshops offered, on how to do journal work or other forms of introspective dialogue. I recommend Natalie Goldberg's books on writing practice, *Writing Down the Bones* (Shambhala, 1986) and *Wild Mind* (Bantam Books, 1990), as well as Anne Lamott's *Bird by Bird* (Anchor Books, 1995).

Working with Dreams: A Dream Incubation

The night dreams speak Wild Woman's Language. She is there broadcasting. All we have to do is take dictation.

—Clarissa Pinkola Estés

You can learn to work with your dreams actively and learn to consult them about specific problems in your life. The process of asking for a dream for guidance is known as dream incubation.[24] I worked on my dreams regularly for seven years with Doris E. Cohen, Ph.D., clinical psychologist and author of *Dreaming on Both Sides of the Brain: Discover the Secret Language of the Night* (Hampton Roads, 2017). The basic process is outlined below. (To listen to a radio show I did with Dr. Cohen that explains this process in more detail, check this out: www.drnorthrup.com/audio/dream-interpretation-doris-e-cohen.)

HOW TO WORK WITH, REMEMBER, AND INTERPRET YOUR DREAMS

1. Set your intention to remember your dreams. Just say out loud or to yourself something like, "I have amazing dream recall. I always remember my dreams." Have a pen, paper, a flashlight, or a recording device by your bedside table. (I use the voice memo app in my iPhone.)

2. Ask a question that you would like to have answered in your dream. Ask that the imagery be easy to understand and interpret. Then let go and drift off to sleep.

3. If a dream awakens you in the middle of the night, it usually has an important message, so jot down just a few details before going back to sleep. Trust me on this—you *must* pull yourself out of your sleepy state to do this. You will resist it, but if you don't record the dream in some way, you will forget, even though in the moment you are certain that you won't.

4. As soon as you awaken, lie in bed for a moment, remembering the details of the dream before they slip away. Write them down or dictate them.

5. Give the dream a title—like a headline in a newspaper. This will encapsulate the wisdom of the dream and bring it all back to you clearly when you go back to review.

6. Check for recurrent themes in your dreams, as well as for any animals. I always look up the symbology of animals from my dreams in *Animal Speak* (Llewellyn, 1993) by Ted Andrews or in *Medicine Cards* (St. Martin's Press, 1999) by Jamie Sams and David Carson. There are also many online inter-

pretation sites. (Use these as a guide, but remember that you are the ultimate authority for what any dream symbol means for *you*.)

Dr. Cohen points out that clothing and shoes in dreams represent the roles we play in life. The hair on your head represents the thoughts in your head. So a new hairdo or color represents a new way of thinking. Cars represent the self—and so do houses. Each room in the house represents how you live in a certain area of your life. The basement is the unconscious. When you find new rooms you didn't know were there, you are opening up new areas in your unconscious.

7. Larry Burk, M.D., radiologist and imagery specialist and coauthor with Kathleen O'Keefe-Kanavos of *Dreams That Can Save Your Life: Early Warning Signs of Cancer and Other Diseases* (Findhorn Press, 2018), suggests that you ask yourself, "What does the dream want?" Listen for the very first thought that comes into your head. He suggests that the spirit world may have a question it wants you to answer.

8. Share the dream with someone. When you recount a dream to a trusted friend, you will quite often remember aspects of it that you hadn't noticed before.

Note: Very often, later in the day, you will remember a dream from the night before. Don't dismiss it. If a dream bothers you, just go back into the dream and change the outcome. Dreams come from the unconscious, but once the unconscious has gotten our attention through the dream, we can use our conscious mind to go back and engage with the material. In other words, we are not victims of our dreams. Dreams are helping us co-create our reality.

Here's an example of a dream I had a while ago and how I was able to use Doris's techniques to tap into what it was trying to tell me. In the dream, I am at Regena Thomashauer's apartment (Regena is also known as Mama Gena, founder and CEO of Mama Gena's School of Womanly Arts). A poster hangs on the wall from a lonely man who has written all about himself on it. I am *very* interested in him and I feel as though I have known him before. It's late at night, and when I leave the building, I find that the man's car is parked in a no-parking zone. I go up to him, and there is instant chemistry between us. He tells me he is sick and dying. We kiss. And then he simply leaves his car where it is and we walk back to Regena's, where it turns out he has a bedroom. He tells me that he has always wanted to date me but "didn't have the stones" to ask me. I am excited.

Then the dream changes. The next time I see him he is well and he feels great. He's now in the kitchen of my childhood home. We flirt. The television is on, and some guy named Danny is selling his Lighten Up brand of weight-loss foods. I turn off the television and say that I almost never have it on. My guy now turns into Tom Selleck. I'm getting ready to leave to go to work. My guy is there with me. I am so happy. We are just at the beginning.

I called this dream "Love Brings Man Back from the Brink." Doris teaches that everyone in a dream is an aspect of yourself, so when I looked at my dream, I could see that it was about befriending and falling in love with my inner male aspect (my animus), a task I'd been actively engaged in for the prior decade. When I went through my divorce, my most fervent wish was to replace my husband with another man who would come and rescue me—financially, sexually, and socially. Little did I know that my soul had other plans—plans that first and foremost included developing the male skills of financial literacy and business savvy as well as learning how to become the kind of woman who would attract the kind of man who interested me (hence the dream's setting at Mama Gena's School of Womanly Arts). In retrospect, I see that I had to make what Carl Jung called the *hieros gamos,* or sacred marriage between the inner masculine and inner feminine parts of the self. In short, I had to become the man I wanted to marry. This dream signified that I had made great progress in that area. I woke up very excited!

Betty, one of my friends, found herself in a painful social situation in which she felt that two of her colleagues were blaming her for the fact that they were being passed over for job promotions. Betty is very bright and creative and is always able to come up with new approaches to her work that are fun, innovative, and productive. Her colleagues through the years have often been jealous of these abilities. Because she loves working with people and has great difficulty with interpersonal conflict, this latest situation was very painful for Betty. She contemplated quitting her job and moving across the country, even though her work was very fulfilling. When she became aware of the hostility of her colleagues in this current situation, the feeling this evoked in her was old and all too familiar. She had been unfairly black-balled, picked on, and scapegoated similarly by others. It had happened over and over again at other jobs and in several other settings, both personal and professional. Completely fed up with being thus victimized by others, she wanted to choose another way to live with her gifts and talents. She decided to do a dream incubation to ask for guidance in changing whatever unconscious patterns kept attracting situations in which she ended up as the victim of other people's inadequacies. After noting all the different situations in which she'd been victimized and allowing herself to feel fully how disgusted she was by the whole thing, she asked for a dream that would help her clarify her situation. She wrote, "Why do I keep re-creating situations in my life in which people pick on me?"

That night she had the following dream: A very good friend was seated to her left. The friend reached over to help a porcupine, and the porcupine shot its quills at her. Betty's friend took the quills and embedded them in

Betty's arm—then looked in her face to see what her reaction would be. Betty simply sat there and allowed the quills to be painfully embedded in her arm. So the same friend took a handful of needles and pins and began sticking them in Betty's arm. Meanwhile, Betty continued to say nothing—simply sitting there with the pain of this. Finally, Betty decided to do something about her pain. She began taking the needles out herself. When she did this, a great deal of blood started pouring out of all the needle holes in her arm. Overwhelmed with the pain and the extent of the bleeding, Betty then decided to complain to her friend, telling her it was not okay to stick quills and needles in her arm. Betty then looked to her right side and saw her mother, father, and sister all sitting there.

When Betty awakened, she realized that throughout her childhood, these family members had insulted and even physically beaten her. Betty had never complained and had never said anything. Instead, she simply put up with the pain and allowed herself to bleed. (Remember, blood is symbolic of family.) As she reflected on her dream, Betty realized that she didn't need to move or change jobs; she needed to change the way she responded when people expressed their resentment of her. She could no longer allow psychic, emotional, or other barbs to accumulate without saying anything. She knew that she had come to the point of "bleeding to death" from the accumulation of a lifetime of hurts that she had never acknowledged or complained about. Because of her upbringing, she had been led to believe that if she complained, she'd simply get beaten more. Now Betty realized that she had to stand up for herself at the first sign of discomfort in her relationships. She saw how deeply the victim mentality had been drummed into her in childhood. She had used her considerable gifts and talents to escape her family of origin—only to have the original family pattern recur in all her later relationships. Having become very clear about her part in creating victim situations by refusing to defend herself, Betty now speaks up for herself at the first sign of discomfort. She also realizes that if a colleague has problems with her abilities, this is not something that she has to fix. The colleague herself must deal with her own inner sense of jealousy and inadequacy to see what it is teaching her. Betty cannot do this for another.

FALLING IN LOVE ENHANCES OUR BRAINS

Falling in love has a reputation for making us appear more scattered and distracted, but powerful evidence shows that it actually helps us think better. Stephanie Cacioppo, Ph.D., a neuroscientist at the University of Chicago, has used neuroimaging to explore what happens in our brains when we're in love. Her data show that romantic love has an effect on the regions of the brain involved in higher-level intellectual activities and cognition (including an area called the angular gyrus), so being in love helps you think faster, better anticipate others' thoughts and behavior, express creativity, and even recuperate faster from illnesses. So not only is love good for our emotions but it's good for our brain as well.

Focusing on reclaiming the fullness of your mind has never been as important as it is now. We simply must realize that we can do much on our own to achieve optimal health in this area. While I certainly respect the field of psychiatry, I find it interesting that at a time when scientific research has still not yielded any confirmed genetic or biological scientific explanation for mental disease, drug companies continue to market more and more psychotropic drugs. For example, while the number of people suffering from depression is not on the decline, more and more people take antidepressants. In Iceland, which reports the highest amount of antidepressants taken per capita, the suicide rate has not changed in the last decade.

In 2013, when the American Psychiatric Association released the latest issue of the *Diagnostic and Statistical Manual of Mental Disorders* (*DSM-5*), considered the psychiatrists' bible, it caused quite a furor among psychiatrists around the world because for the first time it defined certain patterns of behavior and mood as illnesses, which many professionals saw as overmedicalizing mental health. It's not surprising that eighteen out of the twenty-seven members of the task force that produced the *DSM-5* (that's 67 percent) had direct links to the pharmaceutical industry.[25] Prescription drugs certainly have their place, but it's time we took our power back. Let's not rely on pharmaceuticals to do the work we can do so much better on our own, with some guidance.

An inspiring example of what is possible comes from psychiatrist Kelly Brogan, M.D., who wrote a case study for a professional journal about a woman with a host of psychiatric issues.[26] The woman had endured torture as a child, which led to psychotic behavior, suicidal thoughts, and posttraumatic stress disorder, not to mention alcoholism and an eating disorder. Initially, her doctors prescribed antidepressants, and when those didn't work, they diagnosed her with bipolar disorder and prescribed up to fifteen medications over the next several years, some of which caused disabling side effects including fibromyalgia and irritable bowel syndrome.

Then the woman read Dr. Brogan's *New York Times* bestseller, *A Mind of Your Own: The Truth About Depression and How Women Can Heal Their Bodies to Reclaim Their Lives* (HarperCollins, 2016). After one month of following the recommendations in the book—including dietary change, detox, and meditation—the woman enrolled in Dr. Brogan's Vital Mind Reset online program. Using this protocol, she was able to resolve all her symptoms (both physical and psychiatric), and her doctor noted in her medical record that she no longer exhibited bipolar disorder. At the time Dr. Brogan published the case study, the woman had been symptom free for a full year.

STEP EIGHT: GET HELP

We do not believe in ourselves until someone reveals that deep inside us something is valuable, worth listening to, worthy of our trust, sacred to our touch. Once we believe in ourselves we can risk curiosity, wonder, spontaneous delight, or any experience that reveals the human spirit.

—e.e. cummings

Setting aside the time and money to go and talk with a skilled listener can be invaluable. This person may be a therapist, a minister, a life coach, or other trustworthy individual. These sessions can be a way to stop, reassess your life, and give yourself a much-needed focus on a regular basis. Many therapists have helped people begin to look at their lives differently and effect change. A good therapist should be like a midwife, standing by while someone gives birth to what's best in herself. My eleven years of dream therapy with Dr. Cohen have been invaluable. So have the numerous intuitive readings I've received through the years. My only caveat here is that if you are living with an individual who is narcissistic or has borderline personality disorder, you really need a therapist who understands the dynamic. Otherwise you can spend years and years turning yourself into a pretzel trying to get your narcissist to wake up and change—which they almost never do. Check out www.survivortreatment.com for resources in this area.

When I was around fourteen and upset about something that I can't even remember now, my father told me how important it was to express what I was feeling and "get it off my chest." (The phrase "get it off your chest" is an accurate anatomic description of dealing with fourth-chakra issues, such as sadness, which tend to affect the shoulders, breast, and heart.) He told me, "I notice a tendency in you to clam up and not say what's going on. When you do this, you prevent others from helping you." It was good advice, and something I've had to address for decades. We all can use a reassessment of our lives and a skilled listener on a regular basis. Support of this nature should be built into the culture. Community has been largely lost since the Industrial Revolution and the ensuing split between work, home, private, and public. In an ideal world it wouldn't be necessary for us to go to individual therapists or to create separate support groups for those with cancer, those suffering from loneliness, or even those who want to flourish.

There are many different kinds of therapists. The entire field has been changing in response to evolving knowledge about addiction, recovery, personality disorder, PTSD, and the influence of childhood trauma. Specific populations are even being addressed in new, supportive ways. For example, Joy Harden Bradford, Ph.D., is an Atlanta psychologist who founded the website Therapy for Black Girls (www.therapyforblackgirls.com), which presents a wide range of mental health topics in a way meant to counteract the taboo she says exists around seeking therapy in many African American communities.

Therapy is not something that should go on for years, in my view. I much prefer methods like eye movement desensitization and reprocessing (EMDR), tapping, and Divine Love petitions that get to the root of the problem and solve it using the individual's own power and connection with inner wisdom. The old Freudian psychoanalysis model where you go for years and years without making actual changes in your behavior can be itself an addictive process—not much different from the alcoholic/enabler duality. All relationships, therapeutic or otherwise, work best when the participants see each other as essentially whole beings with inner resources and strengths, though sometimes in temporary need of assistance.

EMOTIONAL FREEDOM TECHNIQUE (TAPPING)

The Emotional Freedom Technique, also referred to simply as tapping, combines elements of both Chinese acupressure and modern psychology. It's a scientifically proven and very practical way to decrease stress hormones and facilitate healing. The method consists of tapping your fingertips on eight specific acupressure points along the energy meridians delineated in traditional Chinese medicine while talking about whatever you want to transform—painful memories, difficult emotions, limiting beliefs, or even physical conditions. Acknowledging the symptom or emotion and concentrating on accepting yourself despite the situation as you activate the meridians clears energy blocks and resets your body's natural physiological response. Activating the meridians in this way sends a calming signal to your brain, reducing the stress response the emotion or situation elicits. Also, because the energy meridians you are tapping on are each linked to a specific organ or system, you are facilitating the flow of energy directly to that meridian and so to those body systems and parts.

Sometimes you can release the energy blocks in just one session, while bigger issues may require more sessions. The end result is that you will restore your energy to a balanced state. Once the stress response (and its associated inflammatory chemicals) has been turned off in this way, you will also have more access to your inner wisdom, which will guide you to the solution and also allow your body to heal. Here's how you do it.

Remove any eyeglasses as well as jewelry that is easy to take off (both so that you have clear access to tapping points and also because certain gemstones can electromagnetically interfere with your efforts). Decide on the negative emotion or the unresolved problem you want to work on and assess your current level of physical or emotional discomfort on a scale of 1 to 10. State your tapping affirmation by saying the following sentence out loud, filling in the appropriate blank with the single issue you've chosen: "Even though I [name the problem—for example, 'feel unappreciated by my partner,' 'didn't get the raise I wanted,' 'feel overwhelming anxiety,' 'have migraine headaches'], I deeply and completely love and accept myself." Be as specific as possible.

Begin tapping firmly with the tips of your index and middle fingers (using both hands or just one) on the first tapping point, which is on the crown of your head, and after tapping about five to nine times, move to the second tapping point (the beginning of your eyebrow, near the bridge of your nose), and tap there the same number of times. (If you are tapping with two hands, simultaneously tap on the right side of the body with the right hand and the left side with the left hand.) Continue this process until you've tapped on each of the other points (below your eyebrow at the outer side of your eye, underneath your eye, underneath your nose, on your chin below your lips, on the edge of your collar bone below your throat, and at the base of your armpit). As you tap, repeat a word or phrase as a reminder of the issue, such as "this fear," or "this feeling of failure," or "this headache." The tapping should be firm but not painful. After you tap on all eight points, move back to the first tapping point and repeat the entire process a second time.

Then reassess your level of discomfort, again on a scale of 1 to 10, and see if it has improved. This way, even though you may still be feeling discomfort, you can see your progress. Continue tapping until the issue is cleared. If you reach a plateau, stop and tap again later.

Beginning with a setup statement is often helpful. To do that, say your tapping affirmation as you tap what's called the karate chop point (the fleshy part of the outer edge of your hand on the opposite side of your thumb; it's the part you'd use to deliver a karate chop) with the four fingers of your opposite hand. Repeat the tapping affirmation three times as you continue to tap on this spot. Then follow the sequence outlined above for the eight main tapping points.

A fair amount of research shows that tapping is indeed effective. To begin with, a study at Harvard Medical School proved that stimulating the body's meridian points reduces the stress response produced in the area of the brain called the amygdala.[27] This is the response that floods the body with the stress hormone cortisol.

Dawson Church, Ph.D., an expert on tapping, did a study at the Foundation for Epigenetic Medicine in Fulton, California, to specifically measure tapping's effect on this hormone. He measured the cortisol levels of three groups—one that did a single tapping session, one that received a single session of traditional talk therapy, and a control group that received no treatment at all. The talk therapy group and the control group experienced no significant reduction in cortisol, while the tapping group had an average cortisol drop of 24 percent, with some subjects reducing cortisol levels by as much as 50 percent.[28]

Australian psychologist Peta Stapleton, Ph.D., has tested tapping for food cravings and weight loss. One of her most impressive studies, not yet published, looked at eighty-nine obese women who tapped for about two hours each week for eight weeks (an average of just more than fifteen minutes a day). By the end of the study, they'd lost an average of sixteen pounds by tapping alone—without dieting or exercising. When Dr. Stapleton followed up with them at least six months later, even though most had stopped tapping when the study was over, most had also maintained their weight loss.

For more information about this powerful practice, read *Tapping Solution: A Revolutionary System for Stress-Free Living* (Hay House, 2013) by Nick Ortner or visit his website at www .thetappingsolution.com. You can also find a number of YouTube videos online that will take you through the sequence.

EYE MOVEMENT DESENSITIZATION AND REPROCESSING (EMDR)

Eye movement desensitization and reprocessing (EMDR) is a psychotherapy treatment developed in the 1990s that is designed to alleviate the stress response triggered by traumatic memories. It's been shown to be particularly good for post-traumatic stress syndrome, although it works on many different issues. EMDR is based on the idea that during trauma, the brain processes and stores memories incorrectly, in such a way that when we recall the event, it can feel like it's happening in present time. EMDR allows the brain to restore these memories in their proper place so when the incident is recalled, it loses its charge.

While the eight-phase process is rather complex, the core element involves a trained therapist asking the patient to track the therapist's hand as it moves rapidly across the patient's field of vision while the patient is recalling—in small doses—the incident that triggered the trauma. The idea behind this is that if your attention is diverted by the eye movements, the memory is not as triggering and so the typical stress response is lessened and eventually eliminated. The brain is then able to process the experiences more effectively without the stress response, so it is stored properly in the brain. One theory is that the experience is connected with the biological mechanisms involved in the rapid eye movement period of sleep, when we dream (thought to be a time when the subconscious processes various emotions and experiences). The insights the patient gains in EMDR therapy are not from the therapist's interpretation and guidance but from the patient's own mental processes. This is much more empowering than standard talk therapy, and it usually works more quickly. Some problems can be treated in a single session, while others require several sessions.

The EMDR Institute notes that more than thirty controlled studies show positive results with EMDR therapy, some of which report that 84 to 90 percent of single-trauma victims no longer have PTSD after three 90-minute EMDR sessions.[29] A study of sixty-seven PTSD patients funded by Kaiser Permanente found that 100 percent of single-trauma victims and 77 percent of multiple-trauma victims no longer had PTSD after six 50-minute EMDR sessions.[30]

For more information, see the EMDR Institute's website at www .emdr.com.

Though individual therapy is often a first step for many women, group work of some kind, such as a twelve-step group or a skills training group, can be powerful in that this setting helps us see that our problems are shared by so many others. A member of Overeaters Anonymous once told me, "Addiction recovery is God's answer to community." Group work certainly is one answer that is helping millions. The practical wisdom contained in the twelve steps of Alcoholics Anonymous is a blueprint for how to live a life based on inner guidance. Many other twelve-step fellowships use AA's steps and simply take out the word *alcohol* or *alcoholic* if it's not applicable, substituting something more relevant.

Groups help rid us of our "myth of terminal uniqueness," as a therapist friend calls it, while individual therapy, especially for wounds such as incest, can isolate a woman further because it "privatizes" what is in fact a cultural and even global problem. Part of the wounding power of addictions, incest, or other sexual abuse is due to the secrecy with which we approach them. Imagine the relief of participating in a group of women in which all of them are saying, "That happened to you, too? I always thought I was the only one!"

It has been my experience that women with histories of trauma recover most effectively in a type of group therapy known as cognitive behavioral therapy. This form of therapy focuses more on helping people develop the skills necessary to live productive, healthy lives in the present than on the traumas of the past. It is generally not helpful to spend a great deal of time revisiting the past, where it is too easy to get stuck in pain and immobility. Instead, women with trauma histories need to have their wounds witnessed and validated, and then learn the coping skills that they never developed in childhood. Cognitive behavioral therapy training teaches women to answer the following questions and then to take effective, balanced action.

What am I feeling?

What is the purpose of this feeling? What unmet need is it signaling?

What do I need to do for myself to get this need met?

I have seen more improvement in women's lives with this model than with most others. These skills are practical and helpful for everyone, not just for those with histories of trauma, because they reprogram old subconscious programming.

Many people with chronic or life-threatening illness also come together regularly to share not only their tears but also their joy and their laughter. This grassroots movement of support groups throughout the country has been a source of growth, comfort, and hope to many. I regularly refer people to support groups of all kinds in our community, and have participated myself. Dr. David Spiegel has clearly demonstrated that women with metastatic breast cancer who participated in a support group characterized by emotional openness and sharing lived twice as long as those who didn't participate.[31] If a drug had been shown to have this effect, you can bet it would be widely used. But to date, most women diagnosed with breast cancer are not encouraged to seek the health benefits of this group model.

For many women, it is important to spend time regularly in women-only settings. When we gather together as women, we each hold a piece of the whole story. Together we heal faster than we would if we remained isolated and separate, and group members hold up a mirror for us so that we can see ourselves more clearly.

In the early stages of self-awareness, women often don't tell the whole truth if there's even one man in the room. The same may be true for men. We've been socialized to tailor our conversations to accommodate the other gender. In order to become self-aware, we need environments in which we can truly be ourselves. For many, that means women-only settings until you can tell the truth about any given experience without changing your story to protect the men who are present. This process has taken me years to master.

Annie Rafter, a nurse practitioner colleague from my past, tells the following story: One summer she and a group of women friends crewed together on a sailboat and participated in races. They began to notice that if a man came on their boat, they automatically deferred to him—handing him the tiller or expecting him to chart the right course—before they even knew whether or not he was a good sailor.

Noticing this behavior in themselves, the women decided that for one season, they needed to sail with no men on the boat so that they could become a cohesive crew. So for that one season, they stuck by their agreement and learned to trust one another. By the next sailing season, it didn't matter who came on the boat—the women crew trusted themselves, one another, and their sailing skills. They no longer automatically deferred to men.

In the early days of my practice at Women to Women, we often referred back to Annie Rafter's story about "no men on the boat." Like her crew, we needed to learn to trust one another and to learn how to maintain that trust, no matter who came into the building. Back then, I found that working in a women-only environment gave me the time and space to talk out my problems in a way that simply didn't work with my husband. We women have been mistakenly taught that our mates should be our best friends and our primary source of emotional support. Occasionally this works, but not often. When we rely on men to support us emotionally, we often end up disappointed. I'd find that when I'd had my "process" time with other women, I didn't need my husband to be there for me to go over the details of my day and give me advice or support. When I went home, we met more as partners to share the events of our day in a way that was totally different from the way I shared them with one of my women friends. By having plenty of women-only time and support, I learned not to burden my primary male-female relationship with needs that probably weren't meant to be filled in that relationship in the first place.

Meetings and support help people to get out of denial. Twelve-step and other programs have helped millions of people recover inner strength and serenity—this should be the first step in moving on in their lives. In order to heal fully, however, each of us must get to a point in which we're not overly identified with our wounds. This is not easy, because "we learn the language of wounds as our first language and we use our wounds to create intimacy," as Caroline Myss says. People don't heal fully and move on with their lives as long as they continue to take what has happened to them too personally and identify themselves solely as victims. When a woman's identity becomes bound up with her role as a victim, she may lash out at anyone who dares to suggest that she has the inner wisdom to change. Be careful of your language. Though it may be appropriate to label yourself as an incest survivor or breast cancer survivor initially, eventually this identification with your wound may prevent you from becoming the healthy, whole person you were meant to be. At some point, you'll find that you'll be better served by something like "I am a woman who has experienced breast cancer or incest"—this expands your options, while the label "survivor" may limit them. Be sensitive to when it's time to leave your group and move on. Eventually each of us must take responsibility for our own lives and stop laying the blame for our circumstances on external factors—as valid as this may be—whether they be incest and abuse, illness, addiction, the political system, race, gender identity, or the environment. Seeing our dysfunctional patterns, working on them, and letting them go is a most empowering practice.

HOW TO END THE FIGHT AGAINST CANCER— OR ANYTHING ELSE

Our society generally encourages cancer patients to do battle against the disease, thinking such a fighting attitude will help the patient survive. But what if the mental state necessary to wage war, and the stressful emotions that go along with it, actually do more harm than good? Research suggests that emotional acceptance following a cancer diagnosis may well lead to less distress and better outcomes. This doesn't mean sitting back and accepting a death sentence. Far from it. Emotional acceptance involves allowing all emotions—both positive and negative—to surface, acknowledging them, and then letting them naturally dissipate without trying to control, change, or reject them.[32]

Researchers at the University of Arizona taught 136 women diagnosed with various stages of breast cancer an emotional regulation technique and then measured its effects on various aspects of their physiology.[33] When a woman's emotional acceptance scores were low, the researchers noted, she displayed more symptoms of sickness and her levels of pro-inflammatory cytokines were higher. But as her emotional acceptance scores increased, her cytokines generally went down (important because some cytokines can trigger further inflammatory cascades that actually increase the chance of the cancer metastasizing).[34] Even more intriguing, high levels of emotional acceptance were associated with fewer symptoms of being sick, even in those women whose cytokine levels were high. Not surprisingly, by the way, previous research shows that just being diagnosed with cancer creates a surge of cytokines.[35] Because it stands to reason that anything that can reduce cytokines should lead to a greater chance of survival, this approach is well worth considering.

STEP NINE: WORK WITH YOUR BODY

For most of us, talking things out is simply not enough. "I know all of the things that happened to me as a child and with my husband," said one woman, "but talking about it just doesn't change a thing. I seem to be going in circles." When this happens, we often obsess and seem to spin our wheels. It's easy to get locked into "thought addiction"—a kind of gerbil wheel in the brain that keeps us going around in circles.

Much of the information we need to heal is locked in our muscles and other body parts. Getting a good massage will often release old energy blockages and help us cry or get rid of chronic pain from "holding the world on our shoulders." There are many types of bodywork, ranging from polarity therapy to the Feldenkrais Method, that are beneficial. Bodywork can be divided into two different types: physical bodywork (like Rolfing, classical osteopathy, and massage) and energetic bodywork (like Reiki, acupuncture, and therapeutic touch). Though I will not be discussing these separately, I wanted to make this distinction.

Working on and with the body can be an opportunity for understanding and experiencing the unity of our bodymind. These therapies are often deeply relaxing and give our bodies a chance to rest and sleep, a time when much of the body's repair work goes on. Acupuncture works well for all kinds of problems that aren't easily treated through conventional means. I would like to see it and the many other kinds of physical and energetic bodywork used in conventional hospitals.

I've referred hundreds of patients for bodywork of different kinds over the years and am very gratified by the results. I personally get a full body massage once a week. I regard it as part of my general health maintenance program—with good reason. Massage both decreases stress hormones and increases oxytocin (the so-called bonding or love hormone, produced during childbirth and breast-feeding, as well as during giving or receiving acts of loving-kindness, including touch and hugging).[36] In one study at the University of California San Diego Medical Center, researchers measured blood levels of oxytocin as well as adrenocorticotropin (ACTH)—a hormone that stimulates the adrenal glands to secrete the stress hormone cortisol—before and after a fifteen-minute massage.[37] Oxytocin levels increased by 17 percent and ACTH decreased by 20 percent. A control group that just rested showed a 9 percent decrease in oxytocin and a 30 percent increase for ACTH.

I also do Pilates twice per week—a bodywork practice that has been transformational. I know that without it I would have needed a hip replacement by now. I have also used acupuncture a great deal, as well as foot reflexology, shiatsu massage, myofascial release, Thai massage, and resistance stretching (see chapter 18, on exercise). All these types of bodywork help keep the connective tissue, known as fascia, well hydrated and supple.

Schedule at least a shoulder or foot massage sometime this month. You can also trade massages with a friend. Eventually, work up to a full massage regularly.

STEP TEN: GATHER INFORMATION

Currently, more books of interest to women are available than at any other time in history. I recommend going online, to your bookstore, or to your local library and using your inner guidance to help you make a choice. Acknowledge that you have the wisdom to choose the right book at the right time. Just sit with the books for a while and look over a few titles. See which ones speak to you. Choose the ones that feel right and have appeal. You cannot make a mistake.

It is a powerful experience for women to begin to reclaim our forgotten history by reading about our bodies, menstruation, childbirth, goddesses, and women's lives, all written from a woman's point of view. One of the greatest gifts of the feminist movement of the 1970s was the deconstructing of the patriarchal mindset, which was seen for centuries as "the truth" or "just the way it is." Ursula Le Guin, for example, pointed out that 50 percent of writers are women, but 90 percent of what we call "literature" has been written by men. As I mentioned in chapter 8, Meryl Streep noted in 2015 that the movie review site Rotten Tomatoes, which represents the "perceived wisdom" of what is good to watch, was outrageously tilted toward male reviewers.

Books ranging from *Our Bodies, Ourselves* (Simon & Schuster, 1973; revised by Touchstone, 2005), by the Boston Women's Health Book Collective, which heralded a much-needed reevaluation of women's healthcare, to *The Chalice and the Blade* (Harper, 1990) and *Sacred Pleasure* (HarperSanFrancisco, 1995), by Riane Eisler, have helped the baby boom generation rethink our history and how it has affected our lives.[38] As a result, the younger generation of women now coming of age have been raised by mothers who are far more conscious than our mothers before us—and those before them. And on it goes, as we all evolve and grow. I was recently at a yoga class in Miami taught by a lovely young woman whose mother has the first edition of this book. It delights me to see how the work I did back in the 1980s and 1990s has impacted my daughters' generation. Through the power of the pen, we receive support for our journey together. It has been a great pleasure to include the work of many of these women in these pages, such as Tami Lynn Kent, author of *Wild Creative* (Atria Books, 2014), a physical therapist who was inspired by my work long ago.

The many new volumes on the mind-body connection are also of great help to women in reinforcing their own experience. Hay House, a company started by the late Louise Hay when she was sixty years old, has been a leader in publishing transformational books such as *The Biology of Belief* (Hay House, 2008) by Bruce Lipton, Ph.D., a cellular biologist and former research scientist at Stanford University School of Medicine. Dr. Lipton's work is particularly relevant and helpful, as it documents the science of how thought and emotions affect cells in an easily understood manner that is both convincing and entertaining. (For more information, see www.brucelipton .com.) Everything ever written by the late Louise Hay continues to be relevant, particularly the classic *You Can Heal Your Life* (Hay House, 1987), as well as the updated and revised edition of *Empowering Women* (Hay House, 2019). Every day I receive manuscripts from women all over the world who are writing empowering and uplifting books for other women on topics ranging from health and childbearing to creating sacred space and sacred relationships. It is thrilling to me to see the blossoming of women writers and healers at this time in history.

Books are great companions for many otherwise-isolated women who have not yet found one another or come together in communities. Reading and gathering information is a very nonthreatening first step on the journey to flourishing. Many women spend years secretly reading everything that they can get their hands on before they feel ready to join a group or seek other support and sisterhood. Of course, once they do, they find many others who share their beliefs!

A word about discernment and media literacy: When you're gathering information, take a careful look at who is making what claims and how they are backing them up. After all, even M.D.'s get fooled! Case in point: In 2009, it was revealed that Wyeth, the drug company that makes Premarin and Prempro, had paid a medical communications firm to write twenty-six papers emphasizing the benefits and minimizing the risks of synthetic hormones. The papers—which did not disclose that Wyeth initiated and paid for the work—were submitted and eventually published in eighteen different professional journals between 1998 and 2005, influencing untold numbers of researchers, doctors, and the public in favor of Wyeth's products. Wyeth's investment initially paid off—in 2001 alone, the company's sales of hormone drugs reached nearly $2 billion. But the party was over the following year when the government suddenly halted its famous Women's Health Initiative study on hormone therapy because the women in the study who took Prempro ended up with an alarmingly higher risk of heart disease, stroke, and invasive breast cancer.

Fast-forward to 2009, when a personal injury lawsuit against Wyeth disclosed evidence of what had gone on behind the scenes. Court documents revealed that after being hired by Wyeth, the medical communications company outlined the articles, drafted them, and then sought prestigious doctors to sign their names to the studies, despite the fact that many of these doctors did little or none of the actual article writing. Wyeth insisted that the papers were "scientifically sound" and had been subjected to rigorous review by outside experts, claiming that this was common practice in the industry. Yet *The New York Times* quoted Joseph S. Ross, M.D., an assistant professor of geriatrics at Mount Sinai School of Medicine in New York and one of the professionals who did research on the medical ghostwriting, as saying, "It's almost like steroids and baseball. You don't know who was using and who wasn't; you don't know which articles are tainted and which aren't."[39]

The practice isn't confined to Wyeth—court documents show that the same thing has happened with many drugs made by other pharmaceutical companies as well, including tamoxifen. The actual studies on tamoxifen from the National Cancer Institute show that though it does decrease recurrence rates of breast cancer, it doesn't affect mortality at all. In other words, taking tamoxifen doesn't save lives. As the *Times* notes, the incident reveals "that the level of hidden industry influence on medical literature is broader than previously known." This isn't anything new; it's just that people are starting to wake up and smell the deception! Back in 2000, the editor in chief of the famed *New England Journal of Medicine,* Marcia Angell, M.D., stepped down from her esteemed position when she could no longer tolerate the degree of drug company interference in the practice of medicine and the research that supports it. Her book *The Truth About the Drug Companies: How They Deceive Us and What to Do About It* (Random House, 2004) points out that Big Pharma spends more than $12 billion per year on tactics designed to get both doctors and patients to rely more and more on drug solutions. She teamed up with another former *New England Journal of Medicine* editor in chief, Arnold Relman, M.D., to coauthor an article for *The New Republic* in 2002 in which Dr. Relman (also known for coining the term "medical-industrial complex") wrote, "The medical profession is being bought by the pharmaceutical industry, not only in terms of the practice of medicine but also in terms of teaching and research. The academic institutions of this country are allowing themselves to be the paid agents of the pharmaceutical industry. I think it's disgraceful."[40]

Here's another example. In their book *Spontaneous Evolution* (Hay House, 2009), Bruce Lipton, Ph.D., and Steve Bhaerman point out that "when the pharmaceutical industry needed to increase the profit margin by selling more and more blood pressure medications, it simply got the medical industry to change the definition of high blood pressure. For years, hypertension was considered to be blood pressure that measured above 140/90. In 2003, however, a new condition called pre-hypertension was introduced to describe patients whose blood pressure lies between 120/80 and 140/90. Voilà! The world now has a new condition that can be treated with the same old drugs, and the pharmaceutical industry has a brand-new market with many more new customers."[41] In 2017, blood pressure guidelines changed yet again, with prehypertension now called "elevated blood pressure" and high blood pressure redefined as starting at 130/80 and split into two categories—stage one, which is 130/80 to 139/89, and stage two, which is 140/90 and higher. With this change, an additional 31.1 million Americans became classified as hypertensive, and the percentage of the population with hypertension climbed from 31.9 to 45.6 percent—in other words, from less than one-third to approaching half of all Americans! While medication is recommended for most people starting only with stage two hypertension (with lifestyle changes recommended for those with stage one hypertension and those with elevated blood pressure), the high blood pressure label will no doubt have an effect of its own. It's also worth noting that the 2017 decision was controversial even within the medical community. While the new definition was set by eleven groups that included the American Heart Association and the American College of Cardiology, other groups disagreed. The American College of Physicians and the American College of Family Physicians set the high blood pressure threshold for the systolic reading (the top number) at 150 for people age sixty and older.

Similarly, serious and potentially dangerous side effects are often downplayed, including those associated with some extremely popular medications, even though the FDA requires this information to be included in the prescribing information. For example, antidepressants and the stimulant drugs prescribed for ADHD can cause aggressive and violent behavior in some people.

In a study done at the Institute for Safe Medication Practices in Alexandria, Virginia, researchers identified 1,527 cases of violence disproportionately reported for thirty-one drugs, including eleven antidepressants, six sedatives, three ADHD medications, and a drug used to help people quit smoking.[42] (For more on the dangers of these commonly prescribed drugs, read *Medication Madness: The Role of Psychiatric Drugs in Cases of Violence, Suicide, and Crime* [St. Martin's Press, 2008] by Peter R. Breggin, M.D.) In many of the horrific crimes reported in the news today, including school shootings and high-profile cases of parents killing their children, the perpetrators were reportedly taking such drugs. Clearly, the vast majority of people taking these medications are not affected in this way. But with 35 million Americans currently taking antidepressants, that means thousands of patients are vulnerable.

In the highly entertaining 2005 feature film *Side Effects,* with actress Katherine Heigl, when a drug company rep finally wakes up to the tactics her company is using, her conscience can no longer tolerate her continuing to participate. The movie was written and directed by Kathleen Slattery-Moschkau, who spent a decade working as a drug sales representative for the pharmaceutical industry. She documented her experience and wrote the screenplay when she left. (By the way, many drug reps are absolutely charming people. Drug companies are very smart. They recruit good-looking and personable individuals, many of whom are former cheerleaders—individuals to whom it's difficult to say no if you're an overworked doctor). As Carl Elliott of the Center for Bioethics at the University of Minnesota wrote in a 2006 article in the *Atlantic,* "It is probably fair to say that doctors, pharmacists, and medical-school professors are not generally admired for their good looks and fashion sense. Against this backdrop, the average drug rep looks like a supermodel, or maybe an A-list movie star. Drug reps today are often young, well groomed, and strikingly good-looking. Many are women. They are usually affable and sometimes very smart. Many give off a kind of glow, as if they had just emerged from a spa or salon. And they are always, hands down, the best-dressed people in the hospital. . . . Many reps are so friendly, so easygoing, so much fun to flirt with that it is virtually impossible to demonize them. How can you demonize someone who brings you lunch and touches your arm and remembers your birthday and knows the names of all your children?"[43] Having been visited by scores of drug reps over the years, I can attest to the accuracy of those comments.

Big Pharma also has a lot of influence on most mainstream television news as well as the mainstream news magazines. As a result of this influence, safe, cheap approaches to health are almost always downplayed and even ridiculed in the press, while the latest drug treatment is big news. I feel the film *Side Effects* should be a must-view in all public schools as an intellectual immunization against the belief that there is a pill for every ill. The bottom line: Consumer beware!

One more word of caution about gathering information. Genetic testing has become extremely popular with people who want to learn if they are at risk for various conditions and diseases. While there are times when such testing may indeed be appropriate, the decision should be made carefully. Just because you have a genetic risk for something doesn't mean you will end up with that condition, and as a 2019 Stanford University study shows, just being told you're at risk can alter your actual risk.[44] In this study, researchers found that regardless of people's actual genotype, if they were told their genes reflected a higher risk, they performed worse. Those told their genes made them less prone to obesity produced two and a half times more of the fullness hormone than they had while eating the exact same meal the week before, while those told they were genetically prone to obesity showed no hormonal change. Similarly, people told they had a gene that made them respond poorly to exercise did much worse on a challenging treadmill test than they had the week before, while those told they had the protective gene performed about the same. In this case, knowledge was not power but produced a self-fulfilling prophecy.

Indeed, once we become convinced of something, it can be extremely hard to change our mindset—even if we're shown facts to the contrary. In their book *The Enigma of Reason* (Harvard University Press, 2017), authors Hugo Mercier, Ph.D., and Dan Sperber, Ph.D., write about a fascinating experiment Dr. Mercier helped conduct that showed exactly that. In the experiment, participants answered a series of reasoning problems. Afterward, the researchers asked them to explain their responses and gave them a chance to change their answers if they discovered mistakes. Fewer than 15 percent made changes. Later, they were shown their original answer as well as the answer of another participant who came to a different conclusion—although the researchers switched the two answers, so that the participant's answer was labeled as someone else's. The participants were again given the opportunity to change their responses. Half of them realized the answers had been switched, but in the group that didn't recognize the switch, almost 60 percent rejected their own reasoning in favor of someone else's, thinking they were sticking with their own.

STEP ELEVEN: FORGIVE

We must let ourselves feel all the painful destruction we want to forgive rather than swallow it in denial. If we do not face it, we cannot choose to forgive it.
                                        —Kenneth McAll, *Healing the Family Tree*

Forgiveness frees us. It heals our bodies and our lives. Mario Martinez, Psy.D., puts it like this: "Forgiveness is a liberating act of self-love." The resolution comes from reclaiming the power we gave the offender rather than having to forgive the offender. Please reread this and fully digest it. The power in this statement can't be overestimated.

Pastor Nadia Bolz-Weber says it this way in her 2018 *Forgive Assholes* video, which went viral: "Forgiveness isn't just a pansy way of saying 'It's okay.' It's instead a way of wielding bolt cutters to snap the chain that links you to the act. A way of saying, 'What you did is so not okay that I refuse to be connected to it anymore.' Forgiveness is about being a freedom fighter."[45]

Forgiveness doesn't mean that what another person did to you was right or just. It simply means that you've decided to release the other person as a gift to yourself. It takes a great deal of energy to keep someone (including ourselves) out of our hearts. When we forgive those who have hurt us, both of us are freed. Forgiveness and making amends are completely linked. Holding a grudge and maintaining hatred or resentment hurts *us* at least as much as it hurts the other person. Many times, the person who is hardest to forgive is yourself. Forgiveness means not allowing something from the past to adversely affect you in the present.

Forgiveness moves our energy to the heart area, the fourth chakra. When the body's energy moves there, we don't take our wounds so personally—and we can heal. Forgiveness is the initiation of the heart, and it is hands down the most powerful force for attracting vibrant health that I know. Fred Luskin, Ph.D., of the Stanford Forgiveness Project and author of *Forgive for Good* (HarperSanFrancisco, 2002), has demonstrated that forgiveness can improve the health and quality of life even in those who've experienced enormous wounding. After Dr. Luskin gave a weeklong forgiveness training workshop for seventeen residents of Northern Ireland, each of whom had had a primary family member murdered in the violence there, symptoms of stress (such as dizziness, headaches, and stomachaches) decreased by 35 percent, depression dropped 20 percent, and anger dropped by 12 percent. In addition, participants' physical vitality (including energy level, appetite, sleep patterns, and general well-being) improved significantly.[46] (For more on forgiveness, including Dr. Luskin's Nine Steps to Forgiveness and information about his research, visit his website at https://learningtoforgive.com.)

Forgiveness, quite simply, is good medicine. It has a positive effect on the heart, opening it and allowing appreciation to flow in. (Resentment, on the other hand, closes the heart and has a negative effect on heart health.) Scientific studies have shown that when we think with our hearts by taking a moment to focus on someone or something we love unconditionally—like a puppy or a young child—the rhythm of our hearts evens out and becomes healthier. Hormone levels change and normalize as well. When people are taught to think with their hearts regularly, they can even reverse heart disease and other stress-related conditions. The electromagnetic field of the heart is sixty times stronger than the electromagnetic field produced by the brain; to me, this means that every cell in our bodies—and in the bodies of those around us—can be positively influenced by the quality of our hearts when they are beating in synchrony with the energy of forgiveness and appreciation.[47]

An inspiring example comes from Bill Worth, a guest on my Hay House Radio program *Flourish!*, who used the power of forgiveness to assist him in healing multiple sclerosis. When he was diagnosed thirty years ago, Bill refused to take any of the drugs his neurologist recommended and instead embarked on a journey that included learning about forgiveness, making lifestyle changes (like exercise and diet), and focusing on living an enriching life that included becoming an ordained Unity minister and writing two metaphysical novels. When Bill last had an MRI and visited a neurologist, in December 2015, the doctor could find no evidence of active MS in Bill's brain. (For more details, read Bill's book *Outwitting Multiple Sclerosis: How Forgiveness Helped Me Heal My Brain by Changing My Mind* [Next Century Publishing, 2017].)

When I think back on my breast abscess, I feel great compassion and forgiveness *for myself*. How could I have known what I was doing? I had no role models of women in ob-gyn for balance between work and motherhood. I have forgiven myself, and because of that I have also forgiven my colleagues at the time.

It has taken years for me to come to grips with the concept of forgiveness. When I first wrote this chapter, I didn't even think of putting this crucial step in. When we forgive someone because we think it is the right thing to do, we're merely jumping through a socially acceptable hoop that changes nothing. Psychologist Alice Miller, Ph.D., states that when children are asked to forgive abusive parents without first experiencing their emotions and their personal pain, the forgiveness becomes another weapon of silencing. Leaping to forgive under these circumstances is not really forgiveness—it is just another form of denial. Many women think that forgiving someone who hurt them is the same as saying that what happened to them was okay and that it didn't hurt them. Nothing could be further from the truth. Many women have been brainwashed into submission by the misunderstanding of forgiveness. To get to forgiveness, we first have to work through the painful experiences that require it. Forgiveness is completely premature when a woman doesn't even acknowledge that she has an emotional abscess, let alone that it needs to be drained. Forgiveness doesn't mean that what happened to us was okay. It simply means that we are no longer willing to allow that experience to adversely affect our lives. Forgiveness is something we do, ultimately, for ourselves.

True forgiveness changes us at a core level. It changes our bodies. It is an experience of grace. As I write about this concept, I'm moved to tears by the holiness of what forgiveness really is. I experienced this profoundly a number of years ago when I was reported to the medical board in Maine by a general surgeon. One of this man's patients had come to me for a consultation. Three months before, she had gone to this surgeon because of abdominal pain, weight loss, and narrowing stool caliber. He had attempted a colonoscopy (a test in which a fiber-optic scope is put into the colon to examine the inside and check for conditions such as cancer), but he had been unable to get the instrument all the way up her colon. He told her that she would need to have surgery to remove part of her colon, since he was virtually certain she had a cancer that was causing her symptoms.

She had gone home, changed her diet completely to a macrobiotic approach, and over a three-month period regained the weight she had lost, was free of abdominal pain, and had normal stools once again. All of this had taken place before she saw me. When I first saw her, she was healthy, vital, and committed to avoiding surgery. Since she was so much better, she wanted to know if I thought she still needed the surgery.

I told her that no one could be sure if she did or didn't have cancer without further testing. She had already taken a risk by not having the surgery earlier, but on the other hand, the actions she had taken had certainly reversed all the symptoms for which she had initially sought care. It was possible that she didn't have cancer and that her symptoms had been from diverticulitis (an infection of the colon that can mimic cancer) that was now healed. She decided to continue doing what she was doing with her diet, then have her colonoscopy repeated in a few months. After all, it was her body and she was feeling better than she had in years.

She understood that this decision was in direct conflict with what her surgeon suggested, but at this point he wasn't aware of her striking improvement. I felt sure that once he saw her, he'd agree to postpone her surgery and repeat her tests. Because I believe that people do best when they are cared for by a medical team that is informed, I sent a copy of our discussion to her surgeon.

As it turned out, he was furious with me for not "forcing" her to have surgery, and so he reported me to our state medical board. I had to submit a report of my end of the story and wait for the board to call me for a hearing. They met only every three months, so I had plenty of time to stew about this situation. I felt sure that a doctor-initiated complaint against me would be taken quite seriously, and I was terrified.

This event was the most difficult learning experience of my career. I had spent my whole life in the pursuit of good grades, respectability, and worthiness. I came from a family tradition of "good" doctors. Yet here was the manifestation of my worst fear: The authorities were going to say that I was a "bad" doctor, that I couldn't practice medicine in a way consistent with my own beliefs about healing, and worse, that my patients didn't have the choice with their own bodies, either! I worked with and felt my fear daily for weeks.

If I could change how I felt on the inside, I knew, something would change in the world outside. This had always been part of my belief system. Now I had to put it to a very practical test.

Part of any healing is "letting go," relinquishing the illusion of control. For me, the letting-go was this conclusion: If I couldn't practice medicine in a way that was consistent with the healing power of the human body and individual free choice, then I would willingly give up my license. I was helped and supported during this process by colleagues and patients who told me that they'd accompany me to my hearing if necessary. Nancy Coyne, M.D., a local physician, told me that if I had to go, she'd make sure that the place was "packed with feminists" in support of me. For that, I will be forever grateful.

One day while doing my writing practice, I spontaneously began a letter to this surgeon who had reported me: *Dear Dr. M., I know your fears. I know why you are upset. . . .* As I continued, I felt compassion for this man. I knew who he was. I felt him as a frightened man fighting for control—and I forgave him. As I continued writing, I felt the fear in my solar plexus lift for the first time in weeks. It was a physical feeling, not an intellectual exercise. And at the same time, I knew that everything would be all right, *regardless of the board's decision.*

The next day, one of my colleagues who served on the board at the time saw me in the hospital and told me, "By the way, the board unanimously decided to drop your case. They felt that that surgeon was way out of line!" I never had to go before the board or plead my case in any way. They had upheld my patient's right to informed care and my right to give it.

My ordeal was over. The most striking thing about this experience was the physical feeling of release in my solar plexus area when my fear finally healed and I felt compassion for my adversary. From this I learned that forgiveness is organic and that it is physical as well as spiritual and emotional. My intent had been to heal my own situation, not necessarily to forgive the surgeon. But I subsequently learned that the only way to heal the situation was to withdraw my energy from it and to forgive my accuser. I learned that forgiveness comes unbidden, by itself, when we are committed to vibrant health. To experience forgiveness, however, we must first make a commitment to healing and to making amends, when they are needed.

I never intended to feel compassion and forgiveness toward that surgeon. What I did want to do was get rid of the knot in my solar plexus. This I did by being willing to stay with the knot, to be in dialogue with it, and to learn from it. I believed at a deep level that I could learn from this experience, and that in fact I must learn from it, so that I wouldn't have to repeat it, in another way or another form.

Though I don't recommend being reported to a medical board as a way of achieving personal growth, it was one of the most freeing experiences of

my life. I had faced one of my worst fears, stayed with it, and transformed it.
The patient's tests were repeated at another hospital two months later. Her
colon was perfectly normal, with no sign of a tumor. She had probably never
had cancer in the first place, just an inflammation of the colon. She continues
to be well. My former husband suggested that I report the surgeon to his
board in Massachusetts and ask if it is the standard of care in his state to
remove a normal colon. I said, "No. The war needs to stop somewhere. It's
stopping with me." I did, however, write Dr. M. a note with copies of the
patient's normal tests and remarked, "Isn't the healing ability of the human
body miraculous?"

The late Stephen Levine taught us that the quality of forgiveness is miraculous for bringing balance. Most of us, he reminded us, have been given
nothing in our training to help us work with resentment. Levine offered us
the following meditation.[48]

Close your eyes. . . .
For a moment just reflect on what the word *forgiveness* might really
mean. What is forgiveness?
And now, very gently—no force—just as an experiment in truth—just for a
moment—allow the image of someone for whom you have much
resentment—someone for whom you have anger and a sense of distance—let
them just gently—gently, come into your mind—as an image, as a feeling.
Maybe you feel them at the center of your chest as fear, as resistance.
However they manifest in your mind-body, just invite them in very gently
for this moment—for this experiment.

And in your heart, silently say to them, "I forgive you.
I forgive you for whatever you have done in the past that caused me
pain, intentionally or unintentionally.
However you have caused me pain, I forgive you."
Speak gently to them in your heart with your own words—in your own way.
In your heart, say to them, "I forgive you for whatever you may have
done in the past, through your words, through your actions, through
your thoughts that caused me pain, intentionally or unintentionally, I
forgive you. I forgive you."
Allow . . . Allow them to be touched . . . just for a moment at least . . . by
your forgiveness.
Allow forgiveness.
It is so painful to hold someone out of your heart. How can you hold on
to the pain, that resentment even a moment longer?
Fear, doubt . . . let it go . . . and for this moment, touch them with your
forgiveness.
"I forgive you."

Now let them go gently, let them leave quietly. Let them go with your
blessing.

Now picture someone who has great resentment for you. Feel them maybe in
your chest, seeing them in your mind as an image—a sense of
their being. Invite them gently in. Someone who has resentment, anger—
someone who is unforgiving toward you.
Let them into your heart.
And in your heart, say to them, "I ask your forgiveness, for whatever I may
have done in the past that caused you pain, intentionally or unintentionally—
through my words, through my actions, through my thoughts. However I
caused you pain, I ask your forgiveness. I ask your forgiveness.
Through my anger, my fear, my blindness, my laziness. However I
caused you pain intentionally or unintentionally—I ask your forgiveness."

Let it be. Allow that forgiveness in. Allow yourself to be touched by their
forgiveness. If the mind rises up with thoughts like self-indulgence or
doubt, just see how profound our mercilessness is with ourselves and
open to the forgiveness.
Allow yourself to be forgiven.
Allow yourself to be forgiven.
"However I caused you pain, I ask for your forgiveness." Allow yourself to
feel their forgiveness.
Let it be.
Let it be.
And gently . . . gently . . . let them go on their way in forgiveness for you—
in blessings for you.

And turn to yourself in your own heart and say, "I forgive you" to you.
Whatever tries to block that—the mercilessness and fear—
let it go.
Let it be touched by your forgiveness and your mercy.
And gently, in your heart, calling yourself by your own first name, say,
"I forgive you" to you.
It is so painful to put yourself out of your heart.
Let yourself in. Allow yourself to be touched by this forgiveness.
Let the healing in.
Say, "I forgive you" to you.

Let that forgiveness be extended to the beings all around you.
May all beings forgive themselves.
May they discover joy.
May all beings be freed of suffering.

May all beings be at peace.
May all beings be healed.
May they be at one with their true nature.
May they be free from suffering.
May they be at peace.
Let that loving kindness, that forgiveness, extend to the whole planet—to
every level of existence, seen and unseen.
May all beings be freed of suffering.
May they know the power of forgiveness, of freedom, of peace.
May all beings seen and unseen, at every level of existence, may they
know their true being.
May they know their vastness—their infinite peacefulness.
May all beings be free.
May all beings be free.

STEP TWELVE: ACTIVELY PURSUE
PLEASURE AND PURPOSE

By pursuing your allurements, you help bind the universe together.
The unity of the world rests on the pursuit of passion.

—Brian Swimme

When my younger daughter was nine, she reminded me how beautifully
we are equipped with the innate capacity to live life fully, appreciating it as
we go along. On Easter Sunday, she came bounding downstairs and ex-
claimed, "Don't you love it when you feel good, and you look good, and
your room's clean, too?"

Watch children for a while, and you will begin to see what qualities you
need to embody to wake up your soul and your immune system regularly.
Most young children know exactly what they want. We are all born with an
innate ability to know what we want. We are then socialized to believe that
we can't have what we want, and so we gradually dismiss our innermost
desires, our lives' passions, to avoid disappointment. But I have come to the
conclusion that feminine desire is the most powerful force for good on the
planet.

David Ehrenfeld, M.D., Ph.D., wrote in *The Arrogance of Humanism*
(Oxford University Press, 1978, updated 1981):

Our civilization is coming to equate the value of life with the mere
avoidance of death. An empty and impossible goal, a fool's quest for
nothingness, has been substituted for a delight in living that lies latent in

all of us. When death is once again accepted as one of many important parts of life, then life may recover its old thrill, and the efforts of good physicians will not be wasted.[49]

Get out a piece of paper and write on the top of it, "I desire . . ." or "I choose . . . ," then write in what you want. For example, "I desire a strong, healthy body" or "I choose a strong, healthy body." Notice that the word *desire* or *choose* feels effortless. You just have to allow it to come. This is the feminine receptive mode, so often lacking in our culture. Now write down exactly why you want what you want, so that you can literally feel the excitement generated by your enthusiasm. Remember: By the law of attraction, you attract your vibrational equivalent. It is the feeling and the vibration of the feeling that have the power to attract circumstances to you. In one example: "A healthy, strong body makes me feel powerful and vibrant. I desire my body to be an instrument that is highly attuned to my needs. I desire a body that is a reflection of the beauty that is inside me. I choose a body that is capable of getting me where I want to go. I choose a body that has lots of energy and stamina so that I may enjoy my life more fully."

The positive emotional energy generated by this experience literally begins to draw the experience of health to you. Focus on and think often about what you desire, and you will be setting up an invisible magnetic field that begins to draw health to you, unless you keep blocking it with other thoughts such as "Well, I want it, but I'll never get it." (Review step one and see if your future self has anything to tell you here.) Your thoughts and your emotions need to line up on this one. You can't get around subconscious programming simply with affirmations. If you say you want a healthy body, but deep inside you don't feel that you are worthy of it or that illness is a punishment of some kind, you will be creating a mixed message, and your results won't be nearly as good. Your intention in the affirmation must be in congruence with your unconscious beliefs and thoughts. One way to shine some light on what may be behind an affirmation that isn't working is to ask yourself what the payoff is. What do you get—or what do you not have to give up—if you keep things the way they are? Then you at least have a starting point for beginning to change those unconscious thoughts.

Every day, spend just a few minutes focusing on appreciating what brings you pleasure now. Make appreciation a habit. Keep an appreciation journal. What you pay attention to expands. Spend time noticing what is working and what you like right now. You will never be able to feel happy or fulfilled in the future unless you can feel how that would feel right now. Over time this process will change every cell in your body.

For thirty consecutive nights, just before falling asleep, say to yourself, "I am peace. I am beauty. I am vibrantly healthy. I am prosperous." During sleep, the intellect is quieted and your inner guidance takes over. Your intent to attain or maintain pleasure and peace will be programmed into your body-mind as you sleep. Just try this and see what happens.

As you move through your day, use the power of intent to clear a path for yourself. Say, "I am divinely irresistible to joy and freedom." Or use Gay Hendricks's Ultimate Success Mantra, as put forth in his book *The Big Leap* (HarperCollins, 2009): "I expand love, success, and health every day while inspiring others to do the same." Change the words if you like.

Post affirmations at strategic places around your home and workplace to program your subconscious for more pleasure, health, and purpose. Take the time to really listen to good music and really take in beauty and pleasure.

Make it a habit to concentrate on what is working in your life. Cultivate the habit of noticing what is good and appreciating it. A teacher named Abraham says, "Appreciation is the strongest emotion we have for attracting what we want."[50] When you look for people, places, and things to appreciate and learn to appreciate all of the aspects of your life that are working well, you'll attract more of what you like and less of what you don't. Start noticing little things, like how good the bedsheets feel on your toes at night or how good the pillow feels under your head.

The benefits of this advice have been scientifically proven. The Heart-Math Institute, a nonprofit research and education organization based in Boulder Creek, Colorado, has been studying what is known as heart co-herence for more than two decades (see www.heartmath.org). The heart is coherent when its beat-to-beat rhythms produce a stable, sine-wave-like pat-tern, which happens when we sustain positive emotions like gratitude, love, appreciation, compassion, inspiration, and joy. When the heart is in this co-herent state, the heart, brain, and nervous system all work in harmony, re-ducing stress and improving mental clarity and cognitive function (among many other benefits). While most of us have been taught that the brain rules supreme, sending signals and instructions to all parts of the body, the Heart-Math researchers have found that the heart communicates with the brain as well, through the electromagnetic field that heart rhythms create. In fact, emotions actually move faster than thoughts, affecting heart rhythms *before* they affect brain waves.

One of HeartMath's many studies showed that those achieving heart coherence by focusing on feelings of appreciation and compassion while ra-diating those feelings out into the world increased the crystal structure in their saliva.[51] The higher the level of coherence, the more orderly and com-plex the crystal patterns became. This is particularly notable because about 60 percent of the human body (and one-half of the volume of each of our organs) consists of water. The researchers believe this study demonstrates the effect heart coherence may have on the information embedded in *all* our bodily fluids—and so on our entire physical bodies.

For similar reasons, I strongly recommend that you avoid watching the news on television, hearing it on the radio, or reading about it in the papers for at least thirty days. Instead of waking up to the news or to people talking on the radio, wake up to music. When you do this, you will be removing a major impediment to tuning in to your inner guidance—negative information overload. If you wake up to soft music or silence each morning, you will also be better able to remember your dreams. Over time, you will notice that you don't miss much by avoiding the news. Media-savvy individuals are well aware of how thoroughly the news is manipulated to be as attention-getting as possible, whipping you into a frenzy of worry and fear so that you will feel more vulnerable and therefore buy what the advertisers are selling in order to feel better. The culture being what it is, someone will always tell you what is going on "out there." You'll always find out what applies to you and what you need to know. But you'll have the advantage of a much more intimate relationship with yourself than most people have. I've been on a mostly news-free diet for over a decade. I cannot believe the difference it has made in my thoughts, dreams, and general state of well-being. Now, when I watch television or read the paper, I don't take it very seriously and I'm very selective. I have proved to myself, beyond any doubt, that my ability to create the life I want by selectively choosing what I will give my attention to is the most powerful creative force in my life.

MUSIC AS MEDICINE

Music does more than just make us happy, lessening stress and anxiety in the process. It can also directly improve our physical health. I highly recommend incorporating it into your efforts to bring more pleasure into your life. Most notably, music can alleviate many kinds of chronic pain, including eye pain, urinary pain, gynecological pain, angina, and even post-surgical pain. Studies show those listening to music decrease their use of pain medications as well as lower their levels of cortisol and blood glucose.[52] Music has also been shown to improve various brain disorders by helping the brain to create new cells and additional neural connections.[53] One particularly fascinating study shows that music can have a similar effect to adaptogenic herbs, increasing steroid hormones in those with low hormone levels and reducing the same hormones in those with high hormone levels.[54] What kind of music works best? Generally, whatever music you prefer; many of these benefits are governed by your personal preference.

Write down your short-term and long-term goals for the coming year, as already described on page 741. The very process of writing them down and thinking about them sets something magical into motion. The magical "something" is the power of intent—the power of our thoughts to create. Benjamin Hardy, author of *Willpower Doesn't Work: Discover the Hidden Keys to Success* (Hachette, 2018), explains that the key to goal-setting isn't having the discipline to make it happen or even having a specific skill set (as many people assume). Instead, it's having faith, which he defines as a belief or hope in something you can't see or that doesn't currently exist. You must also believe you can get what you want. Much of our success in achieving goals boils down to whether we have a growth mindset, with positive learning habits, or a fixed mindset, with negative learning habits, he adds. Put more simply, it has much less to do with our specific strengths or weaknesses and much more to do with how we see ourselves. If you believe, he says, you can learn anything. But if you believe you can't, then you won't. These are empowering guidelines to keep in mind.

Another key to understanding this is the reticular activating system (RAS), a bundle of nerves in the brainstem that filters out unnecessary information. It's been compared with a nightclub bouncer for your brain, letting in only the sensory information you can handle so you don't go into overwhelm. The RAS uses your own beliefs as a filter system, so it basically lets in the information that validates what you already believe. We can use this to our advantage by learning to train the RAS through visualizing what we want—creating a mini-movie in our minds of what achieving our goals will look, sound, and feel like (the more detail, the better). This helps us believe the intention is indeed possible because we've already "seen" it happen. Setting intentions with visualizations in this way calls on the power of both our subconscious thoughts and our conscious thoughts to manifest what we desire.

An obvious way to bring more pleasure into your life is to hang around with positive, happy people more often. Happiness can spread through social networks, so you can "catch" happiness from the friend of a friend of a friend, and your happy mood can "infect" countless others in the same way.[55] Researchers also discovered that living within a mile of a happy friend gave people a 25 percent greater chance of becoming happy themselves over the twenty-year period of the study. And finally, a study of British students showed that those with happier friends were happier themselves, and those whose friends were often in bad moods were also more likely to report moodiness.[56] This doesn't necessarily mean that you should ditch all your friends who are less than jovial. But it does mean being conscious about whom you choose to surround yourself with is a very good idea.

Finally, get in the habit of noticing what you want—that is how you find your passion. Maybe you need to walk in the sun more, dig in the dirt more, wear skirts that swing more. When you allow yourself to feel more joy, your life will be filled with more abundance on all levels. I guarantee that somewhere inside you, you already know what it is you need and want.

I hope that going through this section has:

~ Jogged some stuck places in you that needed readjustment

~ Reassured you that you are right on track

~ Touched your anger

~ Brought up tears

~ Made you laugh

~ Inspired you

That's what life is: growing, changing, moving, creating—every day. A thirteenth-century Japanese Zen master, Dogen Zenji, once said that life is one continuous mistake.[57] I love that. It's so freeing to know that you can't get it right—and you'll never get it wrong, either.

Maybe you need to sing; maybe you need to run. Don't wait. This life is not an emergency, but it also doesn't offer any guarantees about going on forever. How do you want to feel? Imagine feeling that way often. What action do you need to take right now to live your life more fully? . . . Got it?

Now take a step toward it!

Blessed be.

16
Getting the Most
Out of Your Medical Care

Wellness that is being allowed, or the wellness that is being denied, is all about the mindset, the mood, the attitude, the practiced thoughts. There is not one exception, in any human or beast; because, you can patch them up again and again, and they will just find another way of reverting back to the natural rhythm of their mind. Treating the body really is about treating the mind. It is all psychosomatic. Every bit of it, no exceptions.

—Abraham, via Esther Hicks

The nature of most people who go into healthcare is they are wonderful human beings who want to help other human beings.

—Susan Frampton, Ph.D.

WHY YOU MUST TAKE RESPONSIBILITY
FOR YOUR HEALTHCARE

One of the most powerful tools for flourishing and healing is knowing how to get the right kind of support at the right time. To do that, you must stand up for yourself and for what you know and feel—and you must absolutely believe that you have the ability to attract what you need as well as be willing to receive it. In the United States, we spent $3.5 trillion, or $10,739 per person, on healthcare in 2017—this is a huge industry, and as discussed in chapter 15, very powerful special interests control mainstream healthcare and the insurance that covers it. In an April 10, 2018, report for biotech clients, Goldman Sachs analysts pointed out that one-shot cures for illness are bad for business. Better to keep people chronically ill—it's more profitable.

> "The potential to deliver 'one shot cures' is one of the most attractive aspects of gene therapy, genetically engineered cell therapy, and gene editing. However, such treatments offer a very different outlook with regard to recurring revenue versus chronic therapies. . . . While this proposition carries tremendous value for patients and society, it could represent a challenge for genome medicine developers looking for sustained cash flow. . . .
>
> "[The] rapid rise and fall of [biotech company Gilead Sciences'] hepatitis C franchise highlights one of the dynamics of an effective drug that permanently cures a disease, resulting in a gradual exhaustion of the prevalent pool of patients," the analysts wrote. The report noted that diseases such as common cancers—where the "incident pool remains stable"—are less risky for business.[1]

You must also assume responsibility for your end of the healthcare partnership. Your healthcare provider has a body of knowledge. What you have is knowledge of your body. Both are necessary. But right now, your knowledge of your body and your willingness to do what it takes to truly flourish no matter what your current state of health are more crucial than ever. We can no longer afford to assume a childlike role and simply turn our health over to the current mainstream medical system without our own very active participation.

David Riley, M.D., the editor in chief of *Alternative Therapies in Health and Medicine,* summarizes this nicely in this editorial on healthcare reform:

> To comprehend the insanity of our current situation, consider this: if we were able to demonstrate that a lifestyle change could prevent most cardiovascular disease in this country, we would bankrupt most if not all the hospitals in the United States and cause a massive gridlock in the healthcare industry. Providing health is not the goal of our current system; managing disease is the name of the game. Hospitals are built around very expensive (and reimbursable) treatments, often of cardiovascular disease with stents and bypass surgery, often without evidence that they are indicated in most of the patients who receive these services.[2]

The late Barbara Starfield, M.D., a revered public health expert at the Johns Hopkins School of Public Health, noted in an editorial published in the year 2000 in the *Journal of the American Medical Association* that there are 225,000 deaths in this country each year from iatrogenic causes (e.g., adverse drug reactions, poor surgical outcomes, etc., that are caused unintentionally by the actions of healthcare providers), an estimate she considered conservative. (Johns Hopkins reports that number has since gone up to 250,000, although other studies claim the number is as high as 440,000.) "In any case," she wrote, "225,000 deaths per year constitutes the third leading cause of death in the United States, after deaths from heart disease and cancer."[3] She broke the figure down into the following categories: 12,000 deaths annually from unnecessary surgery, 7,000 from hospital medication errors, 20,000 from other hospital errors, 80,000 from infections that originated in hospitals, and 106,000 from adverse effects of correctly prescribed prescription drugs.

Bottom line: You won't find health in the conventional medical system. Most doctors already know this. This is why so many of us don't use mainstream medicine much. I also don't expect my health insurance to cover much of anything related to my health—and I have good insurance. I figure that my health insurance is designed to take care of a major medical emergency such as a car accident. That's it. My actual healthcare consists, first and foremost, of knowing that my health comes from deep within and that my thoughts and emotions are hands down the most powerful forces for flourishing that are available to me. I pay out of pocket for massage, vitamins and minerals, and Pilates and yoga classes. My "primary care provider" is my massage therapist and acupuncturist. I also keep a journal, have a solid social support network, read a lot of books, eat organically grown whole foods whenever possible, exercise regularly, get outside, dance, play music, and keep learning new things. I know that I can attract the resources I need when I need them (some of which have indeed been in mainstream hospitals, such as when I had my fibroid removed and when I had my breast abscess treated). When you are truly ready to assume responsibility for your health, you, too, will find the resources you need.

Choosing the Right Healers for You

To flourish, you must own your power to seek out doctors, other healthcare practitioners, and environments that actually increase health. You should begin by finding a healthcare provider whom you trust and believe in. And the healthcare you select must be based on your needs and values. This is as much a part of your health and healing as any mode of treatment you might choose. (I hope that in the not-too-distant future this kind of healthcare will be covered by insurance, or at least we'll have a plan in which individuals like me could use our health insurance money to pay for health-enhancing modalities.)

One of the most common questions I'm asked is "Is there a doctor like you in New York?" or California, or elsewhere. Many patients value an approach that honors their inner wisdom, acknowledges the message an illness holds, and combines Western medicine with other modalities. A new "third line" of healthcare providers who are open to this approach is rapidly emerging. Everywhere I go, I meet doctors and medical students who are interested in and actively practicing what is now known as complementary, integrative, or functional medicine—the coming together of the best of both conventional (allopathic) medicine and so-called alternative medicine, which acknowledges the body as an energy system. Many other healthcare practitioners trained in different disciplines also share this approach. There are scores of deeply committed, caring physicians practicing in the United States and around the world who don't necessarily call themselves holistic. In fact, the doctor you're working with now may well be open to your ideas about your illness and may be willing to follow along with your new path—once you discuss what you want. In fact, for many, it will be a relief to work with someone who is willing to engage in a true partnership.

Here are some steps to help you find the right healthcare practitioner for you.

Get Referrals. When seeking a specialist or other type of healthcare provider, there are two kinds of referrals to consider: those from satisfied patients (or clients) and those from doctors and other medical personnel. However, if a healthcare provider works with alternative medicine modalities, he or she might or might not work within the mainstream medical community. For this reason, your family physician may not know of a good acupuncturist or massage therapist. But that does not mean that there aren't any. Often the best healthcare providers are found through word of mouth—women talking to other women. So ask your friends whom they see and why. And when it comes to doctors in your area, see if you can find a nurse who has worked with the local doctors at your favorite hospital to give you a recommendation. Believe me, the nurses know who is good and who isn't.

If you're looking for an alternative healthcare practitioner, a good place to start other than friends is your local health food store. Many times the staff at these places knows who is available in your area. They may also have a bulletin of listings available. And more and more, alternative practitioners are teaching classes at Y's, high schools, colleges, and adult education programs around the country. Taking a yoga, massage, tai chi, or other class is a very good way to find out who is doing what in your area, because those interested in complementary medicine tend to know one another. Of course, the Web has revolutionized networking to the point where you need only type in "acupuncturist" to find someone in your area. Still, the best referrals are from someone who knows the practitioner personally. And many of the best practitioners are too busy doing what they do to bother much with social media, so you have to seek them out.

Look at Credentials. Board certification is evidence that a doctor has passed a number of qualifying exams that measure competence to practice in his or her chosen field. Having been through the process, I can attest to the rigor involved. Of course you'll want to know a specialist's training—and almost everyone has this information available online. Credentialing varies widely in the alternative healthcare field and in some cases is not yet in place, though this is changing rapidly.

The Academy of Integrative Health and Medicine (AIHM), an organization formed in 2014 in a merger of the American Holistic Medical Association and the American Board of Integrative Holistic Medicine, has a specialty board to certify holistically trained physicians using the same rigorous criteria that other specialties have employed. (For more information, visit the AIHM's website at www.aihm.org.) The Institute for Functional Medicine also has a tab on its website (www.ifm.org) to help you find a functional medicine practitioner in your area. Functional medicine is not a specialty or a separate discipline but rather an approach to medicine that focuses on treating the whole person instead of a set of symptoms and on prevention instead of diseases. Many mainstream physicians are now getting trained in functional medicine. Unfortunately, most of those treatments are not covered by insurance. In addition, Planetree, a nonprofit organization that works with medical practices that want to improve their patients' experiences by focusing on patient-centered care, lists more than 130 healthcare organizations that are members on its website (www.planetree.org).

Ask Yourself Whether the Person Feels Like a Good Fit for You. A healthcare provider can have all the credentials in the world and still be the wrong person for you. Or vice versa. So, having checked out someone's credentials with your intellect, you'll ultimately have to trust your heart and your gut before you let that person care for you or operate on you, no matter how highly he or she has been recommended. I went to see a spine surgeon at New England Baptist Hospital in Boston recently with a friend who was looking into having cervical spine surgery. I was so impressed by the surgeon and the way he went over all the MRIs with us that I trusted him immediately, including trusting him in the operating room. My friend went through the surgery and had a very positive experience and a good outcome. The best healthcare providers are those who are aware of how powerful their words are. The cloak of the shaman rests on their shoulders—whether they realize it or not. Their words have the power to heal or to destroy, because of the powerful impact of beliefs on the body, especially in a person who is vulnerable and afraid. Professionals' words must be truthful and at the same time chosen to support healing.

When my daughter needed oral surgery, I knew before I met him that the oral surgeon had impeccable credentials. But I was not willing to allow him to do anything to my daughter until I had had a chance to experience his interpersonal skills and what I've come to call his "healer quotient." (See next point.) If either of those elements hadn't been there, I would have left the office—and so should you.

In a similar vein, cardiologist John Mandrola, M.D., has been outspoken about the productivity scale used to evaluate many doctors, who are assigned relative value units (RVUs) for the medical procedures they perform in the office.[4] Doctors receive no credit, however, for listening to and counseling patients, examining them, doing research, teaching colleagues, or even reading medical research. "This is the milieu in which a younger generation of clinicians is learning the craft," Dr. Mandrola writes. "I was shocked to learn that a major teaching center (which will remain nameless) compensates its teaching faculty solely on the basis of productivity. Imagine that. Educators whose paychecks are determined by the number of RVUs they generate rather than the bedside skills they impart to learners." He also tweeted this: "Productivity and the RVU have no place in medical care. There needs to be a different system of valuing the care of people with disease."

Assess the Person's "Healer Quotient." Does your healthcare provider feel like a healer? Do you leave the office feeling reassured and uplifted? Do you feel like you're in good hands? A healer knows how to assist you in eliciting your own inner guidance and will not try to talk you out of your gut feeling about a drug or a procedure that doesn't feel right to you.

Over my many years in medicine, I've found that true healers work everywhere, regardless of the tools they use. (This can include the custodial staff at the hospital, by the way!) Though I already knew this, the lesson was brought home to me in a big way when my then-husband and I went to a gifted intuitive in Vermont for a reading. This woman told my husband that he had a great deal of healing energy in his hands and asked him whether or not he did any healing work with them. He said that he didn't, and she suggested to him that he might consider looking into massage or chiropractic. Later, as we were driving home and he was thinking about the reading, he said to me, "Do you suppose that orthopedic surgery counts as doing healing work with my hands?" Then we both laughed, because my husband—as well as much of our culture—has assumed that "healing" is not part of mainstream medicine. He assumed that because he was a pretty mainstream orthopedic surgeon and quite skeptical of much of alternative medicine, he must not be a healer—that healers are those people who use herbs and massage. How wrong he was. My heart is continually warmed by the caring, compassion, and true healing that I see happening every day, regardless of the setting.

On the other hand, when your healthcare provider is aloof, trying to be objective—giving only facts—only the intellect of the patient gets taken care of, and that is not enough. I once had a patient with breast cancer who told her oncologist, "Coping with the cancer is no problem, but recovering from

my visits with you takes me about two weeks." She was referring to his detached manner and her perception that he didn't care. She didn't expect a
miracle, but she longed for some reassurance and an occasional touch. After
she conveyed this to him, their relationship improved. Such improvement
often happens when you let your doctor or other healthcare provider know
what you need.

Another of my patients who came in for a checkup complained about
one of her other doctors: "She doesn't think she can take care of me without
filling the pages with all these little numbers," she said. "I know she's a good
technician, but I don't feel heard."

One of my friends told me that while her doctor was looking at her ovaries via a sonogram during a failed cycle of IVF, he remarked, "What do you
have growing in there? Grass?" She complained about this to the head of the
hospital's ob-gyn department. His response? "Oh, Brenda, quit being so sensitive. Your doctor felt bad and was trying to make light of it." There's not
much that's "light" about a failed IVF cycle that just cost you $10,000!

I continue to hear too many stories like these because our healthcare
system is itself sick. Unfortunately, fixing a patient through the manipulation
of blood chemistry or the repair of broken bones is the main focus of allopathic health education. This has been what medical students get graded
on—not how well they communicate with the patient or how well their very
presence elicits the placebo effect. Though this is changing in medical schools
today, most doctors now in practice were taught the skills of curing, not caring. The really empathic ones too often end up confusing caring with carrying the burdens of their patients, thus leading to burnout. We all need to
realize that compassion is the key, now more than ever. We, as a society,
need to open our hearts to one another. The heart and the intellect need to
work in partnership in all of us.

THE POWER OF PLACEBO

As the late Norman Cousins wrote, "The doctor knows that it is the
prescription slip itself, even more than what is written on it, that is
often the vital ingredient for enabling a patient to get rid of whatever
is ailing him. Drugs are not always necessary. Belief in recovery always is. And so the doctor may prescribe a placebo in cases where
reassurance for the patient is far more useful than a famous-name
pill three times per day."[5] The placebo effect is *physical*.[6] A very
striking example of this (and there are many) was in a study reported
in the *New England Journal of Medicine* in 2002 of people with severe knee pain. Bruce Moseley, M.D., an orthopedic surgeon from

Baylor College of Medicine in Houston, wanted to know just what part of his surgery was the most effective. He divided the study patients into three groups. One group had arthroscopic surgery in which the cartilage was shaved. Another group had the knee flushed out to remove material thought to cause inflammation. The third group was put to sleep and the standard incisions were made in their knees, but no surgery was done. The results were amazing. The first two groups, who actually received surgery, improved. But the truly shocking finding was that the third group—who had no surgery—improved just as much. (I've seen this same thing happen with intractable pelvic pain and laparoscopy. The very act of doing something—along with the patients' belief in the procedure—often effected a cure even though I didn't do much to the pelvis!)[7] The placebo effect in these situations is not "nothing." It is a powerful anti-inflammatory and hormone-balancing effect most likely resulting from the high levels of nitric oxide produced by the lining of the blood vessels in situations in which there is hope and positive expectation. Going to a healthcare provider who inspires hope is therefore a crucial part of your healthcare.

The average ob-gyn in this country has been sued for alleged malpractice at least twice. I am no exception. The emotional toll of this experience is heavy and has served, unfortunately, to put doctors and patients at odds. And it's getting worse, which makes some physicians less willing to go against the standard treatment used in their communities, even when better and safer ones have been shown to work. One of the ways to get around this is for women to include a signed statement in their medical chart indemnifying the physician against any potential litigation should they choose alternatives to standard conventional care. (Malpractice insurance now costs many ob-gyns more than $100,000 per year—and in some states more than $200,000.) Though this is not an ironclad guarantee against a lawsuit, it helps many physicians feel more comfortable with approaches that weren't covered in medical school. If we are to get to a partnership between doctors and patients, we have to start from where we are, and both sides have to be honest about their needs and fears.

Because of my willingness to help patients avoid surgery, I've had the experience of watching conditions such as ovarian cysts go away with such modalities as emotional and dietary change. I've learned many things about the female body that were not included in my training. My general optimism, coupled with the courage and forthrightness of my patients, allowed us both to collect a body of clinical information that many gynecologists wouldn't necessarily see. This is only possible, however, with patients who are truly willing to take responsibility for themselves and their choices. To create health we must all step out of the "blame" model.

Hold Up Your End of the Healthcare Partnership. I know how tempting it is to want someone to intuit exactly what is going on with you and to give you the precise prescription that will cure you no matter what your problem. Each of us harbors this childlike fantasy of finding a doctor whose advice we can unquestioningly follow. The bad news is that this outer authority simply does not exist. The good news is that each of us has a still, small voice within— our inner guidance and authority—that will guide us where we need to go if we are willing to do the disciplined work of gathering the information that our inner wisdom needs before it can help us make a decision or take action.

It's true that it's much easier to transfer responsibility for our health onto someone else rather than assume it ourselves. Blaming someone else for our problems is a default setting for many. But ultimately the rewards of trusting ourselves and knowing that we have the ability to get our needs met are much more satisfying than any fleeting relief that comes from forgoing responsibility and transferring it to someone else.

I was reminded recently of how deep the "trance" is that keeps people locked in to the expectations that their doctors should be able to cure them without their participation. At a workshop in the Northeast, I shared with the audience all of the latest research on how to enhance bone health, including optimal levels of vitamin D, mineral supplementation, weight training, and so on. At the end of the workshop, during the question-and-answer session, a woman got up to say that every year, no matter what treatments her doctor prescribed, her osteoporosis got worse and worse. She wanted to know my opinion on an IV injection that she was now getting that wasn't working, either. She was very concerned about this because her mother had died from complications of osteoporosis.

I asked her if she had ever had her vitamin D level checked. She said no, she hadn't. I asked if she did any weight-bearing exercise. The answer was no. Then I asked if she took minerals. Again, she said no. I wondered if she had heard a word of what I had so passionately said earlier in the workshop. Her mentality (and physical stance) were typical of the victim who waits for some outside expert to hand her the next experimental treatment to save her. I told her that she needed to start by getting a backbone and learning how to stand up for herself. She needed to apply the information I had provided or at least vet it for herself. I also suggested that she call on her mother for support from the other side. Her entire body came alive when I made that suggestion!

It is crucial that you educate yourself about all your choices and then tune in to your inner guidance when it comes to making decisions about surgery, drugs, and procedures. I cannot stress this enough: No one is going to come from the outside and save you when it comes to your health. You must save yourself.

As you consider your options, understand that different physicians often have very different training and interests. As a physician who "walks between the worlds," I see the good that can be done by a variety of approaches. If patients could listen in on the amount of disagreement even among the ob-gyns in a small city such as Portland, Maine, about how to treat a certain condition, they would appreciate how vital their own input is in creating an optimal outcome. Each patient must therefore become her own authority and learn how to assess information from various sources.

BECOME AN ADULT

Many people turn into little children in the doctor's office, giving all their power away. I've seen this repeatedly. When a friend of mine was at the doctor's recently, her blood pressure reading was high. Luckily, she had her husband with her. "Ruth," he said to her, "you're currently eight years old!" (Ruth's mother was sick a lot when she was eight. Ruth didn't have a voice then, although now, at the age of forty-five, she does.) As soon as her husband reminded her, Ruth became an adult and realized that the blood pressure was an indication that she was scared. This was a feeling she needed to acknowledge in the moment. She could then act like an adult and get proper care by asking the right questions.

Women have been taught for years not to make waves or rock the boat. When one of my friends had surgery, I asked her if she had talked with her anesthesiologist beforehand and asked her or him to use healing statements (see the section on how to prepare for surgery) when she would be going under and coming out of anesthesia. She said to me, "No. I was too embarrassed." Her statement summarizes a huge problem in healthcare: Women are too often afraid to ask for what they need. If this is a problem for you, too, take someone with you who will help you speak up when you find yourself getting caught like a deer in the headlights or acting like a child who can't speak up for herself.

On a very practical level, it's important for you to go to your healthcare practitioner fully prepared with a list of questions that he or she can reasonably answer in the time allotted to you. And be aware that you may need to schedule another appointment if your situation is unusually complex.

Changes in the medical system will come about as all of us begin to take responsibility for our own health. (After all, the vast majority of health problems are related to lifestyle choices—this is no exaggeration. A new study from the American Cancer Society shows that half of the deaths from cancer each year are caused by poor lifestyle choices.)[8] And when, despite our best efforts, we do need help, it's good to have a competent doctor with whom we can work in partnership.

Use the Law of Attraction. In part one, I mentioned the law of attraction. Basically, this powerful law of the universe states that we attract to ourselves that which is like ourselves. This means that how you really feel deep inside determines what kind of experience you are likely to attract to yourself. For instance, if you believe that you will be able to get your needs met in any given situation, you will most likely attract to yourself what you need. There are no exceptions to the law of attraction, so please begin to make note of it in your daily life.

Having said that, I also acknowledge that far too many women's health-care needs have not been met well in the medical offices of this country. Medicine, like every other area of society, is drenched in gender bias. The end result of this—and of women's waking up to it—has been a backlog of mistrust of healthcare professionals, particularly doctors, that tends to color the relationship between healthcare provider and patient from the outset. And, because of the law of attraction, this can create a kind of downward spiral that serves no one.

So before going to a new doctor, please ask yourself the following questions and answer them honestly:

~ In general, do I trust doctors? Do I feel that doctors, for instance, charge too much money and are just in this business to get rich?

~ Do I believe that doctors won't listen to me no matter how I state my concerns?

~ Do I believe that drugs and surgery are inherently bad and that it's always better to treat illnesses with alternatives to these modalities?

~ Am I afraid, ashamed, or embarrassed to ask my doctor to be a partner with me in my healthcare decisions?

~ Am I really willing to trust my inner guidance, even if it's different from what my doctor suggests?

~ Am I willing to suggest a compromise position with my doctor so that I can have the advantages of her or his care while taking some responsibility myself?

If you've answered honestly, you may have uncovered some of the beliefs that are keeping you from having a fulfilling and satisfying relationship with a good healthcare provider.

To turn this situation around, I'd like you to think about the fact that there are literally thousands of different healthcare providers practicing in the United States and around the world who can help you help yourself. I'd like you to spend a moment or two each day visualizing how great it will be to have a healthcare team you trust, feel safe with, and feel empowered by. Feel how exhilarating it is to know that no matter where you travel, you have the ability, through your thoughts and feelings, to be able to attract just the circumstances you need for healing.

Acknowledge the Power to Choose. Over the years I've heard many patients tell me that they couldn't take a supplement or get a massage, or whatever it was, because their insurance wouldn't pay for it. Almost invariably, these people have had poorer health than the ones who say things like "I don't care what it takes, I'll find a way to get what I need. Where there's a will, there's a way. I'm not sure how I'm going to do this, but I know I can work it out." Please think for a moment about what it means when you tell yourself that you can't do something for your health because of the rules and regulations that a bunch of insurance executives have come up with. To whom are you giving your power?

I have come to see that one of the leading causes of chronic ill health in this country is the belief that your insurance—or the government, or someone else besides you—is responsible for your healthcare choices. Culturally, we need a big shift in consciousness around this issue. In my view, we should abolish the term "health insurance" and call it what it ought to be called, which is "crisis insurance" or "disease insurance." The business of creating health and staying healthy is our responsibility (and yes, it should also be public policy), and because none of us is perfect at this (and because we've been duped into becoming sheep when it comes to our healthcare system), we need a backup in case of catastrophic illness or an accident. That's what our disease insurance should be for.

So for now, while the entire old system is breaking down, I suggest that you get the highest possible deductible that you can afford and then put the amount of your deductible away in a money market account or, if available to you, a health savings account. (These accounts are becoming increasingly common, but they still have a long way to go. I'm also aware of the plight of those with no health insurance, many of whom simply can't afford the ever-increasing cost of the policies available today.) Then, with the considerable savings that you aren't putting into the pockets of the insurance executives, you will be able to afford all kinds of good food, gym memberships, or massages. These suggestions might sound overly simplistic—and for some people with very limited incomes, they are. But for many others, they are a ticket to true healthcare choice and freedom, in contrast to the sheep mentality that is so prevalent and disempowering.

We are moving toward a time of unprecedented choices and ways to flourish daily in our lives. But until we as a nation start addressing lifestyle issues and make solving them part of public policy, we'll continue to have to pay the enormous cost of bailing people out of situations that could have been prevented in the first place! Why not be a recipient of the healthcare of the future, starting today? You can do this by working with a great paradox: You have to create health yourself, but you don't have to do it alone.

Please acknowledge your power to flourish in your life daily, and understand that healing often comes to us through our connection with others.[9]

KEEPING COPIES OF YOUR MEDICAL RECORDS

Given the current state of healthcare, at least in the United States, I would suggest keeping copies of all your medical records yourself, either electronically or in a notebook. This includes pathology reports, Pap test reports, lab results, and so on. Don't rely so much on the system. I once saw a nun from an order called the Little Sisters of the Poor. The sisters of this order did lots of mission work and traveled around the world. Because of this, she and the other nuns kept all their medical records in perfect order in a spiral-bound notebook that she brought with her to her appointment. I will never forget how easy it was to figure out exactly what she needed as a result. Though we now have electronic patient portals where all our records are supposed to be kept, I have found these systems often lacking as well. Worse yet, artificial intelligence systems comb your records for mention of any problems, regardless of whether that problem was actually diagnosed. The AI systems keep a record of these conditions, seeing them as possible problems, so that it ends up looking like your health is worse than it is. An example of this is a friend of mine who went to a dermatologist for a skin lesion. The doctor wrote "rule out melanoma" on the report. There was never a melanoma. But now my friend has "melanoma" on his medical record! And as you know, once you have an inaccuracy in your file in a computer, it is very difficult to get it fixed.

We're all brought up to give far more credit to the medical system than we should. When we step up and take responsibility for our own history, including our test results, we assume the role of cocreator of our health—not hapless victim of the system.

CHOOSING A TREATMENT:
FROM SURGERY TO ACUPUNCTURE

If you are seriously ill, treat the critical symptoms first, by whatever means are the most appropriate for you. Look for insights later. Conventional medicine is unparalleled in its ability to deal with emergencies and severe symptoms. Though there are many alternative treatments in addition to drugs and surgery, conventional medicine is sometimes necessary and helpful.

After a thorough assessment of a patient's situation has been made and she has been informed of the standard recommended treatments for her situation—like hysterectomy for a large fibroid uterus—then the patient herself must decide what "feels" right. For one, the choice will be the hysterectomy. Another with the same problem might be more comfortable trying dietary change, castor oil packs, or myomectomy first. The Internet has helped women become far better informed about their options, but it has also made things more confusing. The only way out is in—into your own inner wisdom.

Once a treatment program has been recommended to you, regardless of what it is, let the information sink in for a few days or more. See if it feels right in your body. If it doesn't, give it more thought, get another opinion, ask for a dream, or turn it over to your inner guidance. If surgery has been recommended, I'm a very big fan of getting second and even third opinions. Very few conditions are such an emergency that you have to make a decision on the spot, and that includes a diagnosis of cancer. If you sit with a decision for a while, you'll be much more trusting of the treatment you eventually decide upon.

Which Treatment Is Best?

How a woman chooses to treat a condition will depend on her own needs at the time. I say this while acknowledging both the power of the medical-pharmaceutical industry to sway public opinion and the cultural biases I've already explored.

People often have prejudgments about treatments. Those who are oriented toward natural therapies sometimes see surgery or the use of drugs as a failure and the use of vitamins for the same problem as a triumph. One of my friends who finally had an endometrial ablation procedure for heavy menstrual bleeding and chronic anemia said the following: "I realize now that I sort of reverse-discriminated against conventional medicine. Because I was so against surgery and only interested in 'natural' options, I almost missed doing something that was really the right option for me." To those who are more familiar with conventional drugs and surgery, the very notion that an herb or dietary change could help seems preposterous. I teach women that there are many choices and they need not exclude entire categories that could help them—either conventional or alternative.

Eating brown rice, tofu, and vegetables is appropriate for some women who want to decrease symptoms related to excess estrogen, for example, while taking a progesterone preparation is the best option for others with the same problem. Sometimes a woman needs both. Many women are confused about these points and need to understand that they have options.

To approach illness without using the diagnostic tools of modern medicine where they are appropriate is as dualistic and harmful to patients as saying to someone with arthritis, "We've completed your tests. You have arthritis. It is a lifelong, chronic, debilitating disease, and you might as well learn to live with it"—without suggesting that she explore the effects of nutrition, stress, and lifestyle. Because mystery is a constant part of life, we can never be sure how anything will turn out; we can never be sure that a medical condition is hopeless because there are well-documented spontaneous remissions from just about everything! Mark Hyman, M.D., medical director at Cleveland Clinic's Center for Functional Medicine (and ten-time *New York Times* bestselling author), recently wrote a blog post about what he calls "the myth of diagnosis," making the point that having a diagnosis does not lead to a clear path for treatment. In truth, he writes, "diagnoses are just a name we associate with a collection of symptoms. This name has *nothing* to do with *why* you have those symptoms—with the root cause of the 'disease.'"[10] He gives the example that depression may be caused by gluten in one person and by a vitamin B_{12} deficiency in another. It doesn't necessarily mean you should be taking antidepressants. That's why functional medicine is so important—it takes all an individual's factors into account and is the opposite of "one size fits all" medicine. There is never one right answer that fits all people all the time.

A thirty-eight-year-old artist came in for her annual checkup once. She had been trying to decide whether to go on Prozac, an antidepressant, for her periodic depressions. Philosophically she didn't like the idea, but her condition wasn't getting any better. She had had an intuitive reading with a well-respected person in our area who had encouraged her to try the drug. She finally decided that the only way to know whether the drug would help was to give it a trial. She told me afterward, "One of the most helpful things about coming to you was being able to tell you about my intuitive reading and understanding that I could tailor my medical care around how I was feeling about that information. That you were willing to listen to all the different parts of my story is precious to me."

When I saw her three months later, she said that she was feeling wonderful and that the drug seemed to be a "missing link" for her. "I can't believe how my life has changed around," she reported. "Now the universe seems to be providing for me. My artwork is selling well, and I am much more creative. I'm also claiming my power and energy as my own and am not nearly so worried about what other people think or whether I'm better than or worse than anyone else [as an artist]. I have more energy than I've ever had before." Taking the drug became a turning point for her, but before she could accept it, she had had to release her prejudgment about it. Though the drug definitely helped, she also dealt with the issues from her past—childhood sexual abuse—that were core issues in her depression.

Six months later, she stopped taking Prozac because she felt that it was creating "an artificial euphoria" that didn't feel right to her. What had worked well at one point was no longer appropriate. She continues to feel well, powerful, and creative without the drug. (Interestingly, the data on antidepressants versus placebos show that placebos are just as effective. That means that sometimes antidepressants work just because we believe in them.)[11] As a general rule, women are prescribed far too many psych meds— all of which are highly addictive. Not only has antidepressant use in the United States soared almost 65 percent in the past fifteen years (from about 8 percent to 13 percent of Americans age twelve and up), but women are about twice as likely as men to take them—16.5 percent of American women (compared with 8.6 percent of men) are currently on antidepressant medications.[12] These statistics are sobering, considering that people taking antidepressants are 33 percent more likely to die from any cause.[13] (The International Coalition for Drug Awareness has cataloged an enormous number of SSRI nightmares online at www.ssristories.net.) Yet when a woman tries to get off antidepressants, she may well find herself experiencing withdrawal symptoms that mimic the symptoms for which she was prescribed the med. My good friend and colleague Kelly Brogan, M.D., a holistic psychiatrist, has made it her life's work to assist women in avoiding psychiatric medication in the first place or getting off it. Her book *A Mind of Your Own: The Truth About Depression and How Women Can Heal Their Bodies to Reclaim Their Lives* (HarperCollins, 2016) is a must-read for all women suffering from mental symptoms of any kind.

There are many ways to heal. The right way for you is the way that feels best for you at a particular time. We must learn to see ourselves as processes— changing and growing over time. *Eventually, any externally imposed guidelines for how to become well must be consistent with our own inner guidance system. Eventually, we must learn to support ourselves through self-respect— not through restrictive regimens filled with* shoulds *and* oughts *that feel punitive.*

Externally imposed regimens such as dietary improvement are often a first step in healing. These regimens often help women feel good enough to

get on with their real work of finding out both about their deepest woundings and about the self-nourishing things they can do to help them heal their
wounds. These two quests go hand in hand. We can't skip over the parts of
our lives that hurt or are disturbing in an attempt to "follow our bliss." But
when we commit to following our bliss, the healing of our wounds begins
spontaneously.

Analysis Can Cause Paralysis

*We are running around looking for knowledge, but we are drown-
ing in information.*
                                                —Karl-Henrik Robèrt

Information gathering is only a first step to flourishing. Sooner or later,
you have to close your eyes, go inside, and listen for *your* answer, not *the*
answer. Many people, equating techniques, medicines, and even vitamins
with health, stop at this level. I've seen women with a variety of different
conditions go to scores of healthcare practitioners of all types but come no
closer to healing than they were before. Often, the more facts they have, the
more confused they become. This information dilemma is common and can
immobilize us.

In people who are trying to heal a condition with diet, for example, there
often comes a time when trying to control the amount and quality of everything they put into their mouths dominates their lives: "How many greens
should I have? One cup or a half cup? Should they be cooked? How about
my bowel movements—should they sink or float? If they sink, does it mean I
should add fiber? What about water—two glasses or three? And is it okay to
have an orange? One a day or two?"

It is simply not possible to know and understand the effects of everything. This approach becomes very problematic when we are dealing with a
living, breathing, ever-changing human body. The answers are always in
your heart, not your mind.

Hormone therapy is another common situation in which women can
work themselves into a real frenzy if they rely on intellect alone. No amount
of studies on hormone therapy, mineral intake, or exercise will ever be able
to take into account all the variables that affect a woman's life around menopause.

Sometimes we have to take a step back from our intellect and laugh at it,
running around in circles, chasing its tail. Writer Natalie Goldberg calls this
"monkey mind." Regardless of what the issue is, once you've read all the
books and consulted all the experts, only your inner guidance, of which the
intellect is just one part, can give you the right answer.

Please remember, too, that Divine Love is the most powerful healing force on the planet and that no disease is incurable. (Information on the World Service Institute and the petitions is in chapter 15 and at www .worldserviceinstitute.org.)

TREATING SLEEP APNEA MORE EFFECTIVELY WITH ENERGY PSYCHOLOGY

More than 18 million Americans have sleep apnea, an involuntary cessation of breathing while asleep—sometimes hundreds of times each night and often for a minute or longer. While those with apnea often snore, not all do. Their body wakes them up in time to breathe (frequently with a loud snort). Although this disturbs sleep cycles, preventing those affected from getting a good night's rest, most people don't fully wake up when this happens, so they often don't know they have the condition. Untreated sleep apnea can cause serious complications, including high blood pressure, heart disease, stroke, diabetes, depression, memory problems, headaches, weight gain, and daytime sleepiness and fatigue (which itself can cause car accidents when someone falls asleep while driving).

Obstructive sleep apnea (OSA) is the most common type of apnea and is caused by the soft tissue in the back of the throat collapsing and blocking the airway. For those who have central nervous system apnea (CNSA), the brain doesn't send the signal for the body to breathe. In mixed sleep apnea, both problems are present. The best way to diagnose the condition is to spend a night in a sleep lab, although home sleep studies using special monitors are also an option.

Once apnea is diagnosed, the patient may be fitted with a special dental appliance similar to a mouth guard to be worn during sleep. The appliance holds the lower jaw forward just enough to keep the airway open. More serious cases require the patient to use a positive airway pressure (PAP) machine during sleep. To use these machines, the patient wears a mask over their nose and/or mouth, while air is forced into their throat through flexible tubing connecting the mask to the machine. Such machines are expensive, uncomfortable, and difficult to get used to, although they can save lives when they are the only option available.

Fortunately, other treatments do exist. Damaris Drewry, Ph.D., a psychologist who specializes in treating patients with sleep apnea, has broken new ground in the treatment of CNSA. Dr. Drewry found that those most likely to have undiagnosed CNSA include combat veterans, people who were given ether as an anesthetic, and survivors of car accidents, near-drownings, and childhood abuse. Connecting the dots, she suspected that the underlying cause may be energy that had been frozen in the body in response to various traumatizing events. Her experience has borne out this hypothesis.

The key, she says, is that when these individuals originally experienced the trauma, their subconscious programmed their autonomic (involuntary) nervous system to stop breathing as part of the fight-flight-freeze response. (Psychology has recently added "freeze" to the description of this protective mechanism.) You'll recognize this as the sharp inhale of breath we all take when we see or experience a trauma we're helpless to escape or change, followed by involuntarily holding our breath for a few seconds. When this happens, a cascade of stress chemicals is then released. Dr. Drewry explains that during this freeze response, the experience and the meaning we give it (that we're about to die or be seriously hurt) is stored in cellular memory. After the trauma has passed, if it remains unresolved, the stop-breathing neurotransmitter patterns in the body can still play out during sleep, so we reexperience the trauma as though it is still happening—a form of post-traumatic stress disorder. To heal this response and stop the subconscious programming, Dr. Drewry notes, the physical body, the mental body, and the emotional body must all agree that the threat no longer exists. To this end, she has developed a treatment that combines Emotional Freedom Technique (EFT, commonly called tapping) and neuro-linguistic programming (NLP) to reprogram the autonomic nervous system.

In a published study on the technique, she reports that 35 percent of clients experienced immediate cessation of CNSA after the first session and remained free of it.[14] Another 30 percent experienced immediate relief from apnea but lapsed back into it when they did not complete the treatment. Her method won't work for apnea caused by obstruction, and while those with a combination of OSA and CNSA can't be fully cured, she reports that they do benefit from the treatment by feeling they have more control over their own lives and can make better life choices. To learn more about Dr. Drewry's Beyond Talk Therapy practice, visit her website at www.beyond talktherapy.com.

HOLISTIC DENTISTRY

Dentistry is about much more than merely cleaning teeth or fixing cavities. Poor oral health may be a risk factor for conditions such as diabetes, heart disease, and stroke. When you're choosing a dentist, consider finding one with a holistic practice that considers not only your physical health but also your emotional and even spiritual health.

Holistic dentists (whether or not they label their practice as such) use both natural and conventional therapies. They take fewer X-rays and use digital X-ray equipment, which exposes patients to substantially less radiation. They use composite resin instead of metal to fill cavities, and they use natural antibacterial agents during dental procedures. Most are against fluoride treatments, believing fluoride can cause long-term health problems (and doesn't actually prevent tooth decay, despite what most of us have been led to believe).

In treating gum disease, holistic dentists may use highly effective lasers and ozone treatments to clear gums of bacteria. They may also use an iodine irrigation system to prevent bacteria from entering the gums. Finally, holistic dentists may prescribe herbal remedies to promote faster, natural healing.

Nine Ways to Keep Your Mouth Healthy

1. *Try oil pulling.* This is an ancient Ayurvedic dental technique that involves swishing a tablespoon of oil (usually coconut, sesame, or olive oil) inside your mouth for ten to twenty minutes before spitting it out. Ayurvedic practitioners believe oil pulling draws out toxins from the body, but at the very least it's a great replacement for mouthwash because it doesn't kill all of the good bacteria in your mouth. It may also help to remove plaque and whiten your teeth.

2. *Eat less sugar.* Plaque uses sugar as fuel, and then releases acid as a waste product (which can lead to tooth decay).

3. *Have acupuncture.* Each tooth is at the end of an acupuncture meridian, meaning stimulation of that meridian from having a filling or some other acute tooth trauma can cause chronic stimulation of whatever organs are associated with the same meridian. Similarly, chronic tooth problems can indicate an imbalance in an organ or system along the same meridian. Acupuncture restores such imbalances.

4. *Quit smoking.* Smoking not only yellows your teeth over time but is also an important cause of gum disease because it makes plaque stickier.

5. *Use natural toothpaste.* As mentioned previously, fluoride doesn't necessarily prevent cavities and can cause other health problems (as can artificial ingredients commonly found in toothpaste, including sodium lauryl sulfate). But the act of brushing your teeth is still beneficial because it helps remove plaque. Good natural brands of toothpaste include Earthpaste, Tom's of Maine, and Dr. Bronner's.

6. *Floss your teeth.* Flossing helps keep your gums healthy and removes bacteria and food from between your teeth (which can cause plaque to form). Choose between conventional floss and a rechargable air flosser.

7. *Eat a balanced diet.* Just like the rest of your body, your teeth need nutrients to stay healthy. Calcium, phosphorus, vitamin D, and magnesium are especially important for building and strengthening tooth enamel and protecting your teeth.

8. *Drink water.* This helps to wash away food and bacteria left in your mouth after you eat. Water also neutralizes acid that can erode tooth enamel. Even if you don't brush after every meal, at least rinse your mouth out with water.

9. *Don't ignore dental symptoms.* Tooth sensitivity or discoloration, bleeding gums, and oral pain are all reason to make an appointment with the dentist. These symptoms may have underlying causes that can more easily be solved sooner than later.

A note about amalgam fillings: Historically, most dental fillings were done with amalgam, which contains more than 50 percent mercury and can damage your central nervous and immune systems. But don't panic if you've had these types of fillings, because not everyone has a problem with them. I recommend having regular checkups to make sure amalgam fillings aren't leaking. If you experience muscle and joint pain, stiffness and cramping, chronic fatigue, chemical or food sensitivities, or significant neurological symptoms that mimic multiple sclerosis or other neurological diseases, talk to your dentist about removing your amalgam fillings.

To find a holistic dentist, visit the website for the International Academy of Oral Medicine and Toxicology at www.iaomt.org or the website of the Holistic Dental Association at www.holisticdental

.org. For more information about oral wellness, visit www.ora wellness.com. Finally, I recommend the book *Whole-Body Dentistry: A Complete Guide to Understanding the Impact of Dentistry on Total Health* (Quantum Health Press, 2011) by Mark Breiner, D.D.S.

CREATING HEALTH THROUGH SURGERY

At some point in their lives, many women are faced with the prospect of surgery. More than 51 million people in the United States have inpatient surgery each year,[15] and 53.3 million outpatient procedures are performed annually, either in hospitals or in freestanding ambulatory (outpatient) surgery centers.[16] About 58 percent of surgery patients are women, according to the National Center for Health Statistics. I've watched many women put their lives on hold for months or even years while trying to cure "naturally" a condition that is very amenable to conservative, organ-sparing surgery. Surgery to repair the pelvis is totally different from surgery to remove everything in the pelvis. Surgery should always be considered along with other healing modalities. I like to help heal the negativity often associated with surgery by renaming the experience "creating health through surgery." Surgery can be approached as a healing ceremony. Jeanne Achterberg, Ph.D., Barbara Dossey, and Leslie Kolkmeier give full instructions for how to do this in their book *Rituals of Healing* (Bantam Books, 1994).

The Second Opinion

Before having an elective surgery—or any other surgery, for that matter—get a second opinion if you have any doubts whatsoever. I've seen countless women for second opinions regarding hysterectomy. The second opinion gives women time to think about their decision, and it exposes them to the vast differences in thinking that exist even within the conventionally trained medical profession about treating a particular problem. Some women see as many as five or six different specialists before they decide on a course of action. Ultimately, they have to tune in to their inner guidance to come up with the best answer for them, since no doctor can provide it.

Often when I've rendered a second opinion, I've agreed with the referring surgeon's rationale for the hysterectomy; heavy, irregular bleeding that has resulted in anemia, for example, is a conventional reason for hysterectomy. Though there are many ways to treat the problem besides surgery, if surgery feels like the right solution to the woman, she should go with that. If, on the other hand, she is open to alternatives such as dietary change, she should give those a try. The main thing to be aware of is that there are often many different choices—all of which have merit.

Women who have taken the time to read and gather information embark upon a chosen course of therapy or a surgical procedure from a place of strength and knowledge, not because some authority figure said they should. This is a great place to be! No one should ever have elective surgery if she feels she doesn't have permission to speak up, disagree, or get more information.

Finally, understand that this surgery is a choice. If you want to cancel at the last minute because you've rethought the whole thing or it suddenly feels wrong, then go ahead and cancel it. There are two times when a woman needs to grant herself full permission to change her mind: one is at the altar before her wedding, and another is before having elective surgery. (This doesn't apply to lifesaving surgery in emergencies.)

BANK YOUR BLOOD AHEAD OF TIME

Four to six weeks before major surgery such as a hysterectomy or myomectomy, donate two units of your own blood (unless you're too anemic) in case there is any risk of blood loss requiring transfusion. The needle used by the Red Cross for blood donation is large. I suggest you ask your doctor for a prescription for either EMLA or Lidoderm (15 percent lidocaine cream), transdermal anesthetic creams that can be applied to the antecubital fossa of the arm (the area where the blood is drawn) one hour before your blood will be drawn, then covered with a plastic bandage known as Tegaderm. It makes the procedure painless.

PROLONGED FASTING BEFORE SURGERY IS AN OUTDATED PRACTICE

If you had surgery before 1999, you were told to have nothing to eat or drink after midnight the night before the procedure. However, it's fairly likely you've been told the same thing even if you've had surgery more recently. While the American Society of Anesthesiologists modified its fasting-before-surgery practice in 1999, many doctors still give their patients outdated advice.

The new guidelines allow for having a light meal six hours before a surgical procedure and then having only clear fluids—such as water, pulp-free juices, or black coffee or tea—until two hours prior to the operation. The fast begins at that time, not before. The distinction is important because prolonged fasting can lead to dehydration, hypoglycemia, and electrolyte imbalance, which can make some patients more anxious (and so require more drugs). Some patients additionally report headaches and nausea before surgery when they have fasted more than two hours. Furthermore, putting an IV into a patient is much easier for the technician and less painful for the patient when the patient is hydrated.

Surgery Is Not Failure but a Healing Opportunity

Too often, women think they've failed if they require surgery for their problem. This is an example of dualistic, black-and-white thinking. One woman with a fourteen-week-size fibroid uterus said to me through tears, "I'm so ashamed. I keep thinking that I should have been able to prevent this or at least to have made it go away by myself." Further questioning revealed that she had the type of family background in which she had repeatedly heard the phrase "Don't cry, or I'll give you something to cry about." She felt that asking for help and having needs were signs of weakness. Many people grew up this way.

Gail, whose ovarian cyst healing was covered in chapter 7, said, "As a good 'New Age person,' surgery was my last resort. With classic New Age hubris, I felt I should have been able to heal myself, and if I chose surgery, I was a failure. So I tried a gamut of holistic approaches—acupuncture, herbs, castor oil packs, working with a friend who is a channel, and visualization. All of these methods were helpful and were surely healing on certain levels. But I realized that this cyst was too dense, both physically and spiritually, to be melted even by acupuncture needles. It needed to be cut out."

Another patient of mine, June, had a persistent ovarian cyst and very much wanted to avoid surgery. She spent three months doing visualizations, emotional cleansing, and dietary change to heal her cyst. I told June that I felt that surgery was her best option. Her cyst was large—ten centimeters—and had failed to go away on its own after three months. Though she wanted to believe that the cyst was gone and that she could avoid surgery, she had had the following dream: "I went to get my car from the repair shop, and it wasn't ready yet. [Recall that in dreams, the car commonly represents the body.] This dream recurred several times. I started to wonder if the cyst was indeed gone.

I never had felt that the cyst posed any real danger to me, but even though I felt that I had completed my work"—she had developed a great deal of clarity about what the cyst represented in her life and had experienced a great deal of grieving and sadness about this—"I wondered if maybe the cyst was still there. I rarely admitted that thought to myself at all, choosing instead to think positively that it must be gone because I had completed what I thought was my healing work."

A few weeks before her scheduled surgery, June had dinner with a woman she had just met who was fascinated with myths, dream work, and art therapy as tools to help people heal themselves. "When she heard about my car dreams," June later wrote, "she started to push hard. She asked if I knew what was wrong with my car. She said I should have found out what was broken and called in a specialist to tell me how to fix it." This was to be done in a dream state. "She was horrified that I was going to let someone take my ovary without trying harder to keep it. The implication was that if I did not try things her way, I wasn't trying hard enough. I answered her questions seriously. The questions felt so heroic, so guilt-ridden.[17] I am responsible, and this cyst must be what I want. After I left her place, I felt dirty, sort of emotionally raped. Later I realized that searching endlessly for a nonsurgical cure is addictive, that I could keep the cyst and be addicted to the process, or I could just let it go and be done with it." June had the inner strength and wisdom to recognize that sometimes the proponents of alternative modalities can be just as arrogant and intransigent as those who believe in the conventional healthcare system. Although June was briefly intimidated by this woman's insistence, she quickly realized that the feelings she was left with after their dinner were a sign that she was being manipulated in a way that was toxic to her.

An Opportunity to Heal Old Fears

For many women, particularly those who are drawn to natural methods of healing, surgery is terrifying. My patient Gail, after her cyst surgery, said, "That cyst helped me uncover several powerful patterns I hadn't been aware of. My terror around my body, disease, doctors, and hospitals was a result of my mother's long, mysterious heart disease, which led to her death. Throughout parts of my childhood she was in and out of hospitals, never seeming to get better, and the doctors never seeming to know what was wrong with her. What caused even more suffering on my part was the feelings everyone in my family was experiencing around her illness that were never discussed."

Many women have transformed their fears of the hospital and surgery, however, by using such experiences as a "spiritual initiation"—a time to face their fears and walk through them, as well as a chance to reverse old patterns that no longer serve them. Gail wrote, "As I contemplated my upcoming surgery it was absolutely clear to me that I had a wonderful opportunity to confront my childhood terror of hospitals and all they represented. I could experience that my story was totally different from my mother's story. I learned some wonderful lessons. Reversing my family pattern, I shared my fears and concerns with my husband and dear friends and asked for their support. Their outpouring of love and support was a precious gift that I shall treasure for a long time."

Giving yourself permission to let another individual help you can be a profoundly healing experience. When surgery is the best treatment choice, surrendering to the skills of the anesthesiologist, your surgeon, your nurses, and your inner guidance can be a true growth experience. If you received the message in childhood that your physical and emotional needs for support and comfort don't deserve to be met, asking for support during surgery or a hospitalization is an opportunity to reverse this message.

Healing energy is available in hospitals. The nurses and staff can be seen as healing angels. The people who work in hospitals—whether they be nurses, nursing assistants, or orderlies—are often in these settings because they are naturally drawn to healing. When you stop fighting those who are there to help, it's quite a relief.

Take a friend or family member to the preoperative visit if you're having surgery. Your friend can then accompany you to the hospital to meet the anesthesiologist and go through the pre-op phase in the hospital setting. After surgery, these friends or others can provide support at home through cooking, cleaning, or backrubs. Women must learn how to ask for this support. Getting it is a skill. Sometimes we need help learning this.

June wrote the following about getting support: "On my way home after finding out that I needed surgery, I knew I could not be alone that whole weekend, so I stopped at my friend Carol's house. I think Carol became afraid when she saw how depressed I looked. She delivered a strong lecture about how important I am to my son, and to her, and to many other people. I never had acknowledged my importance to any of those people except my son. She made a very strong case for going forward and letting myself be supported by my friends. She told me that I was to recover at her house so that I wouldn't have to cook or shop, or do any other of those details for myself. She helped me immeasurably."

In preparation for her surgery, June went to see a hypnotist and had three sessions. Her hypnotist produced two tapes for her to use—one to prepare her for a healthy experience and a quick recovery, and a second to help her move on afterward. She used these tapes many times during the two weeks prior to surgery.[18] She also began work with a physician who understood and taught qi gong, an ancient Chinese art that teaches us to circulate our life energy through movement, massage, and the breath.

A New Generation of Hospitals

After spending fifteen years as CEO of various hospitals, Kelly Mather was convinced there was a much better way to help people and communities concentrate on getting and staying healthy. So in 2006, she founded an organization called Harmony Healing House, designed to partner with hospitals around the country to encourage them to take a more wellness-based, global perspective.

Mather developed a scientifically proven, low-cost, and simple model to take hospitals beyond the first level of healing (illness and rescue care) and through three additional levels: creating a culture of health via a staff wellness program; creating a healing environment that promotes physical, mental, emotional, and spiritual improvement techniques to patients and visitors; and taking the message beyond the hospital walls and out into the community by partnering with schools, wellness centers, and the like to promote health.

Hospitals that achieve all four levels will receive a "Healing Hospital" designation and will be listed on the organization's website (www.harmonyhealinghouse.com).

Planetree, a nonprofit organization mentioned earlier in this chapter, has a similar certification program for excellence in person-centered care at healthcare organizations around the world (www.planetree.org). Angelica Thieriot founded Planetree in 1978 after her own traumatic experience being treated for a rare viral infection at a prominent teaching hospital in California where the clinical care was excellent but she felt totally dehumanized as a patient. Planetree's goal is personalizing, demystifying, and humanizing patients' experiences, and the result is a higher quality of care, improved patient outcomes, lower readmission rates, and shorter hospital stays. Healthcare organizations benefit as well, with increased employee satisfaction and retention and a noticeably more healing and comforting environment for caregivers and staff as well as for patients and their families.

How to Prepare for Surgery
(or Chemotherapy) and Heal Faster

Peggy Huddleston, M.S., is the author of *Prepare for Surgery, Heal Faster: A Guide of Mind-Body Techniques* (Angel River Press, 1996), a remarkable step-by-step guide to help people get the most out of their surgical experiences (see www.healfaster.com, which also carries her audio record-ings designed to facilitate lasting healing). Her healing statements and steps to prepare for surgery have been clinically proven to decrease blood loss and pain and speed recovery. Her book and the program it outlines are being used in many major hospitals all over the country. I personally used her heal-ing statements when I had my fibroid surgery years ago, and they worked like a charm. Having done surgery for years, I can assure you that nothing is more gratifying to a surgeon than having a patient who will work with her or him in partnership—each trusting the input of the other—so that optimal results can be obtained.

The techniques that Peggy uses have succeeded in helping many of my patients and thousands of people around the world achieve the following benefits:

- Feel calmer before surgery

- Have less pain after surgery

- Use from 23 to 50 percent less pain medication

- Strengthen the immune system

- Save money on medical bills (a study in California reported that pa-tients who prepared for abdominal surgery with the healing state-ments plus guided imagery left the hospital 1.5 days earlier and saved $1,200 per person in hospitalization; because this study was done more than twenty years ago, the cost savings would be much higher now)[19]

Whether you're having a minor outpatient procedure or a major opera-tion, Peggy's approach can help you. And by the way, her techniques, which are described below, can also be used to help you get through radiation and/or chemotherapy.

Step One: Relax to Feel Peaceful

Eighty-five percent of all medical problems are associated with unre-solved tension and stress held in the body. This chronic response to tension results in a cascade of physiologic changes that can and do affect your health adversely. What's the antidote? Learn the skill of deep relaxation and prac-tice it often so that you know you can call up a deep sense of peace at will. Learning deep relaxation and visualization is easy, and there are a number of different ways to do it. For the purpose of preparing for surgery, I'd recom-mend using an audio recording prepared specifically for this purpose. In ad-dition to Peggy's recordings, described above, I also recommend *A Meditation to Promote Successful Surgery* from my colleague Belleruth Naparstek (www

.healthjourneys.com) as well as the Surgical Support series developed by the
Monroe Institute (www.hemi-sync.com). Both of these last two products include not only meditations to be used to prepare for surgery but also music
designed for you to listen to during the procedure itself. Don't be surprised
if, when you are first starting to learn to relax, strong emotions emerge, such
as sadness, anger, or whatever. Feel them fully, cry as long as you need to,
don't hold back—allow whatever you feel to wash through you. Welcome
those intense emotions. They've probably been waiting within you for a long
time trying to get expressed.

Studies have shown that relaxation improves the immune system, calms
the central nervous system, and often cures tension headache, migraine, hypertension, and anxiety, as well as helping you prepare for your surgery.
Many hospitals now offer "prepare for surgery" programs as well.

Step Two: Visualize Your Healing

Visualize your ideal surgical outcome. Imagine as vividly as you can that
your operation is now over and you are comfortable, filled with peace, and
healthy in every respect. Feel yourself surrounded by healing light, or sound,
or a feeling of deep peace. The more you can imagine an ideal outcome in
great detail, the faster you will heal. Your intuitive wisdom will provide you
with the images that seem most healing. Visualize, visualize, visualize: Five
times a day for five minutes each time is more effective than a single twenty-
five-minute session.

Step Three: Organize a Support Group

Surgery is a wonderful time to reach out for support. Make sure that
someone will be with you when you arrive for your surgery, will visit you
daily while you're in the hospital, if necessary, and will help you at home for
as long as you require that assistance. (For abdominal surgery, that's at least
two weeks.) Many women simply don't realize how vulnerable they may feel
post-op, so prepare for this so you can be in a healing cocoon as long as
needed. This will allow you to receive the caring and loving thoughts of your
friends and family. This aspect of preparing for surgery can be especially
healing for those of you who feel that "to get anything done right, I have to
do it myself." You will have the opportunity to allow others to give to you
and provide for you. You'll learn skills of receiving, which for many women
is a major challenge.

When you're in the hospital and/or after you're home, I'd recommend
having at least one Reiki, therapeutic touch, or massage session. A daily
treatment for the first two or three days would be ideal. Both Reiki and
therapeutic touch are energy medicine treatments that are completely safe
and have been shown scientifically to speed the healing process. Ask your
doctor or nurse if they know anyone who is trained in these therapies. Many

healthcare professionals as well as laypeople have this training. (To find a Reiki practitioner, visit www.reikialliance.org; to find a therapeutic touch practitioner, visit www.therapeutictouch.org.)

Step Four: Meet Your Anesthesiologist

You will be entrusting your consciousness to this doctor, so you'll want to meet him or her before surgery. In these days of same-day surgery, it is common to meet your anesthesiologist just before your procedure, but with some effort on your part, it's still possible to schedule a meeting in advance. A study at Harvard showed that meeting the anesthesiologist well before surgery significantly decreased patients' preoperative anxiety. Ask your surgeon to arrange this for you. This is no time to worry about "making waves." Your doctors will remember you and give you more individualized care if you've established yourself as someone who asks respectfully to have your total being taken care of during surgery.

OPIOIDS: SHOULD YOU TAKE THEM?

The opioid crisis has exploded in recent years, not only because these potent drugs relieve pain so effectively but also because when doctors began widely prescribing opioids in the late 1990s, the drug companies assured them their patients would not become addicted. We now know these drugs are in fact highly addictive, *even when taken as prescribed*. People have even overdosed on medications prescribed to them by their doctors.[20]

Research shows that 21 to 29 percent of patients prescribed opioids for chronic pain misuse these drugs,[21] and the misuse is so serious that between 8 and 12 percent of them develop an opioid-use disorder.[22] In 2017, an estimated 1.7 million Americans suffered from such a disorder.[23] One study that covered fifty-two geographic areas in forty-five states showed that opioid overdoses increased an incredible *30 percent* from July 2016 through September 2017.[24] These statistics are more than sobering. They're downright frightening.

The simple truth is that there's no risk-free dose of opioids. Of course, the more you take, the higher your risk, but even at the standard prescription amount—5 to 10 mg of oxycodone every six hours, for example—people can become addicted and sometimes even die of overdoses. One reason is that many medical professionals rely too heavily on what's considered the morphine milligram equivalent (or MME), the dose that would deliver the same amount of pain relief if the patient was taking morphine. If the physician doesn't take into consideration a host of other risk factors, even that dose might prove to be way too much. For example, one study showed that those taking the MME of opioids still had a 2 percent chance of overdose, which is simply unacceptable, especially considering the number of people taking these medications today.[25] Physicians must consult the Risk Index for Overdose or Serious Opioid-Induced Respiratory Depression (RIOSORD), an opioid-overdose calculator developed by researchers who analyzed a huge number of variables in a group of 18.4 million patients on such medication.[26]

A colleague of mine experienced this physician-patient disconnect herself after having chest surgery a few years ago. She went home from the hospital with a prescription for opioids to be taken every four hours. She didn't want to become dependent on them, however, so she took only a few. At her first post-op appointment, she asked the surgeon's nurse for a secondary and even a tertiary plan for pain relief that would not involve taking so much medication.

"The nurse looked at me with a totally blank expression," she told me, "as if no one had ever asked her that question before—and, more concerning, as if she'd never even considered any other option than one pill every four hours. When I pressed her, she said, 'Well, you could try taking Tylenol.' She had no advice for any kind of intermediate plan. Just one opioid every four hours or good luck with over-the-counter pain meds. She didn't even suggest cutting the pills in half. Opioid dependency is a huge problem where I live, and I could see that this attitude by medical professionals—even at the renowned teaching hospital where I had my surgery—was part of the problem. I didn't take any more of the prescription. Without solid guidance, I wasn't willing to risk it. And I was fine without them."

A 2019 animal study from the University of Colorado at Boulder on the effects of opioids on post-surgical pain shows she made the right decision. Rats given repeated doses of morphine experienced inflammation and pain for three weeks longer than rats given only a saline solution.[27] The researchers further found that opioids had the effect of "priming" certain spinal cord cells to become more sensitive to pain. The longer the rats received morphine, the longer they were reactive to pain. Senior study author Linda Watkins, Ph.D., noted of the study that it showed "there is another dark side of opiates that many people don't suspect. It shows that trauma, including surgery, in combination with opiates can lead to chronic pain."[28] The immune system takes a double hit, she added—first with the surgery, and then with the medication.

Similar studies back this up. Yet another animal study done a few years previously showed that even after only a few days of taking opioids for chronic nerve pain, the pain not only intensified but was also prolonged for months due to an increase in systemic inflammation.[29]

Fortunately, other excellent options do exist. A 2016 study of 300 emergency-room patients with acute pain shows that acupuncture was more effective, worked faster, and caused fewer side effects than intravenous morphine.[30]

If you are at all concerned about becoming dependent on opioids after surgery, make sure your doctor listens to your concerns and adequately addresses them. Do not assume that just because they're prescribed by a doctor, opioids are safe. If you do decide to take them, take the least amount that does the job, and then get off them as soon as possible.

Step Five: Use Healing Statements

There are four healing statements that you'll want your surgeon or anesthesiologist to say to you during your operation. Research has shown that these statements are associated with having less pain, fewer complications, and faster healing. Make three copies of these statements; give one to your surgeon and one to your anesthesiologist, and tape one on your hospital gown so it's visible as you go into surgery. Do not let any embarrassment prevent you from asking your doctors to do this for you. Believe me, most doctors have gone into medicine because they want to be healers. Ask them to do their job. I've never once seen a surgeon or anesthesiologist scoff at a patient's request for these statements. If they do, go to someone else. If your consciousness isn't safe with them, then your body won't feel safe, either—and your healing won't be as rapid as it otherwise could be.

Here are the statements:

AS I AM GOING UNDER ANESTHESIA, PLEASE SAY:

"Following this operation, you will feel comfortable and you will heal very well." (Repeat five times.)

After saying the statements, please put on my earphones and start my MP3 player.

AT THE CONCLUSION OF THE SURGERY, PLEASE SAY:

1. "Your operation has gone very well." (Repeat five times.)

2. "Following this operation, you will be hungry for _____. You will be thirsty and you will urinate easily." (Repeat five times.)

3. "Following this operation, _____." (Ask your surgeon to fill this in with positive predictions about recovery, such as "You will be able to exercise and be back to full activity within four weeks," and so on. And add some of your own goals. If you're currently a smoker, for example, you might ask that your anesthesiologist add the following: "You will be a nonsmoker who detests the taste of cigarettes" or "You will be free of the desire to smoke." Anecdotally, I've seen this work.)

As you prepare your MP3 player for surgery, adjust the volume so that you can barely hear the music. Then stick some tape on the volume control so that it can't be increased. When you are under anesthesia, the tiny tissues involved in hearing will be very relaxed and any sound will be amplified. You don't want to risk damaging your hearing by playing the music too loudly during this vulnerable time. If the hospital will not allow you to use earbuds during surgery, you can buy wireless headphones containing a microchip that's preloaded with music, which you can change (available from Surgical Serenity Solutions at www.surgicalserenitysolutions.com/patient-products). A growing number of hospitals make surgical headphones available for patients, so be sure to ask. When a friend of mine recently had surgery, her surgeon did not want her to wear headphones during the operation. But her doctor was more than happy to play her music in the operating room during the procedure. So she arrived with a recording of her favorite songs.

Bernie Siegel, M.D., a famous Yale-trained pediatric surgeon, found that the music that works best for surgery is the music that a patient likes best. That can be anything from the Beatles to Mozart (a popular choice because his music has been found to enhance immune response). Adagio movements are especially good. But anything you love will work, including country and western!

Step Six: Use Supplements to Speed Healing

The following supplements have been shown to speed healing (but be sure to discuss them with your surgeon beforehand):

~ *Vitamin A*. The suggested dose is 25,000 IU daily (unless you are pregnant). Numerous studies have shown the beneficial effects of vitamin A on healing after surgery. It also helps boost the immune system. Start one week before surgery and continue three to four weeks thereafter.

~ *Bromelain*. This supplement, derived from pineapple, helps prevent bruising and also relieves the swelling associated with surgery. Take 1,000 mg per day starting several days before surgery and continuing for about two weeks postoperatively.

~ *Vitamin C.* The suggested dose is 2,000 mg per day. Vitamin C is essential for collagen synthesis, which is part of normal wound healing. Your need for it will increase after your surgery. Start at least a month before your procedure and continue for one month postoperatively.

~ *Zinc, magnesium, B complex.* These supplements have been shown to promote wound healing. The recommended dose is zinc picolinate, 100 mg; magnesium, 800 mg; and 25 to 50 mg B complex, taken in a good-quality supplement that includes at least 800 mcg of folic acid per day.

~ *Vitamin E.* Postoperatively, apply vitamin E oil (d-alpha-tocopherol) onto the incision daily as soon as the surgical dressing is removed (if your surgeon agrees that there is no contraindication to this). This speeds healing and decreases scarring. Some women prefer aloe vera gel, calendula ointment, or other herbal treatments for this purpose.

~ *Homeopathy.* Take Arnica Montana 30X, three or four pellets twice per day (dissolved under the tongue) on the day before surgery and also as soon before surgery as possible. You can take these just before being wheeled into the operating room. Then take them as soon as possible once you get into the recovery room. Your anesthesiologist can help with this, or you can wait until you're back in your room. Take the same dose daily for a week following surgery. Arnica is very good at preventing ill effects from any kind of physical trauma. Many other homeopathic remedies are available that can be used for specific types of surgery. Consult with a trained practitioner.

~ *Herbs.* The Chinese herb known as yunnan baiyao is excellent for promoting wound healing and enhancing the ability of blood to clot. Many of my patients have used this successfully to speed their recovery from surgery. It results in decreased swelling and bruising. Dose is one tablet four times per day for one week prior to surgery, and continuing one month postoperatively. Start as soon after surgery as you can take things by mouth.

Step Seven: Say a Special Prayer for Surgery

When a friend of mine recently had surgery, clinical psychologist and healer Doris Cohen, Ph.D., helped come up with the following list of things for my friend to pray for (and to ask his friends and family to pray for on his behalf) before the surgery. It worked beautifully.

~ A skilled anesthesiologist who monitors me perfectly

~ A body that responds well to the anesthesia

⌐ A skilled surgeon whose hands are steady and who is able to easily and quickly _____ [state what specifically it is the surgeon will be removing, repairing, replacing, or inserting]

⌐ That my unique spirit—and only my unique spirit—comes back into my body when the anesthesia wears off

⌐ That I wake up easily and quickly after surgery

⌐ That my body functions return to normal with no pain

⌐ That this surgery allows me to heal on *all* levels—physical, emotional, and spiritual

HEALING WITH DIVINE LOVE

Whenever one of my loved ones is undergoing surgery or facing a challenge, I always get together with at least one other person and ask to be a channel for Divine Love. Here's the prayer (or petition) that I use, based on the work of Robert Fritchie: "With my soul, I surrender my will to Divine Will. I acknowledge _____ [state the problem here and also the intent for the outcome, such as 'I acknowledge that my sister is having shoulder surgery today and my intent is that she have a completely healed, functional, and comfortable shoulder as a result of this surgery']. I ask that any fears or problems be dissolved with Divine Love according to the Creator's will."

Then I sit with my arms and legs uncrossed, hands in an upright, receiving position. I take a deep breath, hold it for a second, focus on my thymus gland (just under the breastbone), and simply ask to be a channel for Divine Love and send that to my sister (or to whomever I'm praying for). For more information, see the discussion on Divine Love petitions in chapter 15, and visit the website for the World Service Institute (www.worldserviceinstitute.org).

Because the thought of surgery is so terrifying for many people, it can be used as a sort of wake-up call—a time to reprioritize your life. If you approach it with an open mind and an open heart, and if you go through the steps above sincerely—with a sense of surrendering yourself to the process— you may actually heal on your own and find that your surgery will no longer be necessary. I've witnessed this several times in my practice, and Peggy Huddleston gives some examples of this in her book. But don't go through the steps in order to avoid surgery. The key to healing on all levels is that you must proceed with complete willingness to go through with the procedure if necessary. In twelve-step programs they refer to this as "letting go, and letting God." It can work miracles.

After your surgery, notice and acknowledge whatever feelings arise. When a part of your body is removed or when the integrity of your body surface is marred through an incision of any kind, you may need to grieve the loss of your former state.[31] None of us likes surgical scars on our body. It matters little whether you ever did or ever will wear a bikini. We *all* care about how our bodies look.

NEURAL THERAPY: HEALING AFTER SURGERY

Neural therapy can be a huge help in stimulating healing after surgery—even years later. Developed in Germany in the early 1900s, this medical procedure involves the injection of small amounts of an anesthetic such as procaine or lidocaine, usually into a scar, to reestablish the body's natural energy flow, since that flow is disrupted by both the surgery itself and the resulting scar. Neural therapy is also effective for chronic pain, infections, traumas, or conditions such as multiple sclerosis.[32] It works by correcting dysfunctions in the body's autonomic nervous system caused by disturbances in the electrochemical or electromagnetic energy flow within the affected tissues.[33] Neural therapy can restore the energy flow for older scars, too. In fact, some scars will indefinitely block or slow energy unless the flow is repaired. While sometimes one treatment is enough, more than one treatment may be required.

To find a practitioner knowledgeable about neural therapy, visit the doctor search page on the website for the American Association of Orthopaedic Medicine (www.aaomed.org/orthopaedic-doctor).

Old memories may surface after surgery that have been stored in the tissue itself. Surgery has the potential to bring cellular memory to conscious awareness. Incest or other abuse memories may arise in the recovery room or in the days or weeks following surgery. These memories won't surface until you're ready to deal with them, so you need not worry about this. The body's wisdom about when to release information is exquisite.

Allowing yourself to feel emotions connected with surgical removal of tissue is important. Caroline Myss teaches: "When you pull cell tissue out before any of the data have been finalized, the body gets out of synchronicity." Many people have most of their energy tied up in the past and very little available in the present for healing. When an organ or cell tissue is removed and the body messages associated with it are not acknowledged or processed, then part of our energy will remain in the past like an unpaid account— a part of our personal unfinished business. So if any emotions or other data surface before or after surgery, feel them fully and let them work their way through your system.

When one of my patients had her fibroids removed, she wanted to be awake during the procedure, so she was given a spinal anesthetic. It turned out that she had severe adenomyosis, a benign condition in which the endometrial glands inside the uterus grow in the uterine wall, causing excessive bleeding. A hysterectomy was the optimal treatment for this. Her doctor gave her the choice of stopping the operation and leaving the uterus in, since there was no malignancy.

She had been chronically anemic from her condition and experienced some pain. She had tried dietary change and acupuncture without much success. As a mother of three relatively young children, her time for taking optimal care of herself was limited, and so she wouldn't have time to prepare again for a further surgery. She realized that it was time she let go of trying to save her uterus.

Before the uterine removal began, she asked the staff to hold up a mirror for her so that she could see her uterus. She then thanked it for providing her with three healthy children, blessed it, blessed *herself* for trying to preserve it, then said goodbye. Only then did her surgeon begin the hysterectomy. She later told me that the process of letting go and being able to thank her uterus was a key part of her healing. She ended up feeling empowered by this surgery, not devastated.

June, who had the ovarian cyst, also had a spinal and was awake during her surgery. "The operation took less than an hour," she wrote. "I had a spinal block so that I could be fully aware during the surgery. I had a mirror hooked up so that I could watch. It was fabulous. My body is healthy-looking and young for my age [forty-two]. Being able to see the very good condition of my body did me a lot of good. I had lost a lot of confidence in my ability to assess what was going on in my body. [This was because she hadn't realized that her cyst was growing larger. She couldn't feel it.] This showed me what was right about it. The cyst was almost as large as a softball, but instead of being inside my ovary, it was just on the outside wall. Chris said my ovary looked perfect, and asked me if I wanted to try to save it. She did."

Postoperatively, June's friend Carol spent the day and evening with her. June wrote, "She was so supportive and caring. I am so glad she was there. On her way out, she gave me permission to cry. And I did. It was great."

After two and a half weeks of recovery at Carol's house, June's body yielded yet another piece of healing information. She wrote: "Finally I made it home. I still had one more related realization to make and feel. One night I was touching the numbness above the incision, feeling unspeakably sad about the loss of feeling, when I started to cry. Chris had said that if this should happen, to stay with it and explore the feelings. I was crying about the feeling that no man has ever loved me for being the person I really am. Suddenly I realized I was crying about my father. The only two men who have ever loved me for the real me are my cousin and my father. And it was my father who was always there for me. I had never grieved this loss when he died. So I did."

Acknowledging grief and loss is only one part of creating a healthy surgery. Another equally important step is looking forward to a life free from the problem that required surgery. Think of the surgical loss as a cutting away of the old so that there is space for the new to grow.

Another patient of mine, a highly intuitive artist, had a hysterectomy for a large fibroid uterus when she was about forty-four. She had visualized the energy in her pelvis and fibroids as very erratic and unhealthy. Postoperatively in the recovery room, she told me that she realized that the static energy in her pelvis was gone. In its place she sensed an even spiral of healthy energy, a vortex in her pelvis. This surgery was a healing for her.

But I Had Surgery Years Ago and Didn't Know About This

If you've had surgery in the past, reading through this chapter may cause you to feel sad for missing the opportunity to be more fully involved in your healing process. (Stay with this feeling—it is not too late.) Many women who have had hysterectomies had few choices available to them for alternative treatments. The choices for treatment that I've mentioned were not nearly so available even a decade ago as they are now. Each year anesthesia becomes safer, and the techniques to preserve pelvic organs have improved—largely through infertility surgery techniques.

It is natural for women who have had unavoidable surgery in the past to feel some loss, especially now that things have changed. But remember, there is no time limit in the unconscious. What happened in the past can be healed in the present. I can't prevent you from feeling grief over events that are past and organs that have been removed. I do know, however, that it's never too late to grieve properly and fully over your loss, if this comes up for you. If you are feeling sad now, stop reading, lie down, and see what comes up. Stay with your emotions or whatever you are feeling in your body. This is the way you process data in your body and bring all of your cells into the present so that you can finally heal. Remember, part of what keeps us stuck in our lives is thinking that we should have known years ago what we now know—and beating ourselves up for not knowing it at the time.

Removing an organ doesn't necessarily heal the energy blockage associated with the problem in the first place, though it can be a step in the right direction. Some women, years after surgery, still have energetic attachments to tissue that was removed and have not grieved fully. These attachments can still be read in their energy fields. The electromagnetic field of the body contains a pattern of the whole, even after a physical part is gone.

Our healing ability is not limited by time or space. We can heal our past at any time, even fifty years later. Our past waits in our bodies until we're ready. Learning about the female energy system in the body can bring up delayed feelings that a woman never dealt with at the time of her hysterectomy or other surgery. Better late than never. That's the nice thing about understanding energy and medicine. Healing on the energetic level is always a possibility, regardless of what has gone on at the purely physical level and regardless of how long ago it happened. (To get you started, do the womb clearing exercise provided by Tami Lynn Kent in chapter 12—see page 592.)

A powerful example of what this clearing looks and feels like is described in a personal letter sent to me by Doreen Martin, who had a hysterectomy in the 1990s. Her surgeon removed her uterus, cervix, and fallopian tubes but left her ovaries. Eight years later, she had the following experience:

On a beautiful Sunday morning, in my kitchen preparing coffee, I was suddenly overwhelmed with an emotion that felt as if it was moving up through my body from my pelvis. I gripped the sink and held on for I didn't know what. I began to sob uncontrollably until I dropped to my knees and lay on the floor in a fetal position, crying from a deep wounded place. From within, I began to ask, "What is this? Please tell me, what is this?" The best way I can describe what happened next is that it seemed like a symphony of "quiet voices" that were not voices as we know them. I asked this time, "What are you trying to tell me?" The response was, "We miss them." I asked, "Them who?" The response was, "The ones that were taken!"

Something like a flash glowed in my mind. I was vividly aware that my other internal organs were grieving the loss of my reproductive ones. I continued to sob with them, after which came a peace, very soothing, like a smile.

My mentor, Rev. Dr. Eloise Oliver, during many of her lessons on Sunday mornings, speaks to the life within, teaching that all living organs are "alive" with intelligence, skills, and power. My own knowledge of science confirms that as well. My experience that Sunday morning revealed to me the exactness of that truth, and also exposed a deeper, more complex truth. Each and every organ within the human body has a specific function that it joyously performs without knowing why. It just does. Each function is independent. Simultaneously, these individual organs all know their unique functions for the interdependence of the entire body. These organs form a relationship, a connectedness of some sort. When loss occurs, there is a voice and an awareness that each remaining organ experiences, resulting, I think, in reduction, depletion, overproduction, and depression.

I share this with you in hope and prayer that doctors will prepare other women who may for whatever reason need a procedure such as mine so they can receive some form of counseling and support surrounding the overall impact this surgery and other types of surgeries will have in and on their lives.

The few doctors who have a spiritual foundation and who embrace this know that it is not they who do the work. It is the divine presence within them. I pray that they will, as you do, come forth and educate their peers, colleagues, and patients about the miraculous spiritual presence within us all and its relationship with the physical body temple— and, more important, the active, live, intelligence expressed through and from every physical body part.

This powerful story illustrates the mysterious nature of healing and time, as well as how the body's intelligence makes itself known in individual and unique ways. Removal of an organ need not cause depression or depletion. It all depends upon the consciousness that you bring to the situation.

Understand that many healthcare options and choices are available to you. Know that there is no one monolithic "right" way to care for your body. Most important, I hope I have encouraged you to listen to your inner guidance when choosing partners in healthcare. Albert Schweitzer once said, "It's a trade secret, but I'll tell you anyway. All healing is self-healing."

17

Eat to Flourish

If women are truly to enjoy food, it must become one of life's freely experienced sensuous pleasures. By eating well, women take care of themselves on the most basic level.

—Dr. Karen Johnson

No matter how developed you are in any other area of your life, no matter what you say you believe, no matter how sophisticated or enlightened you think you are, how you eat tells all. Bummer.

—Geneen Roth

The act of mindfully enjoying high-quality, delicious, health-sustaining food is one of the simplest and most powerful ways to flourish on a daily basis. Our bodies evolved over millennia to assimilate foods that are found in the natural world. Therefore, we function at our best when we eat these natural foods—not packaged, processed, chemically altered imitations and substitutes with a prolonged shelf life—as often as possible. In the process of eating well and nourishing ourselves optimally with high-quality food, we all have an opportunity to honor our own bodies, as well as the body of the planet as a whole. My father, who was a holistically inclined dentist, kept the classic work of Weston A. Price, D.D.S., *Nutrition and Physical Degeneration* (originally published in 1939), on his reading table. Price and his wife traveled the world back in the 1930s and 1940s, studying the diets of different groups—none of whom had the degenerative diseases we see so commonly today. They were all free of heart disease, diabetes, arthritis, and high blood pressure. But each group ate differently, according to the food found in their areas. Hence the Inuit diet was mostly animal fat and protein with almost no carbohydrates—a diet that was adaptive for their climate and way of living. The Polynesians ate lots of tropical fruit and foods made from coconut. And Swiss herders ate raw-milk cheeses and whole-grain breads. Every group thrived on its diet. There was no "one size fits all." And there was none of the "food fundamentalism" we see today, where proponents of vegan, keto, or paleo diets offer completely contradictory views and the evidence to support them. Bottom line: There is no one "right diet" that works for everyone.

What *is* true is this: Whole, natural food is loaded with energy and information. It brings to our bodies far more than just vitamins, fats, carbohydrates, and proteins. Health researcher Sayer Ji, founder of www.Green MedInfo.com, illuminates the science of exosomes—plant genes that interact with the human microbiome. This is an entirely new area of nutrition that is far beyond conventional food science. This field restores food to its rightful place as an opportunity to profoundly commune with nature and become healthy. It is now well documented that eating whole foods instantaneously sends a message to your microbiome, which begins to turn on the genes associated with health and turn off those that are associated with disease. Food is indeed medicine. In his book *Life-Changing Foods* (Hay House, 2016), medical medium Anthony William delineates the kinds of energy that certain foods impart to us when we eat them. An example is the wild Maine blueberry. Maine blueberries grow in very harsh, rocky soil where nothing else grows. They survive killing frosts and being burned each fall as the blueberry farmers clear the land. Eating wild Maine blueberries imbues our bodies with the imprint of survival, what it takes to hang on. Likewise, the lowly potato, a staple food for so many, is associated with humility. When you begin to appreciate food and the information it contains in this way, food prep and eating become a magical adventure, not an exercise in weighing and measuring (although there is a place for that along the way).

How you digest and assimilate your food is profoundly influenced by the following seven factors:

- Your emotional state, including past or present stressors

- Family lineage and learned behaviors

- Macronutrient intake (proteins, fats, carbohydrates)

- Micronutrient intake (vitamins and minerals)

- Exercise habits

- Environment and timing

- Food *chi* (food energetics)

Nourishing yourself optimally means paying attention to each of these areas, which I will cover in the steps that follow.

CREATING OPTIMAL BODY COMPOSITION
AND VIBRANT HEALTH

Reaching or maintaining healthy body composition and vibrant health through the right food choices happens in your mind, body, and spirit simultaneously. I've spent decades studying nutrition and its effects on women's bodies, minds, and spirits—both personally and professionally. My interest began in childhood. I was raised on organic food and my parents studied the work of Adelle Davis, author of *Let's Eat Right to Keep Fit* (Harcourt, Brace, 1954), and Robert Rodale. But eating whole-grain bread, homemade yogurt, and seven-grain cereal as a child didn't prevent me from feeling the need to go on my first weight loss diet at the age of twelve. I had read in a fashion magazine that a girl of my height (5'3") should weigh 115 pounds, a weight I could never maintain no matter how much I starved myself. (My natural weight by the eighth grade was 125 pounds—heavier than most of the girls in my class at that time. This was back in the day when we were all lined up and weighed, and the weight was shouted out for all to hear.) Thus began a personal war with my size and weight that lasted through my forties, when I finally learned the secrets of lifelong weight maintenance and health that I share with you here. Being born with a body that my parents termed "solid," having had to work consciously at accepting my size and weight for most of my life, and having worked with thousands of women with the same problem, I can assure you that I know what works and what doesn't. And yes, I've had my genetics tested. The report said, "Genetic tendency to gain weight or regain it after losing it." Bingo. What this means is that from the age of twelve onward, I constantly struggled to keep my appetite and weight "under control," an approach that virtually guarantees being at war with the body.

Though I had grown up knowing about the healing power of food, it wasn't until I met Michio Kushi, the founder of the American macrobiotic movement, that I really saw, up close and personal, how effective diet was at reversing chronic disease. At the end of my residency training in Boston, I met Michio and sat with him while he used techniques similar to those of traditional Chinese medicine to diagnose and treat everything from heart disease to cancer in people who came from all over the world. Because they came with voluminous medical records, I could easily see that they'd gone through the gauntlet of Western medicine and had exhausted its ability to help. Macrobiotics was their last hope. In those who followed Michio's dietary recommendations, the changes I witnessed in the ensuing months were nothing short of miraculous. A simple diet of whole grains, beans, and vegetables helped heal heart disease, cancer, and other diseases. It also produced such striking changes in people's faces that they were often barely recognizable two months later when they'd come back for follow-up. I was so impressed with these results that I realized I had to incorporate this approach in my medical practice when possible. And I also knew I had to adopt it myself. I read everything I could get my hands on about the health benefits of vegetarian diets. I also took cooking classes and became a very proficient macrobiotic cook. My daughters were "imprinted" with this diet, which is what I ate when I was pregnant with them and also what I served up until they were about ten years old. Now, as adult women, they remember their childhood "comfort" foods as being brown rice and miso soup.

Though macrobiotics was not the panacea I had originally hoped it would be, it was a great start for discovering how powerful food is for healing. A mostly vegetarian diet rich in whole grains, beans, and vegetables became the cornerstone of my approach to PMS, endometriosis, menstrual cramps, and other women's health problems for years. And for those who followed it, this diet resulted in vast health improvements.

Many other physicians have, likewise, seen the enormous healing potential of food as medicine. These include my colleagues Kelly Brogan, M.D., Dean Ornish, M.D., Neal Barnard, M.D., David Ludwig, M.D., Ph.D., Steven Gundry, M.D., the late Nick Gonzales, M.D., William Davis, M.D., David Perlmutter, M.D., John Douillard, D.C., Ph.D., Mark Hyman, M.D., Jason Fung, M.D., and Sara Gottfried, M.D. Each of these individuals has a slightly different approach. And some of the advice they offer (and the evidence to back it up) contradicts the advice (and evidence) offered by someone else. An example is Neal Barnard, M.D., author of many books including *Dr. Neal Barnard's Program for Reversing Diabetes* (Rodale, 2007), and T. Colin Campbell, Ph.D., coauthor of the widely publicized *China Study* (BenBella Books, 2005), which stated that cancer and heart disease rates were highest in those who ate the most meat, protein, and dairy. Those books and the documentaries *Forks Over Knives* (2011) and *What the Health* (2017) would make nearly anyone think that becoming vegan is the way to go. This information also lines up with my early experience with macrobiotics. So the holy grail must be to become vegan, right? Not so fast. Those who have crunched the raw data of the *China Study* point out that the conclusions don't hold water. If you're interested in diving into the epidemiological data yourself, check out the work of health and nutrition writer Denise Minger (www.deniseminger.com/the-china-study).

Enter William Davis, M.D., author of *Wheat Belly* (Rodale, 2011), a cardiologist who gained thirty pounds and became diabetic on a vegan diet! His dietary approach—which follows that of cardiovascular surgeon Steven Gundry, M.D., author of *Dr. Gundry's Diet Evolution: Turn Off the Genes That Are Killing You and Your Waistline* (Three Rivers Press, 2008)—favors limiting or eliminating grains, fruit, and starchy vegetables. And nephrologist Jason Fung, M.D., champions intermittent fasting and keeping insulin levels low as the way to go.

My colleague and good friend Kelly Brogan, M.D., a holistic psychiatrist who is also board certified in integrative holistic medicine, notes that many women recover from their depression and anxiety when they eliminate gluten but also add red meat. Her Vital Mind Reset program (www.kellybroganmd .com/vital-mind-reset-interest/) has helped hundreds of women come home to themselves mentally, emotionally, and physically. She also regularly gets praise from people all over the world for the life-changing benefits of her morning smoothie (see page 863).

Moreover, holistic neurologist David Perlmutter, M.D., points out in his book *Grain Brain* (Little Brown, 2013) how effective diet is in reversing all manner of neurological symptoms, like facial tics, symptoms of Parkinsonism, and even seizures. His dietary approach, like Dr. Brogan's, also includes animal fat and protein.

Finally, my colleague David Ludwig, M.D., Ph.D., an endocrinologist at Boston Children's Hospital and the author of *Always Hungry* (Hachette, 2016), has conducted an enormous amount of research on the endocrinologic effects of food. The program he outlines in his book cracks the weight loss, blood sugar, and insulin code that finally allows the body to shed excess pounds and also reverse type 2 diabetes. Dr. Ludwig's work with obese children is especially promising.

So what are you supposed to eat? My friend and colleague Mark Hyman, M.D., wrote a book entitled *Food: What the Heck Should I Eat?* (Little, Brown, 2018). The bottom line is that for most people, a diet that is rich in plant foods with a little dairy and meat is the way to go. And fat is simply not the enemy that the sugar industry spent forty years trying to convince us that it was.

All that aside, instead of looking outside yourself to an expert, consider this: We each have an innate sense within us of what our bodies need—once we eliminate junk food, which hijacks our innate body wisdom, from our diets. Once we reset our bodies with whole foods, we actually begin to crave what we really need.

I learned this years ago. When my daughter Kate was four (at that time we were macrobiotic vegans), she tucked into a Cornish game hen that I had prepared as a special treat for Christmas dinner, saying, "I love this codfish!" It was the first time she had ever eaten animal protein and she didn't know chicken from fish. She ate like a starving animal, finally satisfying her body's innate needs. Several years later, she said to me, "I'm not going to be vegetarian when I grow up." She clearly needed more animal protein to look and feel her best, and I finally got the message and lightened up my "food fundamentalism." Her sister, on the other hand, loved being vegan and to this day is more drawn to that way of eating. They are very different people with very different bodies. What works for one doesn't work for the other. Keep that in mind, and don't let the "food police" try to tell you any different.

How to End the War with Food and Create Vital Health

Having spent my entire career trying to figure out the "right" diet and the "right" foods to eat—and having read almost every nutrition book ever written and tried virtually every diet ever presented (keto, paleo, juice cleanses, Ayurvedic cleanses), all in an attempt to lose a few pounds or maintain my weight—I have finally discovered the keys to vibrant health and a stable, healthy weight, give or take ten pounds either way. If you follow the steps I've listed below, I guarantee you that you'll lose weight for good, keep it off, and never have to buy another diet book or go on another "diet" again. Simple. Not easy.

Know this: It's possible to achieve a healthy, vital body that has the right amount of body fat and also looks wonderful. You can begin to move toward this right now, no matter what your current state of health or the number on the scale. You have this power within you once you invite it in. Read through this section and commit to doing as much of it as you feel comfortable with now, even if that means simply taking a walk once a week, enjoying your breakfast more slowly, or starting a vitamin supplement. Each step you take will make it that much easier to begin the next one. Remember, you don't need to go from A to Z in a week. Just go from A to B!

Be easy with yourself and integrate these steps to nourishment gradually. When you change your attitude about self-nourishment, your body composition and body image will also be transformed. This begins with understanding that your body is shaped by your beliefs. To change your body permanently, you must change your beliefs—and you must do this with compassion and love. As my friend the late Louise Hay put it, "Changes that are loved into being are permanent." But changes that are shamed or blamed into being—or that are achieved through deprivation—are fleeting at best (which is why diets simply don't work long term). Like so many women who have gained and lost the same ten pounds repeatedly, I can assure you that the only path to sustaining an optimal weight and size is to slowly integrate new behaviors and a new self-concept. Research has shown that people who have been obese their whole lives, for instance, and then lose weight quickly often continue to have a distorted body image and literally can't see what they really look like even after their size is normal.[1]

Step One: Understand That Self-Respect and Self-Acceptance Are the Cornerstones of Optimal Size and Body Image

Regardless of how you feel right now, the first step toward optimal health is deciding to respect the body you have. It's a big stretch for many women to love their bodies. *Psychology Today* reports that body hatred among women is epidemic (like any of us needs a study to tell us this). The extreme pressure on women to be thin often has crippling consequences for their self-confidence and lives. You'll note that when there's a news story about a woman, her appearance often leads. When the same story is about a man, no one is commenting on his clothing or hair. It's all about his credentials and accomplishments. According to statistics reported by this organization, American women and girls get an average of forty negative messages a day about their bodies.[2] No wonder we're unhappy with what we look like!

Common Sense Media published a 2015 study revealing that 80 percent of ten-year-old girls have already been on a diet, while more than half of girls (and one-third of boys) ages six to eight want thinner bodies.[3] The average age a girl begins dieting is now eight, according to the Eating Disorder Foundation (compared with age fourteen in 1970). This occurs at a time when the nutritional foundation for peak bone mass and breast health is being laid down. One of my friends (now in her fifties), whose mother was obsessed with weight, routinely dumped her lunch down the storm drain every day on her way to school when she was only nine—because she, like me, was told that she was "solid." But dieting isn't such a great idea for adults, either, considering that 87 percent of the people who go on diets end up gaining weight in the long term.

Here's the first step. Talk to your body with compassion and respect, not disgust or anger. Would you talk to a small child or loved one in the way you routinely talk to yourself about your body? Probably not. So let's start right there. Look deeply into your eyes in the mirror and tell yourself out loud, "I respect you and I will take care of you today." Address yourself as though you were an innocent baby of three months old. I'm serious. A commitment to talk to yourself nicely is an essential step toward feeling and looking your best. Respecting yourself will actually help you reach your optimal size. That's because the feelings associated with self-respect create a metabolic milieu in your body that is conducive to optimal fat burning. By contrast, unresolved emotional stress tends to keep excess body fat firmly in place because the stress hormones cortisol and adrenaline drastically affect metabolism.

Jon Gabriel, founder of the Gabriel Method (www.thegabrielmethod .com), has helped hundreds of people all over the world to lose weight and finally keep it off. His method is based on his own experience of weighing more than 300 pounds and failing at every diet he ever tried, including vegan, fasting—you name it. In fact, Jon and I share the distinction of having been yelled at and shamed by the late Robert Atkins, M.D., when his high-fat, low-carb diet failed to work for us. Finally, in 2001, when Jon was working in the financial industry and under tremendous stress, he pulled over on the New Jersey Turnpike with a revelation: As long as his body did not want to lose weight, no diet would ever work.

So Jon decided to focus on getting healthier instead of on losing weight. He stopped dieting for good and just began to concentrate on adding healthy foods to his diet—gradually. He also visualized the body he wanted to have. Over time, his body morphed into the incredibly fit body he currently enjoys today. Jon points out that most overweight people are actually starving for more nutrients. They're often under so much stress that the elevated cortisol levels in their bodies cause intense sugar cravings that are impossible to resist. But when you begin cherishing your body, engaging your parasympathetic nervous system (the part that allows the body to rest and restore), and feeding your body nutrient-rich food, everything changes.

Though I've never been significantly overweight, I can completely relate to Jon's experience. I've personally gone on diets of 500 calories per day for two weeks straight and not lost a pound (and have even *gained* weight), which defies everything we're supposed to believe about the obsolete "eat less and exercise more" doctrine of standard nutrition—advice that is just plain wrong.[4] Some of my closest friends have experienced the same thing. We've all been able to finally "crack the code" by stopping food restriction and feeding ourselves as the precious human beings we are.

Step Two: Eat to Flourish—Stop Dieting

Having tried everything from Atkins to macrobiotics to the Zone diet, I can assure you that there is a kernel of truth in every one of them. But every "diet" out there is doomed to eventual failure unless you understand what kinds of foods your body was designed to function best with and then begin to enjoy them fully. As a matter of fact, eating a chocolate brownie slowly and with gusto and enjoyment does your body more good than gnawing on celery sticks while feeling deprived and resentful. I'm not telling you anything you don't already know.

Many studies comparing different diets bear this out, but one 2018 study was particularly telling. Researchers at Stanford University randomly assigned either a healthy low-carb or a healthy low-fat diet to more than 600 volunteers. After one year, the average weight loss was the same for both groups (thirteen pounds), although there was a lot of individual variation.[5] The big takeaway was that those from either group who had lost the most weight had changed their relationship to food, becoming more thoughtful about what they ate. That, rather than the food choices themselves, were the key to weight loss.

Studies have shown that weight loss and regain and the "diet mentality" have negative health consequences independent of one's actual weight.[6] And only a very small percentage of women achieve permanent weight loss by dieting, despite the multibillion-dollar diet industry. We need to look honestly at our behavior around this and commit to change. Rather than going on a "diet," you want to make slow and permanent changes in your eating that become a way of life.

DO YOU HAVE THE "DIET MENTALITY"?

~ Do you avoid eating all day so that you can binge at dinner?

~ When you're standing before a buffet, do you routinely tell yourself that you can't have what you really want?

~ Do you weigh yourself several times throughout the day?

~ If you step on the scale and weigh a pound or more than usual, do you routinely beat yourself up for it? Do you let it ruin your day and influence what you eat?

~ Do you allow yourself to get so hungry that you gulp whatever is available, rarely even tasting it?

~ Do you say, "I'll eat this now, but I'll start on a diet on Monday," or after New Year's?

~ Do you routinely drink coffee or caffeinated diet drinks during the day as a substitute for food?

~ Do you know the calorie count of almost every food?

If you answered yes to any of these questions, you probably have inherited the "diet mentality." Bob Schwartz, Ph.D., author of *Diets Don't Work* (Breakthru Publications, 1996), did a study of people who had no problems with their weight or with their food intake to determine whether the "diet mentality" could be created by food restriction. The study subjects were placed on weight-loss diets to lose ten pounds each. In the process of dieting to lose weight, many of these formerly "diet-free" individuals actually developed a "diet mentality." They became obsessed with food, often for the first time ever. After losing the required ten pounds, many gained back not only the weight that they had lost but an additional five pounds besides. These additional five pounds were even harder to lose than the original ten had been. By the very process of food restriction and dieting, these formerly thin people had been transformed into people with a weight problem.

My very first diet firmly implanted this "diet mentality"—and my body responded rebelliously with a physiologic "starvation response" mechanism that decreased metabolic rate, thus making each later attempt at caloric restriction that much more difficult.[7] After reading about Dr. Schwartz's study, I finally understood why I had been fighting the same ten to fifteen pounds since I was thirteen. I vowed then and there to stop, and for the next six years, I never weighed myself (except for an insurance physical). During that time, I began breaking free from a destructive cycle of body abuse started many years before. I, like so many, had allowed the number on a bathroom scale to tell me that I was good or bad and allowed it to determine the entire quality of my day. If I weighed less than 140 (or whatever my ideal was at the time), it was a good day; if I weighed more than that, it was a bad day. Now I don't weigh myself at all. I rely on how my clothes fit as a gauge for size.

Most women cannot reach the stage of eating to nourish themselves until they've made some progress moving away from this diet mentality. But once you tap in to your inner guidance about food, you will find that the foods that are good for you and the foods you want to eat will become the same. Several years ago, I interviewed psychologist Gay Hendricks, Ph.D., on my Hay House radio show, *Flourish!* I knew that Gay had been a fat kid, and I asked him how he changed all that. He told me that back in the late 1950s, it was rare for kids to be fat. So his parents took him to many specialists—without results. Then one day in his twenties, weighing in at 300-plus pounds and smoking two packs of cigarettes a day, he fell on the ice here in New England and hit his head. Lying there stunned, he somehow connected for the first time with the part of himself that was permanent and healthy—his soul. He told me that from that moment on, he decided to stay in touch with that changeless part of himself, not the 300-pound, chain-smoking part. So before eating anything, he would check in with his soul. And if his soul wanted that particular food, he ate it. If not, he didn't. At the end of a year, he had lost 100 pounds, and he's never gained it back. He also gave up smoking. I know that each of us has access to that kind of power if and when we're ready to use it.

Sometimes we are motivated by an immediate health problem. A thirty-nine-year-old artist, a former patient of mine, improved her diet in order to help heal her chronic vaginitis. She said to me, "I feel lighter when I eat this way—and cleaner. My nose doesn't run all the time. And I've lost eight pounds since I last saw you. I don't feel deprived at all. I know that I can eat whatever I want. You told me to eat only whole foods and to experiment after avoiding all dairy foods for one month. So I went back to eating cheese after about one month, but I found that I didn't like the way it felt in my body. I stopped eating it, and I feel better. *Increasingly, what I want is also what makes me feel best.* This isn't a punishment—it's just a different way of looking at things. It's a complete change of philosophy for me."

This patient underwent a paradigm shift in the way she looked at food. Weight loss was a side effect. She changed her diet to create health—not to lose weight. By changing her diet to create health, she not only lost weight but eventually came to the point where the food she wanted the most was also the food that made her feel the best. She is now in tune with the wisdom of her body, and her former war against herself is over.

Nutritional improvement and regular exercise are powerful ways to create health. Most women are amazed by how much better they feel when they eliminate most refined foods, excessive sugar, and excessive starch from their diets, following a relatively low-glycemic-index diet instead. The glycemic index is a measure of how much a food raises your blood sugar level. When you eat high-glycemic-index carbohydrates—which in general are starchy and sugary foods such as cookies, candies, soda, alcohol, and white bread, as well as almost all other refined, processed foods—your body quickly metabolizes them into sugar, which causes a spike in insulin levels. But when you eat low-glycemic-index carbohydrates, your body breaks them down slowly, which means your blood sugar and your insulin levels stay relatively steady over a longer period of time.

The link between diet and the health of female organs is impressive. A study in Italy, for example, found a direct association between breast cancer risk and the consumption of sweet foods with a high glycemic index.[8] Our trans-fatty-acid-rich, refined-carbohydrate-rich, fiber-poor, nutrient-poor diet and its effects on blood sugar are part of the reason that breast cancer, endometriosis, and uterine fibroids are on the increase, affecting millions of women. (This same refined-carb-heavy diet has been implicated in heart attacks as early as the 1950s, when Benjamin Sandler, M.D., wrote *How to Prevent Heart Attacks* [Lee Foundation for Nutritional Research, 1958] about his great success in preventing fatal heart attacks in angina patients by prescribing a no-sugar, no-starch food plan that kept blood sugar levels stable.)[9] Sixty percent of all cancers of the breast, ovary, and uterus have to do with diet,[10] with both benign and malignant conditions of the breast, ovary, and uterus related to diets that cause estrogen levels to be too high.[11] Diets that are high in refined carbohydrates are one culprit because they raise blood sugar, and high blood sugar results in increased levels of metabolically active circulating estrogens (because the high triglyceride levels produced by a high-refined-carbohydrate diet displace estrogen from the steroid-binding globulins that render it metabolically inactive). On the other hand, a diet high in a variety of vegetable fibers can lower a woman's estrogen levels, thereby decreasing her risk of breast cancer, because the vegetable fibers change the metabolism of estrogen in the bowel so that less is available for absorption into the bloodstream and more is excreted.

Women who start their menstrual cycles earlier and their menopause later are at greater risk for breast cancer because of their longer exposure to high levels of estrogen. Here, too, diet plays a role. Because of their diet, American women typically start menstruating early (at age twelve or thirteen—and increasingly, as early as eight) and enter menopause late.[12] But women who follow diets consisting of unrefined natural foods, such as the rural Chinese and the !Kung of southern Africa, typically start their menstrual periods at age sixteen or seventeen. These women also begin menopause earlier. Their breast cancer rates are very low.[13] The same was true for hunter-gatherer societies, which had diets that were rich in meat and fat and lacked refined carbohydrates, and which were characterized by high levels of physical activity. This high level of physical activity is also typical of the Chinese and the !Kung. Exercise helps balance hormones and lower an individual's percentage of body fat and risk of breast cancer.

Step Three: Understand the Blood Sugar/ Inflammation Connection

To understand how we as a culture got to where we are now in terms of the foods we're eating and the problems so many are having with them, it helps to go back in time. Our species adapted to a Paleolithic hunter-gatherer diet over a period of more than 100,000 years before agriculture was widely adopted. Their diet consisted of lots of wild bitter greens rich in pharmacologically active plant chemicals that have well-documented anti-inflammatory and other properties. They also ate wild fruits and berries in season, as well as meat from game that ate the same wild foods. Archaeological evidence shows that hunter-gatherers also ate a lot of nutrient-rich organ meats such as brain, kidneys, liver, and heart. Concentrated sweets, other than occasional honey, were simply not available. And though there were a few wild grains in the diet, these bore almost no resemblance to the modern corn, rice, and wheat that are staple foods today. One of the most important things to remember when deciding what is healthy to eat is this: We still have the metabolisms and physiologies of the Paleolithic hunter-gatherers.[14]

Agriculture was introduced about 10,000 years ago, a mere blip on the screen of evolutionary time. To put this in perspective, for 99.8 percent of our time on earth as *Homo sapiens,* we ate exclusively wild foods.[15] Selective breeding practices since that time have increased the starch and sugar content of fruits, vegetables, and grains as well as markedly changed the biochemical composition of the meat we eat. And in the last seventy years, scores of chemical additives and nonfoods such as trans fats, preservatives, and flavor enhancers have been added that our Stone Age metabolisms simply weren't designed to cope with. Soil depletion and the addition of nitrate-based fertilizers after World War II (in response to the need to get rid of the stockpiles of nitrates used for bombs) have further changed the food supply and killed off much of the beneficial bacteria in soil that enhances food quality. In addition, genetically modified foods (termed GMOs) and the addition of pesticides to most conventionally grown produce have created a perfect storm of substandard nutrition.

Excess weight, elevated blood sugar, and elevated blood fats are now the norm as food quantity has far outstripped food quality in most of the developed world. According to the U.S. Department of Agriculture, the average American is now eating 197 pounds of wheat and other grains per year, as well as 141 pounds of sweeteners (including 42 pounds of corn syrup)—significantly more than in previous eras. Processed grains, starches, sugars, and food additives like monosodium glutamate (MSG)—all of which raise blood sugar and lead to addictive eating—are the real culprits when it comes to chronic degenerative diseases such as diabetes, heart disease, and obesity. In his book *The Hacking of the American Mind: The Science Behind the Corporate Takeover of Our Bodies and Brains* (Avery, 2017), Robert Lustig, M.D., points out that food manufacturers and advertisers that sell "pleasure" through consumption are largely responsible for the epidemic rates of depression, anxiety, obesity, and chronic disease in the United States today. I've always been appalled by the fact that fast-food franchises can be found in the lobbies of medical complexes. Dr. Lustig points out that Big Food has deliberately created highly addictive "convenience foods" that raise dopamine levels in our brains. Dopamine makes us feel happy—temporarily. But sustainable contentment is possible only when we have enough serotonin in our brains and bodies. And this is produced by making human connections (including maintaining healthy relationships), contributing to a larger cause (through volunteer work, for example), eating whole foods, and coping with stress in healthy ways. Social media, by the way, can have the same addictive quality—it has been shown that we get a hit of dopamine when we get a "like" on Facebook or Instagram. Even using FaceTime, though a direct social connection, does not have the same positive effect on the body and brain as face-to-face contact. In other words, you can't fool the body. It knows and responds to what is real and sustainable.

It's little wonder that the resources of our healthcare system are being crushed under the weight of the chronic diseases that are the result of this profound shift in the human diet. But that doesn't mean it's impossible to eat a healthy diet these days. In fact, it's getting easier and easier. Here's all you need to know.

Stable Blood Sugar Is the Answer

The most important key to lifelong weight maintenance and vibrant health is knowing how to keep your insulin levels low. Pure and simple. Low insulin levels and stable blood sugar throughout the day are also the keys to preventing or reversing the diseases that are associated with cellular inflammation. (Note: Most of the vast changes in the hunter-gatherer diet that we evolved with are associated with chronic disruptions in blood sugar as their final common pathway.) High blood sugar from eating foods that raise blood sugar quickly (high-glycemic-index foods such as candy, soda, white bread, etc.) signals the pancreas to release the hormone insulin. Insulin is a storage hormone that takes sugar out of the blood and stores it in cells until it can be burned as fuel. If this energy is not needed right away, the excess energy gets stored as fat. Excess stress, in and of itself, raises cortisol levels. And this, in turn, tends to lock fat in to the cells. Keep in mind, however, that there are wide variations among individuals in their blood sugar response to food. Some people's blood sugar spikes after they eat rice but not after they eat ice cream—and vice versa. (The only way to know for sure is to use a glucose meter to test your blood sugar; this can show you what your own personal response is to a given food.)

Stable blood sugar and optimal insulin levels result from eating the right amount of protein, the right kind of carbohydrates, and the right kinds and amounts of fats at the right time for your individual body. It has taken me more than forty-five years of research and clinical experience to figure this out. Back in the late 1980s and early 1990s, like many health-conscious people, I was still eating a mostly grain-based, low-fat diet. And I—like so many—was gaining weight. At about four or five o'clock each afternoon, I would come home from work famished, stand in front of the fridge, and begin my evening "grazing," which didn't end until I went to bed hours later. I craved sweets and had a difficult time controlling my appetite. My patients complained about the same thing. We also noticed that our waistlines seemed to be disappearing when we hit forty. What had gone wrong with the low-fat, high-complex-carbohydrate, vegetarian diet that so much research said should be keeping us healthy and slim?

At about this time, the popular Zone diet of Barry Sears, Ph.D., came out, followed by the work of family physicians Mary Dan Eades, M.D., and Michael Eades, M.D., authors of *Protein Power* (Bantam Books, 1996) and colleagues of Sears's. I read the research that their books were based on. It made sense. Too many refined carbs raise insulin levels, which makes the body store excess calories as fat. Conversely, enough protein increases glucagon, which jump-starts the body into burning fat. Moreover, the right kinds of fats are necessary building blocks for the cellular hormones that fight inflammation and create optimal cellular metabolism (these hormones are known as eicosanoids, and the inflammatory cytokines and prostaglandins are part of this group; see the section on fats, below).

Based on this research, I dutifully added more protein to my diet and cut way back on grains and high-glycemic-index foods. (I didn't want to, though, and it was hard. As a friend once said to me, "I never met a carb I didn't like!") Impressed with my newfound energy and a decrease in sugar cravings, I suggested the same to my patients. We felt better, but my cravings were not gone. I simply couldn't seem to give up my refined carbs, and I was still having a hard time losing weight. So like thousands of others, I decided to carry things a step further. If carbs were bad, why not eliminate them completely for a week or two to see if I'd lose weight? So I went on the Atkins induction program. But that didn't work, either. Though I ate fewer than 20 grams of carbs per day, my body absolutely refused to go into ketosis, the state in which your body begins to burn fat for energy and ketone bodies are eliminated in the urine. My body was holding on to its fat for dear life, it seemed. And my weight had crept up to an all-time high of 148 pounds. (I weighed 150 when I was at the end of my pregnancies!) When I called the late Robert Atkins, M.D., to discuss this with him, he couldn't explain it except to say, "Well, you're menopausal." He insinuated that I wasn't following his diet correctly—a standard "If it isn't working, blame the patient" approach. That explanation didn't work for me. I also didn't like eating all that meat and bacon. It had felt infinitely better to eat more fruits, vegetables, and grains.

The Missing Link: Glycemic Stress and Insulin Resistance

Finally I was introduced to the work of Ray Strand, M.D., author of *Healthy for Life: Developing Healthy Lifestyles That Have a Side Effect of Permanent Fat Loss* (Real Life Press, 2005), a family doctor who, like me, had spent more than twenty-five years seeing the same people and watching them slowly but surely develop expanding waistlines, high cholesterol, high blood pressure, cancer, hypertension, and other illnesses. Dr. Strand's research documents the fact that the conditions known as glycemic stress and excessive insulin secretion begin in childhood and are the result of eating a diet that is far too high in nutrient-poor refined foods that raise blood sugar (and insulin levels) too quickly. This is true even in those who will never get diabetes. Unfortunately, high-glycemic-index foods are the "comfort" foods most people crave, including white bread, cookies, cakes, and bagels. (Remember, these foods quickly raise dopamine levels in the brain.) Eating too many high-glycemic-index foods on a daily basis results in glycemic stress and inflammation of the blood vessels because of the free-radical damage that ensues when blood sugar is too high. Over time, the blood vessel lining thickens, making it more and more difficult for the insulin to get out of and into the cells. As Dr. Strand points out, insulin resistance actually begins in the blood vessels of the skeletal muscles, the place where blood sugar is designed to be burned most efficiently. Glycemic stress and inflammation set the stage for hardening of the arteries and also full-blown insulin resistance or metabolic syndrome (also known as syndrome X—see the list on page 855). Depending upon your genetics, metabolic syndrome results in either diabetes or heart disease or both. Many researchers, like Gary Taubes, author of *The Case Against Sugar* (Knopf, 2016), have since documented the fact that it is sugar, not fat, that is the culprit in our diets.

Just about every cell in our bodies is affected by wide fluctuations in insulin levels, which also results in the production of excess inflammatory chemicals—the basis for all chronic disease, including headaches and insomnia. No wonder Kenneth Cooper, M.D., once said, "We die not so much of a particular disease, as from our entire lives." No kidding. Finally I knew why I had had sweet cravings my entire life, why my HDL cholesterol had been dangerously low when I was in my thirties, and why I was having so much trouble losing weight at midlife. It was all that high-glycemic-index food. (Many vegetarians eat way too many sweets, pastas, and breads, which results in high blood sugar. I was no exception.) The link between glycemic stress, wide fluctuations in insulin levels, and cellular inflammation is why everything from headaches to PMS and high blood pressure often improves when you eat to stabilize your blood sugar and get your insulin levels down.

Over time, as blood sugar levels continue to be too high, the insulin receptors on the cells actually lose their ability to respond to high blood sugar. The wrong kinds of dietary fats also change the insulin receptors on the cell membrane itself, thus contributing to the problem. Micronutrient deficiencies such as too little chromium can contribute to the problem as well. (See the section on micronutrients, page 897.) Over time, the pancreas loses its ability to produce insulin and the cells lose their sensitivity to it. Some of this is simply mechanical—the excess fat stored in the pancreas itself causes the islet cells (which secrete insulin) to malfunction. They literally get crowded out by fat cells. Type 2 diabetes is the result. Fatty liver, from excess sugar, is also now epidemic in our culture.

But there's more. Fat cells themselves produce inflammatory chemicals, which is another reason why obesity is a risk factor for cancer. Body fat is loaded with insulin receptors. The fatter you get, the more insulin it takes to get blood sugar into your cells. And because insulin is a storage hormone, the higher its levels, the harder it is for the body to release fat as fuel. Insulin actually locks fat in place!

HIGH- AND LOW-GLYCEMIC-INDEX FOODS

The following foods are generally regarded as high-glycemic-index (high-GI) or low-glycemic-index (low-GI) foods, but be aware that these are just general guidelines. How a food is prepared makes a big difference. For instance, sweet potatoes are low-GI, but candied sweet potatoes are certainly not! And while pasta is low-GI because it's harder to digest than most flour products, overcooked pasta has a much higher GI than al dente pasta. Steamed white potatoes can be a healthy food—especially when cooled after cooking and reheated before eating. Same with rice. They contain what is known as resistant starch, which passes through the small intestine without being broken down and then ferments in the large intestine. As it ferments, it functions as a prebiotic—food that feeds the microbiome, the good bacteria in our gut. Most women need resistant starches to feel their best—which is why following a strict low-carb diet doesn't work well over time for most women. Also, adding lemon juice, lime juice, or vinegar lowers the GI of a dish, giving potato salad a lower GI than a baked potato.

There's variation among categories, too. Most breads (including the more processed whole-wheat breads) are high-GI, for example. But all sourdough breads (which include pumpernickel) have a low glycemic index, in part because the bacteria in the sourdough starter digest fructans, a type of sugar in grain. If the sourdough is made from whole grains, that's even better. There can even be variation among the foods in a more specific category, such as bran cereal. All-Bran, for instance, is low-GI, while the same manufacturer's bran flakes are high-GI.

Jennie Brand-Miller, Ph.D., of the University of Sydney, one of the world's leading authorities on the glycemic index, says you don't have to avoid high-glycemic-index foods altogether; instead, plan around them. It's fine to have a high-GI food on your dinner menu, for example, as long as the other foods you serve are low-GI. The net effect on blood sugar levels will be lower. This concept is called glycemic load, which takes into consideration both the GI of the food(s) being consumed along with how many total carbohydrates the food or meal contains.

For more information on the glycemic index (including a database of foods and their GI values), visit www.glycemicindex.com, a website maintained by the GI Group of the University of Sydney in Australia. Also see any of the numerous books written or cowritten by Dr. Brand-Miller, including *The New Glucose Revolution: The Authoritative Guide to the Glycemic Index* (Marlowe, 2007), *The New Glucose Revolution: Low GI Eating Made Easy* (Marlowe, 2005), and *The Low GI Diet Cookbook* (Marlowe, 2005), to name just a few.

High-Glycemic-Index Foods

White potatoes (especially
    when served mashed or
    baked)
Corn
Watermelon
White rice (including instant
    white rice)
White breads, rolls, bagels,
    pastries, and doughnuts

Waffles
Puffed wheat, puffed rice,
    rice cakes
Tapioca pudding
Hard candy
Regular (non-diet) soda
Sports drinks
Wine, beer, hard liquor

Low-Glycemic-Index Foods

Broccoli
Cauliflower
Spinach
Zucchini
Beans and peas
Hummus
Sweet potatoes
Sweet corn
Apples
Oranges
Berries
Dried apricots
Meat and fish
Eggs

Milk and yogurt
Ice cream (full-fat)
Cream cheese
Cheddar, mozzarella,
    Parmesan, ricotta, and
    feta cheeses
Cottage cheese
Sourdough and pumper-
    nickel bread
Peanuts, other nuts and
    seeds
Dark chocolate
Salad greens

Stages of Insulin Resistance

1. Glycemic stress. Eating too many foods with a high glycemic load leads to blood vessel inflammation. Many individuals at this stage actually experience hypoglycemia, in which their blood sugar becomes too low after eating a meal with a high glycemic load combined with caffeine (the standard American breakfast of a doughnut or bagel and a cup of coffee).

SIGNS OF WIDE FLUCTUATIONS IN INSULIN LEVELS AND EARLY GLYCEMIC STRESS

Carbohydrate cravings and uncontrollable hunger (the munchies)

Emotional eating

Nighttime eating

Slowly expanding waistline

Increasing resistance to weight loss

Fatigue and possibly shaky weakness following a meal

2. Beginning of insulin resistance. Beta cells of the pancreas are stimulated to produce more insulin to get it across the thickened blood vessel walls and into the cells to store the excess sugar. High insulin levels result in high triglycerides, abnormal estrogen metabolism, low HDL cholesterol (the so-called good cholesterol), high blood sugar, cardiovascular disease, increased risk of diabetes, and an increased risk of many cancers. Once insulin levels are raised, a chain reaction is triggered that results in so many metabolic changes, it can't be stopped without significant lifestyle changes. (When I was a macrobiotic vegetarian—and also eating too much bread—my HDL cholesterol was a dangerous 35. I was only thirty-two years old. Now it is at a healthy 70!) Muscles are the first place to become insulin resistant. Once they do, blood sugar gets redirected to your fat cells, primarily in your abdomen. That means that when you eat a meal with a high glycemic load, it goes right to your tummy and seems to bypass your muscles entirely! (Over time, skeletal muscles also become marbled with fat.) This is the stage at which you and your doctor should be looking for signs of insulin resistance (high triglycerides and low HDL are often the first signs of glycemic stress and early insulin resistance). Don't wait. The sooner you change your diet, the better. You'll then be able to reverse and prevent all kinds of problems, and also reach a healthy weight.

SIGNS OF EARLY INSULIN RESISTANCE

Nighttime eating

Central weight gain (expanding waistline)

Slow weight gain without change in diet

Low HDL cholesterol

Increased triglycerides

Heartburn

Increased fatigue following a high-GI meal or snack (you eat lunch and can't keep your eyes open at work or school)

Menstrual irregularities

Hypoglycemia

Craving sugar and high-GI carbohydrates

Insomnia

3. Full-blown metabolic syndrome. Inexorably, if diet and lifestyle aren't changed, insulin resistance leads to full-blown metabolic syndrome, which includes high blood pressure, high cholesterol, obesity, increased fibrinogen in the blood (a clotting factor), and a whole host of other problems, including increased risk of cancer.

CONDITIONS RELATED TO INSULIN RESISTANCE (SYNDROME X OR METABOLIC SYNDROME)

Type 2 diabetes

Increased levels of fibrinogen (increased blood clotting)

Central obesity (apple-shaped figure)

High blood pressure

Abnormal cholesterol levels

Sleep apnea

Cardiovascular disease, including stroke

Heavy menstrual periods

Most forms of polycystic ovary disease

Anovulation and fertility problems

Hirsutism

Male pattern baldness

Breast, colon, and other cancers

Depression and anxiety

Dementia

Given the high prevalence of wide fluctuations in insulin levels and glycemic stress, I can guarantee you that there's no way you can learn to trust your body's instincts around food until you go on a program that stabilizes your blood sugar and resets your metabolism. You simply have to eliminate all refined carbohydrates, eat low-glycemic-index carbs, and eat the right amount of protein, healthy fats, and micronutrients. This requires a significant reeducation for most people. Think of it as a reboot for your system. There are many different ways to do this, depending on what you're drawn to. The main thing is this: Don't make the mistake of thinking there is only one path. There are many. But regardless of what you choose, when you begin to reverse insulin resistance and glycemic stress, your body automatically starts to release stored fat, particularly the fat around the abdomen that is so metabolically active and difficult to lose on conventional low-calorie and low-fat diets.

Once you've finished a dietary reset, you'll know what it feels like to be free of physical cravings and have stable blood sugar. (You may still desire the taste of chocolate, but you'll be able to stop eating it after a few bites!) You will also notice that you sleep better and have a lot more energy. A wide variety of health problems improve considerably when you get your blood sugar and insulin under control. Resetting your metabolism puts you in a much better position to continue eating for health.

What to Eat

Your diet should consist of 80 percent low-glycemic-index fruits, vegetables and other foods and high-quality fats (see below and also box). Food should be sustainably or organically grown whenever possible. Some people can tolerate grains and others can't. Eliminating all grains from the diet for one month or so can work wonders. Then add a few back and see how you do. The same goes for other high-glycemic-index foods. Eliminate them entirely, then bring them back in small amounts and assess how you feel. Depending on your recovery from sugar addiction, you may or may not be able to tolerate some dessert now and then.

RESET YOUR METABOLISM WITH ONE OF THE FOLLOWING CHOICES

1. *The Whole 30.* For thirty days you eat meat, fish, vegetables, high-quality fats (like olive oil), and some fruit. No dairy, no grains, no legumes, no sugar, no sweeteners. And no gluten-free but high-carb foods like paleo pancakes, either. Full instructions and lots of recipes are online. Start with www.whole30.com/whole30-program-rules.

2. *Kelly Brogan, M.D.'s Vital Mind Reset course.* I highly recommend this online program. Dr. Brogan has worked with women from all over the world—many of whom have been diagnosed with psychiatric conditions such as depression and anxiety. Almost all of them have been able to get off their meds and come home to themselves. For details about the program, see www.kellybroganmd.com/vital-mind-reset-interest.

3. *Always Hungry* by David Ludwig, M.D., Ph.D. Dr. Ludwig's clinically proven program, outlined in this book, is designed to reset your metabolism in about two weeks. As with the other programs listed here, it involves eating only whole foods. It is suitable for everyone, including vegetarians. His companion cookbook, *Always Delicious* (cowritten with his wife, chef Dawn Ludwig) is filled with delicious recipes. For more information, see www.drdavidludwig .com.

4. *The Colorado Cleanse* by John Douillard, D.C., Ph.D. In this two-week program, Dr. Douillard (who lives in Boulder, Colorado—hence the name) uses the ancient science of Ayurveda to cleanse the liver and reset the body. I have done this cleanse twice and always get great results. It is entirely different from the other approaches in that it involves nonfat vegan eating, specific herbs, and increasing amounts of clarified butter during the second week. The cleanse ingredients vary depending upon the season. For more information, see www.lifespa.com/cleansing/colorado-cleanse.

GLUTEN INTOLERANCE

Approximately one in three people suffers from an intolerance to gluten, a protein found in grains, including oats, wheat, kamut, rye, and barley. That means that gluten is found in staples of the American diet such as wraps, breads, pasta, pizza, and rolls. About one in a hundred individuals has full-blown celiac disease (an autoimmune disorder of the small intestine characterized by an inability to digest gluten), which is conventionally diagnosed with an intestinal biopsy (for years, the only way to positively diagnose celiac disease and gluten intolerance). The vast majority of people with gluten intolerance don't even know they have it. In his book *Eat Wheat* (Morgan James, 2017), John Douillard, D.C., Ph.D., points out that wheat has been a staple of the human diet for centuries, and few had any trouble digesting it. However, in the past fifty years or so, pesticides like glyphosate (the active herbicide in Roundup) have increasingly been used to clear fields on large industrial wheat farms. This is a big reason why today's wheat is quite different from the ancient grains (such as einkorn, a type of wheat) we evolved to digest properly.

Research shows glyphosate to be harmful to our gut bacteria, setting us up for disease.[16] Moreover, because of the processed food diet that so many people consume, the ability of many to digest today's wheat has become limited. The end result is gas, bloating, and weight gain. As already stated, certain kinds of grains and breads (like whole-wheat sourdough and pumpernickel) are more digestible for many.

A large Swedish study found that people with diagnosed, undiagnosed, and "latent" celiac disease or gluten sensitivity have a higher risk of death, mostly from heart disease and cancer.[17] This study, which followed 30,000 patients from 1969 to 2008, found that there was a 39 percent increased risk of death in those with celiac disease, a 72 percent increased risk of death in those with gut inflammation related to gluten, and a 35 percent increased risk of death even in those who were sensitive to gluten but did not have a positive intestinal biopsy indicating celiac disease. Again, no one knows if it is the gluten that is the problem or other factors, such as glyphosate.

Gluten sensitivity masquerades as a host of other disorders including osteoporosis, constipation, inflammatory bowel disease, anemia, cancer, fatigue, canker sores, rheumatoid arthritis and other autoimmune disorders, migraines, and even anxiety and depression.[18] According to functional medicine authority Mark Hyman, M.D., one of the reasons gluten intolerance is more common now than ever before is that American strains of wheat have a much higher gluten content than those traditionally found in Europe because high-gluten wheats are needed to make the fluffy white bread and giant bagels that are so popular here.[19]

The best way to test for gluten sensitivity is to eliminate all gluten from your diet for two to four weeks and then reintroduce it. But since it can be hidden in soups, salad dressings, sauces, and many other foods, you have to be knowledgeable about what foods contain it. For those with true gluten sensitivity, even a little soy sauce containing gluten will cause symptoms. (For a complete list of gluten-containing foods, go to www.celiac.com.) An interesting study done in Europe in 2017 showed that in some people who were gluten intolerant, what they were actually sensitive to was not gluten itself but fructans—the sugar chains found in wheat, barley, and rye.[20] These people will be able to eat soy sauce and sourdough bread, both of which are low in fructans, without having problems.

Gluten sensitivity can also be diagnosed by a blood test that looks for specific antigluten antibodies. Such tests are available through Quest Diagnostics (see www.questdiagnostics.com) or Lab-Corp (see www.labcorp.com). Quite frankly, it's far more practical to simply eliminate gluten from your diet and see how you feel. Don't be fooled by all of today's gluten-free foods, however, like cookies and breads. When you read the labels, you'll often find that the gluten has been replaced by high-glycemic-index starches like potato starch or tapioca, and by cane sugar—thus spiking your blood sugar. Read labels.

Here are a few tips for going gluten-free:

Shop the perimeter of the grocery store. The healthiest foods are found here, including fruits, vegetables, lean meats, and eggs (among others). Packaged foods (including packaged sauces and salad dressings) often contain gluten, so consider making your own. Also be wary of baked goods labeled "gluten-free" because they often contain potato starch and tapioca, high-glycemic-index starches that can spike blood sugar.

Read labels. Avoid foods that list wheat, rye, spelt, barley, or kamut—all grains that contain gluten. But also be wary of foods that list spices, flavoring, modified food starch, maltodextrin, glucose syrup, and citric acid, all of which may contain gluten.

Use alternative grains. Alternative grains such as quinoa, teff, buckwheat, and millet do not contain gluten. However, some people can be cross-reactive to certain grains, and their symptoms won't resolve until they eliminate *all* grains temporarily. Once you've done that, then try introducing the alternative grains back into your diet, one at a time, to see if you are sensitive to any of them. Also remember that while oats don't contain gluten, they are often contaminated with gluten during processing, so look for oats labeled "gluten-free."

Consult good references. Check out some of the many websites that offer gluten-free recipes, and look for gluten-free cookbooks and magazines. Many even tell you how to make your own gluten-free bread. You can also find apps focusing on gluten-free living with information on grocery shopping and choosing meals when you eat out in restaurants.

I also recommend the previously mentioned books *Grain Brain* (Little, Brown, 2013) by David Perlmutter, M.D., and *Wheat Belly* (Rodale, 2011) by William Davis, M.D.

INTERMITTENT FASTING

I used to believe that breakfast was the most important meal of the day. And back when I had young children and was always trying to juggle work and home duties, it probably was. More recently I have discovered the benefits of intermittent fasting. It takes twelve hours after eating for insulin levels to fall to zero. And when they do, your body will begin to burn fat as fuel. So on many days, I fast from the end of dinnertime to noon the next day—breaking my fast with lunch. This easily gives me twelve to sixteen hours of fasting time. Over time, as my body has adjusted to this, I find it not only easy but also very convenient. I don't have to deal with figuring out what's for breakfast. And my exercise goes much better on an empty stomach.

The current go-to expert on intermittent fasting is Jason Fung, M.D., a nephrologist from Toronto who spends much of his time doing dialysis on people who are in renal failure, mostly from diabetes. His fasting programs reverse this problem very conveniently. As Dr. Fung explains, fasting works whether you are paleo, vegan, keto, or whatever, because you're not eating. He also points out that fasting has been a part of every major world religion (including the religions of indigenous cultures).

Contrary to accepted conventional wisdom, Dr. Fung explains, merely reducing calories does not work. Study after study looking at these diets shows no sustained weight loss over time because the body's metabolism goes into so-called starvation mode and shuts down. Any weight lost tends to go right back on when calorie consumption returns to a normal level. A study he cites from the United Kingdom, for example, showed that conventional caloric restriction diets failed 99.5 percent of the time, succeeding for only 1 in 210 obese men and 1 in 124 obese women.[21] In the famous Minnesota Starvation Experiment in the 1950s, Ancel Keys, Ph.D., found that when he reduced volunteers' caloric intake by 30 percent, their metabolic rate also decreased by the same percentage.[22] When they went back to their typical diet, they gained all the weight back.

Dr. Fung says that obesity is caused not by an imbalance in the number of calories we eat but instead by an imbalance in hormones—the key hormone here being insulin. Insulin is what tells your body to either burn energy or store it as fat. When insulin rises (which happens when we eat, especially when we eat carbohydrates), the body stores fat. When insulin falls, the body begins to burn fat. In people who are insulin resistant, however, insulin levels stay high even when they're not eating—unless they go through sustained periods of having low insulin, which is what happens with intermittent fasting. Dr. Fung says fasting lowers insulin more powerfully than anything else, giving the body what he describes as a massive jumpstart in normalizing insulin. With insulin normalized, your body can metabolize fat effectively. In fact, the body's metabolic rate goes up by about 10 percent with intermittent fasting. Growth hormone levels also rise, helping to maintain lean body mass.

One 2016 study he cites is particularly telling. It compared alternate-day fasting with classic caloric restriction in a group of obese adults over a period of twenty-four weeks.[23] The fasting group ate no calories on the fasting days but ate normally every other day, while the other group ate 400 fewer calories per day than their normal intake. The fasting group lost almost twice as much visceral fat (the dangerous kind of fat around internal organs that raises risk of heart disease) and were four times better at preserving lean body mass than the other group. The group that restricted calories experienced almost two and a half times more metabolic slowdown than the fasting group, and their levels of ghrelin (the hormone that tells you that you're hungry) went up, unlike those who fasted. The researchers also concluded that alternate-day fasting was not associated with an increased risk for weight regain.

Intermittent fasting also gives you more energy. For one, you're not really hungry during a fast because your body is not being deprived—it's burning fat stores for the energy it needs, so it's satisfied. But in addition, fasting also increases noradrenaline, which has a stimulant effect. It revs you up, keeping metabolism high. There is no question that fasting leads to more mental alertness and clarity. It also favors autophagy, a process by which the body digests old proteins and cells and renews itself. So regular fasting actually leads to a more youthful body. Recent research from Harvard shows fasting not only enhances fat metabolism but also increases longevity and promotes healthy aging.[24] I don't advocate prolonged fasts, but they can be safely done if you're not on medication that would make them contraindicated. Pregnant women and women who are breastfeeding (as well as children, of course) should never fast.

Dr. Fung discusses several different fasting protocols (from twelve-hour fasts through forty-two-hour fasts and beyond) in his book *The Complete Guide to Fasting* (Victory Belt Publishing, 2016), coauthored with Jimmy Moore. His first book, *The Obesity*

Code (Greystone, 2016), also contains helpful information, including details on the relationship between insulin and weight gain. (Also see Dr. Fung's website, www.intensivedietarymanagement.com.)

Even when you're fasting, you can begin your morning with black coffee or tea (without sugar) if you like. Many people add high-quality fat (such as one tablespoon Bulletproof Brain Octane Oil, coconut oil, or butter from grass-fed cows). You simply whip up your morning coffee in a blender with the fat—it's almost like a cappuccino.

In her book *Glow 15* (Houghton Mifflin, 2018), skin care expert Naomi Whittel points out the benefits of green tea, Earl Grey tea (which is flavored with bergamot), and Ceylon cinnamon. All of these ingredients promote autophagy and beautiful skin.

Here's how to make the delicious morning drink Whittel recommends, which she calls Autopha Tea: Fill a mug with 10 to 12 ounces of boiling water and add one organic green tea bag, one Earl Grey tea bag, and a Ceylon cinnamon stick. Let the tea steep for at least three minutes. Then add a tablespoon of raw coconut oil and stir with the cinnamon stick for 20 to 30 seconds. (I save the cinnamon sticks and just grate them to provide a fresh surface for the next cup). I choose to sweeten mine with stevia or trehalose, a type of sugar that is far less sweet than sucrose and that also contributes to autophagy.

Whittel shares more about the benefits of this tea at www.naomiwhittel.com/rejuvenate-the-body-with-autophagy-tea. (On the shop tab, she also sells Autopha Tea tea bags that contain all the ingredients but the coconut oil.)

Breakfast. Some people are really hungry in the morning and need breakfast. If that's you, then eat a breakfast that contains some fat, some protein, and not much sugar. That could be eggs with avocado and a piece of fruit. Or slow-cooked oatmeal with some protein powder and a little healthy fat, like ghee or coconut oil. Or make a smoothie. My colleague Kelly Brogan, M.D., gets more fan mail about her breakfast smoothie than just about anything else she has done. This smoothie not only provides stable blood sugar but also is healing for the brain. She describes it as going from hungry to peaceful, one meal at a time. Here's the recipe:

KB's Breakfast Smoothie

Blend together:

½ cup frozen organic cherries (or berries)
1 cup fermented coconut water, coconut water, or filtered water
3 tablespoons collagen hydrolysate (as a protein base)
1 tablespoon sprouted nut butter
3 egg yolks (from pastured hens)
1 tablespoon coconut oil
1–2 tablespoons ghee
1–2 tablespoons raw cacao powder

There is no question that beginning the day with this kind of meal will set you up for a day of stabilized blood sugar, an uplifted mood, and a lot of energy. Remember this: It is far better to eat no breakfast than to have a meal of cereal, a bagel, or a donut and coffee, which has a high glycemic load. That will set you up for an all-day appetite and high blood sugar, and you are likely to feel the brunt of the effects of this at what I call "arsenic hour" (4:00 to 5:00 P.M., when stress hormone levels are at their peak and when all the stresses of the day seem to accumulate at once). You will tip right over into wanting to eat the wallpaper off the wall at this point.

Lunch. Make sure to have some kind of protein in the form of fish, chicken, meat, or vegetarian alternatives such as tofu. Include lots of low-glycemic-index vegetables such as bok choy, kale, salad greens, and so on. Note: Vegetables like carrots have a relatively high glycemic index, but their glycemic load is low. They are fine! Other alternatives include bean or lentil soup and a salad. Kitchari (an Indian dish typically made with mung dal—split mung beans—and basmati rice) or beans and brown rice can also work well.

Dinner. Same as lunch.

Snacks. Choose fruits and cheese, various low-GI nutritional bars, or a small handful of nuts.

A Note About Timing

Far too many women make the mistake of "saving up" their calories for dinner by starving themselves during the day. This pattern inevitably leads to erratic blood sugar and is a setup for weight problems, too. It has been scientifically demonstrated that people who ate 2,000 calories' worth of food in the morning lost about two pounds of weight per week, while those who consumed this amount of calories after 6:00 P.M. gained weight.[25] It's ideal to wait for three hours after eating before going to bed, though this will not work for everyone.

Controlling Blood Sugar and Insulin Levels Is Not a "Diet," It's a Sustainable Way of Life

Learning to control your blood sugar and cravings is a lifelong job for the 75 percent of the population (like me) who are prone to excess consumption of refined carbohydrates. There are times that you will fall off the wagon. But then you get right back on. Don't expect carbs to stop "singing" to you. They won't. That's just part of being human, although over time you'll find it fairly easy to ignore that singing. But until you get there, expect a few slips. Here's an experience I had a while back. On a trip to New York City for a holiday weekend with my daughters, we went to a French restaurant for breakfast, where I felt compelled to order the basket of croissants and rolls because they looked so good. After enjoying these refined carbohydrates thoroughly, I later paid the price: I got so tired from rebound low blood sugar that I felt like lying down on the sidewalk to take a nap! (And this was in November, so it was cold.) It took me a total of twenty-four hours to fully recover from the metabolic effect of eating two rolls and two croissants—even though I also had a protein-rich omelet, which theoretically should have helped prevent the blood sugar swings. (Protein and fat eaten at the same meal as refined carbs help blood sugar remain stable.) Once you really feel the effect of excessive amounts of high-glycemic-index food on your blood sugar, you can never go back to mindless eating again!

Craving high-glycemic-index carbs is not a character flaw and it's not because of lack of willpower. We were designed to crave foods that put on weight quickly—which are invariably foods with a high glycemic index. The simple truth is that for the vast majority of human history, it was a survival advantage to be able to gain weight quickly during times of plenty in order to make it through lean times. It's interesting to note that certain groups with more recent hunter-gatherer ancestors (e.g., Native Americans, Inuits) have significant trouble with high-glycemic-index foods and also grains. (Note: About 25 percent of people, usually but not always Caucasians, are what I call genetic celebrities, who appear to be able to eat anything they want and never gain a pound. Interestingly, however, these individuals really don't crave refined carbohydrates like the rest of us. Many don't even like chocolate! Imagine.)

GETTING LIGHT ENERGY—FROM EATING LEAFY GREENS!

We all learned about photosynthesis in school, the process by which plants get energy directly from sunlight, thanks to the chlorophyll contained in their leaves. It turns out that we may be able to directly capture the ambient energy from sunlight as well. Researchers at

Columbia University Medical Center recently found that certain mammals that eat vegetables containing chlorophyll can directly convert light into energy that their bodies can use.[26] The study concluded that the metabolites of chlorophyll from the plants eaten by the animals entered the animals' circulation and were then present in the animals' body tissues. When those tissues were exposed to light, researchers found, they had higher concentrations of adenosine triphosphate (ATP), the principal molecule for storing and transferring energy in the body's cells. It makes sense that if some mammals can do this, then we probably can, too. Additional research indicates that some intriguing properties of melanin, which gives our skin color and darkens our skin with sunlight exposure, may be a central part of this process of converting sunlight into energy for our bodies.[27]

Step Four: Be Completely Honest About the Food/Emotion Connection

Guilt is one of the worst foods for the intestines.

—Bill Tims

The inescapable reality is that food creates chemical changes that affect our emotions, and our emotions create chemical changes that affect our food cravings—creating a cycle that can be amazingly enlivening or devastatingly incapacitating for body, mind, and spirit.

—Deborah Kern, Ph.D.

Many women gain weight when they are upset and lose weight easily when they are happy or newly in love. The tendency to eat when emotionally upset can cause you first to retain fluids and then to add body fat, partly because of the action of the hormone cortisol, which is secreted in greater amounts when you are under what you perceive as inescapable stress. Cortisol is a steroid, and if you've ever taken steroids or seen someone balloon up on prednisone, you know what I'm talking about. Scientific studies have shown that unexpressed and unresolved emotional stress results in changes in metabolism that inhibit fat breakdown—comparable to what happens on prednisone. Eating fat-laden, refined-carbohydrate foods while under stress not only results in excess fat storage but also sets the stage for many other illnesses in your body.[28] I once gave a party for my daughter after her first formal dance. This required staying up until 3:00 A.M. following a hectic day of preparation. Though I ate my usual amount of food, I gained two and a half pounds, which took four days to go away. The same thing happened to one of my friends who was helping me out at the time. I've experienced this pattern repeatedly over the years. On the other hand, I've also gone on vacations where I've eaten more than usual and have actually lost weight because there was no stress. Many women have this same experience in France and Italy, where eating well is a stress-free, pleasurable ritual. My younger daughter (who has pretty much the same body and metabolism as I do) once enjoyed pizza and croissants regularly on a trip to Paris and lost weight. A miracle.

Excess fat and fluid can also be our body's armor against feeling what we don't want to feel. I have seen women release emotions held for a long time and literally lose five or more pounds overnight from a good crying (or laughing) session. Many of you have also experienced the fact that when you are in love you don't need to eat much because you feel so full of life energy. This life energy is always available to us whenever we are doing work we love—even when we're not "in love" with another person. This is yet another reason to follow your heart as a way to create health in your life.

Look honestly at how you use food and how much of it you really eat. Include when, why, and how. If you really want to make peace with food, for two weeks or more write down everything you eat, where you ate it, and how you were feeling at the time. This exercise breaks through denial and will help you come to terms with your real relationship with food. My clinical experience has taught me that those women who write down what they eat in order to get clear with themselves have a much better chance of successfully changing their health.

If you eat primarily for emotional comfort and haven't developed the skills necessary to stay present with your pain body and "feel it to heal it," then you're not apt to give up what most of us call comfort foods (usually foods that raise blood sugar quickly and are addictive). That's okay. You may just have to wait for the right time and circumstances. When that time comes, choose one of the reset approaches listed above and do it!

One of my former patients who was obese until the age of twenty-one told me that she always knew she would lose weight once she moved away from home and stopped caring for her mentally ill mother and younger siblings. Though her parents took her to doctor after doctor and put her on a series of diets, she knew that she required food to keep from feeling the pain of her circumstances. Once these changed, she lost weight.

We cannot apply *any* information about improving our relationship with food until we've looked squarely at our nourishment issues and have committed to making peace with them. For that reason, please go through the steps to healing in chapter 15 before or at the same time as you decide to improve your nutrition.

If your compulsive overeating is out of control, I highly recommend that you follow a structured eating plan such as that of Overeaters Anonymous. Or try Bright Line Eating (see box below).

IF YOU'RE A SERIOUS FOOD ADDICT

There is a subgroup of individuals who require a very strict program if they are to recover from their food addiction. For them, certain foods are a trigger to overeat, just as the first drink is a trigger for an alcoholic. The solution for these individuals is called Bright Line Eating, founded by neuropsychologist Susan Peirce Thompson, Ph.D. She calls it "the science of eating happy, free, and thin." Dr. Thompson was a cocaine addict in her early teens and struggled with all kinds of addictions for years until she discovered her current approach. It has helped thousands of people get a "right-size" body when all other programs have failed. (For more information, see www.brightlineeating.com.)

Plans like Bright Line Eating work as an external control system as you learn what your internal triggers to overeating are. Many women have not yet established the link between their emotional pain and how they are using food to control it. Others may have so much stress in their lives that their immune and metabolic systems are adversely affected. For these women, even small amounts of sugary, yeasty, salty, or fatty foods set off binge eating. Most women will fall into one of two broad categories: those who binge on fat-laden sweets such as ice cream and those who binge on salty, fat-laden foods such as potato chips. For these women, sugary or salty fat-laden food is like alcohol to an alcoholic. Sugar-addicted women have told me that once they start, they become light-headed, feel drunk and disoriented, and develop an insatiable desire to eat more and more sugary foods. The same thing can apply to fatty and salty binge food. When women avoid these "trigger foods," their eating returns to normal. Food cravings also lessen considerably when you eat a diet without food additives (especially factory-created glutamates) that is adequate in protein and fat and low in refined carbohydrates. Monosodium glutamate (MSG) is a very common additive associated with weight gain (see the following box, and also see "Step Nine: Rehabilitate Your Metabolism," page 877).[29]

Once a woman has dealt with the emotional causes of overeating and has also improved her diet to reduce cravings, she will often no longer require a food plan as an "external authority." She will know what to eat and when.

BEWARE OF FREE GLUTAMATES

Factory-created glutamates, such as MSG, are found in many processed foods. They're associated with obesity and a variety of other side effects. Below is a list of other names for glutamates.[30] Read labels and avoid these products when possible.

Monopotassium glutamate
Glutamate
Autolyzed plant protein
Sodium caseinate
Vegetable protein extract
Glutamic acid
Yeast extract
Autolyzed yeast
Calcium caseinate
Textured protein

Eat in Good Company

Just about everyone who has ever improved her lifestyle knows one thing: When you begin to adopt healthier habits, you're bound to have friends and family members who will try to sabotage your efforts. This is because your desire for better health (or anything else) will hold up a mirror to them and make them question their own behavior, which they may not want to change. So you're perceived as a threat. Expect this. Resistance to change is normal. On the other hand, however, very encouraging research has documented what each of us has already experienced: Good health habits are also contagious and affect everyone around us. In fact, in a landmark study of smoking cessation, researchers found that when one person stops smoking, that decision affects the smoking behavior of entire groups connected to that person, both directly and indirectly, at up to three degrees of separation.[31]

You can be a powerful influencer of others—particularly your own children. Make every effort to spend time with people who are on the same lifestyle path as you and with whom you can find support for the inevitable times when you feel as though a hot fudge sundae is the solution to your problems!

Nourishment is not just the food that we put in our mouths. It is also the environment around us: the people we're with, the sunlight and starlight from the skies, and the color of our walls. These things affect how food is metabolized in our bodies. You need to reevaluate any friendships you have that support unhealthy eating. If you always spend time with those who use eating to suppress their emotions or as their only form of entertainment, you will quite literally feel and act heavier around these people—and you are apt to gain excess fat. You may need to make some new friendships. On the other hand, when you eat with people who enjoy food fully and without any guilt, you may well find that you feel more satisfied than in the past.

For example, many women notice that they eat much less when they go out to eat than when they're at home. The entire process of being served and having to wait between courses results in a very different digestive process and an enhanced sense of well-being.

THE UNEXPECTED PHYSICAL EFFECTS OF STRESS AND PTSD

Our bodies are designed to deal with acute stress with what we've come to call the "fight-or-flight" response, where the stress hormone cortisol (among other stress hormones) is released to give the body the energy and focus needed to deal with an emergency. Normally, once the event is over and the danger has passed, cortisol levels return to normal. But when the threat doesn't go away (as in chronic stress or PTSD), then the benefits of cortisol become harmful.

For example, higher cortisol levels are related to weight gain and fat storage, as well as cravings for food high in sugar and fat. Fat cells in the stomach have four times more cortisol receptors than fat cells elsewhere in the body, so weight gain associated with stress is more likely to lead to belly fat. Another way stress can lead to weight gain is the antidiuretic properties of cortisol—it causes the body to retain sodium, increasing water retention.

Problems with digestion—including indigestion, bloating, and gas as well as heartburn and acid reflux—are more noticeable in those under chronic stress. Irritable bowel syndrome can also be exacerbated, as can food allergies.

Other unexpected side effects stress can cause include various skin issues, such as dry skin, increased scarring, and eczema; ringing in your ears (tinnitus); increased sensitivity to pain; cold hands and feet; more frequent yawning; and excess sweating.

Step Five: Update Your Cultural Programming

Eighty-five percent of women report that they bear the primary responsibility for taking care of their families, including planning, shopping for, and preparing meals, according to *The Shriver Report: A Woman's Nation Changes Everything* (Center for American Progress, 2009). We therefore have tremendous power over the food we and our families eat and the potential to have a significant impact on the health of ourselves and our loved ones.

Women's roles as traditional mothers—providing the "tribal foods"—is out of date because women are now working outside the home in greater numbers than ever. When my daughters were in college, most of their friends couldn't wait to get home to Mom's home cooking. However, my daughters weren't brought up on much of my home cooking. I had help. And so the chain of mother as the sole provider of food was broken with them. Neither of them expects much more than my company in the food department. Even at Thanksgiving, we used to go out for an organic dinner at a lovely local inn—which, up until recently, had been an annual ritual. Now, with grandchildren running around, we're back to cooking at home. But everyone pitches in. What a relief!

Many men's nutritional and emotional needs have been met by women since birth, which is how mothers program their sons to expect women to serve them. When they marry, their wives have often taken over where their mothers left off. If such a man cooks the occasional meal or volunteers to take care of the children to give his wife a break, it's not culturally expected, and so it is almost always regarded as a gift, as something extra that he does for the family. When a woman tells me that she's exhausted from cooking three separate dinners every night because of all the various food preferences in her family, I immediately do some consciousness-raising. Cooking separate meals for people who don't appreciate the effort—who take it for granted as their due—is a classic form of "othering," putting the needs of others before your own. (If, on the other hand, a woman is well rewarded for her efforts and loves to cook, and she and her family have all agreed on the arrangement, no problem.)

It took me years to become aware of my own programming in the cooking and cleaning department. In the early days of my marriage, when I arrived home before my husband, I was very aware that he expected me to clean up the house and start dinner before he got home from work, even though we both worked long hours at the same job. I also sometimes got resentful when my husband would innocently ask me, "What are we doing for dinner?" I used to think that he was *making* me plan the meals, shop for food, and prepare the meals. He didn't understand why I became irritable.

For a while, neither did I. Then it became clear to me that I was automatically assuming that feeding him was my responsibility.

Once I became conscious of my programming (which, like many other women in my baby boomer generation, I brought into my marriage as surely as I brought my hopes and dreams), I stopped blaming him for *the fact that I felt compelled* to cook and clean against my wishes. I also started to change my behavior. For example, I didn't necessarily pick up unless I wanted to. At the same time, he also began to take a look at his programming—with some help from me. He came to see that he *expected* me to do the jobs that his mother had always done. Once both of us made conscious our unconscious expectations about food, cooking, and cleaning, our relationship improved in this area. (In most relationships the unspoken *shoulds* and *oughts* for both members need to be articulated. I don't pretend that this is easy.)

Increasingly, I'm finding that young men are being brought up to perform household tasks like cooking, cleaning, and laundry. This stems directly from mothers who have changed the cultural programming. Interestingly, the boyfriends (and a husband) that my daughters have chosen have all been skilled in the kitchen, which makes me—and them—really happy! Many people now also take advantage of delivery services when it comes to mealtime.

I encourage you to review some of the subtle and not-so-subtle ways in which you have been conditioned. You cannot make any dietary improvement until you've mapped out your personal food minefield (from childhood to the present) and have honestly examined your assumptions about being the chief cook and bottle-washer or about not being able to take the time to prepare and enjoy good food for yourself. Especially now that the majority of women are working outside of the home, our expectations of ourselves when it comes to food preparation need considerable updating from our mothers' day.

Ask yourself the following questions:

- Do you feel personally responsible for thinking about, shopping for, and preparing the family meals?

- If the refrigerator is empty when family members are hungry, do you feel guilty? Inadequate?

- Have you ever discussed this with your spouse? Your children? Your other loved ones?

- Do you enjoy preparing food?

- Do you prepare delicious meals for yourself even when you're alone? If the answer is no, do you make healthy choices when you eat out or when others prepare food for you?

The women's movement of the late 1960s gave unprecedented numbers of women the impetus and means to support themselves financially for the first time. Women no longer need to marry for economic survival. This makes true partnerships between men and women a viable reality. *The Shriver Report* documented the fact that the war between the sexes is over. Both men and women are negotiating everything in new ways. It's time for women to change their outmoded conditioning about who should do what—and also to lower our standards rather than criticize when a man cleans and cooks but doesn't do it the same way we would. If you value yourself, know what you want, and ask for what you want without anger, guilt, or self-doubt, you'll find that many men will knock themselves out to please you.

Step Six: Make Peace with Your Size and Shape

Excess weight is dreams in storage. There's a myth that we can store up time. Primitive cultures store up for the winter. We store up time in our hips.

—Paulanne Balch, M.D.

Countless women over the years have asked me, "How much should I weigh?" Though all of us have been weighed and measured since birth and compared with the cultural ideal, each individual woman has a natural weight at which her body will stay, for the most part, if she is eating according to physical need and exercising regularly. A woman's weight will often fluctuate by two to four pounds in any given week, and it will also vary with her monthly cycle or annual cycle. This fluctuation is almost always due to changes in fluid levels, not fat or muscle, and is normal. A woman's natural, healthy weight may not match the weight tables of any insurance company or doctor's office, and it may not be related at all to clothing size.

Weight as a measure of health doesn't address body composition and is therefore misleading and ambiguous. The concept of "ideal" body weight is not only extremely destructive for many women but also an obsolete way of thinking about health. A much more meaningful measure is your percentage of body fat, which I will cover on page 876, and also body mass index (BMI). To determine your BMI, simply find your height and weight in figure 23. A BMI under 25 is considered ideal, while a BMI of 30 or above is defined as obese and carries an increased risk of death and disease. A BMI between 25 and 29.9, though not ideal, does not necessarily increase health risk.

Though I've told you that weight is an obsolete measure of health, almost all women (myself included) have been brainwashed at some point in their lives about what they should weigh. So each of us lives our life, usually beginning in adolescence, with an ideal weight etched deeply in our brains.

This ideal weight is almost invariably five to ten pounds less than what we really weigh.

DETERMINE YOUR BODY FRAME SIZE

To reach optimal health and your optimal body composition, you may need to rehabilitate how you have been programmed to think about your size. To determine whether your frame size is small, medium, or large, take your thumb and third finger and encircle your opposite wrist with them right at the point where you would normally wear a watch or bracelet. If the tips of your fingers overlap, you have a small frame. If they just meet, you have a medium frame. If your thumb and third finger don't touch, you have a large frame. Finger length has nothing to do with this—your finger length will be proportionate to your wrist size. Studies have shown that large frame size in and of itself is often associated with repeated unnecessary and unsuccessful attempts at dieting. So if you have a large frame, bless it and get on with your life. (I'm talking to myself here.) You will probably never weigh 115 pounds and there's no reason to think that you ever should—being too thin is not healthy, either.

If we are to constantly judge ourselves by the ideals of our media, we will always be at war with our bodies. The average Miss America's weight dropped from 134 pounds in 1954 to 117 pounds in 1980. An educational website providing information about mental health, www.pyschguides.com, analyzed height and weight data from Miss America winners over the years, comparing it with data from the average American woman. They found that the only decades when Miss America fell into the same range as the average U.S. woman was the 1940s and 1950s. Since that time, Miss America has become increasingly thinner, while the average U.S. woman has become progressively heavier. Their research showed that nearly a third of Miss America winners are considered underweight (a BMI below 18.5), which "can perpetuate an unrealistic expectation for the average female's body."[32] It should come as no surprise, then, that the ideal fashion model twenty-five years ago weighed 8 percent less than the average American woman at that time, but today the ideal fashion model weighs 25 percent less than the average American woman.[33] Thus, the current media image of the "ideal" body is unachievable for most women—unless they take laxatives daily, are anorexic, or use exercise addictively as a form of weight control.

Magazines written for teenage girls are full of dieting and weight information that simply serves to hook young women into a lifetime obsession

FIGURE 23: BODY MASS INDEX CHART

Height (Feet and Inches)

Weight (Pounds)	5'0"	5'1"	5'2"	5'3"	5'4"	5'5"	5'6"	5'7"	5'8"	5'9"	5'10"	5'11"	6'0"	6'1"	6'2"	6'3"	6'4"
100	20	19	18	18	17	17	16	16	15	15	14	14	14	13	13	12	12
105	21	20	19	19	18	17	17	16	16	16	15	15	14	14	13	13	13
110	21	21	20	19	19	18	18	17	17	16	16	15	15	15	14	14	13
115	22	22	21	20	20	19	19	18	17	17	17	16	16	15	15	14	14
120	23	23	22	21	21	20	19	19	18	18	17	17	16	16	15	15	15
125	24	24	23	22	21	21	20	20	19	18	18	17	17	16	16	16	15
130	25	25	24	23	22	22	21	20	20	19	19	18	18	17	17	16	16
135	26	26	25	24	23	22	22	21	21	20	19	19	18	18	17	17	16
140	27	26	26	25	24	23	23	22	21	21	20	20	19	18	18	17	17
145	28	27	27	26	25	24	23	23	22	21	21	20	20	19	19	18	18
150	29	28	27	27	26	25	24	23	23	22	22	21	20	20	19	19	18
155	30	29	28	27	27	26	25	24	24	23	22	22	21	20	20	19	19
160	31	30	29	28	27	27	26	25	24	24	23	22	22	21	21	20	19
165	32	31	30	29	28	27	27	26	25	24	24	23	22	22	21	21	20
170	33	32	31	30	29	28	27	27	26	25	24	24	23	22	22	21	21
175	34	33	32	31	30	29	28	27	27	26	25	24	24	23	22	22	21
180	35	34	33	32	31	30	29	28	27	27	26	25	24	24	23	22	22
185	36	35	34	33	32	31	30	29	28	27	27	26	25	24	24	23	23
190	37	36	35	34	33	32	31	30	29	28	27	26	26	25	24	24	23
195	38	37	36	35	33	32	31	31	30	29	28	27	26	26	25	24	24
200	39	38	37	35	34	33	32	31	30	30	29	28	27	26	26	25	24
205	40	39	37	36	35	34	33	32	31	30	29	29	28	27	26	26	25
210	41	40	38	37	36	35	34	33	32	31	30	29	28	28	27	26	26
215	42	41	39	38	37	36	35	34	33	32	31	30	29	28	28	27	26
220	43	42	40	39	38	37	36	34	33	32	32	31	30	29	28	27	27
225	44	43	41	40	39	37	36	35	34	33	32	31	31	30	29	28	27
230	45	43	42	41	39	38	37	36	35	34	33	32	31	30	30	29	28
235	46	44	43	42	40	39	38	37	36	35	34	33	32	31	30	29	29
240	47	45	44	43	41	40	39	38	36	35	34	33	33	32	31	30	29
245	48	46	45	43	42	41	40	38	37	36	35	34	33	32	31	31	30
250	49	47	46	44	43	42	40	39	38	37	36	35	34	33	32	31	30

☐ Underweight ▨ Weight Appropriate ☐ Overweight ▦ Obese

with weight and food that keeps their energy and their power tied up until they finally find the courage and the guidance to get off this road to nowhere, freeing up enormous creative energy in the process. The statistics on eating disorders speak for themselves. At least 30 million Americans of all ages, genders, socioeconomic backgrounds, and ethnicities have eating disorders, according to the National Association of Anorexia Nervosa and Associated Eating Disorders.[34] Currently, just under 1 percent of American women suffer from anorexia nervosa at some point in their lifetime.[35] This condition is one of the most common psychiatric diagnoses in young women and has one of the highest death rates of any mental health condition, according to the National Eating Disorders Association.[36] Bulimia, which consists of binge eating, self-induced vomiting, laxative use, diuretic use, or exercise to try to lose weight, is present in up to 20 percent of college students. It occurs mostly in young women age thirty or younger. Less than 5 percent of cases are in males.[37] Even so, most bulimics don't lose excessive weight but weigh slightly more than they would like to.

The medical profession reinforces these addictive behaviors by serving as "weight police," having women weigh in and admonishing them to lose weight year after year without actually telling them how to do it and without addressing the complexities of self-nourishment for women. I once heard Robert Lustig, M.D., on a YouTube lecture talking about the fallacy of the "eat less and exercise more" approach that has been the staple advice of dieticians and doctors for decades. He said something like, "If I hear of another dietitian giving this advice, I'm coming after you." I laughed out loud at the sad truth of this.

Most women have bodies that are meant to be larger than the cultural ideal. Women's bodies have more fat on them than men's, nature's way of ensuring that the energy needs of childbearing and lactation will be met even during times of famine. The much larger amount of testosterone men's bodies produce contributes to a leaner body and a much higher metabolic rate than women have. Men also have proportionately more muscle than women, which is another factor that leads to a higher metabolic rate. Since cultural expectations of women are that we can never be too thin, and since being thin is associated with self-control, a lifelong struggle with food and body weight is a cultural norm. Our bodies and their weights are the barometers by which society measures how good we are, how attractive we are, how worthy we are.

How much self-control and body abuse must women go through before it dawns on us that there is something deeply wrong with our entire approach to the "weight problem"? Willpower and self-control are exactly the opposite of what we need. We need to see media images of normal, healthy women who are strong and lean but not anorexic. Of course, we are seeing more images of healthy larger women—enter the plus-size model. And body acceptance is now far more common than ever. But make no mistake: Being significantly overweight is a health risk, pure and simple. And childhood obesity is a growing global problem, an epidemic that is fueled by junk food manufacturers.

Regardless of our body size, self-respect and self-acceptance are the starting points for making peace with our size. We must know that we have the power to get off the conventional weight treadmill and start enjoying our lives, no matter where we are. Like Jon Gabriel, mentioned earlier, you really do have to start with loving yourself "right there"—regardless of your size. And at the same time realize that making an effort to eat nutrient-rich foods and move your body regularly will greatly add to your health span and your quality of life.

I find it fascinating, and also poignant, that I and many other women age fifty and older now like our bodies more than we ever did in our twenties. This is a great reason for celebration! Healing one's body image is definitely possible regardless of the cultural messages.

Step Seven: Find Out If You're Fit or Fat

Excess body fat is not just unsightly but also a serious health risk. But weight itself is truly a meaningless measure of health. Why? Because lean body mass weighs much more than fat. Muscles are 80 percent water, while fat is only 5 to 10 percent water. Muscle is more than eight times heavier than the equivalent amount of fat.[38] An individual can be at "normal" weight, or even less than that, and be overfat. Others may weigh far more than they "should" according to the weight tables, yet be at an ideal body fat percentage. Some women will actually gain weight when they start to build muscle (which is lean body mass), but at the same time they will lose inches. This is because six pounds of fat takes up almost a gallon of space—much more space, proportionally, than muscle occupies.

One of my patients, whom I'll call Jennie, was a former marathon runner who had believed for years that she was shaped "like a knockwurst." Although Jennie wore a size 8, exercised regularly, and looked wonderful in her clothes, I could not convince her that she should stop trying to get down to 125 pounds. Her friends always thought she weighed a lot less than she did because she had a very significant amount of lean muscle mass. It wasn't until we measured Jennie's body composition—which revealed that her body fat percentage was only 25 percent—that it finally began to dawn on her that her weight range of 136 to 140 pounds was both healthy and ideal for her.

Get your body fat measured. It's one of the most helpful steps you can take to break out of the "I weigh too much" tyranny. You can do this at many doctors' offices, or at almost any fitness center or Y. You can also purchase devices that measure body fat. A healthy percentage of body fat for women ranges from 20 to 32 percent. Currently, the average American woman has 40 percent body fat.[39]

For the sake of comparison, female competitive runners' average body fat is 18 percent, while anorexic women may be as low as 10 percent—so low that their bodies must consume their internal organs as fuel. On the other hand, a healthy body fat percentage for men is 15 percent, and competitive male athletes may be as low as 3 or 4 percent. Body fat percentage is one area where it can be deadly to imitate men, because a woman's normal hormonal cycle can be interrupted at body fat percentages lower than 17 to 18 percent. (This is the level of body fat required to have "washboard" abs or a "six-pack"; it is altogether too low for many women and girls.)

If your body fat is currently in a healthy range, congratulate yourself and keep on doing what you're doing. If it is too high, know that by reducing it, you will not only look and feel better but also lower your risk for high blood pressure, high cholesterol, cancer, type 2 diabetes, heart disease, and fluid retention. In fact, increasing your lean body mass and decreasing your body fat percentage is one of the best treatments for these conditions if you already have them.

Step Eight: Retrain Your Eyes

We're all aware that the cultural icons of beauty—today's supermodels—seem thinner than almost anyone we know or see regularly. We also know that the images in magazines are airbrushed and manipulated so much that even the supermodels don't look like themselves. How can any of us feel attractive at a healthy body fat percentage when all the supermodels must be about 18 percent body fat or less?

The answer is that we all have to retrain our eyes to see the beauty inherent in a healthy woman with a healthy body composition, whose image is not an airbrushed, computer-enhanced, quasi-anorexic body that looks something like that of an adolescent boy with big breasts. Once you start looking for it, you'll see this kind of beauty everywhere—I sure do!

Step Nine: Rehabilitate Your Metabolism

Exercise

As women grow older, muscle mass often decreases and fat increases. Exercise reverses the trend toward fat gain and muscle loss no matter at what age you start. Women who exercise regularly can look forward on average to twenty more years of productive living than those who don't exercise. Regular exercise also decreases insulin resistance, which helps your body burn carbohydrates more efficiently, making fat storage much less likely. Because glycemic stress begins in skeletal muscles, regular exercise helps prevent it. The best way to increase your lean muscle mass is by doing weight-bearing exercise regularly. Miriam Nelson, Ph.D., has shown that a weight-training program that exercises all the major muscle groups for forty minutes twice a week helps women lose excess fat and gain significant muscle mass—thus resulting in a higher metabolic rate and ability to burn calories effectively.[40] Weight training—whether once per week or five times per week—also lifts depression and anxiety.[41]

Aerobic exercise also increases your metabolic rate. (See chapter 18.) The more exercise you do, the faster your metabolism speeds up. Fast walking works very well, as do stair climbing, bike riding, treadmills, and similar forms of exercise. The increase in metabolic rate lasts for up to twenty-four hours after exercise is finished. My favorite kind of aerobic exercise—and the kind that provides the most benefit in the shortest amount of time (twenty minutes, two or three times per week) is known as high-intensity interval training, or HIIT. More on that in the next chapter.

Hydrate the Right Way

Optimal hydration is crucial to your health and performance on all levels. The right kind of hydration can reduce or eliminate headaches, fatigue, weight gain, and even digestive issues. Research by the late Fereydoon Batmanghelidj, M.D., author of *Your Body's Many Cries for Water* (Global Health Solutions, 1995), indicates that most of the pain and sickness we experience is actually the result of chronic dehydration. For many of us, he believed, the caffeine and sugar in the beverages we drink (including coffee, tea, soda, and juice) actually deplete the body's water supply because they draw water from the body's reserves as well as cause us to lose our natural thirst for water. (For more information, visit Dr. Batmanghelidj's website at www.watercure.com.) The chronic dehydration that results commonly leads to fatigue (particularly in midafternoon), as well as conditions including dyspepsia (heartburn), arthritic pain, back pain, headache (including migraine), colitis pain and associated constipation, pain from angina (from the heart), and leg pain (when walking). One of my longtime colleagues, an internationally known expert in food and healing, told me that her chronically splitting fingernail problem healed with one month of starting to drink more water!

You've no doubt heard that the amount of water you should drink is eight 8-ounce glasses per day. For most of us, all this does is increase the amount of time we spend in the bathroom. New research has shown that there is a much better way to hydrate. Groundbreaking studies from the University of Washington's Pollack Laboratory and other sources led internal medicine specialist Dana Cohen, M.D., and Hydration Foundation founder

Gina Bria to put the science of hydration all in one place—a book called *Quench: Beat Fatigue, Drop Weight, and Heal Your Body Through the New Science of Optimum Hydration* (Hachette, 2018). Dr. Cohen prescribes "eating" your water instead of drinking it and suggests that in as few as five days, you'll probably notice major benefits. So what does "eating" water actually mean? It means you increase your intake of hydrating fruits and vegetables, which are more than 80 percent water but in which the water is held in cellular structures. This results in the right kind of hydration in your body.

The Top 12 Hydrating Veggies

Vegetable	Percentage of Water by Volume
Cucumber	96.7%
Romaine lettuce	95.6%
Celery	95.4%
Radish	95.3%
Zucchini	95%
Tomatoes	94.5%
Peppers	93.9%
Cauliflower	92.1%
Spinach	91.4%
Broccoli	90.7%
Carrots	90%
Sprouts	86.5%

The Top 12 Hydrating Fruits

Fruit	Percentage of Water by Volume
Starfruit	91.4%
Watermelon	91.4%
Strawberries	91%
Grapefruit	90.5%
Cantaloupe	90.2%
Pineapple	87%
Raspberries	87%
Blueberries	85%
Kiwi	84.2%
Apple	84%
Pear	84%
Grapes	81.5%

Water-rich foods are also packed with nutrients. But cutting-edge science has shown that water that contains electrolytes (like magnesium, chloride, sodium, and potassium) creates optimal electrical function in our bodies. Quite simply, water conducts electricity—which enhances mood, cognition, judgment, and energy. As Dr. Cohen puts it, "Remember that the quality of our hydration has everything to do with the quality of electrical conduction. We can't say it enough: Water conducts electricity, and hydration runs our electrical function. This shifts water from being simply wet, simply moisturizing, or even just cleansing, to being fuel. And get this: Because of the fiber in plants, the water stays in our system longer because we absorb it more slowly. It's a triple play of health: pure water, absorbent fiber, and not only needed nutrients, but electrolytes."[42]

Bottom line: Plants hydrate better than plain water alone—possibly twice as much, according to Dr. Cohen.

The Right Salt: Another Hydration Superstar

Regular table salt (sodium chloride), which is the kind of sodium that processed foods are loaded with, is dehydrating. It moves fluid out of the cells (the intracellular space) and into the area around the cells (the extracellular space). This is why after eating pizza or a highly processed meal containing lots of sodium, you may gain a couple of pounds of water weight or feel bloated. Not that table salt is particularly dangerous; it's just that there are better options. Naturally occurring salt has a mixture of electrolytes (including potassium, magnesium, calcium, and trace minerals) with a much healthier effect on the body. This type of salt actually makes water more hydrating, not less. It helps the cells retain fluid in the right place—inside the cell. Hence it helps enhance the electrical function of water in your body. Try adding a pinch of sea salt (such as Celtic), Himalayan salt, or rock salt labeled as edible to your drinking water or to a smoothie.

If you're worried using salt will cause or exacerbate high blood pressure, don't be—the latest studies show that restricting salt intake actually raises blood pressure. So salt is not the villain it's been made out to be.[43] For more on this issue, see *The Salt Fix: Why the Experts Got It All Wrong—and How Eating More Might Save Your Life* (Harmony Books, 2017) by James DiNicolantonio, Pharm. D.

The following foods are dehydrating. So if you use them, make sure you compensate with more water to replenish your body:

Alcohol
Sugar
Grains and starches
Meats
Cheeses
Any and all processed foods (read labels—you'll find a lot of sodium)
Coffee and tea

If you're an athlete, staying adequately hydrated also protects your joints and tissues. That's because adequate hydration also keeps the connective tissue known as fascia in peak condition. As you will recall, fascia is a semisolid malleable crystalline structure that encases every organ and muscle in our bodies, sending electrical signals throughout our tissues that enhance function.

Here's a good rule of thumb: Drink (or eat) half your body weight in ounces of water per day. If you weigh 140 pounds, for example, you need to drink (or eat) the equivalent of 70 ounces of water each day. A great way to hydrate is to add a tablespoon of chia seeds and a pinch of good mineral-rich salt to water. Let it sit for ten minutes or so, until the chia seeds swell, and then drink it. You'll be amazed at what this does, not only for optimal hydration but also for bowel function.

Regular movement, like yoga or stretching, also enhances hydration and keeps fascia supple and functional (see chapter 18, on exercise).

Eat the Right Carbohydrates

As already stated, eating high-glycemic-index foods leads to a spike in blood sugar—and a temporary, unsustainable boost in the brain chemicals serotonin and endorphin. The problem is that these high blood sugar levels rapidly fall, thus prompting the consumption of more foods that raise blood sugar quickly once again. Chasing the blood sugar high by eating refined or high-sugar carbohydrates is very addictive. Some individuals are more susceptible than others. If you are prone to seasonal affective disorder (SAD) or other forms of depression, you will crave carbohydrates more than most people in order to boost your serotonin to adequate levels. But the reasons for carb cravings are many. Alcoholics and those who crave alcohol often have underlying blood sugar problems as well.

It has been my clinical experience that families in which there are several alcoholics invariably have members who are addicted to sugar, even if they are not prone to excessive alcohol intake themselves. These addictions tend to flip-flop. Any veteran of Alcoholics Anonymous will tell you that sugary snacks are a staple at meetings, as individuals substitute sugar for alcohol.

This observation has been confirmed by the work of Kathleen DesMaisons, Ph.D., a specialist in nutrition and addiction and author of *Potatoes Not Prozac* (Simon & Schuster, 1999), who was able to achieve a 90 percent success rate in rehabilitating repeat-offender drunk drivers by teaching them how to eat in order to stabilize their blood sugar and brain chemistry. Her research, which matches my clinical experience, revealed that individuals who crave either alcohol or sugar—or both—have an increased need (probably inborn) for the brain chemicals serotonin, dopamine, and beta-endorphin. The key to gaining control over their addictive, and often destructive, eating or drinking behaviors is for them to learn to balance their brain chemicals by understanding the food-mood connection.

Dr. DesMaisons has a simple test to help you decide whether you're sugar-sensitive. When you were a kid and went out with your family on summer nights for ice cream, what part of the trip do you remember most? The car, the feel of the night air, your family members, or the ice cream itself? If ice cream comes first in your recollections, you're probably sugar-sensitive.

We know that having enough of the brain chemical serotonin is key to feeling calm and focused, which is why antidepressants such as Prozac, Paxil, and Zoloft, all of which enhance serotonin, have become so popular. (My colleague Kelly Brogan, M.D., has fully researched the effects of nutrition on serotonin and mood and found that a change in diet works far better than psych meds—which can be incredibly difficult to wean yourself from. Here's just one stunning example: Research has shown that the curcumin found in turmeric is *just as effective* as Prozac in treating patients with major depressive disorder—*without* the side effects![44] Check out Dr. Brogan's Vital Mind Reset program, mentioned earlier in this chapter.)

Luckily, you can learn how to enhance and balance your own serotonin without help from drugs. Serotonin is manufactured in the brain from the amino acid tryptophan, which is found in protein. In order for tryptophan to enter your brain from the bloodstream, your body requires insulin—which means you need to eat some carbohydrates as well. You want just enough insulin to do the job, but not so much that you get rebound low blood sugar.

Beta-endorphins are also mood elevators, and they're why we crave the refined carbohydrates we call "comfort foods." Macaroni and cheese, garlic mashed potatoes with plenty of butter, french fries, pancakes, waffles, cakes, and cookies all raise blood sugar quickly, thus increasing our levels of beta-endorphins. Unfortunately, continually eating "comfort foods" eventually wreaks havoc with just about every system in the body, leading to cellular inflammation and chronic degenerative disease. So much for long-term comfort. Happily, there are other ways to boost your serotonin and balance your brain chemicals. Exercise, natural light, the right diet, and meditation are all good.

The bottom line is that growing up in an alcoholic or otherwise dysfunctional family—which I've come to see is true for the majority of us—is stressful. The imprint of that stress continues to affect how we feel about ourselves. We use food as a drug to soothe us. Sugar addiction is an addiction like any other. It needs to be treated like one. Susan Peirce Thompson, Ph.D.'s Bright Line Eating program, mentioned earlier, tackles this head-on with a very effective eating plan. Another classic is *Holy Hunger: A Memoir of Desire* (Knopf, 1999), by Margaret Bullitt-Jonas, a brilliant Episcopal priest. She never touches sugar anymore, is at peace with food, and writes the following words of wisdom: "The first step in the long process of recovery, and the foundation of a food addict's subsequent well-being, is putting down the fork, putting down the food, one day at a time. No insight into self, however subtle; no analysis of the dynamics of addiction, however accurate; no understanding of the nature of desire, however sophisticated or enlightening—none of these fine things can substitute for action. The healing of addiction depends, first and foremost, not on what we know, nor on what we feel, but on what we do—a fact that remains as stubbornly true of 'old timers' as it does for newcomers."[45]

Get Enough Protein

What is "enough protein"? Well, experts disagree. Some feel that all we need is about 30 grams per day (which is a mere ounce); others suggest higher amounts. Though some Americans get more protein than they need, others—and that includes a lot of women—don't get enough to feel their best. This is one area in which I've changed my mind over the past decade based on newer research and both clinical and personal experience.

I, like many, used to think that it was possible for everybody to get all the protein they required for optimal health from grains, beans, and vegetables. Now I realize that while a diet high in complex carbohydrates from whole foods is great for some—the metabolically gifted, who have no problem with insulin—it is not the answer for everyone. I used to erroneously believe that a diet containing protein and fat was invariably associated with an increased risk of losing calcium in the urine, thus increasing the risk of osteoporosis. However, a review of the current literature has shown that this is not always true.[46] It depends on the quality of the protein and fat, and also on how much insulin is hanging around.

Whether you choose to improve your diet on your own or follow the recommendations in one of the many books on diet and nutrition, make sure you are getting an amount of protein every day that is adequate to maintain (or build) your lean body mass—the part of you that burns fat most efficiently. Not every diet proclaimed to be high-protein will provide sufficient amounts of protein. (See table 9 to determine the appropriate amount of protein.)

TABLE 9

CALCULATING YOUR DAILY PROTEIN REQUIREMENT

To determine the daily protein amount required to preserve your lean body mass (LBM), you must first measure your percentage of body fat. (See page 874.) I'll use Carol, a former marathon runner, as an example. She weighs 138 pounds and has a body fat measurement of 25 percent.

1. Multiply your weight in pounds by your percentage of body fat expressed as a decimal. This tells you the weight of your body fat. (For Carol: 138 × 0.25 = 34 pounds.)

2. Subtract the weight of your body fat from your total weight. This tells you your lean body mass. (For Carol: 138–34 = 104 pounds LBM.)

3. Now multiply your LBM by the cofactor that best describes you.
   Sedentary (you do no physical exercise whatsoever): You need 0.5 grams (0.017 oz.) of protein per pound of lean body mass. Multiply your LBM by 0.5.
   Moderately active (you do twenty to thirty minutes of exercise two to three times per week): You need 0.6 grams (0.021 oz.) of protein per pound of lean body mass. Multiply your LBM by 0.6.
   Active (you participate in organized physical activity for more than thirty minutes three to five times per week): You need 0.7 grams (0.024 oz.) of protein per pound of lean body mass. Multiple your LBM by 0.7.
   Very active (you participate in vigorous physical activity lasting an hour or more, five or more times per week): You need 0.8 grams (0.030 oz.) of protein per pound of lean body mass. Multiply your LBM by 0.8.
   Athlete (you are a competitive athlete in training doing twice-daily heavy workouts for an hour or more): You need 0.9 grams (0.320 oz.) of protein per pound of lean body mass. Multiply your LBM by 0.9. (Carol has an LBM of 104 pounds and is moderately active. Therefore, her daily protein requirement is 62 grams, or 2.18 oz.—considerably less than when she was training for marathons.)

   Source: This method for calculating protein requirements is based on *Protein Power* (Bantam, 1996) by Michael Eades, M.D., and Mary Dan Eades, M.D.

As you can see, the terms *high-protein* and *low-protein* are completely meaningless when your dietary approach is individualized. I now believe that most women do better with some animal protein in their diets. Though I appreciate the sentiments of animal-rights activists and the problematic environmental impact of the current meat production industry, I don't feel that it is healthful or necessary for everyone to become a vegetarian. (There is no question, however, that the vast majority of the population needs more vegetables, fruit, nuts, seeds, legumes, and whole grains. But whole grains may need to be limited or avoided if an individual is gluten intolerant [see page 857].) Organic methods of producing animal food that respect the soil, the water, and the animal itself can overcome the environmental concerns posed by the meat industry. You can now buy meat from grass-fed animals raised without chemicals and antibiotics. This meat tends to be leaner, to have smaller amounts of pesticide residues in it, and to have an optimal essential fatty acid profile—meaning more omega-3 fats and less omega-6s. It turns out that the effects of grass-fed beef on blood cholesterol and other lipids are no different from those of fish and chicken.[47] The problem with most commercially produced beef is that it is heavily marbled with the wrong kind of fat as a result of cattle being fed too much grain. So it has the same inflammatory chemical imbalance that many humans have.

ARE YOU SENSITIVE TO ARACHIDONIC ACID?

There is no question that some individuals are very sensitive to arachidonic acid (AA), which is found in all animal products—especially organ meats, red meat, and egg yolks. In fact, this sensitivity to AA is what causes most of the problems that have been commonly attributed to saturated fat and cholesterol. Arachidonic acid is higher in the modern meat supply than in the past because the grain that is fed to livestock results in the same eicosanoid imbalance in animals as it does in humans—that is, it results in more inflammatory chemicals than is healthy. (By the way, arachidonic acid is far less likely to be a problem if no refined carbs are eaten with it.) The symptoms of arachidonic acid sensitivity are chronic fatigue, poor and restless sleep, grogginess upon awakening, brittle hair, brittle nails, dry and flaking skin, minor rashes, and arthritis. It seems clear that some of the health advantages we've attributed to a vegetarian diet are simply the result of lowering the AA content of the diet. To find out if you are susceptible to AA, eliminate all red meat and egg yolks from your diet for one month. Then eat a meal of steak and eggs and see if your symptoms return. To avoid excess AA, eat only low-fat meat (AA is mostly stored in animal fat), or switch to wild game or free-range livestock, which has much lower levels of AA. Look for free-range chickens and the eggs from them. Excess consumption of carbohydrates (particularly refined ones) also increases AA levels.

It's not necessary to eat meat in order to increase your protein intake. You can get adequate protein from veggie burgers, tofu, seitan, and tempeh. Eggs, whey powder, soy powder, and milk products are good sources of protein if you're not sensitive to them. Many vegetarian protein powders, including those made from whole soy or hemp, are readily available. The nutritional quality of soy protein has been studied in depth (see box below). Studies have shown that nitrogen balance, digestibility, and protein utilization are similar between beef, milk, and soy proteins.[48] Other studies show that soy protein can support nitrogen balance[49] and provides adequate amounts of the amino acid methionine, which is important for growth and development.[50] Therefore, the addition of soy to the diet can be a good way to meet your protein requirements.

IS SOY A HEALTHY CHOICE?

Over the last several years, there's been a lot of anti-soy information out there, and it's little wonder women are confused. Long touted for its healthful properties (from helping with hot flashes to reducing breast cancer risk), suddenly soy is being accused of *promoting* breast tumor growth. It actually does just the opposite. It's time to retire the hype, so let me give you the facts.

Soy protein is a nutritionally complete, high-quality protein that contains all the essential amino acids. Amino acids are building blocks of protein. Soy contains all of the essential amino acids, which means that soy is a complete protein—though it is not particularly rich in one amino acid, methionine.[51] However, it contains enough methionine to meet most people's requirements under most circumstances.[52] Soy protein is considered nutritionally excellent by nutritional researchers and the scientific community, especially when compared with other proteins using the Protein Digestibility Corrected Amino Acid Score (PDCAAS).

Dairy, nut, and wheat allergies are far more common than soy allergies. Some people are unquestionably very sensitive to soy. (Soy does appear on the Food and Agriculture Organization's list of the eight most prevalent food allergens. The list also includes milk, eggs, fish, crustaceans, wheat, peanuts, and tree nuts. Together, these foods account for about 90 percent of all food allergies.)

That said, in comparison with milk and nut proteins, soy is a relatively uncommon allergen—milk and peanut allergies are each five to six times more prevalent than soy allergies.[53] In fact, the true incidence of soy allergy is quite low—it's less than 1 percent of children and 0.1 percent of adults, according to double-blind, placebo-controlled studies.

Compared with other food allergies, soy reactions tend to be far milder. In a summary report of clinical food challenge studies, they were noted as minimal to mild 80 percent of the time, with the remaining 20 percent being moderate. No severe allergic reactions to soy were reported. In comparison, milk and peanut allergens produced minimal to mild symptoms in 50–70 percent of cases, moderate symptoms in 20–30 percent of cases, and severe symptoms in 10–15 percent of cases.

In my experience, the vast majority of people with food allergies are sensitive to wheat and dairy foods, not soy. And reactions to wheat and dairy often trigger crossover reactions to other foods.

Bloating and gas from soy don't indicate an allergy. Some people are sensitive to the nondigestible sugars and fiber in soy. These can cause the same abdominal bloating and gas that you'd experience from ingesting the sugars and fibers in beans—or even the lactose in milk.[54] Whenever you add legumes of any kind to your diet, the bowel flora take a while to adjust. But you don't have to suffer—take digestive enzymes and probiotics to keep the intestines in good form and reduce discomfort.

Phytates are part of a healthy diet. If you've read any anti-soy literature, you've probably heard that soy is high in phytates, which can inhibit absorption of important nutrients from the gut. This is a half-truth. Plants store phosphorus (an essential nutrient for plants and animals) in their seeds to support the growth of young seedlings. This phosphorus is stored in the form of phytate (inositol hexametaphosphate). Plant phytates are considered by some to be anti-nutrients, because phytates consumed in the human diet can compete with essential minerals (for example, iron and zinc) and inhibit absorption in the gut.

However, phytates are also important food constituents that not only act as natural food-preserving antioxidants but also help to reduce risks of heart disease and cancer in those who consume whole grains, beans, seeds, and nuts.

Though soybeans contain significant amounts of phytate, so do whole grains, beans, and seeds. There's a robust scientific literature supporting the fact that these foods are important constituents of a healthy diet. So avoiding soybeans to avoid phytates doesn't make sense. That said, isolated soy protein contains far less phytate than whole soybeans.

Both nonfermented and fermented soy products have their place. Soy foods fall into two broad categories: nonfermented and fermented. Nonfermented soy foods include soy nuts, edamame (whole soybeans), soy milk, and tofu (bean curd). Fermented soy products include tamari, soy sauce, miso, tempeh, and natto.

Though opinions vary widely, tending to favor fermented soy over nonfermented, there is no scientific consensus on which is better. Here's why:

~ Fermenting soy foods increases isoflavone bioavailability. However, fermenting a soybean also decreases the actual isoflavone content of the food. That's why typical intakes of nonfermented soy foods result in a higher intake of isoflavones.

~ Fermented soy foods can be easier for some to digest, but taking digestive enzymes and probiotics, as mentioned earlier, can easily make nonfermented soy more digestible if this is a problem for you.

~ Fermented soy products have lower phytate levels than nonfermented soy. But as I said above, phytates aren't necessarily bad for you. Mineral levels of people consuming a healthy mixed diet made up of soy and other phytate-containing foods have not been found to be adversely affected.

~ Fermented soy products can be quite high in sodium, a known risk factor for stomach cancer. A review of soy intake and stomach cancer indicated that risk did increase with intake of fermented soy foods (mainly miso) but decreased with intake of nonfermented soy foods (mainly tofu).

Soy has well-documented health benefits. Many studies have strongly suggested that soy protein has benefits for the cardiovascular system, bones, and overall health, including conferring a decreased risk of some kinds of cancer, among them breast cancer. In a review of twenty-six animal studies of experimental carcinogenesis in which researchers used diets containing soy or soybean isoflavones, 65 percent reported protective effects, while none reported any increased risk of tumors. Soy protein has also helped many women find relief from menopausal symptoms.

Yet the hundreds of studies done on soy are hard to interpret and to use as a basis for specific recommendations because some used whole soy, some isolated isoflavones, and some fermented soy in foods such as miso and tempeh. It's also fairly difficult to tell whether the health benefits associated with soy are a result of overall dietary improvement from decreasing animal protein in the diet and adding more vegetables or whether they're strictly from soy. Here are some highlights:

Cancer/breast cancer. Consumption of nonfermented soy products, such as soy milk and tofu, tended to be either protective against both hormone- and non-hormone-related cancers or not at all associated with cancer risk. In large population studies, soy consumption has been associated with a decreased risk of prostate, breast, and colon cancers.[55] Soy products contain five known classes of anticancer agents, including isoflavones (phytoestrogens, which are present in many foods, but uniquely high in soy), protease inhibitors, phytate, phytosterols, and saponins, as well as other potential anticarcinogens such as phenolic acids, lecithin, and omega-3 fatty acids. Isoflavones are currently the most intensively researched soy phytochemical with respect to breast cancer, although a growing body of literature supports protease inhibitors as anticarcinogens. Also, the Bowman-Birk protease inhibitor (BBI), found in soy, has been shown to be nontoxic and to prevent and suppress carcinogenesis in animal models. A concentrated form of BBI (referred to as BBIC) is now being used in studies on humans.[56]

Soy contains two primary isoflavones, genistein and daidzein. Both appear to be cancer-protective. They are antioxidants that help to neutralize cellular inflammation within the body, a known precursor for cancer. Isoflavones are also estrogen modulators, dampening the potentially harmful impact of not only the more potent estrogens produced by the body but also environmental substances that have estrogen-mimicking properties (xenoestrogens).

Several epidemiological studies have specifically examined the association between soy consumption and the incidence of breast cancer. Many, but not all, have shown that soy intake can be protective. In a study involving 200 Singapore Chinese women with breast cancer and 420 matched controls, a decreased risk of breast cancer was associated with high intakes of soy products in premenopausal women.[57]

A case-control study done at the University of Southern California interviewed 597 Asian American women with previous incidence of breast cancer and 966 controls.[58] Risk of breast cancer decreased with increasing frequency of tofu consumption in both pre- and postmenopausal women. A 2003 study of 21,852 Japanese women ages forty to fifty-nine found that women with the highest intake of soy isoflavones reduced their risk of breast cancer by up to 54 percent compared with women with the lowest intake of soy isoflavones.[59] Looking at an even larger group, researchers at Vanderbilt University analyzed data from the 73,223 Chinese women who participated in the Shanghai Women's Health Study and found that women who consumed a high amount of soy foods consistently during adolescence and adulthood had a substantially reduced risk of premenopausal breast cancer.[60]

Perhaps the breast cancer debate can be best summed up by the conclusions of an international group of nearly twenty researchers from around the world, sponsored by the Council for Responsible Nutrition, who met in Milan in 2009 to evaluate the research on isoflavones and their implication in cancer. The research presented there overwhelmingly supported the idea that isoflavones do not have an effect on established markers for breast cancer risk. In fact, the data instead showed that soy may improve the prognosis of breast cancer patients.[61]

Cardiovascular disease. Soy protein consumption has been linked to a small (3–5 percent) decrease in LDL (bad) cholesterol.[62] Also, because of their antioxidant and estrogenic activities, soy isoflavones may benefit cardiovascular function. But the significance of all this has yet to be studied thoroughly.

Osteoporosis. Fracture rates in Asian populations that consume far more soy than is typical in the United States are significantly lower. Animal studies show the genistein in soy works better than alendronate, raloxifene, and estradiol for preserving bone mineral density and strength.[63] Though soy should not replace getting optimal vitamin D, calcium, magnesium, and weight-bearing exercise, it's well worth consuming as part of your overall bone health strategy.

Soy doesn't disrupt thyroid function in those with normal thyroid function and adequate iodine. The relationship between soy and thyroid function has been studied for more than seventy years. Since then, fourteen human clinical trials have studied the effects of soy foods and soy isoflavones on thyroid function. All involved presumably healthy subjects, and with few exceptions, the soy product used was isolated soy protein. Now here's the important part. With only one exception, all of the studies showed either no effects or minor and clinically irrelevant effects of soy on thyroid function.[64] The one trial that noted marked antithyroid effects (and the one that is often cited in anti-soy literature) involved Japanese adults who were fed roasted soybeans that had been pickled and stored in rice vinegar. It is not known what the soy protein or isoflavone content of this food was. And the study was not controlled. So no firm conclusion can be drawn.

Considering the number of women who are first diagnosed with thyroid problems at midlife, I was particularly reassured by a study of thirty-eight postmenopausal women between the ages of sixty-four and eighty-three who were given daily doses of 90 mg of soy isoflavones or a placebo.[65] Thyroid hormone levels were tested at the beginning of the study and again at 90 and 180 days. After six months, the differences in thyroid hormones between the groups were statistically indistinguishable. Given all this, most experts agree that soy foods and isolated soy protein have little if any effect on thyroid function in normal, healthy adults who consume soy at moderate levels as part of a well-balanced diet.

However, soy isoflavones, especially in high doses, can disrupt thyroid function in those who are iodine deficient (estimated to be 13 percent of the population) and in those who have compromised thyroid function.

Moderation is key. Oscar Wilde once said, "Nothing succeeds like excess." And in our culture, if something has been found to be beneficial, Americans tend to overdo it. That is the case with soy, too. Some people think that if some is good, then more is better, leading them to subsist mainly on soy protein.

Soy foods (and other isoflavones) appear to have protective and healthful effects when consumed as part of a healthful, well-balanced diet beginning in childhood. Healthy dietary intakes of soy isoflavones, as reflected in Asian diets, appear to be in the range of 20–90 mg per day.

In summary, both the scientific evidence and my years of experience strongly support the role of a moderate amount of soy protein (as soy protein isolate, fermented soy, or nonfermented soy) in the diets of the vast majority of people.[66] In addition to being far more ecologically sound to produce—it takes twenty pounds of soybeans to make one pound of beef—soy protein also confers a number of well-documented health benefits.

As always, it's the quality of the food that counts. So look for soy that is non-GMO and, if possible, organically grown. Don't spend your time reacting to extreme views on anything. This, in and of itself, is a health risk. There are far more important matters in life—such as forgiveness, laughter, and joy—than being afraid of soy.

Eat the Right Kinds of Fats

Our bodies can produce most fatty acids from the carbohydrates that we eat. However, there are two fatty acids, known as essential fatty acids, that our bodies cannot produce and that we must therefore get in our diets. These two acids are linoleic acid (LA), an omega-6 fatty acid, and alpha-linolenic acid (LNA), an omega-3 fatty acid. LNA is the starting material for the biosynthesis of eicosapentaenoic acid (EPA) and docosahexaenoic acid (DHA), two important polyunsaturated fatty acids. LNA, EPA, and DHA are the main members of the omega-3 family of fatty acids.

For the majority of human evolution, omega-6 fats (especially corn oil, peanut oil, soy oil, and safflower oil) and omega-3 fats have been consumed in a ratio of about 2:1. But because of all the omega-6 oils that have been used in cooking or prepared food over the past sixty years or so, that ratio has shifted so that it is now anywhere between 10:1 and 20:1. We have also decreased our intake of omega-3 fats considerably. To flourish we need both, but in the right amounts. The majority of us get more than enough omega-6 fats, so we need to concentrate on necessary intake of omega-3 fats.

The essential fatty acids are converted in our bodies into two important classes of eicosanoids—leukotrienes and prostaglandins. These compounds are hormone-like substances that influence a huge number of metabolic processes. An overabundance of the wrong kinds of eicosanoids leads to—you guessed it—cellular inflammation. Eating enough omega-3 fats (1,000–5,000 mg per day) helps prevent cellular inflammation, which is what causes menstrual cramps, joint pain, breast pain, PMS, and a host of other problems.[67] (Note: Many pharmaceutical drugs, such as Celebrex and Advil, work in part by suppressing cellular inflammation from free radical damage and imbalanced eicosanoids.)

Omega-3 fats (found in fish and fish oil, egg yolks, dark green leafy vegetables, flaxseed and its oil, macadamia nuts and their oil, hemp seed oil, and sea algae) are essential for the optimal functioning of every cell membrane in the body. As a result, getting enough of this nutrient is highly beneficial to your immune system, cardiovascular system, brain, and eyes. A deficiency in omega-3 fats can lead to dry skin, cracked nails, brittle hair, fatigue, depression, memory problems, hormone imbalances, achy joints, arthritis, and a poor immune system. Hundreds of studies have shown the health benefits of increasing your intake of omega-3 fats while also decreasing refined carbohydrates, saturated fats, trans fats, and omega-6 fats.

A body of evidence suggests that our current epidemic of heart disease began in the last eighty years, when partially hydrogenated fats (trans fatty acids), the foods containing them, and refined foods devoid of antioxidant vitamins were introduced into the mainstream diet. Trans fats are not found in nature, so our bodies haven't evolved to deal with them. Produced instead by a chemical process in which hydrogen is added to naturally occurring polyunsaturated fat at extremely high temperatures, these fats are solid at room temperature and have an extremely long shelf life (making them useful for margarine, as well as just about every processed food product you can think of, including cookies, crackers, baked goods, and even baby formula). Processed foods containing trans fats often replace foods in which naturally occurring essential fatty acids are found, such as almost all unprocessed nuts, whole grains, and many vegetables.

BENEFITS OF "GOOD" FATS

⁓ People with higher blood levels of omega-3 fats have lower BMIs, narrower waists, and smaller hip circumferences. In fact, cell membranes of overweight and obese people are nearly 14 percent lower in omega-3 fats than are those of people with healthy weights.[68]

⁓ Omega-3 fatty acids (in the form of fish oil supplements) lower cholesterol better than the statin drugs[69] and also lower triglyceride levels.[70] Several prospective cohort studies have found an inverse association between fish consumption and risk of cardiovascular disease.[71] Essential fatty acids also decrease hardening of the arteries by reducing the "stickiness" of blood cells, so they cling less to artery walls.[72]

⁓ Other studies have shown that the essential fatty acids can moderate the cancer-causing effects of radiation and certain chemicals because of their ability to balance inflammatory chemicals.[73] The right dietary oils may also help inhibit the development of breast and other forms of cancer by regulating immune system function in the body.[74]

⁓ Omega-3 fats (particularly DHA) support brain function. Studies have shown that sufficient amounts of DHA for fetuses and infants have been linked to higher IQs, while deficiencies have been associated with learning disabilities such as attention deficit/hyperactivity disorder (ADD, ADHD) and dyslexia.

⁓ DHA can stabilize your moods. Deficiencies are a contributing factor to depression, postpartum depression, preeclampsia, and various postmenopausal conditions.

⁓ Fish oil supplements have been shown to be effective in supporting healthy joints.[75]

⁓ Omega-3 fats increase the feeling of fullness after eating a meal.[76]

⁓ Essential fatty acids can lessen the symptoms of autoimmune diseases. Multiple sclerosis patients in one study who remained on a diet high in naturally occurring essential fatty acids and low in saturated fats had only minimal disability for as long as thirty years. But for patients who discontinued this therapeutic diet, their disease was reactivated and their symptoms increased dramatically.[77]

~ Fish oil has been shown to lessen menstrual cramps even in those who didn't change other aspects of their diets.[78]

~ Research from Italy indicates that taking fish oil may lessen the frequency and severity of hot flashes by 25 percent over twenty-four weeks.[79]

~ Studies show that fish oil's anti-inflammatory properties can help reduce the body's negative response to psychological stress.[80]

RISKS OF "BAD" FATS

~ Partially hydrogenated fats are associated with higher cancer rates than are saturated fats.[81]

~ These artificial fats inhibit normal fatty acid metabolism in our bodies, decrease HDL (the good cholesterol), and increase LDL (the bad stuff), increasing the chance for heart disease.

~ Excess trans fatty acids (as well as sugar, cortisol, alcohol, and inadequate levels of magnesium, zinc, vitamin B_3, vitamin B_6, and vitamin C) inhibit the conversion of essential fatty acids to cellular hormones that are needed for the optimal health of the female body. This can result in water weight gain (edema), increased blood clot formation, arthritis, and increased uterine cramps and pelvic pain.[82]

~ Diets that are high in trans fats and omega-6 fats have been found to significantly alter insulin efficiency and glucose response and to contribute to insulin resistance. These types of fats have also been found to increase the accumulation of storage triglyceride in skeletal muscles (leading to marbling). Marbling of skeletal muscles leads directly to insulin resistance in these muscles, and it also reroutes triglycerides directly to abdominal fat storage sites. In order to burn glucose effectively, the cellular membrane must be flexible. Cell membranes consist of the kind of fat we eat. The more "unsaturated" a cell membrane, the more effectively glucose is utilized and the better our overall health. (Remember, the cell membrane is the "brain" of the cell—and it must be flexible and be composed of the right fats in order to function optimally. The more saturated and "stiff" the membrane, and the more trans fats are incorporated into it, the more deleterious the effect on insulin efficiency and other cell functions as well.)

Fat is not the enemy it has been made out to be in the last fifty years or so. When sugar and insulin levels are kept normal and the diet is adequate in the right balance of omega-3 and omega-6 fats and micronutrients, then there's no need to worry about the impact of your fat intake on overall health. By the way, olive oil is an omega-9 fat, which has a neutral effect. And virgin coconut oil, which is a medium-chain fatty acid, has been found to have many health benefits, including an ability to fight infection.[83] Using organic coconut oil in cooking can be a very healthy part of your diet. Avocados and avocado oil are other good sources of healthy fats. You can safely use some butter and some saturated fat in your diet, too. But everyone needs to severely limit their intake of foods that include large amounts of refined carbs combined with large amounts of fat, such as macaroni and cheese, doughnuts, and pastries.

Calories Count, but Don't Count Them

Though calories do count in a broad general way, using the calorie counts of foods to determine what to eat completely ignores how food is metabolized in the body for optimal health. Though you may be able to lose weight on 1,200 calories a day from bread and pasta, your body won't be able to build the lean muscle mass you need to burn fat efficiently, and your body—in response to the insulin levels generated to metabolize the starch— will tend to go into conservation mode.

Get Enough Sleep

There's a connection between getting enough sleep and maintaining a healthy weight. A study published in 2005 by Columbia University psychotherapist James Gangwisch, Ph.D., found that those who sleep four hours a night or less are 73 percent more likely to be obese than people who sleep seven to nine hours each night.[84] Those who got five hours of sleep were 50 percent more likely to be obese, and those who got six hours were 23 percent more likely to be obese. One explanation is that when you don't get enough sleep, your body produces less leptin (a hormone that signals the body that you're full) and more ghrelin (a hormone that tells the body you're hungry). This delivers a one-two punch: The higher levels of ghrelin make you feel hungrier, but the lower levels of leptin keep you from feeling satisfied. (Leo Galland, M.D., wrote a book called *The Fat Resistance Diet* [Broadway Books, 2005] to specifically address fighting leptin resistance for weight loss.)

Sleep is also, hands down, the most effective way to quell free radical damage to the body and restore the tone of the parasympathetic system (which promotes rest and restoration). For many years it was my go-to medicine—exactly what my body required to recover from my many years of night call. I could easily sleep for twelve hours straight, and sometimes more, especially after traveling across time zones or doing lectures and book signings that lasted beyond 10:00 P.M. The important thing was that I allowed my body to get this sleep. And now, years later, I feel quite rested on the normal eight hours of sleep. But if I need more, I take it—with no guilt whatsoever.

Step Ten: Ensure Optimal Nutrition

For more than twenty-five years, I've recommended nutritional supplements to my patients, friends, and family, and I have taken them regularly myself. There is a profound shift going on in the scientific community concerning nutrition. We're now realizing that there's a huge difference between adequate nutrition (enough to prevent deficiency diseases) and optimal nutrition (the amount that results in peak function).

Nutritional supplements bridge the gap between adequate and optimal nutrition. And this is what really makes a difference. Today, we're living longer, and we all want to be active and healthy into our seventies, eighties, and even nineties. Receiving the right amount of nutrients from food sources and nutritional supplements can help everyone achieve this goal. The Recommended Dietary Allowances (RDAs) were first established in 1941 by the Food and Nutrition Board (FNB) and have been updated only a few times in the last sixty years. At the time, the board looked at large populations to determine how to prevent diseases due to gross vitamin deficiencies. Based on their studies, the FNB set the RDA for vitamin C at 60 mg—the amount needed every day to prevent scurvy—and determined the RDA for vitamin D to be 400 IU (international units)—the amount required to prevent rickets. While it seems obvious that those levels are antiquated by today's standards, many still hold on to the belief that you can get all the nutrition you need from a healthy diet. Although you were meant to get the nutrients your body needs from what you eat, it's nearly impossible to do so today—even if you eat a diet of whole foods with lots of organic fruits and vegetables. That's because over the last sixty-five years, the soil has been depleted of nutrients—especially minerals—due to overfarming, chemical fertilization, and other practices. As a result, the nutritional value of many foods has declined. In addition, our fruits and vegetables are rarely eaten straight from the garden. Instead, they're picked, shipped, and stored—losing nutrients along the way. (One of the reasons that the food tastes so good in Italy and France is that produce tends to be picked at the height of freshness and eaten very soon thereafter!)

Nowadays, we're also exposed to many more environmental hazards, including pollution, pesticides, and chemicals in cleaning products. Your body must detoxify these assaults—and it requires the right nutrients to get the job done properly. Toxins that remain in the body can cause a variety of health problems and lead to DNA damage. When the DNA in your cells is altered, your risk of chronic degenerative diseases (such as heart disease, certain cancers, arthritis, macular degeneration, osteoporosis, and Alzheimer's) increases significantly. Studies have shown that taking the right nutrients can protect you from this type of cellular damage.[85] Although the RDA classifications are still used as the basis for nutritional supplements (not to mention being upheld by many mainstream medical organizations), the emphasis at the FNB has changed over the last few years. They're now looking at nutrition as a way to reduce the risk of chronic disease, as opposed to just preventing vitamin and mineral deficiencies. Focusing on optimal versus adequate nutrition is a giant step in the right direction, since there can be a huge difference between the two.

Vitamins and minerals, also known as micronutrients, can help do all of the following:

- Enhance your immune system[86]

- Reduce oxidative stress and damage from free radicals

- Support healthy brain function

- Protect your cardiovascular system and lower risk of death from heart disease[87]

- Lessen joint pain and enhance the health of your bones and joints

- Promote radiant skin and prevent wrinkling

- Increase your metabolism and help stabilize blood sugar

- Support your vision

A good supplement provides nutritional support in four basic categories: antioxidants, omega-3 fats, B vitamins, and minerals. (See the table on page 915 for a list of important nutrients from each category.) Providing specific information for every vitamin or mineral on this list would take an entire library, but I will cover the basics.

Antioxidants

Sometimes referred to as "antiagers," antioxidants help protect the body at the cellular level by ridding it of free radicals. Free radicals are unstable molecules that are released when you eat poorly, are under considerable amounts of stress, and are exposed to environmental pollutants, as well as through normal body functions. To understand free radical damage, just imagine some apple slices that are left on the counter for a couple of hours. They turn brown—that's free radical damage. But if you add lemon juice right after you slice them, the antioxidant activity of the lemon juice prevents the browning effect. Same goes with guacamole!

Smoking of all kinds (including marijuana), drinking alcohol, taking drugs, consuming caffeine, and eating high-glycemic-index foods are all stressful for the body and produce free radical damage. If left unchecked, free radicals can damage cell membranes and change the way DNA is expressed, thus accelerating aging and putting your health at risk. The most common antioxidants are vitamins A, C, and E, although there are many others, including glutathione, coenzyme Q_{10}, and alpha lipoic acid. One of my all-time favorites is oligomeric proanthocyanidins (OPC). Often called pycnogenol, it's made from grape seeds or pine bark. Many people have taken it successfully to reduce arthritis symptoms because of its anti-inflammatory properties. And since OPC enhances the suppleness of collagen throughout the body, it's also good for hair, skin, and nails. Antioxidants work together synergistically—thus OPC also boosts the body's vitamin E levels, which can thwart free radical damage, such as oxidation of LDL (bad) cholesterol. (See the box that follows for a note on vitamin E.) This in turn helps protect the cardiovascular system and boost the immune system.

Cancer patients undergoing chemotherapy are typically told to stop taking antioxidants because it's thought that they interfere with chemotherapy's effectiveness, although several studies show that on the contrary, antioxidants may indeed *enhance* chemotherapy, while also helping to lessen the side effects.[88]

For those who have inflammation problems, start off with approximately 1 mg of OPC per pound of body weight in divided doses throughout the day. For example, a 140-pound woman would start with about 140 mg of OPC (40–50 mg three times per day with meals) for two weeks to load the tissues. (Tablet size varies, so shoot for a daily loading dose that's within 20–30 mg of your total weight in pounds.) After that, you can reduce the dose to 30–90 mg per day. Take more or less depending upon the amount your body requires. (Many brands of OPC are available at natural food stores. I use Proflavanol brand from USANA Health Sciences.)

VITAMIN E IS SAFE AND IMPORTANT

A 2005 study presented at the American Heart Association meeting in New Orleans by Edgar Miller, III, M.D., Ph.D., and coworkers received a totally overblown amount of publicity and scared people into thinking that vitamin E isn't safe. Just the opposite is true. Dr. Miller's study, which was a meta-analysis of previous studies—many of which were small and dissimilar—suggested that high-dose vitamin E supplementation may increase mortality in adults.[89] Many studies that could have been included in the analysis were eliminated because total mortality rates were low. And many of the studies that were included were conducted with older adults who already had advanced chronic degenerative disease. In other words, most studies that Dr. Miller included were not conducted on normal, healthy adults. And he left out many of the studies showing the most benefit for vitamin E! Many of the studies he did include were small, involving fewer than a thousand people. More important, only the smaller studies showed significant adverse effects. None of the larger (and therefore more powerful) studies, involving several thousand subjects each, showed a statistically significant impact on mortality of vitamin E supplementation. Moreover, the researchers' secondary analysis showed that differences in death rates were statistically insignificant, and that at the highest dose, risk of death was actually lower!

This is a perfect example of how the mainstream media manipulates scientific data in confusing ways. Years of clinical research have shown that vitamin E supplementation is effective and safe.[90] For example, the famous Nurses' Health Study, which involved thousands of women over many years, showed that vitamin E from supplementation (but not from food) reduced the risk of heart attack by 30 percent.[91] In the Iowa Women's Health Study, it was associated with a significant reduction in bowel cancer.[92] Vitamin E has also been shown to reduce the risk of dementia.[93] And a recent study from Tufts showed that this powerful antioxidant slows the development of cataracts.[94] Vitamin E should be part of a comprehensive supplementation program.

It's well worth noting the huge discrepancy between the different nutritional guidelines for these powerful substances. For example, the government's RDAs for the antioxidants vitamin C (75–90 mg), vitamin E (15 mg), and selenium (0.055 mg) total only about 100 mg a day. But if you follow the advice of the most current USDA dietary guidelines suggesting we eat a classic Mediterranean-style diet rich in fruits and vegetables (five to nine servings daily), whole grains, legumes, and nuts, you'd be consuming roughly 1,500 mg of these antioxidants each day. However, taking into consideration all the current research, the total amount of the various antioxidants we need daily for optimal health is at least 2,000 mg.[95]

Omega-3 Fats
See page 892.

B-Complex Vitamins

The right levels of B vitamins can bolster your energy level and stamina. Women who take birth control pills or hormone therapy, who are under a lot of stress, or who experience hormonal changes are likely to require additional B vitamins. The liver needs this nutrient to metabolize hormones. When estrogen isn't metabolized properly, too much of it stays in the bloodstream, especially in relation to progesterone levels, resulting in estrogen dominance. Estrogen dominance leads to an imbalance of the neurotransmitters norepinephrine, serotonin, and dopamine, which makes you prone to anxiety, nervous tension, and PMS symptoms. In addition, B vitamins support the adrenal glands, which are often strained during stressful periods.[96]

Over the past ten years, we've learned a lot about the benefits of folic acid, one of the B vitamins. It's one of the B's that helps metabolize hormones in the liver. It also can support cardiovascular health by lowering homocysteine levels.[97] Many individuals are genetically predisposed to having high homocysteine levels, an independent risk factor for heart disease, and taking enough folic acid (800–1,000 mcg a day) effectively metabolizes homocysteine and eliminates risk.[98] Perhaps more important, 800 mcg a day can help prevent birth defects, such as cleft lip, spina bifida, and neural tube defects, when taken before conception. It's important to take folic acid with the other B vitamins because they work synergistically. Along this same line, research has shown that taking multivitamins prior to conception significantly reduced the risk of prematurity. It also enhances fertility.[99]

A body of literature suggests that about 15 percent of the population is unable to methylate folic acid properly. In functional medicine circles, a huge emphasis is placed on this. Genomic testing can determine if you're in this group; I've had it done and I am apparently one of those who have a problem with this. However, I have never had a problem with regular folic acid. For certain people, though, taking methylated folate can make a big difference. But that doesn't mean that regular folic acid is a health risk—which is what some are led to believe.

Minerals

A variety of minerals, but especially calcium and magnesium, are typically associated with bone health, but they're responsible for so much more. Magnesium, for example, can mitigate neuromuscular pain, lessen the severity and frequency of migraines, and keep your heart healthy. (See "The Wonders of Magnesium," page 906.) Further, copper and selenium support the immune system, chromium and vanadium can help stabilize blood sugar, and manganese can boost the antioxidant process. Of course, calcium is needed for strong bones, but it doesn't act effectively on its own. It needs to be taken along with all the other bone-building minerals, including magnesium, boron, zinc, manganese, and copper. Enough vitamin D must also be present. Most menstruating women need iron. Craving ice is a sign of deficiency. I know—I used to have this symptom! The usual amount of iron to take is 30 mg per day, and this is especially important during pregnancy. The mineral chromium has been found to increase the metabolic rate. Chromium is in short supply in nine out of ten American diets, and it is absolutely essential for normal insulin function.[100] Ingestion of 200 mcg of chromium daily has been shown to support optimal blood sugar.[101] Sometimes it is necessary to increase chromium up to 1,000 mcg per day in problem cases. Look for it in the form of chromium polynicotinate.

THE ELEMENT IODINE AND HEALTHY THYROID FUNCTION

Healthy metabolism and optimal thyroid function go hand in hand. Many women have thyroid problems due to iodine deficiency and don't know it. When iodine levels are ideal (which you can reach by taking between 3 and 12.5 mg of iodine per day, either in drops, in tablets, or by eating iodine-rich seaweed), metabolism and thyroid function often normalize on their own. If you are taking iodine as a supplement, you also have to make sure that you are getting selenium (200 mcg per day is a good target amount). However, some women will still need supplemental thyroid hormone. In many cases, supplementing with only T4 (Synthroid) is not enough. You also need T3. You get this by taking prescription thyroid medication containing both T3 and T4 (e.g., Nature-Throid or Armour Thyroid) or by having a compounding pharmacy provide you with the right balance. Many women are able to restore optimal thyroid function through dietary change and taking TG 100 Natural Glandulars by Allergy Research Group (available at www.allergyresearchgroup .com or on Amazon).

When you have your thyroid function tested, your TSH should be 3.0 or below, although some experts (including myself) recommend a limit of 2.5. Higher levels indicate subclinical hypothyroidism. Likewise, if your free T3 and free T4 levels are in the very low range of normal, you might need thyroid supplementation. (See chapter 14, and also the discussion of iodine in chapter 10.)

Calcium and the Dairy Foods Question

My siblings and I didn't drink bottled milk growing up and my children didn't drink it, either, which many authorities would have you believe meant that we didn't get adequate calcium. When my sister once told a pediatrician friend that my children didn't drink milk, her response was, "They'll die." This is not a scientific evaluation. It is pure emotion, and a typical response.

My children were breast-fed until almost age two. Human milk, a living, dynamic food, is designed for the optimal growth and development of baby humans. Cow's milk, very different in composition from human milk, is designed for the optimal growth and development of baby cattle. Children are bigger today than they used to be. Cow's milk produces rapid growth in children, just as it does in cattle. This is one of the reasons why the American children of relatively small immigrants are so much bigger than their parents. In this country we associate bigger with better.[102]

But conventionally produced milk can be a problem food for many children and adults. The late Frank Oski, M.D., former chief of pediatrics at Johns Hopkins Medical School, published a great little book entitled *Don't Drink Your Milk* (Mollica Press, 1983), which documented the link between dairy foods and allergy, eczema, bed-wetting, and ear infections in children.[103] Countless children are needlessly treated with antibiotics for repeated ear infections that would go away if they were taken off dairy foods. Dr. Oski's honesty about the adverse health effects of dairy foods is a much-appreciated contribution. Since you will find so little cultural support for removing conventionally produced milk from the diet of your children, it is helpful to have good information.

Over the years, I have seen many problems associated with dairy foods: benign breast conditions, chronic vaginal discharge, acne, menstrual cramps, fibroids, chronic intestinal upset, and increased pain from endometriosis. Consumption of dairy foods has been implicated in both breast and ovarian cancers.[104] I can't help but think that there might be some correlation between overstimulation of the cow's mammary glands, through the use of certain hormones intended to increase milk production, and subsequent overstimulation of our own. Nursing babies as well as their mothers are affected by what the mothers eat. They sometimes develop symptoms of cow's milk allergy when their mothers are consuming a lot of cow's milk.

Like most Americans, I was taught that milk was necessary for getting enough calcium, even though three-quarters of the world's population manages to maintain health without drinking milk after infancy. (Many do, however, consume other kinds of dairy foods, usually fermented forms, such as cheese and yogurt, often made from sheep's or goat's milk.) Stopping dairy foods or substituting organically produced dairy foods often improves menstrual cramps, endometriosis pain, allergies, sinusitis, and even recurrent vaginitis. Because an entire generation of baby boomers has been raised on cow's milk instead of human milk, the cow at some deep level is now associated with "mother" and "nourishment." The very notion of eliminating dairy products causes heart palpitations in some people; they cannot conceive of living without milk.

By contrast, dairy foods produced organically, without bovine growth hormone and antibiotics, have a very different effect on the body. Some of my patients with gyn problems related to dairy have had complete remission of these problems when they have switched to organically produced (and often raw) milk products, which are now widely available. One of my community members in Indiana even went so far as to buy a milk cow for her family's milk supply. They have no health problems at all. On the other hand, some people continue to have an allergic-type reaction even to organic cow's milk.

People often wonder, "If I don't drink milk, where will I get my calcium?" Though milk is generally a good source of calcium, there are non-dairy sources as well—for example, dark green leafy vegetables such as kale, collard greens, and broccoli. These sources of calcium can be just as effective for bone health.[105] Most of the world's population, including inhabitants of China, which has almost no breast cancer and no osteoporosis in rural areas, gets its calcium from greens. Studies also show that while the Chinese consume only half the calcium of Americans, osteoporosis is uncommon in China despite an average life expectancy of about seventy-six years—only two years less than ours.[106]

African Bantu women eat no dairy foods, but they consume 150 to 400 mg of calcium daily through the foods they do eat. This is half the amount of calcium consumed by the average American woman. Yet osteoporosis is essentially unknown among the 10 percent of female Bantus who reach more than sixty years of age. Genetic protection was considered the reason but has been ruled out: When relatives of these same Bantu people migrate to more affluent societies and adopt rich diets, osteoporosis and diseases of the teeth become more common.[107]

The current recommended daily allowance (RDA) for calcium in the United States is 1,000 mg a day for women age nineteen to fifty and 1,200 mg a day for women age fifty-one and older. Fully 50 percent of American women do not consume this RDA and are thus at increased risk for osteoporosis. The average Chinese, who has a very low risk of osteoporosis, consumes 328 mg of calcium each day.[108]

The calcium supplement and dairy industries have been so effective at offering us an osteoporosis "fix" that we think we can reduce the complexity of bone physiology to a formula as simple as taking calcium pills. But bone is affected by a whole host of factors (see chapter 14), and bone health is profoundly affected by our daily food and exercise choices. Caffeine, alcohol, sugar, and tobacco also have a negative effect on bone health and contribute to osteoporosis. With lifestyle improvement on all levels, our bones would stay healthy on relatively less calcium, as long as we also exercised, cut back on refined foods, and got enough vitamin D.

Update on Vitamin D

The most recent research reveals that calcium is virtually useless without enough vitamin D, which plays a crucial role in maintaining bone health. Studies now show that women with osteoporosis typically have less vitamin D in their systems than women with healthy bones. In fact, the RDA of this vitamin (600 IU per day for women ages eighteen to seventy) is not even half the amount that is actually necessary to maintain optimal bone health!

By the way, the benefits of vitamin D go way beyond helping you achieve healthy bones. The Vitamin D Council, a nonprofit educational organization, reports on its website (www.vitamindcouncil .org) that current scientific research "has implicated vitamin D deficiency as a major factor in the pathology of at least 17 varieties of cancer as well as heart disease, stroke, hypertension, autoimmune diseases, diabetes, depression, chronic pain, osteoarthritis, osteoporosis, muscle weakness, muscle wasting, birth defects, periodontal disease, and more." (A 33 percent reduction in type 2 diabetes has been reported in those taking 800 IU of vitamin D a day plus calcium, as well as a 78 percent reduction in type 1 diabetes in children taking 2,000 IU a day in the first year of life).[109] Vitamin D deficiency has been linked with bacterial vaginosis, a vaginal infection associated with premature birth.[110] Researchers have also found a correlation between higher vitamin D levels and reduced risk of being overweight, although vitamin D supplements haven't been found to promote weight loss except in those on very low-calorie diets.[111] A 42 percent reduction in multiple sclerosis has been reported for women taking more than 400 IU of vitamin D a day.[112] There's even research showing that vitamin D can ward off influenza.[113] The public health organization Grass Roots Health (www.grassrootshealth .net) has recently published a study showing that women whose vitamin D levels are in the optimal range (60 ng/ml or higher) have a 78 to 82 percent lower risk of breast cancer than those whose levels are in lower ranges.[114] Moreover, optimal vitamin D levels greatly reduce the incidence of preeclampsia, postpartum depression, and premature birth.[115]

To get adequate amounts of vitamin D, I recommend moderate, safe sunlight exposure. A thirty-minute sunbath over most of your body without sunscreen will provide 10,000 IU of vitamin D, but most people don't get outside enough and leave too little skin exposed to the sun when they do. For the average Caucasian living in the United States, exposing the hands, face, and arms for fifteen to twenty minutes to midmorning or late-afternoon sun three days a week provides sufficient UVB radiation to produce vitamin D during the months of March through October. For those who live from about Washington, D.C., north (from latitudes around the mid-30 degrees and higher), an eight- to ten-minute sunbath in a tanning booth once a week will provide you with adequate UVB radiation to make vitamin D during the winter months. Women who live nearer to the equator will have an easier time meeting their vitamin D needs from sunlight. I also recommend taking vitamin D supplements (absorption is higher if you take the supplement with a meal containing some fat) and getting your vitamin D level checked as a baseline. Optimal blood levels are between 40 and 100 ng/ml. If your levels are low, you may need to start by taking 5,000 to 10,000 IU per day. Once you reach a healthy level, you can maintain it by taking anywhere from 2,000 to 5,000 IU a day depending on sun exposure.[116]

The famous Women's Health Initiative Study on calcium and vitamin D supplementation showed that women who took both calcium and vitamin D experienced a 29 percent reduction in the risk of hip fracture over a period of seven years as compared with the placebo group, but no decrease in vertebral fractures—which may have been because study participants took 1,000 mg of calcium per day and only 400 IU of vitamin D, which most experts believe is not a high enough dose. The other limitation to the study was the fact that most women didn't start taking the supplement until they were over sixty years old—after many had probably already lost considerable bone mass.[117] Though there was an increased risk of kidney stones in those who took the calcium, that would probably have been greatly reduced by including adequate magnesium to balance the calcium. (For more about the importance of vitamin D and also sunlight, read *Dr. Lani's No-Nonsense Sun Health Guide: The Truth About Vitamin D, Sunscreen, Sensible Sun Exposure and Skin Cancer* [Turner Publishing, 2019] by Lani Simpson, D.C.; also see the discussion of vitamin D in chapter 10, page 435.)

Bone health is affected by many factors other than calcium.[118] Television advertising promotes the use of antacids because of their calcium content. But antacids such as Tums (calcium carbonate) decrease the acidity of the stomach, which can lead to decreased absorption of calcium, since hydrochloric acid in the stomach is necessary for assimilation of calcium.[119] Given that studies have shown that about 40 percent of postmenopausal women are already deficient in stomach acid, using an antacid such as Tums to supplement calcium doesn't make sense. In addition, it has been shown that people with insufficient stomach acid can absorb only about 4 percent of an oral dose of calcium given as calcium carbonate, while a person with normal stomach acid can absorb about 22 percent. Those with low stomach acid secretion need a soluble, ionized form of calcium such as calcium citrate, succinate, malate, aspartate, or fumarate.[120] Also, the strong alkaline nature of carbonate combined with the calcium that is absorbed can set the stage for kidney stones, especially if milk products are a regular part of the diet. Calcium citrate can act as a good antacid if you need one, even though it isn't marketed as such.

Colas and root beer also contribute to osteoporosis, because the coloring agent and the phosphoric acid used in these drinks interfere with calcium metabolism.[121] Depression is also a significant contributor to osteoporosis because high levels of epinephrine and cortisol, produced by the adrenal glands in greater quantities in depressed individuals, can increase calcium loss in the urine and also cause breakdown of bone.[122]

The best approach to building bone health is a holistic one in which we look at all the dietary, environmental, and genetic factors related to osteoporosis development and improve those areas in which we have some control. (See chapter 14.) Note the following points about calcium sources:

~ The nutritional content of food is dependent upon where the food was grown, when it was harvested, the quality of the soil, and so on.

~ There can be wide variation in the mineral content of foods, depending upon soil mineralization.

~ Organically grown vegetables have higher nutritional content.

~ Calcium is only one of the minerals needed for optimal nutrition.

~ Nondairy sources of calcium are particularly rich in the other minerals needed for health. Some argue that plant oxalates, found in spinach and some other greens, interfere with calcium absorption. The same argument has been used for phytates in grain. Newer data suggest that this absorption issue has been highly overemphasized and is not very significant. So keep eating your spinach.

THE WONDERS OF MAGNESIUM

Magnesium requires its own section because it is so often overlooked and is so important for women's health. This mineral is in much shorter supply than calcium in our diets because of poor dietary choices (refined grains and too few dark green leafy vegetables), soil erosion, and overuse of chemical fertilizers instead of organic farming methods. I was first introduced to the wonders of magnesium during my obstetrical training, where I saw, up close and personal, how effective magnesium sulfate was in preventing seizures and restoring normal blood pressure in pregnant women suffering from toxemia. Years later, I often gave my patients magnesium intravenously (along with a series of other vitamins) as part of an IV mix known as the Myers formula (or Myers cocktail). I found that this mixture frequently relieved muscular pain and also helped speed healing from surgery, sprained ankles, and so on. It also appeared to boost immunity, which is why I often had a colleague give me an IV of it myself when I was coming down with something. Worked like a charm!

An astounding number of studies have documented the effectiveness of IV magnesium in helping prevent cardiac damage and even death following a heart attack. The reason for this is that 40 to 60 percent of sudden deaths from heart attack are the result of spasm in the arteries, not blockage from clots or arrhythmias.[123] And magnesium helps coronary artery muscles (and all other muscles) relax. Recent research also shows that higher magnesium intake is associated with healthier insulin levels (which affects heart health).[124] Carolyn Dean, M.D., N.D., author of *The Magnesium Miracle* (Ballantine Books, 2003; most recently updated in 2017), reports that she's seen magnesium improve patients' PMS, painful periods, chronic fatigue, fibromyalgia, depression, and anxiety—not to mention improving their enjoyment of sexual pleasure. Dr. Dean notes that magnesium is necessary for between 700 and 800 enzyme systems in the body that control thousands of chemical interactions. No wonder it's so important!

Most of us don't require intravenous magnesium, of course. We can get all the benefits we need just by making sure that we have enough of it in our diets or through supplements. Here's what everyone needs to know about getting optimal benefits from this essential (but often overlooked) mineral.

Why We Need Enough Magnesium

Magnesium is essential for the functioning of 700 to 800 different enzyme systems in the body, particularly those that produce, transport, store, and utilize energy. Magnesium is essential for the following:

~ Protein synthesis. DNA and RNA in our cells require magnesium for cell growth and development.

~ Sparking of the electrical signals that must travel throughout the miles of nerves in our bodies (including our brain, heart, and other organs).

~ Normal blood pressure, vascular tone, transmission of nerve cell signals, and blood flow.

~ Functioning of all nerves and muscles.

~ Release and binding of adequate amounts of serotonin in the brain.

In short, living with suboptimal levels of magnesium is like trying to operate a machine with the power turned off.

The Magnesium/Calcium Connection

Though the role of calcium has received an enormous amount of attention, very few people realize that without its partner magnesium, calcium doesn't serve the body nearly as well as it should. In fact, too much calcium can actually impede magnesium's uptake and function, creating further imbalance. When it comes to building healthy bones, magnesium is as important as calcium and vitamin D!

Magnesium and calcium are designed to work together. For example, magnesium controls the entry of calcium into each and every cell—a physiological event that happens every time a nerve cell fires. Without adequate magnesium (which is also a natural calcium channel blocker) too much calcium gets inside the cell. This can result in muscle cramping, blood vessel constriction, migraine headache, and even feelings of anxiety.[125]

Magnesium also keeps calcium dissolved in the blood so that it won't produce kidney stones. In fact, taking calcium without magnesium for osteoporosis can actually promote kidney stone formation!

Magnesium Deficiency on the Rise

Up to 50 percent of Americans are deficient in magnesium.[126] There are a number of reasons for this:

~ **Food processing depletes magnesium,** and the vast majority of Americans eat mostly processed foods. When wheat is refined into white flour, 80 percent of the magnesium in the bran is lost; 98 percent is lost when molasses is refined into sugar. Similarly, magnesium is leached out of vegetables boiled in water or blanched before freezing them. Additives such as aspartame and MSG, as well as alcohol, also deplete magnesium stores.

~ **Indigestion and antacid use.** Insufficient stomach acid impedes magnesium absorption. Unfortunately, a refined-food diet is a potent recipe for indigestion. Antacids, the number one over-the-counter consumer drug in the United States, further deplete hydrochloric acid in the stomach.

~ **Conventional farming practices** have depleted magnesium and other minerals from much of the soil in which we grow produce.

~ **Medications.** Many drugs including common diuretics, birth control pills, insulin, tetracycline and other antibiotics, and cortisone cause the body to waste magnesium.

SELECTED FOODS RICH IN MAGNESIUM

Food	Mg per 100 grams (3½ ounces)
Kelp	760
Wheat bran	490
Wheat germ	336
Molasses	258
Dulse	220
Almonds	270
Peanuts	175
Collard greens	57
Cooked beans	37
Tofu	111
Millet	162

In general, organically grown whole grains and vegetables are rich in magnesium. So are good-quality sea salt and sea vegetables.

THE IMPACT OF MAGNESIUM DEFICIENCY

The following is a partial list of health conditions associated with magnesium deficiency. These conditions may be helped by increasing magnesium intake.

~ **Anxiety and panic attacks.** Magnesium helps keep adrenal stress hormones under control and also helps maintain normal brain function. In her book *The Magnesium Miracle* (which includes a foreword written by magnesium researchers Burton Altura, M.D., and Bella Altura, M.D., authors of more than a thousand research papers on this vital mineral), Dr. Dean points out that the rate of depression has gone up every decade since World War II. It's quite possible that this is related to magnesium depletion.

~ **Asthma.** Magnesium helps relax the muscles of the bronchioles in the lungs.

~ **Constipation.** Magnesium helps keep bowels regular by maintaining normal bowel muscle function. Milk of magnesia has been used for decades to help constipation.

~ **Diabetes.** Magnesium helps insulin transport glucose into the cell. Without this, glucose builds up in tissue, causing glycemic stress and damage.

~ **Heart disease.** Magnesium deficiency is common in those with heart disease. It's an effective treatment for heart attacks and cardiac arrhythmias.

~ **Hypertension.** Without adequate magnesium, blood vessels constrict and blood pressure increases.

~ **Infertility.** Magnesium can relax spasms in fallopian tubes that prevent the implantation of a fertilized egg in the uterus.

~ **Insomnia.** Magnesium helps regulate melatonin, a hormone essential for normal sleep and wakefulness cycles.

~ **Nerve problems.** Magnesium helps eliminate peripheral nerve disturbances that can lead to migraines, leg and foot cramps, gastrointestinal cramps, and so on.

~ **Obstetrical problems.** Magnesium can prevent premature labor (because it calms contractions) as well as eclampsia. It also greatly reduces the risk of cerebral palsy and SIDS in newborns.

~ **Osteoporosis.** Without magnesium, calcium may actually contribute to osteoporosis.

Still other conditions associated with magnesium deficiency include blood clots, bowel disease, cystitis, depression, detoxification, fatigue, hypoglycemia, kidney disease, migraines, musculoskeletal conditions, Raynaud's syndrome, and even tooth decay.

Supplementing with Magnesium

The ratio of calcium to magnesium in the diet for the majority of human history was 1:1, a ratio that's considered optimal. Anywhere from 1:1 to 2:1 is adequate (for example, 800 mg of calcium to 400 mg of magnesium). Unfortunately, today's diets contain an average of ten times more calcium than magnesium.

In addition to eating a nutritious diet, I recommend that you use supplements that contain magnesium. There's considerable variation among individuals as to the ideal amount of magnesium to take. Although for adult women, the Recommended Daily Allowance (RDA) for magnesium is 310–320 mg per day, here's what I recommend: With a calcium intake between 800 and 1,400 mg per day, add enough magnesium to balance it. For example, if you take 1,000 mg of calcium per day, you need at least 500–800 mg of magnesium. But start gradually. If you're healthy, start with 200 mg of magnesium twice a day. If you have any of the conditions mentioned in the box above, you may want to start higher: 500 mg twice a day. You'll know when you've reached your limit—you'll develop loose stools. It's best, of course, to take your magnesium in divided doses throughout the day. You can take it either on an empty stomach or with meals. You can also add Epsom salts (magnesium sulfate) to your baths. It's absorbed through the skin and will help replenish magnesium stores. (A great excuse to read a good book in the tub!)

Magnesium comes in many other forms. Magnesium oxide or chloride is fine, but chelated magnesium is preferred. Capsules usually contain 250–500 mg of magnesium. You can also use a calcium/magnesium supplement. Dr. Dean recommends angstrom magnesium, a form that is completely and instantly absorbed through the cell wall because of its incredibly tiny size. Because of its high absorption, the dose for this form is about ten times lower than most other types. (Another plus: If you have IBS, Crohn's disease, or colitis, you can safely use angstrom magnesium without affecting your bowels.) I highly recommend (and use) the ReMag and ReMyte formulations of Carolyn Dean, M.D., N.D., which you can take in water with a little natural salt. This gives you the benefits of excellent hydration as well as improved electrical conduction throughout your body. These supplements come with a dosing schedule: You start with a low amount and work up. She also sells a wonderful transdermal magnesium lotion (see www.rnareset.com).

Testing for proper levels of the nutrient is difficult (as Dr. Dean puts it, magnesium is "its own worst enemy") because its serum concentration is so low that it's hard to get an accurate picture of how much is in the whole body just by testing what's in the blood. Only 1 percent of the body's magnesium is in the blood, and the body will take it from bones and tissues if that level drops. That means that a blood test could easily show a normal reading, even when the rest of the body is very deficient.

If you want to learn more (and I think that everyone should), I recommend that you read Dr. Dean's *The Magnesium Miracle*. Quite frankly, this book should be in everyone's home library. The information could surely save your—or a loved one's—life! (Dr. Dean is also the medical director of

the Nutritional Magnesium Association; for more information about magnesium, visit the association's website at www.nutritionalmagnesium.org; see
also www.rnareset.com.)

YOU MAY BE BURNING MORE NUTRIENTS THAN YOU ARE GETTING

Whenever a woman tells me she's been getting good results from a
supplement for a while but then it suddenly seems to stop working,
it is generally because her stress level—and therefore her need for
more B vitamins and also magnesium—has increased. That is because the increased production and subsequent breakdown of stress
hormones (cortisol and epinephrine) via the liver actually require an
increase in specific nutrients as co-factors in the metabolic processes
involved. That is, her nutrient burn rate has increased. The following
kinds of stress increase your burn rate and therefore also increase
your need for additional B vitamins and magnesium (as well as some
other nutrients that work well with magnesium, such as vitamin D):

Physical stress: intense exertion or a new method of working out,
manual labor, lack of sleep, travel (particularly across time zones and
in airplanes or heavy traffic), bad weather, lack of sunlight
Chemical stress: drugs, alcohol, marijuana, caffeine, nicotine, environmental pollutants such as cleaning chemicals or pesticides
Mental stress: perfectionism, worry, anxiety, long work hours, visiting
with difficult family members, working with difficult colleagues
Emotional stress: anger, guilt, loneliness, sadness, fear, helplessness
Nutritional stress: food allergies, vitamin and mineral deficiency, suboptimal levels of vitamin D (see below)
Traumatic stress: injuries or burns, surgery, illness, infections, extreme
temperatures
Psycho-spiritual stress: troubled relationships, financial or career pres-
sures, challenges with life goals, spiritual alignment, or happiness

If any of these apply to your situation, do what you can to address and relieve the specific stresses that may be affecting you. This
alone will decrease your nutrient burn rate considerably. In the
meantime, pay particular attention to your intake of magnesium.
You can get plenty of magnesium by putting Epsom salts (magnesium sulfate) in your bathwater so your body can absorb it through
your skin. Add two cups to a warm bath and soak for twenty minutes at least three times per week. Lotions containing magnesium for

the skin can also be effective. Many different kinds of magnesium supplements are available. Most people need 800–1,000 mg/day. You can't overdose because any excess is eliminated in the stool. For additional magnesium information, see www.rnareset.com.

CREATING A SUPPLEMENTATION PROGRAM

When starting a supplementation program, a well-rounded approach is best. Some people mistakenly think that vitamins should be taken to treat a medical condition. For example, they read that vitamin E can help reduce the occurrence of breast cysts and their painful symptoms, so they take a bunch of vitamin E. This method equates to conventional medicine's practice of writing a prescription for a pharmaceutical drug to suppress your symptoms. Instead, start with a good foundation and add other supplements according to your individual needs. But take care not to distort the foundation. Think of it this way: Adding a little extra sugar to a cake may not change it significantly, but adding a whole lot will throw everything else out of proportion. Please understand that optimal supplementation requires at least four to five tablets or capsules per day. In other words, the "one-a-day" mentality is inadequate—you can't get optimal supplementation from one pill a day. (See Resources.)

Once you've found a balanced approach, stick with it for at least three months before switching to another product or adding additional supplements. Sometimes the results are dramatic; more often they're not so remarkable in the first few weeks. But over a period of six weeks to three months (sometimes up to six months), you'll notice that you've had fewer colds, that you recover much faster after strenuous activity, and that you just feel better as some of your minor complaints lessen or go away altogether. You may also experience more vitality and a better ability to "go with the flow." Often when you're feeling good, it's hard to remember how far you've come. Here's a tip for measuring your progress: Make a list of your complaints when you start your supplementation program and then review this list every three weeks. This is a great way to chart your advancement.

Tips for Choosing a Supplement

Check out the latest news on supplements provided by the Council for Responsible Nutrition at www.crnusa.org. Also consider the following tips:

⁓ Pick a high-quality supplement program from a manufacturer that meets Good Manufacturing Practice (GMP) standards. They use pharmaceutical-grade (as opposed to food-grade) ingredients to ensure quality and efficacy.

⁓ Good supplements cost money. Like organic produce, more expensive products represent the real price of high-quality nutrients.

⁓ Folic acid is an expensive ingredient. If your multivitamins contain 800 mcg or more of this nutrient (instead of 400 mcg), this is often an indication that the manufacturer isn't skimping on other ingredients in their product.

⁓ A formula with a combination of antioxidants, such as rutin, bioflavonoids, grapeseed extract, and olive extract, is often more effective than a product containing only one or two antioxidants.

⁓ Make sure that your supplement program has both natural vitamin E (d-alpha-tocopherol as opposed to dl-alpha-tocopherol) and tocotrienols. These are all part of the vitamin E family—and you get the most benefit when they're all present.

⁓ Always take a vitamin B complex, as opposed to just one or two of the Bs.

⁓ Choose chelated minerals when possible. These are wrapped in an amino acid when manufactured to ensure proper absorption.

⁓ If you're taking a well-balanced formula, you don't have to worry about megadosing.

Remember that supplements are not a substitute for a diet of whole, organic foods. The quality of the food you eat is still the cornerstone of good health! But more and more, research is clearly showing that a commitment to supplementing, day in and day out for your entire life, can make an amazing difference in your health. And remember the old saying "An ounce of prevention is worth a pound of cure."

Recommended Supplement Dosages

Here is my list of recommended daily supplements for adults. There really isn't that much difference between the nutritional needs of men and women (except for iron) unless a woman is pregnant or nursing. So these recommendations can also be used for the men in your life. (Note that this program will require about six tablets a day.)

TABLE 10

RECOMMENDED DAILY SUPPLEMENTATION

Vitamins	
Vitamin C	1,000–5,000 mg
Vitamin D_3	2,000–5,000 IU
Vitamin A (as beta-carotene)	25,000 IU
Vitamin E (as mixed tocopherols)	200–800 IU
Alpha-lipoic acid	10–100 mg
Coenzyme Q_{10}	10–100 mg

Omega-3 Fats	
DHA	200–2,500 mg
EPA	500–2,500 mg

B Complex Vitamins	(total of 1,000–5,000 mg)
Thiamine (B_1)	8–100 mg
Riboflavin (B_2)	9–50 mg
Niacin (B_3)	20–100 mg
Pantothenic acid (B_5)	15–400 mg
Pyridoxine (B_6)	10–100 mg
Cobalamin (B_{12})	20–250 mcg
Folic acid	1,000 mcg
Biotin	40–500 mcg
Inositol	10–500 mg
Choline	425 mg

Minerals (should be bound as amino acid chelates for optimal absorption)	
Calcium	500–1,200 mg
Magnesium	400–1,000 mg
Potassium	200–500 mg
Zinc	6–50 mg
Manganese	1–15 mg
Boron	2–9 mg
Copper	1–2 mg
Iron	15–30 mg
Chromium	100–400 mcg
Iodine	3–12.5 mg*
Selenium	50–200 mcg
Molybdenum	45 mcg
Vanadium	50–100 mcg
Trace minerals from marine sources	

* Please refer to iodine discussion in chapter 10.

OTHER COMMON CONCERNS

Can Diet Help Irritable Bowel Syndrome and Other Digestive Problems?

Many women have taken numerous courses of antibiotics for acne, urinary tract infections, and upper respiratory infections. Chronic use of antibiotics kills the normal bowel flora that are necessary for a healthy, functioning colon—a place in the body in which essential bacteria play an important role in nutrient absorption and manufacture. In addition, chronic use of aspirin and other nonsteroidal anti-inflammatory medicines, or NSAIDs—such as ibuprofen (the active ingredient in Advil)—has also been shown to affect both the stomach's and the intestines' physiological function. (One-half to two-thirds of patients who use NSAIDs chronically show evidence of inflammation of the small intestine.)[127] More than 56,000 emergency-room visits per year are due to acetaminophen overdoses; a hundred die annually from overdosing on this drug, which is also the leading cause of liver failure in the country.[128]

Because of our national penchant to overuse antibiotics and NSAIDs, to eat a refined-food diet, and to have a high-stress lifestyle, many women have digestive difficulties, such as chronic constipation, excess gas, frequent diarrhea, and lower abdominal distress. All of these conditions may result from an imbalance in normal intestinal bacteria, intestinal parasites of various kinds, overgrowth of intestinal yeast, and an increase of intestinal permeability (leaky gut syndrome). These conditions are collectively known as intestinal dysbiosis. Intestinal dysbiosis is often related to and may result in chronic vaginitis, migraines, arthritis, autoimmune diseases, and food allergy.

This problem is diagnosed either clinically, from symptoms such as chronic gas or diarrhea, or by sending stool cultures to a lab that specializes in this testing. Intestinal parasites are often diagnosed as well. As with nearly every other disease, chronic cellular inflammation is caused in part by a diet too high in refined carbohydrates and too low in nutrients, fiber, and omega-3 fats. So the first step—and often the only one necessary—is to follow the dietary guidelines outlined in this chapter. Additional supplements known as probiotics (as opposed to antibiotics) such as acidophilus and bifidobacteria, as well as digestive enzymes and hydrochloric acid, also often help restore normal bowel flora and get the yeast under control. A yeast-free diet is prescribed for some, but it has been my repeated experience that this type of rigorous dietary restriction is not necessary once your metabolism, emotions, supplement levels, and food choices become optimal. Once they do, the yeast—and often parasites as well, if present—will go away by themselves.

Another very common related problem, irritable bowel syndrome (IBS), often responds well to probiotics, dietary change, and enteric-coated peppermint. The last of these is available in natural food stores; I have prescribed Integrative Therapeutics' Mentharil or Nature's Way Pepogest peppermint oils with good success.[129] The newest research on IBS sheds more light on our understanding of this condition. Researchers at the University of California, Los Angeles, discovered an association between our gut microbiome and the regions of the brain involved in IBS.[130] They believe analyzing gut bacteria may become a routine screening technique for people with IBS, allowing doctors to tailor treatment with specific dietary recommendations and probiotics as well as recommendations for practices like mindfulness meditation, which have been shown to make changes in the brain regions associated with IBS. The researchers also found that those who suffered childhood trauma display structural and functional brain changes that alter the gut microbiome.

What About Food Allergies?

Intestinal dysbiosis is often accompanied by food allergies.[131] Many women are sensitive to certain foods, which can result in symptoms ranging from intestinal distress to weight gain. More than 90 percent of all food allergies are to dairy, gluten (found in wheat and other grains), corn, or eggs. Once you eliminate one or more of these, negative reactions to other foods often simply disappear. I've also noticed that allergies to cat fur also seem to disappear when individuals stop eating foods that they are allergic to, especially dairy. It appears that the cat allergy is triggered, in part, by the inflammation started by the original allergen.

There are a number of ways to diagnose food allergies, the most common being a blood test known as an IgG ELISA assay. This test should be ordered by a physician familiar with this type of testing and should be performed by a lab that specializes in it.[132] A special diet is then prescribed based on the results. Rather than go through all that, however, I recommend that you just eliminate all gluten, egg, and dairy products for a week and eat mostly lean proteins, fruits, and vegetables. You'll be amazed by how much better you feel. Then, after a week or so, add one of the food groups that you eliminated and see what happens. Many people are amazed that their headaches, runny noses, and other "allergies" return immediately when they resume dairy, or gluten, for example.

Women with multiple food allergies that are resistant to simple dietary change often have a history of abuse of some type, or they are continuing to live in dysfunctional relationships or to stay in overly stressful jobs. When this is the case, dietary change alone won't address the problem over the long term. There is a dramatic synergy between lifestyle choices, stress, and the parts of the immune system that maintain bowel and vaginal health.[133] Supporting your body nutritionally while you learn to support yourself emotionally and psychologically can help enormously. Studies have shown that this normalizes immune system response. I refer to it as "replenishing the soil."

Nambudripad's Allergy Elimination Techniques, known as NAET, is a very effective method of clearing allergies of all types, including those to foods. NAET was developed by Devi Nambudripad, M.D., Ph.D. (who is also a licensed acupuncturist and chiropractor), who discovered through personal and clinical experience that allergies are often associated with certain physical, emotional, and nutritional patterns, all of which require reprogramming in order for them to be eliminated. Her technique uses a process known as kinesiology (muscle testing) to pinpoint the offending allergens and the accompanying emotional pattern, followed by stimulating specific acupuncture or acupressure points to clear the patterns from the body. Until the pattern is cleared, she recommends temporary elimination of the allergen as well. I have referred many patients to practitioners trained in NAET, and I highly recommend this revolutionary approach. (For more information, visit www.naet.com.)

Do I Have to Give Up Caffeine?

Caffeine is a very popular drug worldwide, perhaps the most popular. The average American drinks some thirty-two gallons of caffeinated soft drinks and twenty-eight gallons of coffee a year, and more than a thousand proprietary drugs list caffeine as an ingredient. Ninety-five percent of pregnant women consume caffeine during their pregnancies.[134]

Caffeine stimulates the central nervous system and affects the heart, skeletal muscles, kidneys, and adrenals. Because of the boost of adrenaline that comes from caffeine, it is associated with increased mental acuity initially. However, it may also result in rebound confusion once the effect has subsided. Caffeine also results in an increase in blood sugar followed by a rather sudden drop. When it's combined with a sweet pastry or other "white" food such as a bagel, the blood sugar drop is even worse—and is a setup for out-of-control cravings later in the day. In some women caffeine is a factor in breast pain and cysts. An occasional woman is so sensitive to it that one piece of chocolate (which contains both caffeine and theobromine, a related substance) will cause breast tenderness premenstrually during the month in which she eats that chocolate. Caffeine has also been implicated in cellular inflammation.

However, studies done since 2000 have shown that coffee, like wine, is not harmful in moderation. One of the latest such studies, done in Germany and published in 2018, showed that four cups of coffee a day is enough to signal the production of a protein that helps protect and repair the heart.[135] Once again, you need to consult your own body wisdom.

Sleep disorders often disappear when people stop using caffeine—and so does urinary frequency. Some studies have shown that the effects of caffeine on females may vary according to the level of estrogen in their system.[136] Even decaffeinated coffee can be a breast and bladder irritant for some. Some women are so sensitive that a cup of coffee in the morning will cause insomnia and even bladder symptoms that same night.

Here's a test to see if you're addicted to caffeine: Go without it for three days. If you get a headache, you are addicted. If you don't, it probably doesn't affect you much. Withdrawal from caffeine takes only two or three days. The headache and the fatigue that accompany this withdrawal, however, can be quite debilitating. I recommend that women plan to withdraw over a weekend, or whenever they have time to rest and nurture themselves in other ways. During caffeine withdrawal, drink plenty of water and three to four cups of chamomile tea per day. This tea is considered a "nervine" (nerve tonic) and helps maintain alertness. Many of my patients noted that their tolerance to caffeine decreased over the years. Those who have stopped caffeine and try it again often notice that the drug affects them quite dramatically.

Eliminating caffeine may be a step in the right direction for you. Certainly you will want to do this if you are planning a pregnancy.

Can I Have Diet Soft Drinks or Other Foods with Artificial Sweeteners?

Saccharin (found in the pink artificial sweetener packets), aspartame (in the blue packets), and sucralose (in the yellow packets) have all been associated with adverse health effects. The worst offender of the three is aspartame, a combination of two naturally occurring amino acids (aspartic acid and glutamic acid) that can be toxic when combined. These amino acids trigger nerve cells to fire, and although some nerve cell firing is needed for alertness, too much overstimulates them and causes them to release free radicals. This causes brain cell death. Aspartame consumption has been linked to headache, blurry vision, slurred speech, and memory loss. Some people are particularly susceptible to the toxic effects of aspartame. They include people who have the following conditions (or family histories of these conditions): neuropsychiatric challenges including depression, anxiety attacks, obsessive-compulsive symptoms, manic-depression, or schizophrenia; a history of head injury; blurred vision; memory loss; chronic fatigue syndrome or fibromyalgia; tinnitus (ringing in the ears); spasms, shooting pains, or numbness; attention deficit disorder or hyperactivity disorder; spinal cord injury; multiple sclerosis; Lou Gehrig's disease; migraine headaches; spinal disc problems; Parkinson's disease; or Alzheimer's disease. Many are reporting adverse effects from Splenda (sucralose) as well as saccharin. There's no need to use any of these anymore. The best noncaloric sweetener currently available is stevia, an all-natural sweetener from the stevia plant. Research shows stevia has "pharmacological and therapeutic properties, including antioxidant, antimicrobial, antihypertensive, antidiabetic, and anticancer."[137] I like NuStevia by NuNaturals (www.nunaturals.com). But stevia is also widely available as Truvia, which is also being used to sweeten noncaloric sodas. I predict that stevia will soon replace all other noncaloric sweeteners. I certainly hope so.

Can I Drink Alcohol?

Excessive alcohol consumption is associated with increased risk of breast cancer, menstrual irregularities, osteoporosis, and birth defects. I ask women who drink alcohol regularly to become conscious of why and how they are using alcohol. If they feel the need to have two or more drinks every single night "to relax" (whether at home or out), I seriously question that behavior. Meditation, listening to music, making love, or taking a long bath are good alternatives.

I point out that two drinks of alcohol at night effectively wipe out rapid eye movement (REM) sleep, the type of sleep associated with dreaming. Dreaming is part of your inner guidance system. Why wipe it out with alcohol? Having two drinks a day also increases the risk of breast cancer. In the Nurses' Health Study, for example, researchers found that the risk of breast cancer was 60 percent higher in those who had one or more drinks per day compared with those who didn't drink.[138]

The amount of alcohol a woman takes in has very little to do with whether she has a problem with alcohol. What determines an alcoholic is her relationship to alcohol. One of my patients realized that she felt much more comfortable when she had her bottle of sherry by her bedside. She rarely drank it, but she realized that if it wasn't there, she'd feel agitated. For that reason, she checked out a few Alcoholics Anonymous meetings and found that she did indeed have a tendency toward alcoholism. (Note: Alcohol abuse is common and begins early. The latest data from the University of Michigan's Monitoring the Future study show that 30 percent of twelfth graders have had at least one drink in the past month, and 14 percent had five or more drinks in a row at least once in the past two weeks.[139] This binge drinking gets worse in college.)

Many women hold the "cocktail hour" as a sacred ritual. When I suggest that they drink spring water or sparkling cider as an alternative, in order to see what effect the alcohol is having on them, the reaction I get gives me a few clues about their relationship to alcohol. One woman said, "But my husband

and I look forward to this hour. We have such fun we often forget to eat dinner." (!) Another said that she couldn't substitute a nonalcoholic drink for herself because if she did, "everyone else would start to look stupid." (Hmm-mmm.) On the other hand, having a single drink or a glass of wine at the end of the day can be a health-enhancing ritual of pleasure, as so beautifully illuminated by the work of Mario Martinez, Psy.D., in his studies of healthy centenarians, most of whom enjoy some kind of ritual of pleasure regularly.

Please be good to yourself. Examine your relationship to alcohol and make adjustments if necessary. If you feel you can't go without your evening wine or cocktail, you have a problem.

Note also that when you take in enough B vitamins, decrease sugar, and increase protein, you may find that your craving for alcohol decreases. Also, please remember that drinking alcohol dehydrates tissue. So make sure you follow your alcoholic drinks with some glasses of water with a pinch of natural salt. This will make up for the dehydrating effect.

CAGE SCREEN FOR DIAGNOSIS OF ALCOHOLISM

Doctors typically use the following screening tool to diagnose alcoholism. Two or three positive responses indicates a high suspicion, while four positive responses is considered diagnostic.[140]
Have you ever:

C Thought you should CUT back on your drinking?

A Felt ANNOYED by people criticizing your drinking?

G Felt GUILTY or bad about your drinking?

E Had a morning EYE-OPENER to relieve hangover or nerves?

A WORD ABOUT SMOKING

I Know I Should Stop Smoking . . .

I don't lecture smokers because they generally want to quit anyway. But sometimes a few facts help them to make the decision. The next time you start obsessing about something like swine flu, for example, think about these statistics:

~ More deaths are caused each year by tobacco use than by all deaths from HIV, illegal drug use, alcohol use, motor vehicle injuries, suicides, and murders combined, according to CDC statistics.[141]

~ Fortunately, the number of all eighth graders who smoke is steadily declining, with the rate for 2018 down by 90 percent over its recent peak in the mid-1990s.[142] However, tobacco companies have historically targeted adolescent girls as their number one market for cigarettes because this group has been found to have the lowest self-esteem and is therefore the most likely to start smoking as a result of peer pressure. In fact, the monthly rate of cigarette smoking for eighth-grade girls rose by more than 40 percent between 1991 and 1996, thanks in part to the effectiveness of the tobacco companies' advertising combined with girls' vulnerability . . . not to mention the desire to be thin!

~ While the number of teens who smoke has declined, it is still unacceptably high, and the use of e-cigarettes is dramatically rising. The latest data from the Monitoring the Future study shows that while just under 2 percent of eighth graders reported smoking traditional cigarettes at least once in the last month, 9.7 percent of twelfth graders had.[143] In 2018, almost 21 percent of high school students (and almost 5 percent of middle school students) said they'd smoked e-cigarettes at least once in the previous month.[144]

~ While the leading cause of death among all Americans remains heart disease, cancer is the leading cause of death among women ages forty-five through eighty-four—and the leading cause of cancer deaths for women is lung cancer, according to the Centers for Disease Control.

~ People who smoke are up to four times more likely to suffer blindness later in life from age-related macular degeneration than nonsmokers, according to a 2004 study published in the *British Medical Journal*.

~ Tobacco costs the American public more than $300 billion a year, including more than $156 billion in lost productivity and nearly $170 billion in direct healthcare expenditures (an average of more than $4,000 per adult smoker).[145]

~ One out of every five deaths in the United States is related to tobacco, which is the leading preventable cause of death in this country.[146]

~ Smoking increases the risk of stroke by 300 percent.

~ More than 16 million Americans have at least one serious illness caused by smoking. So for every person who dies of a smoking-related disease, at least thirty additional people suffer from at least one serious illness that is associated with smoking.[147]

~ Tobacco companies know that once hooked, females are less likely to quit than males.

⁓ Cigarettes are more addictive than heroin because taking smoke into the lungs immediately produces a profound drug effect in the brain. It's like mainlining the most addictive substance in the world. Some kids are hooked after only one cigarette.

⁓ More than 4,000 chemicals, including 200 known poisons such as DDT, arsenic, formaldehyde, and carbon monoxide, are housed in tobacco.

Smoking and Specific Women's Health Problems

The power of addiction and denial is nowhere more striking than the case of a pregnant patient who, despite a history of infertility, continues to smoke throughout her pregnancy. Consider the following data:

⁓ Smokers have a miscarriage rate that is twice as high as that of non-smokers. These miscarriages are often of genetically normal fetuses.

⁓ Infants whose mothers smoke run double the risk of dying of SIDS.[148] Secondhand smoke is also estimated to cause more than 202,000 asthma episodes and 790,000 pediatrician visits for middle ear infections.[149]

⁓ Smoking in pregnancy accounts for an estimated 20 to 30 percent of low-birth-weight babies, up to 14 percent of preterm deliveries, and some 10 percent of all infant deaths, according to the American Lung Association. Even full-term, healthy-looking babies of smokers have been found to have narrowed airways and reduced lung function at birth.[150]

⁓ Adult nonsmokers suffer from exposure to secondhand smoke as well, including 7,330 who die of lung cancer and 33,950 who die of heart disease annually in the United States.[151]

⁓ Smokers are at increased risk for cervical cancer, vulvar cancer, and abnormal Pap tests, possibly because smoking depletes vitamins C and A and beta-carotene, antioxidants that are somewhat protective against cancer.[152] Smoking literally poisons the ovaries.

⁓ Smoking ages the skin more quickly than normal.

⁓ As of 2012, lung cancer has passed breast cancer as the number one cancer killer of women. (You *have* come a long way, baby!)

⁓ Smokers are at increased risk for osteoporosis, premature aging, and heart disease.

Dr. Andrew Weil points out that there are tobacco leaves carved on the pillars of the Capitol in Washington, D.C.—testimony to the entwined interests of the government and the tobacco companies. Since the handwriting is on the wall for smoking in the United States, however, tobacco growers are now targeting the almost limitless market overseas in such places as China.

How to Quit Smoking

~ Know that every attempt at quitting increases your chances of success next time. Give yourself credit for trying. Remember that 50 million Americans have successfully become smoke-free.

~ For now, when you smoke, try to become very conscious of your smoking. Go outside, breathe in deeply, and pay attention to your lungs.

~ Ask your lungs for permission to smoke. Check in with this part of your body and see how it feels.

~ When you smoke, just smoke. Try to get as much pleasure from the cigarette as possible. The idea here, as with food, is to change your consciousness around smoking. Doing so will stop the "robot" approach that is the basis for this habit.

~ When you decide to quit, keep a smoking log for a week in which you write down where you smoked, when, whom you were with, and how you felt. This will help you identify your smoking "triggers."

~ Develop a list of alternative behaviors to smoking that you can have ready at your "trigger times." These may include taking five deep breaths, going for a short walk in the fresh air, eating some strongly flavored hard candy such as cinnamon, or drinking a glass of water.

~ Understand that when you stop smoking you won't just be giving up cigarettes, you'll also be giving up your identity as a smoker. That means that your entire social network, which is so often organized around smoking, will undergo changes. Because so many women are relational in nature, this part of smoking cessation may be the hardest part. When I look at the groups of smokers hanging around outside nonsmoking buildings these days, I see how bonded smokers, who may have nothing else in common, have become during their smoking breaks. One of my newsletter readers wrote, "The only reason I wanted to quit smoking was that I never knew where I could smoke anymore and I wanted to be considerate of others who are sensitive to smoke."

~ Prepare to feel fully. All addictions numb feelings. Smoking in particular shuts down the energy of your heart and makes it difficult to feel the depth of your passion and joy—even if it does temporarily help you feel less grief, anxiety, or anger. One newsletter subscriber who successfully quit said,

"I felt that smoking was numbing me in a certain way and that if feelings or parts of myself were numbed, then they were unavailable to me. I was ready to quit when I became unwilling to live any longer with missing parts or inaccessible feelings because they were numbed or smoke-screened. It took me a while to get there, but at that point it became more important to have all of me available to myself in life than to smoke."

~ Don't worry about weight gain. This is not an inevitable consequence of smoking cessation. The only reason women gain weight is that they are substituting one addiction for another. (The dictum to be thin is so great that many smokers would rather risk lung cancer and death than risk being overweight. A few very honest smokers have told me this.)

~ Get support. You can find a support group or smoking cessation program through almost any hospital. For referrals to local groups, you can also call the American Lung Association, 800-586-4872, www.lung.org; or the American Cancer Society, 800-227-2345, www.cancer.org. Smokers Anonymous, a twelve-step program, is available through AA (just look online for meetings in your area). Another good resource is Nicotine Anonymous (NicA), 877-879-6422, www.nicotine-anonymous.org. Also see the extensive information at the Foundation for a Smokefree America's website at www.anti-smoking.org.

~ Try hypnosis. I've been sending smokers for hypnosis for years—often with very good results.

~ Use acupuncture. Acupuncture and traditional Chinese medicine are known to be of benefit in helping with withdrawal from cigarettes and other addictive substances. In New York City, the March of Dimes and Columbia-Presbyterian Hospital advocate acupuncture-based treatment for addicted clients. One three-year study involving 2,282 cases demonstrated that acupuncture had a 90 percent success rate in a nicotine detoxification program.[153] Generally it takes only one treatment. An added benefit is that acupuncture lessens your chance of gaining weight after you stop.

If all else fails, try pharmacological help. Some women have been helped by nicotine gum or the nicotine patch; both are available over the counter and have been heavily promoted as a way to "taper off" smoking. The short-term success rate of each is comparable, and both work better when combined with psychological support. The data on long-term outcomes are mixed. My own preference is for the programs listed above. You want to get rid of nicotine in your system as soon as possible, and these simply draw out the process. If you do try them, follow the package directions precisely, or you could actually overdose on nicotine.

APPRECIATE THE ENERGY OF FOOD

The energy of food has emotional and psychological consequences. Foods aren't broken down completely into anonymous fats, carbohydrates, and proteins when they're digested—they retain some of their original energy.[154] Like humans, food is more than the sum of its parts. It is affected by the way it is raised, processed, handled, and cooked. In short, food has its own unique energy field, *prana,* or *chi.* In ancient monasteries, only the most enlightened monks were allowed to cook and handle the food, because it was felt that their energy field affected the food.

On a couple of trips to Italy, I have been simply amazed at how good the locally grown food tastes there. There is, of course, a rich food tradition in this area of the world. Food is locally grown on mineral-rich soils, harvested at the peak of freshness, and enjoyed in season among family and friends. Eating there is an entirely different experience from gulping fast food in the United States. I believe that this approach to food and eating, as much as anything else, is responsible for the healing benefits of the Mediterranean diet.

A number of studies have documented the link between food, behavior, and mood. Studies on schoolchildren and the observations of many parents have supported the fact that foods that are low in nutrients and high in sugar, caffeine, and food additives sometimes produce erratic behavior. Alexander Schauss has documented the link between diet, crime, and delinquency, showing the connection between diets high in sugar and preservatives and subsequent erratic behavior.[155] On the other hand, if you were sitting on a beach in Hawaii reading novels, you could eat almost anything you wanted and suffer few ill effects—even from foods that usually give you problems (provided, of course, that you like Hawaii and the beach). But when you're under stress, hurried, or unhappy, digestion and food assimilation are adversely affected because of the adverse effect of stress hormones on insulin, blood sugar, and digestive function. This link is important to understand.

Digestion, absorption, and assimilation of our food are also dependent upon our state of consciousness. So if you're eating brown rice and vegetables out of guilt or as a way to beat yourself up, chances are they won't have nearly the beneficial effects that they're capable of providing.

A now-famous study on heart and blood vessel disease was conducted at Ohio State University on rabbits. These rabbits were all genetically bred to develop atherosclerosis (hardening of the arteries) and coronary artery disease. The investigators fed the rabbits an atherogenic diet to speed up the disease process. At the end of the study, when the rabbits were sacrificed, the researchers found that more than 15 percent of the rabbits had almost no coronary artery disease—their arteries were clean. After much head-scratching, they discovered that the bunnies with the clean arteries were the ones whose cages were at waist level. The female graduate student who fed the rabbits used to take these ones out of their cages and pet and play with them awhile before their feeding.[156] This study has been repeated several times, mostly because no one could believe it initially, but the results were the same. Studies like this fly in the face of what we normally believe is going on. My advice: If you're going to eat doughnuts, get a massage—or pray over them first.

The pioneering work of the late Masaru Emoto of Japan, author of *The Hidden Messages in Water* (Beyond Words, 2004), has documented the remarkable effects that emotions have on the crystalline structure of water. Given that our bodies are 60 to 70 percent water (not to mention that one-half of the volume of each of our organs is water), and given that food is largely water as well, it behooves us to prepare and consume our food lovingly, as well as to give thanks for it—regardless of its quality. This alone can transform its effects. In his book *Surviving Chaos: Healing with Divine Love* (World Service Institute, 2009), engineer Robert Fritchie points out that the healing energy of Divine Love has the ability to nullify the adverse effects of toxic food and water if we simply open to that energy before eating. (For more information, see www.worldserviceinstitute.org.)

Another example of the effect of consciousness on how food is assimilated in the body is the fact that people with multiple personality disorder can be very allergic to a food while they are in one personality, yet the same food doesn't affect them a bit when they are in another personality—in the exact same body. Clearly, more is going on with food and nourishment than simply fat, carbohydrates, proteins, vitamins, and calories. When all is said and done, diet is only one factor in creating health, albeit a very powerful one. According to numerous investigators, dietary patterns associated with low cancer and heart disease risk are usually present in those individuals who have other lifestyle factors associated with a low risk of cancer. These include lower consumption of alcohol and fast food, more exercise, and an optimistic worldview.

Commit to the joy and pleasure of eating whole organic food most of the time. But also understand that your consciousness around a food can change that food's effect on your body. For me, the pleasure of eating out at a restaurant where I can relax and be served almost always outweighs the damage of any partially hydrogenated fat in the salad dressing or on the fish. Melvin Morse's study of long-term survivors of near-death experiences showed that they eat better than controls and in general take better care of themselves. They do this not to avoid dying but because, as a result of their near-death experience, they value their lives more than ever before. Eating well is a way of valuing and nourishing ourselves.[157]

The late comedian George Burns, who lived until he was 100, once said, "If I had known I was going to live so long, I'd have taken better care of myself." Part of George Burns's longevity secret was his sense of humor. Don't lose yours—and don't eat without it! Keep food in perspective.

18

The Power of Movement

Our body creates our soul as much as our soul creates our body.
—David Spangler

Very little is known in our day of the magic that resides in movement, and the potency of certain gestures. The number of physical movements that most people make through life is extremely limited. Having stifled and disciplined their movements in the first stages of childhood, they resort to a set of habits, seldom varied. So, too, their mental activities respond to set formulas, often repeated. With this repetition of physical and mental movements, they limit their expression until they become like actors who each night play the same role. With these few stereotyped gestures, their whole lives are passed without once suspecting the world of dance which they are missing.

—Isadora Duncan

O ur bodies were designed to move, stretch, and run. Exercise is natural for children, and it should be natural for all of us at every age. It feels wonderful to have a strong, flexible body—including a strong heart for endurance. Physical exercise or regular movement of some kind is a vital part of flourishing. The latest USDA food pyramid (much of which I disagree with) includes exercise as an important part of a healthy lifestyle. Even women who are disabled or confined to a wheelchair can benefit from strengthening their upper bodies and increasing their cardiovascular fitness. The bottom line is this: If you want to reach and maintain your health and vitality throughout your life span, you simply must move your body regularly in ways that enhance and maintain your aerobic capacity, your strength, and your flexibility. There are no shortcuts here.

Movement needs to be part of your commitment to yourself. It's easy to put it off until the house is clean, more work is done, or you've gone through the mail. But the endless household and work duties will always be there, even after you're dead. Think of it this way: Given that exercise adds an average of seven years to your life, you're *saving* time by exercising. If we wait to take care of ourselves until everything else is done, there will never be time for exercise. We have to create exercise time, or move in ways that enhance our health while going about our daily duties. Exercise is an essential part of not only maintaining cardiovascular, brain, and joint health, but also maintaining a healthy weight. Though I have a family history of heart disease, I don't exercise because I'm afraid of heart disease; I do it because it feels good and my body loves it! The old feminist adage "How you do it is what you get" applies to exercise just as it does to any other area of life. Getting to this point took me more than forty years. First I had to overcome the "no pain, no gain" legacy that I grew up with. And that was no small matter.

OUR CULTURAL INHERITANCE

Many women have to heal their early perceptions of themselves and their physical capabilities before they can become comfortable with physical activities. Ever since their school days, they've felt bad about their physical prowess simply because they weren't "good" at sports. John Douillard, D.C., Ph.D., author of *Body, Mind, and Sport* (Three Rivers Press, 2001) and a pioneer in the field of fitness and consciousness, cites a Louis Harris poll disclosing that upward of 50 percent of Americans experience their first major feeling of failure in sports! The reason many girls don't have the skills to succeed in sports is that no one ever taught them. One of my friends who was a pro baseball player told me that when boys are first learning to throw, they also throw "just like a girl." Boys learn to "throw like a boy" from practicing over and over again with those who are more skilled than they. It's part of their cultural heritage.

Are you someone who was never picked for the school softball team? Did you feel you had to quit playing sports with the boys when you started to grow breasts? Check to see if your history and any messages you received as a girl are preventing you from enjoying physical activity now—especially if you have no interest in sports. If they are, bring them to consciousness so you can experience them fully, then let them go. Of course, even if you still don't enjoy sports, there are many other ways to stay fit. Being good at batting a ball and being physically fit by engaging in yoga, Pilates, or dance are not necessarily related. Brian Swimme, Ph.D., physicist and author of *The*

Universe Is a Green Dragon (Bear, 1985), said it best: "To exercise actually means to bring into action. When we exercise, we bring into action our ancestral memories. Our bodies remember that we lived in trees and forests. We need to crawl and climb and run if we are to develop our intellectual, emotional, and spiritual capacities. . . . We tend to think of exercise as losing weight, as trimming off the fat. But to exercise is to enable the body to remember its past, so that it can stretch out with all its intertwined powers of being and thought and reflection."[1] I love this quote; it always makes me feel good!

Many of the bodily changes we associate with getting older have nothing to do with our age per se. Decreased muscle mass and increased fat may be normal in this culture, but these conditions are not necessarily natural—and we needn't expect them. They are caused by inactivity and the cumulative effects of glycemic stress and insulin resistance, accompanied by a mindset that expects us to grow weaker as we grow older. That mindset is a belief, not a scientific truth. I am actually more flexible and fit now than when I was in my twenties! And when it comes to Pilates and dance, I just keep improving each year.

Unfortunately, our culture teaches us that we are supposed to fall apart when we hit fifty. That's when we're told we need to start all manner of disease screening like colonoscopy. It's as though you're fine when you go to bed at forty-nine, but when you wake up on the morning of your fiftieth birthday, you now need to worry. Age fifty, like age thirty-five for a reproductive-age woman, is another one of those "cultural portals" Mario Martinez, Psy.D., talks about in *The MindBody Code* (Sounds True, 2014). Cultural portals teach us what to expect at certain ages and stages. Because we profoundly affect one another's biology with shared beliefs, our bodies actually manifest the evidence of these beliefs. We have no culturally supported tradition that teaches us that we can improve with age, especially physically. Though countless exceptions to this rule exist, we still suffer under the collective delusion about what happens to our bodies as we grow older. All you have to do is step out of the illusion and decide that these beliefs need not apply to you.

BENEFITS OF EXERCISE

Joanne Cannon, a wellness educator, defines physical prowess as "the ability to meet the physical demands of one's day, plus one emergency." I like that definition because it is so individualized. Feeling strong and capable is an essential ingredient in building health. Studies show that women who are moderately physically active enjoy the following benefits more than sedentary women:[2]

⁓ Lower levels of C-reactive protein, a sign of inflammation that has been linked to a number of health problems, including heart disease and some cancers.[3]

⁓ Lower overall cancer rates and better immune system function (more white blood cells and increased levels of immunoglobulins).[4]

⁓ Decreased risk of breast cancer (women who exercise at least four hours per week have been shown to have a 37 percent reduction in risk for breast cancer[5] and those with a lean body mass index—less than 22.8—who regularly exercise have 72 percent less risk of breast cancer).[6] This holds true even for relatively light exercise such as walking, gardening, and dancing.

⁓ A life expectancy that is on average seven years longer.[7] A 2005 study in the *New England Journal of Medicine* showed that asymptomatic women who weren't fit had twice the risk of premature death of those who were fit.[8]

⁓ Significant reduction in heart attack and stroke risk, because of the beneficial effect of exercise on blood vessel function.[9]

⁓ Less depression and anxiety, and better mental efficiency and speed (higher IQ scores are associated with exercise in some studies).[10]

⁓ Improved cognitive function in middle age and beyond.[11]

⁓ More relaxation, more assertiveness, more spontaneity and enthusiasm; a better attitude about their bodies and better self-acceptance.[12]

⁓ Stronger bones: increased bone thickness, increased bone mass, and increased ability of the bone to resist mechanical stress and fracture.[13]

⁓ More restful sleep.[14]

⁓ Higher self-esteem.[15]

⁓ Much more satisfying sex.[16]

Three British studies of older recreational cyclists who averaged 400 miles per month and had been cycling for decades showed that exercise can keep both muscles and immune systems healthy.[17] The older cyclists' reflexes, memories, balance, and metabolic profiles were closer to those of healthy thirty-year-olds than to those of a control group of sedentary older subjects. They also had almost as many new T cells (important for immunity) in their blood as did the younger group, and high levels of other immune cells that help prevent autoimmune reaction. Those who covered the most mileage had biologically younger muscles, no matter what their age.

Another benefit of physical exercise is that it increases insulin sensitivity and can therefore prevent glycemic stress, insulin resistance, and type 2 diabetes.[18] Remember from chapter 17 that insulin resistance begins in skeletal muscles. Regular exercise is an essential part of controlling blood sugar and weight. It is also energizing. If you're always tired, it may be because you don't move enough. (But sometimes it's because you need to rest. You'll have to check this out for yourself.) For women with PMS, exercise often alleviates symptoms.[19] And pregnant women who exercise moderately have decreased constipation, hemorrhoids, varicose vein complications, and morning sickness.[20] As mentioned in chapter 12, regular exercise during pregnancy reduces the chances of giving birth to overweight newborns.[21] Moving during labor also has many benefits. It is estimated that being upright and mobile during labor is a no-cost intervention that could save $785 million in the United States by decreasing the likelihood of having a C-section and subsequent complications that can result in uterine rupture and maternal death.[22]

Exercise also helps the brain stay young, vibrant, and resilient, in part because it can boost the formation of new brain cells.[23] John Ratey, M.D., associate clinical professor of psychiatry at Harvard Medical School and the author of *Spark: The Revolutionary New Science of Exercise and the Brain* (Little, Brown, 2008), notes that exercise facilitates this process more than any other type of activity or drug that we know of. His book explores the connection between exercise and the brain's performance and shows how even moderate exercise supercharges mental circuits by reducing anxiety, stress, and depression; increasing memory and the capacity for learning new things; and improving motor function and auditory attention in healthy older adults. His research shows that even those who are overweight can see improvements in mood and cognition after following an exercise program for just twelve weeks. In *Spark,* he discusses the fact that exercise improves depression symptoms as well as or better than prescription medication. (For more information, see www.johnratey.com.)

This has been backed up by other research as well. A large-scale review published in 2016 involving more than 1 million subjects showed that being physically fit substantially reduces the risk of developing clinical depression.[24] Other studies show resistance training also protects against depression.[25]

Exercise and Intuition

The mind pervades the body. Moving your body rhythmically and repetitively helps you tap in to your intuition, and more of your mind becomes available to you—the mind in your legs, your heart, and in your biceps. Exercising is a necessary process for fully digesting thoughts. Raising your heartbeat brings into play more of yourself. Your body wakes up—and so does your mind. During your workouts insights arise spontaneously. When you don't do it, you eventually find that your body craves it! However, for sedentary people, that first couple of weeks of any exercise—be it walking or yoga—can be very challenging. As with all things, including dietary improvement, you have to first move through the resistance to the new behavior. That requires the inner muscle known as will: You just make a decision and follow through. Thankfully, we can develop our will by committing to an exercise program and doing it. No excuses.

Studies have shown that repetitive movement increases alpha waves in the brain—and the alpha state is associated with enhanced intuition. Exercising hard is the perfect balance for the mental activity so often required in modern life. But by that I don't necessarily mean running a marathon or doing a hundred push-ups. There are far more effective, more sustainable, and less fascia-damaging ways to achieve balance.

People have very different approaches to exercise and physical activity, and these differences need to be honored, not judged. Each of us has an innate sense of what feels right for our bodies. Some are born soccer players. Others are dancers, yoginis, or equestrians. As a scholar in a family of "jocks," I had to find my own truth about what works best for me. This took decades because I had come to associate pushing myself physically with feeling tortured. Enjoying the exhilaration of feeling strong and capable in my body while doing activities that I love is one of my life's great pleasures now that I have uncoupled being physical from the feeling of being tormented. A lot of this uncoupling was the result of learning how to breathe through my nose while exercising and not pushing myself beyond where I could maintain nose breathing (see below).

Whatever your movement and exercise history, you, too, must find a way to incorporate regular pleasurable movement into your life. You absolutely must move your body through the gravitational field of the earth. Your quality of life depends on it. If you doubt this, look around next time you are at an airport—at least in the United States. The number of wheelchairs lined up for a flight is rather discouraging. And though people do require this kind of assistance from time to time, most of what lands someone in a wheelchair is preventable.

Your truth about movement will not necessarily be what any outside authority tells you is "the right way to do it." And different approaches to exercise work best at different times in people's lives. For some, a twenty-minute walk three times a week is all that is necessary. For others, aerobics, weight training, or dancing feels the best. (In fact, research shows that aerobic dance is just as beneficial as walking or jogging.)[26] Above all, exercise and body movement should be joyful and fun.

Ways to Move the Body

Aerobic Fitness: What Is It and Why Is It Important?

Kenneth Cooper, M.D., coined the term *aerobics* back in the 1960s and developed the Cooper 12-Minute Run, a test to determine an individual's maximum oxygen uptake (VO_2 max). VO_2 max refers to the amount of oxygen someone is capable of utilizing in one minute and is a measure of cardiorespiratory fitness and ability to endure prolonged exercise. Dr. Cooper's test, essentially determining how far you can run or walk in twelve minutes, is pretty accurate and requires very little equipment. A number of other fitness tests that use a treadmill can also measure cardiorespiratory fitness. The main thing to know is that nearly everyone can improve their fitness level through regular exercise of some kind.

The physical activity guidelines from the U.S. Department of Health and Human Services include both aerobic activity and strength training. Here are the key points.

Aerobic Activity. Aerobic activity means that your heart rate is in your training zone—see below on how to calculate this. Get at least 150 minutes of moderate activity or 75 minutes of vigorous activity (or a combination of both) per week. (The research on the high-intensity interval training known as Peak 8—thirty seconds of maximal exercise effort followed by a ninety-second recovery period, repeated eight times; see box below for an example—suggests that two 20-minute sessions per week will do the same thing.) Moderate aerobic activities include brisk walking, swimming, mowing the lawn, dancing, paddling, and so on.

Strength Training. Do strength training on all the major muscle groups at least twice per week. Aim for a single set of each exercise using a weight or resistance level that tires your muscles after twelve to fifteen repetitions. Alternatively, you can do three sets of fifteen reps with lighter weights. Strength training can include using your own body weight (activities such as rock climbing use body weight, too), resistance bands, or resistance paddles in water.

As a general goal, aim for at least thirty minutes of physical activity every day. It doesn't have to be all at once. Even three bouts of ten minutes each will be highly beneficial. That means taking the stairs at work instead of the elevator and parking farther away from your workplace than normal. Make fitness part of your daily life. And don't get too complicated. You can put on some of your favorite music and dance around while doing household activities such as folding laundry, ironing, doing dishes, sweeping, or vacuuming.

Why You Need Both Aerobic and Strength Training

Aerobic exercise plus weight training is more effective than aerobics alone because weight training increases the amount of muscle in the body relative to fat and does so much more effectively than aerobics alone.[27]

Studies show that as we grow older, we create an average of one and a half pounds of fat per year. We also lose a half pound of muscle each year if we don't exercise regularly. Muscle loss results in fat gain. Weight training prevents the muscle loss that too often accompanies aging. Aerobic exercise plus weight training produces more muscle gain on an average than aerobics alone. It also shapes muscles, resulting in a healthier appearance. The increase in muscle strength that comes with weight training is very beneficial to women, who are often weaker in their upper bodies. It also makes older women less likely to fall and break a hip; a 2008 study in Vancouver showed that a group of people age seventy and up who followed a home-based regimen combining walking twice a week with strength training and balance exercises had 36 percent fewer repeat falls after one year.[28]

The reason a combination of aerobic exercise and weight training results in more fat loss is that one pound of muscle requires thirty to fifty calories a day just to stay alive, but one pound of fat needs fewer calories for maintenance. Remember, fat is covered with insulin receptors that tend to lock it into place, while muscle helps burn fat. People with more muscle have higher metabolic rates. This is one reason that overweight women with lots of body fat often maintain their weight even when eating relatively little. To change their metabolic rate, they need to increase their physical activity and also reduce or eliminate high-glycemic-index carbs. This results in the body resetting its metabolism and releasing fat more easily. Strength training is important as well because it provides cognitive benefits—even more than aerobic exercise does.[29]

It is well known that bone mineral content increases with physical activity.[30] Putting vertical vectors of force on bones through weight-bearing exercise such as walking, jogging, biking, weight training, or stair climbing sets up a mini electrical current in the bone, known as a piezoelectric effect. Yoga and Pilates also do this. This current actually draws in calcium, magnesium, and other minerals we need for bone density and strength. Miriam Nelson, Ph.D., former director of the Center for Physical Activity and Nutrition at Tufts University, has been able to demonstrate significant gains in bone density in postmenopausal women who did two 40-minute sessions of weight training twice a week. None of the women were on estrogen replacement. A wonderful side effect of this training was that as the women in the program increased their self-confidence and strength, they also felt more empowered in the world and tended to go out more and get involved in life.[31]

Also, the mindset with which you approach exercise has a profound effect on your results. For example, in her book *Counterclockwise: Mindful Health and the Power of Possibility* (Ballantine, 2009), Harvard professor Ellen Langer, Ph.D., describes a study she did with housekeepers in a hotel chain. She divided them into two groups, measuring their blood pressure, weight, and other health indicators. She told one group that their work every day vacuuming, making beds, and so on constituted optimal exercise according to the Surgeon General. The other group wasn't told anything positive about their work each day. At the end of the study, the group that was told that their daily work constituted optimal exercise had lost weight and experienced a drop in blood pressure. The control group, who did exactly the same amount and type of work, remained virtually unchanged with no appreciable benefits at all. Now that is the power of mindfulness!

The Target Heart Rate Zone

Aerobic activity is defined as exercise in which the heart rate is elevated for fifteen to twenty minutes into what is called "the target zone."

To calculate your target rate according to the conventional recommendations:

1. Subtract your age from 220.

2. Subtract your resting heart rate (beats per minute) from this figure.

3. Multiply the remainder by your "exercise quotient." This is 0.6 for a beginner or 0.8 for an advanced exerciser.

4. Add your resting heart rate to the figure from step 3. This number is your target heart rate in beats per minute. You can divide by 6 to find out your heart rate for a ten-second interval.

Example: Your age is thirty-two. Your resting heart rate is 60, and you are a beginner. Hence: 220–32 = 188. 188–60 = 128. 128 × 0.6 = 76.8. 76.8 + 60 = 136.8. Your target heart rate is 137 beats per minute or 23 beats for a ten-second interval. You will easily reach this by walking briskly.

If you go to a gym, you will likely notice that many of the cardio machines have a display where you can input your age as a way to tailor your workout. What that means is that there's a kind of "planned deterioration" plugged right into the fitness industry. I always put in my age as forty, and I haven't noticed any deterioration in my aerobic capacity over the years. Also, please note that target heart rate and aerobic capacity do not necessarily decrease with age. A good friend who is a master's-level competitive swimmer in his sixties was having trouble with some cardiac arrhythmias this past year (all of which he fixed by increasing his intake of magnesium). On the treadmill test that he did to determine his cardiovascular health, his fitness level was the same as someone in his thirties. So much for inevitable deterioration! Just something to keep in mind. (For more of this kind of approach and thinking, read my book *Goddesses Never Age: The Secret Prescription for Radiance, Vitality, and Well-Being* [Hay House, 2015].)

Nose Breathing: Rethinking the Target Heart Rate and Everything Else

John Douillard, D.C., Ph.D., director of the Invincible Athlete program and LifeSpa in Boulder, Colorado, has found that the target heart rate and most other "fitness truths" don't necessarily apply to individuals who breathe fully through their noses while exercising and consciously tune in to what their bodies are comfortable with. When you learn how to do this, you can easily go through a workout with a heart rate and breathing rate that are much slower and more comfortable than expected. Dr. Douillard's insights have revolutionized the way I approach all sports and exercise and have enhanced my enjoyment of physical activity immeasurably. (For more information, see Dr. Douillard's website at www.lifespa.com.)

Take a moment right now and take three slow, deep breaths through your mouth. When you are finished, stop for a moment and take three full, deep breaths through your nose, allowing the air to go all the way down to the lower lobes of your lungs. Notice which type of breathing gives you the fullest amount of air in your lungs. The nose breathing wins by a mile, even though it may seem harder at first. Infants normally breathe through their noses, and so do all animals. (Have you ever seen a racehorse breathing through its mouth?) In fact, mouth breathing is a sign of stress. Nose breathing is associated with parasympathetic and sympathetic balance in the body. It creates what is called cardiac coherence, in which the beat-to-beat variability of the heart rate is optimal. Exercising at a pace at which you can comfortably breathe through your nose creates a meditative and blissful state and enhances the balance between the right and left hemispheres of the brain. When you train yourself to breathe through your nose during exercise, your lungs become much more efficient and you can achieve higher levels of fitness than ever before with much less effort.

PEAK 8 WORKOUT WITH NOSE BREATHING

Nose breathing while engaging in the interval training known as Peak 8 or HIIT (high-intensity interval training) is an incredibly efficient and pleasurable way to get the benefits of aerobic exercise in a short period of time. Peak 8, also called Sprint 8, was developed by coach Phil Campbell, who found that this type of workout gives you the same cardiovascular benefits as much longer workouts in the gym. I have personally found this to be true.

Here's a sample Peak 8 (HIIT) workout with nose breathing:

1. Prepare to go for a walk or a run, or to use an exercise bike, treadmill, or elliptical trainer.

2. Begin by walking briskly and breathing only through your nose for two minutes. (Or you can warm up for longer if you like—say, for ten to fifteen minutes. If you're on a treadmill, set the intensity to 6 or so with no incline.)

3. Then pick up the pace and push yourself to walk or run faster for thirty seconds. Go as fast as you can but not so fast that you have to open your mouth and gasp for air. Keep breathing through your nose.

4. Then fall back to a slower walking pace so that you are fully recovered in a minute and a half.

5. Then do another thirty-second full-out run or brisk walk (or on the treadmill, increase the speed or add an incline). Do not exert yourself beyond where you can breathe through your nose. You may have to do what Dr. Douillard calls "Darth Vader" breathing— forcibly exhaling through your nose while exerting yourself. But at no time do you resort to mouth breathing, because that will create free radical damage throughout your body and will feel awful (see "Your Breath, Your Life," page 939.).

Do eight sets of thirty-second exertion followed by a slower recovery pace for a minute and a half. This is a standard Peak 8 or HIIT approach. There are many other ways to do this; to find them, just do an Internet search for Peak 8 or HIIT.

REST-BASED TRAINING

If you find high-intensity interval training too difficult, consider an alternative called Rest-Based Training (RBT), developed by brothers Keoni Teta, N.D., and Jade Teta, N.D., both integrative physicians and co-founders of the health and fitness program Metabolic Effect (www.metaboliceffect.com).

RBT is more intuitive and individual than the typical "five sets of ten reps" type of workout. Instead of pushing to hit a magic number, you tune in to your own body and rest whenever you need to for as long as you need to in between bouts of full-on effort. Focusing on the rest period, the Teta brothers found, actually produces higher-intensity workouts and better metabolic results (meaning you burn more fat). And because it puts you in control, it's more motivating and more empowering. It also makes effective training possible for anyone at any fitness level.

The RBT motto is "Push until you can't, rest until you can." Here's how it works: Choose one exercise to do and decide on an overall time period, say five minutes. Do as many reps as you can until you simply can't do any more keeping good form. Then rest for as long as you need, even if you're in the middle of a set—don't push through to finish a certain number of reps. As soon as you feel you can do more, start again. At the end of your time period, you can move to a new exercise with a different muscle group.

With RBT, you may prefer to take lots of shorter rests, or you could take fewer but longer rest periods. It's totally up to you. You'll probably find that with each successive period of exercise, you'll do fewer reps, but the number you do overall will be the same or even more than you would have done in a traditional "five sets of ten reps" type of workout. Even if the number is the same, remember that you're getting a better metabolic effect.

The reason RBT is more effective is that when you give your body exactly as much rest as it needs to recover from maximum output, you can regain the intensity for the next interval. If you go into the next interval without being fully recuperated, you are not able to reach true maximum intensity, and so you don't get results that are as good. The more you rest, the harder you can push yourself. And the harder you push yourself, the more need you'll have to rest and recoup. RBT uses rest strategically to maximize your effort and your results.

Your Breath, Your Life

Consider also the larger implications of breathing fully through your nose. We breathe 28,000 times a day. If our breaths are shallow, taken in through our mouth, and confined mostly to the upper lobes of our lungs, our body gets the message that we're facing an emergency. Heart rate increases;

the body chemicals associated with stress increase. The majority of illnesses are stress-related, and we can choose to decrease or increase stress every time we breathe. When we learn how to breathe fully through our nose, aerating our lower lungs and allowing our rib cage a full expansion, our body relaxes and we experience a sense of peace. Paradoxically, our body also operates much more efficiently. Just breathing properly has the potential to cure sinusitis, chronic colds, snoring, allergies, coughing, and even asthma. It also can dramatically improve sports performance.

Dr. Douillard's research on athletes who use nose breathing while riding a stationary bike show there was no significant difference in heart rate, but the number of breaths per minute and the perceived exertion was lower using nose breathing, while endurance was significantly higher.[32] In addition, the parasympathetic nervous system was more activated, while the sympathetic nervous system (the one involved in the fight-or-flight response, when a threat is perceived) was less activated with the nose breathing, indicating the subject was "in the zone," a highly pleasurable, focused, almost meditative state. Alpha brain waves (those associated with deep relaxation) were significantly higher with nose breathing, and brain waves were more coherent.

In traditional sports and fitness training, however, we are taught that the kind of stress-free exercise that nose breathing promotes is counter to our "no pain, no gain" ethos. When my daughter was running track in high school, her coach told her that she wasn't working hard enough if she finished a run feeling good and energized! There is evidence of this philosophy in every gym I've ever been in. Because exercise done this way is so unpleasant, people use loud music or TV programs to distract themselves from the way their bodies feel.

But once you start breathing properly and enjoying the meditative state that results, you'll find yourself tuning in to and respecting your body's ability rather than trying not to notice how it's feeling. You'll realize clearly that the "no pain, no gain" adage is physiologically incorrect. And you'll also discover that exercise, sports, or any workout becomes a very personal time of tuning in and getting strong. What was once a chore becomes a joy. That's certainly what has happened for me. Now, instead of a forced march to the standards of someone else, my exercise is just between me and myself. That doesn't mean that I don't strive for improvement. I do. Carolyn Dean, M.D., N.D., says our bodies know intuitively when to rest and when to exercise, maintaining their own unique state of healthy equilibrium. This has certainly been my experience.

BUTEYKO BREATHING

I urge everyone to improve their breathing. To that end, I highly endorse the work of the Buteyko Institute of Breathing and Health. The late Konstantin Pavlovich Buteyko, M.D., Ph.D., was a Ukrainian physiologist and physician who found that by changing the breathing patterns of his patients, he was often able to help them reverse chronic disease. Since that time, the institute he founded has published a number of scientific studies on the benefits of nose breathing and proper breathing in general. In his book *Close Your Mouth: Buteyko Breathing Clinic Self Help Manual* (Buteyko Books, 2004), author Patrick McKeown outlines the basic program. One of my favorite techniques is taping my mouth shut at night. I use 3M micropore paper tape, which is very easy on the skin and lips. When I first did it, I had a slight moment of panic. So I just put the tape on about fifteen minutes before turning off the light. Nothing to fear, I discovered. Then I got used to doing this. And here's what happens. By blocking the exit to mouth breathing, your body naturally goes into "rest and restore" sleep, which is deeper and more restful. You will find you won't wake yourself up snoring. Over time, this approach actually restructures your nasal and sinus passages. The Buteyko method has been very well studied and has helped thousands throughout the world recover from asthma, hay fever, allergies, panic attacks, heart palpitations, snoring, restless legs, dry mouth, noisy breathing, waking with a gasp or snort during sleep, teeth grinding, and so on. (See both www.buteyko.com and www.buteyko.info.) I'm convinced that everyone should adopt this method of breathing not only for exercise but also for daily living.

Gentle Approaches to the Body

Fitness involves more than strength, endurance, and proper breathing. It also must include flexibility and proper alignment. The effects of gravity over time and buckling under to life's stresses quite literally wear us down and change the sheath of connective tissue known as fascia that encases every muscle, nerve, and organ.[33] As my Pilates teacher Hope Matthews puts it, "It's not your age, it's your fascia." There is such truth to that. If we don't regularly hydrate and stretch our fascia, our bodies get distorted. (See the box later in this chapter, written by Hope and her partner Chris Renfrow, on how to rejuvenate your fascia. I've worked personally with Hope and Chris for a number of years and believe they have the most comprehensive take on fascia and how to work with it that I have yet found.)

I can surely attest to the wisdom of this. Every year, through regular Pilates and through contracting and stretching my muscles in classic yoga asana patterns, I've found that my body becomes more and more functional. If we don't learn to move in the ways that our bodies were designed for, then back pain, joint deterioration, chronic pain, and limitation are inevitable.

Unless we practice good posture—what Esther Gokhale of the Gokhale Method calls Primal Posture—our muscles, fascia, flexibility, and alignment will deteriorate over time. This actually starts in children as young as four if they sit too much or spend too much time bent over screens. Yoga, the Feldenkrais Method, Pilates, the Alexander Technique, and the Gokhale Method (see below) are all wonderful ways to relax, stretch, and gently stimulate the muscles and internal organs. Proper alignment also keeps the spine and joints supple. The work of Esther Gokhale combines the best of many of these methods, including Iyengar yoga.

There's now more scientific research than ever that shows why these practices are vital to our total body health. Helene Langevin, M.D., now director of the National Center for Complementary and Integrative Health, did some exciting studies in her former position at the Department of Neurology at the University of Vermont College of Medicine on a group of cells known as integrins.[34] Integrins provide a physical link between the cell and the tissues that surround it. She found that cells interact with their physical support and the stresses on them in ways that produce either health or disease. In other words, when you sit slumped in front of a computer all day, you're putting abnormal forces on your fascia. Over time, this will lead to impairment throughout your entire body because the fascia is loaded with receptor membranes that communicate with all your body's other receptor membranes. But if you instead engage in practices that keep your fascia moving freely and normally, such as improving your alignment, getting regular massages, having acupuncture, or even massaging the bottoms of your feet with a tennis ball on a regular basis, you're actually rewiring the signals that go through the fascia to the rest of your body, thus correcting the impairment and improving the health of your entire body.

Esther Gokhale—who experienced excruciating back pain at the age of twenty-one and was told she'd never be able to have more children, and who also had to have disc surgery—went on to study native peoples the world over. She studied those who work with their bodies to make a living, those who bend and gather and carry heavy weights on their heads, yet never have back pain. By studying their postural and movement patterns and learning from them, she not only cured her own back problem but went on to develop a system of foundational training for posture that is now taught throughout the world. In fact, in November 2016, when a crowd-sourced website called Health Outcomes rated the best treatments for back pain, the Gokhale Method ranked right on top—and was found to be far more effective than most back surgery.[35] Esther realized that people don't get back pain when they live and work in ways that maintain proper posture and alignment—which includes a gentle J-shaped spine (straight with a curve from the lowest vertebra in the low back to the highest of the vertebrae in the sacrum, the triangular bone at the base of the spine just above the tailbone), allowing our tailbones to stick out a bit, like a duck with its tail out behind it, not like a dog tucking its tail between its legs. Esther notes the ease with which women in other cultures walk while carrying heavy weights on their heads, thanks to their perfect spinal alignment. I urge you to check out Esther's website (www.gokhalemethod.com) to see the compelling pictures of what natural and unnatural alignment look like and to learn how to correct your own alignment. I know that doing this—through training with Esther and also through Pilates, which I've been doing twice per week for twenty years—I have avoided a hip replacement.

Many Westerners are taught to "tuck your pelvis" or "tuck your tailbone." This puts far too much stress on our lower backs. We can all learn to sit, stand, and move with far more ease once we learn the principles of Primal Posture. I've covered this earlier when discussing optimal pelvic floor function (see chapter 6). Many times when we are told to "sit up or stand up straight," we simply stick our chest out and pull our shoulder blades back. This is counterproductive. Instead, we want to dip our chins ever so slightly, pull our abdominal muscles in and up—to create an inner corset of support (without pulling our shoulders up to our ears), and then simply roll our shoulders back slightly—one at a time. When we sit, we should have a folded towel under our sitz bones so that our pelvis is tilted downward—think of it like a bowl that is tipped so water pours out and down the front of your legs. I highly recommend that everyone learn the principles of Primal Posture either by reading the book Esther coauthored with Susan Adams, 8 Steps to a Pain-Free Back (Pendo Press, 2008) or, better yet, by taking a Primal Posture workshop with one of her many certified teachers throughout the world (see www.gokhalemethod.com).

I've seen women totally transform their bodies through Pilates, the Gokhale Method, and the right kind of yoga—myself included. My experience has convinced me that it's possible to grow stronger, more fit, and more flexible with age—not the opposite.

THE PSOAS MUSCLE

In my early thirties, I often experienced right hip pain and the inability to walk normally for several minutes after getting up from prolonged sitting. I'd have to swing my right leg back and forth for a bit to get the leg to work properly. My then-husband, an orthopedic surgeon, ordered hip X-rays, which were, of course, normal. Now after ten years of Pilates, I no longer have this pain and dysfunction because I have learned how to stretch, strengthen, and relax both my psoas muscles. Hip pain and limitation run in my family, and I know that if I hadn't learned how to work with my psoas muscles, I would most likely have had a hip replacement by now. Hip and low back pain are remarkably common in women, and many times the problem lies in a contracted psoas muscle—the place in the body that we tend to store tension. My massage therapist said she's been told that the psoas muscle is where we store the effects of doing the emotional work of others, and I've found that to be an extremely accurate statement.

The psoas is a huge muscle that is about sixteen inches long, stretching from the rib cage and trunk to the legs. It passes through the pelvis and over the ball and socket of the hip joint and attaches at the inner side of the femur. Most hip pain in women originates in a tight psoas muscle, a muscle that is right in the center of the body and very sensitive to our emotions. It contracts when we are afraid, and it helps us move freely when relaxed and toned. By learning how to relax and release my psoas, I have a stronger core and more aligned hips than ever before. I urge you to get in touch with your psoas for a lifetime of joyful movement. To do this, you can work with a physical therapist, a neuromuscular therapist, a classically trained Pilates instructor, or a yoga teacher. Or you can simply read and do the exercises in *The Psoas Book* (Guinea Pig Publications, 1981, revised 1997) by Liz Koch (see www.coreawareness.com).

THE IMPORTANCE OF FASCIA
By Hope Matthews and Christopher Renfrow

Exercise is not a thing that we are supposed to "do." It is movement that should be an inherent, integrated, and natural activity in our lives. To be human is to move. We are born knowing how to move our bodies. Modern humans have drifted so far away from our instinctive natural movement that we now need to schedule "exercise" into our lives.

The American College of Sports Medicine says we need to exercise for twenty minutes a day. What does that mean? What kind of exercise? Many of us have enslaved ourselves to the gym, spending countless hours in a variety of classes and on treadmills, elliptical machines, recumbent bikes, and other pieces of equipment that have left us with pain and injury, little result, and the insurmountable feeling of going nowhere. What if there's more to fitness than just exercise and weight loss, counting calories, or building muscles and losing fat? The missing ingredient is a type of tissue that we have overlooked—a tissue that plays a vital role in everything we do, feel, and think. It's called fascia.

Fascia is an all-encompassing tissue, running from head to toe. It weaves its way throughout our bodies, connecting and protecting every muscle, bone, tendon, ligament, nerve, vessel, organ, and gland. In fact, it connects every part of our bodies, right down to each and every cell. Fascia is similar to connective tissue in that it is partly made up of collagen protein. But it's more than that. It is a softer, flexible tissue that has the tensile strength to keep us physically together and make us whole.

The complex, dynamic nature of this tissue is just starting to be appreciated. Until very recently, fascia was thought of merely as a protector, insulator, and packing material for our muscles and organs. But a revolutionary new body of research has demonstrated that fascia is actually a communication network that transmits energy, frequency, and vibration to all organs, tissues, and cells in the body in a way that's similar to how the fiber-optic cables used in computer networking and communication work.[36] This aspect of fascia exists because of a type of gel-like collagen protein known as a liquid crystalline matrix. This dynamic matrix is the medium through which all biological material in the body communicates.

The liquid crystalline matrix of fascia stores and retains frequencies, including memories. In fact, massive amounts of memories and information are stored in the body, not just in the brain. Fascia holds our life stories, including emotional traumas that become imprinted, physicalized memories within our tissues—imprints that literally hold us back from living and moving optimally. Thoughts that have become too rigid, critical, or extreme also become imprinted on the fascia. This imprinting causes the fascia's liquid crystalline matrix to morph into a non-pliable and energetically stagnant substance. Over time this leads to scarring of the tissue, which blocks both movement and energy. This impairment has a cascading effect across the entire body, involving not just movement and mechanics of the tissue but also energy flow, electrical conduction of impulses, and optimal hydration. The result is limited movement, pain, and increased susceptibility to disease.

There is also a quantum intelligence stored in our etheric or finer bodies outside of the dense, physical body. Ancient philosophies use terminology like *subtle matter* and *aura* to describe what is outside of the body, but there is much more to it than that. In our experience, these are forms of fascia and have the same communication and memory capabilities as our internal fascia. These capabilities explain why and how information travels between all beings.[37] Information exists not only in our contemporary timeline but also dips into the past and the future—and possibly even into alternate timelines or universes.

In summary, fascia plays a vital role in our health and well-being by physically stabilizing and aligning our posture, optimally hydrating our tissues, and distributing nourishment and hormones throughout the entire body. The discovery of its liquid crystalline matrix is key to understanding our bodies' ability to communicate and function optimally as whole beings and as part of a greater whole known as the universe. The health of your fascia dictates whether you are skinny or fat, stiff or flexible, painful or pain-free, stuck or unstuck, healthy or unhealthy, happy or sad, present or indifferent, and connected or disconnected. Every thought you think, every emotion you feel, and every move you make impacts your fascia, which, fortunately, can *always* be morphed and changed for the better.

At the Center for Intuitive Movement Healing, we've developed a trademarked method called FasciaRehab that integrates many modalities in reconditioning fascia and releasing stored information on the physical cellular level as well as in the emotional body, the mental body, and even the spiritual body outside the physical plane. You can reclaim your inherent ability to see, feel, and use the properties of this internal and external material. To learn more, visit the center's website at www.thecenterforimh.com.

Martial Arts

Martial arts training such as aikido or tai chi combines the body, mind, and spirit very consciously. This approach also increases strength, endurance, and flexibility simultaneously. Studies of individuals who do tai chi regularly, for example, have found that tai chi modifies their biological function via their nervous and hormonal systems. It has been shown to be effective in the treatment of heart disease, hypertension, insomnia, asthma, and osteoporosis. It decreases depression, tension, anger, fatigue, confusion, and anxiety.[38] A more recent study of 200 people over the age of seventy found that tai chi decreased the risk of falls—a major factor in hip fracture.[39]

When I was in college, I got a green belt in jujitsu. Though that's not a high ranking, I did have to spar with a couple of big guys from Cleveland Heights in order to earn it. From that, I learned that I have the strength and the will to fight someone in self-defense if I need to. Studies of men who rape show that they tend to go after women who seem the most vulnerable. The self-confidence and resulting self-confident stance that come from knowing you can fight for yourself is conveyed in the energy field around you and is one way to decrease your chances of being raped. (Rape culture is part and parcel of patriarchy, so I don't pretend that this alone will prevent rape.) Martial arts can also help you discover your voice.[40]

EXERCISE AND ADDICTION

Just about anything can be used addictively, and exercise is no exception. The call to use physical activity as a way to disconnect from our feelings saturates our culture. Some people have actually had to go to rehab for running addiction. You might think running could not possibly be a health problem. In fact, it is well documented that endurance sports such as marathon running actually depress immunity and increase the risk of premature death. This is, in part, because of the free radical damage done by overexercising without adequate antioxidant intake or rest.[41] There is also the issue of extreme wear and tear on joints, which results in the need for so many knee and hip replacements in runners who continue the activity despite increasing pain and dysfunction. (If you are a runner, please take care of your joints by making sure that you restore and hydrate your fascia regularly. And run on trails as much as possible, not pavement.)

Several years ago, I visited a popular spa to give some lectures. One of the women in the group spent three hours per morning on a treadmill, worked out with a personal trainer most of each afternoon, and then went out every evening to buy alcohol, which she'd imbibe until drunk! Though she looked good, I knew that at the rate she was going, her health and her beauty were both in jeopardy. When we use exercise to run away from the stress in our lives or to disconnect from our deepest selves, it is no different from the addictive use of Valium. It may be a healthier choice initially, but it is still an addiction.

Though exercise can blow off steam, if it's used primarily for this purpose it can become a "fix" anytime you feel stressed; you'll use exercise to medicate your emotional pain. It's much better to deal with the source of the stress than to use exercise as a fix. On the other hand, a ten- to fifteen-minute brisk walk will often elevate your mood and help you put things in perspective. It also helps the body get rid of the effects of stress hormones that often trigger overeating. When you experience stress, your body makes the hormone cortisol to mobilize you to move in response to a perceived threat. When you go for a ten- to fifteen-minute walk (or even climb stairs at work), you will be metabolizing the cortisol—and using up the extra calories that your body wanted to consume in response to running away from the stress (which our Stone Age bodies rarely do anymore). The stresses today are different from those of the ancient past, but the body's response is the same: mobilize all resources and prepare to run. When you actually do move, you'll find that the short period of exercise will decrease your appetite and take away the munchies.

Unfortunately, many women use exercise as a fix to run away from stress or as a way to keep their weight down. While exercise does accomplish both of these goals, you'll never establish a healthy relationship with exercise and your body if you do the exercise strictly for stress and/or weight control.

EXERCISE, AMENORRHEA, AND BONE LOSS

Studies have repeatedly shown that many female athletes have stopped having menstrual cycles and suffer from premature bone loss.[42] In the past, I feared that these data would be used to scare women away from choosing to use their bodies as fully and powerfully as men. Follow-up studies, however, have shown that many women athletes stop having periods for the same reason as women who go on stringent diets or become anorexic: They don't eat enough, and their total body fat drops to a level that is too low. This results in loss of periods (amenorrhea) and early osteoporosis.[43] In one study, when women who had developed amenorrhea from exercise ate 500 to 700 calories more per day, their periods returned. (Most competitive women runners won't do this.)

One of my friends, a former competitive bodybuilder, told me that competitors in women's bodybuilding actually look forward to losing their periods and consider it a sign of adequate training. Competitive runners have told me the same thing. Hormonal shutdown of this nature is actually a training goal! Clearly, this is a sign of unhealthy behavior. It's not surprising that drug use in the form of anabolic steroids is the norm rather than the exception in high-level competitions.

Studies indicate that women marathon runners who exercise to the point of becoming amenorrheic often have bone densities comparable to those of osteoporotic women who are much older. There is no definite point at which running may begin to have deleterious effects on a woman's body, although in competitive runners it appears to begin at about fifty miles of training per week.

Still another reason these women become amenorrheic is that, as studies have shown, leanness *combined* with chronic concern about becoming overweight is associated with brain changes that lead to disturbed menstrual cycles.[44] Women athletes are just as influenced by the cultural desire to be thin as other women. For that reason, their caloric intake is often lower than it has to be for the level of activity in which they participate. Eating disorders are as common in athletic women as they are in nonathletic women, but athletic women sometimes use the training as a form of weight control. They exercise heavily—then they don't eat. This is no different from other forms of anorexia.

Since resumption of menses can take some time, progesterone therapy to help restore bone mass is often helpful. Once ovulatory periods have resumed, bone mineral density also begins to improve.[45]

Not all women are at risk for losing their periods from extreme amounts of exercise. In a study by Nancy Lane, M.D., amenorrhea from excessive exercise was primarily a problem of young, childless women. After a woman has had children, she is less likely to develop this problem because childbearing appears to make her hormonal system difficult to suppress via extreme exercise. Her monthly cycling becomes harder to turn off. That's why women runners in their thirties and forties who've had children rarely become amenorrheic.[46] I believe that there's another reason why women who have had children are at less risk for exercise-induced amenorrhea: They are much less likely to maintain ruthless competitiveness, and this shift is associated with an opening of the heart that changes body chemistry. Having a child changes a woman in very fundamental ways—emotionally, psychologically, physically, and spiritually. Her priorities about what's really important change. (By the way, having a baby uses your body as fully and powerfully as any athletic event I can think of, but we can't do this routine every week!)

GETTING STARTED

Step One: Choose an Exercise Program

It is just as healthy to discard the concept of the "ideal" amount of exercise as it is to discard the concept of the "ideal" weight. When people ask me what exercise program is best, I reply, "The one that you'll actually do."

Women can find joy and fitness by participating in a very wide variety of activities, ranging from yoga, tai chi, and dance to teaching Outward Bound courses.

Try this: Recall a time in childhood when you were outside playing—skipping, jumping rope, swimming, or throwing a ball just for fun. Or perhaps you remember dancing—twirling around till you fell on the ground dizzy. Play with this memory in your mind for a while, and feel how it felt. Smell how it smelled. Feel the sun or wind on your face. Feel how good it felt to move your body with joy and energy, stretching it to its full capacity.

When you are ready, bring yourself back into the present. Begin moving your body the way you used to. See how it feels now. Be in your body. Enjoy it, appreciate it. Experiment with moving it. Did any type of movement come to mind as something that felt really good? What was it? How could you incorporate that into your life now?

How Much and What Kind Is Enough?

In October 2008, the government's Health and Human Services Department released the new Physical Activity Guidelines for Americans, based on the first thorough review of research conducted on physical activity and health in more than ten years.[47] (These same recommendations were repeated in the second edition, published in 2018.)

The guidelines allow you lots of flexibility, giving you a total amount of time to shoot for each week instead of a certain amount of exercise per day. You can parcel out your exercise into stints of at least ten minutes at a time, which allows you to fit in many short activities that add up (like taking the stairs at the office) instead of committing to a longer workout. The guidelines also give different suggestions based on the intensity of exercise you prefer. There are two basic options:

~ Two and a half hours a week of moderate exercise, defined as activity that's easy enough to allow you to carry on a conversation, but not so easy that you could sing (such as brisk walking, water aerobics, ballroom dancing, or gardening).

~ One hour and fifteen minutes a week of vigorous exercise, defined as enough exertion so that you can only say a few words at a time without stopping to catch your breath. This includes activities such as racewalking, jogging, swimming laps, jumping rope, or hiking uphill with a heavy backpack.

The recommendations further suggest an additional two days a week of muscle-strengthening activities, such as weight training, push-ups, sit-ups, or heavy gardening.

The expert panel that designed the guidelines noted that such regular physical activity reduces the risk of early death, coronary heart disease, stroke, high blood pressure, type 2 diabetes, colon and breast cancer, and depression. The panel also noted that the suggested program can improve cognitive ability in older adults as well as the ability to engage in activities needed for daily living.

Step Two: Make a Commitment to Move Your Body

Commit to moving your body in some way or in some form three to five times a week for twenty to thirty minutes. Make exercise as simple as possible for yourself. For me, that used to mean keeping the NordicTrack all set up in the family room and keeping my weights arranged on the floor, ready to go—I didn't have to do any elaborate setup. I didn't worry about leaving it out all the time; after all, the house was for me to live in, not to look perfect in case company came. Sometimes I used to go to a gym, especially when traveling. But most of the time, I preferred to be home. Now that the children are gone, I have a room I've converted into an exercise studio. I also do Pilates one-on-one with a classically trained Pilates teacher twice per week. This has truly transformed my body over the past couple of decades.

Commit to doing an exercise program for one month. Within that time your body will probably come to look forward to exercise. If you drop out for a while, let yourself know that you will get back to it when you can. Don't spend a minute beating yourself up. Better yet, make a fitness pact with a buddy. Then on the days when one of you wants to opt out, the other one can cheer you on. Peer pressure can be very healthy.

Step Three: Learn How to Breathe Through Your Nose

Go slowly. Learn the yoga routine Salute to the Sun and go through it to learn how to pace your breath. (For full instructions, see the book *Body, Mind, and Sport* [Three Rivers Press, 2001] by John Douillard, D.C., Ph.D. The postures can also be found online or in many yoga texts or videos.) Don't exert yourself beyond the level at which you can comfortably keep your breathing steady through your nose. If you're already a regular exerciser, you'll notice that it will probably take you three weeks or more to get back to your former level of achievement while breathing properly. Take your time. Once you've trained your body to use oxygen efficiently, you'll find that you'll soon be running farther—or walking faster—with less exertion than you ever dreamed possible. Your rib cage will also become much more flexible and your breathing more efficient. Note: You'll need to take tissues with you when you breathe in and out through your nose because this form of breathing will really keep your nasal passages and sinuses clear and draining. Especially when you exert yourself, you'll be doing what Dr. Douillard calls "Darth Vader" breathing—short, forceful exhalations through the nose that clean it out very effectively!

Step Four: Watch Out for Self-Sabotage

One of the most common reasons that women stop exercising is that they do too much too soon (addictive behavior). Having been out of shape for three years, they vow that they'll run three miles a day for a week and get in shape fast. A much better approach is to do less each day than you are capable of—at least for a while. This will give your body the message that it can trust you to take care of it and not push it to exhaustion. Your body will get the idea that exercise is fun! Dogs love to go for their walks—and we would be just as enthusiastic if we followed our instincts as well as animals do.

If you never push yourself, on the other hand, and always do less than is expected or needed, then you need to push past your current limit. It's good to know your body is capable of the long haul when necessary.

Don't ever use exercise as a way to beat your body into submission or to punish it for not looking perfect. (Anne Wilson Schaef once said that she thinks addiction to self-abuse is probably the most common addiction in our culture, and I would agree.)

If you hate your exercise program and have to manipulate or force yourself into doing it, you'll just build up resistance. You'll eventually quit or manage to get injured, or you'll make the exercise program into an external authority controlling you—and you'll sabotage yourself to get out of doing it. So make sure you're doing something you like!

Step Five: Enjoy Yourself

When one of my former patients was an art teacher in her forties, she started going to a gym for weight lifting. She had a great time pumping iron. Newly divorced and on her own, her muscle strengthening reflected the strengthening she was doing in other areas of her life as well. She began to look and feel wonderful—and powerful. She was living proof that exercise releases naturally occurring substances called endorphins, which are related to morphine and the other opiates. Endorphins produce a feeling of well-being.

Recall that the fascia is a sheath of connective tissue that encases every muscle, organ, and nerve in our bodies and also acts as a kind of hydraulic pump to circulate water and fluids throughout your body. When you move your body consciously, you are pumping vital water throughout your system, stimulating every cell in a positive and healthy way. Your fascia is the way that your cells communicate with each other—from the top of your head to the bottom of your feet. When you move regularly and are well hydrated with the right kind of fluids (see chapter 17)—you remain physically vibrant and healthy—as well as preventing restriction, disease, and pain. If you want to truly flourish, you simply must exercise regularly—starting in childhood and continuing until the day you take your last breath. David Spangler said it well: "Our body creates our soul as much as our soul creates our body." I couldn't agree more.

19

Healing Ourselves, Healing Our World

If you bring forth what is within you,
What you bring forth will save you.
If you do not bring forth what is within you,
What you do not bring forth will destroy you.
　　　　　—Jesus, in *The Gospel According to Thomas*

The world is awakening to a powerful truth: Women and girls aren't the
problem; they're the solution.
　　　　　—Nicholas D. Kristof and Sheryl WuDunn

We have now arrived at what shamanic astrologer Daniel Giamario calls "the turning of the ages." Everywhere we look, all over the planet, old, outmoded, unsustainable ways of thinking—and living—are dying. Dozens of studies have documented the fact that our thoughts can and do affect others in profound and measurable ways. Since 1975, for example, thirty-three studies have been published in peer-reviewed journals reporting that the Transcendental Meditation (TM) program and its advanced variant, the TM-Sidhi Program, when practiced by various groups meditating twice per day, have been associated with a measurable decrease in the number of violent crimes, suicides, terrorist attacks, fires, and conflict in the areas being studied.[1] The late Maharishi Mahesh Yogi, founder of the TM movement, predicted that when 1 percent of the population changed their fields of consciousness through meditation to the degree that they had greater coherence (sort of like the tight focus of a laser beam), then we'd see a measurable positive effect on society as a whole. This has indeed been happening, especially since 2012—the date that was associated with the end of the Mayan calendar. While it was widely touted as "the end of time," obviously this doomsday prophecy was a misinterpretation of what indigenous cultures have taught for centuries. And it is this: If we made it past 2012, we would be in a new era—an era called the Age of Aquarius—in which increasing cooperation, sustainability, and the end of wars would be the norm. And that is exactly what is happening. Mass consciousness—created by the individual consciousness of each of us, a concept Carl Jung called "the collective unconscious," can be thought of as a giant energy field around the earth. British biologist Rupert Sheldrake, Ph.D., named it the "morphogenic field." British author, journalist, and lecturer Lynne McTaggart simply refers to it as "the field." Whatever you call it, it is clear that this field is shifting and changing . . . in a positive direction.

McTaggart is now well known for her large-scale intention experiments, scientifically controlled, Internet-based events that test the power of many people holding the same intention at the same time. In these experiments, McTaggart instructs a large group of people that may be gathered physically in the same place as well as others who join via the Internet to simultaneously send healing energy to a specific area on the planet. As she describes in her book *The Intention Experiment* (Free Press, 2007), the effects can be profound.

McTaggart's Middle East Peace Intention Experiment, which took place on November 9, 2017, is a particularly moving example. McTaggart led the experiment from a studio in the United Kingdom, using video screens to connect with thousands of Israelis gathered for a peace event in a stadium in Jerusalem as well as eight groups of Arabs gathered in hotel conference rooms in various cities in Saudi Arabia, Kuwait, Abu Dhabi, Oman, Bahrain, Jordan, and Tunisia. These nine groups and McTaggart could all see one another simultaneously. In addition, thousands of people from every inhabited continent joined in live via McTaggart's YouTube channel. McTaggart chose the Old City of Jerusalem as the target for the intention because of the symbolic meaning it held as the spiritual heart of the Jewish, Muslim, and Christian faiths. During the experiment, the Arabs and Jews began sending love and forgiveness to each other. The effect was felt not only by them but also by those participating in other countries. It was also enough to measure a strong change in the output from the random event generators maintained by the Global Consciousness Project in Princeton, New Jersey. These machines are designed to generate a completely unpredictable sequence of zeroes and ones, yet during events of intense emotion, the pattern becomes more orderly, indicating a change in the unified field of consciousness surrounding the planet.

One of the most fascinating outcomes McTaggart has experienced with her various intention experiments is that not only does the target—those receiving the energy—benefit, but the senders themselves also benefit, showing significant improvements in health, relationships, professional careers, and more. More recently, she's begun teaching how people can start smaller intention groups (ideally of eight people, but it could be any number, either in the same geographic location or while connected virtually via the Internet) to direct healing energy to a specific person or situation. She gives instructions for this in her book *The Power of Eight* (Atria Books, 2017).

In 2015, McTaggart studied a group of 250 volunteers who agreed to participate in these Power of Eight groups. Almost all of those who met regularly reported major life transformations, healing depression and other mental health issues, improving long-term physical conditions, landing their dream jobs, or receiving money at a time when it was sorely needed. She credits the energy of altruism for these bounce-back effects, noting that research shows displaying altruism activates the vagus nerve, the longest cranial nerve in the body. Activating this nerve has many effects, including triggering the release of the bonding hormone oxytocin (which increases compassion and caring) as well as strengthening the response of the immune system. Interestingly, the vagus nerve response is strongest when people feel a connection to all of humanity, not when they're feeling a strong connection to a particular group they identify with. It turns out that we humans are actually designed to be compassionate and altruistic. The effects are physical, emotional, mental, and spiritual. Dacher Keltner, Ph.D., codirector of the Greater Good Science Center at the University of California at Berkeley, details the science behind this in his book, *Born to Be Good: The Science of a Meaningful Life* (W. W. Norton, 2009).

Work like McTaggart's shows how far we have come in understanding the effects of consciousness on matter and our health in the twenty-five years since this book was first published. Researchers such as neuroscientist Candace Pert, Ph.D. (author of *Molecules of Emotion: Why You Feel the Way You Feel* [Scribner, 1997]), and stem cell biologist Bruce Lipton, Ph.D. (author of *The Biology of Belief* [Hay House, 2008]), published groundbreaking studies on the mind-body connection, showing irrefutable evidence that what we think and feel affects our physical bodies in profound ways. We are not, they have shown us, victims of our DNA; we can actually learn to call the shots. The field of epigenetics—the study of how our genes are influenced by signals coming from *outside* our cells—has lent a whole new level of legitimacy to mind-body medicine.

This in turn has opened the door to the idea that we are responsible in a larger way than we ever imagined for the fate of humanity, not to mention the planet we live on. Leaders in the New Thought movement such as Gregg Braden (author of *Human by Design* [Hay House, 2017]) have effectively bridged science and spirituality, showing how science has borne out the spiritual principles of most if not all indigenous populations concerning the interconnectivity of everything on earth. Futurist Barbara Marx Hubbard famously declared in the years before her death in 2019 that humans are consciously evolving into a new species she called *Homo universalis* that is driven to pave the way to a planetary awakening. These ideas take what we have learned in mind-body science to a new level, furthering a new kind of spiritually based science, promoted by teachers such as McTaggart and Joe Dispenza, D.C. (author of *Becoming Supernatural* [Hay House, 2017]), based on the idea that what goes on in our heads and hearts affects not only our individual physical bodies but also the electromagnetic field surrounding the planet—and with that, everything in our universe.

The Old Energy Dies Hard

For millennia, the many have been controlled by the interests of the few. Going down that rabbit hole is beyond the scope of this book, but suffice it to say that there is an enormous amount of evidence that Big Pharma, Big Food, big banks, the military-industrial complex, and some religions have had an agenda that has controlled the masses for centuries. I call this collective energy "darkness"—the institutions and systems that keep people enslaved by manipulation and fear. The mainstream media—like mainstream medicine—have been overly focused on everything that can go wrong, thus instilling fear and convincing everyone that they require medicine for life. The old "prescription drugs for seniors" political campaign was a good example, reinforcing the notion that as we grow older, we all need prescription medication—which is very often not the case at all if other lifestyle alternatives are offered. Both medicine and the media have also been financed by forces that are not interested in global or personal health. For example, network television in the United States gets a large proportion of its revenue from Big Pharma's advertising dollars (a staggering $69.8 billion in 2018),[2] and so it's produced content that has kept people afraid and therefore easy to manipulate. Fortunately, this is shifting somewhat now with the advent of subscription television like Netflix.

Consciousness on the planet is now changing—slowly but inexorably. And the old energy that has held sway for millennia (preparing for war or recovering from war) is now fighting for its life. It is pulling out all the stops with 24/7 bad news piped right into your mobile devices, complete with compelling music and imagery designed to keep you hooked and enslaved to fear. I liken this time in our planetary history as akin to the incision and drainage of an abscess. The body can live with an abscess deep within for many years because we have defense mechanisms that wall it off and keep the rest of the body protected to some degree. But we still pay a price for this chronic, low-grade inflammation that the body can't quite get rid of. Sooner or later, the abscess comes to the surface, where it can be drained. In surgery you incise the abscess, and the pus comes out all over the place. Then you must reach deep down and break up what are called loculations—thin walls of tissue in the abscess that keep blood and nutrients from getting in. After that, the abscess cavity is left open to drain. And it heals from deep inside to the surface—from the inside out. What we are currently seeing on planet Earth is the incision and drainage stage of healing—the pus is everywhere you look. But all this pus is not new. It's just been buried deep within, creating a kind of chronic low-grade inflammation for decades. Now it's out where you can see it. But make no mistake—deep healing is already taking place, pushing up healthy tissue from within.

Think about it. Before the #MeToo movement, the subjugation of women (and that which is feminine in men) was just the way of things—everywhere. Same with hitting children to keep them in line. If mass consciousness and the quantum field of energy and information surrounding all of us hadn't changed, the #MeToo movement would never have gotten any traction. Neither would the civil rights movement. Recall that many of the founding fathers of the United States were slave owners. The Bill of Rights they crafted, with its assertion that all men are created equal and entitled to life, liberty, and the pursuit of happiness, applied only to white men. Women, children, and people of color were left out. That is all changing. It is the change in mass consciousness that has finally resulted in so many perpetrators being brought to justice.

The Netflix special *Nanette,* starring the comedian Hannah Gadsby, is another profound example of the global change in consciousness. Gadsby is a lesbian from Tasmania whose award-winning comedy special swept the world in 2018, changing the genre forever. She has said that she will no longer use self-deprecation as a form of humor—because for marginalized populations, self-deprecation is humiliation. And her healing from her own internalized homophobia is not helped by humiliation—nor is it for anyone else. She also used her art history degree ingeniously to call out Picasso on his behavior toward women, letting the world know in no uncertain terms that we are no longer willing to give someone credit for their creative work—no matter how good it is—if they abuse others in their personal lives. I watched the special three times, and each time, I stood up and cheered. What a sea change!

Very few individuals who have been abused by a parent or had a spiritual experience outside of what we consider "normal" are ever going to speak up unless they feel safe to do so. But as soon as one person does it, the quantum field changes, making it easier for the next, and the next, and the next. And that is exactly what we are seeing. We are now living in a time when it is increasingly safe to tell the truth about your experience. Remember that the first stage in any healing process is validation and acknowledgment:

"Yes, that happened to you. And it is not okay." Do we have a ways to go? Absolutely. But there is nothing to be gained by always focusing on the negative; it just gives darkness more power. Instead, let us acknowledge the enormous size of the changes that have taken place in the last few decades. Remember, women didn't even get the right to vote until 1920, and 100 years is a mere millisecond of time compared with the thousands of years during which patriarchy has held most of the planet in its grip.

In many ways, time is speeding up. We get more bits of information in ten minutes via our cellphones than our grandparents got in a year. Our global connectivity has made it far more difficult for those in power to control us. At this time in our history, the human race is waking up. We are rapidly approaching that critical 1 percent of people who have raised their consciousness. This changes everything.

One of my thirtysomething colleagues recently wrote the following: "I have been feeling like I am in a psychic battle with some other energy or presence these days. It doesn't exactly feel like my mom or dad, but it's connected to them. Maybe it's an ancestral energy of fear and darkness. It feels like a battle I have no choice but to win. I don't know how to explain it." I know exactly what she is describing.

From time to time I have had the very vivid experience of entering a place inside myself that I call "the pain of all women." The first time it happened, at an intensive with Anne Wilson Schaef, I felt my consciousness going backward in time, as layers and layers and centuries and centuries of denial peeled away. My entry into this process was when Anne said to me, "You're so tired," and then suggested I lie down on a mat to see "what comes up." Having a woman, a mentor at that time, acknowledge my tiredness instead of demanding more sacrifice was one of the most profound experiences of my life. At first, as she sat with me and told me to stay with myself, I felt how strongly my body resisted feeling what I was feeling. I experienced how good I was at pushing down my tears and getting on with whatever I had to do. But eventually, as Anne suggested that I simply stay with myself, I felt my consciousness go backward through all the times when I had never rested: when I'd had my children, during residency, during medical school, during college, during high school. Backward, backward, through my childhood— "Don't ask for a lighter pack, ask for a stronger back," I heard my mother say. And I wept for myself and for that part of me that so needed rest. When I had finished crying all the tears that I had never cried for myself, I began to weep for my mother—for all the times that she had not been allowed to feel or to rest, for all the pain of her own childhood, for all the times she was up all night with a sick child, for the endless grief of losing two children.

And when that was over, I felt the grief of my grandmother, raised by her twelve-year-old sister after her own mother had died in childbirth. When that was complete, I went backward further still—until I was wailing for all women, for all the pain, for all the labors unattended, for all the injustice, for so many thousands of years. What had started as very personal became universal: not my pain, but *the* pain.

When it was over, several hours later, I knew exactly why I was on the earth and what my mission was: to work toward transforming this collective pain into joy. I knew in a flash that there are no mistakes, that I had been destined to become an obstetrician-gynecologist, and that no other path would have served as well. I knew why I had cried so many years before in medical school, when I had first witnessed the birth of a baby: I had tapped in to the field of women's experience—including all of the pain and fear. Seeing the birth had brought up emotions for me that I had no words for back in 1973. I only knew at the time that I had been moved beyond all reason by this birth and that there was no other specialty in medicine for me except the care of women.

Two days after the experience I had at the intensive, I got my period, confirmation for me that our deepest material often comes to consciousness premenstrually—the time when the veil between the worlds of the conscious and unconscious is thinner. And about a week later, as I was relating my experience of this deep process to my mother, I heard a long silence at the other end of the phone line after I had finished. Then she said, "I was sexually abused. I remember the room, I remember the smell of his pipe. I can see it as though it were happening now. It was old Bill, the man who rented a room from my mother. He told me never to tell anyone. I felt dirty. I was eight years old."

My mother, who was sixty-three at that time, had not remembered this part of her history before that moment. Somehow I had broken into the family memory bank with my process—and suddenly the contents were easier for her to access as well. A few months prior to this, she had been having a recurrent dream in which there were horrid growths on her body. She'd awaken in terror. She now knew that these dreams were related to her long-suppressed abuse; the growths on her skin were symbolic of material coming up to consciousness "just under the surface"—ugly material, horrid material.

Mom was alone in her cabin when I called and she remembered her abuse. I asked her if she would be all right after we hung up. She said she would but that she'd call back if she needed support. I suggested that she be willing to stay with that which was "not acceptable." She prayed for guidance and let herself experience the sickening feeling that had surfaced with the sexual abuse memory. She then went to bed. Her loft window was open—it was a warm autumn night—and she later told me that three blue lights came in the window, followed by a large gleaming sphere of white light. The next thing she knew, it was morning. She awakened feeling profoundly at peace, knowing that she had had an experience of grace.

OUR MOTHERS: OUR CELLS

Our memories are stored up in our bodies. Incest memories often surface after a uterine biopsy, and sadness often arises after pelvic surgery, all for a reason. We carry our personal history in the tissue that our consciousness co-creates. It remains there like data banks until we transform it. But we carry much more than what is simply personal. On some level, we carry everyone and everything—the collective—all there within and around our very cells.

It's known that mitochondrial DNA, the DNA that carries out the daily activities of the cytoplasm of the cells, is inherited strictly through the maternal line. The entire human race can be traced back to a group of females in Africa.[3] This fact lends biological credence to my experiences and those of everyone who has entered into realms of experience that don't fit logical thinking. Sometimes body symptoms are the doorway not only into our own individual pain but into the collective pain of others. Insights from quantum physics have now proved that the consciousness of one of us affects all of us.

An old Sufi saying captures the essence of what this means and what each of us must do with it:

> Overcome any bitterness that may have come to you because you were not up to the magnitude of the pain that was entrusted to you.
>
> Like the mother of the world who carries the pain of the world in her heart, each one of us is part of her heart and therefore endowed with a certain measure of cosmic pain. You are sharing the totality of that pain.
>
> You are called upon to meet it in joy instead of self-pity. The secret is to offer your heart as a vehicle to transform cosmic suffering into joy.

The late Stephen Levine taught me that the work we do to let go of our suffering diminishes the suffering of the whole universe. When we have room in our hearts for our own pain, we have room for the pain of others and our compassion helps lighten the suffering of others. And then something magical happens: We find that beneath our pain and suffering lie unending joy, connection, and bliss.

A RITUAL OF RECLAIMING

Years ago, Brenda, a close friend from childhood, decided that she'd like to have her IUD removed in order to get pregnant. She'd been using IUDs for contraception for almost eighteen years with no problem, but now, at the age of forty, she had met a man with whom she wanted to share her life and have children. Because this decision was a major turning point in her life, she wanted someone close to her to share it. So she asked me to remove the IUD while she was here visiting in Maine.

We decided to do a simple ceremony prior to the procedure—to bring intent and consciousness to the process of removing the IUD and inviting in a child. So on a glorious Sunday afternoon in autumn, with the trees ablaze with color, we went over to Women to Women, set up a circle of cloth on the carpet in my office, picked a geranium from an office plant, and gathered a few seashells to place in our circle. We filled a shell with water, lit some candles, and then, sitting around our small circle, acknowledged the forces of nature, God, and the mysteries of life, and invited them to be present with us.

We called Brenda's fiancé on the phone (he was at work in another state at the time). I asked each of them to speak about their fears and hopes for a child, which they did. The fiancé had already had a child many years before, but he was eager for a chance to participate more fully in the process this time. His support and love for Brenda were very evident and clear as he spoke; he had no doubts about his willingness to participate in parenthood. His commitment to support her was strong and inspiring. Their relationship felt like the very embodiment of the masculine at its best when it is in full support of the feminine.

Brenda herself, though eager to have a baby, voiced a concern that she wouldn't know how to give birth. Despite her fear, she was ready to proceed with the IUD removal. We said goodbye to her fiancé, promising to call back as soon as we had completed the procedure.

Now we moved into one of my exam rooms, and I placed a small amount of local anesthetic in the cervix. Once Brenda felt ready, I asked her to cough while I pulled out the IUD. (Coughing while something is going into or coming out of the cervix often interferes with pain pathways and thus makes the procedure more comfortable.)

I told her that she would feel the visceral sense of her uterus as the IUD was pulled out and that this would be a good time for her to tune in to the information stored in there. I told her that the body holds memories and that these sometimes come to the surface during an office procedure such as an endometrial biopsy or an IUD removal. I explained that I would be taking some time after the procedure to "put her energy field back together" by placing my hands over the uterus. Her job was to simply pay attention to any thoughts or feelings that came up.

The IUD came out with no difficulty. I then took Brenda's heels out of the stirrups, had her lie flat, and ran my hands over her body from head to toe several times, doing therapeutic touch. When finished, I laid my hands over her lower abdomen. She began to cry and laugh at the same time as her body released the tension and the emotional charge associated with this sort of procedure. I encouraged her to do whatever she had to do for herself. And I reminded her to simply stay with whatever was coming up.

After crying for a bit, Brenda closed her eyes and then began to laugh. She spoke of being in a forest, with light shining down through the tall trees. She described herself as being young, too young. Then she became frightened again. At this time, I didn't know exactly what was going on, but I simply remained with my hands over her lower abdomen. She told me that having my hands there felt good and she wanted me to keep them there.

She continued to recount being a young girl, alone in the woods. She was pregnant there, without the support of anyone. Her body began to go through what looked like labor. She kept saying, "It's too soon. I don't know how to do this." She began to go through contractions and then pushing. (I've sat with enough women in labor to know what a laboring woman's body goes through.) After about ten minutes she looked down at what sounded like a thirty-week-size stillborn child when she described it. And she asked me, "What is that white rope-like thing going into my vagina?" She was describing the umbilical cord. I told her what it was and said that she'd have to deliver the placenta. Her body then went into another contraction and went through the motions of pushing out a placenta. Brenda had never seen a thirty-week premature baby, a placenta, or a white translucent umbilical cord, but she was able to describe them perfectly—but with the curiosity of a young girl who didn't know exactly what was happening to her, not a worldly forty-year-old.

At this point, the energetic labor and delivery complete, Brenda began to laugh and also to chant, "O-ne-an-ta, O-ne-an-ta." It sounded like a Native American language. During this time she said, "I know the whole language." I wish I had had a recording device—we might have figured out what language it was.

We stayed in the exam room awhile longer while Brenda returned to the twentieth century and stretched her legs. Both of us were amazed by what had just happened. I reminded her that her body did in fact know how to give birth—she had just gone through it, though not on what we'd conventionally call a physical level. Nevertheless, her body now "knew" or "remembered" what labor and delivery were like, and her fear of the process was gone. We returned to my office, sang a lullaby together, and blew out the candles. When she was ready, she called her fiancé and related the experience.

Brenda had tapped in to the collective unconscious, had gained access to some ancient memory that still lived on in her cells. It was an extraordinary experience. I believe that in taking out her IUD and allowing her process to unfold, we were able to heal something deep, on a level that is available to all of us but that we rarely allow ourselves to touch or acknowledge.

Martha, when she had the stomach pain described in chapter 2, did the same thing. *Our bodies contain information that is beyond our mind's capacity to understand. We are much more than we think we are.* And most of our illnesses get their start as emotional pain—with an ensuing negative judgment about ourselves—that gets stuck in the body. When we acknowledge and then release our pain, our bodies and our lives become joyous and healthy. Martha has never had stomach pain again. And Brenda conceived three months after I removed the IUD, and eventually gave birth to a healthy son. The work we do to transform our pain into joy heals the whole world.

TRANSFORMING OUR FEAR OF OUR SHAMAN PAST

It is estimated that in the Middle Ages, up to 9 million women, many of them midwives and healers, were imprisoned, tortured, burned alive, or otherwise murdered as witches. This witch craze, fueled by the Catholic Church, lasted for about 500 years and has been well documented.[4] In her book *Wicca Made Easy: Awaken the Divine Magic Within You* (Hay House, 2019), Phyllis Curott—an attorney and founder of the Temple of Ara, the world's oldest shamanic Wiccan congregation—outlines just how well sanctioned this behavior was. In 1484, she notes, Pope Innocent VII published a papal edict authorizing the use of torture to get women to confess to using witchcraft—an edict that has never been rescinded. Soon after, a pair of German monks published an anti-woman screed called *Malleus Maleficarum,* describing how to carry out the papal edict. Then in 1542, Pope Paul III established the Holy Office of the Inquisition, which also still exists. (My friend Alberto Villoldo, Ph.D., told me that there is an official Office of Inquisition in Lima, Peru.) During this dark period, which Curott says is often referred to as the women's holocaust, women lost their autonomy. They were not allowed to learn to read or to go to school. They were also not permitted to own or inherit property. In fact, they themselves were considered the property of their husbands, fathers, or brothers. Curott writes, "Their traditional roles as shamans and healers, midwives and wise women who were central to the spiritual and physical wellbeing of their villages either disappeared, went underground or shape-shifted into a more socially acceptable form, as it did for their male counterparts and their traditions."

It's not uncommon for women who are reclaiming their power or speaking their personal truths to have terrifying dreams of being burned. I have heard this countless times in my work. Many women reexperience being burned at the stake during sacred spot massage or internal pelvic work. This doesn't surprise me. The energy of love and light always makes space for our deepest sorrow and fear to surface and be released.

The burning times have been suppressed for centuries but are now, at this time of increasing light, surfacing in our consciousness to be cleared and transformed so that the feminine and masculine energies can move into true partnership within each of us and men and women can co-create as equals. When I first wrote about this fear of our past, I had no idea how powerfully I, too, carried it. Only after the first edition of this book was published and I started having nightmares about being murdered every night for a week did I see how prophetic my own words were.

When a woman enters into the work of healing her body and speaking her truth, she must break through the collective field of fear and pain that is all around us and has been for the past 5,000 years of dominator society. It is a field filled with the fear of rape, of beating, of abandonment.

Rupert Sheldrake, Ph.D., a British biologist, posits that all the knowledge of the earth's past exists all around us as electromagnetic fields of information, or "morphogenic fields."[5] As already mentioned, Jung called it the "collective unconscious." Quantum physics calls it the "unified field." When an athlete first breaks a world record, Dr. Sheldrake notes, he or she often has to work for years to do it and is often told that it can't be done—that it is not humanly possible. It was once felt, for example, that no one would ever be able to run a mile in under four minutes. But once Roger Bannister did it, athletes all over the world were able to do it, too. The same is true for many other athletic feats. Dr. Sheldrake explains that the morphogenic field around this world record is changed by the first person who breaks it, thus making it easier for others to equal that performance by tapping in to the new morphogenic field. (For more information, see Dr. Sheldrake's website at www.sheldrake.org.)

Women (and men) all over the planet are finding the courage to break through the collective morphogenic field of shame, fear, and pain. This usually takes the form of rocking the boat of the status quo in one's family. For example, years ago, one of my patients went home to tell her father what it was like to grow up in a household in which he had sexually abused her sisters and herself for years. She stood there and told all of it, not to change him but to break the years of silence. She later told me, "I am ready to go on national television with my father's name. He not only ruined my girlhood but also abused almost every girl in my neighborhood!" She finally had found the courage to feel her anger and pain. This is a first step toward transformation. True forgiveness can't come until a woman takes this step. By releasing the secrets that kept her trapped, she is saying, "No more!" All over the world, women like this are changing the morphogenic field of fear and silence. From Africa, where women are speaking out about female genital mutilation and rape, to India, where selective abortion of females is being addressed, to the United States, where we no longer tolerate intimate violence—silence is everywhere being broken and healing abounds!

Breaking the silence takes courage. I know of no woman who has tapped her inner source of power without going through an almost palpable veil of fear, often feeling as though her very life would be threatened by telling the truth. The journalist Vivian Gornick says, "For a woman, coming off fear is like an addict coming off drugs." I don't know any way around this fear except to name it and then go through it with the help of others who've also experienced it and come out on the other side. Millions of women healers and wise women, and the men who have supported them, have been killed for telling the truth. It is little wonder, given the collective history of women and the feminine, that we have been afraid. When we deny this fear or discount its presence in others, we only give it more power. Experiencing the fear we collectively hold is a very important step toward healing—we need not judge it in others or in ourselves.

But as each of us acknowledges, feels, and moves through her fear, it becomes that much easier for the next woman to heal, and the next one after her, just as when a world record is broken. We are changing the morphogenic field together, as thousands of women the world over break through their fields of fear at the same time. The first women who told the truth about their incest were accused of making it up. Now, when a woman remembers and speaks—no matter what the indignity she has suffered—support, books, the Internet, and meetings are available for her. She need no longer feel alone, like she's crazy or the only one this has happened to.

And then the magic starts. As you allow the life force to guide your life, the exhilaration comes. Once you break through this fear and begin living your life according to your inner wisdom, you find you have everything you need to create a life for yourself that is based on freedom, joy, and opportunity. I have seen this repeatedly and have experienced it myself. So take heart. There is great hope, joy, and love—all around us, all the time—when we clear ourselves of past habits, change our thinking, and embrace our power.

In 1993, I wrote the following: "I often think of myself as standing on the shoulders of all the strong women who came before me and being supported by them, women who had the courage to speak their truths even in the face of great opposition. I reassure myself with the thought, 'They can't burn me this time. There are too many of us this time. This time I am safe.'" Back then, I never expected that my work would be accepted in my lifetime. When the first edition of this book came out, I was terrified to go into the hospital and face my colleagues. I kept moving forward anyway. Now, years later, I am not only safe but also freer and happier than I have ever been in my life. I have more abundance, more love, and more joy than I ever dreamed possible. I look back on where I was in 1993, and I smile with compassion for who I was then. And I want you to know that I see my own journey reflected daily in the lives of women the world over.

OUR DREAMS: EARTH'S DREAMS

Women are rising like yeast all over the planet.

—Sonia Johnson

As we heal, through feeling our grief and our joy, the earth heals. Part of the rise of the feminine that I see happening all over the world is the strengthening of ties between women. Gwendolyn, one of the women we met earlier, said that as a result of her healing, "What has come into my life are beautiful female relationships. This never happened before because I put so much energy into men. Now a sisterhood is starting to happen. When you take the time to tune in to yourself and your needs, the sisterhood starts happening." I see the bonds between women—all women—growing stronger and more powerful every day. I feel more supported by women both locally and globally now than ever before in my life. My daughters are experiencing the same thing. The more we support other women, the more we all thrive. There doesn't need to be competition. When I see a beautiful woman, I feel uplifted by her beauty. She's part of me and I'm part of her.

I couldn't do the work I do without the support of my sisters throughout the world. My women friends and colleagues sustain me. I feel supported and blessed. Brian Swimme, Ph.D., once wrote that we humans are the space where the earth dreams through us. Our heart's desire is the desire of the earth—it is what She is asking you to do. The dominator system has told us that "if it doesn't hurt, it is not worth doing—no pain, no gain." But often just the opposite is true. If what you are doing gives you no joy, no pleasure, no sense of purpose, no sense of fulfillment, it is not worth doing. Your state of health is the barometer of this. Your cells know what you need to do—listen!

Every cell in your body responds to your inner dreams and to pleasure. All children know this. Joy and pleasure are necessary for your health and for that of our planet. The dreams the earth dreams through you are different from the ones She dreams through me. But I need to hear your dreams, and you need to hear mine—otherwise we don't have the whole story. The dominator system has had a vested interest in keeping us from hearing one another for centuries. But our time has come. Let's listen to one another.

Personal Healing Is Planetary Healing

For all of written history, the earth and the natural world have been viewed as feminine, with "virgin resources" to be "exploited." What happens to individual women and what happens to our planet are linked. Our personal and collective degradation of nature, women, and the feminine is drawing to a close, one person at a time.

Outmoded Newtonian science will not save us because it is obsolete. It lacks the voice of intuition, the feminine voice, the voice that speaks from our bodies. We require balance now. We require embodied wisdom that is filtered through all of us—including what the mind of our bodies and our inner guidance is telling us.

I recall a cover of *Ms.* magazine showing a crowd of women with the headline *RAGE + WOMEN = POWER.*[6] This message made me uncomfortable until I saw the potential embedded in it. The anger and rage of silenced women, when used as fuel for positive change, is indeed power. But it must be power from within, power that is fully grounded and centered—not rage directed *against* someone or something. Rage *transformed* is power. Rage *transformed* is strength. It can be likened to fire—fire can destroy your house, or it can cook your dinner. It all depends on how you use it!

To name your work "political," especially when it comes to your body and to things that are womanly, is an act of power. If you are a mother, believe me, your work is political. If you are a nurse, a childcare worker, or anything else, your work is political. If you're healing a fibroid tumor or remembering your incest, you are doing political work. Breast-feeding is political.

How refreshing to see our body's healing as political. Let us give it the importance that it deserves! Gloria Steinem once said, "Any woman who is up off her ass is part of the women's movement." I like that a lot—it leaves room for a wide range of interpretations. We have many choices. No one but you gets to define your healing or your politics for you. Do you need to take six weeks off from work to heal from pelvic surgery? Think of it as political. And then when you've learned from it, see if you can channel future energy outward from your body into work that is positive and life affirming. Or if you need to take six weeks off just to enjoy and get in touch with yourself, that, too, is political!

In the epilogue to her book on her recovery from breast cancer, *A Burst of Light* (Firebrand Books, 1998), the late poet Audre Lorde writes, "I had to examine in my dreams as well as in my immune function tests the devastating effects of overextension. Overextending myself is not stretching myself. I had to accept how difficult it is to monitor the difference. Caring for myself is not self-indulgence, it is self-preservation, and that is an act of political warfare."[7]

In a political system that has not represented womanly values, each woman must represent herself and become a lobbyist for her own needs. Caring for yourself as well as you possibly can, *whether or not* you are sick, is indeed an act of political warfare.

Physician, Heal Thyself—Revisited

My inner guidance came to me through the mind of my uterus while I was in the process of writing the original edition of this book. I was diagnosed with a fibroid tumor that made my uterus about thirteen-week size. I had no symptoms. I had been eating an essentially dairy-free, low-fat diet for years. (I didn't know then that my intake of bread and high-glycemic-index foods was probably contributing to the problem.) At first I was saddened and didn't want anyone to know about it. I grieved for the loss of my "normal" uterus. When one of my colleagues did a pelvic exam and told me about the fibroid, the first thought I had was, "I better get this book finished, because I'm sure this growth is related to it." I felt intuitively that it had started to grow in the early stages of my writing process, two years before. I also thought, "Damn, I've been hanging around too many women with fibroids. Maybe I caught one."[8]

I felt as though I had done something wrong, as though I had somehow failed. I was reminded that our emotions don't always match our level of intellectual development. I was humbled. Later that night, as I lay in my bed, I put my hands over my lower abdomen and said to my uterus, "Okay, now I have to take my own medicine and tune in to what you're telling me." My uterus gave me the following message: "This fibroid is a reminder that you need to learn how to move energy through your body more efficiently. If you take care of yourself now and pay attention, you'll avoid more serious problems in the future. This is also a wonderful opportunity to teach other women by example. Remember, the work you're doing with others applies to you. You've always believed that it is possible to dematerialize fibroids. Here's your chance." I meditated on creativity and what was needing to be birthed through me. As is so often the case, I was clueless about why I really manifested the fibroid. I just knew the territory as it applied to others.

The next day I began a regimen of castor oil packs, and I started a course of acupuncture, something I'd been wanting to do as a general preventive measure for a long time. My acupuncturist told me that my kidney and triple warmer meridians were very low and had been for some time. This was related to overwork and stress and adrenal exhaustion. I was reminded of a chronic energy pattern that Oriental medicine refers to as "stuck blood" or "stuck *chi*," on the right side of my body. My previous migraine headaches had been on my right side; Caroline Myss had once diagnosed energy leaking out of my right hip, manifesting as a hip problem on the right; my breast abscess had been on the right; and now I had a fibroid on the right side of my uterus. All were on the right side of my body—the "masculine" or yang side—and all were related in an energy sense. What that meant to me was that it had been important to develop a strong foundation for my work and to take it out into the world—that was my "masculine" task. Up until the late 1980s I had been afraid of doing so fully because of my perception that the world wasn't ready to hear it and that it would be dangerous for me. Hence, the repeated "wounds" on my right side. The fibroid was simply the latest manifestation—and a timely one at that, given my life's work with women. And despite an ongoing recovery from "othering"—paying more attention to others' needs than to my own—I also realized how much I still wanted the approval of others. I saw how powerless I was—and am—over what people think of me, a lesson that I've finally mastered only this year. This past summer I sat down and read all the reviews for *Dodging Energy Vampires* on Amazon—something I had never done before for any of my books, including this one. Most were positive. A couple were downright nasty—complete character assassinations. In the past, I would have let those negative reviews stop me dead in my tracks for weeks; I would have beaten myself up for not having written the book properly or in a way that someone could read it. Not anymore. I now realized that being that critical of me and my work had far more to do with the person who wrote the review than with me. Revelation.

But back then when I discovered the fibroid, I finally had to realize that it was about more than the book and the depleted acupuncture meridians. After several months of acupuncture and castor oil packs, it seemed to get larger, not smaller. My learning had to go much deeper. What did I need to learn?

I knew that fibroids are related to pouring your creativity into dead-end relationships or jobs. I assumed that mine was related to my work. I realized that my entire relationship with my office and with my profession needed to change—that I was in bondage to an obsolete form. While my heart wanted to write, lecture, and teach women a whole new way of being in relationship with their bodies, my intellectual sense of responsibility dictated that I continue to practice medicine in the way I had been trained: see patients, do surgery, and do my share of emergency calls like everybody else (back then I called this my relationship addiction in yet another guise). I realized that I needed more freedom. I needed to change my practice to teach more of the material in this book. I needed to be responsible to my deepest dreams and my innermost wisdom.

Women's health will never change substantially unless large groups of women begin to reclaim the wisdom of their bodies collectively. For me to do this meant letting go of being "the doctor" to the hundreds of women I'd enjoyed working with so much over the years. I didn't want to leave the practice of medicine—I wanted to transform it. I knew that I could no longer do primary care with all of its cultural assumptions, assumptions that were chaining me to limits that I could no longer tolerate.

I wanted to reinvent the practice of medicine. I realized at a deeper level than ever before that one-on-one healthcare, though valuable, tends to isolate each woman's problem and doesn't allow physicians the time necessary to educate a woman fully about all the issues that can affect her body and how she has the power to transform them. So I began to move toward teaching women in groups how to create health on a daily basis.

I wrote a letter to my patients that said, "I am not leaving the practice of medicine. I am redefining it and expanding into new areas that are critical to truly improving women's health over the long term." I told them that disease screening (which my training had prepared me for) and creating health (where my heart was taking me) were two different things. I needed to concentrate on a new form now. In my letter I asked my patients to consider the following questions. I ask you to do the same.

~ What would it be like if you reclaimed the wisdom of your body and learned how to trust its messages?

~ What would your life be like if you no longer feared germs or cancer?

~ How would your life be different if your body were your friend and ally?

~ How would your life be different if you learned how to love and respect your body as though it were your own precious creation, as valuable as a beloved friend or child? How would you treat yourself differently?

~ What would it be like to know, in the deepest part of you, that every part of your anatomy and each process of your female body contained wisdom and power?

Unbeknownst to me, I was in the early stages of articulating a new vision of women's health that required me first to truly flourish in my own life, then to teach this to others. I didn't realize, however, the extent to which I'd have to walk through fire to do it.

Though I was sure that the fibroid would start to shrink once I finished this book, that wasn't the case. It persisted and tended to wax and wane in size. I asked it to teach me. I had dialogues with it. I tried to love it. I then realized that my relationship to work was only one part of my life. I had to reevaluate every relationship I was in, including those with my husband and immediate family. I saw yet another pattern emerging: I tended to put my emotional and creative needs on hold until the needs of my husband and children were met. I allowed them to interrupt me in my home office and during my work, and I didn't set clear boundaries. My husband and I especially had to begin the process of renegotiating every part of our relationship. I also uncovered the deep belief that if I truly moved into my full potential, those closest to me would feel threatened and would leave me. I would be alone. And so I often made myself "less than," so that no one else would feel "less than" because of my success.

Just before Christmas 1996, the fibroid got bigger. An ultrasound documented that it was causing backup of urine in my left kidney. I found that I had gradually adjusted my life (and my wardrobe) around my fibroid. Though my periods were never a problem, and I had no symptoms, I simply got tired of having a protruding abdomen. I decided that it was time to let go of my dream of dematerializing my fibroid. I saw that I, too, had a belief that it was "good" to use "natural" methods to shrink the fibroid, but "bad" to seek the help I had so often offered to others. I had run headlong into my own addictive thinking. So I decided to schedule surgery—the path I had tried to avoid (and therefore energized) for four years. I called a trusted pelvic surgeon, a man to whom I have referred many patients, and made an appointment in which we scheduled the fibroid removal. I told almost no one, deciding that it would be best for me to contain my energies, thoughts, and feelings about this. I also started on a GnRH agonist (Synarel) to shrink the fibroid so that the incision would be smaller. (By now the fibroid had reached the size of a very large cantaloupe.) I experienced hot flashes on the Synarel and decided that for me, at least, these were not "power surges"— they were uncomfortable, sweaty disturbances in my day. But other than that, I had no problems, and the fibroid shrank nicely.

My surgery time arrived. I asked both my surgeon and my anesthesiologist to say the four healing statements to me. (See the section on how to prepare for surgery in chapter 16.) And in addition to the four healing statements, I asked the anesthesiologist to say the following and repeat it several times: "When you awaken, you will have released the emotional pattern associated with this fibroid." My surgery went well; there was only one large fibroid on the right side of the uterus, embedded in the wall; my recovery was easy, with very little pain; and I left the hospital the day after surgery. For the next three weeks I took naps, had acupuncture, watched movies, and rested. I wanted this to be a total rebirth for me—a time to receive care, not give it. The surgery and recovery were a peak experience for me in many ways. I had faced something I had tried to avoid—the healing path of surgery—and in facing and moving through it I had found care, compassion, skill, and great healing there for me. Though I had wanted to write that I had dematerialized my fibroid in a blinding flash of insight, I came to see that in my case that wasn't to be, and my attachment to that as an "ideal" and "superior" path was just a case of spiritual materialism. (I still know it's possible, however, for women to dematerialize fibroids; I've seen it.)

Looking back on what I originally wrote about that fibroid in 1993 and again in 1998 with the first revision, I have to laugh at myself. I wrote about "carrying the creations" of others, needing to change my work, and on and on. All true to some extent. The truth was that I was circling around and around the real issue but was blind to it because I didn't want to go there. I didn't want to change the very thing that most needed change: my marriage, the thing that was right in front of my eyes. This is so often the case. Be careful what you ask for, the saying goes, because you'll probably get it! Sure enough, once my surgery was completed, those magic words that were whispered to me during anesthesia—"When you awaken, you will have released the emotional pattern that led to this condition"—began to work their magic. My marriage of twenty-four years ended about a year and a half later. Like everything else of significance in life, this was a process, not an event. And as so often happens, I wasn't happy about taking this particular dose of healing medicine. I wanted to be married until death do us part. But the price was getting to be too high. And my body wouldn't let me forget it. I knew too much. If you don't pay attention the first time, you get hit by a bigger hammer: a fibroid today, breast cancer tomorrow. The pain of that time was the impetus for writing the first edition of my second book, *The Wisdom of Menopause*. And the process of writing it transformed me.

My fibroid, like all the conditions in our bodies, was a great teacher. Through my midlife divorce, I learned up close and personal that you can't create anything for another person, only for yourself. I also learned that when we face our worst fears and work through them, the process transforms us in miraculous and unpredictable ways. You can't take another person where he or she doesn't want to go, no matter how skillful, loving, and compassionate you are! But you can take yourself where you've been afraid to go. Personal growth and fulfillment are inside jobs. Ultimately each of us must tap in to the Source of creativity, wellness, and joy that is our birthright. Each of us has that ability. It gets strengthened through intent, faith, and the courage to choose pleasure over pain. And it never fails. My divorce forced me to grow in ways that I never dreamed possible. It forced me to take dominion over my life and my finances in ways I never would have otherwise. It forced me to really trust myself on all levels for the first time in my life. Though it was enormously painful at the time, I now feel nothing but gratitude! It made me into a wise, fulfilled, and happy woman. My former husband is a hero in this story. On a soul level, I believe that he signed up to help me become who I am today.

We can't create a new world if we believe that we must remain small and ineffective on any level in order for others to love us and want to be with us. When we dim our light so that others appear to shine brighter, the whole world gets darker. I have had to apply this learning to my marriage, to my friendships, and even to my relationships with entire institutions such as hospitals and financial institutions. The issues in each situation, large or small, are always the same. And they boil down to the same fear: Will I be loved if I become everything I was meant to be? Let me be the first to report to you from the front lines of this process. The answer is a resounding *yes*! But this love must begin with yourself first. When you become more loving toward yourself, more loving toward your body and its processes, and more appreciative of yourself, your vibration changes. Your point of attraction changes. If you wait for someone else to make the first move here, you'll be stuck in the painful, powerless, victim mode—complete with all its longing, pining, and health problems—endlessly. I've been there. It's hell. But when you have the courage to say yes to yourself, yes to your soul, and yes to life, and begin to realize that you deserve a heavenly, wonderful life right now, then fulfillment beyond your wildest dreams will start coming your way. And the world will open up to you in ways that you never before dreamed possible. Old, outmoded ways of being and living, and old, outmoded relationships, will fall away. And this can be very painful. Just think of it as the natural process of labor through which you are birthing your new self—a self that reflects who you really are and who you were always meant to be. It's always worth it.

MAKING THE WORLD SAFE FOR WOMEN: START WITH YOURSELF

The Pulitzer Prize–winning journalist team of Sheryl WuDunn and Nicholas D. Kristof, authors of *Half the Sky: Turning Oppression into Opportunity for Women Worldwide* (Alfred A. Knopf, 2009), points out that focusing on the needs of women and girls is *the* issue of this century. Discussing why educating and empowering women is a good idea for society as a whole in a 2009 article for *The New York Times,* Kristof and WuDunn share what they call "the dirty little secret of global poverty": "Some of the most wretched suffering is caused not just by low incomes but also by unwise spending by the poor—especially by men. Surprisingly frequently, we've come across a mother mourning a child who has just died of malaria for want of a $5 mosquito bed net; the mother says that the family couldn't afford a bed net and she means it, but then we find the father at a nearby bar. He goes three evenings a week to the bar, spending $5 each week."[9] Their research has found that wherever girls and women are educated, terrorism lessens, and economic development increases in ways that benefit men, women, and children alike. This is reminiscent of an old African proverb I once read: To educate a boy is to educate an individual, but to educate a girl is to educate a whole nation. Kristof and WuDunn's research takes this sentiment out of the realm of the proverbial and proves it.

On their website (www.halftheskymovement.org), WuDunn and Kristof write, "We hope to recruit you to join an incipient movement to emancipate women and fight global poverty by unlocking women's power as economic catalysts. It is a process that transforms bubbly teenage girls from brothel slaves into successful businesswomen. You can help accelerate change if you'll just open your heart and join in."

The entire planet is finally waking up to this truth: Self-development for women is the answer to many, if not most, of the world's problems. But you needn't go to Africa or Afghanistan to support the development of women. The emancipation and education of all women start with your own emancipation and education. As astrologer and writer Rob Brezsny puts it so eloquently, "The quality of your consciousness is crucial in determining whether you'll be able to attract the resources that are essential to your dreams coming true. In order to get what you want, you have to work on yourself at least as hard as you work on the world around you." I couldn't agree more.

If we are ever to create safety in the outside world for ourselves, we must first create safety for ourselves *right in our own bodies.* If, as we undress for bed, we look in the mirror and beat ourselves up for our breast size or our cellulite, we are not walking our walk. *We are not safe with ourselves.* If we can't create a safe space *within ourselves* for our own bodies—their shapes, their sizes, their natural functions, and their weights—if we are forever putting down our own flesh and blood, starving our bodies, and giving them adverse messages, how can we ever expect to flourish? You can't flourish when you are carting around your own internal terrorist!

The truth is that we can change only ourselves, not anyone or anything else. This is such good news and such a relief! After centuries of being told that someone else could, should, and would take care of us, we now know that we can take care of ourselves—together. We can create fulfilling lives on our own terms. A past Boston Women's Fund brochure said it best: "The people we've been waiting for are us." Aren't you energized just reading that? We can start saving ourselves now. We can start living our own lives now. This is the starting point for true partnership and communion with others—including men.

The late Marshall Rosenberg, Ph.D., founder of the Center for Nonviolent Communication, identified three stages in the way we relate to others that most of us work through as we progress in our personal developments. The first is emotional slavery, seeing ourselves as responsible for what other people feel. For example, we put others' needs before our own because we don't want to disappoint or hurt anyone. The next stage, he says, is being obnoxious. In this stage, we allow ourselves to feel and express the anger we experience because we no longer want to be saddled with the weight of the enormous responsibility we were previously so eager to accept. In this stage, we're likely to think (and often say) that if others don't like our actions or our ideas, tough luck! We're putting our own needs ahead of the needs of others so we won't be held down or hurt anymore. The final stage, Dr. Rosenberg notes, is emotional liberation, where we take responsibility for our intentions and actions and for meeting our own needs. Finally, in this stage, we feel free to be gracious and compassionate toward others without compromising our own integrity and well-being. At this final stage of evolution, we move together in a cooperative effort to share responsibility in a true partnership. And this partnership, I might add, resembles a grand dance, filled with beautiful, passionate, and joyful rhythmic movement that ultimately moves the world forward.

When we change ourselves *inside* by allowing ourselves to experience and own our long-suppressed emotions and woundings as well as our hopes and dreams for ourselves, our families, and our planet, the conditions of our lives change on the *outside*. Working for social changes must go hand in hand with the willingness to heal within ourselves all the internalized messages of blame, self-doubt, and self-hatred that are encoded in our very cells. Otherwise, our actions originate out of unhealthy places within us and simply re-create polarization and pain. Being led by the Spirit means living in tune with our inner guidance. Listen quietly. What do you need to do next? Perhaps just being still for a moment is the best way to heal or to serve. Perhaps there's nothing you need to do right now. There is no one "right way" to heal your body. The same goes for any area of life. You must find the way yourself. Emerson once wrote, "The essence of heroism is self-trust." Self-trust is more than the essence of heroism. It is also the basis for trusting our intuition and the healing voice of our cells. Sorting out the genuine messages from our innermost selves (and cells) is no small task. It is indeed the work of heroes.

It takes courage to learn to respect yourself and your body, regardless of how wounded you've been, regardless of your current weight, regardless of whom you married or what your sexual preference is. Several years ago, I met a true hero who is the very embodiment of my message: When you change conditions inside yourself, the conditions outside yourself change in response. This hero is named Immaculée Ilibagiza, author of *Left to Tell* (Hay House, 2006), about the Rwandan holocaust. A beautiful woman with peace and divinity shining out of every pore, Immaculée, along with seven other women, was forced to hide in a small bathroom for three months during the Rwandan genocide. Her entire family was murdered. Her weight dropped to 65 pounds, she was covered with lice, and she couldn't move or talk for fear of being discovered and killed by her former friends and neighbors, who repeatedly came to the door, demanding her death. Amid conditions of unimaginable suffering, she reached deep into herself with faith and conviction and found the living presence of God in her heart. By tapping in to this Source, she manifested miraculous events that saved her life and allowed her to eventually create a joyous life in the United States despite the loss of her family and country. Meeting this woman and reading her story have taken my faith to a new level. If she was able to face what she faced and not only survive but also thrive, the rest of us can do the same.

I was nearing the completion of the second edition of this book during my second Saturn return around the time of my birthday. The second Saturn return signals the time in life when one moves from merely surviving to truly thriving and living life from one's soul. As I was planning my birthday celebration, a good friend asked me if I wanted to join her in going to a lecture by a famous monk. I simply didn't want to go! I didn't care how holy and inspiring he was. What I really wanted to do was have a private tango lesson and get my first pair of tango shoes. (I got them. They were black with very sexy three-inch-tall red lacquered heels. And I did not go to see the monk.)

I had already mastered the joy of selfless service. Continuing to do it in the same old way would be like getting four Ph.D.'s in the same field. I will continue to enjoy the intoxicating joys of serving others, but from the fullness of myself, not from a "give until it hurts" place of burnout. My ability to experience sustainable pleasure through dance, music, and art is just as healing for me and for others as is direct service. In fact, at the level at which all humans are one, the happier and more joyful I become, the easier it will be for the next woman to find that place within herself, too.

Several days before my birthday weekend, I wrote an email about the monk decision to my colleague Sandra Chiu, a New York City Chinese medicine physician and licensed acupuncturist (who also dances tango). She summarized my feelings precisely when she wrote:

> I could not agree with you more about going to see monks. I used to do that and it was good heart energy, but I'm over that—it doesn't turn me on a lick. And you're right—like we as women need a lesson in how to be selfless. Those things sometimes end up making a woman even more pathologically selfless. But if it were a Vietnamese nun stripping out of her robes to do a pole dance in a corset—*that* kinda monk/nun I'd see!
>
> We've got to go out there and cultivate life force. I'm over world peace and Zen compassion. Let's go gyrate, lady! This is exactly what you're about—spreading the word about how life force and health are enhanced by fun and pleasure. We need a respected woman and M.D. like you to say, "Hey, it's not only okay to make sure you get hits of fun and pleasure in your life—it's crucial." I'm your accomplice 100 percent in this mission.

Sandra's response reminded me of the truth embodied in the famous quote from civil rights leader and writer Howard Thurman that I shared earlier: "Don't ask yourself what the world needs; ask yourself what makes you come alive. And then go and do that. Because what the world needs is people who have come alive."

Women are the source of life force. Of Shakti. And when we've tapped in to our pleasure, we turn on the world. We are the force for good that the world has been waiting for. Whatever you call the inner power that Immaculée tapped in to—God, Goddess, Source, the Universe, or your Higher Power—know that it lives in each and every cell in your body. I believe it's the force that American writer Frederick Buechner was talking about when he wrote, "The place God calls you to is the place where your deep gladness and the world's deep hunger meet." This power is the one thing that we can count on always. I call it God. The women whose stories I've shared with you are ordinary women; they are healing women. They have all tapped in to this source of goodness and miracles. Their stories are the stories of transforming pain into joy. These women are my heroes.

Self-healing is a highly personal and individual process. Self-healing requires personal disarmament, refusing to be at war any longer with a part of your body or your life that's trying to tell you something. Let war end with you. One of my former patients, a fifteen-year member of Alcoholics Anonymous, summed this up beautifully: "Each morning I pray for willingness to do whatever it is I must do. *And I also pray to remain teachable.* There have been times in my life when no one could teach me anything. I thought I knew it all. I never want to be there again." Commit to creating heaven on earth for yourself. Know that it takes great courage to be as happy and fulfilled as you can be. It takes great courage to resist the voices of doubt and fear that inevitably crop up in our minds and hearts when we decide to become as magnificent as we really are. Be courageous anyway.

Commit to living your dreams—one day at a time. This is the process that is required to create vibrant health in our families, our communities, and our planet. May you go forth now, to take a nap, to embrace a child, to feel the sun on your face, or to eat a good meal slowly, knowing deep within you that the next step for healing and living joyfully is already there, waiting for you to listen to it, waiting to be born into the world—through you, dear woman.

Resources

This resources section is updated with subsequent printings of this book. For the most up-to-date information, visit Dr. Northrup's website at www.drnorthrup .com.

Christiane Northrup, M.D., F.A.C.O.G.
P.O. Box 199
Yarmouth, ME 04096
www.drnorthrup.com

Dr. Northrup's website (www.drnorthrup.com) is the best place to find regularly updated blogs, articles, videos, podcasts, and other content, as well as information about her lectures and other resources, including her many books, courses, and products. Answers to many of her readers' most frequently asked questions can also be found here.

In addition, Dr. Northrup stays in touch with her large and growing community worldwide through her Facebook page (Facebook.com/DrChristianeNorthrup), Instagram (@drchristianenorthrup), Twitter (@DrChrisNorthrup), and her biweekly e-newsletter (to subscribe, sign up at www.drnorthrup.com).

BOOKS
Dodging Energy Vampires: An Empath's Guide to Evading Relationships That Drain You and Restoring Your Health and Power (Hay House, 2018).

In this book, Dr. Northrup explores the phenomenon of energy vampires (also known as personality-disordered individuals) and shows how to spot them, dodge their tactics, and take back your own energy. She draws on the latest research, along with stories from her global community as well as her own life. She delves into the dynamics of vampire-empath relationships to discover how vampires use others' energy to fuel their own dysfunctional lives. Once you recognize the patterns of behavior that mark these relationships, you'll be empowered to identify the vampires in your life, too.

A Daily Dose of Women's Wisdom (Hay House, 2017).

For decades, Dr. Northrup has been helping women navigate their lives with grace and joy. This elegant, compact volume offers her trademark wisdom in a fresh form, filled with pointed reminders "to help you develop a deeper respect for, and connection to, your own body and its exquisite guidance system to create a vibrantly healthy body, mind, and spirit." Each beautifully designed black-and-white page carries a quote that touches on a topic of deep significance—including heart-listening, epigenetics, and the importance of knowing that your decisions about medical treatment are not irreversible.

Making Life Easy: How the Divine Inside Can Heal Your Body and Your Life (Hay House, 2016).

In this joyfully encouraging book—as useful for men as it is for women—Dr. Northrup explores the essential truth that has guided her ever since medical school: Our bodies, minds, and souls are profoundly intertwined. Making life flow with ease, and truly feeling your best, is about far more than physical health; it's also about having a healthy emotional life and a robust spiritual life. When you view your physical well-being in isolation, life can become a constant battle to make your body "behave." When you acknowledge the deep connection between your beliefs and your biology and start to tune in to the divine part of yourself, it's a whole new ball game—and the first step in truly making your life easy.

Goddesses Never Age: The Secret Prescription for Radiance, Vitality, and Well-Being (Hay House, 2015).

Though we talk about wanting to "age gracefully," the truth is that when it comes to getting older, we're programmed to dread an inevitable decline: in our health, our looks, our sexual relationships, and even the pleasure we take in living life. But as Dr. Northrup shows us in this profoundly empowering book, we have it in us to make growing older an entirely different experience, for both our bodies and our souls.

In chapters that blend personal stories and practical exercises with the latest research on health and aging, Dr. Northrup lays out the principles of ageless living, including rejecting processed foods, releasing stuck emotions, embracing our sensuality, and connecting deeply with our divine Source. She brings it all together in a fourteen-day Ageless Goddess Program, offering tools and inspiration for creating a healthful and soulful new way of being at any stage of life.

Beautiful Girl: Celebrating the Wonders of Your Body (Hay House, 2013).

For years, Dr. Northrup has taught women about health, wellness, and the miracle of their bodies. Now, in her first children's book, she presents these ideas to the youngest of girls. *Beautiful Girl* presents this simple but important message: that to be born female is a very special thing and carries with it magical gifts and powers that must be recognized and nurtured. Dr. Northrup believes that helping girls learn at a young age to value the wonder and uniqueness of their bodies can have positive benefits that will last throughout their lives. By reading this lovely book, little girls will learn how their bodies are perfect just the way they are, the importance of treating themselves with gentle care, and how changes are just a part of growing up.

The Wisdom of Menopause: Creating Physical and Emotional Health and Healing During the Change (Bantam, 2012).

In this *New York Times* bestselling book, Dr. Northrup shows women how they can make menopause a time of personal empowerment and positive energy—emerging wiser, healthier, and stronger in both mind and body. The "change" is not simply a collection of physical symptoms to be "fixed," this book explains, but a mind-body revolution that brings the greatest opportunity for growth since adolescence. Dr. Northrup outlines how the choices a woman makes now—from the quality of her relationships to the quality of her diet—have the power to secure her health and well-being for the rest of her life.

The Wisdom of Menopause Journal (Hay House, 2007).

This companion book to Dr. Northrup's bestselling book *The Wisdom of Menopause* helps you focus on the "me" in menopause. Designed to help you both navigate and document this important transitional time, the journal is packed with action-oriented, practical advice for your mind and body.

This journal gives you everything you need to create vibrant health in midlife on all levels—not just in your heart, bones, pelvic organs, breasts, and brain, but also in your sex life, your relationships, and even your beauty regimen! It enables you to record your current health and concerns, as well as the steps you want to take to achieve your goals in each area. You'll also find powerful affirmations, inspiring quotes, and plenty of blank pages for journaling, so you can create a record of your thoughts and feelings during this important time.

The Secret Pleasures of Menopause (Hay House, 2008).

This book delivers a breakthrough message that will help perimenopausal and menopausal women understand that at menopause, life has just begun. It's the beginning of a very exciting and fulfilling time, full of pleasure beyond your wildest dreams!

The Secret Pleasures of Menopause Playbook (Hay House, 2009).

This companion volume to *The Secret Pleasures of Menopause* serves as a personal guide to the territory of life-giving pleasure, with space provided to write down and commit to your own personal pleasure plan.

Mother-Daughter Wisdom: Understanding the Crucial Link Between Mothers, Daughters, and Health (Bantam, 2005).

Dr. Northrup explains how the mother-daughter relationship sets the stage for our state of health and well-being for our entire lives. Because our mothers are our first and most powerful female role models, our most deeply ingrained beliefs about ourselves as women come from them. And our behavior in relationships—with food, with our children, with our mates, and with ourselves—is a reflection of those beliefs. In this book, Dr. Northrup shows how once we understand our mother-daughter bonds, we can rebuild our own health, whatever our age, and create a lasting positive legacy for the next generation.

ONLINE RESOURCES
The Dr. Christiane Northrup E-Newsletter

Dr. Northrup's free biweekly newsletter is sent directly to subscribers' email addresses. It contains the most updated information on a wide variety of topics guaranteed to enhance your health on all levels. With links to take readers directly to relevant and the most up-to-date content and resources, the e-newsletter is one of the best ways to stay on track with your health. Available at www.drnorthrup .com/newsletter.

DrNorthrup.com

Dr. Northrup's website, www.drnorthrup.com, houses a wealth of information, designed to both inform and uplift users. With content covering the latest medical research and trends as well as hundreds of archived health-related articles, blog posts, online seminars, inspirational audio downloads, videos, and podcasts, this is the perfect go-to resource for anyone wanting to be healthy in mind, body, and spirit.

AUDIO/VIDEO PROGRAMS

Dr. Northrup's audio and video programs are all available through www .drnorthrup.com or through Hay House (800-654-5126; www.hayhouse.com).

Dodging Energy Vampires: An Empath's Guide to Evading Relationships That Drain You and Restoring Your Health and Power. Audio download.

In this program, Dr. Northrup explores the phenomenon of energy vampires and shows how to spot them, dodge their tactics, and take back your own energy. She draws on the latest research, along with stories from her global community as well as her own life. She delves into the dynamics of vampire-empath relationships to discover how vampires use others' energy to fuel their own dysfunctional lives. Once you recognize the patterns of behavior that mark these relationships, you'll be empowered to identify the vampires in your life, too.

Making Life Easy. Audio Download.

In this program, Dr. Northrup explores the essential truth that has guided her ever since medical school: Our bodies, minds, and souls are profoundly intertwined. Making life flow with ease, and truly feeling your best, is about far more than physical health; it's also about having a healthy emotional life and a robust spiritual life. When you view your physical well-being in isolation, life can become a constant battle to make your body "behave." When you acknowledge the deep connection between your beliefs and your biology and start to tune in to the Divine part of yourself, it's a whole new ball game—and the first step in truly making your life easy. Drawing on fields as diverse as epigenetics, past-life regression, and standard Western medicine, Dr. Northrup distills a brilliant career's worth of wisdom into one comprehensive user's guide to a healthy, happy, radiant life.

Goddesses Never Age. Audio Download.

Though we talk about wanting to "age gracefully," the truth is that when it comes to getting older, we're programmed to dread an inevitable decline: in our health, our looks, our sexual relationships, and even the pleasure we take in living life. But as Dr. Northrup shows us in this profoundly empowering audio program, we have it in us to make growing older an entirely different experience, for both our bodies and our souls.

Inside-Out Wellness. Audio download by Christiane Northrup, M.D., and Dr. Wayne W. Dyer.

Dr. Northrup and Dr. Dyer team up for this inspirational and informative program that discusses how to transform the old habits, traditional beliefs, and everyday thoughts that keep you from becoming all that you can be. Topics include how to rewire your thought patterns and let go of your past so you can cultivate pleasure instead of stress, reawaken your passions, follow your bliss, and create the life you want.

Menopause and Beyond. Audio CD and audio download.

With cutting-edge medical information and guidance, Dr. Northrup invites midlife women to embrace their inner wisdom and transform the second half of their lives in this program, based on her bestselling book, *The Wisdom of Menopause.* The program focuses on heart health, hormone therapy, diet, and sexuality. Dr. Northrup also presents a five-step program that guarantees weight loss.

The Power of Joy. Audio CD and audio download.

Life is meant to be joyous! We are pleasure-seeking creatures by nature. Joy makes you younger, smarter, more intuitive, and healthier, with better hormonal balance and immune-system functioning. Joy even positively affects your metabolism. On this audio program, Dr. Northrup prescribes a ten-step process for overcoming habitual patterns of negative thinking, guilt, and pain in order to evoke the power of joy in your life every day.

The Secret Pleasures of Menopause. Audio download.

Dr. Northrup believes that it's about time menopausal women came out of the closet and learned to enjoy the best years of their lives! Even though studies show that menopause does not decrease libido, ease of reaching orgasm, or sexual satisfaction, the majority of menopausal women are not experiencing the pleasure and sexual satisfaction that is their birthright. In this audio program, Dr. Northrup delivers a breakthrough message that will help millions of perimenopausal and menopausal women throughout the world understand that at menopause . . . life has just begun! It is the beginning of a very exciting and fulfilling time, full of pleasure beyond your wildest dreams!

Mother-Daughter Wisdom. Online video.

In the course of this journey to self-realization, Dr. Northrup covers a rich range of topics that are designed to bring mothers and daughters to greater consciousness, including the five facets of feminine power, how to end the mother-daughter "chain of pain," the power of forgiveness, and how to deal with a difficult mother or daughter.

The Empowering Women Gift Collection. Audio download.

This program includes inspiration and knowledge for women of all ages from Dr. Northrup, Louise L. Hay, Caroline Myss, and Susan Jeffers, Ph.D.

Dodging Energy Vampires Online Course

In six powerful, jam-packed lessons, Dr. Northrup teaches you how to recognize and rid yourself of energy-vampire relationships so that you can quickly separate from people who are using your energy to fuel their dysfunctional lives. Along the way, she interviews top experts from the field of personality disorders and offers simple, clear strategies and healing practices so that you can address the wounds that are keeping you stuck.

Ageless Goddess Online Course

Growing older is inevitable, but making the decision to stay fully active and engaged in life is a choice. In this online course, Dr. Northrup incorporates women's health and wellness that expands well beyond emotional, mental, and physical well-being. This innovative course teaches you a new way to view growing older that brings excitement and joy to your life, no matter your chronological age or your current quality of life. When you have the right information and guidance, youthful living can be yours and you can continue to thrive, create, and engage in your life for years to come.

Women's Bodies, Women's Wisdom Online Course—An Owner's Guide to Flourishing in Your Body for a Lifetime

For ages, women have been shamed and misinformed about their bodies—and this legacy has been handed down to us for millennia. This permeates not only our culture at large but also the entire medical system, where normal functions of the female body have become pathologized and medicalized. We have been alienated from understanding our bodies, and our beliefs about our worthiness have taken a plunge. Dr. Northrup is here to change that and to help you radically transform your health. "I walked a very fine line for many years," she says about her medical career, before breaking from mainstream medicine to speak the truth about women's wellness. And in this online course, she pulls no punches. She dives straight into the truth about women's health and everything you need to know to not only maintain your physical body but also to flourish throughout your life. In these comprehensive and mesmerizing lessons, Dr. Northrup will discuss everything you ever wanted to know—and absolutely need to learn—about your body.

OTHER

Amata Life by Dr. Christiane Northrup

After extensive research and development, Dr. Northrup formulated an array of drug-free products designed to relieve symptoms related to hormonal imbalance, including *Pueraria mirifica*. The products are distributed via www.amatalife.com.

General Resources

Holistic Healthcare Organizations

Academy of Integrative Health and Medicine (858-240-9033; www.aihm.org)

Founded in 1978 as the American Holistic Medical Association, this organization merged with the American Board of Integrative Holistic Medicine in 2013 to become AIHM. It is an organization of licensed medical doctors (M.D.s), doctors of osteopathic medicine (D.O.s), and medical students studying for those degrees. Physicians from every specialty are represented. The AIHM website contains both an online physician referral directory as well as a guide to choosing a holistic practitioner.

Institute for Functional Medicine (800-228-0622; www.ifm.org)

Functional medicine is an approach to medicine that treats the whole person instead of a set of symptoms and focuses on prevention instead of disease. Practitioners come from a variety of specialties and disciplines. The IFM website gives information about functional medicine and offers a directory of functional medicine practitioners.

Citizens for Health (www.citizens.org)

Citizens for Health was formed by a group of ordinary people who believe that good health is a right, not a benefit that should be determined by government or based on economic or social status. This idea grew into a movement and is now a national and international network of thousands of individuals, young and old, at every level of society, who want to exercise their rights to make informed choices regarding their healthcare.

Homeopathy

National Center for Homeopathy (856-437-4752; www.homeopathycenter.org)

The NCH website has a wealth of information and resources, including an interactive directory to help you find a homeopath in your area.

Natural Health Supply (888-689-1608; https://a2zhomeopathy.com)

This company sells a wide range of homeopathic remedy kits—including kits suitable for beginners, families, students, travelers, and practitioners—in various strengths and sizes.

Formulary Pharmacies

International Academy of Compounding Pharmacists (800-927-4227 or 281-933-8400; www.iacprx.org)

IACP (formerly known as Professionals and Patients for Customized Care, or P2C2) is a nonprofit organization made up of more than 4,000 pharmacists, technicians, students, and members of the compounding community nationwide. The IACP website has a locator feature that can help you find a compounding pharmacy in your area.

Diagnostic Laboratories

My Med Lab (888-696-3352; www.mymedlab.com)

This direct-to-consumer lab service allows you to order any of various medical tests without having to first schedule an appointment with your doctor just to get the test ordered. Here's how it works: After ordering your test online or over the phone, an in-house physician in your state reviews and approves the order, and the company uploads a digital lab order to your My Med Lab account and notifies you via email. You log on to your account, print the order, and search the listing of almost 2,000 patient service centers to see which is most convenient. You take the order to the service center of your choice to have your samples taken—you don't need a prior appointment. My Med Lab typically posts the results to your account within twenty-four to forty-eight hours, notifying you by email when they are ready.

The results include a brief explanation and a direct link to the National Library of Medicine for more detailed result information. If the results are abnormal, you should schedule an appointment with your doctor to discuss the findings. (Test results will not show up on your permanent medical record unless you share them with your doctor.) Although this form of testing is not generally covered by health insurance, prices are extremely reasonable.

Botanicals and Herbs

Emerson Ecologics (800-654-4432 or 603-656-9778; www.emersonecologics.com)
Emerson Ecologics provides high-quality nutritional supplements, antioxidants, vitamins, minerals, herbs, standardized herbal extracts, green foods, and essential fatty acids from the world's leading manufacturers of professional supplements.

NutraMedix (800-730-3130 or 561-745-2917; www.nutramedix.com)
NutraMedix uses a proprietary extraction and enhancement process in manufacturing its liquid extracts, resulting in a highly bio-available whole-plant, broad-spectrum, cost-effective extract. The company also offers high-quality powdered capsule products, many of which have been designed to enhance the effectiveness of its liquid extracts.

Essential Oils

Essential Oils Database (http://dr-lobisco.com/essential-oils-database)
Sara LoBisco, N.D., is a licensed naturopathic doctor and certified functional medicine practitioner who has compiled an online database containing numerous detailed articles on a wide variety of specific essential oils. The database is indexed by the type of oil as well as by health topic. In addition to her medical practice, Dr. LoBisco offers essential oil consultations by phone.

Multivitamin-Mineral Supplements

USANA (888-950-9595 or 801-954-7200; www.usana.com)
USANA makes a superior line of nutritional supplements using pharmaceutical-grade ingredients.

Verified Quality, available through Emerson Ecologics (800-654-4432 or 603-656-9778; www.emersonecologics.com). I also recommend this brand.

Intuitive Guidance

Doris Cohen, Ph.D. (216-556-1781; www.drdorisecohen.com)
Dr. Cohen, lecturer, workshop leader, and author of *Dreaming on Both Sides of the Brain* (Hampton Roads, 2017) and *Repetition: Past Lives, Life and Rebirth* (Hay House, 2008), has been a clinical psychologist and psychotherapist in private practice for more than thirty years. She is also a certified psychic and medical intuitive, known for her uncanny accuracy and insightful psychic readings.

Deena Spear (607-387-7787; www.singingwoods.org)

Deena is a vibrational and acoustical healer with a degree in neurobiology from Cornell University who combines twenty-nine years of experience as a violin maker with her training as an energy healer from the Barbara Brennan School of Healing.

Diane Goldner (323-813-8593; www.dianegoldner.com)

Diane went from being a skeptical reporter spending four years interviewing hundreds of people who have healed in unconventional ways to being a healer herself. She is the author of *Yes, You Can Heal* (Golden Spirit Books, 2018), *Awakening to the Light* (Golden Spirit Books, 2018), and *How People Heal: Exploring the Scientific Basis of Subtle Energy in Healing* (Hampton Roads, 2003). Diane has a hands-on healing practice in Los Angeles and New York and also does long-distance healing via telephone.

Julie Ryan (https://askjulieryan.com)

Julie is a medical intuitive who also works with energy fields to facilitate healing. She is a spiritual medium as well, and has identified twelve phases of transition we all go through at death, when angels and loved ones come to escort us to the other side. Julie works with families throughout the dying process to explain what's happening on the spirit level. She's the author of *Angelic Attendants: What Really Happens as We Transition from This Life into the Next* (Clement, 2017).

Chapter 1: The Patriarchal Myth: The Origin of the Mind/Body/Emotion Split

Anne Wilson Schaef, *When Society Becomes an Addict* (Harper & Row, 1987).

Riane Eisler, Ph.D., *The Chalice and the Blade: Our History, Our Future* (Harper & Row, 1987).

Riane Eisler, Ph.D., *Sacred Pleasure: Sex, Myth, and the Politics of the Body* (HarperSanFrancisco, 1995).

Chapter 3: Inner Guidance

Jerry and Esther Hicks, *The Vortex: Where the Law of Attraction Assembles All Cooperative Relationships* (Hay House, 2009); *Money, and the Law of Attraction: Learning to Attract Wealth, Health, and Happiness* (Hay House, 2008); *The Astonishing Power of Emotions: Let Your Feelings Be Your Guide* (Hay House, 2007); *The Law of Attraction: The Basics of the Teachings of Abraham* (Hay House, 2006); *The Amazing Power of Deliberate Intent: Living the Art of Allowing* (Hay House, 2006); *Ask and It Is Given: Learning to Manifest Your Desires* (Hay House, 2004). Also see www.abraham-hicks.com.

Chapter 5: The Menstrual Cycle

Lara Owen, *Her Blood Is Gold: Celebrating the Power of Menstruation* (Archive Publishing, 2009).

The Red Web Foundation (415-596-5356; www.theredweb.org)
The Red Web is dedicated to creating a positive view of the menstrual cycle (in its entirety from menarche through menopause) for girls and women through education and community. The group is also committed to women rediscovering meaning in their cycles because, as their website states, "when we learn how to live wisely with life-cycles, we learn to ground our self-esteem in profound internal wisdom. Body image and menstrual cycles are interlinking facets of women's total health and well-being."

For castor oil packs, please see resources for "Dysfunctional Uterine Bleeding (DUB)," later in the resources for this chapter.

Menastil
Menastil (available from Claire Ellen Products, 508-366-6411; www .bestpainrelief.com) is an effective and fast-acting topical roll-on product made from an extract of calendula petals and other essential oils, and clinically tested under FDA guidelines.

Acupuncture
Contact the American Association of Acupuncture and Oriental Medicine (www.aaaomonline.org) to locate an acupuncturist near you.

Bupleurum (Xiao Yao Wan)
For menstrual cramps, Easy Wanderer Plus from Emerson Ecologics contains Xiao Yao Wan. (800-654-4432 or 603-656-9778; www.emersonecologics.com).

Indole-3-carbinol from Longevity Science is available through Emerson Ecologics (800-654-4432 or 603-656-9778; www.emersonecologics.com).

FLO Living (www.floliving.com)
FLO Living offers in-person, over-the-phone, and online programs to help women heal their period problems and hormonal issues naturally without drugs or surgery.

OnOurMoon
This Instagram site founded by Alex Damour is a virtual red tent experience, aiming to normalize conversations about shame through vulnerable storytelling. See www.instagram.com/onourmoon as well as a listing of events available on the OnOurMoon website (www.onourmoon.com).

Premenstrual Syndrome (PMS)

Seasonal Affective Disorder/Light Therapy
To purchase a full-spectrum light, contact Sunshine Sciences (800-468-1104 or 303-834-9161; www.sunshinesciences.com).

Progesterone Cream

Progesterone cream 2 percent is available from a number of different sources. I have personally used Emerita's Pro-Gest, which is widely available through pharmacies, natural food stores, and on Amazon. Natural progesterone capsules are available by prescription through any formulary pharmacy. (See General Resources, above.)

Dysfunctional Uterine Bleeding (DUB)

Castor Oil Packs

Castor oil packs are wonderful for healing menstrual problems, urinary tract infections, joint aches and pains, and abdominal distress. Applied to the upper chest, they also can relieve a cough. The usual treatment frequency is one hour three to five times a week. (Don't use them during the heaviest days of the menstrual period.) Used once per week, they are also good preventive medicine. They have been shown to increase immune system functioning.

A castor oil pack is wool flannel saturated with castor oil, applied directly to the skin. A plastic sheet goes over the pack to keep the castor oil from going all over the place, and a heat source is then applied on top of the plastic. We highly recommend a hot water bottle for this purpose; though a heating pad can be used, a nonelectrical source of heat is preferred. Once a castor oil pack is made up, it can be stored for months in a plastic bag and reused over and over, simply adding more oil as necessary.

Castor oil and wool flannel are available from Emerson Ecologics (800-654-4432 or 603-656-9778; www.emersonecologics.com).

Preparing Our Daughters

See page 988 for information on the Red Web Foundation.

Joan Morais, *A Time to Celebrate: A Celebration of a Girl's First Menstrual Period* (Lua Publishing, 2003); www.joanmorais.com.

Chapter 6: The Uterus

Endometriosis

The Endometriosis Association (800-992-3636 or 414-355-2200; www.endometriosisassn.org)

This is a networking and educational organization for those with endometriosis.

Endometriosis Treatment Center (888-256-7705 or 408-358-2511; www.vitalhealth.com)

This center specializes in the education of patients with endometriosis and in treatment plans ranging from lifestyle changes to surgery when necessary.

Fibroids

Many medical centers have divisions devoted to the treatment of fibroids. Here are several examples.

Cleveland Clinic's Center for Menstrual Disorders, Fibroids and Hysteroscopic Services (800-223-2273, ext. 46601 or 216-444-6601; http://my.clevelandclinic.org/departments/obgyn-womens-health/depts/menstrual-disorders)

This arm of the famed Cleveland Clinic was designed to give women minimally invasive options to treat menstrual aberrations and alternatives to hysterectomy. The center also gives patients access to groundbreaking clinical trials, clinical research opportunities, and education programs.

Johns Hopkins Fibroid Center (443-997-0400; www.hopkinsmedicine.org/gynecology_obstetrics/specialty_areas/gynecological_services/treatments_services/fibroid_treatment.html)

This fibroid treatment center specializes in state-of-the-art therapies and the rapid application of new research (such as magnetic resonance imaging and guided high-intensity ultrasound), with an emphasis on minimally invasive techniques.

Center for Fibroid Biology and Therapy at Duke University Medical Center (855-855-6484 [appointments]; www.dukehealth.org/treatments/obstetrics-and-gynecology/fibroids)

Duke's cutting-edge fibroid center explores all nonsurgical and medical treatment options. Treatments offered include minimally invasive surgical options, drug therapies, and noninvasive MRI-guided focused ultrasound treatment.

See page 155 for natural progesterone and page 988 for how to find an acupuncturist.

See General Resources above for formulary pharmacies.

Hysterectomy

See chapter 14 resources for labs that perform salivary hormone testing.

Posture

Esther Gokhale, a pioneer in postural alignment and creator of the Gokhale Method, is the author of *8 Steps to a Pain-Free Back* (Pendo Press, 2008). Her work is based first on her own experience of having to have back surgery to fuse some vertebrae in her lower back. After traveling the world and studying the posture of people in cultures that do not experience back pain or joint problems, she rediscovered the posture we are all born with and then put all of her findings into her foundation's Primal Posture training (https://gokhalemethod.com). She has trained individuals throughout the world in this method, and it has saved thousands from having to have back surgeries (as well as other surgeries).

Gokhale also designed a desk chair that facilitates what she calls stretchsitting and stacksitting, two techniques that transform sitting into a comfortable position and something that heals you rather than hurts you. To order the chair, see https://shop.gokhalemethod.com/products/gokhale-pain-free-chair.

Chapter 7: The Ovaries

Genetic Counseling

If you've had a family member with ovarian cancer, you may want to determine whether or not you are at a high genetic risk. I'd recommend consulting with a genetic counselor or contacting the Familial Ovarian Cancer Registry at the Roswell Park Cancer Institute (800-767-9355 or 716-845-2300; www.ovariancancer .com).

Chapter 8: Reclaiming the Erotic

Mike Lousada and Louise Mazanti, Ph.D., *Real Sex: Why Everything You Learned About Sex Is Wrong* (Hay House, 2017); www.mazantilousada.com.

Multiples.com

Jack Johnston, who manages the website www.multiples.com, has discovered that sexual energy can be greatly increased in the body through deep relaxation and the use of a special sound (detailed on his website). The site also includes a very supportive online community that is safe and has integrity. The orgasmic sound-trigger approach is also very therapeutic and healing for anyone who has had a history of sexual trauma. The twenty-minute practice of using this sound is deeply meditative. I highly recommend this unique approach for optimizing one's sexual energy.

Keggel: The Yoni Egg Practice (https://keggel.org)

Keggel offers yoni egg sets made from certified semiprecious gemstones, beginning with starter kits and going all the way to mastery sets. Each kit comes with instructions, as well as a ten-milliliter bottle of organic French lavender essential oil for sterilizing the egg before and after using it.

Rosie Rees (www.rosierees.com)

Rosie Rees is the founder of Women's Nude Yoga and the creator of Yoni Pleasure Palace, an online boutique that sells excellent-quality yoni eggs, among other products.

Jade Eggs Global (http://jadeeggsglobal.com)

This woman-owned company selling jade yoni eggs includes a downloadable program with each purchase to guide you through a yoni egg practice.

Kim Anami (www.kimanami.com)

Holistic sex and relationship coach Kim Anami offers sex and relationship instruction and advice via online videos available on her website. She also leads intimacy retreats in Bali and Mexico. Her coaching is a spiritual synthesis of two decades of tantra, Taoism, Osho, transpersonal psychology, philosophy, and a host of quantum growth-accelerating practices.

Isa Herrera's Female Pelvic Alchemy S.T.A.R.R. System (www.pelvicpainrelief.com)

Licensed physical therapist and pelvic floor specialist Isa Herrera created this eight-module online program, which includes video lectures (with live-model demos), downloadable PDF diaries and checklists, and mastery sheets that help you review the most important information. The ninety-day program—which addresses pelvic pain, leaking, and prolapse and is appropriate for women of all ages, whether or not they have experienced childbirth—has a 100 percent success rate (for those who do the exercises).

Anne Davin, Ph.D. (www.annedavin.com)

Depth psychologist, life coach, and teacher Anne Davin, Ph.D., offers several online home study courses, including her signature Feminosity intensive (which teaches a five-stage process for turning your desires into your destiny). The tools and practices she teaches draw from the collective wisdom of earth-based mother cultures as well as somatic and Jungian principles. Her approach includes dream analysis, myth and imagination, hypnotherapy, cognitive behavior therapy, and somatic psychotherapy techniques. Her work is focused on the unconscious and the cultivation of an inner wholeness, which creates a deeper connection with self, others and one's deepest purpose.

Tami Lynn Kent, Expert Pelvic Floor Physical Therapist (www.wildfeminine.com)

Tami Lynn Kent is a women's health physical therapist who has trained many other physical therapists around the world. She has done pioneering work on the pelvic bowl and creativity and has also helped hundreds of women with pelvic health problems.

Chapter 9: Vulva, Vagina, Cervix, and Lower Urinary Tract

Isa Herrera, *Ending Female Pain: A Woman's Manual* (BookSurge Publishing, 2009); www.endingfemalepain.com.

Vulvodynia

For a PDF containing an excellent chart of the oxalate content of various foods, see www.urinarystones.info/resources/Docs/Oxalate-content-of-food-2008.pdf. Low-oxalate recipes are available from the VP Foundation (336-226-0704; www .thevpfoundation.org).

National Vulvodynia Association (301-299-0775; www.nva.org) provides a newsletter, support groups, and information services.

Nambudripad's Allergy Elimination Techniques (NAET), Devi S. Nambudripad, M.D., D.C., L.Ac., Ph.D. (714-523-8900; www.naet.com)

Dr. Nambudripad is an acupuncturist and chiropractor who has had extensive experience both personally and professionally treating allergies. She has developed a system of allergy treatment that "reprograms the brain" so that one can get rid of allergies without avoiding allergens completely. She has written a book called *Say Goodbye to Your Allergies* (Delta, 1993) and actively trains healthcare practitioners in her innovative techniques. NAET has also been reported to help fibroids, endometriosis, and numerous other conditions. Write or call to find a practitioner in your area.

Urinary Tract: Chronic, Recurrent UTI, or Interstitial Cystitis

See information above about NAET, which works well for interstitial cystitis.

femiNature (https://hmslaboratories.com)
This supplement helps prevent UTIs. It contains inulin (a natural prebiotic that helps rebalance intestinal flora), cranberry extract (which balances the pH level in the urinary tract to stop *E. coli* bacteria from sticking to the bladder walls and urinary tract lining), D-mannose (a natural antibiotic and pain reliever), phellodendron extract (a Chinese herb used to fight bacteria), and MSM (methylsulfonylmethane—a mineral that fights pain). The product is completely vegan and non-GMO. You can also download a free UTI prevention guide from their website.

Stress Urinary Incontinence

See information above about pelvic floor physical therapy.

Kegel Exercises
Weighted vaginal cones (including sets of cones having graduated weights) can be used for Kegel-type exercises to help alleviate urinary stress incontinence.

A wide variety of vaginal weights (also called Kegel weights) are available online.

Proanthocyanidins

These powerful antioxidants are found in grape pips and pine bark. Start with 1 mg per pound of body weight per day, divided into three doses. After two weeks, cut back to 40–80 mg per day. I recommend:

Proflavanol and Proflavanol 90, available from USANA (888-950-9595 or 801-954-7200; www.usana.com).

OPC Pine Gold and OPC Grape Gold, manufactured by Primary Source and available from Emerson Ecologics (800-654-4432 or 603-656-9778; www.emersonecologics.com).
Many excellent brands of OPCs are also available at pharmacies and natural food stores.

See page 985 for formulary pharmacies.

Herpes

Pink Tent (www.pinktent.com)
Kelly Martin Schuh, D.C., is the creator of Pink Tent, an online community where she shares holistic information about decreasing herpes. Included are meditations and exercises designed to assist with overcoming grief and practicing forgiveness. Dr. Schuh, who has had herpes herself for more than two decades, offers personal coaching as well as an online course. She is also the author of *Live, Love and Thrive with Herpes: A Holistic Guide for Women* (Create Space, 2013).

HPV Vaccine

SaneVax (http://sanevax.org)

This website—the first international HPV vaccine information clearinghouse—promotes only safe, affordable, necessary, and effective vaccines and vaccination practices through education and information. SaneVax's goal is to provide consumers with the science-based information necessary for them to make informed decisions about their health and well-being. SaneVax also provides referrals to helpful resources for those who have experienced vaccine-related injuries.

Following Vaccinations (www.followingvaccinations.com)

In 2010, Joan Campbell started an inquiry among parents of autistic children, compiling a list of those who had been adversely affected by any vaccine. She published the list online. The list has thousands of entries and is still growing. She asks those submitting information to include the vaccine the child took, a description of the child's reaction, how the child's health is at the time of submission, and the municipality where the vaccine was administered.

Chapter 10: Breasts

For castor oil packs, see chapter 5 resources.

National Lymphedema Network (800-541-3259; www.lymphnet.org)

A nonprofit information and networking organization to help those with lymphedema, either primary (the kind one is born with) or secondary (the kind one gets after an operation or injury, notably mastectomy and lymph node dissection). They publish a very helpful newsletter.

Breast Cancer

John Voell and Cynthia Chatfield, *The Cancer Report: The Latest Research in Psychoneuroimmunology (How Thousands Are Achieving Permanent Recoveries)* (Change Your World Press, 2005).

For more information on this research, visit www.cancerreport.com.

Catherine Guthrie, *Flat: Reclaiming My Body from Breast Cancer* (Skyhorse, 2018).

This memoir of a thirty-eight-year-old women's health journalist diagnosed with breast cancer makes a strong point about the need for breast cancer patients to take their power back over their bodies and their healthcare decisions, considering their own pleasure first in making reconstructive choices based on what they value and how they want to live in their bodies instead of being pressured into aligning with cultural norms.

Sanoviv Medical Institute (800-726-6848; www.sanoviv.com)

This fully licensed medical facility along the Baja Coast of Mexico (about an hour from San Diego) combines both traditional and complementary medicine practices to treat the whole person, addressing physical, mental, and spiritual health. It offers everything from surgery to spa facilities. Although Sanoviv helps cancer patients, it also treats those with autoimmune diseases, including lupus, multiple sclerosis, diabetes, chronic fatigue, and neurodegenerative diseases such as Parkinson's and Alzheimer's.

The Radical Remission Project, Kelly Turner, Ph.D. (www.radicalremission.com)

Dr. Turner has researched those who survive cancer against all odds and has identified nine practices they all have in common. I highly recommend her book and program for anyone diagnosed with cancer.

COENZYME Q$_{10}$

I recommend Enzymatic Therapy's coenzyme Q$_{10}$. Each softgel contains 100 mg of this important antioxidant. Available from Emerson Ecologics (800-654-4432 or 603-656-9778; www.emersonecologics.com).

D*action Breast Cancer Prevention Project (https://daction.grassrootshealth.net)

This is the world's largest project designed to solve vitamin D deficiency. When you order a kit to test your vitamin D levels, you will receive access to information on specific health topics as they relate to vitamin D as well as access to the MyData-MyAnswers online health portal. Here, you can track your test results as well as any lifestyle changes you may make along with the outcome. You can take just one vitamin D test or enroll in the full five-year project, which involves filling out an extended health questionnaire and having your vitamin D levels checked every six months for the five-year period.

Chapter 11: Our Fertility

Candace De Puy and Dana Dovitch, *The Healing Choice* (Simon & Schuster, 1997).

I highly recommend this compassionate and enlightened book to all those who are seeking guidance and more in-depth healing information concerning abortion.

Trudy M. Johnson, *CPR: Choice Processing and Resolution* (Outskirts Press, 2009).

Trudy is a licensed marriage and family therapist with twenty years of experience counseling women who are grieving what she calls VPT (voluntary pregnancy termination). Her website (www.missingpieces.org) also offers other resources and support.

Redemption Circle (www.redemptioncircle.org)

Founded by Sara Avant Stover, Redemption Circle is a nonprofit global movement to heal the stigma of abortion and create a support network to empower women to heal—physically, mentally, emotionally, and spiritually.

Fertility

Randine A. Lewis, *The Infertility Cure: The Ancient Chinese Wellness Program for Getting Pregnant and Having Healthy Babies* (Little, Brown, 2004).

Julia Indichova, *Inconceivable: A Woman's Triumph over Despair and Statistics* (Broadway Books, 2001).

Niravi B. Payne, M.S., and Brenda Lane Richardson, *The Whole Person Fertility Program: A Revolutionary Mind-Body Process to Help You Conceive* (Three Rivers Press, 1997).

The PCOS Revolution (www.floridacompletewellness.com/podcasts)

Licensed acupuncture physician and reproductive Oriental medicine practitioner Farrar Duro, D.O.M., has spent nearly twenty years helping patients with PCOS. She's also healed the condition in her own body. In her weekly *PCOS Revolution* podcasts, she interviews PCOS experts as well as women who have the condition and are dealing with it successfully. More information on PCOS is available on Dr. Duro's website (www.thepcosrevolution.com) and her Facebook page (The PCOS Revolution).

FertilityHour podcast (www.fertilityhour.com)

This weekly natural fertility podcast offers video interviews with leading experts in the fields of natural fertility, integrative and functional medicine, and preconception care. The content includes evidence-based strategies and complementary and alternative therapeutic approaches to improving fertility and treating infertility holistically. The podcast is hosted by San Francisco Bay area acupuncturist and fertility specialist Charlene Lincoln and is co-produced by the team from Natural Fertility Prescription, a group of naturopaths in the field of natural fertility since 2007.

Julie Von, O.M.D. (www.drjulievon.com)

Dr. Von works with women (and men) all over the world to restore fertility. Her book *Spiritual Fertility* (Hay House, 2019) is inspiring, practical, and supportive as are her online and in-person program.

Calm Birth (www.calmbirth.org)

Calm Birth is a form of childbirth preparation that uses proven mind-body and breathing techniques to help create an atmosphere of calmness that decreases fear, pain, and complications for both pregnancy and childbirth. This very powerful program can also help couples with infertility. In addition to practitioners, Calm Birth also offers a CD called *Calm Birth,* as well as a postnatal program called *Calm Healing.*

Natural Family Planning

OVULATION METHOD

Fertility Care Centers of America (FCCA) (www.fertilitycare.org). This international, nonprofit organization promotes the services of the Creighton Model FertilityCare System.

Billings Ovulation Method Association (651-699-8139; www.boma-usa.org)

Pregnancy Loss

Lorraine Ash, *Life Touches Life: A Mother's Story of Stillbirth and Healing* (NewSage, 2004).

The following websites offer a wide range of support options and resources for further information geared to women who have lost a child:

Empty Cradle (www.emptycradle.org)

Silent Grief (www.silentgrief.com)

Chapter 12: Pregnancy and Birthing

Doulas

Marshall Klaus, M.D., John Kennell, M.D., and Phyllis Klaus, C.S.W., *The Doula Book: How a Trained Labor Companion Can Help You Have a Shorter, Easier, and Healthier Birth* (Addison-Wesley, 1993). (Formerly titled *Mothering the Mother.*)

Professional labor support professionals—or doulas—usually work well within the medical system. To locate one in your area, ask your doctor or midwife, or call the labor and delivery unit of your local hospital. You can also contact the organizations listed below.

DONA International (formerly known as Doulas of North America) (888-788-3662; www.dona.org)

Labor Assistant Training and Certification Organization (formerly known as the Association of Labor Assistants and Childbirth Educators, or ALACE) (804-320-0607; www.tolabor.com)

Pregnancy and Childbirth Education

Ina May Gaskin, *Ina May's Guide to Childbirth* (Bantam Books, 2003).
Also see Ina May's website, www.inamay.com.

CIMS (www.motherfriendly.org)
The Coalition for Improving Maternity Services (CIMS), a United Nations–recognized NGO, is a collaborative effort of numerous individuals, leading researchers, and more than fifty organizations representing 90,000-plus members. CIMS promotes a wellness model of maternity care that will improve birth outcomes and substantially reduce costs; CIMS developed the Mother-Friendly Childbirth Initiative in 1996. A consensus document that has been recognized as an important model for improving the healthcare and well-being of children beginning at birth, the Mother-Friendly Childbirth Initiative has been translated into several languages and is gaining support around the world.

International Childbirth Education Association (919-674-4183; www.icea.org)
The International Childbirth Education Association (ICEA) is a professional organization that supports educators and other healthcare providers who believe in freedom of choice based on knowledge of alternatives in family-centered maternity and newborn care. Their website features a directory of certified doulas.

Orgasmic Birth (www.orgasmicbirth.com)
Orgasmic Birth is an eighty-five-minute documentary examining the sexual nature of birth. The film, which has been featured on ABC's *20/20*, shows couples talking about their ecstatic and even orgasmic birth experiences, as well as medical and birthing experts (including Dr. Northrup) explaining how that can be possible. (A big key to this is the increased levels of oxytocin, prolactin, and beta-endorphins—what Dr. Northrup calls the molecules of ecstasy—in a birthing mother's body.) The film's goal is to educate and inspire expectant parents to con-

sider all their options, so they can make truly informed decisions about the birthing experience they want.

Ecstatic Birth (www.ecstatic-birth.com)
Ecstatic birth advocate and trainer Sheila Kamara Hay offers an online program for ecstatic birth preparation as well as training on ecstatic birth for midwives, doulas, and childbirth educators. For a directory of ecstatic birth practitioners in your area, see www.ecstatic-birth.com/practitioner-directory.

Pregnancy and Fitness

Elizabeth Jones-Boswell, M.Ed., *Exercise for Pregnancy and Beyond: A Pilates-Based Approach for Women* (Jones-Boswell, Inc., 2006).
For more information about this program to ease pregnancy's discomforts through Pilates, contact Elizabeth (509-499-1435; www.elizabethjonesboswell.com), a mother of four and a Pilates master teacher.

Shiva Rea's Prenatal Yoga (www.shivarea.com)
Legendary yoga instructor and mother Shiva Rea has designed a yoga program specifically for pregnancy to increase energy and stamina and develop concentration for labor and delivery. Her pregnancy routine includes safe stretching and strength building, with modifications for each trimester.

Birthfit (www.birthfit.com)
This organization offers support and education through in-person and online programs that focus on fitness, nutrition, chiropractic wellness, and mindset. They offer a six-week preconception program, a thirty-six-week prenatal program, a fifteen-week postpartum program, and two different six-week core and pelvic floor courses, one for mothers who have delivered vaginally and another for those who had cesareans. I highly recommend their offerings.

Belly Dancing and Pregnancy

Maha Al Musa (www.mahaalmusa.com)
Al Musa is a belly dance instructor and doula who lives in Australia and has both Lebanese and Palestinian roots. Both her book, *Dance of the Womb: The Essential Guide to Belly Dance for Pregnancy and Birth* (Maha Al Musa, 2008), and her DVD, *Dance of the Womb: A Gentle Guide to Belly Dance for Pregnancy and Birth,* give beginners a great introduction to using this ancient art as a tool for empowered birth.

Chapter 13: Motherhood: Bonding with Your Baby

Attachment Parenting

Attachment Parenting International (www.attachmentparenting.org)
This nonprofit organization is dedicated to educating and supporting all parents in raising secure, joyful, and empathetic children in order to strengthen families and create a more compassionate world. The organization's website covers the basics of healthy attachment, including co-sleeping, wearing your baby, evaluating

childcare, and so on, and has a link to a page detailing the API's Eight Principles of Parenting.

API cofounders Barbara Nicholson and Lysa Parker are also the authors of *Attached at the Heart: 8 Proven Parenting Principles for Raising Connected and Compassionate Children* (Health Communications, 2013).

Dr. Shefali Tsabary, Ph.D. (www.drshefali.com)

Dr. Tsabary is a clinical psychologist with a private practice in Great Neck, New York. Her work on parenting is most unusual and helps parents connect with their child's soul. You can sign up for coaching consultations on her website, which also offers online courses and videos. Dr. Tsabary gives lectures and workshops internationally and is the author of *The Awakened Family* (Penguin, 2016).

Postpartum Depression

Postpartum Support International (800-944-4773 or 503-894-9453 (text); www .postpartum.net)

Postpartum Support International is an education, referral, and advocacy group devoted to increasing awareness about and discussion of postpartum depression. Its website has lots of background information, as well as a bookstore, Internet forums, and chat rooms, links to local support groups across the country, and a self-assessment test.

Vaginal Dryness

A number of excellent natural lubricants are available to supplement vaginal moisture during times of hormonal shifts, such as postpartum and perimenopause. Good over-the-counter options include K-Y Jelly, Sylk, Probe, and Good Clean Love. Organic coconut oil also works very well.

Vaginal moisturizer made with *Pueraria mirifica* is available from Amata Life (www.amatalife.com).

Circumcision

Ronald Goldman, Ph.D., *Circumcision: The Hidden Trauma* (Vanguard Publications, 1997).

Ronald Goldman, Ph.D., *Questioning Circumcision: A Jewish Perspective* (Vanguard Publications, 1988).

Kristen O'Hara, *Sex as Nature Intended It* (Turning Point Publications, 2002).

Thomas J. Ritter, *Say No to Circumcision: 40 Compelling Reasons Why You Should Respect His Birthright and Keep Your Son Whole* (Hourglass Book Publishing, 1996).

National Organization of Circumcision Information and Resource Centers (415-488-9883; www.nocirc.org)

Doctors Opposing Circumcision (DOC) (www.doctorsopposingcircumcision.org)

A nonprofit organization providing publications, videos, and a newsletter in order to educate practitioners and parents on how to stop perpetuating the practice of circumcision.

Circumcision Resource Center (www.circumcision.org)

Focuses on circumcision as an American cultural practice and as a religious practice.

Intact America (www.intactamerica.org)

This organization works to protect newborns from the pain and sequelae of routine circumcision through social media, education, and activism.

Breast-feeding

La Leche League International (800-LALECHE or 919-459-2167; www.llli.org)

This organization provides accurate information and grassroots practical support for successful breast-feeding.

International Lactation Consultant Association (888-452-2478 or 919-861-5577; www.ilca.org)

This organization of health professionals specializes in promoting, protecting, and supporting breast-feeding worldwide.

Happy Ducts lactation support (www.wishgardenherbs.com)

This herbal tincture made by WishGarden Herbs provides short-term herbal support for nursing mothers. It's designed to nurture healthy lymph nodes and breasts and can be taken the minute you feel as though you may be getting mastitis. Relief is often immediate. Order Happy Ducts from the WishGarden website or on Amazon or look for it in many natural food stores.

Chapter 14: Menopause

See also General Resources for formulary pharmacies and chapter 5 resources, particularly for 2 percent progesterone cream.

Christiane Northrup, M.D., *The Wisdom of Menopause* (Bantam Books, 2012).

Dr. Northrup's interactive website (www.drnorthrup.com) is the best place to find regularly updated information on her lectures and other resources.

Barbara Hand Clow, *The Liquid Light of Sex: Kundalini, Astrology, and the Key Life Transitions* (Bear, 1991).

Pueraria mirifica

Pueraria Mirifica Plus (which contains *Pueraria mirifica* extract along with a few additional supplements that optimize its benefits) and Pueraria Mirifica Pure (containing only *Pueraria mirifica*) are both excellent supplements for help lessening menopausal symptoms. Available from Amata Life (www.amatalife.com).

Hormonal Testing

The DUTCH Test (www.dutchtest.com)

This the gold standard for urinary and salivary hormone testing, and it can be done in your own home. The original DUTCH (dried urine test for comprehensive hormones) test measures urinary hormones, including cortisol and sex steroids, over a twenty-four-hour period. The DUTCH Plus test adds a salivary evaluation of how your cortisol levels change throughout the day. The tests are available from Precision Analytical, Inc.

Individualized Hormonal Support

Many physicians and formulary pharmacists work in partnership with their patients to provide individualized hormone replacement solutions. Ask your physician about this kind of customized care; he or she can call a local formulary pharmacy to consult with a knowledgeable pharmacist.

Flax

The Flax Council of Canada (204-982-2115; www.flaxcouncil.ca) endeavors to provide general flax facts of interest to consumers, as well as more specialized information for nutritionists, dietitians, food producers, manufacturers, and flax growers.

Whole Flax Seed from Cathy's Country Store is organically grown golden flax. Available from Emerson Ecologics (800-654-4432 or 603-656-9778; www .emersonecologics.com).

Dakota Flax Gold is an organic flaxseed grown at Heintzman Farms in South Dakota (800-333-5813; www.heintzmanfarms.com). A "starter kit" is available that consists of three one-pound bags of flaxseed and an electric grinder.

Chapter 15: Steps for Flourishing

Futures Without Violence (formerly known as the Family Violence Prevention Fund) (415-678-5500; www.futureswithoutviolence.org)

Their website has research, statistics, and resources such as a detailed Personal Safety Plan.

National Center for Victims of Crime (202-467-8700; www.victimsofcrime.org)

This organization is the leading resource and advocacy organization for crime victims in the United States. The center's website offers a comprehensive collection of online resources for crime victims in addition to an extensive database of service providers for referrals.

Therapy for Black Girls (www.therapyforblackgirls.com)

Atlanta psychologist Joy Harden Bradford, Ph.D., founded this website dedicated to encouraging the mental wellness of African American women and girls. The site presents a wide range of mental health topics in a way that feels more accessible and relevant to those who may feel constrained by the taboo that surrounds seeking therapy in many African American communities.

Chapter 16: Getting the Most Out of Your Medical Care

Guidance for Alternative Medical Care

Institute for Health and Healing (www.sutterhealth.org/services/holistic-integrative
-medicine/institute-health-healing)

Created in 1994 as part of California Pacific Medical Center Foundation, the
Institute for Health and Healing is now a national leader in integrative medicine.
This physician-led hospital department includes many Western-trained practition-
ers who are also experts in complementary therapies.

Preparing for Surgery

Jeanne Achterberg and Barbara Dossey, *Rituals of Healing* (Bantam Books, 1994).

Successful Surgery. Guided-imagery audio program by Belleruth Naparstek. Available from Health Journeys (800-800-8661 or 216-675-0496; www.healthjourneys
.com).

Belleruth Naparstek's audiobooks combine healing imagery, powerful music,
and the most current understanding of the mind-body connection to engage the
imagination in the healing process. Topics include asthma, cancer, chemotherapy,
depression, diabetes, general wellness, grief, headache, PMS, pain, stress, stroke,
surgery, weight loss, and more.

Prepare for Surgery, Heal Faster. Book and relaxation/healing audio program by
Peggy Huddleston (781-864-2668; www.healfaster.com), available separately or
as a combination.

Chapter 17: Eat to Flourish

See chapter 5 PMS resources for information about full-spectrum lighting.

See chapter 9 resources for information about NAET.

See chapter 14 resources for information about hormone testing.

Tommy Rosa and Stephen Sinatra, M.D., *Health Revelations from Heaven and
Earth* (Rodale, 2015).

Ocean Robbins, *The 31-Day Food Revolution: Heal Your Body, Feel Great, and
Transform Your World* (Grand Central Publishing, 2019).

Joseph Mercola, D.O., *Fat for Fuel: A Revolutionary Diet to Combat Cancer,
Boost Brain Power, and Increase Your Energy* (Hay House, 2017).

The World's Healthiest Foods (www.whfoods.com)

This website, maintained by the nonprofit George Mateljan Foundation, offers
a list of the 100 healthiest foods (along with their criteria), more than a hundred
quick, easy, and healthful recipes (which can be prepared and cooked in twenty
minutes or less), and a treasure trove of information designed to help you eat and
cook for optimal health.

Pharmaceutical-Grade Multivitamins

USANA (888-950-9595 or 801-954-7200; www.usana.com)

USANA offers state-of-the-art vitamins and mineral supplements. Their Essentials combined with Proflavanol compose an excellent basic nutritional program. I also recommend their convenient HealthPak, which is a combination of Essentials and Optimizers and includes an exclusive bioflavonoid complex.

Emerson Ecologics (800-654-4432 or 603-656-9778; www.emersonecologics.com)

Emerson Ecologics is a full-service distributor of high-quality nutritional and health products, with education support for healthcare practitioners.

Notes

Chapter 1: The Patriarchal Myth

1. R. Eisler, *The Chalice and the Blade* (Cambridge, MA: Harper & Row, 1987); M. Gimbutas, *The Civilization of the Goddess* (HarperSanFrancisco, 1991).

2. J. Highwater, *Myth and Sexuality* (New York: Penguin, 1988), pp. 8–9.

3. Common Sense Media, *Children, Teens, Media, and Body Image: A Common Sense Research Brief,* January 2015, https://www.commonsensemedia.org/research/children-teens-media-and-body-image#.

4. A. Wilson Schaef and D. Fassel, *The Addictive Organization* (HarperSanFrancisco, 1988), p. 58.

5. "What Is 'Victim Shaming'?" DomesticShelters.org, May 27, 2015, https://www.domesticshelters.org/domestic-violence-articles-information/what-is-victim-shaming.

6. M. C. Black et al., "The National Intimate Partner and Sexual Violence Survey: 2010 Summary Report," 2011, http://www.cdc.gov/violenceprevention/pdf/nisvs_report2010-a.pdf.

7. M. J. Breiding et al., "Prevalence and Characteristics of Sexual Violence, Stalking, and Intimate Partner Violence Victimization—National Intimate Partner and Sexual Violence Survey, United States, 2011," *MMWR* 2014; 63(SS-8): 1–18.

8. M. C. Black et al., "The National Intimate Partner and Sexual Violence Survey: 2010 Summary Report," 2011, http://www.cdc.gov/violenceprevention/pdf/nisvs_report2010-a.pdf.

9. P. Tjaden and N. Thoennes, "Extent, Nature, and Consequences of Intimate Partner Violence: Findings from the National Violence Against Women Survey," 2000, https://www.ncjrs.gov/pdffiles1/nij/181867.pdf.

10. B. A. Bailey, "Partner Violence During Pregnancy: Prevalence, Effects, Screening, and Management," *International Journal of Women's Health* 2 (2010): 183–97.

11. M. J. Breiding et al., "Prevalence and Characteristics of Sexual Violence, Stalking,

and Intimate Partner Violence Victimization—National Intimate Partner and Sexual Violence Survey, United States, 2011," *MMWR* 2014; 63(SS-8): 1–18.

12. J. L. Truman and R. E. Morgan, "Nonfatal Domestic Violence, 2003–2012," 2014, http://www.bjs.gov/content/pub/pdf/ndv0312.pdf.

13. M. A. Rodriguez et al., "Screening and Intervention for Intimate Partner Abuse: Practices and Attitudes of Primary Care Physicians," *Journal of the American Medical Association*, vol. 282 (1999), pp. 468–74.

14. World Health Organization, "Global and Regional Estimates of Violence Against Women: Prevalence and Health Effects of Intimate Partner Violence and Non-Partner Sexual Violence," 2013, http://apps.who.int/iris/bitstream/10665/85239/1/9789241564625_eng.pdf; L. Heise, M. Ellsberg, and M. Gotemoeller, "Ending Violence Against Women," Population Reports, Series L, no. 11, Johns Hopkins University School of Public Health, Population Information Program, Baltimore, December 1999; H. M. Bauer et al., "Intimate Partner Violence and High-Risk Sexual Behaviors Among Female Patients with Sexually Transmitted Diseases," *Sexually Transmitted Diseases*, vol. 29 (2002), pp. 411–16; N. Romero-Daza, M. Weeks, and M. Singer, " 'Nobody Gives a Damn If I Live or Die': Violence, Drugs, and Street-Level Prostitution in Inner-City Hartford, Connecticut," *Medical Anthropology*, vol. 22 (2003), pp. 233–59; R. M. Harris et al., "The Interrelationship Between Violence, HIV/AIDS, and Drug Use in Incarcerated Women," *Journal of Associated Nurses AIDS Care*, vol. 14 (2003), pp. 27–40; P. Braitstein et al., "Sexual Violence Among a Cohort of Injection Drug Users," *Social Science and Medicine*, vol. 57 (2003), pp. 561–69. R. J. Peters Jr. et al., "The Relationship Between Sexual Abuse and Drug Use: Findings from Houston's Safer Choices 2 Program," *Journal of Drug Education*, vol. 33 (2003), pp. 49–59.

15. V. Felitti et al., "Relationship of Childhood Abuse and Household Dysfunction to Many of the Leading Causes of Death in Adults," *American Journal of Preventive Medicine*, vol. 14 (1998), pp. 245–58.

16. United Nations, Department of Economic and Social Affairs, Statistics Division, *The World's Women 2015: Trends and Statistics*, no. E.15.XVII.8 (New York: United Nations, 2015).

17. International Labour Organization, *ILO Global Estimate of Forced Labour: Results and Methodology*, 2012, p. 13.

18. UNICEF, *The State of the World's Children 2006: Excluded and Invisible*, December 2005.

19. United Nations Children's Fund, *Female Genital Mutilation/Cutting: A Global Concern* (New York: UNICEF, 2016); United Nations Children's Fund, *Female Genital Mutilation/Cutting: A Statistical Overview and Exploration of the Dynamics of Change* (New York: UNICEF, 2013).

20. H. Goldberg et al., "Female Genital Mutilation/Cutting in the United States: Updated Estimates of Women and Girls at Risk, 2012," Centers for Disease Control Public Reports, January 14, 2016, www.publichealthreports.org.

21. J. Fortin, "Michigan Doctor Is Accused of Genital Cutting of 2 Girls," *New York Times*, April 13, 2017, www.nytimes.com/2017/04/13/us/michigan-doctor-fgm-cutting.html.

22. K. S. Arora and A. J. Jacobs, "Female Genital Alteration: A Compromise Solution," *Journal of Medical Ethics*, vol. 42, no. 3 (2016), pp. 148–54.

23. A. Gentleman, "India Still Fighting to 'Save the Girl Child,'" *International Herald Tribune,* April 15, 2005.

24. T. Rosenberg, "The Daughter Deficit," *New York Times Magazine,* August 23, 2009, p. MM23, www.nytimes.com/2009/08/23/magazine/23FOB-idealab-t.html.

25. F. Faqir, "Intrafamily Femicide in Defence of Honour: The Case of Jordan," *Third World Quarterly,* vol. 22, no. 1 (2001), pp. 65–82; Nicholas D. Kristof and Sheryl WuDunn, *Half the Sky: Turning Oppression into Opportunity for Women Worldwide* (New York: Alfred A. Knopf, 2009); Nicholas D. Kristof and Sheryl WuDunn, "The Women's Crusade," *New York Times Magazine,* August 23, 2009, p. MM28, www.nytimes.com/2009/08/23/magazine/23Women-t.html.

26. Kristof and WuDunn, *Half the Sky;* Kristof and WuDunn, "The Women's Crusade."

27. Q. Wodon et al., "Ending Child Marriage: Legal Age for Marriage, Illegal Child Marriages, and the Need for Interventions," Save the Children and The World Bank, October 2017.

28. World Bank Group, "Women, Business and the Law 2016: Getting to Equal," Washington, D.C., 2015, http://wbl.worldbank.org/~/media/WBG/WBL/Documents/Reports/2016/Women-Business-and-the-Law-2016.pdf.

29. UN Women, "World AIDS Day Statement: For Young Women, Inequality Is Deadly," November 30, 2016, www.unwomen.org/en/news/stories/2016/11/un-women-statement-aids-day.

30. R. C. Dellar, S. Dlamini, and Q. A. Karim, "Adolescent Girls and Young Women: Key Populations for HIV Epidemic Control," *Journal of the International AIDS Society,* vol. 18, no. 2, suppl. 1 (2015), p. 19408.

31. Kristof and WuDunn, "The Women's Crusade."

32. A. Wilson Schaef and D. Fassel, *The Addictive Organization* (HarperSanFrancisco, 1988), p. 58.

33. C. Morgan et al., "Incidence, Clinical Management, and Mortality Risk Following Self Harm Among Children and Adolescents: Cohort Study in Primary Care," *British Medical Journal (Clinical Research Edition),* vol. 359 (October 18, 2017), p. j4351.

34. American Foundation for Suicide Prevention, https://afsp.org/about-suicide/suicide-statistics.

35. Data from Oxfam America, 115 Broadway, Boston, Massachusetts, 02116.

36. B. Grad et al., "An Unorthodox Method of Treatment on Wound Healing in Mice," *International Journal of Parapsychology,* vol. 3 (Spring 1961), pp. 5–24. This well-designed study showed that wound healing in mice was speeded up significantly ($p. < .01$) when a self-styled healer passed hands over the animals' cage.

37. M. T. Stein, J. H. Kennell, and A. Fulcher, "Benefits of a Doula Present at the Birth of a Child," *Journal of Developmental and Behavioral Pediatrics,* vol. 25 (5 Suppl.) (October 2004), pp. S89–92; M. T. Stein, J. H. Kennell, and A. Fulcher, "Benefits of a Doula Present at the Birth of a Child," *Journal of Developmental and Behavioral Pediatrics,* vol. 24, no. 3 (June 2003), pp. 195–98; J. H. Kennell and M. H. Klaus, "Continuous Nursing Support During Labor," *Journal of the American Medical Association,* vol. 289, no. 2 (January 8, 2003), pp. 175–76; M. H. Klaus et al., "Effects of Social Support During Parturition in Maternal and

Infant Mortality," *British Medical Journal*, vol. 293 (1986), pp. 585–87; M. H. Klaus et al., "Maternal Assistance and Support in Labor: Father, Nurse, Midwife, or Doula?" *Clinical Consultation in Obstetrics and Gynecology*, vol. 4 (December 1992); M. Klaus, J. Kennell, and P. Klaus, *Mothering the Mother: How a Doula Can Help You Have a Shorter, Easier, and Healthier Birth* (New York: Addison-Wesley, 1993), p. 25.

38. The Herbal Academy, https://theherbalacademy.com/herbal-history.

39. S. Hall, "Cheating Fate," *Health*, vol. 6, no. 2 (April 1992), p. 38. Every doctor has seen at least a few cases of "spontaneous remission," and every year these cases are reported in the medical literature. Far too often, instead of being studied, they are ignored. Their existence flies in the face of the medical belief system.

40. A. Gawande, "Overkill," *The New Yorker*, May 11, 2015, https://www.newyorker.com/magazine/2015/05/11/overkill-atul-gawande.

41. T. Parker-Pope, "Overtreatment Is Taking a Harmful Toll," *New York Times*, August 28, 2012, p. D1, https://well.blogs.nytimes.com/2012/08/27/overtreatment-is-taking-a-harmful-toll.

42. V. S. Periyakoil et al., "Do unto Others: Doctors' Personal End-of-Life Resuscitation Preferences and their Attitudes Toward Advance Directives," *PLoS One*, vol. 9, no. 5 (May 28, 2014), pp. e98246.

43. J. Kung, R. R. Miller, and P. A. Mackowiak, "Failure of Clinical Practice Guidelines to Meet Institute of Medicine Standards: Two More Decades of Little, If Any, Progress," *Archives of Internal Medicine*, vol. 172, no. 21 (November 26, 2012), pp. 1628–33.

44. National Eating Disorder Association, https://www.nationaleatingdisorders.org/what-are-eating-disorders.

45. C. D. Bethell et al., "A National and State Profile of Leading Health Problems and Health Care Quality for US Children: Key Insurance Disparities and Across-State Variations," *Academic Pediatrics*, vol. 11, no. 3S (May–June 2011), p. S22.

46. K. Hartmann et al., "Outcomes of Routine Episiotomy: A Systematic Review," *Journal of the American Medical Association*, vol. 293, no. 17 (May 4, 2005), pp. 2141–48.

47. K. Gooch, "Though Discouraged by Experts, Episiotomy Rates Still High: How Hospitals Are Responding," *Becker's Clinical Leadership and Infection Control*, July 19, 2016, https://www.beckershospitalreview.com/quality/though-discouraged-by-experts-episiotomy-rates-still-high-how-hospitals-are-responding.html.

48. Association of American Medical Colleges, 2018 Physician Specialty Data Report, Executive Summary, https://www.aamc.org/download/492910/data/2018executivesummary.pdf.

49. A. Wilson Schaef, *When Society Becomes an Addict* (HarperSanFrancisco, 1987), p. 72.

50. C. P. Estes, *Women Who Run with the Wolves: Myths and Stories of the Wild Woman Archetype* (New York: Ballantine Books, 1992), p. 3.

51. A. Cuddy, Ph.D., "Your Body Language May Shape Who You Are," TEDGlobal 2012, Edinburgh, Scotland, June 2012, https://www.ted.com/talks/amy_cuddy_your_body_language_shapes_who_you_are. A. Cuddy, *Presence; Bringing Your Boldest Self to Your Biggest Challenges* (New York: Little, Brown, 2015).

52. P. Reis, "The Women's Spirituality Movement: Ideas Generated and Questions Asked," presentation to feminist seminar, Proprioceptive Writing Center, Maine, December 3, 1990.

Chapter 2: Feminine Intelligence and a New Mode of Healing

1. M. Ho and D. P. Knight, "The Acupuncture System and the Liquid Crystalline Collagen Fibers of the Connective Tissues," *American Journal of Chinese Medicine,* vol. 26, nos. 3–4 (1998), pp. 251–63.

2. F. Murad, "Discovery of Some of the Biological Effects of Nitric Oxide and Its Role in Cell Signaling," *Bioscience Reports,* vol. 19, no. 3 (June 1999), pp. 133–54.

3. S. Field et al., *Science News,* vol. 127, no. 301, reported in *Brain/Mind Bulletin,* December 9, 1985.

4. M. H. Klaus and J. H. Kennell, *Parent/Infant Bonding,* 2d ed. (St. Louis: C. V. Mosby, 1982).

5. L. F. Berman and S. L. Syme, "Social Networks, Host Resistance, and Mortality: A Nine-Year Follow-up of Almeda County Residents," *American Journal of Epidemiology,* vol. 109 (1978), pp. 186–204.

6. J. Achterberg, *Imagery in Healing: Shamanism and Modern Medicine* (Boston: Shambhala, 1985).

7. F. Fang et al., "Suicide and Cardiovascular Death After a Cancer Diagnosis," *New England Journal of Medicine,* vol. 366, no. 14 (April 5, 2012), pp. 1310–8.

8. V. J. Felitti et al., "Relationship of Childhood Abuse and Household Dysfunction to Many of the Leading Causes of Death in Adults. The Adverse Childhood Experiences (ACE) Study," *American Journal of Preventive Medicine,* vol. 14, no. 4 (May 1998), pp. 245–58.

9. A. Tyborowska et al., "Early-Life and Pubertal Stress Differentially Modulate Grey Matter Development in Human Adolescents," *Scientific Reports,* vol. 8, no. 1 (June 15, 2018), p. 9201.

10. M. Gershon, *The Second Brain* (New York: HarperCollins, 1998).

11. C. Pert, *Molecules of Emotion: Why You Feel the Way You Feel* (New York: Scribner, 1997).

12. L. Dossey, *Healing Words: The Power of Prayer and the Practice of Medicine* (HarperSanFrancisco, 1993).

13. Quoted from personal notes of 1991 lecture series, Mystery School Program, at which Jean Houston was the facilitator.

14. A. Moir and D. Jessel, *Brain Sex* (New York: Carol, 1991), p. 195.

15. R. Bly and D. Tannen, "Where Are Women and Men Today," *New Age Journal,* January–February 1992, p. 32.

16. S. J. Schleifer et al., "Depression and Immunity: Lymphocyte Function in Ambulatory Depressed Patients, Hospitalized Schizophrenic Patients, and Patients Hospitalized for Herniorrhaphy," *Archives of General Psychiatry,* vol. 42 (1985), pp. 129–33.

17. J. K. Kiecolt-Glaser et al., "Stress, Loneliness, and Changes in Herpes Virus Latency," *Journal of Behavioral Medicine,* vol. 8, no. 3 (1985), pp. 249–60.

18. The following autoimmune diseases affect women much more frequently than men: Systemic lupus erythematosus—90 percent of sufferers are women. Myasthenia gravis—85 percent are women. Autoimmune thyroid disease—80 percent are women. Rheumatoid arthritis—75 percent are women. Multiple sclerosis—70 percent are women.

19. A. L. Roberts et al., "Association of Trauma and Posttraumatic Stress Disorder with Incident Systemic Lupus Erythematosus (SLE) in a Longitudinal Cohort of Women," *Arthritis and Rheumatology*, vol., 69, issue 11 (November 2017), pp. 2162–9.

20. S. F. Maier et al., "Opiate Antagonists and Long-Term Analgesic Reaction Induced by Inescapable Shock in Rats," *Journal of Comparative Physiology and Psychology*, vol. 4 (December 1980), pp. 1177–83; M. L. Laudenslager, "Coping and Immunosuppression: Inescapable but Not Escapable Shock Suppresses Lymphocyte Proliferation," *Science*, August 1983, pp. 568–70; S. E. Locke et al., "Life Change Stress, Psychiatric Symptoms and Natural Killer Cell Activity," *Psychosomatic Medicine*, vol. 46, no. 5 (1984), pp. 441–53; B. S. Linn et al., "Degree of Depression and Immune Responsiveness," *Psychosomatic Medicine*, vol. 44 (1982), p. 128.

21. R. J. Weber and C. B. Pert, "Opiatergic Modulation of the Immune System," in E. E. Muller and Andrea R. Genazzani, eds., *Central and Peripheral Endorphins* (New York: Raven Press, 1984), p. 35.

22. R. L. Roessler et al., "Ego Strength, Life Changes, and Antibody Titers," paper presented at the annual meeting of the American Psychosomatic Society, Dallas, Texas, March 25, 1979.

23. E. Langer, *Counterclockwise: Mindful Health and the Power of Possibility* (New York: Ballantine Books, 2009), p. 116.

24. B. R. Levy et al., "Longevity Increased by Positive Self-Perceptions of Aging," *Journal of Personality and Social Psychology*, vol. 83, no. 2 (August 2002), pp. 261–70.

25. E. Langer, *Mindfulness* (Reading, MA: Addison-Wesley, 1989), pp. 100–13.

26. M. Guerin, "Psychosocial Lecture Notes," Department of Obstetrics and Gynecology, Michigan State University School of Medicine, Lansing, MI, 1991.

27. E. Kübler-Ross, *On Death and Dying* (New York: Macmillan, 1969).

Chapter 3: Inner Guidance

1. S. Sullivan, "Inhibition of Salivary and Lacrimal Secretion by an Enkephalin Analogue," *American Journal of Psychiatry*, vol. 139, no. 3 (March 1982), pp. 385–86.

2. W. G. Frey et al., "Effect of Stimulus on the Composition of Tears," *American Journal of Ophthalmology*, vol. 92, no. 4 (1982), pp. 559–67.

3. O. and A. Worrall, *The Gift of Healing* (Columbus, OH: Ariel Press, 1985). The work of Olga Worrall, a world-renowned intuitive healer, was studied and documented by physicians at Johns Hopkins School of Medicine. The book is available from Ariel Press, P.O. Box 30975, Columbus, OH 43230. Her work is currently being carried on by Robert Leichtman, M.D. Edgar Cayce is another well-known medical intuitive.

4. M. Ferguson, "Commentary: Waking Up in the Dark," *Brain/Mind and Common Sense,* April 1993, p. 3.

5. M. Stout, *The Sociopath Next Door* (New York, Broadway Books, 2005).

6. E. R. McDonald et al., "Survival in Amyotrophic Lateral Sclerosis: The Role of Psychological Factors," *Archives of Neurology,* vol. 51, no. 1 (January 1994), pp. 17–23.

7. Matthew Fox, quoted in M. Toms, "Renegade Priest: An Interview with Matthew Fox," *The Sun,* issue 89 (August 1991), p. 10.

8. R. Grossinger, *On the Integration of Nature: Post 9-11 Biopolitical Notes* (Berkeley, CA: North Atlantic Books, 2005).

Chapter 4: The Female Energy System

1. G. Bennette, "Psychic and Cellular Aspects of Isolation and Identity Impairment in Cancer," *Annals of the New York Academy of Sciences,* vol. 131 (1972), pp. 352–63.

2. C. E. Wenner and S. Weinhouse, "Diphosphopyridine Nucleotide Requirements of Oxidations by Mitochondria of Normal and Neoplastic Tissues," *Cancer Research,* vol. 12 (1952), pp. 306–7.

3. M. Kirshenbaum, *The Emotional Energy Factor: The Secrets High-Energy People Use to Beat Emotional Fatigue* (New York: Delacorte Press, 2003), p. 4.

4. I am talking about common patterns here. Some illnesses are mysterious—almost archetypal—and don't fit the personal patterns I describe in this section.

5. D. B. Clayson, *Chemical Carcinogenesis* (London: Churchill Publishers, 1962).

6. C. B. Thomas and K. R. Duszynski, "Closeness to Parents and the Family Constellation in Prospective Study of Five Disease States: Suicide, Mental Illness, Malignant Tumor, Hypertension, Coronary Heart Disease," *Johns Hopkins Medical Journal,* vol. 134 (1974), pp. 251–70.

7. C. Dale, *Advanced Chakra Healing: Heart Disease* (Berkeley, CA: Crossing Press, 2007), pp. 6–7.

8. Personal communication from a colleague.

9. See N. Shealy and C. Myss, *The Creation of Health* (Walpole, NH: Stillpoint Publications, 1988), and also C. Myss, *Anatomy of the Spirit* (New York: Harmony Books, 1996), which goes into much more detail on the human energy system. Dr. Shealy, a neurosurgeon who founded the American Holistic Medical Association, has done extensive research on energy medicine with Caroline Myss. A world-renowned medical intuitive, Myss needs to know only the name and age of an individual to be able to give a full diagnostic reading; the individual can be located anywhere in the world. For several years, Caroline assisted me in clinical practice with energy readings on my own patients, whose physical conditions were correlated with energy anatomy. Her concepts formed the original basis for this chapter. In the second edition, I was assisted in updating the material by Mona Lisa Schulz, M.D., Ph.D., who is both a psychiatrist and a behavioral neuroscientist with an extensive research background. She is also a practicing medical intuitive.

10. C. Wallis, "The Real Story on the Chakras: The Six Most Important Things You Never Knew About the Chakras," February 2016, https://tantrikstudies.squarespace.com/blog/2016/2/5/the-real-story-on-the-chakras.

11. G. A. Bachmann et al., "Childhood Sexual Abuse and Consequences in Adult Women," *Obstetrics and Gynecology,* vol. 71, no. 4 (1988), pp. 631–41.

12. R. C. Reiter et al., "Correlation Between Sexual Abuse and Somatization in Women with Somatic and Nonsomatic Pain," *American Journal of Obstetrics and Gynecology,* vol. 165, no. 1 (1991), p. 104; A. Lampe et al., "Chronic Pain Syndromes and Their Relation to Childhood Abuse and Stressful Life Events," *Journal of Psychosomatic Research,* vol. 54, no. 4 (April 2003), pp. 361–67; A. Lampe et al., "Chronic Pelvic Pain and Previous Sexual Abuse," *Obstetrics and Gynecology,* vol. 96, no. 6 (December 2000), pp. 929–33; P. Latthe et al., "Factors Predisposing Women to Chronic Pelvic Pain: Systematic Review," *British Medical Journal,* vol. 332, no. 7544 (April 1, 2006), pp. 749–55.

13. Scientific studies supporting this premise include M. Tarlau and M. A. Smalheiser, "Personality Patterns in Patients with Malignant Tumors of the Breast and Cervix," *Psychosomatic Medicine,* vol. 13 (1951), p. 117. In this study of women with cervical cancer, most of the subjects had uniformly negative feelings toward heterosexual relations. Most of them had a higher incidence of premarital sexual experiences, and nearly 75 percent had had multiple marriages ending in divorce or separation.

14. S. Prasad, B. Sung, and B. B. Aggarwal, "Age-Associated Chronic Diseases Require Age-Old Medicine: Role of Chronic Inflammation," *Preventive Medicine Reports,* vol. 54 (Supplement) (May 2012), pp. S29–37.

15. C. A. Ross, "Childhood Sexual Abuse and Psychosomatic Symptoms in Irritable Bowel Syndrome," *Journal of Child Sexual Abuse,* vol. 14, no. 1 (2005), pp. 27–38; P. Salmon, K. Skaife, and J. Rhodes, "Abuse, Dissociation, and Somatization in Irritable Bowel Syndrome: Towards an Explanatory Model," *Journal of Behavioral Medicine,* vol. 26, no. 1 (February 2003), pp. 1–18; Sarah Payne, "Sex, Gender, and Irritable Bowel Syndrome: Making the Connections," *Gender Medicine,* vol. 1, no. 1 (August 2004), pp. 18–28; J. M. Lackner, G. D. Gudleski, and E. B. Blanchard, "Beyond Abuse: The Association Among Parenting Style, Abdominal Pain, and Somatization in IBS Patients," *Behaviour Research and Therapy,* vol. 42, no. 1 (January 2004), pp. 41–56; D. A. Drossman et al., "Alterations of Brain Activity Associated with Resolution of Emotional Distress and Pain in a Case of Severe Irritable Bowel Syndrome," *Gastroenterology,* vol. 124, no. 3 (March 2003), pp. 754–61; A. Ali et al., "Emotional Abuse, Self-Blame, and Self-Silencing in Women with Irritable Bowel Syndrome," *Psychosomatic Medicine,* vol. 62, no. 1 (January–February 2000), pp. 76–82.

16. "The differences in body image scores between the body-exterior cancer group and the body-interior cancer group seem to reflect basic differences in personality orientation." S. Fisher and S. E. Cleveland, "Relationship of Body Image to Site of Cancer," *Psychosomatic Medicine,* vol. 18, no. 4 (1956), p. 309.

17. M. Stout, *The Sociopath Next Door* (New York: MJF Books, 2012).

18. Tarlau and Smalheiser, "Personality Patterns."

19. J. I. Wheeler and B. M. Caldwell, "Psychological Factors in Breast Cancer: A Preliminary Study of Some Personality Trends in Patients with Cancer of the Breast,"

Psychosomatic Medicine, vol. 17 (1955), p. 96; A. H. Labrum, "Psychological Factors in Gynecologic Cancer," *Primary Care,* vol. 3, no. 4 (1976), pp. 811–24.

Chapter 5: The Menstrual Cycle

1. M. Xiaolong et al., "Endometrial Regenerative Cells: A Novel Stem Cell Population," *Journal of Translational Medicine,* vol. 5 (2007), p. 57.

2. E. Hartman, "Dreaming Sleep (the D State) and the Menstrual Cycle," *Journal of Nervous and Mental Disease,* vol. 143 (1966), pp. 406–16; E. M. Swanson and D. Foulkes, "Dream Content and the Menstrual Cycle," *Journal of Nervous and Mental Disease,* vol. 145, no. 5 (1968), pp. 358–63.

3. F. A. Brown, "The Clocks: Timing Biological Rhythms," *American Scientist,* vol. 60 (1972), pp. 756–66; M. Gauguelin, "Wrangle Continues of Pseudoscientific Nature of Astrology," *New Scientist,* February 25, 1978; W. Menaker, "Lunar Periodicity in Human Reproduction: A Likely Unit of Biological Time," *American Journal of Obstetrics and Gynecology,* vol. 77, no. 4 (1959), pp. 904–14; E. M. Dewan, "On the Possibility of the Perfect Rhythm Method of Birth Control by Periodic Light Stimulation," *American Journal of Obstetrics and Gynecology,* vol. 99, no. 7 (1967), pp. 1016–19.

4. R. P. Michael, R. W. Bonsall, and P. Warner, "Human Vaginal Secretion and Volatile Fatty Acid Content," *Science,* vol. 186 (1974), pp. 1217–19; W. B. Cutler, "Human Sex-Attractant Pheromones: Discovery Research, Development, and Application in Sex Therapy," *Psychiatric Annals,* vol. 29 (1999), pp. 54–59.

5. C. Wira, "Mucosal Immunity: The Primary Interface Between the Patient and the Outside World," in "The ABC's of Immunology," course syllabus, Dartmouth Hitchcock Medical Center, September 20–21, 1996.

6. E. Hampson and D. Kimura, "Reciprocal Effects of Hormonal Fluctuations on Human Motor and Perceptual Skills," *Behavioral Neuroscience,* vol. 102 (1988), pp. 456–59.

7. Wira, "Mucosal Immunity."

8. D. George, *Mysteries of the Dark Moon: The Healing Power of the Dark Goddess* (HarperSanFrancisco, 1992), pp. 70–71.

9. W. Menaker, "Lunar Periodicity in Human Reproduction: A Likely Unit of Biological Time," *American Journal of Obstetrics and Gynecology,* vol. 77, no. 4 (1959), pp. 904–14.

10. Lunar data adapted from Caroline Myss.

11. Hartman, "Dreaming Sleep," and Swanson and Foulkes, "Dream Content."

12. M. Altemus, B. E. Wexler, and N. Boulis, "Neuropsychological Correlates of Menstrual Mood Changes," *Psychosomatic Medicine,* vol. 51 (1989), pp. 329–36.

13. T. Benedek and B. Rubenstein, "Correlations Between Ovarian Activity and Psychodynamic Processes: The Ovulatory Phase," *Psychosomatic Medicine,* vol. 1, no. 2 (1939), pp. 245–70.

14. B. C. Gines, "Cultural Hypnosis of the Menstrual Cycle," *New Concepts of Hypnosis* (London: George Allen Press, 1953).

15. D. Ruble, "Premenstrual Symptoms: A Reinterpretation," *Science,* vol. 197 (July 15, 1977), pp. 291–92.

16. For further information, see R. Eisler, *The Chalice and the Blade: Our History, Our Future* (HarperSanFrancisco, 1988) and M. Gimbutas, *Goddesses and Gods of Old Europe, 7000 to 35 B.C.* (Berkeley and Los Angeles: University of California Press, 1982). The degradation of women's wisdom took place gradually. By the time European settlers arrived in what would become the United States, native tribes were mixed in their approach to women. Some degraded them and their bodily processes, setting them apart in shame, while others revered women's wisdom.

17. T. Buckley, "Menstruation and the Power of Yurok Women," in T. Buckley and A. Gottlieb, eds., *Blood Magic: The Anthropology of Menstruation* (Berkeley, CA: University of California Press, 1998), p. 190.

18. Credit for the term *offices of womanhood* goes to Tamara Slayton. See also B. Medicine Eagle, "Women's Moontime: A Call to Power," *Shaman's Drum,* vol. 4 (Spring 1986), p. 21.

19. L. Owen, *Her Blood Is Gold: Celebrating the Power of Menstruation* (Wimborne, UK: Archive Publishing, 2009).

20. P. L. Brown and W. M. O'Neil, cited in P. Shuttle and P. Redgrove, *The Wise Wound* (New York: Grove, 1986).

21. Quoted by Dr. R. Norris at lecture on PMS (Rockland, ME, November 1982).

22. R. Loudall, P. Snow, and J. Johnson, "Myths About Menstruation: Victims of Our Folklore," *International Journal of Women's Studies,* vol. 1 (1984), p. 70; W. M. O'Neil, *Time and the Calendars* (Manchester, UK: Manchester University Press, 1976); P. L. Brown, *Megaliths, Myths and Men: An Introduction to Astro-Archeology* (London: Blandford Press, 1976).

23. Dr. J. Goodrich, lecture on adolescent gynecology, Maine Medical Center, Portland, ME, July 29, 1992.

24. Quoted from Tampax box insert, given to me by Gina Orlando.

25. A. Yang, "Reflection on SMCR Conference," *The Red Web Foundation Newsletter,* vol. 6, no. 19 (Summer 2009).

26. L. S. Morch et al., "Contemporary Hormonal Contraception and the Risk of Breast Cancer," *New England Journal of Medicine,* vol. 377, no. 23 (December 7, 2017), pp. 2228–39.

27. L. Iversen et al., "Lifetime Cancer Risk and Combined Contraceptives: The Royal College of General Practitioners' Oral Contraception Study," *American Journal of Obstetrics and Gynecology,* vol. 216, no. 6, pp. 580.e1–9.

28. A. H. DeCherney, "Hormone Receptors and Sexuality in the Human Female," *Journal of Women's Health and Gender-Based Medicine,* vol. 9, supplement 1 (2000), pp. S9–13.

29. For an in-depth discussion of postpartum sexuality, please see my book *Mother-Daughter Wisdom* (New York: Bantam Books, 2005), pp. 99–100.

30. W. B. Cutler, "Human Sex-Attractant Pheromones: Discovery, Research, Development, and Application in Sex Therapy," *Psychiatric Annals,* vol. 29 (1999), pp. 54–59.

31. M. K. McClintock, "Menstrual Synchrony and Suppression," *Nature*, vol. 299 (1971), pp. 244–45.

32. M. C. P. Rees et al., "Prostaglandins in Menstrual Fluid in Menorrhagia and Dysmenorrhea," *British Journal of Obstetrics and Gynecology*, vol. 91 (1984), p. 673.

33. Kim Dirke et al., "The Influence of Dieting on the Menstrual Cycle of Healthy Young Women," *Journal of Clinical Endocrinology and Metabolism*, vol. 60, no. 6 (1985), pp. 1174–79.

34. R. A. DeFronzo, "The Triumvirate: B-Cell, Muscle, Liver: A Collusion Responsible for NIDDM," *Diabetes*, vol. 37 (1983), pp. 667–87; G. W. Mitchell and J. Rogers, "The Influence of Weight Reduction on Amenorrhea in Obese Women," *New England Journal of Medicine*, vol. 249 (1953), pp. 835–37.

35. K. M. Fairfield et al., "A Prospective Study of Dietary Lactose and Ovarian Cancer," *International Journal of Cancer*, vol. 110, no. 2 (June 10, 2004), pp. 271–77.

36. M. A. Merritt et al., "Dairy Foods and Nutrients in Relation to Risk of Ovarian Cancer and Major Histological Subtypes," *International Journal of Cancer*, vol. 132, no. 5 (March 1, 2013), pp. 1114–24.

37. M. T. Faber et al., "Use of Dairy Products, Lactose, and Calcium and Risk of Ovarian Cancer: Results from a Danish Case-Control Study," *Acta Oncologica*, vol. 51, no. 4 (April 2012), pp. 454–64.

38. "Government Data Proves Raw Milk Safe: Raw Milk Risk Extremely Small Compared to Risk of Other Foods," Weston A. Price Foundation, June 22, 2011, https://www.westonaprice.org/government-data-proves-raw-milk-safe.

39. B. Lund, T. Baird-Parker, and G. Gould, editors, *The Microbiological Safety and Quality of Food*, vol. 1 (Gaithersburg, MD: Aspen Publishers, 2000), pp. 518–19.

40. T. R. Dhiman et al., "Conjugated Linoleic Acid Content of Milk from Cows Fed Different Diets," *Journal of Dairy Science*, vol. 82 (October 1999), pp. 2146–56; S. Couvreur et al., "The Linear Relationship Between the Proportion of Fresh Grass in the Cow Diet, Milk Fatty Acid Composition, and Butter Properties," *Journal of Dairy Science*, vol. 89, no. 6 (June 2006), pp. 1956–69.

41. R. R. Grummer, "Effect of Feed on the Composition of Milk Fat," *Journal of Dairy Science*, vol. 74, no. 9 (September 1991), pp. 3244–57.

42. G. Loss et al., "The Protective Effect of Farm Milk Consumption on Childhood Asthma and Atopy: The GABRIELA Study," *Journal of Allergy and Clinical Immunology*, vol. 128, no. 4 (2011), pp. 766–73.e4.

43. G. E. Abraham, "Nutritional Factors in the Etiology of the Premenstrual Tension Syndromes," *Journal of Reproductive Medicine*, vol. 28, no. 7 (1983), pp. 446–64.

44. D. Mills, "The Nutritional Status of the Endometriosis Patient," Institute for Optimum Nutrition project, September 1991, reported in Nance Edwards Merrill, *Endometriosis Association Newsletter*, vol. 17, nos. 5–6 (1996).

45. D. M. Lithgow and W. M. Polizer, "Vitamin A in the Treatment of Menorrhagia," *South African Medical Journal*, vol. 51 (1977), p. 191.

46. J. D. Cohen and H. W. Rubin, "Functional Menorrhagia: Treatment with Bioflavonoids and Vitamin C," *Current Therapeutic Research*, vol. 2 (1960), p. 539.

47. T. Fumii, "The Clinical Effects of Vitamin E on Purpura Due to Vascular Defects," *Journal of Vitaminology,* vol. 18 (1972), pp. 125–30.

48. F. Facchinetti et al., "Magnesium Prophylaxis of Menstrual Migraine," *Headaches,* vol. 31 (1991), pp. 298–304; F. Facchinetti et al., "Oral Magnesium Successfully Relieves Premenstrual Mood Changes," *Obstetrics and Gynecology,* vol. 78, no. 2 (August 1991), pp. 177–81; P. Muller, presentation at the First International Symposium of Magnesium Deficit in Human Pathology, 1971; G. E. Abraham, "Nutritional Factors in the Etiology of the Premenstrual Tension Syndromes," *Journal of Reproductive Medicine,* vol. 28, no. 7 (1983), pp. 446–64.

49. Z. Harel et al., "Supplementation with Omega-3 Fatty Acids in the Management of Dysmenorrhea in Adolescents," *American Journal of Obstetrics and Gynecology,* vol. 174 (1996), pp. 1335–38.

50. W. Menaker, "Lunar Periodicity in Human Reproduction: A Likely Unit of Biological Time," *American Journal of Obstetrics and Gynecology,* vol. 77, no. 4 (1959), pp. 905–14; E. M. Dewan, "On the Possibility of a Perfect Rhythm Method of Birth Control by Periodic Light Stimulation," *American Journal of Obstetrics and Gynecology,* vol. 99, no. 7 (1967), pp. 1016–19.

51. Dewan, "On the Possibility of a Perfect Rhythm Method of Birth Control by Periodic Light Stimulation."

52. B. L. Parry et al., "Morning vs. Evening Bright Light Treatment of Late Luteal Phase Dysphoric Disorder," *American Journal of Psychiatry,* vol. 146 (1991). For a full discussion of light therapy, see Jacob Liberman, *Light: Medicine of the Future* (Santa Fe: Bear and Co., 1991).

53. J. M. Helms, "Acupuncture for the Management of Primary Dysmenorrhea," *Obstetrics and Gynecology,* vol. 69, no. 1 (January 1987), pp. 51–56.

54. The diagnosis of "liver stagnation" or "blocked liver *chi*" is supported by the fact that the herbs mentioned have been shown to normalize elevated liver enzymes. Margaret Naeser, "Outline Guide to Chinese Herbal Patent Medicines in Pill Form—with Sample Pictures of the Boxes: An Introduction to Chinese Medicine," available from Boston Chinese Medicine Society, P.O. Box 5747, Boston, MA 02114.

55. I. Goodale, A. Domar, and H. Benson, "Alleviation of Premenstrual Syndrome Symptoms with the Relaxation Response," *Obstetrics and Gynecology,* vol. 75, no. 4 (April 1990), pp. 649–89.

56. Controlled trials of natural progesterone that have been reported in the gynecological literature *do not* bear out my experience here. I think that this is because diet, exercise, and supplements have not been part of these studies, and also because women in these studies have not been taught how to think about their PMS as a signal that their lives are out of balance.

57. A. J. Rapkin, M. Morgan, L. Goldman, D. Brann, D. Simone, and V. B. Mahesh, "Progesterone Metabolite Allopregnanolone in Women with Premenstrual Syndrome," *Obstetrics and Gynecology,* vol. 90, no. 5 (November 1997), pp. 709–14; E. S. Arafat et al., "Sedative and Hypnotic Effects of Oral Administration of Micronized Oral Progesterone May Be Medicated Through Its Metabolites," *American Journal of Obstetrics and Gynecology,* vol. 159 (1988), p. 1203; Andrew Herzog, "Intermittent Progesterone Therapy and Frequency of Complex Partial Seizures in Women with Menstrual Disorders," *Neurology,* vol. 36 (1986), pp. 1607–10.

58. T. A. Lovick et al., "A Specific Profile of Luteal Phase Progesterone Is Associated with the Development of Premenstrual Symptoms," *Psychoneuroendocrinology*, vol. 75 (January 2017), pp. 83–90.

59. Data based on report from independent testing of over-the-counter progesterone and yam creams, performed by Aeron LifeCycles Laboratory, 1933 Davis Street, Suite 310, San Leandro, CA 94577, 800-631-7900.

60. For years, those interested in PMS have batted around the idea of a "menotoxin" present in women around the time of their periods because of this Jekyll-and-Hyde phenomenon and also because skin breakouts were worse premenstrually.

61. A. Barbarino et al., "Corticotrophin-Releasing Hormone Inhibition of Gonadotropin Secretion During the Menstrual Cycle," *Metabolism*, vol. 38 (1989), pp. 504–6; I. Nagata et al., "Ovulatory Disturbances: Causative Factors Among Japanese Women Student Nurses in a Dormitory," *Journal of Adolescent Health Care*, vol. 7 (1986), pp. 1–5; M. R. Soules et al., "Luteal Phase Deficiency: Characterization of Reproductive Hormones over the Menstrual Cycle," *Journal of Clinical Endocrine Metabolism*, vol. 69 (1989), pp. 804–12.

62. T. Oleson and W. Flocco, "Randomized Controlled Study of Premenstrual Symptoms Treated with Ear, Hand, and Foot Reflexology," *Obstetrics and Gynecology*, vol. 82 (1993), pp. 901–11; J. Blum, *Woman Heal Thyself* (Boston: Charles Tuttle, 1995).

63. J. Prior et al., "Conditioning Exercise Decreases Premenstrual Symptoms: A Prospective Controlled Six-Month Trial," *Fertility and Sterility*, vol. 47 (1987), pp. 402–9.

64. M. Imamura et al., "Repeated Thermal Therapy Improves Impaired Vascular Endothelial Function in Patients with Coronary Risk Factors," *Journal of the American College of Cardiology*, vol. 38, no. 4 (2001), pp. 1983–8.

65. T. Laukkanen, H. Khan, F. Zaccardi, and J. A. Laukkanen, "Association Between Sauna Bathing and Fatal Cardiovascular and All-Cause Mortality Events," *Journal of the American Medical Association—Intern Medicine*, vol. 175, no. 4 (2015), pp. 542–48.

66. M. E. Sears, K. J. Kerr, and R. I. Bray, "Arsenic, Cadmium, Lead, and Mercury in Sweat: A Systematic Review," *Journal of Environmental and Public Health*, 2012, p. 184745 (published online February 22, 2012).

67. During the menstrual cycle, excess epinephrine released via stress (known as autonomic overdrive) may disrupt the natural autonomic nervous system balance. E. W. Winenman, "Autonomic Balance Changes During the Human Menstrual Cycle," *Psychophysiology*, vol. 8, no. 1 (1971), pp. 1–6.

68. American College of Obstetricians and Gynecologists (ACOG) 57th Annual Clinical Meeting, papers on current clinical and basic investigation, presented May 4, 2009.

69. There is no uniformly agreed-upon definition of PMS in the medical literature, so many of the studies on the incidence of this disorder disagree. Regardless of medical definition, the experience of thousands of women around their menstrual cycle is one of emotional and physical suffering. F. L. Reid and S. S. Yen, "Premenstrual Syndrome," *American Journal of Obstetrics and Gynecology*, vol. 139 (1981), p. 86.

70. R. Norris, "Progesterone for Premenstrual Tension," *Journal of Reproductive Medicine,* vol. 28, no. 8 (August 1983), pp. 509–15.

71. D. L. Jakubowicz, E. Godard, and J. Dewhurst, "The Treatment of Premenstrual Tension and Mefanamic Acid: Analysis of Prostaglandin Concentration," *British Journal of Obstetrics and Gynaecology,* vol. 91 (1984), p. 78.

72. In one study, PMS patients consumed five times more dairy products than controls without PMS. The excess calcium intake from the dairy products may hinder magnesium absorption. G. S. Goci and G. E. Abraham, "Effect of Nutritional Supplement . . . on Symptoms of Premenstrual Tension," *Journal of Reproductive Medicine,* vol. 83 (1982), pp. 527–31.

73. A. M. Rossignol, "Caffeine-Containing Beverages and Premenstrual Syndrome in Young Women," *American Journal of Public Health,* vol. 75, no. 11 (1985), pp. 1335–37.

74. B. L. Snider and D. F. Dietman, "Pyridoxine Therapy for Premenstrual Acne Flare," *Archives of Dermatology,* vol. 110 (July 1974); G. E. Abraham and J. T. Hargrove, "Effect of Vitamin B on Premenstrual Tension Syndrome: A Double Blind Crossover Study," *Infertility,* vol. 3 (1980), p. 155; M. S. Biskind, "Nutritional Deficiency in the Etiology of Menorrhagia Cystic Mastitis, Premenstrual Syndrome, and Treatment with Vitamin B Complex," *Journal of Clinical Endocrinology and Metabolism,* vol. 3 (1943), pp. 227–334; R. W. Engel, "The Relation of B Complex Vitamins and Dietary Fat to the Lipotropic Action of Choline," *Journal of Biological Chemistry,* vol. 37 (1941), p. 140.

75. D. G. Williams, "The Forgotten Hormone," *Alternatives,* vol. 4, no. 6 (1991), p. 11.

76. B. L. Denrefer et al., "Progesterone and Adenosine 3', 5'-Monophosphate Formation by Isolated Human Corpora Lutea of Different Ages: Influence of Human Chorionic Gonadotropin and Prostaglandins," *Journal of Clinical Endocrinology and Metabolism,* vol. 55 (1982), pp. 102–107.

77. B. R. Goldin et al., "Estrogen Excretion Patterns and Plasma Levels in Vegetarian and Omnivorous Women," *New England Journal of Medicine,* vol. 307 (1982), pp. 1542–47; B. R. Goldin et al., "Effect of Diet on Excretion of Estrogens in Pre- and Post-Menopausal Women," *Cancer Research,* vol. 41 (1981), pp. 3771–73.

78. G. E. Abraham, "Nutritional Factors in the Etiology of the Premenstrual Tension Syndromes," *Journal of Reproductive Medicine,* vol. 28 (1983), p. 446; M. Lubran and G. Abraham, "Serum and Red Cell Magnesium Levels in Patients with Premenstrual Tension," *American Journal of Clinical Nutrition,* vol. 34 (1982), p. 2364; G. E. Abraham and J. T. Hargrove, "Effect of Vitamin B on Premenstrual Tension Syndrome: A Double Blind Crossover Study," *Infertility,* vol. 3 (1980), p. 155; Facchinetti et al., "Oral Magnesium."

79. R. S. Landau et al., "The Effect of Alpha Tocopherol in Premenstrual Symptomatology: A Double-Blind Trial," *Journal of the American College of Nutrition,* vol. 2 (1983), pp. 115–23; M. R. Werback, *Nutritional Influences on Illness* (Tarzana, CA: Third Line Press, 1988).

80. Lubran and Abraham, "Serum and Red Cell Magnesium Levels"; Facchinetti et al., "Oral Magnesium."

81. B. L. Parry et al., "Morning vs. Evening Bright Light Treatment of Late Luteal

Phase Dysphoric Disorder," *American Journal of Psychiatry*, vol. 146 (1991), p. 9.

82. J. Ott, *Health and Light* (New York: Pocket Books, 1978); Z. Kime, *Sunlight Could Save Your Life* (Penryn, CA: World Health Publications, 1980, available by writing to World Health Publications, P.O. Box 400, Penryn, CA 95663); Jacob Liberman, *Light: Medicine of the Future* (Santa Fe: Bear and Co., 1991); M. D. Rao, B. Muller-Oerlinghausen, and H. P. Volz, "The Influence of Phototherapy on Serotonin and Metatonin in Nonseasonal Depression," *Pharmacopsychiatry*, vol. 23 (1990), pp. 155–58; J. E. Blundell, "Serotonin and Appetite," *Neuropharmacology*, vol. 23, no. 128 (1984), pp. 1537–51.

83. M. Steiner et al., "Fluoxetine in the Treatment of Premenstrual Dysphoria," *New England Journal of Medicine*, vol. 332, no. 23 (1995), pp. 1529–34.

84. S. Zuckerman, "The Menstrual Cycle," *The Lancet*, June 18, 1949, pp. 1031–35.

85. Cystic and adenomatous hyperplasia of the endometrium is very common after periods of amenorrhea or anovulation. It is a benign condition if there is no atypia of the cells. A good gynecological pathologist can make a prediction as to how dangerous this condition is, depending upon the nature of the cells present on the specimen.

86. F. Z. Stanczyk, R. J. Paulson, and S. Roy, "Percutaneous Administration of Progesterone: Blood Levels and Endometrial Protection," *Menopause*, vol. 12, no. 2 (March 2005), pp. 232–37.

87. Clomid has an estrogen-like structure. Its presence in the first half of the menstrual cycles causes the hypothalamus to put out increased levels of the hormones LH and FSH, thus stimulating the ovary to produce an egg.

88. A. J. Hartz et al., "The Association of Obesity with Infertility and Related Menstrual Abnormalities in Women," *International Journal of Obesity*, vol. 3 (1979), pp. 57–73.

89. A. E. Jacobson et al., "Patterns of von Willebrand Disease Screening in Girls and Adolescents with Heavy Menstrual Bleeding," *Obstetrics and Gynecology*, May 7, 2018 (published electronically ahead of print).

90. C. Benedetto, "Eicosanoids in Primary Dysmenorrhea, Endometriosis and Menstrual Migraines," *Gynecological Endocrinology*, vol. 3, no. 1 (1989), pp. 71–94; A. Anderson et al., "Reduction of Menstrual Blood Loss by Prostaglandin-Synthetase Inhibitors," *The Lancet*, 1967, p. 774.

91. H. O'Connor and A. Magos, "Endometrial Resection for the Treatment of Menorrhagia," *New England Journal of Medicine*, vol. 335 (1996), pp. 151–56.

92. American Psychological Association Task Force on the Sexualization of Girls, *Report of the APA Task Force on the Sexualization of Girls* (Washington, DC: American Psychological Association, 2007), www.apa.org/pi/wpo/sexualization.html.

93. B. Klettke, D. J. Hallford, and D. J. Mellor, "Sexting Prevalence and Correlates: A Systematic Literature Review," *Clinical Psychology Review*, vol. 34, no. 1 (February 2014), pp. 44–53.

94. S. V. Ng, "Social Media and the Sexualization of Adolescent Girls," *American Journal of Psychiatry Residents' Journal*, vol. 11, no. 12 (December 2016), p. 14.

95. D. M. Szymanski, L. B. Moffitt, and E. R. Carr, "Sexual Objectification of

Women: Advances to Theory and Research," *The Counseling Psychologist*, vol. 39, no. 1 (2011), pp. 6–38.

96. J. M. Stankiewicz and F. Rosselli, "Women as Sex Objects and Victims in Print Advertisements," *Sex Roles*, vol. 58, no. 7 (April 2008), pp. 579–89.

97. J. Kilbourne, *Can't Buy My Love: How Advertising Changes the Way We Think and Feel* (New York: Simon & Schuster, 1999).

98. N. Wolf, *The Beauty Myth: How Images of Beauty Are Used Against Women* (New York: William Morrow, 1991), p. 4.

99. I was introduced to this concept by Tamara Slayton.

Chapter 6: The Uterus

1. While doing the research for this book, I was amazed by the lack of data on the uterus itself, separate from childbearing. The silence on the organ speaks volumes.

2. M. K. Whiteman et al., "Inpatient Hysterectomy Surveillance in the United States 2000–2004," *American Journal of Obstetrics and Gynecology*, vol. 198, no. 1 (January 2008), p. 34.e1–7.

3. Whiteman et al., "Inpatient Hysterectomy Surveillance in the United States."

4. L. Lepine et al., "Hysterectomy Surveillance—United States, 1980–1993," *Morbidity and Mortality Weekly Report*, vol. 46, no. SS-04 (August 8, 1997), pp. 1–16.

5. Centers for Disease Control and Prevention, *Key Statistics from the National Survey of Family Growth*, 2015, www.cdc.gov/nchs/nsfg/key_statistics/h.htm #hysterectomy.

6. Lepine et al., "Hysterectomy Surveillance—United States, 1980–1993."

7. S. Domingo and A. Pellicer, "Overview of Current Trends in Hysterectomy," *Expert Review of Obstetrics and Gynecology*, vol. 4, no. 6 (2009), pp. 673–85.

8. W. Cutler and E. Genovese-Stone, "Wellness in Women After 40 Years of Age: The Role of Sex Hormones and Pheromones," *Disease-A-Month*, vol. 44, no. 9 (September 1998), p. 526.

9. S. J. Glynn, "Breadwinning Mothers Are Increasingly the U.S. Norm," Center for American Progress, December 19, 2016, www.americanprogress.org/issues/ women/reports/2016/12/19/295203/breadwinning-mothers-are-increasingly-the -u-s-norm.

10. J. C. Gambone and R. C. Reiter, "Nonsurgical Management of Chronic Pelvic Pain: A Multidisciplinary Approach," *Clinical Obstetrics and Gynecology*, vol. 33 (1990), pp. 205–11; R. C. Reiter and J. C. Gambone, "Demographic and Historic Variables in Women with Idiopathic Chronic Pelvic Pain," *Obstetrics and Gynecology*, vol. 75 (1990), pp. 428–32.

11. Reiter and Gambone, "Demographic and Historic Variables."

12. Information from Caroline Myss.

13. Dr. I. Schiff, Chairman of the Department of Gynecology at Massachusetts General Hospital, at Grand Rounds, Maine Medical Center, Portland, ME, 1993.

14. N. Petersen and B. Hasselbring, "Endometriosis Reconsidered," *Medical Self Care*, May–June 1987.

15. D. B. Redwine, "The Distribution of Endometriosis in the Pelvis by Age Groups and Fertility," *Fertility and Sterility,* vol. 47 (January 1987), p. 173.

16. Supporting evidence can be found in V. Bancroft, C. A. Williams, and M. Elstein, "Minimal/Mild Endometriosis and Infertility: A Review," *British Journal of Obstetrics and Gynaecology,* vol. 96, no. 4, pp. 454–50. The role of minimal or mild endometriosis in the etiology of infertility remains unclear, but an increased prostanoid content and macrophage activity in peritoneal fluid may exert an effect by a variety of mechanisms, including altered tubal motility, sperm function, and early embryo wastage. Ovarian function may be altered in a variety of ways, including many subtle abnormalities detectable only by detailed investigation. Autoimmune phenomena may also be contributory.

17. J. Sampson, "Peritoneal Endometriosis Due to the Menstrual Dissemination of Endometrial Tissue into the Peritoneal Cavity," *American Journal of Obstetrics and Gynecology,* vol. 14 (1927), pp. 422–69.

18. This theory is based on the work of Dr. David Redwine, who along with Nancy Petersen, R.N., is the founder of the St. Charles Medical Center endometriosis treatment program in Bend, Oregon.

19. Petersen and Hasselbring, "Endometriosis Reconsidered." See also D. Redwine, "Age-Related Evolution in Color Appearance of Endometriosis," *Fertility and Sterility,* vol. 48, no. 6 (December 1987), pp. 1062–63; D. Redwine, "Is Microscopic Peritoneal Endometriosis Invisible?" *Fertility and Sterility,* vol. 50, no. 4 (October 1988), pp. 665–66.

20. N. Gleicher, "Is Endometriosis an Autoimmune Disease?" *Obstetrics and Gynecology,* vol. 70, no. 1 (July 1987); E. Surry and J. Halme, "Effect of Peritoneal Fluid from Endometriosis Patients on Endometrial Stromal Cell Proliferation in Vitro," *Obstetrics and Gynecology,* vol. 76, no. 5, part 1 (November 1990), pp. 792–98; S. Kalma et al., "Production of Fibronection by Peritoneal Macrophages and Concentration of Fibronection in Peritoneal Fluid from Patients With or Without Endometriosis," *Obstetrics and Gynecology,* vol. 72 (July 1988), pp. 13–19; J. Halme, S. Becker, and S. Haskil, "Altered Maturation and Function of Peritoneal Macrophages: Possible Role in Pathogenesis of Endometriosis," *American Journal of Obstetrics and Gynecology,* vol. 156 (1987), p. 783; J. Halme et al., "Retrograde Menstruation in Healthy Women and in Patients with Endometriosis," *Obstetrics and Gynecology,* vol. 64 (1984), pp. 13–18.

21. C. Northrup, *Mother-Daughter Wisdom* (New York: Bantam Books, 2005), p. 234.

22. Conventional insurance is set up to cover only certain treatment modalities and often does not cover relatively inexpensive measures to maintain health. Much has been written about the politics of medical treatment, a topic that is beyond the scope of this book. Though all of us end up paying for very expensive conventional medical treatments such as GnRH agonists, individuals with insurance don't bear this cost *directly* and therefore don't want to pay for modalities that aren't covered by insurance.

23. Food and Drug Administration, "Urogynecologic Surgical Mesh: Update on the Safety and Effectiveness of Transvaginal Placement for Pelvic Organ Prolapse," 2011, http://www.fda.gov/MedicalDevices/Safety/AlertandNotices/ucm262760.pdf.

24. H. Abed et al., "Incidence and Management of Graft Erosion, Wound Granula-

tion, and Dyspareunia Following Vaginal Prolapse Repair with Graft Materials: A Systematic Review," *International Urogynecology Journal,* vol. 22, no. 7 (July 2011), pp. 789–98.

25. C. M. A. Glazener et al., "Mesh, Graft, or Standard Repair for Women Having Primary Transvaginal Anterior or Posterior Compartment Prolapse Surgery: Two Parallel-Group, Multicentre, Randomised, Controlled Trials (PROSPECT)," *The Lancet,* vol. 389, no. 10067 (January 28, 2017), pp. 381–92.

26. E. A. Stewart et al., "Epidemiology of Uterine Fibroids: A Systematic Review," *BJOG: An International Journal of Obstetrics and Gynaecology,* vol. 124, no. 10 (September 2017), pp. 1501–12.

27. A. D. Feinstein, "Conflict over Childbearing and Tumors of the Female Reproduction System: Symbolism in Disease," *Somatics* (Fall/Winter 1983).

28. R. C. Reiter, P. C. Wagner, and J. C. Gambone, "Routine Hysterectomy for Large Asymptomatic Leiomyomata: A Reappraisal," *Obstetrics and Gynecology,* vol. 79, no. 4 (April 1992), pp. 481–84.

29. An entire body of literature on the healing power of sound is available. Each chakra, for example, is associated with a certain vibration. Healers who use sound may suggest that a person sing certain tones or listen to specially designed music. For more information about this treatment, read: W. David, *The Harmonics of Sound, Color, and Vibration: A System for Self-Awareness and Evolution* (Marina del Rey, CA: DeVorss and Co., 1985); Kay Gardner, *Sounding the Inner Landscape* (Stonington, ME: Caduceus Publications, 1990).

30. A. J. Friedman et al. "A Randomized, Double-Blind Trial of Gonadotropin . . . in the Treatment of Leiomyomata Uteri," *Fertility and Sterility,* vol. 49 (1988), p. 404.

31. Progestin hormone, in the form of Provera or Aygestin, can be taken daily on days fourteen to twenty-eight of the menstrual cycle to decrease excess buildup of endometrial tissue inside the uterus. This treatment sometimes works like a D&C and in fact is sometimes called a "medical D&C." I recommend this approach for those women whose heavy bleeding is unaffected by dietary change or for whom dietary change is impractical. It is sometimes used in addition to other therapies, such as acupuncture. Each case is individualized.

32. Alan de Cherney, M.D., chairman of the Department of Obstetrics and Gynecology, Tufts University Medical Center, Boston, is a pioneer in this surgery and has trained physicians throughout the country in this technique.

33. Society of Interventional Radiology, "Minimally Invasive, Less Expensive Treatment for Uterine Fibroids Underutilized: National Study Suggests Many Women Are Not Aware of Benefits of Uterine Fibroid Embolization," *Science Daily,* March 6, 2017, www.sciencedaily.com/releases/2017/03/170306092746.htm.

34. L. Bradley and J. Newman, "Uterine Artery Embolization for Treatment of Fibroids: From Scalpel to Catheter," *The Female Patient,* vol. 25 (2000), pp. 71–78.

35. K. J. Carlson, B. Z. Miller, and F. J. Fowler, "The Maine Women's Health Study: I. Outcomes of Hysterectomy," *Obstetrics and Gynecology,* vol. 83 (1994), pp. 556–65.

36. S. Rako, *The Hormone of Desire* (New York: Harmony Books, 1996).

37. L. Zussman et al., "Sexual Response After Hysterectomy-Oophorectomy: Recent Studies and Reconsideration of Psychogenesis," *American Journal of Obstetrics and Gynecology,* vol. 140, no. 7 (August 1, 1981), pp. 725–29.

38. Carlson, Miller, and Fowler, "Maine Women's Health Study."

39. J. P. Roovers et al., "Hysterectomy and Sexual Wellbeing: Prospective Observational Study of Vaginal Hysterectomy, Subtotal Abdominal Hysterectomy, and Total Abdominal Hysterectomy," *British Medical Journal,* vol. 327, no. 7418 (October 4, 2003), pp. 774–78.

40. B. Ranney and S. Abu-Ghazaleh, "The Future Function and Control of Ovarian Tissue Which Is Retained in Vivo During Hysterectomy," *American Journal of Obstetrics and Gynecology,* vol. 128 (1977), p. 626; N. Siddle, P. Sarrel, and M. Whitehead, "The Effect of Hysterectomy on the Age of Ovarian Failure: Identification of a Subgroup of Women and Premature Loss of Ovarian Function and Literature Reviews," *Fertility and Sterility,* vol. 47 (1987), p. 94.

41. B. J. Parys et al., "The Effects of Simple Hysterectomy on Vesicourethral Function," *British Journal of Urology,* vol. 64 (1989), pp. 594–99; S. J. Snooks et al., "Perineal Nerve Damage in Genuine Stress Urinary Incontinence," *British Journal of Urology,* vol. 42 (1985), pp. 3–9; C. R. Wake, "The Immediate Effect of Abdominal Hysterectomy and Intervesical Pressure and Detrusor Activity," *British Journal of Obstetrics and Gynaecology,* vol. 87 (1980), pp. 901–2: A. G. Hanley, "The Late Urological Complications of Total Hysterectomy," *British Journal of Urology,* vol. 41 (1969), pp. 682–84.

42. J. Mytton et al., "Removal of All Ovarian Tissue Versus Conserving Ovarian Tissue at Time of Hysterectomy in Premenopausal Patients with Benign Disease: Study Using Routine Data and Data Linkage," *British Medical Journal,* vol. 356 (February 6, 2017), p. j372.

43. J. H. Manchester et al., "Premenopausal Castration and Documented Coronary Atherosclerosis," *American Journal of Cardiology,* vol. 28 (1971), pp. 33–37; A. B. Ritterband et al., "Gonadal Function and the Development of Coronary Heart Disease," *Circulation,* vol. 27 (1963), pp. 237–87.

44. S. West, *The Hysterectomy Hoax* (New York: Doubleday, 1994); H. Goldfarb, *The No-Hysterectomy Option* (New York: John Wiley and Sons, 1990).

Chapter 7: The Ovaries

1. M. McLaughlin et al., "Non-Growing Follicle Density Is Increased Following Adriamycin, Bleomycin, Vinblastine and Dacarbazine (ABVD) Chemotherapy in the Adult Human Ovary," *Human Reproduction,* vol. 32, no. 1 (January 2017), pp. 165–74.

2. M. McLaughlin et al., "Metaphase II Oocytes from Human Unilaminar Follicles Grown in a Multi-Step Culture System," *Molecular Human Reproduction,* vol. 24, no. 3 (March 1, 2018), pp. 135–42.

3. O. Hikabe et al., "Reconstruction *in Vitro* of the Entire Cycle of the Mouse Female Germ Line," *Nature,* vol. 539 (November 10, 2016), pp. 299–303.

4. J. H. Nadeau, "Do Gametes Woo? Evidence for Their Nonrandom Union at Fertilization," *Genetics,* vol. 207, no. 2 (October 1, 2017), pp. 369–87.

5. R. H. Asch and R. Greenblatt, "Steroidogenesis in the Postmenopausal Ovary," *Clinical Obstetrics and Gynecology,* vol. 4, no. 1 (1977), p. 85.

6. E. R. Novak, B. Goldberg, and G. S. Jones, "Enzyme Histochemistry of the Meno-

pausal Ovary Associated with Normal and Abnormal Endometrium," *American Journal of Obstetrics and Gynecology,* vol. 93 (1965), p. 669; C. R. Garcia and W. Cutler, "Preservation of the Ovary: A Reevaluation," *Fertility and Sterility,* vol. 42, no. 4 (October 1985), pp. 510–14.

7. K. P. McNatty et al., "The Production of Progesterone, Androgens, and Estrogens by Granulosa Cells, Thecal Tissue, and Stromal Tissue by Human Ovaries in Vitro," *Journal of Clinical Endocrinology and Metabolism,* vol. 49 (1979), p. 687.

8. B. Dennefors et al., "Steroid Production and Responsiveness to Gonadotropin in Isolated Stromal Tissue of Human Postmenopausal Ovaries," *American Journal of Obstetrics and Gynecology,* vol. 136 (1980), p. 997; G. Mikhail, "Hormone Secretion of Human Ovaries," *Gynecological Investigation,* vol. 1 (1970), p. 5; B. B. Sherwin and M. M. Gelfand, "The Role of Androgen in the Maintenance of Sexual Functioning in Oophorectomized Women," *Psychosomatic Medicine,* vol. 49 (1987), p. 397.

9. M. Chia and M. Chia, *Cultivating Female Sexual Energy: Healing Love Through the Tao* (Huntington, NY: Healing Tao Books, 1986), available from Healing Tao Books at www.healingtao.com/b06.html.

10. F. P. Paloucek and J. B. Graham, "The Influence of Psychosocial Factors on the Prognosis in Cancer of the Cervix," *Annals of the New York Academy of Sciences,* vol. 125 (1966), pp. 815–16.

11. I. Gerendai et al., "Unilateral Ovariotomy-Induced Luteinizing Hormone-Releasing Hormone Content Changes in the Two Halves of the Mediobasal Hypothalamus," *Neuroscience Letters,* vol. 9 (1978), pp. 333–36.

12. J. R. Givens, "Reproduction and Hormonal Alterations in Obesity," in P. Bjorntorp and B. Brodoff, eds., *Obesity* (New York: Lippincott, 1992).

13. R. L. Barbieri et al., "Insulin Stimulates Androgen Accumulation in Incubations of Ovarian Stroma Obtained from Women with Hyperandrogenism," *Journal of Clinical Endocrinology and Metabolism,* vol. 62 (1986), p. 904.

14. R. J. Chang et al., "Insulin Resistance in Non-Obese Patients with Polycystic Ovarian Syndrome," *Journal of Clinical Endocrinology and Metabolism,* vol. 61 (1985), p. 946; C. A. Stuart et al., "Insulin Resistance with Acanthosis Nigricans: The Role of Obesity and Androgen Excess," *Metabolism,* vol. 35 (1986), p. 197.

15. P. J. Torres et al.,"Gut Microbial Diversity in Women with Polycystic Ovary Syndrome Correlates with Hyperandrogenism," *Journal of Clinical Endocrinology and Metabolism,* vol. 103, no. 4 (April 1, 2018), pp. 1502–11.

16. K. Kelly et al., "Psychodynamic Psychological Correlates with Secondary Amenorrhea," *Psychosomatic Medicine,* vol. 16 (1954), p. 129; M. M. Gill, "Functional Disturbances in Menstruation," *Bulletin of the Menninger Clinic,* vol. 7 (1943), p. 12.

17. T. B. Clarkson et al., "From Menarche to Menopause: Coronary Artery Atherosclerosis and Protection in Cynomolgus Monkeys," *American Journal of Obstetrics and Gynecology,* vol. 160, no. 5, part 2 (May 1989), pp. 1280–85.

18. T. Piotrowski, "Psychogenic Factors in Anovulatory Women," *Fertility and Sterility,* vol. 13 (1962), p. 11; T. Loftus, "Psychogenic Factors in Anovulatory Women: Behavioral and Psychoanalytic Aspects of Anovulatory Amenorrhea," *Fertility and Sterility,* vol. 13 (1962), p. 20.

19. Though some might argue that all cysts should therefore be removed when they

are first diagnosed and are relatively small, I disagree. Not all cysts grow rapidly, and not all cysts replace all normal ovarian tissue. And of course, some cysts go away on their own.

20. A. Koushik, M. E. Parent, and J. Siemiatycki, "Characteristics of Menstruation and Pregnancy and the Risk of Lung Cancer in Women," *International Journal of Cancer,* vol. 125, no. 10 (November 15, 2009), pp. 2428–33.

21. W. H. Parker et al., "Ovarian Conservation at the Time of Hysterectomy and Long-Term Health Outcomes in the Nurses' Health Study," *Obstetrics and Gynecology,* vol. 113, no. 5 (May 2009), pp. 1027–37.

22. Ibid.

23. C. M. Rivera et al., "Increased Mortality for Neurological and Mental Diseases Following Early Bilateral Oophorectomy," *Neuroepidemiology,* vol. 33, no. 1 (2009), pp. 32–40.

24. W. H. Parker, "Bilateral Oophorectomy Versus Ovarian Conservation: Effects on Long-Term Women's Health," *Journal of Minimally Invasive Gynecology,* vol. 17, no. 2 (March–April 2010), pp. 161–66.

25. Ibid.

26. Ibid.

27. Ibid.

28. B. S. Centerwall, "Premenopausal Hysterectomy," *American Journal of Obstetrics and Gynecology,* vol. 139 (1981), p. 38; R. Punnonen and L. Raurama, "The Effect of Long-Term Oral Oestriol Succinate Therapy on the Skin of Castrated Women," *Annals of Gynaecology,* vol. 66 (1977), p. 214.

29. T. Speroff et al., "A Risk-Benefit Analysis of Elective Bilateral Oophorectomy: Effect of Changes in Compliance with Estrogen Therapy on Outcome," *American Journal of Obstetrics and Gynecology,* vol. 164, no. 1, part 1 (January 1991), pp. 165–74.

30. W. B. Cutler, "Human Sex-Attractant Pheromones: Discovery, Research, Development, and Application in Sex Therapy," *Psychiatric Annals,* vol. 29 (1999), pp. 54–59.

31. J. G. Annegers et al., "Ovarian Cancer: Reappraisal of Residual Ovaries," *American Journal of Obstetrics and Gynecology,* vol. 97 (1967), p. 124; G. V. Smith, "Ovarian Tumors," *American Journal of Surgery,* vol. 95 (1958), p. 336; V. S. Counselor et al., "Carcinoma of the Ovary Following Hysterectomy," *American Journal of Obstetrics and Gynecology,* vol. 69 (1955), p. 538; R. H. Grogan, "Reappraisal of Residual Ovaries," *American Journal of Obstetrics and Gynecology,* vol. 97 (1967), p. 124.

32. T. Sperof, "A Risk-Benefit Analysis of Elective Bilateral Oophorectomy: Effect of Changes in Compliance with Estrogen Therapy on Outcome," *American Journal of Obstetrics and Gynecology* 164, no. 1, pt. 1 (January 1991), pp. 165–74.

33. D. W. Cramer and B. L. Harlow, "Author's Response to Progress in Nutritional Epidemiology of Ovarian Cancer," *American Journal of Epidemiology,* vol. 134, no. 5 (1991), pp. 460–61; D. W. Cramer et al., "Galactose Consumption and Metabolism in Relationship to Risks for Ovarian Cancer," *The Lancet,* vol. 2 (1989), pp. 66–71; D. W. Cramer, "Lactose Persistence and Milk Consumption as Determinants of Ovarian Cancer Risk," *American Journal of Epidemiology,* vol. 130 (1989), pp. 904–10; D. W. Cramer et al., "Dietary Animal Fat and Rela-

tionship to Ovarian Cancer Risk," *Obstetrics and Gynecology,* vol. 63, no. 6 (1984), pp. 833–38.

34. K. L. Terry et al., "Genital Powder Use and Risk of Ovarian Cancer: A Pooled Analysis of 8,525 Cases and 9,859 Controls," *Cancer Prevention Research,* vol. 6, no. 8 (August 2013), pp. 811–21.

35. D. W. Cramer et al., "Ovarian Cancer and Talc: A Case-Control Study," *Cancer,* vol. 50 (1982), pp. 372–76; W. J. Henderson, T. C. Hamilton, and K. Griffiths, "Talc in Normal and Malignant Ovarian Tissue," *The Lancet,* vol. 1 (1979), p. 499.

36. G. E. Egli and M. Newton, "The Transport of Carbon Particles in the Human Female Reproductive Tract," *Fertility and Sterility,* vol. 12 (1961), pp. 151–55.

37. B. L. Harlow et al., "The Influence of Lactose Consumption on the Association of Oral Contraceptive Pills and Ovarian Cancer Risk," *American Journal of Epidemiology,* vol. 134, no. 5 (1991), pp. 445–61.

38. B. V. Stadel, "The Etiology and Prevention of Ovarian Cancer," *American Journal of Obstetrics and Gynecology,* vol. 123 (1975), pp. 772–74.

39. K. Helzisouer et al., "Serum Gonadotrophins and Steroid Hormones and the Development of Ovarian Cancer," *Journal of the American Medical Association,* vol. 274, no. 24 (December 27, 1995), pp. 1926–30.

40. S. E. Hankinson et al., "Tubal Ligation, Hysterectomy, and Risk of Ovarian Cancer: A Prospective Study," *Journal of the American Medical Association,* December 15, 1993; A. S. Whittemore, R. Harris, J. Intyre, and the Collaborative Ovarian Cancer Group, "Characteristics Relating to Ovarian Cancer Risk: Collaborative Analysis of 12 U.S. Case-Control Studies. Part II: Invasive Epithelial Ovarian Cancers in White Women," *American Journal of Epidemiology,* vol. 136 (1992), pp. 1184–1203.

41. U.S. Preventive Services Task Force et al., "Screening for Ovarian Cancer: U.S. Preventive Services Task Force Recommendation Statement," *Journal of the American Medical Association,* vol. 319, no. 6 (February 13, 2018), pp. 588–94.

42. Ibid.

43. C. Granai, "Sounding Board: Ovarian Cancer: Unrealistic Expectations," *New England Journal of Medicine,* vol. 327, no. 3 (1993), pp. 197–200.

44. S. S. Buys et al., "Effect of Screening on Ovarian Cancer Mortality: the Prostate, Lung, Colorectal and Ovarian (PLCO) Cancer Screening Randomized Controlled Trial," *Journal of the American Medical Association,* vol. 305, no. 22 (June 8, 2011), pp. 2295–303.

45. S. Campbell et al., "Screening for Early Ovarian Cancer," *The Lancet,* vol. 1 (1988), pp. 710–11.

46. E. Andolf, E. Svalenius, and B. Astedt, "Ultrasonography for the Early Detection of Ovarian Cancer," *British Journal of Obstetrics and Gynaecology,* vol. 93 (1986), pp. 1286–89.

47. "FDA Clears a Test for Ovarian Cancer," FDA News Release, September 11, 2009, www.fda.gov/NewsEvents/Newsroom/PressAnnouncements/ucm182057.htm.

48. W. Hamilton et al., "Risk of Ovarian Cancer in Women with Symptoms in Primary Care: Population Based Case-Control Study," *British Medical Journal,* vol. 339 (August 25, 2009), www.bmj.com/cgi/content/abstract/339/aug25_2/b2998.

49. Gilda Radner, a well-known comedienne and wife of actor Gene Wilder, died of familial ovarian cancer. To prevent this from happening to others, Wilder has publicized the genetic risk for those who have this disease in their families, usually in first-degree relatives on the mother's side of the family.

50. J. K. Tobachman et al., "Intra-Abdominal Carcinomatosis After Prophylactic Oophorectomy in Ovarian Cancer Prone Families," *The Lancet,* vol. 2 (1982), p. 795; Elvio Silva and Rosemary Jenkins, "Serious Carcinoma in Endometrial Polyps," *Modern Pathology,* vol. 3, no. 2 (1990), pp. 120–22.

51. Denise Grady, "Gain Reported in Combating Ovary Cancer," *New York Times,* January 5, 2006, pp. 1–3.

52. A. A. Wright et al., "Use and Effeciveness of Intraperitoneal Chemotherapy for Treatment of Ovarian Cancer," *Journal of Clinical Oncology,* vol. 33, no. 26 (September 10, 2015), pp. 2841–47.

53. B. O'Regan and C. Hirshberg, *Spontaneous Remission: An Annotated Bibliography* (Petaluma, CA: Institute of Noetic Sciences, 1993).

Chapter 8: Reclaiming the Erotic

1. G. Ogden, *The Return of Desire: A Guide to Rediscovering Your Sexual Passion* (Boston: Trumpeter Books, 2008).

2. D. Amen, *Sex on the Brain* (New York: Harmony Books, 2007), p. 21.

3. D. Weeks and J. James, *Secrets of the Superyoung* (New York: Villard, 1998).

4. H. E. O'Connell, K. V. Sanjeevan, and J. M. Hutson, "Anatomy of the Clitoris." *Journal of Urology,* vol. 174, no. 4 (October 2005), pp. 1189–95; H. E. O'Connell and J. O. L. DeLancey, "Clitoral Anatomy in Nulliparous, Healthy, Premenopausal Volunteers Using Unenhanced Magnetic Resonance Imaging," *Journal of Urology,* vol. 173, no. 6 (June 2005), pp. 2060–3.

5. O'Connell, Sanjeevan, and Hutson, "Anatomy of the Clitoris."

6. P. Foldes and O. Buisson, "The Clitoral Complex: A Dynamic Sonographic Study," *Journal of Sexual Medicine,* vol. 6, no. 5 (May 2009), pp. 1223–31.

7. J. L. Sevely, *Eye's Secrets: A New Theory of Female Sexuality* (New York: Random House, 1987), pp. 89–90.

8. C. Muir and C. Muir, *Tantra: The Art of Conscious Loving* (San Francisco: Mercury House, 1989). The Muirs teach that finding the sacred spot is often difficult for a woman to accomplish alone. Even if she does locate it, it may be very difficult for her to stimulate it herself, which is the only way to access its healing power and its sexual and spiritual potential. Nevertheless, you can try to locate it in the following way: Squat with two fingers inside the vagina, press your fingers upward toward the navel while pressing down on the pubic bone with the other hand. If you can manage to stimulate or massage the area, the spot will swell. You may then be able to feel it between your fingers. For most women, this part of their awakening process requires the loving touch of a partner who respects the vulnerable nature of this spot.

Following the first edition of this book, I received a letter from Robert Svoboda, the first Westerner to graduate from a college of Ayurvedic medicine in India. As a student of the tantric tradition, with a deep understanding of its complexities and subtleties, he pointed out that to equate tantric yoga only with "enjoyable sex," as the Muirs do in their book, is to misunderstand and misrepresent this field. Though I find the Muirs' work helpful, I do not want to mislead my readers into thinking that it represents true tantric yoga. For further reading on tantric yoga, see D. R. Brooks, *The Secret of the Three Cities: An Introduction to Hindu Sakta Tantrism* (Chicago: University of Chicago Press, 1990).

9. Muir and Muir, *Tantra*, p. 74.

10. G. Ogden, *Women Who Love Sex* (New York: Pocket Books, 1994).

11. P. B. Doress-Worters and D. L. Siegal, *Ourselves, Growing Older* (New York: Simon & Schuster, 1987).

12. H. B. Van de Weil et al., "Sexual Functioning Following Treatment of Cervical Cancer," *European Journal of Gynecologic Oncology* (1988), pp. 275–81.

13. A. D'Amour, "Your Soul Was Damaged and Your Body Remembers: I Thought I Knew My #MeToo Story," *On Our Moon*, November 15, 2017, http://onourmoon .com/soul-damaged-body-remembers.

14. A. Glatt, S. Zinner, and W. McCormack, "The Prevalence of Dyspareunia," *Obstetrics and Gynecology*, vol. 75, no. 3 (March 1990), pp. 433–36.

15. "A View from Above: The Dangerous World of Wannabes," *Time*, November 25, 1991, p. 77.

16. Ibid.

17. J. Shifren et al., "Sexual Problems and Distress in United States Women: Prevalence and Correlates," *Obstetrics and Gynecology*, vol. 112, no. 5 (November 2008), pp. 970–78.

18. L. Jaspers et al., "Efficacy and Safety of Flibanserin for the Treatment of Hypoactive Sexual Desire Disorder in Women: A Systematic Review and Meta-analysis," *Journal of the American Medical Association Internal Medicine*, vol. 176, no. 4 (2016), pp. 453–62.

19. P. Orenstein, "What Young Women Believe About Their Own Sexual Pleasure," TEDWomen 2016, https://www.ted.com/talks/peggy_orenstein_what_young_women _believe_about_their_own_sexual_pleasure.

20. D. Herbenick et al., "Pain Experienced During Vaginal and Anal Intercourse with Other-Sex Partners: Findings from a Nationally Representative Probability Study in the United States," *Journal of Sexual Medicine*, vol. 12, no. 4 (April 2015), pp. 1040–51.

21. Centers for Disease Control and Prevention, "U.S. Teenage Birth Rate Resumes Decline," *NCHS Data Brief*, vol. 58 (February 2011), pp. 1–8.

22. D. K. Eaton et al., Centers for Disease Control and Prevention (CDC), "Youth Risk Behavior Surveillance—United States, 2011," *MMWR Surveillance Summary*, vol. 61, no. 4 SS-4 (2012), pp. 1–162.

23. S. Harlap, K. Kost, and J. D. Forrest, *Preventing Pregnancy, Protecting Health: A New Look at Birth Control Choices in the United States* (New York: AGI, 1991).

24. A. Nicholas et al., "A Woman's History of Vaginal Orgasm Is Discernible from Her Walk," *Journal of Sexual Medicine*, vol. 5, no. 9 (September 2008), pp. 2119–24.

25. S. Pilz et al., "Effect of Vitamin D Supplementation on Testosterone Levels in Men," *Hormone and Metabolic Research*, vol. 43, no. 3 (March 2011), pp. 223–25.

26. K. Nimptsch et al., "Association Between Plasma 25-OH Vitamin D and Testosterone Levels in Men," *Clinical Endocrinology,* vol. 77, no. 1 (2012), pp. 106–12.

27. E. M. Chang et al., "Association Between Sex Steroids, Ovarian Reserve, and Vitamin D Levels in Healthy Nonobese Women," *Journal of Clinical Endocrinology and Metabolism,* vol. 99, no. 7 (July 2014), pp. 2526–32.

28. M. Chia and M. Chia, *Cultivating Female Sexual Energy: Healing Love Through the Tao* (Huntington, NY: Healing Tao Books, 1986); available from Healing Tao Books, at www.healingtao.com/b06.html.

29. Women's sense of smell is more acute than men's. A smell can evoke an entire stream of memories, either positive or negative. Smell is the longest-remembered sense. A particular smell evokes associated memories more than the senses of vision, hearing, and touch. The olfactory center is located in the brain in an area that is intimately connected with memory function.

30. Part of normal dolphin life is being sexual with each other. A male dolphin often wraps his penis around a female's lower body playfully—not to procreate but simply to communicate. Male dolphins sometimes do this when they are communicating with humans, too. This happened to my sister once—she described her dolphin encounter as an ecstatic experience.

31. R. Eisler, *Sacred Pleasure: Sex, Myth, and the Politics of the Body* (HarperSanFrancisco, 1995), p. 15.

32. National Geographic Channel, "Totally Wild," May 25, 2005.

33. W. Cutler and E. Genovese-Stone, "Wellness in Women After 40 Years of Age: The Role of Sex Hormones and Pheromones," *Disease-A-Month,* vol. 44, no. 9 (September 1998), p. 526.

34. A. Damasio, "Brain Trust," *Nature,* vol. 435 (June 2, 2005), pp. 571–72.

35. M. E. Melisko et al., "Vaginal Testosterone Cream vs. Estradiol Vaginal Ring for Vaginal Dryness or Decreased Libido in Women Receiving Aromatase Inhibitors for Early-Stage Breast Cancer: A Randomized Clinical Trial," *JAMA Oncology,* vol. 3, no. 3 (November 10, 2016), pp. 313–19.

36. B. Berkeley, *Foreskin: A Closer Look* (Boston: Alyson Publications, 1993), p. 188.

37. J. L. Sevely, *Eve's Secrets: A New Theory of Female Sexuality* (New York: Random House, 1987), p. 17; W. H. Masters and V. E. Johnson, *Human Sexual Response* (Boston: Little, Brown, 1966), p. 46.

38. K. O'Hara and J. O'Hara, "The Effect of Male Circumcision on the Sexual Enjoyment of the Female Partner," *British Journal of Urology,* vol. 83, supplement 1 (January 1999), pp. 79–84.

39. M. L. Sorrells et al., "Fine-Touch Pressure Thresholds in the Adult Penis," *BJU International,* vol. 99, no. 4 (April, 2007), pp. 864–69; K. McGrath, "The Frenular Delta: A New Preputial Structure," in *Understanding Circumcision: A Multi-Disciplinary Approach to a Multi-Dimensional Problem,* Proceedings of the Sixth International Symposium on Genital Integrity: Safeguarding Fundamental Human Rights in the 21st Century, December 7–9, 2000, Sydney, Australia.

40. Barbara Walker points out that the Hebrew Gospels designated Mary by the word *mah,* mistakenly translated as "virgin" but really meaning "young woman." See also E. Harding, *Women's Mysteries, Ancient and Modern* (New York: Rider and Co., 1955).

Chapter 9: Vulva, Vagina, Cervix, and Lower Urinary Tract

1. See the book by the Body Shop Team, *Mamamoto: A Celebration* (New York: Viking, 1992), p. 78.

2. T. R. Nansel et al., "The Association of Psychosocial Stress and Bacterial Vaginosis in a Longitudinal Cohort," *American Journal of Obstetrics and Gynecology,* vol. 194, no. 2 (February 2006), pp. 381–86.

3. R. J. Hafner, S. L. Stanton, and J. Guy, "A Psychiatric Study of Women with Urgency and Urge Incontinence," *British Journal of Urology,* vol. 49 (1977), pp. 211–14; L. R. Staub, H. S. Ripley, and S. Wolf, "Disturbance of Bladder Function Associated with Emotional States," *Journal of the American Medical Association,* vol. 141 (1949), p. 1139.

4. A. J. Macaulay et al., "Psychological Aspects of 211 Female Patients Attending a Urodynamic Unit," *Journal of Psychosomatic Research,* vol. 31, no. 1 (1991), pp. 1–10; D. L. P. Rees and N. Farhoumand, "Psychiatric Aspects of Recurrent Cystitis in Women," *British Journal of Urology,* vol. 49 (1977), pp. 651–58.

5. M. Tarlau and M. A. Smalheiser, "Personality Patterns in Patients with Malignant Tumors of the Breast and Cervix," *Psychosomatic Medicine,* vol. 13 (1951), p. 117. Women with cervical cancer characteristically experienced an early rejection; the patients grew up in homes lacking a male figure due to the death or desertion of the father.

6. J. H. Stephenson and W. Grace, "Life Stress and Cancer of the Cervix," *Psychosomatic Medicine,* vol. 14, no. 4 (1954), pp. 287–94.

7. A. Schmale and H. Iker, "Psychological Setting of Uterine Cervical Cancer," *Annals of the New York Academy of Sciences,* vol. 125 (1966), pp. 807–13.

8. M. H. Antoni and K. Goodkin, "Host Moderator Variables in the Promotion of Cervical Neoplasia: I. Personality Facets," *Journal of Psychosomatic Research,* vol. 32, no. 3 (1988), pp. 327–28.

9. K. Goodkin et al., "Stress and Hopelessness in the Promotion of Cervical Intraneoplasia to Invasive Squamous Cell Carcinoma of the Cervix," *Journal of Psychosomatic Research,* vol. 30, no. 1 (1986), pp. 67–76.

10. A. L. Coker et al., "Psychosocial Stress and Cervical Neoplasia Risk," *Psychosomatic Medicine,* vol. 65, no. 4 (July–August 2003), pp. 644–51.

11. U. S. Preventive Services Task Force, "Screening for Cervical Cancer: U.S. Preventive Services Task Force Recommendation Statement," *Journal of the American Medical Association,* vol. 320, no. 7 (August 21, 2018), pp. 674–86.

12. A. J. Blatt et al., "Comparison of Cervical Cancer Screening Results Among 256,648 Women in Multiple Clinical Practices," *Cancer Cytopathology,* vol. 123, no. 5 (May 2015), pp. 282–88.

13. G. S. Ogilvie et al., "Effect of Screening with Primary Cervical HPV Testing vs Cytology Testing on High-Grade Cervical Intraepithelial Neoplasia at 48 Months: The HPV FOCAL Randomized Trial," *Journal of the American Medical Association,* vol. 320, no. 1 (July 3, 2018), pp. 43–52.

14. J. Buscema, "The Predominance of Human Papilloma Virus—Type 16 in Vulvar Neoplasia," *Obstetrics and Gynecology,* vol. 71, no. 4 (1988), pp. 601–5.

15. R. Kiecolt-Glaser et al., "Stress, Loneliness, and Changes in Herpes Virus Latency," *Journal of Behavioral Medicine,* vol. 8, no. 3 (1985), pp. 249–60.

16. Two studies note that many patients have effectively used hypnosis to relieve warts. See R. H. Rulison, "Warts: A Statistical Study of 921 Cases," *Archives of Dermatology and Syphilology,* vol. 46 (1942), pp. 66–81; and M. Ullman, "On the Psyche and Warts. II: Hypnotic Suggestion and Warts," *Psychosomatic Medicine,* vol. 22 (1960), pp. 68–76.

17. To diagnose warts that aren't visible, or so-called flat warts, the penis must be bathed in vinegar and then viewed through some sort of magnifying lens. Only then will the flat white warts be obvious to those who know what to look for. Treatment issues for men are exactly the same as for women.

18. For more information about podofilox, visit www.watson.com.

19. L. Sadler et al., "Treatment for Cervical Intraepithelial Neoplasia and Risk of Preterm Delivery," *Journal of the American Medical Association,* vol. 291, no. 17 (May 5, 2004), pp. 2100–6.

20. S. Swanick, K. Windstar-Hamlin, and H. Zwickey, "An Alternative Treatment for Cervical Intraepithelial Neoplasia II, III," *Integrative Cancer Therapies,* vol. 8, no. 2 (June 2009), pp. 164–67; K. Windstar, C. Dunlap, and H. Zwickey, "Escharotic Treatment for ECC-Positive CIN3 in Childbearing Years: A Case Report," *Integrative Medicine (Encinitas),* vol. 13, no. 2 (April 2014), pp. 43–49.

21. N. Whitehead et al., "Megaloblastic Changes in Cervical Epithelium: Association of Oral Contraceptive Therapy and Reversal with Folic Acid," *Journal of the American Medical Association,* vol. 226 (1993), pp. 1421–24; J. N. Orr, "Localized Deficiency of Folic Acid in Cervical Epithelial Cells May Promote Cervical Dysplasia and Eventually Carcinoma of the Cervix," *American Journal of Obstetrics and Gynecology,* vol. 151 (1985), pp. 632–35; J. Lindenbaum et al., "Oral Contraceptive Hormones, Eolate Metabolism, and Cervical Epithelium," *American Journal of Clinical Nutrition,* April 1975, pp. 346–53; S. L. Romney et al., "Plasma Vitamin C and Uterine Cervical Dysplasia," *American Journal of Obstetrics and Gynecology,* vol. 151, no. 7 (1985), pp. 976–80; S. L. Romney et al., "Retinoids in the Prevention of Cervical Dysplasia," *American Journal of Obstetrics and Gynecology,* vol. 141, no. 8 (1981), pp. 890–94; S. Wassertheil-Smaller et al., "Dietary Vitamin C and Uterine Cervical Dysplasia," *American Journal of Epidemiology,* vol. 114, no. 5 (1981), pp. 714–24; C. LaVecchia et al., "Dietary Vitamin A and the Risk of Invasive Cervical Cancer," *International Journal of Cancer,* vol. 34 (1985), pp. 319–22; P. Ramsnamy and R. Natarajan, "Vitamin B6 Status in Patients with Cancer of the Uterine Cervix," *Nutrition and Cancer,* vol. 6 (1984), pp. 176–80; E. Dawson et al., "Serum Vitamin and Selenium Changes in Cervical Dysplasia," *Federal Proceedings,* vol. 43 (1984), p. 612.

22. D. Wang et al., "Phenethyl Isothiocyanate Upregulates Death Receptors 4 and 5 and Inhibits Proliferation in Human Cancer Stem-Like Cells," *BMC Cancer,* vol. 14, no. 1 (August 15, 2014), p. 591.

23. L. Hay, *I Love My Body* (Farmingdale, NY: Coleman Publishing, 1985), p. 49.

24. National Vaccine Information Center, "New Gardasil vs. Menactra Risk Report (February 2009): An Analysis by the National Vaccine Information Center of Gardasil & Menactra Adverse Event Reports to the Vaccine Adverse Events Reporting System (VAERS)," February 2009, https://www.nvic.org/vaccines-and -diseases/HPV/gardasilvsmenactra.aspx.

25. R. Rabin, "A New Vaccine for Girls, but Should It Be Compulsory?" *New York Times,* July 18, 2006, p. F5, https://www.nytimes.com/2006/07/18/health/18essa.html.

26. A. Gandey, "Report of Motor Neuron Disease After HPV Vaccine," *Medscape,* October 28, 2009, www.medscape.com/viewarticle/711461.

27. Ibid.

28. I. Sutton et al., "CNS Demyelination and Quadrivalent HPV Vaccination," *Multiple Sclerosis,* vol. 15, no. 1 (January 2009), pp. 116–19.

29. B. A. Slade et al., "Postlicensure Safety Surveillance for Quadrivalent Human Papillomavirus Recombinant Vaccine," *Journal of the American Medical Association,* vol. 302, no. 7 (August 19, 2009), pp. 750–57.

30. A. M. Noone et al. (eds.), *SEER Cancer Statistics Review, 1975–2015,* National Cancer Institute. Bethesda, MD, https://seer.cancer.gov/csr/1975_2015, based on November 2017 SEER data submission, posted to the SEER website, April 2018, https://seer.cancer.gov/statfacts/html/cervix.html.

31. "Death After Cervarix Propels HPV Vaccination into Headlines Again," *Medscape,* last updated October 1, 2009, www.medscape.com/viewarticle/709718.

32. Noone et al. (eds.), *SEER Cancer Statistics Review, 1975–2015.*

33. L. Gavin et al., "Sexual and Reproductive Health of Persons Aged 10–24 Years—United States, 2002–2007," *Morbidity and Mortality Weekly Report,* vol. 58, no. SS-6 (July 17, 2009), pp. 1–58.

34. U.S. Food and Drug Administration, Vaccines and Related Biological Products Advisory Committee (VRBPAC) Background Document: Gardasil HPV Quadrivalent Vaccine. May 18, 2006, VRBPAC Meeting, accessed at re-check.ch/wordpress/wp-content/uploads/2017/03/2006-VRBPAC_Background_Document-422283.pdf.

35. T. C. Wright et al., "The ATHENA Human Papillomavirus Study: Design, Methods, and Baseline Results," *American Journal of Obstetrics and Gynecology,* vol. 206, no. 1 (January 2012), pp. 46e1–46e11.

36. F. Guo, J. M. Hirth, and A. B. Berenson, "Comparison of HPV Prevalence Between HPV-Vaccinated and Non-Vaccinated Young Adult Women (20–26 Years)," *Human Vaccinations and Immunotherapeutics,* vol. 11, no. 10 (2015), pp. 2337–44.

37. W. K. Huh et al., "Final Efficacy, Immunogenicity, and Safety analysis of a Nine-Valent Human Papillomavirus Vaccine in Women Aged 16–26 years: A Randomized, Double-Blind Trial," *The Lancet,* vol. 390, no. 10108 (November 11, 2017), pp. 2143–59; "Six-Year Efficacy Data for Gardasil 9 Presented at EUROGIN 2017 Congress," press release from Merck, October 10, 2017, https://investors.merck.com/news/press-release-details/2017/Six-year-Efficacy-Data-for-GARDASIL-9-Presented-at-EUROGIN-2017-Congress/default.aspx.

38. C. Young, in a letter written to *Obstetrics and Gynecology,* published online April 5, 2008, by VaccineInfo.net, http://www.vaccineinfo.net/immunization/vaccine/hpv/doc_against_HPV.shtml.

39. D. Harper, S. L. Vierthaler, and J. A. Santee, "Review of Gardasil," *Journal of Vaccines and Vaccination,* vol. 1, no. 107 (November 23, 2010), pp. 1000107.

40. See https://youtube/sSdCxgF0blc.

41. E. Rosenthal, "Drug Makers' Push Leads to Vaccines' Fast Rise," *New York*

Times, August 19, 2008, p. A1, https://www.nytimes.com/2008/08/20/health/policy/20vaccine.html.

42. M. Holland, K. Mack Rosenberg, and E. Iorio, *The HPV Vaccine on Trial: Seeking Justice for a Generation Betrayed* (New York: Skyhorse Publishing, 2018), p. xvii.

43. M. A. Steller and T. E. Nolan, "Universal Human Papillomavirus Vaccination: Pro and Con," *The Female Patient,* vol. 32, no. 5 (May 2007), pp. 47–48.

44. American Cancer Society, "Help Prevent Six Cancers with the HPV Vaccine," www.cancer.org/cancer/cancer-causes/infectious-agents/hpv/hpv-vaccines.html.

45. M. Martinez-Lavin and L. Amezcua-Guerra, "Serious Adverse Events After HPV Vaccination: A Critical Review of Randomized Trials and Post-Marketing Case Series," *Clinical Rheumatology,* vol. 36, no. 10 (October 2017), pp. 2169–78.

46. R. Inbar et al., "Behavioral Abnormalities in Female Mice Following Administration of Aluminum Adjuvants and the Human Papillomavirus (HPV) Vaccine Gardasil," *Immunologic Research,* vol. 65, no. 1 (February 2017), pp. 136–49.

47. L. Tomljenovic, J. P. Spinosa, and C. A. Shaw, "Human Papillomavirus (HPV) Vaccines as an Option for Preventing Cervical Malignancies: (How) Effective and Safe?" *Current Pharmaceutical Design,* vol. 19, no. 8 (2013), pp. 1466–87.

48. F. Joelving, "What the Gardasil Testing May Have Missed," *Slate,* December 17, 2017, https://slate.com/health-and-science/2017/12/flaws-in-the-clinical-trials-for-gardasil-made-it-harder-to-properly-assess-safety.html.

49. U.S. House of Representatives Committee on Government Reform, "Conflicts of Interest in Vaccine Policy Making, Majority Staff Report," June 15, 2000; vaccinesafetycommission.org/pdfs/Conflicts-Govt-Reform.pdf.

50. S. H. Lee, "Allegations of Scientific Misconduct by GACVS/WHO/CDC Representatives et al.," January 14, 2016, https://sanevax.org/wp-content/uploads/2016/01/Allegations-of-Scientific-Misconduct-by-GACVS.pdf.

51. Email from R. Pless to H. Petousis-Harris, February 18, 2014, https://sanevax.org/wp-content/uploads/2016/01/WHO-GACVS-emails.pdf.

52. Y. Hu, L. Tornes, and R. Lopez-Alberola, "Two Cases of Pediatric Multiple Sclerosis After Human Papillomavirus Vaccination (P4.353)," *Neurology,* vol. 90 (15 Supplement) (April 25, 2018).

53. N. M. Scheller et al., "Quadrivalent HPV Vaccination and Risk of Multiple Sclerosis and Other Demyelinating Diseases of the Central Nervous System," *Journal of the American Medical Association,* vol. 311, no. 1 (2015), pp. 54–61.

54. K. Hikel, "'One Less' Sucker," Green Mountain Doc, Medscape blog, February 16, 2009, http://boards.medscape.com/forums?128@1005.r24habZseYP@.29efea0e!comment=1.

55. B. Zablotsky, L. I. Black, and S. J. Blumberg, "Estimated Prevalence of Children with Diagnosed Developmental Disabilities in the United States, 2014–2016," *NCHS Data Brief,* no. 291 (Hyattsville, MD: National Center for Health Statistics, 2017).

56. R. L. Winer et al., "Condom Use and the Risk of Genital Human Papillomavirus Infection in Young Women," *New England Journal of Medicine,* vol. 354, no. 25 (June 22, 2006), pp. 2645–54.

57. M. Teymouri et al., "Curcumin as a Multifaceted Compound Against Human

Papilloma Virus Infection and Cervical Cancers: A Review of Chemistry, Cellular, Molecular, and Preclinical Features," *Biofactors,* vol. 43, no. 3 (May 6, 2017), pp. 331–46; P. Basu et al., "Clearance of Cervical Human Papillomavirus Infection by Topical Application of Curcumin and Curcumin Containing Polyherbal Cream, A Phase II Randomized Controlled Study," *Asian Pacific Journal of Cancer Prevention,* vol. 14, no. 10 (2013), pp. S753–59.

58. P. Chayavichitsilp et al., "Herpes Simplex," *Pediatrics in Review,* vol. 30, no. 4 (April 2009), pp. 119–30.

59. G. McQuillan et al., "Prevalence of Herpes Simplex Virus Type 1 and Type 2 in Persons Aged 14–49: United States, 2015–2016," NCHS Data Brief no. 304 (Hyattsville, MD: National Center for Health Statistics. 2018).

60. G. J. Mertz, S. L. Rosenthal, and L. R. Stanberry, "Is Herpes Simplex Virus Type 1 (HSV-1) Now More Common than HSV-2 in First Episodes of Genital Herpes?" *Sexually Transmitted Diseases,* vol. 30, no. 10 (October 2003), pp. 801–2; A. Wald et al., "Oral Shedding of Herpes Simplex Virus Type 2," *Sexually Transmitted Infections,* vol. 80, no. 4 (August 2004), pp. 272–76 [published erratum appears in *Sexually Transmitted Infections,* vol. 80, no. 6 (December 2004), p. 546]; R. Engelberg et al., "Natural History of Genital Herpes Simplex Virus Type 1 Infection," *Sexually Transmitted Diseases,* vol. 30, no. 2 (February 2003), pp. 174–77.

61. A. Wald et al., "Frequent Genital Herpes Simplex Virus 2 Shedding in Immunocompetent Women: Effect of Acyclovir Treatment," *Journal of Clinical Investigation,* vol. 99, no. 5 (March 1997), pp. 1092–97.

62. Ibid.

63. L. Koutsky et al., "Underdiagnosis of Genital Herpes by Current Clinical and Viral-Isolation Procedures," *New England Journal of Medicine,* vol. 326, no. 23 (1992), pp. 1533–39.

64. H. C. Taylor, "Vascular Congestion and Hyperemia," *American Journal of Obstetrics and Gynecology,* vol. 57, no. 22 (1949), p. 22; M. E. Kemeny et al., "Psychological and Immunological Predictors of Genital Herpes Recurrence," *Psychosomatic Medicine,* vol. 52 (1989), pp. 195–208.

65. U.S. Preventive Services Task Force, "Serologic Screening for Genital Herpes Infection: U.S. Preventive Services Task Force Recommendation Statement," *Journal of the American Medical Association,* vol. 316, no. 23 (December 20, 2016), pp. 2525–30.

66. A. Wald et al., "Reactivation of Genital Herpes Simplex Virus Type 2 Infection in Asymptomatic Seropositive Persons," *New England Journal of Medicine,* vol. 342, no. 12 (March 23, 2000), pp. 844–50.

67. Z. A. Brown et al., "Genital Herpes Complicating Pregnancy," *Obstetrics and Gynecology,* vol. 106, no. 4 (October 2005), pp. 845–56.

68. "Current Management of Herpes Simplex Infection in Pregnant Women and Their Newborn Infants: What's Hot and What's Not," *Canadian Journal of Infectious Diseases = Journal Canadien des Maladies Infectieuses,* vol. 14, no. 4 (2003), pp. 197–200.

69. K. M. Stone et al., "Pregnancy Outcomes Following Systemic Prenatal Acyclovir Exposure: Conclusions from the International Acyclovir Pregnancy Registry,

1984–1999," *Birth Defects Research Part A, Clinical and Molecular Teratology,* vol. 70, no. 4 (April 2004), pp. 201–7.

70. Z. A. Brown et al., "Effect of Serologic Status and Cesarean Delivery on Transmission Rates of Herpes Simplex Virus from Mother to Infant," *Journal of the American Medical Association,* vol. 289, no. 2 (January 8, 2003), pp. 203–9.

71. J. J. van Everdingen, M. F. Peeters, and P. ten Have, "Neonatal Herpes Policy in the Netherlands: Five Years After a Consensus Conference," *Journal of Clinical Investigation,* vol. 21, no. 5 (1993), pp. 371–75.

72. M. A. Adefumbo and B. H. Lau, "Allium Sativum (Garlic): A Natural Antibiotic," *Medical Hypothesis,* vol. 12, no. 3 (1983), pp. 327–37.

73. There are a number of brands of garlic on the market: Kyolic (by the Wakunga Company) and Garlicin (by Murdock) are two that Women to Women often recommends.

74. R. H. Wolbling and K. Leonhardt, "Local Therapy of Herpes Simplex with Dried Extract from *Melissa Officinalis,*" *Phytomedicine,* vol. 1 (1994), pp. 25–31; R. A. Cohen et al., "Antiviral Activity of *Melissa Officinalis* (Lemon Balm Extract)," *Proceedings of the Society for Experimental Biology and Medicine,* vol. 117 (1964), pp. 431–34; F. C. Herrmann Jr. and L. S. Kucera, "Antiviral Substances in Plants of the Mint Family *(Labiatae).* II. Nontannin Polyphenol of *Melissa Officinalis,*" *Proceedings of the Society for Experimental Biology and Medicine,* vol. 124, no. 3 (1967), pp. 869–74; Z. Dimitrova et al., "Antiherpes Effect of *Melissa Officinalis* L. Extracts," *Acta Microbiologica Bulgarica* (Sofia), vol. 29 (1993), pp. 65–75.

75. Not all products labeled "tea tree oil" are equally effective. I've used melaleuca oil or Melagel from the Melaleuca Company; see www.melaleuca.com.

76. "Pap Smear Screening for Cervical Cancer," *Maine Cancer Perspectives,* vol. 2, no. 2 (April 1996).

77. A. H. Mokdad et al., "Actual Causes of Death in the United States, 2000," *Journal of the American Medical Association,* vol. 291, no. 10 (March 10, 2004), pp. 1238, 1241.

78. C. L. Murall, C. T. Bauch, and T. Day, "Could the Human Papillomavirus Vaccines Drive Virulence Evolution?" *Proceedngs of the Royal Society B in Biological Sciences,* vol. 282, no. 1798 (January 7, 2015); P. A. Orlando et al., "Evolutionary Ecology of Human Papillomavirus: Trade-offs, Coexistence, and Origins of High-Risk and Low-Risk Types," *Journal of Infectious Diseases,* vol. 205, no. 2 (January 15, 2012), pp. 272–79.

79. L. E. Markowitz et al., "Prevalence of HPV After Introduction of the Vaccination Program in the United States," *Pediatrics,* vol. 137, no. 3 (March 2016), http://pediatrics.aappublications.org/content/pediatrics/137/3/e20151968.full.pdf.

80. J. D. Oriel, "Sex and Cervical Cancer," *Genitourinary Medicine,* vol. 64 (1988), pp. 81–89; C. LaVecchia et al., "Oral Contraceptives and Control Study," *British Journal of Cancer,* vol. 54 (1986), p. 311; J. J. Schlesselman, "Cancer of the Breast and Reproductive Tract in Relation to Use of CC's," *Contraception,* vol. 40 (1989), p. 1.

81. N. Potischman and L. Brinton, "Nutrition and Cervical Neoplasia," *Cancer Causes and Control,* vol. 7 (1996), pp. 113–26.

82. Pap tests are taken even after the cervix has been removed in a hysterectomy. This is especially important for women who have had a prior history of an abnormal Pap test.

83. Therapeutic touch, a system of healing with the hands, has been very well studied, and its beneficial effects have been well documented by Delores Kreiger, Ph.D., a nurse at Columbia University. Marcelle Pick, a cofounder of Women to Women, has studied with Dr. Kreiger.

84. I feel that chlamydia *may* also be a normal inhabitant of the vagina in some women and that it may cause problems only when there's an imbalance. Chlamydia is like the buzzard flying around the dying calf, as far as I'm concerned, though many of my colleagues would disagree.

85. A. Ramirez-Garcia et al., "Candida albicans and Cancer: Can This Yeast Induce Cancer Development or Progression?" *Critical Reviews in Microbiology,* vol. 42, no. 2 (2016), pp. 181–93.

86. C. Wira and C. Kaushic, "Mucosal Immunity in the Female Reproductive Tract: Effect of Sex Hormones on Immune Recognition and Responses," in H. Kiyono, P. L. Ogra, and J. R. McGhee, eds., *Mucosal Vaccines* (New York: Academic Press, 1996), pp. 375–88.

87. Gardiner-Caldwell SynerMed, "The Role of Reduced Regimens in the Management of Vulvovaginitis," *Medical Monitor,* vol. 1, no. 1 (April 1991).

88. M. R. Miles, L. Olsen, and A. Rogers, "Recurrent Vaginal Candidiasis: Importance of an Intestinal Reservoir," *Journal of the American Medical Association,* vol. 238, no. 17 (October 24, 1977), pp. 1836–37.

89. Genova Diagnostics in Asheville, NC, 800-522-4762 or 828-253-0621, www.gdx .net.

90. Miles, Olsen, and Rogers, "Recurrent Vaginal Candidiasis."

91. K. T. Gunsalus et al., "Manipulation of Host Diet to Reduce Gastrointestical Colonization by the Opportunistic Pathogen Candida albicans," *mSphere,* vol. 1, no. 1 (November 18, 2015), pp. e00020–15.

92. D. Steward et al., "Psychosocial Aspects of Chronic, Clinically Unconfirmed Vulvovaginitis," *Obstetrics and Gynecology,* vol. 76, no. 5, part 1 (November 1990), pp. 852–56.

93. S. Mathur et al., "Anti-Ovarian and Anti-Lymphocyte Antibodies in Patients with Chronic Vaginal Candidiasis," *Journal of Reproductive Immunology,* vol. 2 (1980), pp. 247–62.

94. Centers for Disease Control and Prevention, "Diagnoses of HIV Infection Among Adults Aged 50 Years and Older in the United States and Dependent Areas 2011–2016," *HIV Surveillance Supplemental Report 2018,* vol. 23, no. 5 (August 2018), www.cdc.gov/hiv/library/reports/hiv-surveillance.html.

95. Centers for Disease Control and Prevention, *Sexually Transmitted Disease Surveillance 2017* (Atlanta: U.S. Department of Health and Human Services, 2018).

96. C. Fordham von Reyn, M.D., "HIV and Acquired Immunodeficiency Syndrome," lecture, September 21, 1996, Dartmouth Medical School, Lebanon, NH.

97. There are also known cases of persons infected with HIV for over ten years who have no evidence of either declining levels of CD4+ T lymphocytes or AIDS. A. R. Lifson et al., "Long-Term Human Immunodeficiency Virus Infection in Asymp-

tomatic Homosexual and Bisexual Men with Normal CD4+ Lymphocyte Counts: Immunologic and Virologic Characteristics," *Journal of Infectious Disease*, vol. 163 (1991), pp. 959–65.

98. F. Pittman, "Frankly Speaking," *Psychology Today*, September–October 1996, p. 60.

99. Centers for Disease Control and Prevention, "HIV Prevalence Estimates—United States, 2006," *Morbidity and Mortality Weekly Report*, vol. 57, no. 39 (2008), pp. 1073–6.

100. Centers for Disease Control, "Diagnoses of HIV Infection in the United States and Dependent Areas, 2016," *HIV Surveillance Report 2017*, vol. 28 (November 2017); Centers for Disease Control, "Estimated HIV Incidence and Prevalence in the United States, 2010–2015," *HIV Surveillance Supplemental Report 2018*, vol. 23, no. 1 (March 2018).

101. F. J. Palella Jr. et al., "Declining Morbidity and Mortality Among Patients with Advanced Human Immunodeficiency Virus Infection. HIV Outpatient Study Investigators," *New England Journal of Medicine*, vol. 338, no. 13 (March 26, 1998), pp. 853–60.

102. C. Myss, *AIDS, Passageway to Transformation* (Walpole, MA: Stillpoint Publications, 1985).

103. S. M. Hammer, "Clinical Practice, Management of Newly Diagnosed HIV Infection," *New England Journal of Medicine*, vol. 353, no. 16 (October 20, 2005), pp. 1702–10.

104. C. B. Furlonge et al., "Vulvar Vestibulitis Syndrome: A Clinicopathological Study," *British Journal of Obstetrics and Gynaecology*, vol. 98 (1991), pp. 703–6.

105. E. Friedrick, "Vulvar Vestibulitis Syndrome," *Journal of Reproductive Medicine*, vol. 32, no. 2 (February 1987), pp. 110–14.

106. T. Warner et al., "Neuroendocrine Cell-Axonal Complexes in the Minor Vestibular Gland," *Journal of Reproductive Medicine*, vol. 41 (1996), pp. 397–402.

107. C. C. Solomons, M. H. Melmed, and S. M. Heitler, "Calcium Citrate for Vestibulitis," *Journal of Reproductive Medicine*, vol. 36, no. 12 (1991), pp. 879–82.

108. Dr. McNamara's study uses the USANA brands Essential and Proflavanol.

109. D. E. Stewart et al., "Psychological Aspects of Chronic Clinically Unconfirmed Vulvovaginitis," *Obstetrics and Gynecology*, vol. 76 (1990), pp. 852–56; D. E. Stewart et al., "Vulvodynia and Psychological Distress," *Obstetrics and Gynecology*, vol. 84, no. 4 (October 1994), pp. 587–90.

110. E. A. Walker et al., "Medical and Psychiatric Symptoms in Women with Childhood Sexual Abuse," *Psychosomatic Medicine*, vol. 54 (1992), pp. 658–64.

111. H. Glazer, "Treatment of Vulvar Vestibulitis Syndrome with Electromyographic Biofeedback of Pelvic Floor Musculature," *Journal of Reproductive Medicine*, vol. 4, no. 4 (1995), pp. 283–90.

112. Ibid.

113. International Society of Aesthetic Plastic Surgery, "The International Study on Aesthetic/Cosmetic Procedures Performed in 2016," www.isaps.org/wp-content/uploads/2017/10/GlobalStatistics2016-1.pdf.

114. American Society of Aesthetic Plastic Surgery, "Quick Facts: Highlights of the

2017 Stats," www.surgery.org/sites/default/files/ASAPS-Stats2017-Quick-Facts .pdf.

115. American Society for Aesthetic Plastic Surgery, "2015 Cosmetic Surgery National Data Bank Statistics," www.surgery.org/sites/default/files/ASAPS-Stats2015.pdf.

116. J. Mackenzie, "Vagina Surgery 'Sought by Girls as Young as Nine,'" BBC News, July 3, 2017, www.bbc.com/news/health-40410459.

117. J. L. Bercaw-Pratt et al., "The Incidence, Attitudes and Practices of the Removal of Public Hair as a Body Modification," *Journal of Pediatric and Adolescent Gynecology*, vol. 25, no. 1 (February 2012), pp. 12–14.

118. American College of Obstetricians and Gynecologists, Committee on Adolescent Health Care, Committee Opinion No. 686, January 2017, www.acog.org/Clinical -Guidance-and-Publications/Committee-Opinions/Committee-on-Adolescent-Health -Care/Breast-and-Labial-Surgery-in-Adolescents.

119. American Society for Aesthetic Plastic Surgery, "ISAP International Survey on Aesthetic/Cosmetic Procedures Performed in 2017," www.isaps.org/wp-content/ uploads/2018/10/ISAPS_2017_International_Study_Cosmetic_Procedures.pdf, www .isaps.org/wp-content/uploads/2018/10/ISAP2016_17_comparison.pdf.

120. M. M. Karram, "Frequency, Urgency, and Painful Bladder Syndromes," in M. D. Walters and M. M. Karram, eds., *Clinical Urogynecology* (St. Louis, MO: Mosby, 1993), pp. 285–98.

121. E. M. Messing and T. A. Stamey, "Interstitial Cystitis: Early Diagnosis, Pathology, and Treatment," *Urology*, vol. 12 (1978), p. 381.

122. J. M. H. Teichman, "The Role of Pentosan Polysulfate in Treatment Approaches for Interstitial Cystitis," *Reviews in Urology*, vol. 4 (supplement 1) (2002), pp. S21–27.

123. E. Sobota, "Inhibition of Bacterial Adherence by Cranberry Juice: Potential Use for the Treatment of Urinary Tract Infections," *Journal of Urology*, vol. 131 (1984), pp. 1013–16; P. N. Papas et al., "Cranberry Juice in the Treatment of Urinary Tract Infections," *Southwestern Medicine*, vol. 47A (1966), pp. 17–30; D. R. Schmidt and A. E. Sobota, "An Examination of the Antiadherence Activity of Cranberry Juice on Urinary and Non-Urinary Bacterial Isolates," *Microbios*, vol. 55, nos. 224–225 (1988), pp. 173–81.

124. J. Avorn et al., "Reduction of Bacteria and Pyuria After Ingestion of Cranberry Juice," *Journal of the American Medical Association*, vol. 271 (1994), pp. 751–54.

125. V. Frohne, "Untersuchungen zur Frage der Garbdesfuzierenden Wirkungen von Barentraubenblatt-Extracten," *Planta Medica*, vol. 18 (1970), pp. 1–25.

126. R. Raz et al., "A Controlled Trial of Intravaginal Estriol in Post-Menopausal Women with Recurrent Urinary Tract Infections," *New England Journal of Medicine*, vol. 329 (1993), pp. 753–56.

127. N. Bhatia et al., "Urodynamic Effects of a Vaginal Pessary in Women with Stress Urinary Incontinence," *American Journal of Obstetrics and Gynecology*, vol. 147 (1983), p. 876; and A. Diokno, "The Benefits of Conservative Management for SUI," *Contemporary ObGyn*, March 1997, pp. 128–42.

Chapter 10: Breasts

1. C. Chen, "Adverse Life Events and Breast Cancer: A Case-Controlled Study," *British Medical Journal,* vol. 311 (December 9, 1995), pp. 1527–30.

2. S. Geyer, "Life Events Prior to Manifestation of Breast Cancer: A Limited Prospective Study Covering Eight Years Before Diagnosis," *Journal of Psychosomatic Research,* vol. 35 (1991), pp. 355–63.

3. A. Ramirez et al., "Stress and Relapse of Breast Cancer," *British Medical Journal,* vol. 298 (1989), pp. 291–93.

4. In the nineteenth century, the unusual case history studies of Herbert Snow likened breast and uterine cancer with a history of a "troubled mind and chronic anxiety." Particularly evident in the women he studied was the loss of a significant relationship as the precipitating factor in the manifestation of a tumor. See Herbert Snow, *The Proclivity of Women to Cancerous Disease* (London, 1883).

    In this century, M. Tarlau and M. A. Smalheiser found that the typical pattern for women with breast cancer was that their father had been absent psychologically; for women with cervical cancer, the father had been absent due to death or desertion. See M. Tarlau and M. A. Smalheiser, "Personality Patterns in Patients with Malignant Tumors of the Breast and Cervix," *Psychosomatic Medicine,* vol. 13 (1951), p. 117. They also found that women with breast cancer uniformly had negative feelings about their sexuality, had adapted by denying their sexuality, and often had negative feelings about heterosexual relationships as such. Women with cervical cancer, by contrast, had less negative feelings about their sexuality. The breast cancer patients were much more likely to have remained in an unsatisfactory marriage, while many of the cervical cancer patients were divorced or had been married several times.

    A study by Bacon and colleagues found that many women with breast cancer frequently were unable to discharge or deal appropriately with their anger, aggressiveness, or hostility. Often these women covered up such feelings with a facade of pleasantness. Women with breast cancer frequently responded with "denial and unrealistic sacrifice" to resolve hostile conflict with their mothers. See C. L. Bacon et al., "A Psychosomatic Survey of Cancer of the Breast," *Psychosomatic Medicine,* vol. 14, no. 6 (1952), pp. 453–59.

    See also C. B. Bahnson, "Stress and Cancer: The State of the Art," *Psychosomatics,* vol. 22, no. 3 (1981), pp. 207–20.

5. S. Levy et al., "Perceived Social Support and Tumor Estrogen Progesterone Receptor Status as Predictors of Natural Killer Cell Activity in Breast Cancer Patients," *Psychosomatic Medicine,* vol. 51 (1990), pp. 73–85.

6. A. Bremond, G. Kune, and C. Bahnson, "Psychosomatic Factors in Breast Cancer Patients: Results of a Case Control Study," *Journal of Psychosomatic Obstetrics and Gynecology,* vol. 5 (1986), pp. 127–36.

7. K. W. Pettingale et al., "Serum IgA Levels and Emotional Expression in Breast Cancer Patients," *Journal of Psychosomatic Research,* vol. 21 (1977), p. 395.

8. U.S. Preventive Services Task Force, "Screening for Breast Cancer: U.S. Preventive Services Task Force Recommendation Statement," *Annals of Internal Medicine,* vol. 151, no. 10 (November 17, 2009), pp. 716–26, www.annals.org/content/151/10/716.full.

9. D. B. Thomas et al., "Randomized Trial of Breast Self-Examination in Shanghai:

Final Results," *Journal of the National Cancer Institute,* vol. 94, no. 19 (October 2, 2002), pp. 1445–57.

10. V. F. Semiglazov et al., [Interim Results of a Prospective Randomized Study of Self-Examination for Early Detection of Breast Cancer (Russia/St. Petersburg/WHO)], *Voprosy Onkologii,* vol. 45, no. 3 (1999), pp. 265–71.

11. S. M. Love, R. S. Gelman, and W. J. Sile, "Fibrocystic 'Disease' of the Breast: A Non-Disease," *New England Journal of Medicine,* vol. 307 (1982), p. 1010.

12. P. E. Preece et al., "Importance of Mastalgia in Operable Breast Cancer," *British Medical Journal,* vol. 284 (1982), pp. 1299–1300; and L. E. Hughes and D. J. Webster, "Breast Pain and Modularity," in *Benign Disorders and Disease of the Breast* (London: Bailliere Tindale, 1989).

13. G. Plu-Bureau et al., "Cyclic Mastalgia as a Marker of Breast Cancer Susceptibility: Results of a Case Control Study Among French Women," *British Journal of Cancer,* vol. 65 (1992), pp. 945–49; and J. R. Harris et al., "Breast Cancer," part 1, *New England Journal of Medicine,* vol. 327 (1992), pp. 319–28.

14. P. L. Jenkins et al., "Psychiatric Illness in Patients with Severe Treatment-Resistant Mastalgia," *General Hospital Psychiatry,* vol. 15 (1993), pp. 55–57.

15. American Cancer Society, "How Common Is Breast Cancer?," last revised January 8, 2019, www.cancer.org/cancer/breast-cancer/about/how-common-is-breast -cancer.html.

16. U.S. Preventive Services Task Force, "Screening for Breast Cancer: U.S. Preventive Services Task Force Recommendation Statement," *Annals of Internal Medicine,* vol. 151, no. 10 (November 17, 2009), pp. 716–26, www.annals.org/content/151/ 10/716.full.

17. J. S. Mandelblatt et al., "Effects of Mammography Screening Under Different Screening Schedules: Model Estimates of Potential Benefits and Harms," *Annals of Internal Medicine,* vol. 151, no. 10 (November 17, 2009), pp. 738–47, www .annals.org/content/151/10/738.full.

18. P. C. Gotzsche and O. Olsen, "Is Screening for Breast Cancer with Mammography Justifiable?" *The Lancet,* vol. 355, no. 9198 (January 8, 2000), pp. 129–34; P. C. Gotzsche and O. Olsen, "Cochrane Review on Screening for Breast Cancer with Mammography," *The Lancet,* vol. 358, no. 9290 (October 20, 2001), pp. 1340–42.

19. A. Bleyer and H. G. Welch, "Effect of Three Decades of Screening Mammography on Breast-Cancer Incidence," *New England Journal of Medicine,* vol. 367, no. 21 (November 22, 2012), pp. 1998–2005.

20. P. C. Gotzsche and K. Jorgensen, "Screening for Breast Cancer with Mammography," Cochrane Database of Systematic Reviews 2013, issue 6 (June 4, 2013), article number CD001877.

21. P. Zahl, J. Maehlen, and H. G. Welch, "The Natural History of Invasive Breast Cancers Detected by Screening Mammography," *Archives of Internal Medicine,* vol. 168, no. 21 (November 2008), pp. 2311–6.

22. T. Parker-Pope, "Benefits and Risks of Cancer Screening Are Not Always Clear, Experts Say," *New York Times,* October 22, 2009, p. A26, http://www.nytimes .com/2009/10/22/health/22screen.html#; L. Esserman, Y. Shieh, and I. Thompson, "Rethinking Screening for Breast Cancer and Prostate Cancer," *Journal of the American Medical Association,* vol. 302, no. 15 (October 21, 2009), pp. 1685–

92. G. Kolata, "Cancer Society, in Shift, Has Concerns on Screenings," *New York Times,* October 21, 2009, p. A1, www.nytimes.com/2009/10/21/health/21cancer.html#.

23. Parker-Pope, "Benefits and Risks of Cancer Screening Are Not Always Clear, Experts Say."

24. R M. Martin et al., "Effect of a Low-Intensity PSA-Based Screening Intervention on Prostate Cancer Mortality: The CAP Randomized Clinical Trial," *Journal of the American Medical Association,* vol. 319, no. 9 (March 6, 2018), pp. 883–95.

25. For a map of showing which states have notification laws for women with dense breasts, see www.diagnosticimaging.com/breast-imaging/breast-density-notification-laws-state-interactive-map.

26. J. Brodersen and V. D. Siersma, "Long-Term Psychosocial Consequences of False-Positive Screening Mammography," *Annals of Family Medicine,* vol. 11, no. 2 (March–April 2013), pp. 106–15.

27. A. M. D. Wolf, "Share the Burden of Uncertainty with Patients," *Consultant,* vol. 43, no. 9 (August 2003), pp. 1102–3.

28. R. A. Hubbard et al., "Cumulative Probability of False-Positive Recall or Biopsy Recommendation After 10 Years of Screening Mammography: A Cohort Study," *Annals of Internal Medicine,* vol. 155, no. 8 (October 18, 2011), pp. 481–92.

29. T. Quay, "Opinion: Patients Should Be Informed of Mammograms' Negatives," Athena Institute for Women's Wellness website, www.athenainstitute.com/sciencelinks/informedconsentmammograms.html.

30. A. B. Miller et al., "Canadian National Breast Screening Study 2: 13-Year Results of a Randomized Trial in Women Aged 50–59 Years," *Journal of the National Cancer Institute,* vol. 92, no. 18 (September 20, 2000), pp. 1490–9.

31. W. Cutler et al., "Invasive Breast Cancer Incidence in 2,305,427 Screened Asymptomatic Women: Estimated Long Term Outcomes During Menopause Using a Systematic Review," *PLoS One,* vol. 10, no. 6 (June 24, 2015), p. e0128895.

32. P. Autier et al., "Effectiveness of and Overdiagnosis from Mammography Screening in The Netherlands: Population Based Study," *British Medical Journal,* vol. 359 (December 5, 2017), pp. j5224.

33. K. Kerlikowske et al., "Continuing Screening Mammography in Women Aged 70 to 79 Years: Impact on Life Expectancy and Cost-Effectiveness," *Journal of the American Medical Association,* vol. 282, no. 22 (December 8, 1999), pp. 2156–63.

34. J. P. van Netten et al., "Physical Trauma and Breast Cancer," *The Lancet,* vol. 343, no. 8903 (April 16, 1994), pp. 978–79.

35. C. Lagadec et al., "Radiation-Induced Reprogramming of Breast Cancer Cells," *Stem Cells,* vol. 30, no. 5 (May 2012), pp. 833–44; C. Printz, "Radiation Treatment Generates Therapy-Resistant Cancer Stem Cells from Less Aggressive Breast Cancer Cells," *Cancer,* vol. 118, no. 13 (July 1, 2012), p. 3225.

36. C. Baines, "Rethinking Breast Screening—Again," *British Medical Journal,* vol. 331 (2005), p. 1031.

37. Y. Shieh et al., "Breast Cancer Screening in the Precision Medicine Era: Risk-Based Screening in a Population-Based Trial," *Journal of the National Cancer Institute,* vol. 109, no. 5 (January 27, 2017).

38. A. T. Stavros et al., "Solid Breast Nodules: Use of Sonography to Distinguish Between Benign and Malignant Lesions," *Radiology,* vol. 195 (1995), pp. 123–34; E. Staren, "Breast Ultrasound for Surgeons," *American Surgeon,* vol. 62 (1996), pp. 109–12.

39. R. J. Bleicher et al., "Association of Routine Pretreatment Magnetic Resonance Imaging with Time to Surgery, Mastectomy Rate, and Margin Status," *Journal of the American College of Surgeons,* vol. 209 (2009), pp. 180–87.

40. W. Cong, X. Intes, and G. Wang, "Optical Tomographic Imaging for Breast Cancer Detection," *Journal of Biomedical Optics,* vol. 22, no. 9 (September 2017), pp. 1–6.

41. K. Lee, "Optical Mammography: Diffuse Optical Imaging of Breast Cancer," *World Journal of Clinical Oncology,* vol. 2, no. 1 (January 10, 2011), pp. 64–72.

42. J. D. Bronzino, ed., *Medical Devices and Systems (The Biomedical Engineering Handbook)* (Boca Raton, FL: CRC Press/Taylor & Francis Group, 2006).

43. R. Amalric et al., "Does Infrared Thermography Truly Have a Role in Present-Day Breast Cancer Management?" *Progress in Clinical and Biological Research,* vol. 107 (1982), pp. 269–78.

44. N. Arora et al., "Effectiveness of a Noninvasive Digital Infrared Thermal Imaging System in the Detection of Breast Cancer," *American Journal of Surgery,* vol. 196, no. 4 (October 2008), pp. 523–26.

45. M. Gautherie and C. M. Gros, "Breast Thermography and Cancer Risk Prediction," *Cancer,* vol. 45, no. 1 (January 1, 1980), pp. 51–56.

46. H. J. Isard, W. Becker, R. Shilo, and B. J. Ostrum, "Breast Thermography After Four Years and 10,000 Studies," *American Journal of Roentgenology, Radium Therapy, and Nuclear Medicine,* vol. 115, no. 4 (August 1972), pp. 811–21.

47. M. Gautherie and C. M. Gros, "Breast Thermography and Cancer Risk Prediction," *Cancer,* vol. 45, no. 1 (January 1, 1980), pp. 51–56.

48. K. Louis, J. Walter, and M. Gautherie, "Long-Term Assessment of Breast Cancer Risk by Thermal Imaging," in M. Gautherie and E. Albert, eds., *Biomedical Thermology: Proceedings of an International Symposium Held in Strasbourg, France, June 30–July 4, 1981* (New York: A. R. Liss, 1982), pp. 279–301; M. Gautherie, "Thermobiological Assessment of Benign and Malignant Breast Diseases," *American Journal of Obstetrics and Gynecology,* vol. 147, no. 8 (December 15, 1983), pp. 861–69.

49. H. Spitalier et al., "Does Infrared Thermography Truly Have a Role in Present-Day Breast Cancer Management?" in M. Gautherie and E. Albert, eds., *Biomedical Thermology: Proceedings of an International Symposium* (New York: A. R. Liss, 1982), pp. 269–78; R. Amalric et al., "Does Infrared Thermography Truly Have a Role in Present-Day Breast Cancer Management?" *Progress in Clinical and Biological Research,* vol. 107 (1982), pp. 269–78.

50. P. Gamagami, "Indirect Signs of Breast Cancer: Angiogenesis Study," *Atlas of Mammography* (Cambridge, MA: Blackwell Science, 1996), pp. 231–258.

51. J. R. Keyserlingk et al., "Infrared Imaging of the Breast: Initial Reappraisal Using High-Resolution Digital Technology in 100 Successive Cases of Stage I and II Breast Cancer," *The Breast Journal,* vol. 4, no. 4 (July/August 1998), pp. 245–51.

52. Y. R. Parisky et al., "Efficacy of Computerized Infrared Imaging Analysis to Eval-

uate Mammographically Suspicious Lesions," *American Journal of Roentgenology,* vol. 180, no. 1 (January 2003), pp. 263–69.

53. Ibid.; N. Arora et al., "Effectiveness of Noninvasive Digital Infrared Thermal Imaging System in the Detection of Breast Cancer," *American Journal of Surgery,* vol. 196, no. 4 (October 2008), pp. 523–26; E. Y. Ng and E. C. Kee, "Advanced Integrated Technique in Breast Cancer Thermography," *Journal of Medical Engineering and Technology,* vol. 32, no. 2 (March–April 2008), pp. 103–14; D. A. Kennedy, T. Lee, and D. Seely, "A Comparative Review of Thermography as a Breast Cancer Screening Technique," *Integrative Cancer Therapies,* vol. 8, no. 1 (March 2009), pp. 9–16.

54. G. Kolata, "Breast Cancer Screening Under 50: Experts Disagree If Benefit Exists," *New York Times,* December 14, 1993, p. C-1; W. G. Welch and W. Black, "Advances in Diagnostic Imaging," *New England Journal of Medicine,* vol. 328 (April 1993), pp. 1237–42; M. Nielson et al., "Breast Cancer and Atypia Among Young Middle-Aged Women: A Study of 110 Medical-Legal Autopsies," *British Journal of Cancer,* vol. 56 (1987), pp. 814–19. An unpublished autopsy study with similar findings was done at Cook County Hospital in Chicago (personal communication with Kate Havens, M.D.).

55. S. A. Narod et al., "Breast Cancer Mortality After a Diagnosis of Ductal Carcinoma In Situ," *JAMA Oncology,* vol. 1, no. 7 (October 2015), pp. 888–96.

56. L. J. Esserman, I. M. Thompson, and B. Reid, "Overdiagnosis and Overtreatment in Cancer: An Opportunity for Improvement," *Journal of the American Medical Association,* vol. 310, no. 8 (August 28, 2013), pp. 797–98.

57. L. Esserman and C. Yau, "Rethinking the Standard for Ductal Carcinoma In Situ Treatment," *JAMA Oncology,* vol. 1, no. 7 (October 2015), pp. 881–83.

58. G. Kolata, "Doubt Is Raised on Quick Surgery on Breast Lesion," *New York Times,* August 21, 2015, p. A1.

59. V. Ernster et al., "Incidence of and Treatment for Ductal Carcinoma In Situ of the Breast," *Journal of the American Medical Association,* vol. 275, no. 12 (March 27, 1996), pp. 913–18.

60. G. Arpino, R. Laucirica, and R. M. Elledge, "Premalignant and In Situ Breast Disease: Biology and Clinical Implications," *Annals of Internal Medicine,* vol. 143, no. 6 (September 20, 2005), pp. 446–57.

61. C. I. Li et al., "Age-Specific Incidence Rates of In Situ Breast Carcinomas in Histologic Type, 1980 to 2001," *Cancer Epidemiology, Biomarkers and Prevention,* vol. 14, no. 4 (April 2005), pp. 1012–15.

62. C. I. Li et al., "Adjuvant Hormonal Therapy for Breast Cancer and Risk of Hormone Receptor-Specific Subtypes of Contralateral Breast Cancer," *Cancer Research,* vol. 69, no. 17 (August 25, 2009), pp. 6865–70.

63. S. Hwang and K. D. Miller, " 'Cultural Change': Dialing Back the Discussion and Treatment of DCIS," *Medscape,* January 17, 2018, www.medscape.com/viewarticle/891198.

64. A. M. Noone et al. (eds.), *SEER Cancer Statistics Review, 1975–2015,* National Cancer Institute. Bethesda, MD, https://seer.cancer.gov/statfacts/html/breast.html, based on November 2017 SEER data submission, posted to the SEER website, April 2018.

65. National Cancer Institute, "Breast Cancer Risk in American Women," September 24, 2012, www.cancer.gov/types/breast/risk-fact-sheet.

66. Noone et al. (eds.), *SEER Cancer Statistics Review, 1975–2015;* National Cancer Institute, "Breast Cancer Risk in American Women."

67. National Center for Health Statistics, *Vital Statistics of the United States,* 1987, vol. 2, *Mortality, Part A,* DHHS Publication no. PHS 90-1101 (Washington, DC: U.S. Government Printing Office, 1990).

68. The following chemicals have been implicated: the pesticides DDT, heptachlor, and atrazine, several polycyclic aromatic hydrocarbons (PAHs), petroleum by-products, dioxin, and polychlorinated biphenyls (PCBs). See also Janet Ralof, "Ecocancer: Do Environmental Factors Underlie a Breast Cancer Epidemic?" *Science News,* vol. 144 (July 3, 1993), p. 1013.

69. S. Epstein, M.D., letter to Dr. D. Kessler, commissioner of the FDA, February 14, 1994, cited in B. Joseph, *My Healing from Breast Cancer* (New Canaan, CT: Keats, 1996), p. 7.

70. S. Mason, V. Welch, and J. Neratko, "Synthetic Polymer Contamination in Bottled Water," *Frontiers in Chemistry,* vol. 6 (September 11, 2018), p. 407, https://orbmedia.org/sites/default/files/FinalBottledWaterReport.pdf.

71. M. Kosuth et al., "Synthetic Polymer Contamination in Global Drinking Water," *Orb,* May 16, 2017, https://orbmedia.org/stories/invisibles_final_report/multimedia.

72. S. Steingraber, *The Falling Age of Puberty in U.S. Girls: What We Know, What We Need to Know* (San Francisco: Breast Cancer Fund, 2007), http://www.breastcancerfund.org/site/pp.asp?c=kwKXLdPaE&b=3291891.

73. C. Savetsky, "The 'Pink Ribbon' Elicits My Gag Reflex," *Natural Healing for Women* blog, October 29, 2015, www.naturalhealingforwomen.com/the-pink-ribbon-elicits-my-gag-reflex.

74. P. Buell, "Changing Incidence of Breast Cancer in Japanese-American Women," *Journal of the National Cancer Institute,* vol. 51 (1973), pp. 1479–83; L. Kinlen, "Meat and Fat Consumption and Cancer Mortality: A Study of Strict Religious Orders in Britain," *The Lancet,* 1982, pp. 946–49; W. Willett et al., "Dietary Fat and Risk of Breast Cancer," *New England Journal of Medicine,* vol. 316, no. 22 (1987).

75. D. J. Hunter et al., "Cohort Studies of Fat Intake and the Risk of Breast Cancer: A Pooled Analysis," *New England Journal of Medicine,* vol. 334 (1996), pp. 356–61.

76. S. Franceschi et al., "Intake of Macronutrients and Risk of Breast Cancer," *The Lancet,* vol. 347 (1996), pp. 1351–56.

77. I. Romieu et al., "Dietary Glycemic Index and Glycemic Load and Breast Cancer Risk in the European Prospective Investigation into Cancer and Nutrition (EPIC)," *American Journal of Clinical Nutrition,* vol. 96, no. 2 (August 2012), pp. 345–55.

78. P. A. van den Brandt and M. Schulpen, "Mediterranean Diet Adherence and Risk of Postmenopausal Breast Cancer: Results of a Cohort Study and Meta-Analysis," *International Journal of Cancer,* vol. 140, no. 10 (May 15, 2017), pp. 2220–31.

79. S. Seely and D. F. Horrobin, "Diet and Breast Cancer: The Possible Connection with Sugar Consumption," *Medical Hypotheses,* vol. 3 (1983), pp. 319–27; K. K. Caroll, "Dietary Factors in Immune-Dependent Cancer," in M. Winick, ed.,

Current Concepts in Nutrition, vol. 6, *Nutrition and Cancer* (New York: John Wiley and Sons, 1977), pp. 25–40; S. K. Hoeh and K. K. Carroll, "Effects of Dietary Carbohydrate in the Incidence of Mammary Tumors Induced in Rates by 7, 12-Dimethylbenzanthracene," *Nutrition and Cancer,* vol. 1, no. 3 (1979), pp. 27–30; R. Kazer, "Insulin Resistance, Insulin-Like Growth Factor I and Breast Cancer: A Hypothesis," *International Journal of Cancer,* vol. 62 (1995), pp. 403–6.

80. G. C. Kabat et al., "Repeated Measures of Serum Glucose and Insulin in Relation to Postmenopausal Breast Cancer," *International Journal of Cancer,* vol. 125, no. 11 (2009), pp. 2704–10.

81. N. Provinciali et al., "BP129 Insulin Resistance (IR) and Prognosis of Metastatic Breast Cancer (MBC) Patients," *The Breast,* vol. 24, no. 3 (November 2015), p. S66.

82. C. Catsburg et al., "Insulin, Estrogen, Inflammatory Markers, and Risk of Benign Proliferative Breast Disease," *Cancer Research,* vol. 74, no. 12 (June 15, 2014), pp. 3248–58.

83. T. A. Sellers et al., "Effect of Family History, Body-Fat Distribution, and Reproductive Factors on the Risk of Postmenopausal Breast Cancer," *New England Journal of Medicine,* vol. 326, no. 20 (May 14, 1992), pp. 1323–9.

84. B. L. Pierce et al., "Elevated Biomarkers of Inflammation Are Associated with Reduced Survival Among Breast Cancer Patients," *Journal of Clinical Oncology,* vol. 27, no. 21 (July 20, 2009), pp. 3437–44.

85. R. T. Chlebowski et al., "Association of Low-Fat Dietary Pattern with Breast Cancer Overall Survival: A Secondary Analysis of the Women's Health Initiative Randomized Clinical Trial," *Journal of the American Medical Association,* vol. 4, no. 10 (October 1, 2018), p. e181212.

86. C. X. Zhang et al., "Greater Vegetable and Fruit Intake Is Associated with a Lower Risk of Breast Cancer Among Chinese Women," *International Journal of Cancer,* vol. 125, no. 1 (July 1, 2009), pp. 181–88; J. L. Freudenheim et al., "Premenopausal Breast Cancer Risk and Intake of Vegetables, Fruits, and Related Nutrients," *Journal of National Cancer Institute,* vol. 88, no. 6 (March 20, 1996), pp. 340–48.

87. L. E. Carlson et al., "Mindfulness-Based Cancer Recovery and Supportive-Expressive Therapy Maintain Telomere Length Relative to Controls in Distressed Breast Cancer Survivors," *Cancer,* vol. 121, no. 3 (February 1, 2015), pp. 476–84.

88. K. A. Biegler et al., "Longitudinal Change in Telomere Length and the Chronic Stress Response in a Randomized Pilot Biobehavioral Clinical Study: Implications for Cancer Prevention," *Cancer Prevention Research,* vol. 5, no. 10 (October 2012), pp. 1173–82.

89. N. Boyd, "Effect of a Low-Fat, High-Carbohydrate Diet on Symptoms of Cyclical Mastopathy," *The Lancet,* vol. 2 (1988), p. 128; D. Rose et al., "Effect of a Low-Fat Diet on Hormone Levels in Women with Cystic Breast Disease. I: Serum Steroids and Gonadotropins," *Journal of the National Cancer Institute,* vol. 78 (1987), p. 623; D. Rose et al., "Effect of a Low-Fat Diet on Hormone Levels in Women with Cystic Breast Disease. II: Serum Radioimmunoassayable Prolactin and Growth Hormone and Bioactive Lactogenic Hormones," *Journal of the National Cancer Institute,* vol. 78 (1987), p. 627.

90. M. Woods, "Low-Fat, High-Fiber Diet and Serum Estrone Sulfate in Premeno-pausal Women," *American Journal of Clinical Nutrition*, vol. 49 (1989), p. 1179; D. Ingram, "Effect of Low-Fat Diet on Female Sex Hormone Levels," *Journal of the National Cancer Institute*, vol. 79 (1987), p. 1225; and H. Aldercreutz, "Diet and Plasma Androgens in Postmenopausal Vegetarian and Omnivorous Women and Postmenopausal Women with Breast Cancer," *American Journal of Clinical Nutrition*, vol. 49 (1989), p. 433; A. Tavani et al., "Consumption of Sweet Foods and Breast Cancer Risk in Italy," *Annals of Oncology* 17, no. 2 (February 2006), pp. 341–45.

91. M. H. Holl et al., "Gut Bacteria and Aetiology of Cancer of the Breast," *The Lancet,* vol. 2 (1971), pp. 172–73; R. E. Hughes, "Hypothesis: A New Look at Dietary Fiber in Human Nutrition," *Clinical Nutrition,* vol. 406 (1986), pp. 81–86.

92. J. Michnovicz and H. Bradlow, "Altered Estrogen Metabolism and Excretion in Humans Following Consumption of Indole-3-Carbinol," *Nutrition and Cancer,* vol. 16 (1991), pp. 59–66.

93. Rose et al., "Serum Steroids and Gonadotropins."

94. H. Aldercreutz et al., "Dietary Phyto-oestrogens and the Menopause in Japan," *The Lancet,* vol. 339 (1992), p. 1233; H. P. Lee et al., "Dietary Effects of Breast Cancer Risk in Singapore," *The Lancet,* vol. 337 (May 18, 1991), pp. 1197–1200.

95. N. N. Ismael, "A Study of Menopause in Malaysia," *Maturitas,* vol. 19 (1994), pp. 205–9.

96. X. O. Shu et al., "Soy Food Intake and Breast Cancer Survival," *Journal of the American Medical Association,* vol. 302, no. 22 (December 9, 2009), pp. 2437–43.

97. L. J. Lu et al., "Decreased Ovarian Hormones During a Soya Diet: Implications for Breast Cancer Prevention," *Cancer Research,* vol. 60, no. 15 (August 1, 2000), pp. 4112–21; N. B. Kumar et al., "The Specific Role of Isoflavones on Estrogen Metabolism in Premenopausal Women," *Cancer,* vol. 94, no. 4 (February 15, 2002), pp. 1166–74; C. Nagata et al., "Decreased Serum Estradiol Concentration Associated with High Dietary Intake of Soy Products in Premenopausal Japanese Women," *Nutrition and Cancer,* vol. 29, no. 3 (1997), pp. 228–33.

98. T. Hirano et al., "Antiproliferative Activity of Mammalian Lignan Derivatives Against the Human Breast Carcinoma Cell Line ZR-75-1," *Cancer Investigations,* vol. 8 (1990), pp. 595–602.

99. H. Aldercreutz et al., "Excretion of the Lignans Enterolactone and Enterodiol and of Equol in Omnivorous and Vegetarian Women and in Women with Breast Cancer," *The Lancet,* vol. 2 (1992), pp. 1295–99.

100. S. J. Wayne et al., "Breast Cancer Survivors Who Use Estrogenic Botanical Supplements Have Lower Serum Estrogen Levels Than Non Users," *Breast Cancer Research and Treatment,* vol. 117, no. 1 (September 2009), pp. 111–19.

101. Council for Responsible Nutrition, "International Researchers Convene Meeting on Isoflavones," press release, June 17, 2009, www.npicenter.com/anm/anmviewer .asp?a=24304&print=yes.

102. S. Yamamoto et al., "Soy, Isoflavones, and Breast Cancer Risk in Japan," *Journal of the National Cancer Institute,* vol. 95, no. 12 (June 18, 2003), pp. 906–13.

103. H. Chen et al., "Isoflavones Extracted from Chickpea Cicer arietinum L. Sprouts

Induce Mitochondria-Dependent Apoptosis in Human Breast Cancer Cells," *Phototherapy Research,* vol. 29, no. 2 (February 2015), pp. 210–19.

104. A. Eakin et al., "Does High Dietary Soy Intake Affect a Woman's Risk of Primary or Recurrent Breast Cancer?" *Journal of Family Practice,* vol. 64, no. 10 (October 2015), pp. 660–62.

105. S. Qiu and C. Jiang, "Soy and Isoflavones Consumption and Breast Cancer Survival and Recurrence: A Systematic Review and Meta-Analysis," *European Journal of Nutrition,* October 31, 2018 (Epub ahead of print).

106. Personal communication, Margaret Ritchie, Ph.D., June 2009.

107. L. Rosenberg et al., "Breast Cancer and Alcoholic Beverage Consumption," *The Lancet,* vol. 1 (1982), p. 267.

108. W. C. Willett et al., "Moderate Alcohol Consumption and the Risk of Breast Cancer," *New England Journal of Medicine,* vol. 316, no. 19 (May 7, 1987), pp. 1174–80.

109. C. I. Li et al., "Relationship Between Potentially Modifiable Lifestyle Factors and Risk of Second Primary Contralateral Breast Cancer Among Women Diagnosed with Estrogen Receptor-Positive Invasive Breast Cancer," *Journal of Clinical Oncology,* vol. 27, no. 32 (November 10, 2009), pp. 5312–8.

110. I. Kato et al., "Alcohol Consumption in Cancers of Hormone Related Organs in Females," *Japan Journal of Clinical Oncology,* vol. 19, no. 3 (1989), pp. 202–7.

111. D. Bagga et al., "Dietary Modulation of Omega-3/Omega-6 Polyunsaturate Fatty Acid Ratios in Patients with Breast Cancer," *Journal of the National Cancer Institute,* vol. 89, no. 15 (1997), pp. 1123–31.

112. R. S. London et al., "The Effect of Alpha-Tocopherol on Premenstrual Symptomatology," *Cancer Research,* vol. 41 (1981), pp. 3811–16; R. S. London et al., "The Effect of Alpha-Tocopherol on Premenstrual Symptomatology: A Double-Blind Study," *Journal of American College Nutrition,* vol. 3 (1984), pp. 351–56; R. S. London et al., "The Role of Vitamin E in Fibrocystic Breast Disease," *Obstetrics and Gynecology,* vol. 65 (1982), pp. 104–6; A. A. Abrams, "Use of Vitamin E for Chronic Cystic Mastitis," *New England Journal of Medicine,* vol. 272 (1965), pp. 1080–81.

113. R. R. Brown et al., "Correlation of Serum Retinol Levels with Response to Chemotherapy in Breast Cancer," *American Journal of Obstetrics and Gynecology,* vol. 148, no. 3, pp. 309–12.

114. K. P. McConnell et al., "The Relationship Between Dietary Selenium and Breast Cancer," *Journal of Surgical Oncology,* vol. 5, no. 1 (1980), pp. 67–70.

115. L. C. Clark et al., "Effects of Selenium Supplementation for Cancer Prevention in Patients with Carcinoma of the Skin," *Journal of the American Medical Association,* vol. 276 (1996), pp. 1957–63.

116. T. T. Kellis and L. E. Vickery, "Inhibition of Human Estrogen Synthetase (Aromatase) by Flavonoids," *Science,* vol. 255 (1984), pp. 1032–34. The bioflavonoids compete for estrogen as a substrate in fat metabolism.

117. B. Goldin and J. Gorsbach, "The Effect of Milk and Lactobacillus Feeding on Human Intestinal Bacterial Enzyme Activity," *American Journal of Clinical Nutrition,* vol. 39 (1984), pp. 756–61. *Lactobacillus acidophilus* inhibits beta glucuronidase, the fecal bacterial enzyme responsible for deconjugating liver-conjugated estrogen.

118. K. Lockwood et al., "Partial and Complete Regression of Breast Cancer in Patients in Relation to Dosage of Coenzyme Q_{10}," *Biochemical and Biophysical Research Communications,* vol. 199, no. 3 (1994), pp. 1504–8.

119. R. Staud, "Vitamin D: More Than Just Affecting Calcium and Bone," *Current Rheumatology Reports,* vol. 7, no. 5 (October 2005), pp. 356–64.

120. Ibid.; J. J. Cannell and B. W. Hollis, "Use of Vitamin D in Clinical Practice," *Alternative Medicine Review,* vol. 13, no. 1 (March 2008), pp. 6–20; J. J. Cannell et al., "On the Epidemiology of Influenza," *Virology Journal,* vol. 25, no. 5 (February 25, 2008), p. 29; M. F. Holick, "Vitamin D: Importance in the Prevention of Cancers, Type 1 Diabetes, Heart Disease, and Osteoporosis," *American Journal of Clinical Nutrition,* vol. 79, no. 3 (March 2004), pp. 362–71.

121. C. F. Garland et al., "Vitamin D for Cancer Prevention: Global Perspective," *Annals of Epidemiology,* vol. 19, no. 7 (July 2009), pp. 468–83.

122. C. F. Garland et al., "Vitamin D and Prevention of Breast Cancer: Pooled Analysis," *Journal of Steroid Biochemistry and Molecular Biology,* vol. 103, nos. 3–5 (March 2007), pp. 708–11.

123. S. L. McDonnell et al., "Breast Cancer Risk Markedly Lower with Serum 25-Hydroxyvitamin D Concentrations ≥60 vs <20 ng/ml (150 vs 50 nmol/L): Pooled Analysis of Two Randomized Trials and a Prospective Cohort," *PLoS One,* vol. 13, no. 6 (June 15, 2018), p. e0199265.

124. American Society of Clinical Oncology 2008 Annual Meeting, Abstract 511, preview presscast, May 15, 2008.

125. P. J. Goodwin et al., "Prognostic Effects of 25-Hydroxyvitamin D Levels in Early Breast Cancer," *Journal of Clinical Oncology* 27, no. 23 (August 10, 2009), pp. 3757–63.

126. T. Rink et al., "Effect of Iodine and Thyroid Hormones in the Induction and Therapy of Hashimoto's Thyroiditis," *Nuklearmedizin,* vol. 38, no. 5 (1999), pp. 144–49.

127. O. Turken et al., "Breast Cancer in Association with Thyroid Disorders," *Breast Cancer Research,* vol. 5, no. 5 (2003), pp. R110–13; B. Rasmusson et al., "Thyroid Function in Patients with Breast Cancer," *European Journal of Cancer and Clinical Oncology,* vol. 23, no. 5 (May 1987), pp. 553–56.

128. B. V. Stadel, "Dietary Iodine and Risk of Breast, Endometrial, and Ovarian Cancer," *The Lancet,* vol. 1, no. 7965 (April 24, 1976), pp. 890–91.

129. J. H. Kessler, "The Effect of Supraphysiologic Levels of Iodine on Patients with Cyclic Mastalgia," *The Breast Journal,* vol. 10, no. 4 (2004), pp. 328–36; W. R. Ghent et al., "Iodine Replacement in Fibrocystic Disease of the Breast," *Canadian Journal of Surgery,* vol. 35, no. 5 (October 1993), pp. 453–60.

130. Kessler, "The Effect of Supraphysiologic Levels of Iodine on Patients with Cyclic Mastalgia," pp. 328–36.

131. W. R. Ghent et al., "Iodine Replacement in Fibrocystic Disease of the Breast," *Canadian Journal of Surgery,* vol. 36, no. 5 (October 1992), pp. 453–60.

132. B. A. Eskin et al., "Mammary Gland Dysplasia in Iodine Deficiency," *Journal of the American Medical Association,* vol. 200 (1967), pp. 115–19.

133. K. J. Chang et al., "Influences of Percutaneous Administration of Estradiol and

Progesterone on Human Breast Epithelial Cell Cycle in Vivo," *Fertility and Sterility,* vol. 63 (1995), pp. 785–91.

134. P. E. Mohr et al., "Serum Progesterone and Prognosis in Operable Breast Cancer," *British Journal of Cancer,* vol. 73 (1996), pp. 1552–55.

135. A. McTiernan, "Exercise and Breast Cancer—Time to Get Moving?" *New England Journal of Medicine,* vol. 336, no. 18 (May 1, 1997), pp. 1311–2.

136. I. Thune et al., "Physical Activity and the Risk of Breast Cancer," *New England Journal of Medicine,* vol. 336, no. 18 (May 1, 1997), pp. 1269–75.

137. B. Rockhill et al., "A Prospective Study of Recreational Physical Activity and Breast Cancer Risk," *Archives of Internal Medicine,* vol. 159, no. 19 (October 25, 1999), pp. 2290–96.

138. T. M. Peters et al., "Intensity and Timing of Physical Activity in Relation to Postmenopausal Breast Cancer Risk: The Prospective NIH-AARP Diet and Health Study," *BMC Cancer,* vol. 9, no. 1 (October 1, 2009), p. 349.

139. P. K. Verkasalo et al., "Sleep Duration and Breast Cancer: A Prospective Cohort Study," *Cancer Research,* vol. 65, no. 20 (October 15, 2005), pp. 9595–600.

140. E. S. Schernhammer et al., "Rotating Night Shifts and Risk of Breast Cancer in Women Participating in the Nurses Health Study," *Journal of the National Cancer Institute,* vol. 93, no. 20 (October 17, 2001), pp. 1563–68.

141. D. E. Blask et al., "Melatonin-Depleted Blood from Premenopausal Women Exposed to Light at Night Stimulates Growth of Human Breast Cancer Xenografts in Nude Rats," *Cancer Research,* vol. 65, no. 23 (December 1, 2005), pp. 11174–84.

142. E. S. Schernhammer et al., "Urinary Melatonin Levels and Breast Cancer Risk," *Journal of the National Cancer Institute,* vol. 97, no. 14 (July 20, 2005), pp. 1084–87.

143. L. Burk, "Warning Dreams Preceding the Diagnosis of Breast Cancer: A Survey of the Most Important Characteristics," *Explore,* vol. 11, no. 3 (May/June 2015), pp. 193–98.

144. S. Narod et al., "Familial Breast-Ovarian Cancer Locus on Chromosome 17q12a23," *The Lancet,* vol. 338 (July 13, 1991), pp. 82–83.

145. D. Thompson et al., "Cancer Incidence in BRCA1 Mutation Carriers," *Journal of the National Cancer Institute,* vol. 94, no. 18 (September 18, 2002), pp. 1358–65. The Breast Cancer Linkage Consortium, "Cancer Risks in BRCA2 Mutation Carriers," *Journal of the National Cancer Institute,* vol. 91, no. 15 (August 4, 1999), pp. 131–36. National Cancer Institute, "National Cancer Institute Fact Sheet: BRCA1 and BRCA2: Cancer Risk and Genetic Testing," www.cancer.gov/cancertopics/factsheet/Risk/BRCA.

146. National Cancer Institute, "National Cancer Institute Fact Sheet: BRCA1 and BRCA2: Cancer Risk and Genetic Testing."

147. E. R. Copson et al., "Germline BRCA Mutation and Outcome in Young-Onset Breast Cancer (POSH): A Prospective Cohort Study," *Lancet Oncology,* vol. 19, no. 2 (February 2018), pp. 169–80.

148. M. B. Fitzgerald et al., "Germ Line BrCa 1 Mutations in Jewish and Non-Jewish Women with Early Onset Breast Cancer," *New England Journal of Medicine,*

vol. 334, no. 3 (1996), pp. 143–49; F. S. Collins, "BrCa 1: Lots of Mutations, Lots of Dilemmas," *New England Journal of Medicine,* vol. 334, no. 3 (1996), pp. 186–88; A. A. Langston, "BrCa 1 Mutations in Population-Based Sample of Young Women with Breast Cancer," *New England Journal of Medicine,* vol. 334, no. 3 (1996), pp. 137–42.

149. C. B. Begg et al., "Variation of Breast Cancer Risk Among BRCA 1/2 Carriers," *Journal of the American Medical Association,* vol. 299, no. 2 (January 9, 2008), pp. 194–201.

150. U.S. Preventive Services Task Force, "Genetic Risk Assessment and BRCA Mutation Testing for Breast and Ovarian Cancer Susceptibility: Recommendation Statement," *Annals of Internal Medicine,* vol. 143, no. 5 (September 6, 2005), pp. 355–61.

151. R. Semelka, "Imaging X-Rays Cause Cancer: A Call to Action for Caregivers and Patients," *Medscape,* last reviewed February 16, 2007.

152. S. B. Haga et al., "Genomic Profiling to Promote a Healthy Lifestyle: Not Ready for Prime Time," *Nature Genetics,* vol. 34, no. 4 (August 2003), pp. 347–50.

153. National Cancer Institute, "Cancer Stat Facts: Female Breast Cancer," https://seer .cancer.gov/statfacts/html/breast.html.

154. J. A. Sparano et al., "Adjuvant Chemotherapy Guided by a 21-Gene Expression Assay in Breast Cancer," *New England Journal of Medicine,* vol. 379, no. 2 (July 12, 2018), pp. 111–21.

155. S. Johnson, *Wildfire: Igniting the She-volution* (Albuquerque, NM: Wildfire Books, 1990), p. 38.

156. Breast cancer, in the conventional sense, can recur anytime. That's why no conventional doctor would consider Monica "cured." They would say that she is "in remission." Whatever one calls it, I like the way she looks and is living her life.

157. For a fascinating account of the breast implant controversy, see the "Chronology of Silicone Breast Implants" page on the website for the PBS show *Frontline* at www.pbs.org/wgbh/pages/frontline/implants/cron.html.

158. L. A. Brinton et al., "Cancer Risk at Sites Other Than the Breast Following Augmentation Mammoplasty," *Annals of Epidemiology,* vol. 11, no. 4 (May 2001), pp. 248–56.

159. Implant statistics cited in Marsha Angell, "Shattuck Lecture—Evaluating the Health Risks of Breast Implants: The Interplay of Medical Science, the Law, and Public Opinion," *New England Journal of Medicine,* vol. 334, no. 23 (1996), pp. 1513–18.

160. L. A. Brinton et al., "Mortality Among Augmentation Mammoplasty Patients," *Epidemiology,* vol. 12, no. 3 (May 2001), pp. 321–26.

161. D. B. Sarwer, G. K. Brown, and D. L. Evans, "Cosmetic Breast Augmentation and Suicide," *American Journal of Psychiatry,* vol. 164, no. 7 (July 2007), pp. 1006–13.

162. V. C. Koot et al., "Total and Cause Specific Mortality Among Swedish Women with Cosmetic Breast Implants: Prospective Study," *British Medical Journal,* vol. 326, no. 7388 (March 8, 2003), pp. 527–28.

163. J. S. Hasan, "Psychological Issues in Cosmetic Surgery: A Functional Overview," *Annals of Plastic Surgery,* vol. 44, no. 1 (January 2000), pp. 89–96.

164. M. J. L. Colaris et al., "Two Hundred Cases of ASIA Syndrome Following Silicone Implants: A Comparative Study of 30 Years and a Review of Current Literature," *Immunology Research*, vol. 65, no. 1 (February 2017), pp. 120–28.

165. J. W. Cohen Tervaert and R. M. Kappel, "Silicone Implant Incompatibility Syndrome (SIIS): A Frequent Cause of ASIA (Shoenfeld's Syndrome)," *Immunology Research*, vol. 56, nos. 2–3 (July 2013), pp. 293–98.

166. Personal communication from Mona Lisa Schulz, M.D., Ph.D., who researched the area thoroughly prior to having bilateral reconstructions herself after the diagnosis of breast cancer.

167. "Saline-Filled Breast Implant Surgery: Making an Informed Decision," patient labeling for saline-filled breast implants, Mentor Corporation (updated January 2004); "Making an Informed Decision: Saline-Filled Breast Implant Surgery; 2004 Update," patient labeling for saline-filled breast implants, INAMED Corporation (updated November 2004).

168. N. Hurst, "Lactation After Augmentation Mammoplasty," *Obstetrics and Gynecology*, vol. 87, no. 1 (1996), pp. 30–34.

169. A. R. Staib and D. R. Logan, "Hypnotic Stimulation of Breast Growth," *American Journal of Clinical Hypnosis*, vol. 19, no. 4 (April 1977), pp. 201–8; R. D. Willard, "Breast Enlargement Through Visual Imagery and Hypnosis," *American Journal of Clinical Hypnosis*, vol. 19, no. 4 (April 1977), pp. 195–200; J. E. Williams, "Stimulation of Breast Growth by Hypnosis," *Journal of Sex Research*, vol. 10, no. 4 (November 1, 1974), pp. 316–26; L. M. LeCron, "Breast Development Through Hypnotic Suggestion," *Journal of the American Society of Psychosomatic Dentistry and Medicine*, vol. 16, no. 2 (1969), pp. 58–61.

170. Willard, "Breast Enlargement Through Visual Imagery and Hypnosis."

Chapter 11: Our Fertility

1. C. Goldin and L. Katz, "The Power of the Pill: Oral Contraceptives and Women's Career and Marriage Decisions," *Journal of Political Economy*, vol. 110, no. 4 (August 2002), pp. 730–70, www.jstor.org/pss/3078534.

2. D. Chamberlain, *The Mind of Your Newborn Baby* (Berkeley, CA: North Atlantic Books, 1998); see also www.birthpsychology.com.

3. I met a woman ob-gyn physician from China who told me she had performed 20,000 abortions in her career. In China, from 1975 to 2015, only one child per couple was allowed (with a few specific exceptions)—sometimes not even one. During this time, abortion was commonly used for birth control. If a couple had more than one child while this was in force, the parents could have lost a job or have been subject to other sanctions. As a result, many Chinese couples selectively aborted female fetuses until the law was changed. Because of this practice, an entire generation of young men do not have enough women their age for wives— a fact that, although tragic, seems a cruel kind of justice.

4. C. Smith-Rosenberg, *Disorderly Conduct: Visions of Gender in Victorian America* (New York: Oxford University Press, 1986).

5. In a society in which there is so much incest and rape, sexual behavior is often distorted, starting in childhood. Any woman who has recovered from sexual

abuse will tell you that having multiple sexual partners and sexual "acting out" are among the consequences of sexual abuse. I'm not blaming these women. I'm merely suggesting that we need to start the healing process somewhere.

6. Smith-Rosenberg, *Disorderly Conduct*.

7. Smith-Rosenberg, *Disorderly Conduct*, p. 218.

8. D. Grossman and K. Grindlay, "Safety of Medical Abortion Provided Through Telemedicine Compared with in Person," *Obstetrics and Gynecology*, vol. 130, no. 4 (October 2017), pp. 778–82.

9. A. R. A. Aiken et al., "Self Reported Outcomes and Adverse Events After Medical Abortion Through Online Telemedicine: Population Based Study in the Republic of Ireland and Northern Ireland," *British Medical Journal*, vol. 357 (May 16, 2017), p. j2011.

10. N. J. Kassebaum et al., "Global, Regional, and National Levels and Causes of Maternal Mortality During 1990–2013: A Systematic Analysis for the Global Burden of Disease Study 2013," *The Lancet*, vol. 384, no. 9947 (September 13, 2014), pp. 980–1004.

11. D. A. Grimes et al., "Unsafe Abortion: The Preventable Pandemic," *The Lancet*, vol. 368, no. 9550 (November 25, 2006), pp. 1908–19.

12. M. Melbye et al., "Induced Abortion and the Risk of Breast Cancer," *New England Journal of Medicine*, vol. 336 (1996), pp. 81–85.

13. G. T. McGarey, *Born to Live* (Phoenix, AZ: Inkwell Production, 2001), p. 54. For more information, contact Gladys T. McGarey Medical Foundation, 4848 E. Cactus Rd., Suite 505–506, Scottsdale, AZ 85254, 480-946-4544, www.mcgareyfoundation.org.

14. J. Trussell, F. Stewart, F. Guest, and R. A. Hatcher, "Emergency Contraceptive Pills: A Simple Proposal to Reduce Unintended Pregnancies," *Family Planning Perspectives*, vol. 24, no. 6 (November–December 1992), pp. 269–73.

15. R. Hatcher et al., *Contraceptive Technology* (New York: Irvington Publishers, 1991).

16. M. K. Horwitt et al., "Relationship Between Levels of Blood Lipids, Vitamins C, A, E, Serum Copper, and Urinary Excretion of Tryptophan Metabolites in Women Taking Oral Contraceptive Therapy," *American Journal of Clinical Nutrition*, vol. 28 (1975), pp. 403–12; K. Amatayakul, "Vitamin Metabolism and the Effects of Multivitamin Supplementation in Oral Contraceptive Users," *Contraception*, vol. 30, no. 2 (1984), pp. 179–96; and J. L. Webb, "Nutritional Effects of Oral Contraceptive Use," *Journal of Reproductive Health*, vol. 25, no. 4 (1980), p. 151.

17. A. M. Kaunitz, "Oral Contraceptives," in Thomas G. Stovall and Frank W. Ling, eds., *Gynecology for the Primary Care Physician* (Philadelphia: Current Medicine, 1999).

18. I. F. Godsland et al., "The Effects of Different Formulations of Oral Contraceptive Agents on Lipid and Carbohydrate Metabolism," *New England Journal of Medicine*, vol. 323, no. 20 (November 15, 1990), pp. 1375–81.

19. M. Bernier et al., "Combined Oral Contraceptive Use and the Risk of Systemic Lupus Erythematosus," *Arthritis Care and Research*, vol. 61, no. 4 (April 15, 2009), pp. 476–81.

20. C. W. Skovlund et al., "Association of Hormonal Contraception with Depression," *Journal of the American Medical Association Psychiatry,* vol. 73, no. 11 (November 1, 2016), pp. 1154–62; J. Kulkarni, "Depression as a Side Effect of the Contraceptive Pill," *Expert Opinion on Drug Safety,* vol. 6, no. 4 (July 2007), pp. 371–74; M. Gingnell et al., "Oral Contraceptive Use Changes Brain Activity and Mood in Women with Previous Negative Affect on the Pill—A Double-Blinded, Placebo-Controlled Randomized Trial of a Levonorgestrel-Containing Combined Oral Contraceptive," *Psychoneuroendocrinology,* vol. 38, no. 7 (July 2013), pp. 1133–44.

21. T. M. Meiner et al., "Kynurenic Acid Is Reduced in Females and Oral Contraceptive Uers: Implications for Depression," *Brain, Behavior, and Immunity,* vol. 67 (January 2018), pp. 59–64.

22. W. V. Williams, "Hormonal Contraception and the Development of Autoimmunity: A Review of the Literature," *The Linacre Quarterly*, vol. 84, no. 3 (August 2017), pp. 275–95.

23. V. Cogliano et al., "Carcinogenicity of Combined Oestrogen-Progestagen Contraceptives and Menopausal Treatment," *Lancet Oncology,* vol. 6, no. 8 (August 2005), pp. 552–53.

24. Collaborative Group on Hormonal Factors in Breast Cancer, "Breast Cancer and Hormonal Contraceptives: Further Results," *Contraception,* vol. 54, no. 3 suppl. (September 1996), pp. 1S–106S.

25. L. S. Morch et al., "Contemporary Hormonal Contraception and the Risk of Breast Cancer," *New England Journal of Medicine,* vol. 377, no. 23 (December 7, 2017), pp. 2228–39.

26. S. S. Bassuk and J. E. Manson, "Oral Contraceptives and Menopausal Hormone Therapy: Relative and Attributable Risks of Cardiovascular Disease, Cancer, and Other Health Outcomes," *Annals of Epidemiology,* vol. 25, no. 3 (March 2015), pp. 193–200; K. A. Michels et al., "Modification of the Associations Between Duration of Oral Contraceptive Use and Ovarian, Endometrial, Breast, and Colorectal Cancers," *JAMA Oncology,* vol. 4, no. 4 (April 1, 2018), pp. 516–521.

27. C. Panzer et al., "Impact of Oral Contraceptives on Sex Hormone Binding Globulin and Androgen Levels: A Retrospective Study in Women with Sexual Dysfunction," *Journal of Sexual Medicine,* vol. 3, no. 1 (January 2006), pp. 104–13.

28. U.S. Food and Drug Administration, "FDA Updates Labeling for Ortho Evra Contraceptive Patch," November 10, 2005, www.fda.gov/NewsEvents/Newsroom/PressAnnouncements/2005/ucm108517.htm.

29. Y. C. Le, M. Rahman, and A. B. Berenson, "Early Weight Gain Predicting Later Weight Gain Among Depot Medroxyprogesterone Acetate Users," *Obstetrics and Gynecology,* vol. 114 (2 Pt 1) (August 2009), pp. 279–84.

30. Quoted from Joan Morais flyer, used by permission of the author.

31. My introduction to the true scope of science backing natural family planning came when I heard Joseph Stanford, M.D., speak at the 1993 annual meeting of the American Holistic Medical Association in Kansas City, Kansas. The research that is cited in this section was graciously provided to me by Dr. Stanford, who currently teaches in the Department of Family and Preventive Medicine, University of Utah School of Medicine, 375 Chipeta Way, Suite A, Salt Lake City, Utah 84108.

32. Observation of vaginal mucus discharge to determine time of fertility was originally developed by two physicians, John and Evelyn Billings. Hence, this method
is sometimes referred to as the Billings method.

33. T. W. Hilgers, A. I. Bailey, and A. M. Prebil, "Natural Family Planning IV: The
Identification of Postovulatory Infertility," *Obstetrics and Gynecology*, vol. 58,
no. 3 (1981), pp. 345–50.

34. T. W. Hilgers, "The Medical Applications of Natural Family Planning: A Contemporary Approach to Women's Health Care" (Omaha, NE: Pope Paul VI Institute Press, 1991); T. W. Hilgers, "The Statistical Evaluation of Natural Methods
of Family Planning," *International Review of Natural Family Planning*, vol. 8, no.
3 (Fall 1984), pp. 226–64; J. Doud, "Use-Effectiveness of the Creighton Model of
NFP," *International Review of Natural Family Planning*, vol. 9, no. 54 (1985).

35. E. Berglund Scherwitzl, A. Lindén Hirschberg, and R. Scherwitzl, "Identification
and Prediction of the Fertile Window Using NaturalCycles," *European Journal of
Contraception and Reproductive Healthcare*, vol. 20, no. 5 (2015), pp. 403–8; E.
Berglund Scherwitzl et al., "Fertility Awareness-Based Mobile Application for
Contraception," *European Journal of Contraception and Reproductive Healthcare*, vol. 21, no. 3 (June 2016), pp. 234–41; E. Berglund Scherwitzl et al.,
"Perfect-Use and Typical-Use Pearl Index of a Contraceptive Mobile App," *Contraception*, vol. 96, no. 6 (December 2017), pp. 420–25; J. Trussell, "Contraceptive Failure in the United States," *Contraception*, vol. 83, no. 5 (May 2011),
pp. 397–404.

36. M. C. Koch et al., "Improving Usability and Pregnancy Rates of a Fertility Moni-
tor by an Additional Mobile Application: Results of a Retrospective Efficacy
Study of Daysy and DaysyView app," *Reproductive Health*, vol. 15, no. 1
(March 2, 2018), p. 37.

37. M. Duane et al., "The Performance of Fertility Awareness-Based Method Apps
Marketed to Avoid Pregnancy," *Journal of the American Board of Family Medicine*, vol. 29, no. 4 (July–August 2016), pp. 508–11.

38. T. Hilgers et al., "Cumulative Pregnancy Rates in Patients with Apparently Normal Fertility and Fertility-Focused Intercourse," *Journal of Reproductive Medicine*, vol. 37, no. 10 (October 1992), pp. 864–66.

39. Quote taken from lecture handout of J. Stanford, annual meeting of the American
Holistic Medical Association, March 13, 1993. Study is cited in Hilgers, "The
Medical Applications of Natural Family Planning."

40. A. Wilcox and C. Weinberg, "Timing of Sexual Intercourse in Relation to Ovulation: Effects on the Probability of Conception, Survival of Pregnancy, and Sex of
Baby," *New England Journal of Medicine*, vol. 333 (December 7, 1995),
pp. 1517–21.

41. H. Klaus, "Natural Family Planning: A Review," *Obstetrics and Gynecology* Survey, vol. 37, no. 2 (February 1982), pp. 128–50; T. W. Hilgers and A. M. Prebil,
"The Ovulation Method: Vulvar Observations as an Index of Fertility and Infertility," *Obstetrics and Gynecology*, vol. 53, no. 1 (January 1979), pp. 12–22;
World Health Organization, "A Prospective Multicentre Trial of the Ovulation
Method of Natural Family Planning: I. The Teaching Phase," *Fertility and Sterility*, vol. 362 (August 1981), pp. 152–58.

42. T. W. Hilgers, G. F. Abraham, and D. Cavanagh, "Natural Family Planning. I.

The Peak Symptom and Estimated Time of Ovulation," *American Journal of Obstetrics and Gynecology,* vol. 52, no. 5 (November 1978), pp. 575–82.

43. Material for this section was obtained from Dr. Joseph Stanford.

44. J. F. Cattanach and B. J. Milne, "Post-Tubal Sterilization Problems Correlated with Ovarian Steroidogenesis," *Contraception,* vol. 38, no. 5 (1988); J. Donnez, M. Wauters, and K. Thomas, "Luteal Function After Tubal Sterilization," *Obstetrics and Gynecology,* vol. 57, no. 1 (1981); M. M. Cohen, "Long-Term Risk of Hysterectomy After Tubal Sterilization," *American Journal of Epidemiology,* vol. 125 (1987).

45. S. Sumiala et al., "Salivary Progesterone Concentration After Tubal Sterilization," *Obstetrics and Gynecology,* vol. 88 (1996), pp. 792–96.

46. J. Block, "The Battle over Essure," *The Washington Post,* July 26, 2017, www.washingtonpost.com/sf/style/2017/07/26/essure.

47. A. Domar et al., "The Prevalence and Predictability of Depression in Infertile Women," *Fertility and Sterility,* vol. 58 (1992), pp. 1158–63; A. Domar et al., "The Psychological Impact of Infertility: A Comparison with Patients with Other Medical Conditions," *Journal of Psychosomatic Obstetrics and Gynecology,* vol. 14 (1993), pp. 45–52.

48. I. Gerhard et al., "Prolonged Exposure to Wood Preservatives Induces Endocrine and Immunologic Disorders in Women," *American Journal of Obstetrics and Gynecology,* vol. 165, no. 2 (August 1991), pp. 487–88; P. Thompkins, "Hazards of Electromagnetic Fields to Human Reproduction," *Fertility and Sterility,* vol. 53, no. 1 (January 1990), p. 185; *The World Factbook 2009,* Central Intelligence Agency, Washington, D.C., https://www.cia.gov/library/publications/the-world-factbook/rankorder/2127rank.html.

49. A. Stagnaw-Green et al., "Detection of At Risk Pregnancy by Means of Highly Sensitive Assays for Thyroid Autoantibodies," *Journal of the American Medical Association,* vol. 269, no. 11 (September 19, 1990), pp. 1422–25; and O. B. Christiansen et al., "Autoimmunity and Spontaneous Abortion," *Human Reproduction* [Denmark], vol. 4, no. 8 (1989), pp. 913–17.

50. M. Stauber, "Psychosomatic Problems of Childless Couples," *Archives of Gynecology and Obstetrics,* vol. 245, nos. 1–4 (1989), pp. 1047–50.

51. L. Jeker et al., "Wish for a Child and Infertility: A Study of 116 Couples. I. Interview and Psychodynamic Hypotheses," *International Journal of Fertility,* vol. 33, no. 6 (1988), pp. 411–20.

52. D. Sable, "How Entrepreneurs Will Move IVF into the Future," *Forbes,* February 3, 2018.

53. S. Dyer et al., "International Committee for Monitoring Assisted Reproductive Technologies World Report: Assisted Reproductive Technology 2008, 2009 and 2010," *Human Reproduction,* vol. 31, no. 7 (July 2016), pp. 1588–609; V. A. Kushnir et al., "Systematic Review of Worldwide Trends in Assisted Reproductive Technology 2004–2013," *Reproductive Biology and Endocrinology,* vol. 15, no. 1 (January 10, 2017), p. 6.

54. T. Shevell et al., "Assisted Reproductive Technology and Pregnancy Outcome," *Obstetrics and Gynecology,* vol. 106, no. 5 (November 2005), pp. 1039–45.

55. P. Kemeter, "Studies on Psychosomatic Implications of Infertility: Effects of Emo-

tional Stress on Fertilization and Implantation in In Vitro Fertilization," *Human Reproduction,* vol. 3, no. 3 (April 1988), pp. 341–52.

56. F. Facchinetti et al., "An Increased Vulnerability to Stress Is Associated with a Poor Outcome of In Vitro Fertilization—Embryo Transfer Treatment," *Fertility and Sterility,* vol. 67 (1997), pp. 309–14.

57. K. Menninger, "Somatic Correlations with the Unconscious Repudiation of Femininity in Women," *Journal of Nervous and Mental Disease,* vol. 89 (1939), p. 514; Therese Benedek and Boris Rubenstein, "Correlations Between Ovarian Activity and Psychodynamic Processes: The Ovulatory Phase," *Psychosomatic Medicine,* vol. 1, no. 2 (1939), pp. 245–70; A. Mayer, "Sterility in Women as a Result of Functional Disturbance," *Journal of the American Medical Association,* vol. 105 (1935), p. 1474; Kemeter, "Studies on Psychosomatic Implications of Infertility."

58. H. Ellis, *Studies in the Psychology of Sex* (Philadelphia: Davis and Co., 1928); T. H. Van de Veld, *Fertility and Sterility in Marriage* (New York: Covici-Friede, 1931).

59. H. F. Dunbar, *Emotions and Bodily Changes* (New York: Columbia University Press, 1935), p. 595; R. L. Dickerson, "Medical Analysis of 1000 Marriages," *Journal of the American Medical Association,* vol. 97 (1931), p. 529; C. C. Norris, "Sterility in the Female Without Gross Pathology," *Surgery, Gynecology, and Obstetrics,* vol. 15 (1912), p. 706.

60. D. H. Hellhammer et al., "Male Infertility, Relationships Among Gonadotropins, Sex Steroids, Seminal Parameters, and Personality Attitudes," *Psychosomatic Medicine,* vol. 47, no. 1 (1985), pp. 58–66.

61. A. M. Brkovich and W. A. Fisher, "Psychological Distress and Infertility: Forty Years of Research," *Journal of Psychosomatic Obstetrics and Gynaecology,* vol. 19, no. 4 (December 1998), pp. 218–28.

62. A. D. Domar et al., "The Mind/Body Program for Infertility: A New Behavioral Treatment Approach for Women with Infertility," *Fertility and Sterility,* vol. 53., no. 2 (February 1990), pp. 246–49.

63. Reproductive Health Technologies Project, *Ovarian Stimulation and Egg Retrieval: Overview and Issues to Consider,* Washington, DC, 2009, www.rhtp.org/documents/RHTP-OvarianStimulationandEggRetrievalPaperUpdated.pdf.

64. Some of this material was originally published in the June 1997 issue of Christiane Northrup's newsletter, *Health Wisdom for Women.*

65. D. R. Meldrum, "Female Reproductive Aging—Ovarian and Uterine Factors," *Fertility and Sterility,* vol. 59, vol. 1 (January 1993), pp. 1–5; C. Wood, I. Calderon, and A. Crombie, "Age and Fertility: Results of Assisted Reproductive Technology in Women over 40 Years," *Journal of Assisted Reproduction and Genetics,* vol. 9, no. 5 (October 1992), pp. 482–84; S. L. Tan et al., "Cumulative Conception and Livebirth Rates After In-Vitro Fertilisation," *The Lancet,* vol. 339, no. 8806 (June 1992), p. 1390–94.

66. W. J. Kennedy, *Edinburgh Medical Journal,* vol. 27 (1882), p. 1086.

67. Personal communication from Brant Secunda.

68. J. Johnson et al., "Germline Stem Cells and Follicular Renewal in the Postnatal Mammalian Ovary," *Nature,* vol. 428, no. 6979 (March 11, 2004), pp. 145–50.

69. J. A. Martin et al., "Births: Final Data for 2017," *National Vital Statistics Report,* vol. 67, no. 8 (November 7, 2018), p. 4.

70. S. K. Henshaw, "Unintended Pregnancy in the United States," *Family Planning Perspectives,* vol. 30, no. 1 (January–February 1998), pp. 24–29, 46.

71. H. Benson, "Stress, Anxiety and the Relaxation Response," *Behavioral Biology in Medicine: A Monograph Series,* No. 3 (So. Norwalk, CT: Meducation, 1985), pp. 1–28.

72. While the pregnancy rate for other infertile couples seeking medical treatment is between 17 and 25 percent, the pregnancy rate in Dr. Domar's program is 44 percent, with 37 percent taking home a baby (some pregnancies end in miscarriage). "The Goddess of Fertility," *Boston Magazine,* March 1997, pp. 57–117.

73. Facchinetti et al., "An Increased Vulnerability to Stress."

74. H. Fisch with S. Braun, *The Male Biological Clock: The Startling News About Aging, Sexuality, and Fertility in Men* (New York: Free Press, 2005), p. xiii.

75. D. M. Kristensen et al., "Ibuprofen Alters Human Testicular Physiology to Produce a State of Compensated Hypogonadism," *Proceedngs of the National Academy of Sciences of the United States of America,* vol. 115, no. 4 (January 23, 2018), pp. E715–24.

76. J. Pei et al., "Quantitative Evaluation of Spermatozoa Ultrastructure After Acupuncture Treatment for Idiopathic Male Infertility," *Fertility and Sterility,* vol. 84, no. 1 (July 2005), pp. 141–47.

77. Fisch, p. xiv.

78. E. Dewan, "On the Possibility of a Perfect Rhythm Method of Birth Control by Periodic Light Stimulation," *American Journal of Obstetrics and Gynecology,* vol. 99, no. 7 (December 1, 1967), pp. 1016–19. See also notes for chapter 5, "The Menstrual Cycle."

79. J. A. Grieger et al., "Pre-Pregnancy Fast Food and Fruit Intake Is Associated with Time to Pregnancy," *Human Reproduction,* vol. 33, no. 6 (June 1, 2018), pp. 1063–70.

80. E. R. Gonzalez, "Sperm Swim Singly After Vitamin C Therapy," *Journal of the American Medical Association,* vol. 20 (1983), p. 2747; T. R. Haroma et al., "Zinc, Plasma Androgens, and Male Sterility," letter to the editor, *The Lancet,* vol. 3 (1977), pp. 1125–26; M. Igarashi, "Augmentative Effects of Ascorbic Acid upon Induction of Human Ovulation in Clomiphene Ineffective Anovulatory Women," *International Journal of Fertility,* vol. 22, no. 3 (1977), pp. 68–73; D. W. Dawson, "Infertility and Folate Deficiency," case reports, *British Journal of Obstetrics and Gynaecology,* vol. 89 (1982), p. 678.

81. J. Hargrove and E. Guy, "Effect of Vitamin B_6 on Infertility in Women with Premenstrual Tension Syndrome," *Infertility,* vol. 2, no. 4 (1979), pp. 315–22.

82. J. Chu et al., "Vitamin D and Assisted Reproductive Treatment Outcome: A Systematic Review and Meta-Analysis," *Human Reproduction,* vol. 33, no. 1 (January 1, 2018), pp. 65–80.

83. L. M. Westphal et al., "A Nutritional Supplement for Improving Fertility in Women: A Pilot Study," *Journal of Reproductive Medicine,* vol. 49, no. 4 (April 2004), pp. 289–93.

84. D. E. Stewart et al., "Infertility and Eating Disorders," *American Journal of Obstetrics and Gynecology*, vol. 163 (1990), pp. 1196–99.

85. A. Blau et al., "The Psychogenic Etiology of Premature Births," *Psychosomatic Medicine*, vol. 25 (1963), p. 201; Robert J. Weil, "The Problem of Spontaneous Abortion," *American Journal of Obstetrics and Gynecology*, vol. 73 (1957), p. 322.

86. L. Fenster et al., "Caffeinated Beverages, Decaffeinated Coffee, and Spontaneous Abortion," *Epidemiology*, vol. 8., no. 5 (September 1997), pp. 515–23.

87. R. L. Bick and D. Hoppensteadt, "Recurrent Miscarriage Syndrome and Infertility Due to Blood Coagulation Protein/Platelet Defects: A Review and Update," *Clinical and Applied Thrombosis/Hemostasis*, vol. 11, no. 1 (January 2005), pp. 1–13; F. E. Preston et al., "Increased Fetal Loss in Women with Heritable Thrombophilia," *The Lancet*, vol. 348, no. 9032 (October 5, 1996), pp. 913–16.

88. R. Stanford, "Recurrent Miscarriage Syndrome Treated with Acupuncture and an Allergy Elimination/Desensitization Technique," *Alternative Therapies in Health and Medicine*, vol. 15, no. 5 (September–October 2009), pp. 62–63.

89. R. J. Weil and C. Tupper, "Personality, Life Situation, Communication: A Study of Habitual Abortion," *Psychosomatic Medicine*, vol. 22, no. 6 (1960), pp. 448–55.

90. Ibid.

91. E. R. Grimm, "Psychological Investigation of Habitual Abortion," *Psychosomatic Medicine*, vol. 24, no. 4 (1962), pp. 370–78.

92. R. L. VandenBergh, "Emotional Illness in Habitual Aborters Following Suturing of Incompetent Cervical Os," *Psychosomatic Medicine*, vol. 28, no. 3 (1966), pp. 257–63.

93. "Chapter 10: Ectopic Pregnancy," in F. G. Cunningham et al., eds., *Williams Obstetrics*, 22d ed. (New York: McGraw-Hill Professional, 2005), pp. 254–55.

94. U. Chinagozi and C. Nugent, "Adoption-Related Behaviors Among Women Aged 18–44 in the United States: 2011–2015," National Center for Health Statistics Data Brief No. 315, July 2018, www.cdc.gov/nchs/products/databriefs/db315 .htm.

95. Evan B. Donaldson Adoption Institute, "Landmark Study Shows Vast Majority of Americans Support Adoption: Positive Attitudes Toward Adoption Give New Reason for Hope," press release on 2002 National Survey, June 19, 2002, www .adoptioninstitute.org/old/survey/press_release.html.

96. Union of Concerned Scientists, 2 Brattle Square, Cambridge, MA 02238, 617-547-5552, www.ucsusa.org.

97. D. Boyer and D. Fine, "Sexual Abuse as a Factor in Adolescent Pregnancy and Child Maltreatment," *Family Planning Perspectives*, vol. 24, no. 1 (January–February 1992), pp. 4–11, 19.

98. National Center for Health Statistics, *Vital Statistics of the United States, 2003*, vol. 1, *Natality*, www.cdc.gov/nchs/products/vsus/vsus_1980_2003.htm. National Center for Health Statistics, *Natality Public Use Files, 2000–2016*. J. A. Martin et al., "Births: Final Data for 2016," *National Center for Health Statistics National Vital Statistics Reports*, vol. 67, no. 1 (2018).

99. K. Ethier, L. Kann, and T. McManus, "Sexual Intercourse Among High School

Students—29 States and United States Overall, 2005–2015," *Morbidity and Mortality Weekly Report,* vol. 66, nos. 51–52 (January 5, 2018), pp. 1393–97.

Chapter 12: Pregnancy and Birthing

1. Betsey Stevenson as quoted in M. Dowd, "Blue Is the New Black," *New York Times,* September 20, 2009, p. WK9. Betsey Stevenson is coauthor with Justin Wolfers of "The Paradox of Declining Female Happiness," to be published in an upcoming edition of the *American Economic Journal: Economic Policy.*

2. Center for Women's Business Research, "Key Facts About Women-Owned Businesses," 2009; Brad Harrington and Jamie Ladge, "Got Talent? It Isn't Hard to Find," in Heather Boushey and Ann O'Leary, eds., *The Shriver Report: A Woman's Nation Changes Everything* (Washington, DC: Center for American Progress, 2009), p. 206.

3. M. Shriver, "The Unfinished Revolution," *Time,* October 26, 2009; *The Shriver Report: A Woman's Nation Changes Everything* (Washington, DC: Center for American Progress, 2009).

4. T. R. Verny and P. Weintraub, *Tomorrow's Baby: The Art and Science of Parenting from Conception Through Infancy* (New York: Simon & Schuster, 2002), p. 29.

5. P. W. Nathanielsz, *Life in the Womb: The Origin of Health and Disease* (Ithaca, NY: Promethean Press, 1999). L. Szabo, "Aging Well Starts in Womb, As Mom's Choices Affect Whole Life," *USA Today,* June 30, 2009, www.usatoday.com/news/health/2009-06-30-prenatalcover_N.htm.

6. U.S. Department of Health, Education, and Welfare, the National Center for Health Statistics, *Wanted and Unwanted Births by Mothers 15–44 Years of Age: United States, 1973* (Washington, DC: U.S. Government Printing Office, 1973); advance data from *Vital and Health Statistics,* no. 9 (August 10, 1977); National Institutes of Health, Institute of Child Health and Human Development, research reports, November 1992, available from NICHD Office of Research Reporting, building 31, room 2A312, National Institutes of Health, Bethesda, MD 01892, 310-496-5133; M. D. Muylder et al., "A Women's Attitude Toward Pregnancy: Can It Predispose Her to Preterm Labor?" *Journal of Reproductive Medicine,* vol. 37, no. 4 (April 1992); R. Newton and L. Hunt, "Psychosocial Stress in Pregnancy and Its Relationship to Low Birth Weight," *British Medical Journal,* vol. 288 (1984), p. 1191.

7. M. Lobel et al., "The Impact of Prenatal Maternal Stress and Optimistic Disposition on Birth Outcomes in Medically High-Risk Women," *Health Psychology,* vol. 19, no. 6 (November 2000), pp. 544–53.

8. V. L. Katz et al., "Catecholamine Levels in Pregnant Physicians and Nurses: A Pilot Study of Stress and Pregnancy," *Obstetrics and Gynecology,* vol. 77, no. 3 (March 1991), pp. 338–41.

9. S. Guendelman et al. "Maternity Leave in the Ninth Month of Pregnancy and Birth Outcomes Among Working Women," *Women's Health Issues,* vol. 19, no. 1 (January–February 2009), pp. 30–37.

10. C. D. Fryar, M. D. Carroll, and C. L. Ogden, "Prevalence of Overweight, Obesity, and Severe Obesity Among Adults Aged 20 and Over: United States, 1960–1962 Through 2015–2016," National Center for Health Statistics, September 2018, www.cdc.gov/nchs/data/hestat/obesity_adult_15_16/obesity_adult_15_16.pdf.

11. K. M. Rasmussen and A. L. Yaktine, eds., *Weight Gain During Pregnancy: Reexamining the Guidelines* (Washington, DC: National Academies Press, 2009).

12. A. M. Molloy et al., "Maternal Vitamin B_{12} Status and Risk of Neural Tube Defects in a Population with High Neural Tube Defect Prevalence and No Folic Acid Fortification," *Pediatrics,* vol. 123, no. 3 (March 2009), pp. 917–23.

13. A. Merewood et al., "Association Between Vitamin D Deficiency and Primary Cesarean Section," *Journal of Clinical Endocrinology and Metabolism,* vol. 94, no. 3 (2009), pp. 940–45.

14. E. S. N. Husebye et al., "Verbal Abilities in Children of Mothers with Epilepsy: Association to Maternal Folate Status," *Neurology,* vol. 91, no. 9 (August 28, 2018), pp. e811–21.

15. L. M. Bodnar, M. A. Krohn, and H. N. Simhan, "Maternal Vitamin D Deficiency Is Associated with Bacterial Vaginosis in the First Trimester of Pregnancy," *Journal of Nutrition,* vol. 139 (2009), pp. 1157–61.

16. M. L. Mulligan et al., "Implications of Vitamin D Deficiency in Pregnancy and Lactation," *American Journal of Obstetrics and Gynecology,* vol. 202, no. 5 (May 2010), pp. 429.e1–9.

17. C. L. Wagner and R. Lawrence, Pediatric Academic Societies annual meeting, Vancouver, British Columbia, May 1–4, 2010; S. Boyles, "High Doses of Vitamin D May Cut Pregnancy Risks," WebMD, May 4, 2010, www.webmd.com/baby/news/20100504/high-doses-of-vitamin-d-may-cut-pregnancy-risk#2.

18. S. L. McDonnell et al., "Maternal 25(OH)D Concentrations ≥40 ng/mL Associated with 60% Lower Preterm Birth Risk Among General Obstetrical Patients at an Urban Medical Center," *PLoS One,* vol. 12, no. 7 (July 24, 2017), p. e0180483.

19. J. A. McGregor et al., "The Omega-3 Story: Nutritional Prevention of Preterm Birth and Other Adverse Pregnancy Outcomes," *Obstetrical and Gynecological Survey,* vol. 56, no. 5 suppl. 1 (May 2001), pp. S1–13.

20. K. Owe et al., "Association Between Regular Exercise and Excessive Newborn Birth Weight," *Obstetrics and Gynecology,* vol. 114, no. 4 (October 2009), pp. 770–76.

21. M. Perales, R. Artal, and A. Lucia, "Exercise During Pregnancy," *Journal of the American Medical Association,* vol. 317, no. 11 (March 21, 2017), pp. 1113–14.

22. American College of Obstetricians and Gynecologists, "ACOG Committee Opinion No. 650: Physical Activity and Exercise During Pregnancy and the Postpartum Period," *Obstetrics and Gynecology,* vol. 126, no. 6 (December 2015), pp. e135–42.

23. T. Field et al., "Pregnant Women Benefit from Massage Therapy," *Journal of Psychosomatic Obstetrics and Gynaecology,* vol. 20, no. 1 (March 1999), pp. 31–38; T. Field, "Labor Pain Is Reduced by Massage Therapy," *Journal of Psychosomatic Obstetrics and Gynaecology,* vol. 18, no. 4 (December 1997), pp. 286–91.

24. D. A. Oren et al., "An Open Trial of Morning Light Therapy for Treatment of Antepartum Depression," *American Journal of Psychiatry,* vol. 159, no. 4 (April 2002), pp. 666–69.

25. E. B. Da Fonseca et al., "Prophylactic Administration of Progesterone by Vaginal Suppository to Reduce the Incidence of Spontaneous Preterm Birth in Women at Increased Risk: A Randomized Placebo-Controlled Double-Blind Study," *American Journal of Obstetrics and Gynecology*, vol. 188, no. 2 (February 2003), pp. 419–24; P. J. Meis et al., "Prevention of Recurrent Preterm Delivery by 17 Alpha-Hydroxyprogesterone Caproate," *New England Journal of Medicine*, vol. 348, no. 24 (June 12, 2003), pp. 2379–85.

26. E. R. Norwitz, L. E. Phaneuf, and A. B. Caughey, "Progesterone Supplementation and the Prevention of Preterm Birth," *Reviews in Obstetrics and Gynecology*, vol. 4, no. 2 (Summer 2011), pp. 60–72.

27. V. M. Schmouder et al., "The Rebirth of Progesterone in the Prevention of Preterm Labor," *Annals of Pharmacotherapy*, vol. 47, no. 4 (April 2013), pp. 527–36; E. B. da Fonseca et al., "Prophylactic Administration of Progesterone by Vaginal Suppository to Reduce the Incidence of Spontaneous Preterm Birth in Women at Increased Risk: A Randomized Placebo-Controlled Double-Blind Study," *American Journal of Obstetrics and Gynecology*, vol. 188, no. 2 (February 2003), pp. 419–24; P. J. Meis et al., "Prevention of Recurrent Preterm Delivery by 17 alpha-hydroxyprogesterone caproate," *New England Journal of Medicine*, vol. 348, no. 24 (June 12, 2003), pp. 2379–85.

28. R. Romero et al., "Vaginal Progesterone for Preventing Preterm Birth and Adverse Perinatal Outcomes in Singleton Gestations with a Short Cervix: A Meta-Analysis of Individual Patient Data," *American Journal of Obstetrics and Gynecology*, vol. 218, no. 2 (February 2018), pp. 161–80.

29. J. E. Norman et al., "Progesterone for the Prevention of Preterm Birth in Twin Pregnancy (STOPPIT): A Randomised, Double-Blind, Placebo-Controlled Study and Meta-Analysis," *The Lancet*, vol. 373, no. 9680 (June 13, 2009), pp. 2034–40.

30. N. Mamelle et al., "Prevention of Preterm Birth in Patients with Symptoms of Preterm Labor—The Benefits of Psychologic Support," *American Journal of Obstetrics and Gynecology*, vol. 177, no. 4 (1977), pp. 947–52.

31. S. E. Andrade et al., "Prescription Drug Use in Pregnancy," *American Journal of Obstetrics and Gynecology*, vol. 191, no. 2 (August 2004), pp. 398–407.

32. J. G. Donahue et al., "Association of Spontaneous Abortion with Receipt of Inactivated Influenza Vaccine Containing H1N1pdm09 in 2010–11 and 2011–12," *Vaccine*, vol. 35, no. 40 (September 25, 2017), pp. 5314–22.

33. "Pregnancy and Medicine," *WebMD*, article reviewed by Nivin Todd, M.D., on August 5, 2018, www.webmd.com/women/pregnancy-medicine.

34. S. H. Schmitz et al., "Side Effects of AZT Prophylaxis After Occupational Exposure to HIV-Infected Blood," *Annals of Hematology*, vol. 69, no. 3 (September 1994), pp. 135–38; Concorde Coordinating Committee, "Concorde: MRC/ANRS Randomized Double-Blind Controlled Trial of Immediate and Deferred Zidovudine in Symptom-Free HIV Infection," *The Lancet*, vol. 343, no. 8902 (April 9, 1994), pp. 871–81; M. C. Dalakas et al., "Mitochondrial Myopathy Caused by Long-Term Zidovudine Therapy," *New England Journal of Medicine*, vol. 322, no. 16 (April 19, 1990), pp. 1098–105.

35. Institute of Medicine (US) Committee on Reviewing the HIVNET 012 Perinatal HIV Prevention Study, *Review of the HIVNET 012 Perinatal HIV Prevention Study* (Washington, DC: National Academies Press, 2005), https://www.ncbi.nlm.nih.gov/books/NBK22293.

36. E. Cardis and the INTERPHONE Study Group, "Brain Tumour Risk in Relation to Mobile Telephone Use: Results of the INTERPHONE International Case-Control Study," *International Journal of Epidemiology*, vol. 39, no. 3 (June 2010), pp. 675–94.

37. IuG. Grigor'ev, "The Probability of Developing Brain Tumors Among Users of Cellular Telephones (Scientific Information to the Decision of the International Agency for Research on Cancer (IARC) Announced on May 31, 2011)," *Radiatsionnaia Biologila, Radioecologiia*, vol. 51, no. 5 (September–October 2011), pp. 633–38.

38. M. Wyde et al., "Report of Partial Findings from the National Toxicology Program Carcinogenesis Studies of Cell Phone Radiofrequency Radiation in Hsd: Sprague Dawley SD Rats (Whole Body Exposure)," *bioRxiv*, May 26, 2016, modified February 1, 2018, https://doi.org/10.1101/055699.

39. National Institute of Environmental Health Sciences National Toxicology Program, *Peer Review of the Draft NTP Technical Reports on Cell Phone Radiofrequency Radiation*, March 26–28, 2018, https://ntp.niehs.nih.gov/ntp/about_ntp/trpanel/2018/march/peerreview20180328_508.pdf.

40. E. Cardis et al., "The INTERPHONE Study: Design, Epidemiological Methods, and Description of the Study Population," *European Journal of Epidemiology*, vol. 22, no. 9 (2007), pp. 647–64; L. Hardell, M. Carlberg, and D. Gee, "Mobile Phone Use and Brain Tumour Risk: Early Warnings, Early Actions? Late Lessons from Early Warnings: Science, Precaution, Innovation," *European Environmental Agency Report*, no. 1, January 22, 2013, pp. 509–29; G. Coureau et al., "Mobile Phone Use and Brain Tumours in the CERENAT Case-Control Study," *Occupational and Environmental Medicine*, vol. 71, no. 7 (July 2014), pp. 514–22.

41. J. A. Martin et al., "Births: Final Data for 2016," *National Vital Statistics Report*, vol. 67, no. 1, January 31, 2018, p. 8.

42. K. Fuchs and R. Wapner, "Elective Cesarean Section and Induction and Their Impact on Late Preterm Births," *Clinics in Perinatology*, vol. 33, no. 4 (December 2006), pp. 793–801; "Preterm Birth Rate Continues to Rise," *The Medical News*, October 5, 2009, www.news-medical.net/news/20091005/Preterm-birth-rate-continues-to-rise.aspx.

43. R. Meyers, "Maternal Anxiety and Fetal Death," *Psychoneuroimmunology in Reproduction* (New York: Elsevier/North-Holland Biomedical Press, 1979), pp. 555–73.

44. L. E. Mehl et al., "The Role of Hypnotherapy in Facilitating Normal Birth," in P. G. Fedor-Freburgh and M. L. V. Vogel, eds., *Encounter with the Unborn: Perinatal Psychology and Medicine* (Park Ridge, NJ: Parthenon, 1988), pp. 189–207; I. E. Mehl, "Hypnosis in Preventing Premature Labor," *Journal of Prenatal and Perinatal Psychology*, vol. 8 (1988), pp. 234–240; A. Omer, "Hypnosis and Premature Labor," *Journal of Psychosomatic Medicine*, vol. 57 (1986), pp. 454–60.

45. R. L. VandenBerge et al., "Emotional Illness in Habitual Aborters Following Suturing of the Incompetent Cervical Os," *Psychosomatic Medicine*, vol. 28, no. 3 (1966), pp. 257–63.

46. L. B. Finer and M. R. Zolna, "Declines in Unintended Pregnancy in the United States, 2008–2011," *New England Journal of Medicine*, vol. 374, no. 9 (March 3, 2016), pp. 843–52.

47. V. Laukaran and C. van Den Berg, "The Relationship of Maternal Attitude to Pregnancy Outcomes and Obstetric Complications: A Cohort Study of Unwanted Pregnancies," *American Journal of Obstetrics and Gynecology,* vol. 139 (1981), p. 596; R. McDonald, "The Role of Emotional Factors in Obstetric Complications," *Psychosomatic Medicine,* vol. 30 (1968), p. 222; M. D. De Muylder, "Psychological Factors and Preterm Labour," *Journal of Reproductive Psychology,* vol. 7 (1989), p. 55.

48. R. Myers, "Maternal Anxiety and Fetal Death," in L. Zichella and P. Pancheri, eds., *Psychoneuroendocrinocology and Reproduction* (New York: Elsevier, 1979).

49. L. E. Mehl-Madrona, "Psychosocial Prenatal Intervention to Reduce Alcohol, Smoking, and Stress and Improve Birth Outcome Among Minority Women," *Journal of Prenatal and Perinatal Psychology and Health,* vol. 14, no. 3 (2000), pp. 257–79.

50. H. P. Schobel et al., "Preeclampsia: A State of Sympathetic Overactivity," *New England Journal of Medicine,* vol. 335, no. 20 (1996), pp. 480–85; H. J. Passloer, "Angstlich—Feindseliges Verhalten als Prakursor einer Schaumangerschafstinduzierten Hypertonic (SIJ)," *A. Guburtsh Perinat.,* vol. 195 (1991), pp. 137–42.

51. E. Muller-Tyl and B. Wimmer-Puchinger, "Psychosomatic Aspects of Toxemia," *Journal of Psychosomatic Obstetrics and Gynecology,* vol. 1, nos. 3–4 (1982), pp. 111–17; C. Ringrose, "Psychosomatic Influence in the Genesis of Toxemia of Pregnancy," *Canadian Medical Association Journal,* vol. 84 (1961), p. 647; and A. J. Cooper, "Psychosomatic Aspects of Pre-eclamptic Toxemia," *Journal of Psychosomatic Research,* vol. 2 (1958), p. 241.

52. R. L. McDonald, "Personality Characteristics in Patients with Three Obstetric Complications," *Psychosomatic Medicine,* vol. 27, no. 4 (1965), pp. 383–90.

53. C. Cheek and E. Rossi, *Mind-Body Hypothesis* (New York: W. W. Norton, 1989).

54. L. Mehl, "Hypnosis and Conversion of the Breech to the Vertex Position," *Archives of Family Medicine,* vol. 3 (1994), pp. 881–87.

55. Martin et al., "Births: Final Data for 2016," p. 4.

56. Ibid., p. 7.

57. F. Althabe and J. F. Belizan, "Caesarean Section: The Paradox," *The Lancet,* vol. 368 (2006), pp. 1472–73.

58. O. E. Keag, J. E. Norman, and S. J. Stock, "Long-Term Risks and Benefits Associated with Cesarean Delivery for Mother, Baby, and Subsequent Pregnancies: Systematic Review and Meta-Analysis," *PLoS Medicine,* vol. 15, no. 1 (January 23, 2018), p. e1002494.

59. S. M. Taffel, P. J. Placek, and T. Liss, "Trends in the United States Cesarean Section Rate and Reasons for the 1980–85 Rise," *American Journal of Public Health,* vol. 77, no. 8 (1987), pp. 955–59.

60. S. Levy and L. Kane, "Medscape Ob/Gyn Malpractice Report 2017: Real Physicians. Real Lawsuits," *Medscape,* December 5, 2017, https://www.medscape.com/slideshow/2017-obgyn-malpractice-report-6009316#1.

61. American College of Obstetricians and Gynecologists (ACOG), 57th Annual Clinical Meeting, papers on current clinical and basic investigation, presented May 5, 2009.

62. M. J. K. Osterman and J. A. Martin, "Recent Declines in Induction of Labor by

Gestational Age," National Center for Health Statistics Data Brief No. 155, June 2014, p. 1, https://www.cdc.gov/nchs/products/databriefs/db155.htm.

63. T. Postel, "Childbirth Climax: The Revealing of Obstetrical Orgasm," *Sexologies,* vol. 22, no. 4 (October–December 2013), pp. e89–92.

64. L. Crocker, "Can Women Orgasm During Childbirth," *The Daily Beast,* June 9, 2013, www.thedailybeast.com/can-women-orgasm-during-childbirth.

65. A. de Jonge et al., "Perinatal Mortality and Morbidity in a Nationwide Cohort of 529,688 Low-Risk Planned Home and Hospital Births," *BJOG: An International Journal of Obstetrics and Gynaecology,* vol. 116 (August 2009), pp. 1177–84.

66. K. C. Johnson and B. A. Daviss, "Outcomes of Planned Home Births with Certified Professional Midwives: Large Prospective Study in North America," *British Medical Journal,* vol. 330, no. 7505 (June 18, 2005), p. 1416.

67. M. Cheyney, M. Bovbjerg, C. Everson, W. Gordon, D. Hannibal, and S. Vedam, "Outcomes of Care for 16,924 Planned Home Births in the United States: The Midwives Alliance of North America Statistics Project, 2004 to 2009," *Journal of Midwifery and Women's Health,* vol. 59, no. 1 (January–February 2014), pp. 17–27.

68. Centers for Disease Control and Prevention, "State-Specific Maternal Mortality Among Black and White Women—United States, 1987–1996," *Morbidity and Mortality Weekly Report,* vol. 48, no. 23 (June 18, 1999).

69. American College of Nurse-Midwives, "Fact Sheet: CNM/CM-Attended Birth Statistics in the United States," updated March 2016, www.midwife.org/acnm/files/ccLibraryFiles/Filename/000000005950/CNM-CM-AttendedBirths-2014-031416FINAL.pdf.

70. I. M. Gaskin, "Maternal Death in the United States: A Problem Solved or a Problem Ignored?" *Journal of Perinatal Education,* vol. 17, no. 2 (Spring 2008), pp. 9–13.

71. N. J. Kassebaum et al., "Global, Regional, and National Levels of Maternal Mortality, 1990–2015: A Systematic Analysis for the Global Burden of Disease Study 2015," *The Lancet,* vol. 388, no. 10053 (October 8, 2016), pp. 1775–1812.

72. N. Martin, R. Montagne, "U.S. Has the Worst Rate of Maternal Deaths in the Developed World," National Public Radio, May 12, 2017, https://www.npr.org/2017/05/12/528098789/u-s-has-the-worst-rate-of-maternal-deaths-in-the-developed-world.

73. Centers for Disease Control, Pregnancy Mortality Surveillance System, data reported from 2011 to 2014, https://www.cdc.gov/reproductivehealth/maternalinfanthealth/pregnancy-mortality-surveillance-system.htm.

74. New York City Department of Health and Mental Hygiene, Bureau of Maternal, Infant and Reproductive Health, "Pregnancy-Associated Mortality, New York City 2006–2010," https://www1.nyc.gov/assets/doh/downloads/pdf/ms/pregnancy-associated-mortality-report.pdf.

75. E. R. Declercq et al., "Major Survey Findings of Listening to Mothers (SM) III: Pregnancy and Birth: Report of the Third National U.S. Survey of Women's Childbearing Experiences," *Journal of Perinatal Education,* vol. 23, no. 1 (Winter 2014), pp. 9–16; E. R. Declercq et al., "Major Survey Findings of Listening to Mothers (SM) III: New Mothers Speak Out: Report of National Surveys of Women's Childbearing Experiences Conducted October–December 2012 and January–

April 2013," *Journal of Perinatal Education,* vol. 23, no. 1 (Winter 2014), pp. 17–24.

76. New York City Department of Health and Mental Hygiene, "Severe Maternal Morbidity in New York City, 2008–2012," 2016, https://www1.nyc.gov/assets/doh/downloads/pdf/data/maternal-morbidity-report-08-12.pdf.

77. S. H. Meghani, E. Byun, and R. M. Gallagher, "Time to Take Stock: A Meta-Analysis and Systematic Review of Analgesic Treatment Disparities for Pain in the United States," *Pain Medicine,* vol. 13, no. 2 (February 2012), pp. 150–74; K. A. Schulman et al., "The Effect of Race and Sex on Physicians' Recommendations for Cardiac Catheterization," *New England Journal of Medicine,* vol. 340, no. 8 (February 25, 1999), pp. 618–26.

78. ACOG Statement of Policy on Racial Bias, February 2017, www.acog.org/-/media/Statements-of-Policy/Public/StatementofPolicy93RacialBias2017-2.pdf.

79. Building U.S. Capacity to Review and Prevent Maternal Deaths, *Report from Nine Maternal Mortality Review Committees,* 2018, http://reviewtoaction.org/Report_from_Nine_MMRCs.

80. B. Sawyer and S. Gonzales, "How Does Infant Mortality in the U.S. Compare to Other Countries?" Peterson-Kaiser Health System Tracker, July 7, 2017, https://www.healthsystemtracker.org/chart-collection/infant-mortality-u-s-compare-countries.

81. J. Levit, *Brought to Bed: Childbearing in America, 1750–1950* (New York: Oxford University Press, 1988).

82. R. Sosa et al., "The Effect of Supportive Companions on Perinatal Problems, Length of Labor, and Mother-Infant Interaction," *New England Journal of Medicine,* vol. 303 (1980), pp. 597–600; M. H. Klaus et al., "Effects of Social Support During Parturition in Maternal and Infant Mortality," *British Medical Journal,* vol. 293 (1986), pp. 585–87; M. H. Klaus et al., "Maternal Assistance and Support in Labor: Father, Nurse, Midwife, or Doula?" *Clinical Consultation in Obstetrics and Gynecology,* vol. 4 (December 1992).

83. R. M. Sapolsky, *Why Zebras Don't Get Ulcers* (New York: W. H. Freeman, 1994), pp. 116–22.

84. F. T. Kapp et al., "Some Psychological Factors in Prolonged Labor Due to Inefficient Uterine Action," *Comparative Psychiatry,* vol. 4 (1963), p. 9; L. Gunter, "Psychopathology and Stress in the Life Experience of Mothers of Premature Infants," *American Journal of Obstetrics and Gynecology,* vol. 86 (1963), p. 333; A. Davids and S. Devault, "Maternal Anxiety During Pregnancy and Childbirth Abnormalities," *Journal of Psychosomatic Medicine,* vol. 24 (1972), p. 464.

85. Questions provided here are part of the American College of Obstetricians and Gynecologists' Domestic Violence Screening Program.

86. J. J. Oat et al., "Characteristics and Motives of Women Choosing Elective Induction of Labor," *Journal of Psychosomatic Research,* vol. 30, no. 3 (1986), pp. 375–80.

87. Cited in G. H. Peterson, *Birthing Normally: A Personal Approach to Childbirth* (Berkeley, CA: Mindbody Press), appendix 2, p. 181. See also L. Mehl et al., "Complications of Home Delivery: Analysis of a Series of 287 Deliveries from Santa Cruz, California," *Birth and Family Journal,* vol. 2, no. 4 (1975), pp. 123–31; and G. Peterson et al., "Outcome of 1146 Elective Home Births," *Journal of Reproductive Medicine,* vol. 19, no. 3 (1977), pp. 281–90.

88. Data are from the Houston Healthcare Coalition, Houston, TX (1986); personal communications with Dr. Bethany Hays.

89. D. A. Luthy et al., "Effects of Electronic Fetal Heart Rate Monitoring as Compared with Periodic Auscultation on the Neurologic Development of Premature Infants," *New England Journal of Medicine* 322, no. 9 (March 1, 1990), pp. 588–93.

90. E. R. Declercq et al., "Major Survey Findings of Listening to Mothers (SM) III: New Mothers Speak Out: Report of National Surveys of Women's Childbearing Experiences Conducted October–December 2012 and January–April 2013)," *Journal of Perinatal Education,* vol. 23, no. 1 (Winter 2014), pp. 17–24.

91. American College of Gynecologists and Obstetricians, "Practice Bulletin No. 106: Intrapartum Fetal Heart Rate Monitoring: Nomenclature, Interpretation, and General Management Principles," *Obstetrics and Gynecology,* vol. 114, no. 1 (July 2009), pp. 192–202; American College of Gynecologists and Obstetricians, "ACOG Refines Fetal Heart Rate Monitoring Guidelines," press release, June 22, 2009, www.acog.org/from_home/publications/press_releases/nr06-22-09-2.cfm.

92. S. Gardner, "When Your Patient Demands a C-Section," *OBG Management,* November 1991.

93. M. H. Hall, "Commentary: Confidential Enquiry into Maternal Death," *British Journal of Obstetrics and Gynaecology,* vol. 97, no. 8 (August 1990), pp. 752–53; N. Schuitemaker et al., "Maternal Mortality After Cesarean Section in the Netherlands," *Acta Obstetricia et Gynecologica Scandinavica,* vol. 76, no. 4 (1997), pp. 332–34; C. Deneuz-Tharaux et al., *Obstetrics and Gynecology,* vol. 108, no. 3 (part 1) (September 2006), pp. 541–48.

94. E. L. Shearer, "Cesarean Section: Medical Benefits and Costs," *Social Science and Medicine,* vol. 37, no. 10 (1993), pp. 1223–31; American College of Obstetricians and Gynecologists, Task Force on Cesarean Delivery Rates, *Evaluation of Cesarean Delivery* (Washington, DC: ACOG, 2000).

95. S. M. Miovich et al., "Major Concerns of Women After Cesarean Delivery," *Journal of Obstetric, Gynecologic, and Neonatal Nursing,* vol. 23, no. 1 (1994), pp. 53–59.

96. E. R. Declercq et al., *Listening to Mothers: Report of the First National U.S. Survey of Women's Childbearing Experiences* (New York: Maternity Center Association/ Harris Interactive Inc., October 2002); E. Declercq et al., "Mothers' Reports of Postpartum Pain Associated with Vaginal and Cesarean Deliveries: Results of a National Survey," *Birth,* vol. 35, no. 1 (March 2008), pp. 16–24.

97. M. Lydon-Rochelle et al., "Association Between Method of Delivery and Maternal Rehospitalization," *Journal of the American Medical Association,* vol. 283, no. 18 (2000), pp. 2411–16; E. Declercq et al., "Maternal Outcomes Associated with Planned Primary Cesarean Births Compared with Planned Vaginal Births," *Obstetrics and Gynecology,* vol. 109, no. 3 (March 2007), pp. 669–77; H. Goer, M. Sagady Leslie, and A. Romano, "Step 6: Does Not Routinely Employ Practices, Procedures Unsupported by Scientific Evidence," *Journal of Perinatal Education,* vol. 16, no. 1 (Winter 2007), pp. 32S–64S.

98. E. Declercq et al., "Mothers' Reports of Postpartum Pain Associated with Vaginal and Cesarean Deliveries: Results of a National Survey," *Birth,* vol. 35, no. 1 (March 2008), pp. 16–24.

99. J. Jolly, J. Walker, and K. Bhabra, "Subsequent Obstetric Performance Related to Primary Mode of Delivery," *British Journal of Obstetrics and Gynaecology*, vol. 106, no. 3 (1999), pp. 227–32.

100. J. M. Crane et al., "Neonatal Outcomes with Placenta Previa," *Obstetrics and Gynecology*, vol. 93, no. 4 (1999), pp. 541–44.

101. G. C. Smith, J. P. Pell, and R. Dobbie, "Caesarean Section and Risk of Unexplained Stillbirth in Subsequent Pregnancy," *The Lancet*, vol. 362, no. 9398 (November 29, 2003), pp. 1779–84; R. Gray et al., "Caesarean Delivery and Risk of Stillbirth in Subsequent Pregnancy: A Retrospective Cohort Study in an English Population," *British Journal of Obstetrics and Gynaecology*, vol. 114, no. 3 (March 2007), pp. 264–70; R. Kennare et al., "Risks of Adverse Outcomes in the Next Birth After a First Cesarean Delivery," *Obstetrics and Gynecology*, vol. 109, no. 2 (part 1) (May 2007), pp. 270–76; R. Richter, R. L. Bergmann, and J. W. Dudenhausen, "Previous Caesarean or Vaginal Delivery: Which Mode Is a Greater Risk of Perinatal Death at the Second Delivery?" *European Journal of Obstetrics and Gynecology and Reproductive Biology*, vol. 132, no. 1 (May 2007), pp. 51–57; L. K. Taylor et al., "Risk of Complications in a Second Pregnancy Following Caesarean Section in the First Pregnancy: A Population-Based Study," *Medical Journal of Australia*, vol. 183, no. 10 (November 21, 2005), pp. 515–19.

102. T. Rosen, "Placenta Accreta and Cesarean Scar Pregnancy: Overlooked Costs of the Rising Cesarean Section Rate," *Clinics in Perinatology*, vol. 35, no. 3 (September 2008), pp. 519–29.

103. March of Dimes, medical references: preterm birth, http://www.marchofdimes .com/professionals/14332_1157.asp.

104. M. A. Van Ham, P. W. van Dongen, and J. Mulder, "Maternal Consequences of Caesarean Section. A Retrospective Study of Intra-Operative and Postoperative Maternal Complications of Caesarean Section During a 10-Year Period," *European Journal of Obstetrics, Gynecology, and Reproductive Biology*, vol. 74, no. 1 (1997), pp. 1–6.

105. D. J. Annibale et al., "Comparative Neonatal Morbidity of Abdominal and Vaginal Deliveries After Uncomplicated Pregnancies," *Archives of Pediatrics and Adolescent Medicine*, vol. 149, no. 8 (1995), pp. 862–67.

106. E. M. Levine et al., "Mode of Delivery and Risk of Respiratory Diseases in Newborns," *Obstetrics and Gynecology*, vol. 97, no. 3 (2001), pp. 439–42.

107. T. Schlinzig et al., "Epigenetic Modulation at Birth—Altered DNA-Methylation in White Blood Cells After Caesarean Section," *Acta Paediatrica*. vol. 98, no. 7 (July 2009), pp. 1096–99.

108. American College of Obstetricians-Gynecologists, "ACOG Practice Bulletin: Episiotomy: Clinical Management Guidelines for Obstetrician-Gynecologists: Number 71, April 2006," *Obstetrics and Gynecology*, vol. 107, no. 4 (April 2006), pp. 957–62.

109. A. M. Friedman et al., "Variation in and Factors Associated with Use of Episiotomy," *Journal of the American Medical Association*, vol. 313, no. 2 (January 13, 2015), pp. 197–99.

110. P. Shiono et al., "Midline Episiotomies: More Harm Than Good," *American Journal of Obstetrics and Gynecology*, vol. 75, no. 5 (May 1990), pp. 765–70.

111. M. P. R. Walker et al., "Epidural Anesthesia, Episiotomy, and Obstetric Lacera-

tion," *American Journal of Obstetrics and Gynecology*, vol. 77, no. 5 (May 1991), pp. 668–71.

112. F. Vieira et al., "Scientific Evidence on Perineal Trauma During Labor: Integrative Review," *European Journal of Obstetrics, Gynecology and Reproductive Biology*, vol. 223 (April 2018), pp. 18–25.

113. J. Ecker et al., "Is There a Benefit to Episiotomy at Operative Vaginal Delivery: Observations over 10 Years in a Stable Population," *American Journal of Obstetrics and Gynecology*, vol. 176 (1997), pp. 411–14.

114. K. Hartmann et al., "Outcomes of Routine Episiotomy: A Systematic Review," *Journal of the American Medical Association*, vol. 293, no. 17 (May 4, 2005), pp. 2141–48.

115. J. Press et al., "Mode of Delivery and Pelvic Floor Dysfunction: A Systematic Review of the Literature on Urinary and Fecal Incontinence and Sexual Dysfunction by Mode of Delivery," Medscape Ob/Gyn and Women's Health, Clinical Update, posted January 17, 2006, http://www.medscape.com/viewprogram/4989.

116. J. Thorpe et al., "The Effect of Continuous Epidural Anesthesia on Cesarean Sections for Dystocia in Primiparous Patients," *American Journal of Obstetrics and Gynecology*, vol. 161, no. 3 (September 1989); H. Kaminski, A. Stafl, and J. Aiman, "The Effect of Epidural Analgesia on the Frequency of Instrumental Obstetric Delivery," *American Journal of Obstetrics and Gynecology*, vol. 69, no. 5 (May 1987); L. Fusi et al., "Maternal Pyrexia Associated with the Use of Epidural Analgesia in Labour," *The Lancet*, vol. 1, no. 8649 (1989), pp. 1250–51.

117. E. Lieberman et al., "Association of Epidural Analgesia with Cesarean Delivery in Nulliparas," *Obstetrics and Gynecology*, vol. 88 (1996), pp. 993–1000; Shiv Sharma et al., "Cesarean Delivery: A Randomized Trial of Epidural Versus Patient-Controlled Meperidine Analgesia During Labor," *Anesthesiology*, vol. 87, no. 3 (1997), pp. 487–94; David Chestnut, "Epidural Analgesia and the Incidence of Cesarean Section," *Anesthesiology*, vol. 87, no. 3 (1997), pp. 472–76.

118. E. Lieberman et al., "Changes in Fetal Position During Labor and Their Association with Epidural Analgesia," *Obstetrics and Gynecology*, vol. 105, no. 5, Pt. 1 (May 2005), pp. 974–82.

119. E. Lieberman, "Epidural Analgesia, Intrapartum Fever, and Neonatal Sepsis Evaluation," *Pediatrics*, vol. 99, no. 1 (1997), pp. 415–19.

120. "Peter Chamberlen, the Elder." 2010. Encyclopedia Brittanica Online. March 11, 2010.

121. Known as the McRoberts maneuver, this can be demonstrated by bringing your legs up into a squatting position while lying on your back.

122. M. Klaus, J. Kennell, and P. Klaus, *Mothering the Mother: How a Doula Can Help You Have Shorter, Easier, and Healthier Birth* (New York: Addison-Wesley, 1993), p. 25.

123. J. Stenson, "Number of C-Sections Must Be Reduced," *Medical Tribune*, May 2, 1996.

124. S. Bewley, "Obstetricians' Views on Caesarean Section Versus Vaginal Birth," *The Lancet*, vol. 347, no. 9009 (April 27, 1996), p. 1189.

125. S. Tahseen and M. Griffiths, "Vaginal Birth After Two Caesarean Sections (VBAC-2): A Systematic Review with Meta-Analysis of Success Rate and Adverse Outcomes of VBAC-2 Versus VBAC-1 and Repeat (Third) Caesarean Sections,"

British Journal of Gynecology, vol. 117, no. 1 (January 2010), pp. 5–19; American College of Obstetricians and Gynecologists, "Practice Bulletin No. 194: Vaginal Birth After Cesarean Delivery," *Obstetrics and Gynecology,* vol. 130, no. 5 (November 2017), pp. e217-e233.

126. M. B. Landon et al., "Maternal and Perinatal Outcomes Associated with a Trial of Labor After Prior Cesarean Delivery," *New England Journal of Medicine,* vol. 351, no. 25 (December 16, 2004), pp. 2581–89.

127. National Institutes of Health Consensus Development Conference, *Vaginal Birth After Cesarean: New Insights,* March 8–10, 2010, https://consensus.nih.gov/2010/images/vbac/vbac_abstracts.pdf.

128. M. G. Dominguez-Bello et al., "Partial Restoration of the Microbiota of Cesarean-Born Infants via Vaginal Microbial Transfer," *Nature Medicine,* vol. 22, no. 3 (March 2016), pp. 250–53.

129. ACOG Committee on Obstetric Practice, "Committee Opinion No. 725: Vaginal Seeding," *Obstetrics and Gynecology,* vol. 130, no. 5 (November 2017), pp. e274–78, http://journals.lww.com/greenjournal/Fulltext/2017/11000/Committee_Opinion_No_725_Vaginal_Seeding.52.aspx.

130. Membranes rarely rupture from pelvic examinations. Perhaps mine did because of an unusual umbilical cord insertion on the membranes, known as a velamentous insertion. Or maybe they were just ready to go!

131. As we will see, being "distracted" in the middle of a process as important as labor may not be the best approach.

132. V. Noble, *Shakti Woman* (San Francisco: Harper and Row, 1992).

133. A. A. Tobian et al., "Male Circumcision for the Prevention of HSV-2 and HPV Infections and Syphilis," *New England Journal of Medicine,* vol. 360, no. 13 (March 26, 2009), pp. 1298–309.

134. G. A. Millett et al., "Circumcision Status and Risk of HIV and Sexually Transmitted Infections Among Men Who Have Sex with Men: A Meta-Analysis," *Journal of the American Medical Association,* vol. 300, no. 14 (October 8, 2008), pp. 1674–84; D. J. Templeton, G. A. Millett, and A. E. Grulich, "Make Circumcision to Reduce the Risk of HIV and Sexually Transmitted Infections Among Men Who Have Sex with Men," *Current Opinion in Infectious Diseases,* vol. 23, no. 1 (February 2010), pp. 45–52; "Call for Higher Circumcision Rate," BBC News, March 26, 2009, http://news.bbc.co.uk/go/pr/fr/-/2/hi/health/7960798.stm.

135. J. S. Svobada, "Circumcision of Male Infants as a Human Rights Violation," *Journal of Medical Ethics,* vol. 39, no. 7 (July 2013), pp. 469–74.

136. G. Denniston, "Unnecessary Circumcision," *Female Patient,* vol. 17 (July 1992), p. 13.

137. Data on the effects of circumcision are available from the Circumcision Resource Center, 617-523-0088, www.circumcision.org.

138. M. Owings, S. Uddin, and S. Williams, "Trends in Circumcision for Male Newborns in U.S. Hospitals: 1979–2010," Centers for Disease Control and Prevention's Division of Health Care Statistics, August 2013.

139. World Health Organization and Joint United Nations Programme on HIV/AIDS, *Neonatal and Child Male Circumcision: A Global Review,* April 2010, p. 5, www.who.int/hiv/pub/malecircumcision/neonatal_child_MC_UNAIDS.pdf.

Chapter 13: Motherhood: Bonding with Your Baby

1. M. H. Klaus and J. H. Kennell, *Maternal-Infant Bonding* (St. Louis, MO: C. V. Mosby Company, 1976).

2. Ibid.

3. C. M. Huhn et al., "Tactile-Kinesthetic Stimulation Effects on Sympathetic and Adrenocortical Function in Preterm Infants," *Journal of Pediatrics*, vol. 119, no. 3 (1991), pp. 434–40.

4. Actually, the first studies on putting babies in incubators were done on premature babies who weren't expected to live and who therefore had been "discarded" by their mothers. Martin Cooney, a pioneer in neonatal care, put a group of these infants in incubators and toured with them, even to the Chicago World's Fair, where he had an attraction called "Live Babies in Incubator"; its receipts were second only to those of Sally Rand the Fan Dancer. Once he got the babies to a certain weight, he tried to give them back to their mothers, but the mothers didn't want them, having formed no emotional tie with them. This information is from Kennell and Klaus, *Maternal-Infant Bonding*.

5. G. M. Morley, "Cord Closure: Can Hasty Clamping Injure the Newborn?" *OBG Management*, vol. 10, no. 7 (1998), pp. 29–36; S. Kinmond et al., "Umbilical Cord Clamping and Preterm Infants: A Randomised Trial," *British Medical Journal*, vol. 306, no. 6871 (1993), pp. 172–75. If a blood pressure gauge is placed on an unclamped umbilical cord, it will pick up pressure rises as high as 60 mm Hg with each uterine contraction. This indicates that these contractions are intimately involved in the transfer of placental blood through the cord. A striking pressure rise, which persists through the first few hours of life, is also evident in the baby's vena cava and right atrium of the heart. All studies on this indicate a significantly higher systemic pressure in infants who have been clamped late (90 percent in the first nine hours) and conversely, a significant drop in those early-clamped infants (70 percent of systemic by the second hour, and almost 50 percent of systemic by the fourth hour) (A. J. Moss and M. Monset-Couchard, "Placental Transfusion; Early Versus Late Clamping of the Umbilical Cord," *Pediatrics*, vol. 40, no. 1 [July 1967], pp. 109–26). The placental blood normally belongs to the infant, and his or her failure to get this blood is equivalent to submitting the newborn to a severe hemorrhage at birth. The time of cord clamping may be involved in the pathogenesis of idiopathic respiratory distress syndrome (the earlier clamped, the more respiratory distress) (S. Saigal et al., "Placental Transfusion and Hyperbilirubinemia in the Premature," *Pediatrics*, vol. 49, no. 3 [March 1972], pp. 406–19). Placental blood acts as a source of nourishment that protects infants against the breakdown of body protein (Q. B. De Marsh et al., "The Effect of Depriving the Infant of Its Placental Blood," *Journal of the American Medical Association*, vol. 116, no. 23 [June 7, 1941], pp. 2568–73). Studies have shown that immediate cord clamping prolongs the average duration of the third stage and greatly increases maternal blood loss (S. Z. Walsh, "Maternal Effects of Early and Late Clamping of the Umbilical Cord," *The Lancet*, vol. 1, no. 7550 [May 11, 1968], pp. 996–97).

6. E. K. Hutton and E. S. Hassan, "Late vs. Early Clamping of the Umbilical Cord in Full-Term Neonates," *Journal of the American Medical Association*, vol. 297, no. 11 (March 21, 2007), pp. 1241–52.

7. G. Eichenbaum-Pikser and J. S. Zasloff, "Delayed Clamping of the Umbilical Cord: A Review with Implications for Practice," *Journal of Midwifery and Women's Health*, vol. 54, no. 4 (July–August 2009), pp. 321–26.

8. American College of Obstetricians and Gynecologists, "ACOG Committee Opinion No. 684: Delayed Umbilical Cord Clamping After Birth," *Obstetrics and Gynecology*, vol. 129, no. 1 (January 2017), pp. 232–33.

9. H. Rabe et al., "Effect of Timing of Umbilical Cord Clamping and Other Strategies to Influence Placental Transfusion at Preterm Birth on Maternal and Infant Outcomes," *Cochrane Database of Systematic Reviews*, vol. 8 (August 15, 2012), p. CD003248; S. J. McDonald, P. Middleton, T. Dowsell, and P. S. Morris, "Effect of Timing of Umbilical Cord Clamping of Term Infants on Maternal and Neonatal Outcomes," *Cochrane Database of Systematic Reviews*, vol. 7 (July 11, 2013), p. CD004074.

10. S. K. Misri, *Pregnancy Blues: What Every Woman Needs to Know About Depression During Pregnancy* (New York: Delacorte Press, 2005).

11. H. Vinamaki et al., "Evolution of Postpartum Mental Health," *Journal of Psychosomatic Obstetrics and Gynecology*, vol. 18 (1997), pp. 213–19; D. D. Affonso and G. Domino, "Postpartum Depression: A Review," *Birth*, vol. 11, no. 4 (Winter 1984), pp. 231–35.

12. S. K. Dorheim et al., "Sleep and Depression in Postpartum Women: A Population-Based Study," *Sleep*, vol. 32, no. 7 (July 1, 2009), pp. 847–55.

13. K. Dalton, "Successful Prophylactic Progesterone for Idiopathic Post-Natal Depression," *International Journal of Prenatal Studies* (1989), pp. 322–27.

14. D. Sichel et al., "Prophlactic Estrogen in Recurrent Postpartum Affective Disorder," *Society of Biological Psychiatry*, vol. 38 (1995), pp. 814–18.

15. A. Bruno et al., "Inside-Out: The Role of Anger Experience and Expression in the Development of Postpartum Mood Disorders," *Journal of Maternal-Fetal and Neonatal Medicine*, vol. 31, no. 22 (November 2018), pp. 3033–38.

16. J. B. Sperstad et al., "Diastasis Recti Abdominis During Pregnancy and 12 Months After Childbirth: Prevalence, Risk Factors and Report of Lumbopelvic Pain," *British Journal of Sports Medicine*, vol. 50, no. 17 (September 2016), pp. 1092–96.

17. G. Sharma, T. Lobo, and L. Keller, "Postnatal Exercise Can Reverse Diastasis Recti," *Obstetrics and Gynecology*, vol. 123 (May 2014), pp. 171S.

18. S. Ip et al., "Breastfeeding and Maternal and Infant Health Outcomes in Developed Countries," Agency for Healthcare Research and Quality (AHRQ), Evidence Report/Technology Assessment No. 153 (April 2007), pp. 1–186.

19. M. M. Vennemann et al., "Does Breastfeeding Reduce the Risk of Sudden Infant Death Syndrome?" *Pediatrics*, vol. 123, no. 3 (March 2009), pp. e406–10.

20. E. P. Gunderson et al., "Duration of Lactation and Incidence of the Metabolic Syndrome in Women of Reproductive Age According to Gestational Diabetes Mellitus Status: A 20-Year Prospective Study in CARDIA—The Coronary Artery Risk Development in Young Adults Study," *Diabetes*, published online December 3, 2009, http://diabetes.diabetesjournals.org/content/early/2009/11/12/db09-1197.abstract.

21. L. Strathearn et al., "Does Breastfeeding Protect Against Substantiated Child Abuse and Neglect?" *Pediatrics*, vol. 123, no. 2 (2009), pp. 483–93.

22. A. Lucas et al., "Breast Milk and Subsequent Intelligence Quotient in Children Born Preterm," *The Lancet* 339, no. 8788 (February 1, 1992), pp. 261–64.

23. F. Hassiotou et al., "Breastmilk Stem Cells Transfer from Mother to Neonatal Organs," *FASEB Journal,* vol. 28, no. 1 (April 2014).

24. T. Baker et al., "Transfer of Inhaled Cannabis into Human Breast Milk," *Obstetrics and Gynecology,* vol. 131, no. 5 (May 2018), pp. 783–88.

25. J. Heyman, A. Earle, and J. Hayes, *The Work, Family, and Equity Index: Where Does the United States Stand Globally?* (Cambridge, MA: Harvard School of Public Health, Project on Global Working Families, 2004).

26. K. Kendall-Tackett, Z. Cong, and T. W. Hale, "The Effect of Feeding Method on Sleep Duration, Maternal Well-Being, and Postpartum Depression," *Clinical Lactation,* vol. 2, no. 2 (2011), pp. 22–26.

27. L. Feldman-Winter, K. Szucs, A. Milano, E. Gottschilch, B. Sisk, and R. J. Schanler, "National Trends in Pediatricians' Practices and Attitudes About Breastfeeding: 1995–2014," *Pediatrics,* vol. 140, no. 4 (October 2017), p. e20171299.

28. J. Martucci, A. Barnhill, "Unintended Consequences of Invoking the 'Natural' in Breastfeeding Promotion," *Pediatrics,* vol. 137, no. 4 (April 2016), p. e20154154, http://pediatrics.aappublications.org/content/137/4/e20154154.

29. P. O'Mara, "Case Closed: Breast Is Best," *Mothering,* issue 154 (May/June 2009), pp. 8–12.

30. Changing Markets Foundation, "Busting the Myth of Science-Based Formula: An Investigation into Nestle Infant Milk Products and Claims," February 2018, http://changingmarkets.org/wp-content/uploads/2018/02/busting-the-myth-of-science-based-formula.pdf.

31. Changing Markets Foundation, "Milking It: How Milk Formula Companies Are Putting Profits Before Science," October 2017, http://changingmarkets.org/wp-content/uploads/2017/10/Milking-it-Executive-summary-CM.pdf.

32. J. L. Pomeranz, M. J. Romo Palafox, and J. L. Harris, "Toddler Drinks, Formulas, and Milks: Labeling Practices and Policy Implications," *Preventive Medicine,* vol. 109 (April 2018), pp. 11–16.

33. Centers for Disease Control and Prevention, "Breastfeeding—Report Card: United States/2018," www.cdc.gov/breastfeeding/data/reportcard.htm.

34. A solution to this might be the visualization procedure mentioned at the end of the section on breast augmentation in chapter 10.

35. B. Zablotsky, L. I. Black, and S. J. Blumberg, "Estimated Prevalence of Children with Diagnosed Developmental Disabilities in the United States, 2014–2016," *NCHS Data Brief,* no. 291 (Hyattsville, MD: National Center for Health Statistics. 2017).

36. J. Van Cleave, S. L. Gortmaker, and J. M. Perrin, "Dynamics of Obesity and Chronic Health Conditions Among Children and Youth," *Journal of the American Medical Association,* vol. 303, no. 7 (February 17, 2010), pp. 623–30.

37. C. D. Bethell et al., "A National and State Profile of Leading Health Problems and Health Care Quality for U.S. Children: Key Insurance Disparities and Across-State Variations," *Academic Pediatrics,* vol. 11, no. 3 (May–June 2011), pp. S22–33.

38. U. S. Department of Health and Human Services, Health Resources and Services

Administration, National Vaccine Injury Compensation Program Data and Statistics, November 1, 2017, page 9, https://www.hrsa.gov/sites/default/files/hrsa/vaccine-compensation/VICPmonthlyreportNov2017.pdf.

39. S. O. Shaheen et al., "Measles and Atopy in Guinea-Bissau," *The Lancet*, vol. 347, no. 9018 (June 29, 1994), pp. 1792–96; M. R. Odent, "Pertussis Vaccination and Asthma: Is There a Link?" *Journal of the American Medical Association*, vol. 272, no. 8 (1994), pp. 592–93; J. S. Alm et al., "Atopy in Children of Families with an Anthroposophic Lifestyle," *The Lancet*, vol. 353, no. 9163 (May 1, 1999), pp. 1457–58; T. Kemp et al., "Is Infant Immunization a Risk Factor for Childhood Asthma or Allergy?" *Epidemiology*, vol. 8, no. 6 (November 1997), pp. 678–80.

40. Z. Wang et al., "Difficulties in Eliminating Measles and Controlling Rubella and Mumps: A Cross-Sectional Study of a First Measles and Rubella Vaccination and a Second Measles, Mumps, and Rubella Vaccination," *PLoS One*, vol. 9, no. 2 (February 20, 2014), p. e89361.

41. N. Boulianne et al., ["Major Measles Epidemic in the Region of Quebec Despite a 99% Vaccine Coverage"], *Canadian Journal of Public Health*, vol. 82, no. 3 (May–June 1991), pp. 189–90.

42. K. Brogan, *Special Report: Vaccines and Brain Health*, January 2018, https://kellybroganmd.com/wp-content/uploads/2018/01/VaccinesandBrainHealth.pdf; J. M. Warfel, L. I Zimmerman, and T. J. Merkel, "Acellular Pertussis Vaccines Protect Against Disease but Fail to Prevent Infection and Transmission in a Nonhuman Primate Model," *Proceedings of the National Academy of Sciences of the United States of America*, vol. 111, no. 2 (January 14, 2014), pp. 787–92.

43. P. Brodin et al., "Variation in the Human Immune System Is Largely Driven by Non-Heritable Influences," *Cell*, vol. 160, nos. 1–2 (January 15, 2015), pp. 37–47.

44. D. A. Geier et al., "Biomarkers of Environmental Toxicity and Susceptibility in Autism," *Journal of Neurological Sciences*, vol. 280, nos. 1–2 (May 15, 2009), pp. 101–8.

45. R. L. Blaylock, "A Possible Central Mechanism in Autism Spectrum Disorders, Part 1," *Alternative Therapies in Health and Medicine*, vol. 14, no. 6 (November–December 2008), pp. 46–53; R. L. Blaylock, "A Possible Central Mechanism in Autism Spectrum Disorders, Part 2," *Alternative Therapies in Health and Medicine*, vol. 15, no. 1 (January–February 2009), pp. 60–67.

46. C. Exley, "Aluminum Should Now Be Considered a Primary Etiological Factor in Alzheimer's Disease," *Journal of Alzheimer's Disease Reports*, vol. 1, no. 1 (June 8, 2017), pp. 23–35; R. K. Gherardi et al., "Biopersistence and Brain Translocation of Alunimum Adjuvants of Vaccines," *Frontiers in Neurology*, vol. 6 (February 2015), p. 4; C. A. Shaw and L. Tomljenovic, "Aluminum in the Central Nervous System (CNS): Toxicity in Humans and animals, Vaccine Adjuvants, and Autoimmunity," *Immunologic Research*, vol. 56, nos. 2–3 (July 2013), pp. 304–16; L. E. Guimaraes et al., "Vaccines, Adjuvants and Autoimmunity," *Pharmacological Research*, vol. 100 (October 2015), pp. 190–209; G. Morris, B. K. Puri, and R. E. Frye, "The Putative Role of Environmental Aluminum in the Development of Chronic Neuropathology in Adults and Children. How Strong is the Evidence and What Could Be the Mechanisms Involved?" *Metabolic Brain Disease*, vol. 32, no. 5 (October 2017), pp. 1335–55.

47. K. Brogan, "Psychobiology of Vaccination Effects: Bidirectional Relevance of De-pression," *Alternative Therapies in Health and Medicine,* vol. 21, supplement 3 (August 2015), pp. 18–26; D. A. Geier et al., "Thimerosal Exposure and Distur-bance of Emotions Specific to Childhood and Adolescence: A Case-Control Study in the Vaccine Safety Datalink (VSD) Database," *Brain Injury,* vol. 31, no. 2 (2017), pp. 272–78.

48. Y. Shoenfeld and N. Agmon-Levin, "'ASIA'—Autoimmune/Inflammatory Syn-drome Induced by Adjuvants," *Journal of Autoimmunity,* vol. 36, no. 1 (February 2011), pp. 4–8.

49. A. R. Mawson et al., "Pilot Comparative Study on the Health of Vaccinated and Unvaccinated 6- to 12-Year-Old U.S. Children," *Journal of Translational Sci-ence* 3 (2017), https://www.oatext.com/Pilot-comparative-study-on-the-health-of -vaccinated-and-unvaccinated-6-to-12-year-old-U-S-children.php#Article.

50. A. R. Mawson et al., "Preterm Birth, Vaccination and Neurodevelopmental Dis-orders: A Cross-Sectional Study of 6- to 12-Year-Old Vaccinated and Unvacci-nated Children," *Journal of Translational Science* 3 (2017), https://oatext.com/ Preterm-birth-vaccination-and-neurodevelopmental-disorders-a-cross-sectional -study-of-6-to-12-year-old-vaccinated-and-unvaccinated-children.php#Article_Info.

51. S. R. Mostaghim, J. J. Gagne, and A. S. Kesselheim, "Safety Related Label Changes for New Drugs After Approval in the U.S. through Expedited Regulatory Path-ways: Retrospective Cohort Study," *BMJ,* vol. 358 (September 7, 2017), pp. j3837.

52. M. Mold et al., "Aluminum in Brain Tissue in Autism," *Journal of Trace Ele-ments in Medicine and Biology,* vol. 46 (March 2018), pp. 76–82.

53. L. Tomljenovic and C. A. Shaw, "Do Aluminum Vaccine Adjuvants Contribute to the Rising Prevalence of Autism?" *Journal of Inorganic Biochemistry,* vol. 105, no. 11 (November 2011), pp. 1489–99.

54. G. S. Goldman and N. Z. Miller, "Relative Trends in Hospitalizations and Mor-tality Among Infants by the Number of Vaccine Doses and Age, Based on the Vaccine Adverse Event Reporting System (VAERS), 1990–2010," *Human and Experimental Toxicology,* vol. 31, no. 10 (October 2012), pp. 1012–21.

55. G. Crepeaux et al., "Non-linear Dose-Response of Aluminum Hydroxide Adju-vant Particles: Selective Low Dose Neurotoxicity," *Toxicology,* vol. 375 (Janu-ary 15, 2017), pp. 48–57.

56. Committee on the Assessment of Studies of Health Outcomes Related to the Rec-ommended Childhood Immunization Schedule, Board on Population Health and Public Health Practice, Institute of Medicine, *The Childhood Immunization Schedule and Safety: Stakeholder Concerns, Scientific Evidence, and Future Stud-ies* (Washington, DC: National Academies Press, March 2013).

57. "Real-Life Data Show That the CDC Vaccine Schedule Is Causing Harm," Chil-dren's Health Defense, March 19, 2019, https://childrenshealthdefense.org/news/ real-life-data-show-that-the-cdc-vaccine-schedule-is-causing-harm.

58. E. Goodman, "Search for Father Dominating Lives," *Portland Press Herald,* April 10, 1992, syndicated from *Boston Globe.*

Chapter 14: Menopause

1. American Congress of Obstetricians and Gynecologists, *2011 Women's Health Statistics*, p. 33, www.acog.org/-/media/NewsRoom/MediaKit.pdf.

2. T. Slayton, *Reclaiming the Menstrual Matrix: Evolving Feminine Wisdom— A Workbook* (Petaluma, CA: Menstrual Health Foundation, 1990), p. 41.

3. J. C. Prior et al., "Spinal Bone Loss and Ovulatory Disturbances," *New England Journal of Medicine,* vol. 323 (1990), pp. 1221–27.

4. C. Longscope, R. Hunter, and C. Franz, "Steroid Secretion by the Postmenopausal Ovary," *American Journal of Obstetrics and Gynecology,* vol. 138 (1980), pp. 6540–68; C. Longscope, C. Bourget, and C. Flood, "The Production and Aromatization of Dehydroepiandrosterone in Postmenopausal Women," *Maturitas,* vol. 4 (1982), pp. 325–32; C. Longscope, W. Jaffe, and G. Griffing, "Production Rates of Androgens and Oestrogens in Post-Menopausal Women," *Maturitas,* vol. 3 (1981), pp. 215–23.

5. E. Langer, *Counterclockwise* (New York: Ballantine Books, 2009), p. 123.

6. Y. Dunneram et al., "Dietary Intake and Age at Natural Menopause: Results from the UK Women's Cohort Study," *Journal of Epidemiology and Community Health,* vol. 72, no. 8 (August 2018), pp. 733–40.

7. W. M. Jeffries, "Cortisol and Immunity," *Medical Hypotheses,* vol. 34 (1991), pp. 198–208; J. P. Kahn et al., "Salivary Cortisol: A Practical Method for Evaluation of Adrenal Function," *Biological Psychiatry,* vol. 23 (1988), pp. 335–49; M. H. Laudet et al., "Salivary Cortisol: A Practical Approach to Assess Pituitary-Adrenal Function," *Journal of Clinical Endocrinology and Metabolism,* vol. 66 (1988), pp. 343–48; R. F. Vining and R. A. McGinley, "The Measurement of Hormones in Saliva: Possibilities and Pitfalls," *Journal of Steroid Biochemistry,* vol. 27, nos. 1–3 (1987), pp. 81–94.

8. E. Barrett-Connor et al., "A Prospective Study of Dehydroepiandrosterone Sulfate, Mortality, and Cardiovascular Disease," *New England Journal of Medicine,* vol. 315, no. 24 (1986), pp. 1519–24; R. E. Bulbrook et al., "Relation Between Urinary Androgen and Corticoid Excretion and Subsequent Breast Cancer," *The Lancet,* vol. 2, no. 7721 (1971), pp. 395–98; S. E. Monroe and K. M. J. Menon, "Changes in Reproductive Hormone Secretion During the Climacteric and Post-Menopausal Periods," *Clinical Obstetrics and Gynecology,* vol. 20 (1977), pp. 113–22; W. Regelson et al., "Hormonal Intervention: 'Buffer Hormones' or 'State Dependency': The Role of DHEA, Thyroid Hormone, Estrogen, and Hypophysectomy in Aging," *Annals of the New York Academy of Sciences,* vol. 521 (1988), pp. 260–73. A recent study of postmenopausal women age sixty to seventy using DHEA skin cream showed that after a year of treatment, the women experienced a 10 percent decrease in body fat, a 10 percent increase in muscle mass, decreased blood sugar levels, decreased insulin levels, and a decrease in cholesterol. Their vaginal tissue also showed a thickening similar to that seen with estrogen, but there was no increase in stimulation of the uterine lining. There was also an increase in bone density. Unfortunately, these women also experienced a 70 percent increase in the oiliness of their skin, which resulted in acne—an effect that could probably be reduced with somewhat lower doses. See R. Sahelian, "Landmark One-Year DHEA Study," *Health Counselor,* vol. 9, no. 2 (1997), pp. 46–47.

9. R. McCraty et al., "The Impact of a New Emotional Self-Management Program on Stress, Emotions, Heart Rate Variability, DHEA and Cortisol," *Integrative Physiological and Behavioral Sciences,* vol. 33, no. 3 (April–June 1998). An updated "Research Overview" provides more information on the many studies the Institute of HeartMath has done and is presently involved with. Available from the Institute of HeartMath, P.O. Box 1463, Boulder Creek, CA 95006, 931-338-8500.

10. C. Dean, *The Magnesium Miracle* (New York: Ballantine Books, 2007).

11. H. van der Rhee et al., "Sunlight: For Better or for Worse? A Review of Positive and Negative Effects of Sun Exposure," *Cancer Research Frontiers,* vol. 2, no. 2 (May 2016), pp. 156–83, http://cancer-research-frontiers.org/wp-content/uploads/2016/04/CRF-2016-2-156.pdf.

12. M. S. Massoudi et al., "Prevalence of Thyroid Antibodies Among Healthy Middle-Aged Women. Findings from the Thyroid Study in Healthy Women," *Annals of Epidemiology,* vol. 5, no. 3 (May 1995), pp. 229–33.

13. P. Paramsothy et al., "Duration of Menopausal Transition Is Longer in Women with Young Age at Onset," *Menopause,* vol. 24, no. 2 (2017), pp. 142–49.

14. J. Hargrove and E. Eisenberg, "Menopause," *Medical Clinics of North America,* vol. 79, no. 6 (1995), pp. 1337–56.

15. C. B. Coulam, "Premature Gonadal Failure," *Fertility and Sterility,* vol. 38, no. 645 (1982); C. B. Coulam, S. C. Adamson, and J. F. Annegers, "Incidence of Premature Ovarian Failure," *American Journal of Obstetrics and Gynecology,* vol. 67, no. 4 (1986); R. des Moraes et al., "Autoimmunity and Ovarian Failure," *American Journal of Obstetrics and Gynecology,* vol. 112, no. 5 (1972); H. J. Gloor, "Autoimmune Oophoritis," *American Journal of Clinical Pathology,* vol. 81 (1984), pp. 105–9; M. Leer et al., "Secondary Amenorrhea Due to Autoimmune Ovarian Failure," *Australia and New Zealand Journal of Obstetrics and Gynecology,* vol. 20 (1980), pp. 177–79; T. Miyake et al., "Acute Oocyte Loss in Experimental Autoimmune Oophoritis as a Possible Model of Premature Ovarian Failure," *American Journal of Obstetrics and Gynecology,* vol. 158, no. 1 (1988); T. Miyake et al., "Evidence of Autoimmune Etiology in Some Premature Menopause," *ObGyn News,* November 1981.

16. J. Pfenninger, "Sex and the Maturing Female," *Mature Health,* January–February 1987, pp. 12–15.

17. L. Zussman et al., "Sexual Response After Hysterectomy-Oophorectomy: Recent Studies and Reconsideration of Psychogenesis," *American Journal of Obstetrics and Gynecology,* vol. 140, no. 7 (1981), pp. 725–29.

18. A. Koushik, M. E. Parent, and J. Siemiatycki, "Characteristics of Menstruation and Pregnancy and the Risk of Lung Cancer in Women," *International Journal of Cancer,* vol. 125, no. 10 (May 11, 2009), pp. 2428–33.

19. W. H. Parker et al., "Ovarian Conservation at the Time of Hysterectomy and Long-Term Health Outcomes in the Nurses' Health Study," *Obstetrics and Gynecology,* vol. 113, no. 5 (May 2009), pp. 1027–37.

20. C. M. Rivera et al., "Increased Mortality for Neurological and Mental Diseases Following Early Bilateral Oophorectomy," *Neuroepidemiology,* vol. 33, no. 1 (2009), pp. 32–40.

21. T. Speroff et al., "A Risk-Benefit Analysis of Elective Bilateral Oophorectomy:

Effect of Changes in Compliance with Estrogen Therapy on Outcome," *American Journal of Obstetrics and Gynecology*, vol. 164, 1 Pt 1 (January 1991), pp. 165–74.

22. L. C. Swartzman, "Impact of Stress on Objectively Recorded Menopausal Hot Flashes and on Flush Report Bias," *Health Psychology*, vol. 9 (1990), pp. 529–45.

23. F. Grodstein, J. E. Manson, and M. J. Stampfer, "Hormone Therapy and Coronary Heart Disease: The Role of Time Since Menopause and Age at Hormone Initiation," *Journal of Women's Health (Larchmont)*, vol. 15, no. 1 (January–February 2006), pp. 35–44.

24. R. J. Baber, N. Panay, and A. Fenton (the IMS Writing Group), "2016 IMS Recommendations on Women's Midlife Health and Menopause Hormone Therapy," *Climacteric*, vol. 19, no. 2 (April 2016), pp. 109–50.

25. J. Eden, "The Endometrial and Breast Safety of Menopausal Hormone Therapy Containing Micronized Progesterone: A Short Review," *Australian and New Zealand Journal of Obstetrics and Gynaecology*, vol. 57, no. 1 (February 2017), pp. 12–15.

26. A. Fournier, F. Berrino, and F. Clavel-Chapelon, "Unequal Risks for Breast Cancer Associated with Different Hormone Replacement Therapies: Results from the E3N Cohort Study," *Breast Cancer Research and Treatment*, vol. 107, no. 1 (January 2008), pp. 103–11.

27. K. Holtorf, "The Bioidentical Hormone Debate: Are Bioidentical Hormones (Estradiol, Estriol, and Progesterone) Safer or More Efficacious Than Commonly Used Synthetic Versions in Hormone Replacement Therapy?," *Postgraduate Medicine*, vol. 121, no. 1 (January 2009), pp. 73–85.

28. R. Chlebowski et al., "Breast Cancer After Use of Estrogen Plus Progestin in Postmenopausal Women," *New England Journal of Medicine*, vol. 360, no. 6 (February 5, 2009), pp. 573–87.

29. B. R. Bhavnani and A. Cecutti, "Pharmacokinetics of 17b-Dihydroequilin Sulfate and 17b-Dihydroequilin in Normal Postmenopausal Women," *Journal of Clinical Endocrinology and Metabolism*, vol. 78 (1994), pp. 197–204.

30. Kronos Longevity Research Institute, "Plenary Symposium #1—Presidential Symposium: New Findings from the Kronos Early Prevention Study (KEEPS) Randomized Trial," North American Menopause Society 23rd Annual Conference, October 6–12, 2012.

31. S. M. Harmon et al., "Arterial Imaging Outcomes and Cardiovascular Risk Factors in Recently Menopausal Women: A Randomized Trial," *Annals of Internal Medicine*, vol. 161, no. 4 (August 2014), pp. 249–60.

32. H. N. Hodis et al., "Vascular Effects of Early versus Late Postmenopausal Treatment with Estradiol," *New England Journal of Medicine*, vol. 374, no. 13 (March 31, 2016), pp. 1221–23.

33. V. W. Henderson et al., "Cognitive Effects of Estradiol After Menopause," *Neurology*, vol. 87, no. 7 (Aug 2016), pp. 699–708.

34. H. Lyytinen, E. Pukkala, and O. Ylikorkala, "Breast Cancer Risk in Postmenopausal Women Using Estrogen-Only Therapy," *Obstetrics and Gynecology*, vol. 108, no. 6 (December 2006), pp. 1354–60; A. Fournier et al., "Breast Cancer Risk in Relation to Different types of Hormone Replacement Therapy in the E3N-EPIC cohort," *International Journal of Cancer*, vol. 114, no. 3 (April 2005), pp. 448–

54; L. Bergkvist et al., "The Risk of Breast Cancer After Estrogen and Estrogen-Progestin Replacement," *New England Journal of Medicine,* vol. 321, no. 5 (August 3, 1989), pp. 293–97.

35. A. Follingstad, "Estriol, the Forgotten Hormone," *Journal of the American Medical Association,* vol. 239, no. 1 (1978), pp. 29–39; H. Lemon, "Clinical and Experimental Aspects of the Anti-Mammary Carcinogenic Activity of Estriol," *Frontiers of Hormonal Research,* vol. 5, no. 1 (1977), pp. 155–73; H.Lemon, "Estriol Prevention of Mammary Carcinoma Induced by 7, 12-Dimethyibenzathracene and Procarbazine," *Cancer Research,* vol. 35 (1975), pp. 1341–53; H. Lemon, "Oestriol and Prevention of Breast Cancer," *The Lancet,* vol. 1, no. 802 (1973), pp. 546–47; H. Lemon, "Pathophysiologic Considerations in the Treatment of Menopausal Patients with Oestrogens: The Role of Oestriol in the Prevention of Mammary Cancer," *Acta Endocrinologica,* vol. 233, Suppl. (1980), pp. 17–27; H. Lemon et al., "Reduced Estriol Excretion in Patients with Breast Cancer Prior to Endocrine Therapy," *Journal of the American Medical Association,* vol. 196 (1966), pp. 1128–36; B. G. Wren and J. A. Eden, "Do Progesterones Reduce the Risk of Breast Cancer? A Review of the Evidence," *Menopause,* vol. 3, no. 1 (1996), pp. 4–12; M. van Haaften et al., "Oestrogen Concentrations in Plasma, Endometrium, Myometrium, and Vagina of Postmenopausal Women, and Effects of Vaginal Oestriol (E3) and Oestradiol (E2) Applications," *Journal of Steroid Biochemistry,* vol. 4A (1989), pp. 647–53.

36. M. Melamed et al., "Molecular and Kinetic Basis for the Mixed Agonist/Antagonist Activity of Estriol," *Molecular Endocrinology,* vol. 11, no. 12 (November 1997), pp. 1868–78.

37. L. Rajkumar et al., "Prevention of Mammary Carcinogenesis by Short-Term Estrogen and Progestin Treatments," *Breast Cancer Research,* vol. 6, no. 1 (2004), pp. R31–37.

38. S. Granberg et al., "The Effects of Oral Estriol on the Endometrium in Postmenopausal Women," *Maturitas,* vol. 42, no. 2 (June 25, 2002), pp. 149–56.

39. K. Takahashi et al., "Efficacy and Safety of Oral Estriol for Managing Postmenopausal Symptoms," *Maturitas,* vol. 34, no. 2 (February 15, 2000), pp. 169–77; K. Takahashi et al., "Safety and Efficacy of Oestriol for Symptoms of Natural or Surgically Induced Menopause," *Human Reproduction,* vol. 15, no. 5 (May 2000), pp. 1028–36.

40. R. Punnonen and L. Raurama, "The Effect of Longterm Oral Oestriol Succinate Therapy on the Skin of Castrate Women," *Annals of Gynecology,* vol. 66 (1977), p. 214.

41. Hargrove and Eisenberg, "Menopause."

42. Ibid.

43. F. Z. Stanczyk, R. J. Paulson, and S. Roy, "Percutaneous Administration of Progesterone: Blood Levels and Endometrial Protection," *Menopause,* vol. 12, no. 2 (March 2005), pp. 232–37.

44. F. Labrie et al., "Effect of Intravaginal Dehydroepiandrosterone (Prasterone) on Libido and Sexual Dysfunction in Postmenopausal Women," *Menopause,* vol. 16, no. 5 (September–October 2009), pp. 923–31.

45. A. Wright, "An Ethnography of the Navajo Reproductive Cycle," *American In-*

dian Quarterly, vol. 6, nos. 1–2 (Spring/Summer 1982), pp. 52–70; also quote in A. Voda, M. Dinnerstein, and C. R. O'Donnell, eds., *Changing Perspectives on Menopause* (Austin: University of Texas Press, 1982).

46. J. K. Brown and V. Kerns, eds., *In Her Prime: A New View of Middle-Aged Women* (Amherst, MA: Bergin and Garvey, 1985).

47. F. Kronenberg and J. A. Downey, "Thermoregulatory Physiology of Menopausal Hot Flashes: A Review," *Canadian Journal of Physiological Pharmacology,* vol. 65 (1987), pp. 1312–24.

48. R. S. Finkler, "The Effect of Vitamin E in the Menopause," *Journal of Clinical Endocrinology and Metabolism,* vol. 9 (1949), pp. 89–94.

49. C. J. Smith, "Non-Hormonal Control of Vasomotor Flushing in Menopausal Patients," *Chicago Medicine,* vol. 67, no. 5 (1964), pp. 193–95.

50. C. A. B. Clemetson et al., "Estrogens in Food: The Almond Mystery," *International Journal of Gynecology and Obstetrics,* vol. 15 (1978), pp. 515–21; S. O. Elakovich and J. Hampton, "Analysis of Couvaestrol, a Phytoestrogen, in Alpha Tablets Sold for Human Consumption," *Journal of Agricultural and Food Chemistry,* vol. 32 (1984), pp. 173–75.

51. H. Aldercreutz et al., "Dietary Phyto-Oestrogens and the Menopause in Japan," *The Lancet,* vol. 339 (1992), p. 1233; M. J. Messina et al., "Soy Intake and Cancer Risk: A Review of the In Vitro and In Vivo Data," *Nutrition and Cancer,* vol. 21 (1994), pp. 113–31; and G. Wilcox et al., "Oestrogenic Effects of Plant Foods in Postmenopausal Women," *British Medical Journal,* vol. 301 (1990), pp. 905–6.

52. S. Basaria et al., "Effect of High-Dose Isoflavones on Cognition, Quality of Life, Androgens, and Lipoprotein in Post-Menopausal Women," *Journal of Endocrinological Investigation,* vol. 32, no. 2 (February 2009), pp. 150–55.

53. M. Murray, "HRT vs. Remifemin in Menopause," *American Journal of Natural Medicine,* vol. 3, no. 4 (1996), pp. 7–10; G. Warnecke, "Beeinflussing Klimakterischer Beschwerden durch ein Phytotherapeutikum [Influencing Menopausal Symptoms with a Phytotherapeutic Agent]," *Medwelt,* vol. 36 (1985), pp. 871–74.

54. W. Wuttke, D. Seidlová-Wuttke, and C. Gorkow, "The Cimicifuga Preparation BNO 1055 vs. Conjugated Estrogens in a Double-Blind Placebo-Controlled Study: Effects on Menopause Symptoms and Bone Markers," *Maturitas,* vol. 44, suppl. 1 (March 14, 2003), pp. S67–77; G. Hernandez Munoz and S. Pluchino, "*Cimicifuga racemosa* for the Treatment of Hot Flushes in Women Surviving Breast Cancer," *Maturitas,* vol. 44, suppl. 1 (March 14, 2003), pp. S59–65.

55. I. I. Bukham and O. I. Kirillov, "Effect of Eleutherococus on Alarm-Phase of Stress," *Annual Review of Pharmacology,* vol. 8 (1969), pp. 113–21; A. Milewiez et al., "Vitex Agnus Castus Extract in the Treatment of Luteal Phase Defects Due to Hyperprolactinemia: Results of a Randomized Placebo-Controlled Double-Blind Study," *Arzneimittel-Forschung/Drug Research,* vol. 43 (1993), pp. 752–56; D. B. Mowrey, *The Scientific Validation of Herbal Medicine* (New Canaan, CT: Keats, 1986); G. Sliutz et al., "Agnus Castus Extracts Inhibit Prolactin Secretion of Rat Pituitary Cells," *Hormone and Metabolic Research,* vol. 2 (1993), pp. 253–55.

56. S. E. Geller et al., "Safety and Efficacy of Black Cohosh and Red Clover for the Management of Vasomotor Symptoms: A Randomized Controlled Trial," *Menopause* 16, no. 6 (November–December 2009), pp. 1156–66.

57. P. M. Maki et al., "Effects of Botanicals and Combined Hormone Therapy on Cognition in Postmenopausal Women," *Menopause* 16, no. 6 (November–December 2009), pp. 1167–77.

58. J. Tan Garcia et al., "Use of a Multibotanical (Nutrafem) for the Relief of Menopausal Vasomotor Symptoms: A Double-Blind, Placebo-Controlled Study," *Menopause* 17, no. 2 (March 2010), pp. 303–8.

59. J. Manonai et al., "Effects and Safety of *Pueraria mirifica* on Lipid Profiles and Biochemical Markers of Bone Turnover Rates in Healthy Postmenopausal Women," *Menopause,* vol. 15, no. 3 (May–June 2008), pp. 530–35; N. Urasopon et al., "*Pueraria mirifica,* a Phytoestrogen-Rich Herb, Prevents Bone Loss in Orchidectomized Rats," *Maturitas,* vol. 56, no. 3 (March 20, 2007), pp. 322–31.

60. V. Chandeying and M. Sangthawan, "Efficacy Comparison of *Pueraria mirifica* (PM) Against Conjugated Equine Estrogen (CEE) With/Without Medroxyprogesterone Acetate (MPA) in the Treatment of Climacteric Symptoms in Perimenopausal Women: Phase III Study," *Journal of the Medical Association of Thailand,* vol. 90, no. 9 (September 2007), pp. 1720–26.

61. S. Lamlertkittikul and V. Chandeying, "Efficacy and Safety of Pueraria mirifica (Kwao Kruea Khao) for the Treatment of Vasomotor Symptoms in Perimenopausal Women: Phase II Study," *Journal of the Medical Association of Thailand,* vol. 87, no. 1 (January 2004), pp. 33–40.

62. P. Virojchaiwong, V. Suvithayasiri, and A. Itharat, "Comparison of Pueraria mirifica 25 and 50 mg for Menopausal Symptoms," *Archives of Gynecology and Obstetrics,* vol. 284, no. 2 (August 2011), pp. 411–19.

63. J. Manonai et al., "Effects and Safety of *Pueraria mirifica* on Lipid Profiles and Biochemical Markers of Bone Turnover Rates in Healthy Postmenopausal Women," *Menopause,* vol. 15, no. 3 (May–June 2008), pp. 530–35; N. Urasopon et al., "Preventive Effects of Pueraria mirifica on Bone Loss in Ovariectomized Rats," *Maturitas,* vol. 59, no. 2 (February 20, 2008), pp. 137–48; N. Urasopon et al., "*Pueraria mirifica,* a Phytoestrogen-Rich Herb, Prevents Bone Loss in Orchidectomized Rats," *Maturitas,* vol. 56, no. 3 (March 20, 2007), pp. 322–31.

64. S. Suthon et al., "Anti-Osteoporotic Effects of *Pueraria candollei* var. *mirifica* on Bone Mineral Density and Histomorphometry in Estrogen-Deficient Rats," *Journal of Natural Medicines,* vol. 70, no. 2 (April 2016), pp. 225–33.

65. S. Ramnarine, J. MacCallum, and M. Ritchie, "Phyto-oestrogens: Do They Have a Role in Breast Cancer Therapy?" *Proceedings of the Nutrition Society,* vol. 68 (OCE) (2009), p. E93.

66. T. C. Lin et al., "*Pueraria mirifica* Inhibits 17β-Estradiol-induced Cell Proliferation of Human Endometrial Mesenchymal Stem Cells," *Taiwan Journal of Obstetrics and Gynecology,* vol. 56, no. 6 (December 2017), pp. 765–69.

67. T. Hudson, "Maca: New Insights on an Ancient Plant," *Integrative Medicine,* vol. 7, no. 6 (December 2008/January 2009), pp. 54–57.

68. J. R. Lee, *What Your Doctor May Not Tell You About Menopause* (New York: Warner Books, 1996).

69. L. M. Germaine and R. R. Freedman, "Behavioral Treatment of Menopausal Hot

Flashes: Evaluation by Objective Methods," *Journal of Consulting and Clinical Psychology*, vol. 52 (1984), pp. 1072–9; R. R. Freedman and S. Woodward, "Behavioral Treatment of Menopausal Hot Flushes: Evaluation by Ambulatory Monitoring," *American Journal of Obstetrics and Gynecology*, vol. 167 (1992), pp. 436–39; R. R. Freedman et al., "Biochemical and Thermoregulatory Effects of Behavioral Treatment for Menopausal Hot Flashes," *Menopause*, vol. 2 (1995), pp. 211–18; J. H. Irvin et al., "The Effects of Relaxation Response Training on Menopausal Symptoms," *Journal of Psychosomatic Obstetrics and Gynaecology*, vol. 17 (1996), pp. 202–7; K. Wijima et al., "Treatment of Menopausal Symptoms with Applied Relaxation: A Pilot Study," *Journal of Behavior Therapy and Experimental Psychiatry*, vol. 28 (1997), pp. 251–61.

70. A. D. Domar and H. Dreher, *Healing Mind, Healthy Woman* (New York: Henry Holt and Co., 1996), pp. 291–92; Swartzman, "Impact of Stress"; Freedman and Woodward, "Behavioral Treatment of Menopausal Hot Flushes: Evaluation by Ambulatory Monitoring"; L. C. Swartzman, R. Edelberg, and E. Kemmann, "The Menopausal Hot Flush: Symptom Reports and Concomitant Physical Changes," *Journal of Behavioral Medicine*, vol. 13 (1990), pp. 15–30; D. W. Stevenson and D. J. Delprato, "Multiple Component Self-Control Program for Menopausal Hot Flashes," *Journal of Behavior Therapy and Experimental Psychology*, vol. 14, no. 2 (1983), pp. 137–40.

71. J. Manonai et al., "Effect of *Pueraria mirifica* on Vaginal Health," *Menopause*, vol. 14, no. 5 (September–October 2007), pp. 919–24; N. Suwanvesh et al., "Comparison of *Pueraria mirifica* Gel and Conjugated Equine Estrogen Cream Effects on Vaginal Health in Postmenopausal Women," *Menopause*, vol. 24, no. 2 (February 2017), pp. 210–15.

72. N. Carroll et al., "Postmenopausal Restoration of the Estradiol/Estrone Ratio Reduces Severity of Vasomotor Symptoms," presented at the 57th Annual Meeting of the American College of Obstetricians and Gynecologists, May 2009, Chicago, IL.

73. M. Freedman et al., "Twice-Weekly Synthetic Conjugated Estrogens Vaginal Cream for the Treatment of Vaginal Atrophy," *Menopause*, vol. 16, no. 4 (July/August 2009), pp. 735–41.

74. S. Weed, *Menopausal Years: The Wise Women's Way: Alternative Approaches for Women 30–90* (Woodstock, NY: Ash Tree Publishing, 1992).

75. M. Bygdeman and M. L. Swahn, "Replens Versus Dienoestrol Cream in Symptomatic Treatment of Vaginal Atrophy in Postmenopausal Women," *Maturitas*, vol. 23 (1996), pp. 256–63.

76. S. Rako, *The Hormone of Desire: The Truth About Sexuality, Menopause, and Testosterone* (New York: Harmony, 1996).

77. V. L. Handa, "Vaginal Administration of Low-Dose Conjugated Estrogens: Systemic Absorption and Effects of the Endometrium," *Obstetrics and Gynecology*, vol. 84 (1994), pp. 215–18; G. M. Heimer and E. L. E. Englund, "Effects of Vaginally Administered Oestriol on Postmenopausal Urogenital Disorders: A Cytohormonal Study," *Maturitas*, vol. 3 (1992), pp. 171–79; C. S. Iosif, "Effects of Protracted Administration of Estriol on the Lower Urinary Tract in Postmenopausal Women," *Archives of Gynecology and Obstetrics*, vol. 3, no. 251 (1992), pp. 115–20; A. L. Kirkengen et al., "Oestriol in the Prophylactic Treatment of Recurrent Urinary Tract Infections in Postmenopausal Women," *Scandinavian*

Journal of Primary Health Care, June 1992, pp. 139–42; R. Ruz and W. Stamm, "A Controlled Trial of Intravaginal Estriol in Post-Menopausal Women with Recurrent Urinary Tract Infections," *New England Journal of Medicine,* vol. 329, no. 11 (1993), pp. 753–56. M. van Haaften et al., "Oestrogen Concentrations in Plasma, Endometrium, Myometrium, and Vagina of Postmenopausal Women, and Effects of Vaginal Oestriol (E3) and Oestradiol (E2) Applications," *Journal of Steroid Biochemistry,* vol. 4A (1989), pp. 647–53.

78. D. Michaelson et al., "Bone Mineral Density in Women with Depression," *New England Journal of Medicine,* vol. 335, no. 16 (October 17, 1996), pp. 1176–81.

79. C. E. Cann, M. C. Martin, and R. B. Jaffe, "Decreased Spinal Mineral Content in Amenorrheic Women," *Journal of the American Medical Association,* vol. 25, no. 5 (1984), pp. 626–29; J. S. Lindberg et al., "Increased Vertebral Bone Mineral in Response to Reduced Exercise in Amenorrheic Runners," *Western Journal of Medicine,* vol. 146 (1987), pp. 39–42; R. Marcus et al., "Menstrual Function and Bone Mass in Elite Women Distance Runners," *Annals of Internal Medicine,* vol. 102 (1985), pp. 158–63; J. C. Prior, "Spinal Bone Loss and Ovulatory Disturbances," *New England Journal of Medicine,* vol. 323, no. 18 (November 1, 1990), pp. 1221–27.

80. W. S. Browner et al., "Mortality Following Fractures in Older Women: The Study of Osteoporotic Fracture," *Archives of Internal Medicine,* vol. 156 (1996), pp. 1521–25; P. Dargen-Molina et al., "Fall-Related Factors and Risk of Hip Fracture: The EPI-DOX Prospective Study," *The Lancet,* vol. 348 (1996), pp. 148–49.

81. L. Avioli, "Osteoporosis: A Growing National Health Problem," *Female Patient,* vol. 17 (1992), pp. 25–28; W. A. Wallace, "The Increasing Incidence of Fractures of the Proximal Femur: An Orthopaedic Epidemic," *The Lancet,* vol. 1, no. 833 (June 25, 1993), p. 1413.

82. H. Bischoff-Ferrari, "Effect of Extended Physiotherapy and High-Dose Vitamin D on Rate of Falls and Hospital Re-admission After Acute Hip Fracture: A Randomized Controlled Trial," presented at the 31st Annual Meeting of the American Society for Bone and Mineral Research (ASBMR), September 2009, Denver, CO.

83. L. S. Harkness et al., "Decreased Bone Resorption with Soy Isoflavone Supplementation in Postmenopausal Women," *Journal of Women's Health* (Larchmont), vol. 13, no. 9 (November 2004), pp. 1000–7; M. Mori et al., "Soy Isoflavone Tablets Reduce Osteoporosis Risk Factors and Obesity in Middle-Aged Japanese Women," *Clinical and Experimental Pharmacology and Physiology,* vol. 31, suppl. 2 (December 2004), pp. S39–41; M. Mori et al., "Soy Isoflavones Improve Bone Metabolism in Postmenopausal Japanese Women," *Clinical and Experimental Pharmacology and Physiology,* vol. 31, suppl. 2 (December 2004), pp. S44–46; E. Nikander et al., "Effects of Phytoestrogens on Bone Turnover in Postmenopausal Women with a History of Breast Cancer," *Journal of Clinical Endocrinology and Metabolism,* vol. 89, no. 3 (March 2004), pp. 1207–12.

84. N. Urasopon et al., "*Pueraria mirifica,* a Phytoestrogen-Rich Herb, Prevents Bone Loss in Orchidectomized Rats," *Maturitas,* vol. 56, no. 3 (March 20, 2007), pp. 322–31.

85. D. Feskanich, W. C. Willett, and G. A. Colditz, "Calcium, Vitamin D, Milk Consumption, and Hip Fractures: A Prospective Study Among Postmenopausal

Women," *American Journal of Clinical Nutrition,* vol. 77, no. 2 (February 2003), pp. 504–11.

86. H. A. Bischoff-Ferrari et al., "Calcium Intake and Hip Fracture Risk in Men and Women: A Meta-Analysis of Prospective Cohort Studies and Randomized Controlled Trials," *American Journal of Clinical Nutrition,* vol. 86, no. 6 (December 2007), pp. 1780–90.

87. M. Castleman, "The Calcium Myth," *Natural Solutions,* July–August 2009, pp. 57–62, www.naturalsolutionsmag.com/articles-display/15403/The-Calcium -Myth.

88. E. Angin, Z. Erden, and F. Can, "The Effects of Clinical Pilates Exercises on Bone Mineral Density, Physical Performance and Quality of Life of Women with Postmenopausal Osteoporosis," *Journal of Back and Musculoskeletal Rehabilitation,* vol. 28, no. 4 (2015), pp. 849–58; L. C. de Oliveira, R. G. de Oliveira, and D. A. de Almeida Pires-Oliveira, "Effects of Whole-Body Vibration Versus Pilates Exercise on Bone Mineral Density in Postmenopausal Women: A Randomized and Controlled Clinical Trial," *Journal of Geriatric Physical Therapy* 42, no. 2 (April–June 2019), pp. E23–E31; C. S. Kim, J. Y. Kim, and H. J. Kim, "The Effects of a Single Bout Pilates Exercise on mRNA Expression of Bone Metabolic Cytokines in Osteopenia Women," *Journal of Exercise, Nutrition, and Biochemistry,* vol. 18, no. 1 (March 2014), pp. 69–78.

89. M. Sinaki and B. A. Mikkelsen, "Postmenopausal Spinal Osteoporosis: Flexion Versus Extension Exercises," *Archives of Physical Medicine and Rehabilitation,* vol. 65, no. 10 (October 1984), pp. 593–96.

90. Y. H. Lu et al., "Twelve-Minute Daily Yoga Regimen Reverses Osteoporotic Bone Loss," *Topics in Geriatric Rehabilitation,* vol. 32, no. 2 (April 2016), pp. 81–87.

91. M. Hernandez-Avila et al., "Caffeine, Moderate Alcohol Intake, and Risk of Fracture of the Hip and Forearm in Middle-Aged Women," *American Journal of Clinical Nutrition,* vol. 54 (1991), pp. 157–63; D. E. Nelson et al., "Alcohol as a Risk Factor for Fall Injury Events Among Elderly Persons Living in the Community," *Journal of the Geriatric Society,* vol. 40 (1992), pp. 658–61; H. D. Nelson et al., "Smoking, Alcohol, and Neuromuscular and Physical Function of Older Women," *Journal of the American Medical Association,* vol. 272, no. 24 (1994), pp. 1909–13.

92. D. C. Bauer et al., "Factors Associated with Appendicular Bone Mass in Older Women," *Archives of Internal Medicine,* vol. 118, no. 9 (1993), pp. 657–65; D. P. Kiel et al., "Caffeine and the Risk of Hip Fracture: The Framingham Study," *Biological Psychiatry,* vol. 23 (1988), pp. 335–49.

93. M. F. Holick, "Optimal Vitamin D Status for the Prevention and Treatment of Osteoporosis," *Drugs and Aging,* vol. 24, no. 12 (2007), pp. 1017–29.

94. R. Vieth, "The Role of Vitamin D in the Prevention of Osteoporosis," *Annals of Medicine,* vol. 37, no. 4 (2005), pp. 276–77.

95. Feskanich, Willett, and Colditz, "Calcium, Vitamin D, Milk Consumption, and Hip Fractures: A Prospective Study Among Postmenopausal Women."

96. B. Dawson-Hughes et al., "Effect of Vitamin D Supplementation on Wintertime and Overall Bone Loss in Healthy Postmenopausal Women," *Annals of Internal Medicine,* vol. 115, no. 17 (1991), pp. 505–12.

97. H. I. Abdalla et al., "Prevention of Bone Mineral Loss in Postmenopausal Women by Norethisterone," *Obstetrics and Gynecology,* vol. 66 (1985), pp. 789–92; J. Dequeker and E. De Muylder, "Long-Term Progestogen Treatment and Bone Remodeling in Premenopausal Women: A Longitudinal Study," *Maturitas,* vol. 4 (1982), pp. 309–13; R. Lindsay et al., "Comparative Effectiveness of Estrogen and a Progestogen on Bone Loss in Postmenopausal Women," *Clinical Science and Molecular Medicine,* vol. 54 (1978), pp. 93–95; J. McCann and N. Horwitz, "Provera Alone Builds Bone," *Medical Tribune,* July 1987, pp. 4–5; J. C. Prior et al., "Progesterone as a Bone-Tropic Hormone," *Endocrine Reviews,* vol. 11 (1990), pp. 386–98; B. L. Riggs et al., "Effect of Sex Hormones in Bone in Primary Osteoporosis," *Journal of Clinical Investigations,* vol. 48 (1969), pp. 1065–72; F. G. R. Snow and C. Anderson, "The Effect of 17-Beta Estradiol and Progestogen on Trabecular Bone Remodeling in Oophorectomized Dogs," *Calcification Tissue,* vol. 39 (1986), pp. 198–205.

98. A. K. Banerjee, P. J. Lane, and F. W. Meichen, "Vitamin C and Osteoporosis in Old Age," *Age and Aging,* vol. 7, no. 1 (1978), pp. 16–18.

99. F. H. Nielsen, "Studies on the Relationship Between Boron and Magnesium Which Possibly Affects the Formation and Maintenance of Bones," *Magnesium Trace Elements,* vol. 9, no. 2 (1990), pp. 61–91; J. U. Reginster et al., "Preliminary Report of Decreased Serum Magnesium in Post-Menopausal Osteoporosis," *Magnesium,* vol. 8, no. 2 (1989), pp. 106–9.

100. T. L. Holbrook et al., "Dietary Calcium and Risk of Hip Fracture: A 14-Year Prospective Population Study," *The Lancet,* vol. 2 (1988), pp. 1046–49; H. Spencer et al., "Absorption of Calcium in Osteoporosis," *American Journal of Medicine,* vol. 37 (1964), pp. 223–24.

101. F. H. Nielsen et al., "Effects of Dietary Boron on Mineral, Estrogen, and Testosterone Metabolism in Post-Menopausal Women," *Federation of American Societies for Experimental Biology Journal,* vol. 1 (1987), pp. 394–97.

102. C. V. Odvina et al., "Severely Suppressed Bone Turnover: A Potential Complication of Alendronate Therapy," *Journal of Clinical Endocrinology and Metabolism,* vol. 90, no. 3 (March 2005), pp. 1294–301.

103. D. C. Bauer et al., "Change in Bone Turnover and Hip, Non-Spine, and Vertebral Fracture in Alendronate-Treated Women: The Fracture Intervention Trial," *Journal of Bone and Mineral Research,* vol. 19, no. 8 (August 2004), pp. 1250–58; E. B. Kwek et al., "An Emerging Pattern of Subtrochanteric Stress Fractures: A Long-Term Complication of Alendronate Therapy?" *Injury,* vol. 39, no. 2 (February 2008), pp. 224–31; A. S. Neviaser et al., "Low-Energy Femoral Shaft Fractures Associated with Alendronate Use," *Journal of Orthopaedic Trauma,* vol. 22, no. 5 (May–June 2008), pp. 346–50; T. Parker-Pope, "Drugs to Build Bones May Weaken Them," *New York Times,* July 15, 2008, www.nytimes.com/2008/07/15/health/15well.html?partner=rssnyt&emc=rss; R. K. Cheung et al., "Sequential Non-Traumatic Femoral Shaft Fractures in a Patient on Long-Term Alendronate," *Hong Kong Medical Journal,* vol. 13, no. 6 (December 2007), pp. 485–89.

104. P. Alonso-Coello et al., "Drugs for Pre-Osteoporosis: Prevention or Disease Mongering?" *British Medical Journal,* vol. 336, no. 7636 (January 19, 2008), pp. 126–29.

105. 32nd Annual San Antonio Breast Cancer Symposium (SABCS): Abstracts 21 and 27. Presented December 10, 2009.

106. S. L. Ruggiero et al., "Osteonecrosis of the Jaws Associated with the Use of Bisphosphonates: A Review of 63 Cases," *Journal of Oral and Maxillofacial Surgery*, vol. 62, no. 5 (May 2004), pp. 527–34.

107. L. Liu et al., "Association Between Alendronate and Atypical Femur Fractures: A Meta-Analysis," *Endocrine Connections*, vol. 4, no. 1 (March 2015), pp. 58–64.

108. L. Speroff, "Is Long-Term Alendronate Treatment a Problem?" *Ob/Gyn Clinical Alert*, vol. 22, no. 2 (June 1, 2005), pp. 9–10.

109. U. Hartmann et al., "Low Sexual Desire in Midlife and Older Women: Personality Factors, Psychosocial Development, Present Sexuality," *Menopause*, vol. 11, no. 6, pt. 2 (November/December 2004), pp. 726–40; R. Basson, "Recent Advances in Women's Sexual Function and Dysfunction," *Menopause*, vol. 11, no. 6, pt. 2 (November/December 2004), pp. 714–25; *NAMS Supplement—Update on Sexuality at Menopause and Beyond: Normative, Adaptive, Problematic, Dysfunctional*, North American Menopause Society, vol. 11, no. 6 (November 2004), pp. 708–86; P. Sarrel and M. I. Whitehead, "Sex and Menopause: Defining the Issues," *Maturitas*, vol. 7 (1985), pp. 217–24; R. H. van Lunsen and E. Laan, "Genital Vascular Responsiveness and Sexual Feelings in Midlife Women: Psychophysiologic, Brain, and Genital Imaging Studies," *Menopause*, vol. 11, no. 6, pt. 2 (November/December 2004), pp. 741–48.

110. G. Ogden, *The Return of Desire* (Boston: Trumpeter, 2008).

111. L. M. Diamond, *Sexual Fluidity: Understanding Women's Love and Desire* (Cambridge, MA: Harvard University Press, 2008).

112. B. Zumoff et al., "24-Hour Mean Plasma Testosterone Concentration Declines with Age in Normal Premenopausal Women," *Journal of Clinical Endocrinology and Metabolism*, vol. 80, no. 4 (1995), pp. 1429–30.

113. G. A. Bachmann, "Correlates of Sexual Desire in Postmenopausal Women," *Maturitas*, vol. 7, no. 3 (1985), p. 211, cited in D. Youngs, "Common Misconceptions About Sex and Depression During Menopause: A Historical Perspective," *Female Patient*, vol. 17 (1992), pp. 25–28; Pfenninger, "Sex and the Maturing Female"; J. R. Wilson, "Sexuality in Aging," in J. J. Sciarra, ed., *Gynecology and Obstetrics* (Philadelphia: Lippincott, 1987), pp. 1–12.

114. Bachmann, "Correlates of Sexual Desire."

115. H. Fisch with S. Braun, *The Male Biological Clock: The Startling News About Aging, Sexuality, and Fertility in Men* (New York: Free Press, 2005).

116. Personal communication with Dr. Alan Gaby (a specialist in nutritional medicine); personal communication with David Zava, Ph.D., Aeron Lifecycles Lab.

117. M. Chia and M. Chia, *Cultivating Female Sexual Energy: Healing Love Through the Tao* (Huntington, NY: Healing Tao Books, 1986); available from Healing Tao Books, 2 Creskill Place, Huntington, NY 11743.

118. J. K. Meyers, M. M. Weissman, and G. L. Tischler, "Six-Month Prevalence of Psychiatric Disorder in Three Communities," *Archives of General Psychiatry*, vol. 41 (1984), p. 959.

119. S. M. McKinlay, J. B. McKinlay, and D. J. Bramblilla, "Health Status and Utilization Behavior Associated with Menopause," *American Journal of Epidemiology*, vol. 125 (1987), p. 110.

120. S. Hozl, L. Demisch, and B. Gollnik, "Investigations About Antidepressive and

Mood Change Effects of *Hypericum Perforatum*," *Planta Medica*, vol. 55 (1989), p. 643.

121. M. Van Eck McCain, *Transformation Through Menopause* (Amherst, MA: Bergin and Garvey, 1991).

122. M. Holloway, "The Estrogen Factor," *Scientific American*, June 1992.

123. G. A. Greendale et al., "Effects of the Menopause Transition and Hormone Use on Cognitive Performance in Midlife Women," *Neurology*, vol. 72, no. 21 (May 26, 2009), pp. 1850–57.

124. K. J. Chang et al., "Influences of Percutaneous Administration of Estradiol and Progesterone on Human Breast Epithelial Cell Cycle in Vivo," *Fertility and Sterility*, vol. 63, no. 4 (April 1995), pp. 785–91; M. J. Foidart et al., "Estradiol and Progesterone Regulate the Proliferation of Human Breast Epithelial Cells," *Fertility and Sterility*, vol. 69, no. 5 (May 1998), pp. 963–69.

125. J. C. Prior, "Perimenopause: The Complex Endocrinology of the Menopausal Transition," *Endocrine Reviews*, vol. 19, no. 4 (August 1998), pp. 397–428.

126. S. Franceschi et al., "Intake of Macronutrients and Risk of Breast Cancer," *The Lancet*, vol. 347 (1996), pp. 1351–56; A. Tavani et al., "Consumption of Sweet Foods and Breast Cancer Risk in Italy," *Annals of Oncology* 17, no. 2 (February 2006), pp. 341–45.

127. E. Ginsburg et al., "Effects of Alcohol Ingestion on Estrogens in Postmenopausal Women," *Journal of the American Medical Association*, vol. 276, no. 21 (1996), pp. 1747–51.

128. M. Eades and M. D. Eades, *Protein Power* (New York: Bantam Books, 1996). Both the Eadeses and the Hellers have done groundbreaking research on the effects of diet, excessive fat, and insulin on health. Both teams are available for consultation with physicians, and their books are excellent practical guides for patients and physicians alike.

129. J. Jeppesen et al., "Effects of Low-Fat, High-Carbohydrate Diets on Risk Factors for Ischemic Heart Disease in Postmenopausal Women," *American Journal of Clinical Nutrition*, vol. 65 (1997), pp. 1027–33.

130. M. Kearney et al., "William Heberden Revisited: Postprandial Angina Interval—Interval Between Food and Exercise and Meal Consumption Are Important Determinants of Time of Onset of Ischemia and Maximal Exercise Tolerance," *Journal of the American College of Cardiology*, vol. 29 (1997), pp. 302–7.

131. B. M. Altura et al., "Cardiovascular Risk Factors and Magnesium: Relationships to Atherosclerosis, Ischemic Heart Disease, and Hypertension," *Magnesium and Trace Elements*, vol. 10 (1991–92), pp. 182–92; R. DeGronzo and E. Ferrannini, "Insulin Resistance: A Multifaceted Syndrome Responsible for NIDDM, Obesity, Hypertension, Dyslipidemia, and Atherosclerotic Cardiovascular Disease," *Diabetes Care*, vol. 14, no. 3 (1991), pp. 173–94; A. Ferrara et al., "Sex Differences in Insulin Levels in Older Adults and the Effect of Body Size, Estrogen Replacement Therapy, and Glucose Tolerance Status: The Rancho Bernardo Study, 1984–87," *Diabetes Care*, vol. 18, no. 2 (1995), pp. 220–25; J. M. Gaziano, "Antioxidant Vitamins and Coronary Artery Disease Risk," *American Journal of Medicine*, vol. 97 (1994), pp. 3A–18S, 21S; J. Hallfrisch et al., "High Plasma Vitamin C Associated with High Plasma HDL and HDL(2) Cholesterol," *American Journal of Clinical Nutrition*, vol. 60 (1994), pp. 100–5; M. Modan et al., "Hyperinsu-

linemia: A Link Between Hypertension, Obesity, and Glucose Intolerance," *Journal of Clinical Investigation*, vol. 75 (1985), pp. 809–17; H. Morrison et al., "Serum Folate and Risk of Fatal Coronary Heart Disease," *Journal of the American Medical Association*, vol. 275, no. 24 (June 26, 1996), pp. 1893–96; R. A. Riemersma et al., "Risk of Angina Pectoris and Plasma Concentrations of Vitamins A, E, C, and Carotene," *The Lancet*, vol. 337 (1991), pp. 1–5; M. Stampfer et al., "Vitamin E Consumption and the Risk of Coronary Heart Disease in Women," *New England Journal of Medicine*, vol. 328, no. 20 (May 20, 1993), pp. 1444–49; D. Steinberg et al., "Antioxidants in the Prevention of Human Atherosclerosis," *Circulation*, vol. 85, no. 6 (1972), pp. 2338–43; D. A. Street et al., "A Population Based Case Control Study of the Association of Serum Antioxidants and Myocardial Infarction," *American Journal of Epidemiology*, vol. 124 (1991), pp. 719–20.

132. M. Studer et al., "Effect of Different Antilipidemic Agents and Diets on Mortality: A Systematic Review," *Archives of Internal Medicine*, vol. 165, no. 7 (April 11, 2005), pp. 725–30.

133. M. Daviglus et al., "Fish Consumption and the 30-Year Risk of Fatal Myocardial Infarction," *New England Journal of Medicine*, vol. 336, no. 15 (April 10, 1997), pp. 1046–53.

134. R. K. Hermsmeyer et al., "Cardiovascular Effects of Medroxyprogsterone Acetate and Progesterone: A Case of Mistaken Identity?" *Nature Clinical Practice Cardiovascular Medicine*, vol. 5, no. 7 (July 2008), pp. 387–95.

135. Alzheimer's Association, "2018 Alzheimer's Disease Facts and Figures," *Alzheimer's and Dementia*, vol. 14, no. 3 (2018), pp. 367–429, alz.org/media/HomeOffice/Facts%20and%20Figures/facts-and-figures.pdf.

136. D. Snowden et al., "Linguistic Ability in Early Life and Cognitive Function and Alzheimer's Disease in Late Life," *Journal of the American Medical Association*, vol. 275, no. 7 (February 21, 1996), pp. 528–32.

137. Q. Chengxuan and L. Fratiglioni, "Aging without Dementia is Achievable: Current Evidence from Epidemiological Research," *Journal of Alzheimer's Disease*, vol. 62, no. 3 (2018), pp. 933–42; T. Perls, *Experimental Gerontology*, vol. 39, nos. 11–12 (November–December 2004), pp. 1587–93.

138. R. Peters, "Ageing and the Brain," *Postgraduate Medical Journal*, vol. 82, no. 964 (February 2006), pp. 84–88.

139. M. A. Espeland et al., "Conjugated Equine Estrogens and Global Cognitive Function in Postmenopausal Women: Women's Health Initiative Memory Study," *Journal of the American Medical Association*, vol. 291, no. 24 (June 23, 2004), pp. 2959–68.

140. T. L. Loucks and S. L. Berga, "Does Postmenopausal Estrogen Use Confer Neuroprotection?" *Seminars in Reproductive Medicine*, vol. 27, no. 3 (May 2009), pp. 260–74.

141. V. Henderson et al., "Estrogen Replacement Therapy in Older Women: Comparisons Between Alzheimer's Disease Cases and Nondemented Control Subjects," *Archives of Neurology*, vol. 51 (1994), pp. 896–900; H. Honjo et al., "An Effect of Conjugated Estrogen to Cognitive Impairment in Women with Senile Dementia, Alzheimer's Type: A Placebo-Controlled Double Blind Study," *Journal of the Japanese Menopause Society*, vol. 1 (1993), pp. 167–71; T. Ohkura et al., "Evaluation of Estrogen Treatment in Female Patients with Dementia of the Alz-

heimer's Type," *Endocrine Journal,* vol. 41 (1994), pp. 361–71; A. Paganini-Hill and V. W. Henderson, "Estrogen Deficiency and Risk of Alzheimer's Disease in Women," *American Journal of Epidemiology,* vol. 140 (1994), pp. 256–61.

142. J. F. Flood, J. E. Morley, and E. Roberts, "Memory-Enhancing Effects in Male Mice of Pregnenolone and Steroids Metabolically Derived from It," *Proceedings from the National Academy of Sciences,* vol. 89 (March 1992), pp. 1567–71: C. R. Mevril et al., "Reduced Plasma DHEA Concentrations in HIV Infection and Alzheimer's Disease," in M. Kalimi and W. Regelson, eds., *The Biological Role of Dehydroepiandrosterone* (New York: de Gruyter, 1990), pp. 101–5; W. Regelson et al., "Dehydroepiandrosterone (DHEA)—The 'Mother Steroid.' I. Immunologic Action," *Annals of the New York Academy of Sciences,* vol. 719 (1994), pp. 553–63; S. S. C. Yen et al., "Replacement of DHEA in Aging Men and Women: Potential Remedial Effects," *Annals of the New York Academy of Sciences,* vol. 774 (1995), pp. 128–42.

143. L. L. Ekblad, J. Johansson, S. Heilin, M. Viitanen, H. Laine, P. Puukka, A. Jula, and J. O. Rinne, "Midlife Insulin Resistance, APOE Genotype, and Late-Life Brain Amyloid Accumulation," *Neurology,* vol. 90, no. 13 (March 27, 2018), pp. e1150–57.

144. S. M. de la Monte and J. R. Wands, "Alzheimer's Disease Is Type 3 Diabetes—Evidence Reviewed," *Journal of Diabetes Science and Technology,* vol. 2, no. 6 (November 2008), pp. 1101–13.

145. M. Boldrini et al., "Human Hippocampal Neurogenesis Persists Throughout Aging," *Cell Stem Cell,* vol. 22, no. 4 (April 5, 2018), pp. 589–99; Z. Chaker et al., "Hypothalamic Neurogenesis Persists in the Aging Brain and Is Controlled by Energy-Sensing IGF-I Pathway," *Neurobiology of Aging,* vol. 41 (May 2016), pp. 64–72.

146. M. Freedman et al., "Computerized Axial Tomography in Aging," in M. L. Albert, ed., *Clinical Neurology of Aging* (New York: Oxford University Press, 1984); U. Lehr and R. Schmitz-Scherzer, "Survivors and Non-Survivors: Two Fundamental Patterns of Aging," in H. Thomas, ed., *Patterns of Aging* (Basel: S. Karger, 1976); A. L. Benton, P. J. Eslinger, and A. R. Damasio, "Normative Observations on Neuropsychological Test Performance in Old Age," *Journal of Clinical Neuropsychiatry,* vol. 3 (1981), pp. 33–42.

147. P. H. Evans, J. Klinowski, and E. Yano, "Cephaloconiosis: A Free Radical Perspective on the Proposed Particulate-Induced Etiopathogenesis of Alzheimer's Dementia and Related Disorders," *Medical Hypotheses,* vol. 34 (1991), pp. 209–19; I. Rosenberg and J. Miller, "Nutritional Factors in Physical and Cognitive Functions of Elderly People," *American Journal of Clinical Nutrition,* vol. 55 (1992), pp. 1237S–1243S; R. N. Strachan and J. G. Henderson, "Dementia and Folate Deficiency," *Quarterly Journal of Medicine,* vol. 36 (1967), pp. 189–204.

148. J. K. Morris et al., "Aerobic Exercise for Alzheimer's Disease: A Randomized Controlled Pilot Trial," *PLoS One,* vol. 12, no. 2 (February 10, 2017), p. e0170547.

149. Weed, from an introductory flyer for *Menopausal Years.*

Chapter 15: Steps for Flourishing

1. Exercise adapted from a workshop author participated in with Annie Gill-O'Toole.

2. This teaching is from Abraham, who teaches through Esther Hicks. I've consistently found the Abraham teachings to be very practical material for living joyfully. For more information, visit www.abraham-hicks.com.

3. Bruce Lipton, Ph.D., made this comment on the program *Flourish! with Dr. Christiane Northrup*, Hay House Radio, October 21, 2009.

4. N. P. Kellermann, "Epigenetic Transmission of Holocaust Trauma: Can Nightmares Be Inherited?" *The Israel Journal of Psychology and Related Sciences*, vol. 50, no. 1 (2013), pp. 33–39; N. P. Kellermann, "Transmission of Holocaust Trauma—An Integrative View," *Psychiatry*, vol. 64, no. 3 (Fall 2001), pp. 256–67.

5. A. L. Roberts et al., "Women's Experience of Abuse in Childhood and Their Children's Smoking and Overweight," *American Journal of Preventive Medicine*, vol. 46, no. 3 (March 2014), pp. 249–58.

6. R. A. Sansone and L. A. Sansone, "Borderline Personality Disorder in the Medical Setting: Suggestive Behaviors, Syndromes, and Diagnoses," *Innovations in Clinical Neuroscience*, vol. 12, nos. 7–8 (July–August 2015), pp. 39–44.

7. S. Cohen, D. Janicki-Deverts, and W. J. Doyle, "Self-Rated Health in Healthy Adults and Susceptibility to the Common Cold," *Psychosomatic Medicine*, vol. 77, no. 9 (November–December 2015), pp. 959–68.

8. S. R. H. Beach et al., "When Inflammation and Depression Go Together: The Longitudinal Effects of Parent-Child Relationships," *Development and Psychopathology*, vol. 29, no. 5 (December 2017), pp. 1969–86.

9. Leslie Kussman, personal communication, May 6, 1992, before filming *Harbour of Hope*, a documentary about those who have healed from chronic or terminal illness, http://harbourofhope.com.

10. V. Robin and J. Dominguez, *Your Money or Your Life: 9 Steps to Transforming Your Relationship with Money and Creating Financial Independence* (New York: Penguin, 2008).

11. P. Arnstein et al., "From Chronic Pain Patient to Peer: Benefits and Risks of Volunteering," *Pain Management Nursing*, vol. 3, no. 3 (September 2002), pp. 94–103.

12. B. L. Fredrickson et al., "A Functional Genomeic Perspective on Human Well-Being," *Proceedings of the National Academy of Sciences*, vol. 110, no. 33 (August 13, 2013), pp. 13684–89.

13. C. Dann, "Poll: Workplace Equality Stalls for Women Even as Perceptions Improve," NBC News, March 22, 2018, https://www.nbcnews.com/politics/first-read/poll-workplace-equality-stalls-women-even-perceptions-improve-n859206.

14. M. DeWolf, "12 Stats About Working Women," U.S. Department of Labor Blog, March 1, 2017, https://blog.dol.gov/2017/03/01/12-stats-about-working-women.

15. R. Grossarth-Maticek, J. Bastiaans, and D. T. Kanazir, "Psychosocial Factors as Strong Predictors of Mortality from Cancer, Ischaemic Heart Disease and Stroke:

The Yugoslav Prospective Study," *Journal of Psychosomatic Research,* vol. 29, no. 2 (1985), pp. 167–76.

16. B. C. Broom, R. J. Booth, and C. Schubert, "Symbolic Diseases and 'MindBody' Co-Emergence. A Challenge for Psychoneuroimmunology," *Explore,* vol. 8, no. 1 (January–February 2012), pp. 16–25, www.letmagichappen.com/images/uploads/documents/Symbolic_Diseases.Explore_2012.pdf.

17. G. Maté, *When the Body Says No* (Hoboken, NJ: John Wiley & Sons, 2003), p. 257.

18. At one of my workshops a woman from Atlanta told me that her woman's group simply calls this deep work "the process." She had never heard of Anne Wilson Schaef or her work.

19. Naomi Wolf has documented the tragic aspects of this in *The Beauty Myth* (New York: Morrow, 1990).

20. F. S. Shinn, *The Game of Life and How to Play It* (Marina del Rey, CA: DeVorss and Co., 1925).

21. Patricia Reis, author of *Through the Goddess* (Freedom, CA: Crossing Press, 1991), worked with us at Women to Women for four years, teaching us the deep patterns held in women's psyches and bodies.

22. An in-depth approach to this is available in V. Noble, *Shakti Woman* (HarperSan-Francisco, 1992).

23. For more information, write to the Proprioceptive Writing Center, P.O. Box 165, Lake Clear, NY 12945, 423-454-9760, http://pwriting.org.

24. Dream incubation is adapted from the work of Patricia Reis.

25. L. Cosgrove and S. Krimsky, "A Comparison of *DSM*-IV and *DSM*-5 Panel Members' Financial Associations with Industry: A Pernicious Problem Persists," *PLoS Medicine,* vol. 9, no. 3 (March 2012), p. e1001190, https://journals.plos.org/plosmedicine/article/file?id=10.1371/journal.pmed.1001190&type=printable.

26. K. Brogan, "Remote Healing of Bipolar Disorder, Eating Disorder Not Otherwise Specified, Posttraumatic Stress Disorder, Fibromyalgia, and Irritable Bowel Syndrome Through Lifestyle Change," *Advances in Mind-Body Medicine,* vol. 31, no. 4 (Fall 2017), pp. 4–9.

27. J. Fang et al., "The Salient Characteristics of the Central Effects of Acupuncture Needling: Limbic-Paralimbic-Neocortical Network Modulation," *Human Brain Mapping,* vol. 30, no. 4 (April 2009), pp. 1196–206.

28. D. Church, G. Yount, and A. J. Brooks, "The Effect of Emotional Freedom Techniques on Stress Biochemistry: A Randomized Controlled Trial," *Journal of Nervous and Mental Disease,* vol. 200, no. 10 (October 22012), pp. 891–96.

29. B. O. Rothbaum, "A Controlled Study of Eye Movement Desensitization and Reprocessing in the Treatment of Posttraumatic Stress Disordered Sexual Assault Victims," *Bulletin of the Menninger Clinic,* vol. 61, no. 3 (Summer 1997), pp. 317–34; S. A. Wilson, L. A. Becker, and R. H. Tinker, "Eye Movement Desensitization and Reprocessing (EMDR) Treatment for Psychologically Traumatized Individuals," *Journal of Consulting and Clinical Psychology,* vol. 63, no. 6 (December 1995), pp. 928–37; S. A. Wilson, L. A. Becker, and R. H. Tinker, "Fifteen-Month Follow-Up of Eye Movement Desensitization and Reprocessing (EMDR) Treatment for Posttraumatic Stress Disorder and Psychological Trauma," *Journal*

of Consulting and Clinical Psychology, vol. 65, no. 6 (December 1997), pp. 1047–56.

30. S. V. Marcus, P. Marquis, and C. Sakai, "Controlled Study of Treatment of PTSD Using EMDR in an HMO Setting," *Psychotherapy Theory Research and Practice*, vol. 34, no. 3 (September 1997), pp. 307–15; S. V. Marcus, P. Marquis, and C. Sakai, "Three- and 6-Month Follow-Up of EMDR Treatment of PTSD in an HMO Setting," *International Journal of Stress Management*, vol. 11, no. 3 (August 2004), pp. 195–208.

31. D. Spiegel et al., "Effects of Psychosocial Treatment on Survival of Patients with Metastatic Breast Cancer," *The Lancet*, vol. 2 (1989), pp. 888–91; D. Spiegel, "A Psychosocial Intervention and Survival Time of Patients with Metastatic Breast Cancer," *Advances*, vol. 7, no. 3 (1991), pp. 10–19.

32. J. J. Gross, "The Emerging Field of Emotion Regulation: An Integrative Review," *Review of General Psychology*, vol. 2, no. 3 (September 1998), pp. 271–99, http://www.elaborer.org/psy1045d/cours/Gross(1998).pdf.

33. R. G. Reed et al., "Emotional Acceptance, Inflammation, and Sickness Symptoms Across the First Two years Following Breast Cancer Diagnosis," *Brain, Behavior, and Immunity*, vol. 56 (August 2016), pp. 165–74.

34. B. E. Lippitz, "Cytokine Patterns in Patients with Cancer; A Systematic Review," *The Lancet—Oncology*, vol. 14, no. 6 (May 2013), pp. e218–28.

35. M. C. Janelsins et al., "Differential Expression of Cytokines in Breast Cancer Patients Receiving Different Chemotherapies: Implications for Cognitive Impairment Research," *Supportive Care in Cancer*, vol. 20, no. 4 (April 2012), pp. 831–39.

36. K. Uvnas-Moberg, L. Handlin, and M. Petersson, "Self-Soothing Behaviors with Particular Reference to Oxytocin Release Induced by Non-Noxious Sensory Stimulation," *Frontiers in Psychology*, vol. 5 (January 12, 2015), p. 1529; K. Unvas-Moberg and M. Petersson, "Oxytocin, a Mediator of Anti-Stress, Well-Being, Social Interaction, Growth and Healing," *Zeitschrift für Psychosomatische Medizin und Psychotherapie*, vol. 51, no. 1 (2005), pp. 57–80.

37. V. Morhenn, L. E. Beavin, and P. J. Zak, "Massage Increases Oxytocin and Reduces Adrenocorticotropin Hormone in Humans," *Alternative Therapies in Health and Medicine*, vol. 18, no. 6 (November–December 2012), pp. 11–18.

38. Boston Women's Health Book Collective, *The New Our Bodies, Ourselves* (New York: Simon & Schuster, Inc., 1984); Riane Eisler, *The Chalice and the Blade: Our History, Our Future* (HarperSanFrancisco, 1988).

39. N. Singer, "Medical Papers by Ghostwriters Pushed Therapy," *New York Times*, August 5, 2009, p. A1.

40. A. S. Relman and M. Angell, "America's Other Drug Problem: How the Drug Industry Distorts Medicine and Politics," *New Republic*, vol. 227, no. 25 (December 16, 2002), pp. 27–41.

41. J. Law, *Big Pharma: Exposing the Global Healthcare Agenda* (New York: Carroll & Graf, 2006), p. 48; B. Lipton and S. Bhaerman, *Spontaneous Evolution: Our Positive Future (And a Way to Get There from Here)* (Carlsbad, CA: Hay House, 2009), p. 208.

42. T. J. Moore, J. Glenmullen, and C. D. Furberg, "Prescription Drugs Associated with Reports of Violence Towards Others," *PLoS One*, vol. 5, no. 12 (Decem-

ber 15, 2010), p. e15337, http://breggin.com/antidepressant-drugs-resources/
Moore2011-violence-rates-all-drugs-FDA.pdf.

43. C. Elliott, "The Drug Pushers," *The Atlantic,* April 2006, www.theatlantic.com/
doc/200604/drug-reps.

44. B. P. Turnwald et al., "Learning One's Genetic Risk Changes Physiology Independent of Actual Genetic Risk," *Nature Human Behaviour,* vol. 3 (2019), pp. 48–
56.

45. N. Bolz-Weber, "Forgive Assholes: Have a Little Faith," YouTube, posted by
Makers, May 30, 2018, https://www.youtube.com/watch?v=VhmRkUtPra8.

46. F. Luskin and B. Bland, "Stanford–Northern Ireland Hope 2 Project," unpublished manuscript, Stanford University, Palo Alto, CA, February 2001.

47. R. McCraty et al., "The Effects of Emotions on Short-Term Power Spectrum
Analysis of Heart Rate Variability," *American Journal of Cardiology,* vol. 76, no.
14 (November 15, 1995), pp. 1089–93; Doc Lew Childre, *Women Lead with
Their Hearts: A White Paper,* obtainable from the Institute of HeartMath, P.O.
Box 1463, Boulder Creek, CA 95006, 831-338-8500, www.heartmath.org.

48. S. Levine, *Guided Meditations, Explorations and Healings* (New York: Doubleday, 1991), p. 324.

49. D. Ehrenfeld, *The Arrogance of Humanism,* quoted in R. Sandor, "The Attending
Physician," *Sun,* vol. 4 (September 1, 1991), p. 4.

50. Quoted in Hicks and Hicks, *A New Beginning,* parts I and II.

51. A. Deyhle and J. Waterman, "Heart Coherence Increases Order of Crystallization
Patterns in Dried Saliva Study," HeartMath Research Center, Institute of Heart-
Math, Boulder, Colorado, October 2013, https://pdfs.semanticscholar.org/a83f/
4b54e3aa99dcba23676260862e242a52c298.pdf.

52. S. L. Liedliecki and M. Good, "Effect of Music on Power, Pain, Depression and
Disability," *Journal of Advanced Nursing,* vol. 54, no. 5 (June 2006), pp. 553–62.

53. H. Fukui and K. Toyoshima, "Music Facilitate the Neurogenesis, Regeneration
and Repair of Neurons," *Medical Hypotheses,* vol. 71, no. 5 (November 2008),
pp. 765–69.

54. H. Fukui, "The Effect of Music to Sex Hormones of Elderly Person," *Neuroscience Research Supplements,* vol. 55, no. 1 (January 2006), p. S58.

55. J. H. Fowler and N. A. Christakis, "Dynamic Spread of Happiness in a Large
Social Network: Longitudinal Analysis over 20 Years in the Framingham Study,"
British Medical Journal, vol. 337 (December 4, 2008), p. a2338.

56. R. W. Eyre et al., "Spreading of Components of Mood in Adolescent Social Networks," Royal Society Open Science, vol. 4, no. 9 (September 20, 2017),
p. 170336.

57. Dogen Zenji, found in S. Suzuki, *Zen Mind, Beginner's Mind,* ed. T. Dixon (Boston, MA: Shambhala, 2006), p. 30.

Chapter 16: Getting the Most Out of Your Medical Care

1. S. Richter, *The Genome Revolution,* Goldman Sachs, April 10, 2018, https://
www.goldmansachs.com/insights/pages/genome-revolution.html.

2. D. Riley, "Healthcare Reform," *Alternative Therapies in Health and Medicine,* vol. 15, no. 5 (September/October 2009), p. 8.

3. B. Starfield, "Is US Health Really the Best in the World?" *Journal of the American Medical Association,* vol. 284, no. 4 (July 26, 2000), pp. 483–85, www.jhsph .edu/research/centers-and-institutes/johns-hopkins-primary-care-policy-center/ Publications_PDFs/A154.pdf.

4. J. Mandrola, "A Corrosive Force in Medical Care," *Medscape,* October 20, 2017, www.medscape.com/viewarticle/887382.

5. N. Cousins, *Anatomy of an Illness as Perceived by the Patient* (New York: Bantam, 1979), pp. 49–50.

6. H. Benson et al., "The Placebo Effect: A Neglected Asset in the Care of Patients," *Journal of the American Medical Association,* vol. 232, no. 12 (June 23, 1975); A. B. Carter, "The Placebo: Its Use and Abuse," *The Lancet,* October 17, 1973, p. 823; B. Blackwell et al., "Demonstration to Medical Students of Placebo Responses and Non-Drug Factors," *The Lancet,* vol. 2 (June 1972), p. 1279; S. Wolf and H. K. Beecher, "The Powerful Placebo," *Journal of the American Medical Association,* vol. 159 (1955), pp. 1602–6.

7. J. B. Moseley et al., "A Controlled Trial of Arthroscopic Surgery for Osteoarthritis of the Knee," *New England Journal of Medicine,* vol. 347, no. 2 (July 11, 2002), pp. 81–88.

8. F. Islami et al., "Proportion and Number of Cancer Cases and Deaths Attributable to Potentially Modifiable Risk Factors in the United States," *CA: A Cancer Journal for Clinicians,* vol. 68, no. 1 (January 2018), pp. 31–54.

9. These steps adapted from a supplement to C. Northrup's *Health Wisdom for Women* newsletter.

10. M. Hyman, "The Myth of Diagnosis," blog post, May 4, 2018, http://drhyman .com/blog/2018/05/04/the-myth-of-diagnosis.

11. I. Kirsch et al., "The Emperor's New Drugs: An Analysis of Antidepressant Medication Data Submitted to the U.S. Food and Drug Administration," *Prevention and Treatment,* vol. 5, no. 1 (July 15, 2002), p. 23, https://pdfs.semanticscholar .org/15f4/3875a20b1e6e03ca7729070680477ad46e31.pdf.

12. L. Pratt, D. J. Brody, and Q. Gu, "Antidepressant Use Among Persons Aged 12 and Over: United States, 2011–2014," National Center for Health Statistics Data Brief No. 283, August 2017, https://www.cdc.gov/nchs/products/databriefs/ db283.htm.

13. M. M. Maslej et al., "The Mortality and Myocardial Effects of Antidepressants Are Moderated by Preexisting Cardiovascular Disease: A Meta-Analysis," *Psychotherapy and Psychosomatics,* vol. 86, no. 5 (2017), pp. 268–82.

14. D. Drewry, "Central Nervous System Apnea Can Be Caused by Traumatizing Events, and It Can Be Solved," *International Journal of Healing and Caring,* vol. 17, no. 1 (January 2017), pp. 1–11, http://www.wholistichealingresearch.org/wp -content/uploads/2016/12/Drewry-17-1.pdf.

15. Centers for Disease Control and Prevention (CDC), National Center for Health Statistics. *National Hospital Discharge Survey: 2010 Table, Procedures by Selected Patient Characteristics—Number by Procedure Category and Age* (Atlanta, GA: CDC, 2010), www.cdc.gov/nchs/data/nhds/4procedures/2010pro4 _numberprocedureage.pdf.

16. K. A. Cullen, M. J. Hall, and A. Golosinskiy, "Ambulatory Surgery in the United States, 2006," *National Health Statistics Report,* no. 11 (Hyattsville, MD: National Center for Health Statistics, 2009), p. 1, www.cdc.gov/nchs/data/nhsr/nhsr011.pdf.

17. The sense of the word *heroic* in this context is from the philosophy of Susun Weed, a wise woman herbalist who associates the heroic tradition with allopathic medicine.

18. *Gentle Visions: A Pre-Operative Relaxation Program,* 1991, 1992. For more information or to order, write to Healing Images, P.O. Box 2972, Framingham Center Station, Framingham, MA 01701.

19. This entire section is adapted from an article in the April 1996 issue of C. Northrup's *Health Wisdom for Women* newsletter. An extensive bibliography of the studies that support these steps can be found in Huddleston, *Prepare for Surgery* (see Resources for chapter 16).

20. N. E. Morone and D. K. Weiner, "Pain as the Fifth Vital Sign: Exposing the Vital Need for Pain Education," *Clinical Therapeutics,* vol. 35, no. 11 (November 2013), pp. 1728–32; A. Van Zee, "The Promotion and Marketing of OxyContin: Commercial Triumph, Public Health Tragedy," *American Journal of Public Health,* vol. 99, no. 2 (February 2009), pp. 221–27.

21. K. E. Vowles et al., "Rates of Opioid Misuse, Abuse, and Addiction in Chronic Pain: A Systematic Review and Data Synthesis," *Pain,* vol. 156, no. 4 (April 2015), pp. 569–76.

22. P. K. Muhuri, J. C. Gfroerer, and M. C. Davies, "Associations of Nonmedical Pain Reliever Use and Initiation of Heroin Use in the United States," *CBHSQ Data Review,* August 2013, https://www.samhsa.gov/data/sites/default/files/DR006/DR006/nonmedical-pain-reliever-use-2013.htm; T. J. Cicero et al., "The Changing Face of Heroin Use in the United States: A Retrospective Analysis of the Past 50 Years," *Journal of the American Medical Association—Psychiatry,* vol. 71, no. 7 (July 1, 2014), pp. 821–26; R. G. Carlson et al., "Predictors of Transition to Heroin Use Among Initially Non-Opioid Dependent Illicit Pharmaceutical Opioid Users: A Natural History Study," *Drug and Alcohol Dependence,* vol. 160 (March 1, 2016), pp. 127–34.

23. Center for Behavioral Health Statistics and Quality (CBHSQ). *2017 National Survey on Drug Use and Health: Detailed Tables* (Rockville, MD: Substance Abuse and Mental Health Services Administration, 2018).

24. A. M. Vivolo-Kantor et al., "Vital Signs: Trends in Emergency Department Visits for Suspected Opioid Overdoses—United States, July 2016–September 2017," *MMWR Morbidity and Mortality Weekly Report,* vol. 67 (March 9, 2018), pp. 279–85.

25. Y. Liang and B. J. Turner, "Assessing Risk for Drug Overdose in a National Cohort: Role for Both Daily and Total Opioid Dose," *Journal of Pain,* vol. 16, no. 4 (April 2015), pp. 318–25.

26. P. A. Nadpara et al., "Risk Factors for Serious Prescription Opioid-Induced Respiratory Depression or Overdose: Comparison of Commercially Insured and Veterans Health Affairs Populations," *Pain Medicine,* vol. 19, no. 1 (January 1, 2018), pp. 79–96.

27. P. M. Grace et al., "Repeated Morphine Prolongs Postoperative Pain in Male Rats," *Anesthesia and Analgesia,* vol. 128, no. 1 (January 2019), pp. 161–67.

28. University of Colorado at Boulder, "Post-Surgical Opioids Can, Paradoxically, Lead to Chronic Pain: Rats Given Morphine Experienced Pain-Reactivity for Three Weeks Longer, Inflammatory Changes in Spinal Cord," *ScienceDaily,* April 16, 2018, www.sciencedaily.com/releases/2018/04/180416145456.htm.

29. P. M. Grace et al., "Morphine Paradoxically Prolongs Neuropathic Pain in Rats by Amplifying Spinal NLRP3 Inflammasome Activation," *Proceedings of the National Academy of Sciences,* vol. 113, no. 24 (June 14, 2016), pp. E3441–50.

30. M. H. Grissa et al., "Acupuncutre vs. Intravenous Morphine in the Management of Acute Pain in the ED," *American Journal of Emergency Medicine,* vol. 34, no. 11 (November 2016), pp. 2112–16.

31. One summer, while climbing Mount Katahdin, I ran a stick through my shin. Not only did it hurt, it left an ugly gash that I knew would leave a scar. I grieved for my leg, even as my brother joked, "What do you care? You're not a model—you don't need your legs to look good for anything."

32. G. R. Harris, "Effective Treatment of Chronic Pain by the Integration of Neural Therapy and Prolotherapy," *Journal of Prolotherapy,* vol. 2, no. 2 (May 2010), pp. 377–86, www.journalofprolotherapy.com/pdfs/issue_06/issue_06_07_neural_therapy.pdf; R. G. Gibson and S. L. M. Gibson, "Neural Therapy in the Treatment of Multiple Sclerosis," *Journal of Alternative and Complementary Medicine,* vol. 5, no. 6 (1999), pp. 543–52, http://encognitive.com/files/Neural%20Therapy%20in%20the%20Treatment%20of%20Multiple%20Sclerosis.pdf.

33. D. K. Klinghardt, "Neural Therapy," *Explore!,* vol. 11, no. 2 (2002), pp. 25–29, http://www.klinghardtacademy.com/images/stories/neural_therapy/Neural-Therapy-2002.pdf.

Chapter 17: Eat to Flourish

1. During medical school, one of the surgeons I studied with performed intestinal bypass surgery on women (and men) who were morbidly obese. Though they lost weight quickly, postoperatively many were unable to adjust to their new size and continued to think and feel fat.

2. All the statistics in this paragraph are from the National Organization on Women and Body Image, www.womenandbodyimage.com.

3. S. Pai and K. Schryver, *Children, Teens, Media, and Body Image: A Common Sense Media Research Brief,* January 21, 2015, www.commonsensemedia.org/research/children-teens-media-and-body-image.

4. A. Malhotra, T. Noakes, and S. Phinney, "It Is Time to Bust the Myth of Physical Inactivity and Obesity: You Cannot Outrun a Bad Diet," *British Journal of Sports Medicine,* vol. 49, no. 15 (August 2015), pp. 967–68.

5. C. D. Gardner et al., "Effect of Low-Fat vs Low-Carbohydrate Diet on 12-Month Weight Loss in Overweight Adults and the Association with Genotype Pattern or Insulin Secretion: The DIETFITS Randomized Clinical Trial," *Journal of the American Medical Association,* vol. 319, no. 7 (February 20, 2018), pp. 667–79.

6. L. Lissner et al., "Variability of Body Weight and Health Outcomes in the Framingham Population," *New England Journal of Medicine,* vol. 324 (1991), pp. 1839–44.

7. The scenario of the overachieving, driven adolescent girl is a setup for anorexia. It's estimated that 50 percent of prep school girls are bulimic or anorexic to some extent. M. Woodman's *Addiction to Perfection: The Still Unravished Bride* (Toronto: Inner City Press, 1982) is a beautiful exploration of the depth of issues represented by eating disorders.

8. A. Tavani et al., "Consumption of Sweet Foods and Breast Cancer Risk in Italy," *Annals of Oncology* 17, no. 2 (February 2006), pp. 341–45.

9. To read this book online, see www.seleneriverpress.com/media/pdf_docs/0_How_to_Prevent_Heart_Attacks_BEN_SANDLER_MD_1958.pdf.

10. See the extensive bibliography of the medical literature in National Academy of Sciences, *Diet, Nutrition, and Cancer* (Washington, DC: National Academy Press, 1982), pp. 73–105.

11. B. MacMahan et al., "Urine Estrogen Profiles in Asian and North American Women," *International Journal of Cancer,* vol. 14 (1974), pp. 161–67; L. E. Dickinson et al., "Estrogen Profiles of Oriental and Caucasian Women in Hawaii," *New England Journal of Medicine,* vol. 291 (1974), pp. 1211–13; D. A. Snowden, letter to the editor, *Journal of the American Medical Association,* vol. 3, no. 254 (1985), pp. 356–57; D. W. Cramer et al., "Dietary Animal Fat and Relationship to Ovarian Cancer Risk," *Obstetrics and Gynecology,* vol. 63, no. 6 (1984), pp. 833–38; T. McKenna, "Pathogenesis and Treatment of Polycystic Ovary Syndrome," *New England Journal of Medicine,* vol. 318 (1988), p. 558; D. Polson, "Polycystic Ovaries—A Common Finding in Normal Women," *The Lancet,* vol. 1 (1988), p. 870.

12. P. Hill, "Diet, Lifestyle, and Menstrual Activity," *American Journal of Clinical Nutrition,* vol. 33 (1980), p. 1192.

13. A. Sanchez, "A Hypothesis on the Etiologic Role of Diet on the Age of Menarche," *Medical Hypotheses,* vol. 7 (1981), p. 1339; S. Schwartz, "Dietary Influences on Growth and Sexual Maturation in Premenarchal Rhesus Monkeys," *Hormones and Behavior,* vol. 22 (1988), p. 231.

14. C. Leigh Broadhurst, "Nutrition and Non-Insulin Dependent Diabetes Mellitus from an Anthropological Perspective," *Alternative Medicine Review,* vol. 2, no. 5 (1997), pp. 378–99.

15. S. B. Eaton et al., "An Evolutionary Perspective Enhances Understanding of Human Nutritional Requirements," *Journal of Nutrition,* vol. 126, no. 6 (June 1996), pp. 1732–40; S. B. Eaton, S. B. Eaton III, and M. J. Konner, "Paleolithic Nutrition Revisited: A Twelve-Year Retrospective on Its Nature and Implications," *European Journal of Clinical Nutrition,* vol. 51, no. 4 (April 1997), pp. 207–16; Michael Crawford and David Marsh, *Nutrition and Evolution* (New Caanan, CT: Keats Publishing, 1995).

16. A. Samsel and S. Seneff, "Glyphosate's Suppression of Cytochrome P450 Enzymes and Amino Acid Biosynthesis by the Gut Microbiome: Pathways to Modern Diseases," *Entropy,* vol. 15, no. 4 (2013), pp. 1416–63.

17. J. F. Ludvigsson et al., "Small Intestinal Histopathology and Mortality Risk in

Celiac Disease," *Journal of the American Medical Association,* vol. 302, no. 11 (September 16, 2009), pp. 1171–78.

18. R. J. Farrell and C. P. Kelly, "Celiac Sprue," *New England Journal of Medicine,* vol. 346, no. 3 (January 17, 2002), pp. 180–88.

19. M. Hyman, "Gluten: What You Don't Know Might Kill You," *Huffington Post,* January 2, 2010, www.huffingtonpost.com/dr-mark-hyman/gluten-what-you-dont -know_b_379089.html.

20. J. Tap et al., "Identification of an Intestinal Microbiota Signature Associated with Severity of Irritable Bowel Syndrome," *Gastroenterology,* vol. 152, no. 1 (January 2017), pp. 111–23.e8.

21. A. Fildes et al., "Probability of an Obese Person Attaining Normal Body Weight: Cohort Study Using Electronic Health Records," *American Journal of Public Health,* vol. 105, vol. 9 (September 2015), pp. e54–59.

22. A. Keys et al., *The Biology of Human Starvation,* vols. 1–2 (Minneapolis: University of Minnesota Press, 1950).

23. V. A. Catenacci et al., "A Randomized Pilot Study Comparing Zero-Calorie Alternate-Day Fasting to Daily Caloric Restriction in Adults with Obesity," *Obesity,* vol. 24, no. 9 (September 2016), pp. 1874–83.

24. H. J. Weir et al., "Dietary Restriction and AMPK Increase Lifespan via Mitochondrial Network and Peroxisome Remodeling," *Cell Metabolism,* vol., 26, no. 6 (December 5, 2017), pp. 884–896.e5.

25. Studies cited in P. Lipetz's *The Good Calorie Diet* (New York: HarperCollins, 1994), p. 72. This book has more helpful, scientifically documented information on the differences between carbohydrates than anything else I've found.

26. C. Xu et al., "Light-Harvesting Chlorophyll Pigments Enable Mammalian Mitochondria to Capture Photonic Energy and Product ATP," *Journal of Cell Science,* vol. 127, part 2 (January 15, 2014), pp. 388–99; see also A. S. Herrera et al., "Beyond Mitochondria, What Would Be the Energy Source of the Cell?" *Central Nervous System Agents in Medical Chemistry,* vol. 15, no. 1 (2015), pp. 32–41.

27. Herrera et al., "Beyond Mitochondria, What Would Be the Energy Source of the Cell?"

28. R. Melmed et al., "The Influence of Emotional State on the Mobilization of Marginal Pool Leukocytes and Insulin-Induced Hypoglycemia: A Possible Role for Eicosanoids as Major Mediators of Psychosomatic Processes," *Annals of the New York Academy of Sciences,* vol. 296 (1987), pp. 467–76.

29. J. W. Olney, "Brain Lesions, Obesity, and Other Disturbances in Mice Treated with Monosodium Glutamate," *Science,* vol. 164, no. 880 (May 9, 1969), pp. 719–21; K. He et al., "Association of Monosodium Glutamate Intake with Overweight in Chinese Adults: The INTERMAP Study," *Obesity,* vol. 16, no. 8 (August 2008), pp. 1875–80.

30. This list as well as other information about glutamates are available from the Truth in Labeling Campaign at www.truthinlabeling.org.

31. N. A. Christakis and J. H. Fowler, "The Collective Dynamics of Smoking in a Large Social Network," *New England Journal of Medicine,* vol. 358, no. 21 (May 22, 2008), pp. 2249–58.

32. "The Evolution of Miss America," PsychGudies.com, September 2015, www .psychguides.com/interact/the-evolution-of-miss-america.

33. Statistics from K. O'Nell, *The Famine Within* Probes Women's Pursuit of Thinness," review of K. Gilday's film *The Famine Within, Christian Science Monitor,* August 31, 1992.

34. See ANAD, "Eating Disorder Statistics," https://anad.org/education-and -awareness/about-eating-disorders/eating-disorders-statistics.

35. J. I. Hudson et al., "The Prevalence and Correlates of Eating Disorders in The National Comorbidity Survey Replication," *Biological Psychiatry,* vol. 61, no. 3 (2007), pp. 348–58.

36. See www.nationaleatingdisorders.org.

37. J. E. Mitchell et al., "Medical Complications and Medical Management of Bulimia," *Annals of Internal Medicine,* vol. 71 (1987).

38. R. E. Frisch, "The Right Weight: Body Fat, Menarche, and Ovulation," *Baillieres Clinical Obstetrics and Gynecology,* vol. 4, no. 3 (September 1990), pp. 419–39.

39. C. Li et al., "Estimates of Body Composition with Dual-Energy X-Ray Absorptiometry in Adults," *American Journal of Clinical Nutrition,* vol. 90, no. 6 (December 2009), pp. 1457–65.

40. M. Nelson et al., "Effects of High-Intensity Strength Training on Multiple Risk Factors for Osteoporitic Fractures: A Randomized Controlled Trial," *Journal of the American Medical Association,* vol. 272, no. 24 (December 28, 1994), pp. 1909–14.

41. B. R. Gordon et al., "Association of Efficacy of Resistance Exercise Training with Depressive Symptoms: Meta-Analysis and Meta-Regression Analysis of Randomized Controlled Trials," *Journal of the American Medical Association—Psychiatry,* vol. 75, no. 6 (June 1, 2018), pp. 566–76; B. R. Gordon et al., "The Effects of Resistance Exercise Training on Anxiety: A Meta-Analysis and Meta-Regression Analysis of Randomized Controlled Trials," *Sports Medicine,* vol. 47, no. 12 (December 2017), pp. 2521–32.

42. D. Cohen and G. Bria, *Quench: Beat Fatigue, Drop Weight, and Heal Your Body Through the New Science of Optimum Hydration* (New York: Hachette, 2018), p. 64.

43. L. Moore and M. L. Bradlee, "Low Sodium Intakes Are Not Associated with Lower Blood Pressure Levels Among Framingham Offspring Study Adults," Abstract No. 446.6, Proceedings of the 2017 Experimental Biology Conference (Chicago, April 25, 2017).

44. J. Sanmukhani et al., "Efficacy and Safety of Curcumin in Major Depressive Disorder: A Randomized Controlled Trial," *Psychotherapy Research,* vol. 28, no. 4 (April 2014), pp. 579–85.

45. M. Bullitt-Jonas, *Holy Hunger: A Memoir of Desire* (New York: Knopf, 1999), p. 119.

46. Personal communication with Dr. Michael Eades, who has reviewed the existing literature on this topic and shared it with me.

47. "Lean Beef Shown to Be as Healthy as Chicken and Fish," *Food Chemistry News,* vol. 32, no. 39 (1990), p. 6, cited in J. Bland, letter to the editor, *New England Journal of Medicine,* vol. 326, no. 3 (1992), p. 200.

48. A. Wayler et al., "Nitrogen Balance Studies in Young Men to Assess the Protein Quality of an Isolated Soy Protein in Relation to Meat Proteins," *Journal of Nutrition,* vol. 113, no. 12 (December 1983), pp. 2485–91; A. Baglieri et al., "Gastro-Jejunal Digestion of Soya-Bean-Milk Protein in Humans," *British Journal of Nutrition,* vol. 72, no. 4 (October 1994), pp. 519–32; F. Mariotti et al., "Nutritional Value of [15N]-Soy Protein Isolate Assessed from Ileal Digestibility and Postprandial Protein Utilization in Humans," *Journal of Nutrition,* vol. 129, no. 11 (November 1999), pp. 1992–97; C. Gaudichon et al., "Net Postprandial Utilization of [15N]-Labeled Milk Protein Nitrogen Is Influenced by Diet Composition in Humans," *Journal of Nutrition,* vol. 129, no. 4 (April 1999), pp. 890–95.

49. N. Istfan et al., "An Evaluation of the Nutritional Value of a Soy Protein Concentrate in Young Adult Men Using the Short-Term N-Balance Method," *Journal of Nutrition,* vol. 113, no. 12 (December 1983), pp. 2516–23; V. R. Young et al., "A Long-Term Metabolic Balance Study in Young Men to Assess the Nutritional Quality of an Isolated Soy Protein and Beef Proteins," *American Journal of Clinical Nutrition,* vol. 39, no. 1 (January 1984), pp. 8–15.

50. V. R. Young et al., "Evaluation of the Protein Quality of an Isolated Soy Protein in Young Men: Relative Nitrogen Requirements and Effects of Methionine Supplementation," *American Journal of Clinical Nutrition,* vol. 39, no. 1 (January 1984), pp. 16–24; A. Y. Zezulka and D. H. Calloway, "Nitrogen Retention in Men Fed Varying Levels of Amino Acids from Soy Protein With or Without Added L-Methionine," *Journal of Nutrition,* vol. 106, no. 2 (February 1976), pp. 212–21.

51. V. R. Young and P. L. Pellett, "Plant Proteins in Relation to Human Protein and Amino Acid Nutrition," *American Journal of Clinical Nutrition,* vol. 59 (May 1994), pp. 1203S-12S.

52. Istfan et al., "An Evaluation of the Nutritional Value of a Soy Protein Concentrate in Young Adult Men Using the Short-Term N-Balance Method"; Wayler et al., "Nitrogen Balance Studies in Young Men to Assess the Protein Quality of an Isolated Soy Protein in Relation to Meat Proteins"; Young et al., "Evaluation of the Protein Quality of an Isolated Soy Protein in Young Men: Relative Nitrogen Requirements and Effects of Methionine Supplementation."

53. C. T. Cordle, "Soy Protein Allergy: Incidence and Relative Severity," *Journal of Nutrition,* vol. 134, no. 5 (May 2004), pp. 1213S-19S.

54. Baglieri et al., "Gastro-Jejunal Digestion of Soya-Bean-Milk Protein in Humans."

55. M. Cotterchio et al., "Dietary Phytoestrogens Intake Is Associated with Reduced Colorectal Cancer Risk," *Journal of Nutrition,* vol. 136, no. 12 (December 2006), pp. 3046–53.

56. L. L. Lin et al., "Phase I Randomized Double-Blind Placebo-Controlled Single-Dose Safety Studies of Bowman-Birk inhibitor Concentrate," *Oncology Letters,* vol. 7, no. 4 (April 2014), pp. 1151–58.

57. H. P. Lee et al., "Dietary Effects on Breast-Cancer Risk in Singapore," *The Lancet,* vol. 337, no. 8751 (May 18, 1991), pp. 1197–200.

58. A. H. Wu et al., "Tofu and Risk of Breast Cancer in Asian-Americans," *Cancer Epidemiology, Biomarkers and Prevention,* vol. 5, no. 11 (November 1996), pp. 901–6.

59. S. Yamamoto et al., "Soy, Isoflavones, and Breast Cancer Risk in Japan," *Journal of the National Cancer Institute,* vol. 9, no. 12 (June 18, 2003), pp. 906–13.

60. S. A. Lee et al., "Adolescent and Adult Soy Food Intake and Breast Cancer Risk: Results from the Shanghai Women's Health Study," *American Journal of Clinical Nutrition,* vol. 89, no. 6 (June 2009), pp. 1920–26.

61. Council for Responsible Nutrition, "International Researchers Convene Meeting on Isoflavones," press release, June 17, 2009, www.npicenter.com/anm/anmviewer .asp?a=24304&print=yes.

62. K. Taku et al., "Soy Isoflavones Lower Serum Total and LDL Cholesterol in Humans: A Meta-Analysis of 11 Randomized Controlled Trials," *American Journal of Clinical Nutrition,* vol. 85, no. 4 (April 2007), pp. 1148–56.

63. A. Bitto et al., "Effects of Genistein Aglycone in Osteoporatic, Ovariectomized Rats: A Comparison with Alendronate, Raloxifene and Oestradiol," *British Journal of Pharmacology,* vol. 155, no. 6 (November 2008), pp. 896–905.

64. M. Messina and G. Redmond, "Effects of Soy Protein and Soybean Isoflavones on Thyroid Function in Healthy Adults and Hypothyroid Patients: A Review of the Relevant Literature," *Thyroid,* vol. 16, no. 3 (March 2006), pp. 249–58.

65. B. Bruce, M. Messina, and G. A. Spiller, "Isoflavone Supplements Do Not Affect Thyroid Function in Iodine-Replete Postmenopausal Women," *Journal of Medicinal Food,* vol. 6, no. 4 (Winter 2003), pp. 309–16.

66. I. C. Munro et al., "Soy Isoflavones: A Safety Review," *Nutrition Reviews,* vol. 61, no. 1 (January 2003), pp. 1–33; J. Slavin, "Nutritional Benefits of Soy Protein and Soy Fiber," *Journal of the American Dietetic Association,* vol. 91, no. 7 (July 1991), pp. 816–19.

67. J. F. Balch, *Prescription for Nutritional Healing* (New York: Avery Publications, 1990).

68. M. Micallef et al., "Plasma n-3 Polyunsaturated Fatty Acids Are Negatively Associated with Obesity," *British Journal of Nutrition,* May 19, 2009, pp. 1–5 [Epub ahead of print].

69. M. Studer et al., "Effect of Different Antilipidemic Agents and Diets on Mortality: A Systematic Review," *Archives of Internal Medicine,* vol. 165, no. 7 (April 11, 2005), pp. 725–30.

70. T. A. Sanders et al., "Influence of n-6 Versus n-3 Polyunsaturated Fatty Acids in Diets Low in Saturated Fatty Acids on Plasma Lipoproteins and Hemostatic Factors," *Arteriosclerosis, Thrombosis, and Vascular Biology,* vol. 17, no. 12 (1997), pp. 3449–60; M. H. Davidson, "Mechanisms for the Hypotriglyceridemic Effect of Marine Omega-3 Fatty Acids," *American Journal of Cardiology,* vol. 98 (August 21, 2006), pp. 27–33.

71. A. Leaf and P. C. Weber, "Cardiovascular Effects of N-3 Fatty Acids," *New England Journal of Medicine,* vol. 318, no. 9 (March 3, 1988), pp. 549–57; E. B. Schmidt et al., "N-3 Polyunsaturated Fatty Acid Supplementation (Pikasol) in Men with Moderate and Severe Hypertriglyceridaemia: A Dose-Response Study," *Annals of Nutrition and Metabolism,* vol. 36, nos. 5–6 (1992), pp. 283–87; F. B. Hu et al., "Fish and Long-Chain Omega-3 Fatty Acid Intake and Risk of Coronary Heart Disease and Total Mortality in Diabetic Women," *Circulation,* vol. 107, no. 14 (April 15, 2003), pp. 1852–57; P. J. Skerrett and C. H. Hennekens, "Consumption of Fish and Fish Oils and Decreased Risk of Stroke," *Preventive*

Cardiology, vol. 6, no. 1 (Winter 2003), pp. 38–41; A. Zampelas et al., "Fish Consumption Among Healthy Adults Is Associated with Decreased Levels of Inflammatory Markers Related to Cardiovascular Disease: The ATTICA Study," *Journal of the American College of Cardiology,* vol. 46, no. 1 (July 5, 2005), pp. 120–24.

72. R. L. McLennon, "Reversal of Arrhythmogenic Effects of Long-Term Saturated Fatty Acid Intake by Dietary N3 and N6 Polyunsaturated Fatty Acids," *American Journal of Clinical Nutrition,* vol. 51 (1980), pp. 53–58; D. Kim et al., "Dietary Fish Oil Added to Hyperlipidemic Diet for Swine Results in Reduction in Excessive Numbers of Monocytes Attached to Arterial Epithelium," *Arteriosclerosis,* vol. 81 (1991), pp. 209–16; C. J. Diskin et al., "Fish Oil to Prevent Intimal Hyperplasia and Thrombosis," *Nephron,* vol. 55 (1990), pp. 445–47.

73. U. N. Das et al., "Benzo(a)pyrene and Gamma Radiation Induced Genetic Damage in Mice May Be Prevented by GLA but Not Arachidonic Acid," *Nutrition Research,* vol. 5 (1985), pp. 101–5.

74. D. Horrobin et al., "Omega-6 Fatty Acids May Reverse Carcinogenesis by Restoring Natural PGE-1 Metabolism," *Medical Hypotheses,* vol. 6 (1980), pp. 469–86; J. J. Jarkowski and W. T. Cave, "Dietary Fish Oil May Inhibit Development of Breast Cancer," *Journal of the National Cancer Institute,* vol. 74 (1985), pp. 1145–50.

75. J. M. Kremer, "N-3 Fatty Acid Supplements in Rheumatoid Arthritis," *American Journal of Clinical Nutrition,* vol. 71, no. 1 suppl. (January 2000), pp. 349S–51S; D. Volker et al., "Efficacy of Fish Oil Concentrate in the Treatment of Rheumatoid Arthritis," *Journal of Rheumatology,* vol. 27, no. 10 (October 2000), pp. 2343–46; C. L. Curtis et al., "Effects of n-3 Fatty Acids on Cartilage Metabolism," *Proceedings of the Nutrition Society,* vol. 61, no. 3 (August 2002), pp. 381–89.

76. D. Parra et al., "A Diet Rich in Long Chain Omega-3 Fatty Acids Modulates Satiety in Overweight and Obese Volunteers During Weight Loss," *Appetite,* vol. 51, no. 3 (November 2008), pp. 676–80.

77. R. L. Weank et al., "Effect of Low Saturated Fat Diet in Early and Late Cases of Multiple Sclerosis," *The Lancet,* vol. 336 (1990), pp. 1145–50.

78. Z. Harel et al, "Supplementation with Omega-3 Fatty Acids in the Management of Dysmenorrhea in Adolescents," *American Journal of Obstetrics and Gynecology,* vol. 174, no. 4 (1996), pp. 1335–38.

79. C. Campagnoli et al., "Polyunsaturated Fatty Acids (PUFAs) Might Reduce Hot Flushes: An Indication from Two Controlled Trials on Soy Isoflavones Alone and with a PUFA Supplement," *Maturitas,* vol. 51, no. 2 (June 16, 2005), pp. 127–34.

80. M. Maes et al., "In Humans, Serum Polyunsaturated Fatty Acid Levels Predict the Response of Proinflammatory Cytokines to Psychologic Stress," *Biological Psychiatry,* vol. 47, no. 10 (May 15, 2000), pp. 910–20.

81. M. G. Enig et al., "Dietary Fat and Cancer Trends: A Critique," *Federal Proceedings,* vol. 37 (1978), pp. 25–30.

82. G. Abraham, "Primary Dysmenorrhea," *Clinical Obstetrics and Gynecology,* vol. 21, no. 1 (1978), pp. 139–45.

83. H. G. Preuss et al., "Minimum Inhibitory Concentrations of Herbal Essential Oils and Monolaurin for Gram-Positive and Gram-Negative Bacteria," *Molecular and*

Cellular Biochemistry, vol. 272, nos. 1–2 (April 2005), pp. 29–34; H. G. Preuss et al., "Effects of Essential Oils and Monolaurin on *Staphylococcus aureus:* In Vitro and In Vivo Studies," *Toxicology Mechanisms and Methods,* vol. 15, no. 4 (July 2005), pp. 279–85.

84. J. E. Gangwisch et al., "Inadequate Sleep as a Risk Factor for Obesity: Analyses of the NHANES I," *Sleep,* vol. 28, no. 10 (October 1, 2005), pp. 1289–96.

85. B. Villeponteau, R. Cockrell, and J. Feng, "Nutraceutical Interventions May Delay Aging and the Age-Related Diseases," *Experimental Gerontology,* vol. 35, nos. 9–10 (December 2000), pp. 1405–17.

86. T. A. Barringer et al., "Effect of a Multivitamin and Mineral Supplement on Infection and Quality of Life. A Randomized, Double-Blind, Placebo-Controlled Trial," *Annals of Internal Medicine,* vol. 138, no. 5 (March 4, 2003), pp. 365–71.

87. G. Pocobelli et al., "Use of Supplements of Multivitamins, Vitamin C, and Vitamin E in Relation to Mortality," *American Journal of Epidemiology,* vol. 170, no. 4 (August 15, 2009), pp. 472–83.

88. K. N. Prasad, "Multiple Dietary Antioxidants Enhance the Efficacy of Standard and Experimental Cancer Therapies and Decrease Their Toxicity," *Integrative Cancer Therapies,* vol. 3, no. 4 (December 2004), pp. 310–22.

89. E. R. Miller III, "Meta-Analysis: High-Dosage Vitamin E Supplementation May Increase All-Cause Mortality," *Annals of Internal Medicine,* vol. 142, no. 1 (January 4, 2005), pp. 37–46.

90. C. D. Morris and S. Carson, "Routine Vitamin Supplementation to Prevent Cardiovascular Disease: A Summary of the Evidence for the U.S. Preventive Services Task Force," *Annals of Internal Medicine,* vol. 139, no. 1 (July 1, 2003), pp. 56–70.

91. M. J. Stampfer et al., "Vitamin E Consumption and the Risk of Coronary Disease in Women," *New England Journal of Medicine,* vol. 328, no. 20 (May 20, 1993), pp. 1444–49.

92. R. M. Bostick et al., "Reduced Risk of Colon Cancer with High Intakes of Vitamin E: The Iowa Women's Health Study," *Cancer Research,* vol. 53, no. 18 (September 15, 1993), pp. 4230–37.

93. P. P. Zandi, "Reduced Risk of Alzheimer Disease in Users of Antioxidant Vitamin Supplements: The Cache County Study," *Archives of Neurology,* vol. 61, no. 1 (January 2004), pp. 82–88.

94. M. Lu, "Prospective Study of Dietary Fat and Risk of Cataract Extraction Among U.S. Women," *American Journal of Epidemiology,* vol. 161, no. 10 (May 15, 2005), pp. 948–59.

95. J. Higdon, *An Evidence-Based Approach to Vitamins and Minerals* (New York: Thieme, 2003), p. 253; X. Gao et al., "The Maximal Amount of Dietary Alpha-Tocopherol Intake in U.S. Adults (NHANES 2001–2002)," *Journal of Nutrition,* vol. 136 (2006), pp. 1021–6; Q. Jian et al., "Gamma-Tocopherol, the Major Form of Vitamin E in the U.S. Diet, Deserves More Attention," *American Journal of Clinical Nutrition,* vol. 74 (2001), pp. 714–22; P. J. McLaughlin and J. L. Weihrauch, "Vitamin E Content of Foods," *Journal of the American Dietetic Association,* vol. 75 (1979), pp. 647–65; L. C. Nebeling et al., "The Impact of Lifestyle Characteristics on Carotenoid Intake in the United States: The 1987 National Health Interview Survey," *American Journal of Public Health,* vol. 87 (1997),

pp. 268–71; L. C. Nebeling et al., "Changes in Carotenoid Intake in the United States: The 1987 and 1992 National Health Interview Surveys," *Journal of the American Dietetic Association*, vol. 97 (1997), pp. 991–96; A. Scalbert and G. Williamson, "Dietary Intake and Bioavailability of Polyphenols," *Journal of Nutrition*, vol. 130 (2000), pp. 2073S–85S; C. Weber, A. Bysted, and G. Holmer, "Coenzyme Q$_{10}$ in the Diet—Daily Intake and Relative Bioavailability," *Molecular Aspects of Medicine*, vol. 18 (1997), pp. S251–54.

96. C. Northrup, *The Wisdom of Menopause* (New York: Bantam Books, 2001).

97. M. R. Malinow et al., "The Effects of Folic Acid Supplementation on Plasma Total Homocysteine Are Modulated by Multivitamin Use and Methylenetetrahydrofolate Reductase Genotypes," *Arteriosclerosis, Thrombosis, and Vascular Biology*, vol. 17, no. 6 (June 1997), pp. 1157–62.

98. M. F. Bellamy et al., "Oral Folate Enhances Endothelial Function in Hyperhomocysteinaemic Subjects," *European Journal of Clinical Investigation*, vol. 29, no. 8 (August 1999), pp. 659–62; A. Bronstrup et al., "Effects of Folic Acid and Combinations of Folic Acid and Vitamin B-12 on Plasma Homocysteine Concentrations in Healthy, Young Women," *American Journal of Clinical Nutrition*, vol. 68, no. 5 (1998), pp. 1104–10.

99. A. Vahratian et al., "Multivitamin Use and Risk of Preterm Birth," *American Journal of Epidemiology*, vol. 160, no. 9 (November 1, 2004), pp. 886–92.

100. R. A. Anderson and S. Koslovsky, "Chromium Intake, Absorption, and Excretion of Subjects Consuming Self-Selected Diets," *American Journal of Clinical Nutrition*, vol. 41 (1985), pp. 1177–80.

101. W. Mestz et al., "Present Knowledge of the Role of Chromium," *Fedéral Proceedings*, vol. 33 (1974), pp. 2275–83.

102. Interestingly, breast milk contains 300 mg of calcium per quart, while cow's milk contains 1,200 mg per quart. Yet the breast-fed infant absorbs more calcium than the infant fed cow's milk. More isn't necessarily better. Source: W. Manahan, *Eat for Health* (Tiburon, CA: H. J. Kramer, 1988), p. 164.

103. F. A. Oski, *Don't Drink Your Milk* (Brushton, NY: Teach Services, 1996); available from Teach Services, 800-367-1844 or 518-358-3494, or visit www.teachservices.com.

104. D. Cramer et al., "Galatose Consumption and Metabolism in Relation to the Risk of Ovarian Cancer," *The Lancet*, vol. 2, no. 8654 (July 8, 1989), pp. 66–71.

105. A. J. Lanou, S. E. Berkow, and N. D. Barnard, "Calcium, Dairy Products, and Bone Health in Children and Young Adults: A Reevaluation of the Evidence," *Pediatrics*, vol. 115, no. 3 (March 2005), pp. 736–43.

106. T. C. Campbell, Ph.D., quoted in "More on the Dietary Fat and Breast Cancer Link," *NABCO News*, vol. 4, no. 3 (July 1990), pp. 1–2.

107. Manahan, *Eat for Health*. Dentists point out that the first place osteoporosis shows up is in the lower jaw, and that osteoporosis is linked with periodontal disease, the leading cause of adult tooth loss.

108. F. Huang et al., "Dietary Calcium Intake and Food Sources Among Chinese Adults in CNTCS," *PLoS One*, vol. 13, no. 10 (October 2018), p. e0205045.

109. M. F. Holick, "Vitamin D Deficiency," *New England Journal of Medicine*, vol. 357, no. 3 (July 19, 2007), pp. 266–81.

110. L. M. Bodnar, M. A. Krohn, and H. N. Simhan, "Maternal Vitamin D Deficiency Is Associated with Bacterial Vaginosis in the First Trimester of Pregnancy," *Journal of Nutrition,* vol. 139, no. 6 (June 2009), pp. 1157–61.

111. M. Sneve, Y. Figenschau, and R. Jorde, "Supplementation with Cholecalciferol Does Not Result in Weight Reduction in Overweight and Obese Subjects," *European Journal of Endocrinology,* vol. 159, no. 6 (December 2008), pp. 675–84; S. D. Sibley et al., "Plasma Vitamin D: A Predictor of Subsequent Weight Loss Success," presented at the 91st Annual Meeting of the Endocrine Society, Washington, DC, June 11, 2009, www.abstracts2view.com/endo/view.php?nu= ENDO09L_OR14-5.

112. Holick, "Vitamin D Deficiency."

113. J. J. Cannell et al., "On the Epidemiology of Influenza," *Virology Journal,* vol. 5, no. 29 (February 25, 2008), http://www.virologyj.com/content/5/1/29.

114. S. L. McDonnell et al., "Breast Cancer Risk Markedly Lower with Serum 25-Hydroxyvitamin D Concentrations ≥ 60 vs < 20 ng/ml (150 vs 50 nmol/L): Pooled Analysis of Two Randomized Trials and a Prospective Cohort," *PLoS One,* vol. 13, no. 6 (June 15, 2018), p. e0199265.

115. S. L. McDonnell et al., "Maternal 25(OH)D Concentrations ≥40 ng/mL Associated with 60% Lower Preterm Birth Risk Among General Obstetrical Patients at an Urban Medical Center," *PLoS One,* vol. 12, no. 7 (July 24, 2017), p. e0180483.

116. B. Dawson-Hughes et al., "Effect of Vitamin D Supplementation on Wintertime and Overall Bone Loss in Healthy Postmenopausal Women," *Annals of Internal Medicine,* vol. 115, no. 17 (1991), pp. 505–12.

117. R. D. Jackson et al., "Calcium Plus Vitamin D Supplementation and the Risk of Fractures," *New England Journal of Medicine,* vol. 354, no. 7 (February 16, 2006), pp. 669–83.

118. Bone metabolism also requires vitamin C, vitamin D, and a number of trace minerals, including zinc, silica, copper, boron, and manganese. All of these substances, working synergistically, form bone.

119. M. Grossman, J. Kirsner, and I. Gillespie, "Basal and Histalog-Stimulated Gastric Secretion in Control Subjects and Patients with Peptic Ulcer or Gastric Cancer," *Gastroenterology,* vol. 45 (1963), pp. 15–26.

120. R. Recker, "Calcium Absorption and Achlorhydria," *New England Journal of Medicine,* vol. 313 (1985), pp. 70–73; M. J. Nicar and C. Y. C. Pak, "Calcium Bioavailability from Calcium Carbonate and Calcium Citrate," *Journal of Clinical Endocrinology and Metabolism,* vol. 61 (1985), pp. 391–93.

121. Personal communication with Jeffrey Bland.

122. D. Michaelson et al., "Bone Mineral Density in Women with Depression," *New England Journal of Medicine,* vol. 335 (1996), pp. 1176–81.

123. M. J. Eisenberg, "Magnesium Deficiency and Sudden Death," *American Heart Journal,* vol. 124, no. 2 (1992), pp. 544–49; P. D. Turlapaty and B. M. Altura, "Magnesium Deficiency Produces Spasms in Coronary Arteries: Relationship to Etiology of Sudden Death Ischemic Heart Disease," *Science,* vol. 208, no. 4440 (April 11, 1980), pp. 198–200; B. M. Altura, "Sudden Death Ischemic Heart Disease and Dietary Magnesium Intake: Is the Target Site Coronary Vascular Smooth Muscle?" *Medical Hypotheses,* vol. 5, no. 8 (August 1979), pp. 843–48.

124. A. Hruby et al., "Higher Magnesium Intake Is Associated with Lower Fasting Glu-

cose and Insulin, with No Evidence of Interaction with Select Genetic Loci, in a Meta-analysis of 15 CHARGE Consortium Studies," *Journal of Nutrition,* vol. 143, no. 3 (March 2013), pp. 345–53.

125. B. S. Levine and J. W. Coburn, "Magnesium, the Mimic/Antagonist of Calcium," *New England Journal of Medicine,* vol. 310, no. 19 (May 10, 1984), pp. 1253–55.

126. A. M. Uwitonze and M. S. Razzaque, "Role of Magnesium in Vitamin D Activation and Function," *Journal of the American Osteopathic Association,* vol. 118, no. 3 (March 2018), pp. 181–89.

127. M. DeVos, "Articular Disease and the Gut: Evidence of a Strong Relationship Between Spondylarthropathy and Inflammation of the Gut in Man," *Acta Clinica Belgica,* vol. 45, no. 10 (1990), pp. 20–24; P. Jackson et al., "Intestinal Permeability in Patients with Eczema and Food Allergy," *The Lancet,* vol. 1 (1981), p. 1285.

128. A. M. Larson et al., "Acetaminophen-Induced Acute Liver Failure: Results of a United States Multicenter, Prospective Study," *Hepatology,* vol. 42, no. 6 (December 2005), pp. 1364–72.

129. A three-part series on common intestinal problems and holistic treatment for them is available in the April, May, and June 1997 issues of C. Northrup's *Health Wisdom for Women* newsletter.

130. J. S. Labus et al., "Differences in Gut Microbial Composition Correlate with Regional Brain Volumes in Irritable Bowel Syndrome," *Microbiome,* vol. 5, no. 1 (May 1, 2017), p. 49.

131. IgG levels are known to be altered in diseases related to intestinal dysbiosis and food allergies. IgG is an immunoglobulin that is involved with the body's response to outside elements such as pollen, animal dander, grass, wheat, etc., which are not usually harmful to our bodies. However, in those people who are chronically stressed either emotionally or physically, the IgG levels are elevated, creating the possibility for hyperimmune response, which results in reactions to normally occurring environmental substances. In some people, the IgG levels are decreased, resulting in immunosuppression and therefore increased susceptibility to colds, etc.

132. One good lab for this is Immuno Laboratories in Fort Lauderdale, FL, 800-231-9197 or 954-691-2500, www.immunolabs.com.

133. T. Shirakawa et al., "Lifestyle Effect on Total IgG: Lifestyles Have a Cumulative Impact of Controlling Total IgG Levels," *Allergy,* vol. 46 (1991), pp. 561–69; I. Waxman, "Case Records of the MGH: A 59-Year-Old Woman with Abdominal Pain and an Abnormal CT Scan," *New England Journal of Medicine,* vol. 329, no. 5 (July 29, 1993), pp. 343–49.

134. Data from *Brain/Mind Bulletin,* December 1988.

135. N. Ale-Agha et al., "CDKN1B/p27 Is Localized In Mitochondria and Improves Respiration-Dependent Processes in the Cardiovascular System—New Mode of Action for Caffeine," *PLOS Biology,* vol. 16, no. 6 (June 21, 2018), p. e2004408.

136. M. E. Arnold et al., "The Effects of Caffeine, Impulsivity, and Sex on Memory for Word Lists," *Physiology and Behavior,* vol. 41, no. 1 (1987), pp. 25–30.

137. A. Carrera-Lanestosa, Y. Moguel-Ordonez, and M. Segura-Campos, "Stevia Rebaudiana Bertoni: A Natural Alternative for Treating Diseases Associated with Metabolic Syndrome," *Journal of Medicinal Food,* vol. 20, no. 10 (October 2017), pp. 933–43.

138. W. C. Willett et al., "Moderate Alcohol Consumption and the Risk of Breast Cancer," *New England Journal of Medicine,* vol. 316, no. 19 (May 7, 1987), pp. 1174–80.

139. L. D. Johnston et al., *Monitoring the Future, National Survey Results on Drug Use 1975–2018:* Overview, *Key Findings on Adolescent Drug Use* (Ann Arbor: Institute for Social Research, University of Michigan, 2019), p. 37, www.monitoringthefuture.org/pubs/monographs/mtf-overview2018.pdf.

140. J. A. Ewing, "Detecting Alcoholism. The CAGE Questionnaire," *Journal of the American Medical Association,* vol. 252, no. 14 (October 12, 1984), pp. 1905–7.

141. CDC, "Tobacco-Related Mortality," last reviewed January 17, 2018, www.cdc.gov/tobacco/data_statistics/fact_sheets/health_effects/tobacco_related_mortality/index.htm.

142. L. D. Johnston et al., *Monitoring the Future, National Survey Results on Drug Use 1975–2018:* Overview, *Key Findings on Adolescent Drug Use* (Ann Arbor: Institute for Social Research, University of Michigan, 2019), p. 39, www.monitoringthefuture.org/pubs/monographs/mtf-overview2018.pdf.

143. L. D. Johnston et al., *Monitoring the Future, National Survey Results on Drug Use 1975–2017:* Overview, *Key Findings on Adolescent Drug Use* (Ann Arbor: Institute for Social Research, University of Michigan, 2018), p. 39.

144. A. S. Gentzke et al., "Vital Signs: Tobacco Product Use Among Middle and High School Students—United States, 2011–2018," *Centers for Disease Control and Prevention Morbidity and Mortality Weekly Report, 2019,* vol. 68, no. 06 (2019); K. A. Cullen et al., "Notes from the Field: Use of Electronic Cigarettes and Any Tobacco Product Among Middle and High School Students—United States, 2011–2018," *Centers for Disease Control and Prevention Morbidity and Mortality Weekly Report, 2018,* vol. 67, no. 45 (2018), pp. 1276–77.

145. Centers for Disease Control and Prevention, *The Health Consequences of Smoking—50 Years of Progress: A Report of the Surgeon General,* 2014 (Atlanta, GA: U.S. Department of Health and Human Services, Centers for Disease Control and Prevention, National Center for Chronic Disease Prevention and Health Promotion, Office of Smoking and Health, 2014); X. Xu et al., "Annual Healthcare Spending Attributable to Cigarette Smoking: An Update," *American Journal of Preventive Medicine,* vol. 48, no. 3 (March 2015), pp. 326–33.

146. Centers for Disease Control and Prevention, *The Health Consequences of Smoking—50 Years of Progress: A Report of the Surgeon General,* 2014 (Atlanta, GA: U.S. Department of Health and Human Services, Centers for Disease Control and Prevention, National Center for Chronic Disease Prevention and Health Promotion, Office of Smoking and Health, 2014).

147. Centers for Disease Control and Prevention, *The Health Consequences of Smoking—50 Years of Progress: A Report of the Surgeon General,* 2014 (Atlanta, GA: U.S. Department of Health and Human Services, Centers for Disease Control and Prevention, National Center for Chronic Disease Prevention and Health Promotion, Office of Smoking and Health, 2014).

148. B. Haglund et al., "Cigarette Smoking as a Risk Factor for Sudden Infant Death Syndrome," *American Journal of Public Health,* vol. 80, no. 1 (January 1990), pp. 29–32.

149. California Environmental Protection Agency, Proposed Identification of Environmental Tobacco Smoke as a Toxic Air Contaminant, June 2005.

150. U.S. Department of Health and Human Services, *Women and Smoking: A Report of the Surgeon General* (Washington, DC: Public Health Service, 2001).

151. Centers for Disease Control and Prevention, *The Health Consequences of Smoking—50 Years of Progress: A Report of the Surgeon General,* 2014 (Atlanta, GA: U.S. Department of Health and Human Services, Centers for Disease Control and Prevention, National Center for Chronic Disease Prevention and Health Promotion, Office of Smoking and Health, 2014).

152. R. A. Riemersma et al., "Risk of Angina Pectoris and Plasma Concentration of Vitamins A, C, E and Carotene," *The Lancet,* vol. 337 (1991), pp. 1–5.

153. S. E. Moner, "Acupuncture and Addiction Treatment," *Journal of Addictive Disease,* vol. 15, no. 3 (1996), pp. 79–100.

154. S. Miller, *Food for Thought: A New Look at Food and Behavior* (New York: Prentice-Hall, 1979).

155. A. Schauss, *Diet, Crime, and Delinquency* (Berkeley, CA: Parker House, 1980).

156. R. M. Nerem, M. J. Levesque, and J. T. Cornill, "Social Environment as a Factor in Diet-Induced Atherosclerosis," *Science,* vol. 208, no. 4451 (1980), pp. 1474–76.

157. M. Morse, *Transformed by the Light* (New York: Villard, 1992).

Chapter 18: The Power of Movement

1. B. Swimme, *The Universe Is a Green Dragon* (Santa Fe, NM: Bear and Company, 1983), p. 106.

2. Many of the following studies were found in R. A. Anderson, *Wellness Medicine* (Lynnwood, WA: American Health Press, 1987).

3. P. T. Campbell et al., "A Yearlong Exercise Intervention Decreases CRP Among Obese Postmenopausal Women," *Medicine and Science in Sports and Exercise,* vol. 41, no. 8 (August 2009), pp. 1533–39.

4. *Body Bulletin* (Emmaus, PA: Rodale Press, January 1984).

5. I. Thune et al., "Physical Activity and the Risk of Breast Cancer," *New England Journal of Medicine,* vol. 336, no. 18 (May 1, 1997), pp. 1269–75.

6. A. McTiernan, "Exercise and Breast Cancer—Time to Get Moving?" *New England Journal of Medicine,* vol. 336, no. 18 (May 1, 1997), pp. 1311–12.

7. N. B. Belloc and L. Breslow, "Relationship of Physical Health Status and Health Practices," *Preventive Medicine,* vol. 1, no. 3 (1972), pp. 409–21.

8. M. Gulati et al., "The Prognostic Value of a Nomogram of Exercise Capacity in Women," *New England Journal of Medicine,* vol. 353, no. 5 (Aug 4, 2005), pp. 468–75.

9. P. J. Harvey et al., "Exercise as an Alternative to Oral Estrogen for Amelioration of Endothelial Dysfunction in Postmenopausal Women," *American Heart Journal,* vol. 149, no. 2 (February 2005), pp. 291–97.

10. R. J. Young, "Effects of Regular Exercise on Cognitive Functioning and Personal-

ity," *British Journal of Sports Medicine,* vol. 13, no. 3 (1979), pp. 110–17; B. Gutin, "Effect of Increase in Physical Fitness on Mental Ability Following Physical and Mental Stress," *Research Quarterly,* vol. 37, no. 2 (1966), pp. 211–20.

11. K. I. Erickson and A. F. Kramer, "Aerobic Exercise Effects on Cognitive and Neural Plasticity in Older Adults," *British Journal of Sports Medicine,* vol. 43, no. 1 (January 2009), pp. 22–24; M. Angevaren et al., "Physical Activity and Enhanced Fitness to Improve Cognitive Function in Older People Without Known Cognitive Impairment," *Cochrane Database of Systematic Reviews,* vol. 2 (July 16, 2008), CD005381; M. Hamer, E. Stamatakis, and A. Steptoe, "Dose Response Relationship Between Physical Activity and Mental Health: The Scottish Health Survey," *British Journal of Sports Medicine,* April 10, 2008 [Epub ahead of print]; T. Liu-Ambrose et al., "Otago Home-Based Strength and Balance Retraining Improves Executive Functioning in Older Fallers: A Randomized Controlled Trial," *Journal of the American Geriatrics Society,* vol. 56, no. 10 (October 2008), pp. 1821–30; A. Singh-Manoux et al., "Effects of Physical Activity on Cognitive Functioning in Middle Age: Evidence from the Whitehall II Prospective Cohort Study," *American Journal of Public Health,* vol. 95, no. 12 (December 2005), pp. 2252–58.

12. M. S. Bahrke, "Exercise, Meditation and Anxiety Reduction," *American Corrective Therapy Journal,* vol. 33, no. 2 (1979), pp. 41–44; J. W. Collingswood and L. Willet, "The Effects of Physical Training Upon Self-Concept and Body Attitude," *Journal of Clinical Psychology,* vol. 27, no. 3 (1971), pp. 411–12.

13. R. Prince et al., "Prevention of Postmenopausal Osteoporosis: A Comparative Study of Exercise, Calcium Supplementation and Hormone Replacement Therapy," *New England Journal of Medicine,* vol. 325, no. 17 (1991), pp. 1189–204; J. F. Aloia et al., "Prevention of Involution Bone Mass by Exercise," *Annals of Internal Medicine,* vol. 89, no. 3 (1978), pp. 351–58; Consensus Development Conference on Osteoporosis, National Institutes of Health (Washington, DC, 1989).

14. S. J. Griffin and J. Trinder, "Physical Fitness, Exercise, and Human Sleep," *Psychophysiology,* vol. 15, no. 5 (1978), pp. 447–50.

15. J. Morgan et al., "Psychological Effects of Chronic Physical Activity," *Medical Science Sports,* vol. 2, no. 4 (1970), pp. 213–17.

16. D. Hoppe, *Healthy Sex Drive, Healthy You: What Your Libido Reveals About Your Life* (Encinitas, CA: Health Reflections Press, 2010).

17. R. D. Pollock et al., "An Investigation into the Relationship Between Age and Physiological Function in Highly Active Older Adults," *Journal of Physiology,* vol. 593, no. 3 (February 1, 2015), pp. 657–80; N. A. Duggal et al., "Major Features of Immunesenescence, Including Reduced Thymic Output, Are Ameliorated by High Levels of Physical Activity in Adulthood," *Aging Cell,* vol. 17, no. 2 (April 2018), p. e12750; R. D. Pollock et al., "Properties of the Vastus Lateralis Muscle in Relation to Age and Physiological Function in Master Cyclists Aged 55–70 Years," *Aging Cell,* vol. 17, no. 2 (April 2018), p. e12735.

18. S. P. Helmrich et al., "Physical Activity and Reduced Occurrence of Non-Insulin-Dependent Diabetes Mellitus," *New England Journal of Medicine,* vol. 325, no. 3 (July 18, 1991), pp. 147–52.

19. J. Prior, "Conditioning Exercise Decreases Premenstrual Symptoms: A Prospective, Controlled 6-Month Trial," *Fertility and Sterility,* vol. 47, no. 3 (1987), pp. 402–8.

20. B. P. Worth et al., "Running Through Pregnancy," *Runner's World,* November 1978, pp. 54–59.

21. K. Owe et al., "Association Between Regular Exercise and Excessive Newborn Birth Weight," *Obstetrics and Gynecology,* vol. 114, no. 4 (October 2009), pp. 770–76.

22. A. R. Hersh et al., "A Two-Delivery Model Examining Upright Positioning During Labor: A Cost-Effectiveness Analysis [34C]," *Obstetrics and Gynecology,* vol. 131 (May 2018), pp. 39S.

23. A. C. Pereira et al., "An In Vivo Correlate of Exercise-Induced Neurogenesis in the Adult Dentate Gyrus," *Proceedings of the National Academy of Sciences,* vol. 104, no. 13 (March 27, 2007), pp. 5638–43.

24. F. B. Schuch et al., "Are Lower Levels of Cardiorespiratory Fitness Associated with Incident Depression? A Systematic Review of Prospective Cohort Studies," *Preventive Medicine,* vol. 93 (December 2016), pp. 159–65.

25. B. R. Gordon et al., "Association of Efficacy of Resistance Exercise Training with Depressive Symptoms: Meta-Analysis and Meta-Regression Analysis of Randomized Controlled Trials," *Journal of the American Medical Association—Psychiatry,* vol. 75, no. 6 (June 1, 2018), pp. 566–76.

26. C. E. Garber, J. S. McKinney, and R. A. Carleton, "Is Aerobic Dance an Effective Alternative to Walk-Jog Exercise Training?" *Journal of Sports Medicine and Physical Fitness,* vol. 32, no. 2 (June 1992), pp. 136–41.

27. I have found that The Firm aerobic workout with weights is very effective if you have the time to do it. Each workout lasts from forty-five to sixty minutes, and you can feel results in your body after only five or so workouts, doing three workouts per week on average. See www.gaia.com/collections/the-firm. My favorites are volumes 4, 5, and 6. I'd recommend that you begin with volume 6.

28. Liu-Ambrose et al., "Otago Home-Based Strength and Balance Retraining Improves Executive Functioning in Older Fallers: A Randomized Controlled Trial."

29. Y. Mavros et al., "Mediation of Cognitive Function Improvements by Strength Gains After Resistance Training in Older Adults with Mild Cognitive Impairment: Outcomes of the Study of Mental and Resistance Training," *Journal of the American Geriatric Society,* vol. 65, no. 3 (March 2017), pp. 550–59.

30. H. H. Jones et al., "Humeral Hypertrophy in Response to Exercise," *Journal of Bone and Joint Surgery,* vol. 59, no. 2 (1977), pp. 204–8; N. K. Dalen and E. Olsson, "Bone Mineral Content and Physical Activity," *Acta Orthopaedica Scandinavia,* vol. 45, no. 2 (1974), pp. 170–74.

31. M. Nelson et al., "Effects of High-Intensity Strength Training on Multiple Risk Factors for Osteoporitic Fractures: A Randomized Controlled Trial," *Journal of the American Medical Association,* vol. 272, no. 24 (1994), pp. 1909–14. The program Nelson used has been adapted for home use and is available in her book, *Strong Women Stay Young* (New York: Bantam, 1997).

32. F. Travis et al., "Invincible Athletics Program: Aerobic Exercise and Performance Without Strain," *International Journal of Neuroscience,* vol. 85, nos. 3–4 (April 1996), pp. 301–8.

33. P. C. Benias et al., "Structure and Distribution of an Unrecognized Interstitium in Human Tissues," *Scientific Reports,* vol. 8, no. 1 (March 27, 2018), p. 4947.

34. H. M. Langevin et al., "Dynamic Fibroblast Cytoskeletal Response to Subcutane-

ous Tissue Stretch Ex Vivo and In Vivo," *American Journal of Physiology—Cell Physiology,* vol. 288, no. 3 (March 2005), pp. C747–56.

35. "Crowdsourcing Nominates Posture Modification as Best Lower Back Pain Solution," Gokhale Method, November 2016, https://gokhalemethod.com/blog/62650; "Top-Rated Treatments for Lower Back Pain," HealthOutcome, https://www.healthoutcome.org/condition/43/lower-back-pain-treatment.

36. M. W. Ho and D. P. Knight, "The Acupuncture System and the Liquid Crystalline Collagen Fibers of the Connective Tissues," *American Journal of Chinese Medicine,* vol. 26, nos. 3–4 (1998), pp. 251–63.

37. Mae-Wan Ho, "Organism and Psyche in a Participatory Universe," *Meaning of Life and the Universe: Transforming* (Hackensack, NJ: World Scientific, 2017), pp. 80–103, www.i-sis.org.uk/organis.php.

38. Jin Putai, "Changes in Heart Rate, Noradrenaline, Cortisol, and Mood During Tai Chi," *Journal of Psychosomatic Research,* vol. 33, no. 2 (1989), pp. 197–206.

39. S. L. Wolf, H. X. Barnhart, and N. G. Kutner, "Reducing Frailty and Falls in Older Persons: An Investigation of Tai Chi and Computerized Balance Training," *Journal of the American Geriatric Society,* vol. 44 (1996), pp. 489–97.

40. I'm a big fan of "model mugging"—the training that helps women develop a strategy for surviving an attack.

41. W. L. Knez, J. S. Coombes, and D. G. Jenkins, "Ultra-Endurance Exercise and Oxidative Damage: Implications for Cardiovascular Health," *Sports Medicine,* vol. 35, no. 5 (2006), pp. 429–41; J. Finaud, G. Lac, and E. Filaire, "Oxidative Stress: Relationship with Exercise and Training," *Sports Medicine,* vol. 36, no. 4 (2006), pp. 327–58; M. L. Urso and P. M. Clarkson, "Oxidative Stress, Exercise, and Antioxidant Supplementation," *Toxicology,* vol. 189, nos. 1–2 (July 15, 2003), pp. 41–54.

42. R. Markus et al., "Menstrual Function and Bone Mass in Elite Women Distance Runners: Endocrine and Metabolic Features," *Annals of Internal Medicine,* vol. 102 (1985), pp. 158–63.

43. N. A. Rigotti et al., "Osteoporosis in Women with Anorexia Nervosa," *New England Journal of Medicine,* vol. 311 (1989), pp. 1601–5.

44. L. L. Schweiger et al., "Caloric Intake, Stress, and Menstrual Function in Athletes," *Fertility and Sterility,* vol. 49 (1988), pp. 447–50.

45. B. L. Drinkwater et al., "Bone Mineral Density After Resumption of Menses in Amenorrheic Athletes," *Journal of the American Medical Association,* vol. 256, no. 3 (1986), pp. 380–82; J. S. Lindberg et al., "Increased Vertebral Bone Mineral in Response to Reduced Exercise in Amenorrheic Runners," *Western Journal of Medicine,* vol. 146 (1987), pp. 39–47.

46. N. Lane, "Exercise and Bone Status," *Complementary Medicine,* May–June 1986.

47. Physical Activity Guidelines Advisory Committee, *Physical Activity Guidelines Advisory Committee Report, 2008* (Washington, DC: U.S. Department of Health and Human Services, 2008), www.health.gov/paguidelines/Report/pdf/Committee Report.pdf.

Chapter 19: Healing Ourselves, Healing Our World

1. D. W. Orme-Johnson and R. M. Oates, "A Field-Theoretic View of Consciousness: Reply to Critics," *Journal of Scientific Exploration*, vol. 23, no. 2 (2009), pp. 139–66; D. W. Orme-Johnson, "The Science of World Peace," *International Journal of Healing and Caring*, vol. 3, no. 3 (2003), pp. 1–9; D. W. Orme-Johnson et al., "Effects of Large Assemblies of Participants in the Transcendental Meditation and TM-Sidhi Program on Reducing International Conflict and Terrorism," *Journal of Offender Rehabilitation*, vol. 36, nos. 1–4 (2003), pp. 283–302; J. S. Hagelin et al., "Effects of Group Practice of the Transcendental Meditation Program on Preventing Violent Crime in Washington, DC: Results of the National Demonstration Project, June–July 1993," *Social Indicators Research*, vol. 47, no. 2 (1999), pp. 153–201; D. W. Orme-Johnson, C. N. Alexander, and J. L. Davies, "The Effects of the Maharishi Technology of the Unified Field: Reply to a Methodological Critique," *Journal of Conflict Resolution*, vol. 34 (1990), pp. 756–68; D. W. Orme-Johnson et al., "International Peace Project in the Middle East: The Effect of the Maharishi Technology of the Unified Field," *Journal of Conflict Resolution*, vol. 32, no. 4 (1988), pp. 776–812.

2. D. Feldman, "U.S. TV Ad Spend Drops as Digital Ad Spend Climbs to $107B in 2018," *Forbes*, March 28, 2018, www.forbes.com/sites/danafeldman/2018/03/28/u-s-tv-ad-spend-drops-as-digital-ad-spend-climbs-to-107b-in-2018/#13f266a57aa6.

3. C. W. Birky, "Relaxed Cellular Controls and Organelle Heredity," *Science*, vol. 222 (1983), pp. 466–75; M. C. Corballis and M. J. Morgan, "On the Biological Basis of Human Laterality," *Journal of Behavioral Science*, vol. 2 (1978), pp. 261–336; Norman Geschwind and Albert Galaburda, "Cerebral Lateralization, Biological Mechanisms, and Pathology," *Archives of Neurology*, vol. 42, no. 6 (1985), pp. 521–52.

4. *The Burning Times* is a documentary film by Donna Reed (part 2 of her women and spirituality series) that chronicles the burning of 9 million women and their sympathizers as witches during the Middle Ages. To order the DVD, contact Direct Cinema Limited at 310-636-8200, 800-525-0000, or www.directcinema.com. For more information on this subject, see Starhawk, *The Spiral Dance: A Rebirth of the Ancient Goddess* (HarperSanFrancisco, 1979).

5. R. Sheldrake, *The Presence of the Past: Morphic Resonance and the Habits of Nature* (London: Collins, 1988) and *A New Science of Life* (Boston: Houghton Mifflin, 1981). Sheldrake's theory concerns "morphic units," which can be regarded as forms of energy. "Although these aspects of form and energy can be separated conceptually they are always associated with one another. No morphic unit can have energy without form, and no material form can exist without energy." The characteristic form of a given morphic unit is determined by the form of previous similar systems that act upon it across time and space, in a process of "morphic resonance" through "morphogenic fields." This influence depends on the system's three-dimensional structures and patterns of vibration.

   For example, thousands of rats are trained to perform a new task in a laboratory in London. If Sheldrake's theory holds, then at a later time and in laboratories somewhere else, similar rats should be able to learn and carry out the same task more quickly. That's because the initial rats have changed the "morphogenic field" around rat learning. This effect should take place in the absence of any known physical connection or communication between the two laboratories.

Evidence that this effect actually occurs has been reported by W. E. Ager et al., "Fourth (Final) Report on a Test of McDougall's Lamarckian Experiment on the Training of Rats," *Journal of Experimental Biology,* vol. 3 (1954), pp. 304–21.

6. *Ms.* (January–February 1992), cover.

7. A. Lorde, *Burst of Light* (Ithaca, NY: Firebrand Books, 1988), p. 131. According to her book, Lorde had metastases of breast cancer to her liver, diagnosed in 1984. In 1992, she was named the poet laureate of New York State. Usually a tumor that has metastasized to the liver gives the person six months to live. Lorde lived nine years after this diagnosis.

8. This thought had a bit of accuracy in it. Medical students are notorious for starting to experience the symptoms of the patients they are around when they're just learning about different diseases. My personal boundaries were not very well placed in the past, and I have "taken home" too much of what goes on in the office. Since I'm in the energy field associated with fibroids all day long and am quite empathetic with my patients, my energy field has undoubtedly been influenced by theirs—and I still have to take responsibility for this condition and learn and grow from it.

9. N. Kristof and S. WuDunn, "The Women's Crusade," *New York Times Magazine,* August 17, 2009, www.nytimes.com/2009/08/23/magazine/23Women-t.html.

Index

Page numbers of illustrations appear in italics.

Abortion, 7–8, 102, 466–75, 478
  alternate view of, 472–75
  breast cancer and, 470
  emergency contraception in lieu of, 476
  grieving and, 466, 468–71
  guilt and, 92
  gynecological problems and, 164, 201, 233, 236
  healing post-abortion trauma, 469–72
Abraham (teacher), 742, 792, 796
Abrams, Douglas, 307
Abrams, Rachel Carlton, 307
Abuse against women, xxi–xxiv, 4–9, 37, 52, 64, 72, 79, 83, 100, 106, 110, 371, 372, 567
  ACE study and, 33, 84
  cultural shift about, xxi–xxii, 4–5, 9, 109, 110, 288, 958
  cycle of, 532
  helpline for, 567
  illness and, 6, 20, 24, 104, 105, 200
  Inner Child Rescue exercise, 78, 81–82
  protection of predators, 97
  sexual and incest, xxi–xxiv, 6–7, 20, 24, 33, 34, 49, 64, 79, 83, 92, 98, 106, 109, 250, 288, 290, 358–59, 371, 373, 520, 567, 959, 965
  survivors, labor, delivery, and, 567–68
Accidents, message of, 32, 112

Acetaminophen (Tylenol), 547
Acetylcholine, brain levels, 706
Achterberg, Jeanne, 32, 817
Acne, 72–73
ACTH (hormone), 157, 778
Acupuncture or acupressure, 30, *160*, 275, 777, 918, 942
  blood clotting/platelet disorders, 521
  breech presentation, turning, *555, 556*
  chemotherapy and, 665
  depression, 697
  gynecological problems, 152, 159, 178
  healthy teeth, 815
  menopause, 696
  smoking cessation, 925
  thinning hair, 696
  UTIs, 381
Acyclovir (Zovirax), 344
Adams, Susan, 298, 943
Adenomyosis, 181
Adenosine triphosphate (ATP), 865
Adhesions, 158, *158*, 200, *202,* 292, 519–20, 524
Adoption, 528–30
Adrenal glands, 648, 778, 909
  cortisol and, 652–53, 778
  DHEA and, 653–54
  environmental, physical stress and, 652
  key hormones produced by, 652

Adrenal glands (*cont'd*):
  restoration program, 654–60
  tests of, 654
  unresolved emotional stress and,
    651–52
Adrenaline, 652
Adzich, Kathy, 525
Affirmations
  at bedtime, 791
  daily use, 792
  for divine guidance, 718
  for genitals and sexual health, 331, 346
  for gynecological problems, 154, 250
  for HPV, 331
  intention and, 791
  for orgasm, 301
  for sexuality, 297
  spiritual connection, 79–80
  for surgery, healing statements, 827–28
  on time, 739
  Ultimate Success Mantra, 792
Agape International Spiritual Center, 154
Aging
  ageist culture and, 644–47
  author's mother and, 646
  avoidable causes of body changes, 930
  dementia and, 702, 703
  fertility and, 505, *505,* 512
  fitness industry and, 936
  hormone therapy and anti-aging, 672
  lifestyle and, 672
  memory loss, 702–4
  perception, long life and, 46–47, 647,
    705
  reversal of, 646–47
  updating beliefs about, 646
Aikido, 946
Alcohol, 880, 898, 920–21
  abuse, 7, 18, 355, 719
  Alzheimer's prevention and, 706
  bone density and, 688
  breast cancer and, 428, 433, 700
  breast-feeding and, 621–22
  CAGE screen for alcoholism, 921
  cravings, 881
  estrogen replacement therapy and, 700
  fertility and, 517
  interstitial cystitis and, 378
  PMS and, 170–72
  sperm counts and, 504

Alcoholics Anonymous, 774, 881, 920,
    978
Aldara (Imiquimod), 329
Alexander Technique, 942
Allen, Pat, 269, 308
Allende, Isabel, 287
Allergies (food), 886–87, 902, 917–18
All the Single Ladies (Traister), 196
*Alternative Therapies in Health and
    Medicine* magazine, 797
Altura, Burton and Bella, 909
Always Delicious (Ludwig), 857
Always Hungry (Ludwig), 840, 857
Alzheimer's disease, 666, 702–4
Amata Life company, 680
Amen, Daniel, 287
Amenorrhea, 133, 164, 178, 248–49,
    683, 948–49
American Girls (Sales), 183
American Holistic Medical Association,
    800
Amyotrophic lateral sclerosis (ALS or
    Lou Gehrig's disease), 69–70, 112,
    919
Anami, Kim, 736
Andrews, Ted, 764
Androgens, 177, 241, 676–77, 695
  bioidentical, 670
  blood sugar, insulin, and, 696
  ovarian cancer and, 261
  PCOS and, 177, 248
  production sites, 648, 649
  Pueraria mirifica to increase levels, 676
  spironolactone and, 249
Angell, Marcia, 630, 780
Anger, 88, 91, 137, 389–90
  -clearing exercise, 745–46
  as energy, 745–46, 968
  expressing and healing, 83–84, 742–46
  liver meridian and, 22
  at men, 307
  physical symptoms of, 22, 72, 82, 101,
    125, 254, 257–58, 317, 318, 355,
    382–83, 389–90
  premenstrual, 125, 167–70
Anima, 100
Animal Speak (Andrews), 764
"Annapurna Living" (blog), 640
Antibiotics, 145, 207, 344, 364, 379,
    382, 432, 481, 884, 903, 909, 916

routine, in a newborn's eyes, 599–600
vaginitis and, 362–63
Antidepressants, 781–82, 810–11
SSRIs, 441, 811, 882
Antihistamine cream (Eurax), 374
Antioxidants, 331, 354, 378, 434, 701, 705–6, 897–99, 914
in anticarcinogenic protocol, 330
chemotherapy and, 898
proanthocyanidins (pycnogenol, OPC), 331, 354, 372, 705–6, 898
RDA vs. optimal dosage, 899
Antivirals, 344
Anxiety/anxiety attacks, 71, 90–91, 179, 257, 318, 551, 730, 858, 878, 909, 932
Appreciation, 791, 792
Arachidonic acid (AA), 622, 884
elimination diet, 147
Archetypes, 103–5, 108, 201, 252, 258
Armstrong, Alison, 39
Arnica Montana, 829
Aromatherapy, 155, 399
Arrogance of Humanism, The (Ehrenfeld), 790
Art of Deliberate Creation (Hicks), 655
Art of Extreme Self-Care, The (Richardson), 732
ASCUS (atypical squamous cells of undetermined significance), 351–52
Ash, Lorraine, 528
Ask and It Is Given (Hicks), 655
Aspartame, 908, 919
Aspirin, 143, 348, 916
Association for Pre-and Perinatal Psychology and Health, 555, 564
Atalanta, Hilde, 376
Atkins, Robert, 843, 850
Attached (Levine and Heller), 90
Attached at the Heart (Nicholson and Parker), 609
Attachment Parenting International (API), 609
Autism, 627, 629–30, 633
Autoimmune diseases, 41, 42, 96, 207, 361, 378, 379, 456, 479, 522–23, 664, 743, 858, 893–94, 916
Autophagy, 861, 862
Avalon, Arthur, 88

Aygestin, 174, 176, 182
Ayurveda medicine, 12, 857

Bachmann, Gloria, 100
Back pain, 49, 67, 96, 163, 212, 277, 388, 544, 546, 618, 720, 750–51, 878, 942–43, 944
Baines, Cornelia, 409
Baker, Jeannine Parvati, 465, 473
Balch, Paulanne, 124, 872
Bannister, Roger, 965
Bantu women, 903
Barbach, Lonnie, 310
Barnard, Neal, 839
Basal body temperature (BBT), 484, 485, 489–90, 516
charts, 488, 489
Bathroom Key, The (Kassai and Perelli), 383
Baths, 297, 362
for cramps or pelvic pain, 153, 155, 222
Epsom salts, 658, 911
monthly self-care breast massage, 399
Batmanghelidj, Fereydoon, 878
Bayston, Margaret, 6
Beals, Ted, 146
Beauty Myth, The (Wolf), 184, 461
Beckwith, Michael Bernard, 154
Becoming Supernatural (Dispenza), 957
Being at One with the Divine (Fritchie), 758
Beliefs, xxiii, 60
changing, 44–48, 841
examining your own, 728–42
how perceptions become physical, 46–48
as physical, 40–48
unconscious nature of, 43–45, 59
Benedek, Therese, 125
Benn, Christine Stabell, 628–29
Benson, Herbert, 35, 153, 515
Bercov, Kris, 469
Berkovich, A. M., 508
Berman, Laura, 304
Beta-carotene, 331, 460, 542, 688–89, 923
recommended daily dose, 915
Beyer-Flores, Carlos, 559
Bhaerman, Steve, 781

Big Leap, The (Hendricks), 735, 738
Bigtree, Del, 632
Biocognitive Science Institute, 37
Biofeedback, 36, 180, 378, 573, 702
　vaginal, 372–73
Bioflavonoids, 148, 434, 678, 914
Bioidentical Hormone Initiative, 672
Biology of Belief, The (Lipton), 17, 29,
　719, 779, 956
Bird by Bird (Lamott), 763
Birth as We Know It (Tonetti-
　Vladimirova), 561
Birth control pills, 477–78, 479–81, 498
　abnormal Pap test and, 353
　breast pain and, 440, 441
　cancer risk, 479–80
　for DUB, 176
　for endometriosis, 207
　health benefits, 480
　health risks, 135–36, 479–80
　for heavy periods, 182
　implants replacing, 135
　intuition and, 135–40
　loss of sexual desire and, 139, 480,
　　483
　magnesium deficiency and, 909
　medications that interfere with, 481
　menstrual cramps and, 141
　ovarian cancer risk reduced by,
　　260–61
　PCOS treatment, 249
　Seasonale, 135
　smoking and, 480
　supplements recommended, 480, 517
　vaginitis and, 363
Birth defects, 112, 543
Birthfit, 544–45
Birthing. *See* Labor and birth
Birthing Normally (Peterson), 568
Black cohosh, 149, 351, 548
　BNO 1055, 679
　extract, Remifemin, 351, 679, 682
Bladder, 120, 321. *See also* UTIs
Bladder distention or instillation, 379
Blame, 22, 51, 84, 88, 91, 508–9,
　510, 511, 573, 730, 740, 804,
　976
Blessing Way ritual, 709
Block, Jennifer, 535
Blue Fire, A (Hillman), 56

Blum, Jeanne, 159
Bly, Robert, 39
BMI (body mass index), 872, 874
Bodansky, Vera and Steve, 297, 304,
　307, 483
Body, Mind, and Sport (Douillard), 929,
　951
Body image, 5, 288, 751–52, 873,
　875–77
Body work, 777–78. *See also specific
　types*
Bolen, Jean Shinoda, 387
Bolz-Weber, Nadia, 784
Bonding with your baby, 576, 579,
　605–11
　father's, 607–8
Bone health, 684–91, 804, 890
　calcium for, 901–6
　density, 683
　dual-energy X-ray absorptiometry
　　(DEXA), 683–84
　exercise for, 935
　Fosamax, Boniva, and Actonel, 683,
　　685, 690–91
　hip fracture and, 683, 686, 688, 904,
　　947
　low-acid diet for, 685–87
　magnesium/minerals and, 900–901,
　　908
　piezoelectric effect, 935
　program for, 684–89
　Pueraria mirifica for, 680
　testing, 683–84
　vitamin D for, 685, 688, 904–5
　See also Osteoporosis
Book of SHE, The (Stover), 473
Born to Be Good (Keltner), 956
Born to Live (McGarey), 472
Boron, 542, 658, 689, 901, 915
Borysenko, Joan, 464, 639
Boundary violation, 317, 320
Bowman, Katy, 213, 277, 618–19
　DVD and video course, 283–84
Braden, Gregg, 956
Bradford, Joy Harden, 770
Bradley, Marion Zimmer, 300
Brain
　aging and memory, 702–4
　biological vs. chronological age, 703
　-boosting smoothie, 152

chemistry, sugar, serotonin and,
    881–82
exercise benefits, 931
heart communication with, 792
intuitive capacity, 66
mind-body continuum, *138*
neurotransmitters, 173
oophorectomy and dementia, *257*
preservation program, 705–6
women's, 39–40
Brain Sex (Moir and Jesse), 39
Brain That Changes Itself, The (Doidge),
    302
Brand-Miller, Jennie, 852
Breast, xxiii, 387–463
    abscess, author's, 623, 785, 798, 969
    anatomy, 394, *395*
    bra fit and caution, 440
    caring for, 463
    cultural inheritance and, 387–94, 626
    DOT screening of, 412
    encoded wisdom in, 119
    enlargement, natural, 461–63
    genomic (genetic) profiles, 445
    massage ritual for health, 440
    monthly self-care breast massage, 399
    nipple discharge, 388, 399–400, 401
    nourishing yourself and, 463
    nursing and, 623, 626
    program to promote healthy, 397,
        429–43
    talking to, 440
Breast cancer, 424–53, 968
    abortion and, 470
    aftercare, 463
    biopsy, 404
    BRCA genes and, 261, 263, 443–44
    breast pain and, 402
    DCIS, 421–24
    deaths, 405–6, 407, 408, 409
    detection and diagnosis, 404–21
    diet-hormone link to, 425, 427–28,
        432, 700, 846–47, 902
    disappearance without intervention,
        407
    dreams and, 441–42
    emotional acceptance and better
        outcomes, 776–77
    environmental contaminants and,
        425
    estrogen and, 423, 427, 429–30, 668
    fourth chakra issues and, 109
    genetic link, 443–47
    HT and, 666–67, 699–700
    inflammation and, 427, 428
    inner guidance and treatment, 56–57
    LCIS, 422
    limits of early detection, 410
    mammography and, 405–10, 416–18,
        444, 667
    mind/body/soul connection, 392–93
    nipple discharge and, 401
    nutrition and supplements for, 429–43,
        847, 888–90
    online support, 448–49
    personality, emotions, stress, and,
        105–6, 109, 389–94, 433, 739
    pharma industry and pink ribbons,
        426
    postmenopausal women, 699–700
    premenopausal women and, 403
    prevention, 410, 445–47, 620, 680,
        690, 888–89
    progesterone and, 403, 428
    program for healthy breasts, 429–43
    prophylactic mastectomy, 423, 444
    Risk Assessment Tool, 407
    self-exams (BSE), 14, 394–99, *396*
    slow-growing cancers, 407
    tamoxifen and, 780
    thermography, 412–15, 418–20, 421,
        424
    treatment, 422–24, 447–50
    ultrasound screening and MRIs,
        410–11
    wisdom of, 393
    WISDOM study, 409
    women's stories, 391–94, 445–53
Breast Cancer Action (BCA), 426
Breast Cancer Awareness Month, 426
Breast cysts, 108, 391, 401–2, 411
Breast-feeding, xxiv, 16, 606, 619–27,
    902
    alcohol or cannabis and, 621–22
    breast implants and, 460
    iodine and, 437
Breast lumps, 399–400
    biopsy, 404
    mammography and, 405–10
    ultrasound screening and, 411

Breast pain, 399–400, 402–3
  bras and, 440
  cancer and, 402
  causes, 403
  cyclic mastalgia, 400, 403
  drugs to avoid, 440–41
  iodine supplements for, 437–39
  messages (encoded wisdom) in, 403–4
  nutrition and, 403, 429–43
  program for relief, 429–43
Breast surgery, cosmetic, 388, 453–61
  augmentation (implants), 453–57
  breast-feeding and, 456, 460
  cancer risk, 455, 456
  chronic bilateral micromastia, 388
  healing program for implants, 456, 460
  mammography and, 456–57
  reconstruction, 460, 463
  reduction, 460–61
  women's stories, 457–60
Breathing, 939–40
  bioenergetic, 555
  Buteyko breathing, 941
  Calm Birth, 545
  "Darth Vader" breathing, 938
  exercise and, 937, 951–52
  Four-Cycle Breathing, 759–60
  meditative state and, 940
  for menopausal symptoms, 681
  mouth breathing, 938
  nose breathing, 937, 951–52
  Peak 8 Workout and, 937–38
  proper, health benefits, 940
Breggin, Peter R., 782
Breiner, Mark, 817
Brexanolone (Zulresso), 613
Brezsny, Rob, 975
Bria, Gina, 716
Bright Line Eating, 867
Brody, Howard, 83
Brogan, Kelly, 152, 613, 614, 661–62,
  697, 768, 811, 839, 862, 882
  KB's Breakfast Smoothie, 863
  Vital Mind Reset Program, 614, 769,
  840, 856, 882
Bromelain, 828–29
Bromocriptine, 441
Brown, Sandra L., 106, 258, 722
Brownstein, David, 437
Buber, Martin, 48

Building Bone Vitality (Lanou and
  Castleman), 686
Buisson, Odile, 271
Bulletproof Brain Octane Oil, 862
Bullitt-Jonas, Margaret, 882
Burk, Larry, 66, 378–79, 441–42, 765
Burns, George, 927
Burst of Light (Lorde), 968
Burwell, Judith, 494
Bushnell, Laura, 297, 752
Buteyko, Konstantin Pavlovich, 941
BV (bacterial vaginosis), 317, 326, 541,
  543, 904

Cacioppo, Stephanie, 767–68
Caffeine and coffee, 380, 384–85, 521,
  651, 678, 688, 844, 853, 878, 880
  adrenal gland function and, 651, 657
  bone density and, 688, 903
  eliminating, 148, 164, 378, 400, 433,
  918–19
  free radical damage and, 898
  miscarriage and, 521
  ovarian cancer and, 260
Calcium, 900–906
  for bone health, 147, 689
  dairy foods and, 900–906
  kidney stones and, 689, 905, 906,
  908
  magnesium and, 178, 905, 908
  for menstrual problems, 178
  for pregnancy, 542
  RDA vs. optimal dose, 903, 915
  sources, 147, 903
  for vulvodynia, 371–72
Calhoun, Peter, 746
Calm Birth (CD), 545, 584
Calm Healing (CD), 545
Campbell, Phil, 937–38
Campbell, T. Colin, 839
Cancer, 52, 78, 361
  abuse and onset of, 7, 104
  anticarcinogenic protocol, 330
  antioxidants and, 898
  birth control pill and, 479–80
  blockage of energy and, 80, 82
  body fat and, 877
  "cancer energy," 254
  circumcision and penile, 310
  diagnosis, deadly stress of, 32–33

emotional acceptance and better outcomes, 776–77

emotions and, 43, 243–44, 389–94, 743

estrogen-progestin pills and, 480

exercise and reduced risk, 931

fibroid tumors and, 219

"fighting" metaphor and, 11, 74, 776–77

inflammation as preceding, 105, 428

National Cancer Institute website, 265

nutrition and, 839

oophorectomy and increased risk, 256

overdiagnosis, 14, 405, 408

Pap test and, 349, 350

personality influence on, 105–6

research websites, 390

soy foods and, 678, 888–89

vitamin D and, 410, 428, 434, 435–37

See also Breast cancer; specific types

CancerMath, 449

Cancer Report, The (Voell and Chatfield), 390

Cannon, Joanne, 930

Carbohydrates, 881–83

  Alzheimer's and, 704

  breast cancer and, 700

  free radical damage and, 898

  glycemic stress and insulin resistance, 851, 852, 853–54

  high- and low-glycemic foods, 141, 144, 165, 846, 852–53

  postpartum, 613

  program for optimal hormonal balance and pelvic health, 144–48

  stable blood sugar and, 849, 862–63

  sugar addiction, 881–83

  what to eat, 881–83

Carson, David, 764

Case Against Sugar, The (Taubes), 851

Castleman, Michael, 686

Castor oil packs, 154–55

  breast cancer and, 451

  breast pain and, 440

  for cystitis and UTIs, 381, 378

  for gynecological problems, 154–55, 180, 210, 232, 969

Cayce, Edgar, 154, 438

Cellphones, risks for women, 549–50

Cellular inflammation. See Inflammation

Cellular memory, 814, 831, 961

Center for Intuitive Movement Healing, 946

Center for Nonviolent Communication, 11, 975

Center for Partnership Studies, 9

Centripetal energy, 85, 86, 87

Cervarix, 333

Cervical cancer, 18, 108, 243, 318, 354

  birth control pill and, 480

  death rates, 348

  father's loss and, 109

  HPV and, 325–27, 334

  mind/body connection, 720

  Pap test screening, 348–52

  passive coping style and, 105–6, 320

  second chakra issues and, 109

  smoking and, 923

  symptoms, 348

  technologies for cell testing, 352–53

  vaccine, 331–39

Cervical dysplasia, 24, 50, 318, 320, 347–59

  common concerns, 353

  cone biopsy and, 352

  HPV and, 325–27

  Pap test screening, 348–52

  smoking and, 353, 354

  symptoms, 348

  technologies for cell testing, 352–53

  treatment, 352, 353–54

  women's stories, 354–59

Cervicitis, 347

Cervix, 315, 320, 321–22

  miscarriage and, 522, 551

  mucus checks, 484, 487

  as sphincter, 569, 577

  squamocolumnar junction (SCJ), 322, 352

  wisdom of, 120

Cesarean section (C-section), 572–75

  age and, 557

  ART and, 506

  DUB and, 175

  herpes and, 344

  high rate of, 12, 557–58, 572

  hypnosis to reduce incidence of, 555

  injecting scar, 614

  pelvic floor dysfunction and, 577–78

Cesarean section (C-section) (*cont'd*):
  risks, 574–75
  vaginal birth after (VBAC), 574, 582
  vaginal seeding and, 585
  ways to reduce your risk for, 540,
    581–84
Chakras, 86–113, *93*, *98–99*
  archetypes and first three, 103–5
  energy anatomy table, 94–96
  family wounds, 89–91, 96–99
  fifth chakra, 110–11
  first chakra issues, 89–91, 96–99, 236,
    238, 601
  fourth chakra, 105–9, 389
  healing lower-chakra wounds, 110–12
  high heart, low heart and, 106
  lower female centers, 89–92, 96–110,
    197
  second chakra issues, 89–91, 181,
    194–96, 236, 238, 243, 254, 257,
    736
  self-esteem and personal power, 91,
    101–2, 236, 238, 242
  seventh chakra, 111–12
  shame and first three chakras, 105–6
  sixth chakra, 111, 455
  stress and first three chakras, 91–92
  symbolic creative space, 99–101
  third chakra issues, 91–92
  women of color and, 729–30
Chalice and the Blade, The (Eisler), 8,
    779
Chamberlain, Wilt, 293
Chanel, Coco, 752
Charity: Water, 716
Chasteberry, 175, 517, 548
Chatfield, Cynthia, 390
Chelation, 339
Chemotherapy
  artificial menopause and, 665, 745
  preparing for, 822–33
Chia, Maneewan and Mantak, 307, 694
Chia seeds, 881
Childbirth. *See* Labor and birth
Childbirth Connection, 565
Childhood
  abuse, sexual, 6, 8, 20, 24, 33, 34, 49,
    64, 79, 83, 98, 106, 179, 250,
    358–59, 371, 520
  ACE study and, 33, 84

adoption and bloodline memories,
    529–30
  examining your own, 729–30
  fears, 520–21
  "inner child," tubal problems and,
    518
  memories, healing, 513–114
  prenatal influences, 530, 537
Chimerism, 603
China, diet and health in, 847, 903
China Study, The (Campbell), 839
Chinese angelica (dong quai), 548, 679
Chiu, Sandra, 130, 131–32, 159, 977
Chlamydia, 368
Chlebowski, Rowan, 667
Chlorophyll, 864–65
Cholesterol, 47, 98, 441, 653, 851,
    854, 884, 885, 877, 889, 890,
    893, 894
  estrogen and, 671
  statin drugs and, 435, 441, 893
Chopra, Deepak, 46
Chromium, 542, 658, 851, 901, 915
Chronic fatigue syndrome, 26, 41, 361
Church, Dawson, 772
Circumcision, male, 310–13, 600–602
Clear Passage Therapies, 157, 520
Climacteric, 637, 662, 670, 677, 692
Clitoris, 269–72, 300, 307, 311
  "clitoral complex," 269
  website for printing a model of,
    270–71
Clomid, 177, 249
Close Your Mouth (McKeown), 941
Coalition for Improving Maternity
    Services (CMIS), 565, 574, 575
  "Having a Baby? Ten Questions to
    Ask," 565
Codependence, 357–58, 359
Coenzyme Q10 (CoQ10), 434–35, 915
Coffee. *See* Caffeine and coffee
Cohen, Dana, 716, 878–80
Cohen, Doris E., 64, 65, 66, 81, 82, 764,
    765, 766, 769
Cohen, Jon, 523
Colorado Cleanse, The (Douillard), 857
Colposcopy, 326, 327, 352, 352–53,
    357
Cometa, Ariane, 419–20, 421
Cometa Wellness Center, 418–20

Coming to Term (Cohen), 523

Complementary or integrative medicine, 799, 809, 810–11

Complete Guide to Fasting, The (Fung and Moore), 861

Conceiving with Love (Wiesner), 512

Conception, 121, 477–73, 507, 510–11

Condoms, 295, 327, 339, 343, 368, 381, 476, 483, 497

Cone biopsy, 352, 353, 354

Conjugated linoleic acid (CLA), 146

Conquering Infertility (Domar), 515

Conscious Conception (Baker), 472

Consciousness, 3, 17–18, 29, 45, 51, 58, 69, 98, 122, 236, 237, 242, 250, 266, 316, 508, 514, 564, 705, 828, 835, 924, 926, 927, 930, 954, 960, 961, 965, 975

  author's going backward in time, 959

  changing, and changing cells, 714–16

  global change in, 957–60

  intention experiments, 955–56

  naming, healing emotional pain, 18–25

  Step by Step Process for Bringing Dream Wisdom to Consciousness, 65–66

Contraception, 8, 477–73

  barrier methods, 476, 478, 483, 496, 497, 500–501

  choosing method, 478

  Depo-Provera, 478, 482, 503

  emergency, 476

  Essure implant, 492–93

  failure of, 478

  female condom (FC2), 478

  fertility awareness, 478, 483–90, *488, 489,* 496

  implants, 135, 478, 482, 499–500

  injectable progestin, 503

  IUDs, 135, 476, 478, 479, 482–83, 499

  methods compared, 496–503

  NuvaRing, 478, 481, 501

  oral, 479–81, 498 (*see also* Birth control pills)

  outercourse, 483

  Ovulation Method, 484–86

  patches, 478, 481–82, 502–3

  Reality female condom, 497

  spermicides, 499

  STDs and, 368

  tubal ligation, 478, 490–95, 503

  vasectomy, 491, 493, 503

  withdrawal, 503

  women's stories, 493–95

Cook, Andrew, 203, 206

Cooking for Hormone Balance (Wszelaki), 150

Cooper, Kenneth, 851

Copper, 542, 658, 900, 901, 915

Cora company, 129

Cortisol, 42, 317, 652–53, 656, 865, 869, 906

Cosmetic surgery

  breast implants, 411, 453–57

  vaginal, 375–77

Cotinine, 353

Council for Responsible Nutrition, 913

Counterclockwise (Langer), 936

Cousins, Norman, 3, 802

Coyne, Nancy, 787

CPR (Johnson), 468

Cramer, Daniel, 145

C-reactive protein, 428

Creativity, 735–40

  "the birthing field" and, 197–98

  fertility metaphor and, 531–32

  fibroid tumors and, 216–17, 232–36

  labor and birth, 604

  menopause and, 709

  menstrual cycle and, 117, 121

  ovaries and, 244, 254, 256, 266, 740

  second chakra and, 99–101, 106

  uterus and, 237–39, 242

Cronin, Thomas, 454

Crouch, Naomi, 375–76

Crying, 59, 63, 125, 720, 749, 824, 832–33, 959–60

  children, babies, and, 62, 89

  energy flow and, 75

  toxin removal and, 61

Cryocautery, 330, 347

Crystals, 285

cummings, e. e., 769

Curott, Phyllis, 964

Cutler, Winnifred, 257, 308

Cystitis. *See* Interstitial cystitis

Cystoscopy, 378

Dairy foods, 144–47, 902
  allergies, problems with, 902
  BGH or antibiotics in, 145, 425, 432–33
  calcium and, 901–3
  elimination of, 144–45, 164, 432–33
  ovarian cancer and, 145, 259–60
  raw milk and diary, benefits, 146–47
  Real Milk Finder website, 147
Dalai Lama, 56
Dale, Cyndi, 77, 86
Dalton, Katerina, 125
D'Amour, Alexandra, 290
Danocrine (danazol), 208, 440
Davis, Adelle, 838
Davis, William, 839, 859
Days for Girls, 129
DCIS (ductal carcinoma-in-situ), 421–24
  Comparison of Operative to Monitoring and Endocrine Therapy study, 424
  IDLE and, 422
  treatment, 422–23
Dean, Carolyn, 338–39, 361, 651, 657, 907, 909, 911, 940
  ReMag, ReMyte, and, 658–59, 911
Death, 28
  breast cancer and, 393, 424, 444, 455
  cervical cancer and, 348
  child's or stillbirth, 525–28, 541, 617
  emotions of loss, 88, 390, 730, 833
  expressing grief, 525–26, 730, 744
  fear of, 52
  fetal, 551
  healing and, 48
  HIV and, 369
  lung cancer and, 424, 923
  near-death experiences, 112, 927
  ovarian cancer and, 264
  pregnancy, labor, and, 525, 559, 563–65, 575
  premature births and, 550
  smoking and, 541, 921, 923
  spirit and, 31
  Thanatos and, 296
  trauma of loss, and cancer onset, 390
  trauma of loss, and PMS, 164, 730
  women's, top causes, 666, 922, 923, 931

Denniston, George, 601
Dentistry, holistic, 815–17
Depression, 32, 41, 479, 858, 882
  alternative approaches, 810–11
  carbohydrate craving, serotonin, sugar sensitivity and, 882
  energy leaks and, 78–79
  exercise for, 878, 932
  family legacy of, 719
  infertility awareness and, 504
  menopause and, 696–97
  menstrual problems and, 178
  oophorectomy and, 257
  osteoporosis and, 688
  postpartum, 612–17
  SAD, 166–67, 168, 881
  Vital Mind Reset Program, 614, 769, 840, 856, 882
Désilets, Saida, 107
DesMaisons, Kathleen, 881, 882
Detoxification, 159, 161, 338–39, 420, 439, 896, 910, 925
DeVeaux, Alexis, 531
DHEA, 648, 652–63, 669–70, 676
  Alzheimer's prevention and, 704
  cortisol and, 652, 653, 657
  for loss of sexual desire, 231
  menopause and, 675, 676, 694
  source of, 652
  supplement, 659, 676–77
  testing levels, 654
Diabetes, 7, 102, 144, 248, 620, 681, 701, 727–28, 877, 910, 931
  Alzheimer's as Type 3 diabetes, 704
  nutrition and, 836, 840, 850, 854
Diagnostic and Statistical Manual of Mental Disorders (DSM-5), 768
Diastasis recti, 618–19
Diastasis Recti (Bowman), 618
Diet. See Nutrition
Diets Don't Work (Schwartz), 844
Dignity Period, 129
DiNicolantonio, James, 880
Dispenza, Joe, 957
Divine Feminine–Awakened Masculine Institute, 965
Divine Love, 285, 339, 392–93, 757–61, 770, 813, 830, 927
  Healing Statement for One Symptom, 759

Healing Statement to Remove All
Symptom Pop-Ups, 759
meditation, 221
Dixson, Alan F., 230
Dobson, Andrew, 462
Dodging Energy Vampires (Northrup),
68, 127, 258, 306, 553, 723, 970
Doidge, Norman, 302
Do Less (K. Northrup), 736
Domar, Alice, 504, 508, 515
Dominator system, 9–28, 623
characteristics of, 22–23
creativity controlled in, 238
dependency in, 19
film reviewers and, 290–91, 778–79
fundamental beliefs of, 11–17, 60
information overload and, 812
mothering in, 623, 633–36
patriarchy and, xxii, 3–28, 60, 102
pregnancy as illness in, 533–34,
555–58
responsibility vs. blame and, 51–52
sex in, 288–95
spirituality and, 754
See also Western culture
Dominguez, Joe, 736
Don't Call Me Princess (Orenstein),
294
Don't Drink Your Milk (Oski), 902
Dopamine, 30, 302, 614, 656, 848, 881,
900
Dossey, Barbara, 817
Dossey, Larry, 235
DOT (diffuse optical tomography), 412
Douching, 316, 317, 362, 364, 541
Douillard, John, 438, 839, 857, 929,
937, 938, 940, 951
Doula, 12, 566, 577, 580–81, 582
Dreaming on Both Sides of the Brain
(Cohen), 66, 764
Dreams, 64–66, 358, 452–53
alcohol disrupting, 920
breast cancer warning and, 441–42
common symbolism in, 65–66, 765
diagnostic power of, 66, 765
diary for, 442
earth's dreams, 967–74
healing and, 210
as inner guidance, 64, 452–53, 733,
769

lunar information and menstruation,
124
Step by Step Process for Bringing
Dream Wisdom to Consciousness,
65–66
working with, remembering, and
interpreting, 764–69, 819–20
Dreams That Can Save Your Life (Burk
and O'Keefe-Kanavos), 66, 442, 765
Dreher, Henry, 105
Dresser, Sarah, 462
Dressing Your Truth (Tuttle), 752
Drewry, Damaris, 813–14
Beyond Talk Therapy website, 814
Dr. Gundry's Diet Evolution (Gundry),
839–40
*Dr. Lani's No-Nonsense Bone Health
Guide* (Simpson), 684
*Dr. Lani's No-Nonsense Sun Health
Guide* (Simpson), 905
*Dr. Neal Barnard's Program for
Reversing Diabetes* (Bernard), 839
DUB (dysfunctional uterine bleeding),
175–77
PCOS and, 177
Dubner, Stephen, 467
Dumais, Sue, 515
Duncan, Isadora, 928
Durek, Judith, 117
Dynamic Laws of Prosperity, The
(Ponder), 737
Dyspareunia, 203, 291–92

Eades, Mary Dan, 849
Earth
dreams, the earth's and ours, 967–74
effect of the natural world, 755–56
energy, 84–86, 965
first chakra and, 89
healing of, 954–78
menstrual cycle, seasons, and, 121,
166–67, *168*
Eating disorders, 15, 102, 133, 517, 875
Eat Wheat (Douillard), 857
Eberstadt, Mary, 303
Echart, Meister, 533
Ecstasy, 305, 558
birthing, 269, 559–60, 598
Ecstatic Birth program, 546–47
Ectopic pregnancy, 523–24

EFT (Emotional Freedom Technique, Tapping), 374, 375, 378, 770–72, 814

Egypt, ancient, herbal medicine guide, 12

Ehrenfeld, David, 790

8 Steps to a Pain-Free Back (Adams and Gokhale), 278, 298, 943

Einstein, Albert, 3

Einstein Time, 738–39

Eisler, Riane, 4, 8–9, 305, 779

Electrocautery, 330

ELITE (Early Versus Late Intervention Trial with Estradiol), 671

Ella (Fibristal), 476

Elliott, Carl, 782

Elmiron (Pentosan Polysufate Sodium), 379

EMbody Program, 619

EMDR (Eye Movement Desensitization and Reprocessing), 374, 614, 770, 773

Emergence of the Sensual Woman (Désilets), 107

Emerson, Ralph Waldo, 976

EMF (electromagnetic field), 549–50

Emmanuelle (films), 310

Emotional Energy Factor, The (Kirshenbaum), 78

Emotions
  affecting cells, 779
  appreciation, 791, 792
  archetypal forms of wounding and, 37
  behaviors that avoid or deny, 18
  biochemistry of, 21
  blockage of energy and, 80–83
  "breakdown to breakthrough," 720
  cleansing of, 60–63, 745–46
  crying, 59, 61, 63, 75, 125, 720, 744, 749, 824, 959–60
  DHEA levels and, 654, 704
  effect on gastrointestinal system, 58–59
  emotional acceptance of cancer diagnosis and better outcomes, 776–77
  emotional pain, acknowledging and healing, 10, 22, 24–25, 236
  emotional security, 62, 90
  endometriosis and, 201

  energy of, 78
  expression of, 60–61, 62–63, 730
  food/emotion connection, 865–69
  fourth chakra and, 106
  happiness as power, 69–70
  hormones and, 125–26
  infertility and, 505, 513–14
  Inner Child Rescue exercise, 78, 81–82
  intellect seen as superior to, 18
  menopause and, 638–43
  men out of touch with, 75
  miscarriage and, 522–23
  naming, power of, and, 18–21
  negative, health consequences, 32
  obsessive thoughts/behaviors and, 43–44
  ovulation and, 135, 136–40, 150–51
  pelvic pain and, 200
  physical consequences of suppressed, 20, 22, 24–28, 35–37, 41–43, 72, 109, 200, 236, 249–50, 257–58, 316–21, 355–56, 389–90, 403–4, 429, 433, 470–71, 613, 720, 727–28, 730, 741, 743
  positive, heart coherence and, 792
  primal sounds and, 744
  processing, step by step, 73–74
  purpose of, 60
  "radical surrender," 390
  reestablishing cyclic emotional flow, 150–51
  respecting and releasing, 34, 59, 60–63, 75, 80, 82, 742–46, 776–77
  righteous anger, 727–28
  shamanic imprint removal, 746–48
  stuck at childhood level, 81
  symptoms of, 60, 73–74
  whole body and, 35–36
  writing to release, 210

Emoto, Masaru, 31, 927

Empowering Women (Hay), 779

Ending Female Pain (Herrera), 374

Endocrine system, 81, 175

Endometrial ablation, 182, 225

Endometrial hyperplasia, 173–75, 180

Endometriosis, 24, 27, 41, 49, 140, 200–210, *202*, 809
  alternative to hysterectomy, 209–10
  common concerns, 204–6
  cul-de-sac of Douglas and, 203

diagnosis, 203
dietary supplements and, 148
diet-excess weight link, 204
diet-hormone link, 902
emotional conflict and, 201
heavy bleeding and, 181
infertility and, 505
lesions and pain of, 205–6
mind/body connection, 720
neuroendocrine-immune connection, 206–7
Pueraria mirifica for, 208–9
relationships, security, creativity and, 101
symptoms, 202
treatment, 207–9, 374
wisdom of, 211
women's stories, 210–11
Energy fields and energy systems, 29–34, 78, 833–34, 957–60
accessing birth energy, 592–95
altruism as, 956
anger as, 745–46
bodies as energy, 29–34
body as a hologram, 30, 325
chi (life force energy), 30, 242
desire and, 791–92
Earth's, 84–86, 965
EFT for blocks, 770–72
Einstein Time and, 738–39
female energy system, chakras, 77–113
of food, 837, 926–27
healing, 821, 833–35
healing leaks, 80–84, 236
heart's energy field, 85, 784–85, 792
hot flashes and, 681
illness as energy leaks, 78–79
integrins and cellular connection, 30
intention experiments, 955–56
interconnectivity of everything, 956–57
law of attraction and, 30–31, 74, 112, 223, 397, 742–43, 791, 806–7
life force, women as, 978
light energy from leafy greens, 864–65
menstrual cycle and, 121, 123
money and, 196, 736
"narcissistic supply," 108
the old energy (darkness), 957
piezoelectric effect, 935
positive or negative influences, 70–71

potential future selves and, 716
process for positive flow, 73
reading energy fields, 66–67
releasing emotions and, 513–14, 833–34
sexual, 287, 298, 305, 313–14, 694
spirit as, 30
tubal ligation or vasectomy and, 494
vibrational fields, 31–32
vibrational healing, 339
Energy healer, 80
Energy vampires, xxiii, 68, 74, 107, 258, 306, 553, 722
Enigma of Reason, The (Mercier and Sperber), 783
Environmental toxins, 370, 896–97
energy links and, 80
glyphosate, 857–58
health risks, cancer, and, 205, 425, 428, 521, 652
Ephistogram, 513
Epigenetics, 257, 956
Episiotomy, 16–17, 561, 573, 576, 611
Epstein-Barr virus, 41
Ericksen, Melanie, 80
Erotic Interludes (Barbach), 310
Escharotic treatment, 330
Essential oils, 548
Esserman, Laura J., 409, 422
Essure, 492–93
Estes, Clarissa Pinkola, 19, 237, 764
Estradiol (Estrace), 309, 381, 432, 671–72, 673, 682, 700, 704
Estratest, 695
Estriol, 352, 385, 673, 674, 682
Estrogen, *138,* 673, 846
bioidentical, 671–72, 704
body fat and, 165, 177
breast cancer and, 425, 428, 429–30, 440, 674, 846–47
breast pain and, 403, 425, 429
dementia, Alzheimer's, and, 703–4
dominance, 674–75, 900
DUB and, 175
ELITE trial, 671
endometriosis and, 205, 207–8
foods to moderate levels, 144, 429–30
foods to promote production, 846–47
hormone therapies and, 665–66, 667, 669, 670, 681

Estrogen (*cont'd*):
  for hot flashes, 681
  inflammation and, 205
  KEEPS study, 670–71
  libido restoration and, 230
  menopause and, *649, 650*
  menstrual cycle and, 122, 125, 126, 177
  metabolism of, 847, 900
  phytoestrogens and, 678–79
  PMS and, 165
  Premarin and, 385, 665–68, 671, 681, 700, 703–4, 707, 780
  Pueraria mirifica to balance, 149, 157
  salivary testing of, 484
  transdermal or vaginal ring, 681, 682
  types of, natural, 673
  urethral tissue and, 385
  UTIs and, 382
  vaginal creams, 385, 682
  vaginal thinning/dryness and, 309, 352, 682
  vegetarians and, 165
  yogurt and lactobacillus acidophilus to metabolize, 434
  See also Birth control pills
Estrogen Errors, The, (Prior), 644, 675, 699
Estrone, 165, 441, 673, 700
Evans, Leonard, 32
Exercise, 928–53
  addiction and, 947–48, 952
  for adrenal/thyroid/sex steroid restoration program, 659–60
  aerobic, 878, 933, 934, 935–36
  aging and fitness level, 936–37
  Alzheimer's prevention and, 706
  amenorrhea and, 178, 948–49
  amount per day, 945
  for bone health, 683, 687–88, 931
  for brain health, 706
  for breast health, 441, 931
  breathing and, 937, 951–52
  cultural inheritance, 929–30
  for detoxification, 159
  fascia and, 159, 941–42
  flexibility and alignment, 941–43
  getting started, 949–53
  health benefits, 878
  heart disease risk and, 701, 931

HIIT, 878, 937–38
  how much and what kind, 950–51
  insulin resistance and, 930, 935
  intuition and, 932–33
  "no pain, no gain" fallacy, 940
  ovarian breathing, 242
  Peak 8 Workout, 937–38
  pelvic floor, 278–84, 279–83, 298, 384
  PMS and, 161, 169, 171
  preconception program (Before the Bump), 544–45
  for pregnancy, 544–45
  psoas muscle, 943–44
  Rest-Based Training (RBT), 938–39
  squats for prolapse and incontinence, 213
  strength training, 878, 932, 934–36
  stretching, 881
  target heart rate, 878, 936
  weight bearing, 687–88, 878
  Yoni Egg Practice, 285–87, 286
Exosomes, 837
Extended Massive Orgasm (Bodansky), 304, 483

Facial hair (hirsutism), 248, 440, 695, 855
Fallopian tubes
  deep tissue massage for, 519, 524
  ectopic pregnancy, 523–24
  infertility and, 505, 518, 519
  tubal ligation, 478, 490–95
Family legacy, 718–21
  Adverse Health Effects of Cluster B Individuals on Those in Relationships with Them, 721–23
  transgenerational beliefs in DNA, 43, 719
Fascia, 159, 881, 941–42, 944–46
  FasciaRehab method, 945
  liquid crystalline matrix, 945
Fasting, intermittent, 860–62
Fat, body, 841
  BMI and, 872, *874*
  estrogen and, 165, 177, 429, 441
  insulin secretion and, 427–28, 851
  measuring, 876–77
  menstruation and, 133, 177
  stress urinary incontinence and, 384

Fat, dietary, 840, 892–95
  benefits of good fats, 893–94
  breast cancer link, 427
  essential fatty acids, 149, 435, 544,
    621, 892–93, 894
  estrogen and, 429, 441
  healthy fats, 144
  ketogenic diet and, 144
  omega-3 fats and DHA, 149, 428,
    433–34, 456, 460, 544, 613, 678,
    706, 892–93, 915
  omega-6 and -9 fats, 892, 895
  ovarian cancer and, 259–60
  red meat and saturated, 147, 259–60
  risks of bad fats, 894–95
  trans fats, 147–48, 892–93, 894
Fear
  asking for needs and, 805
  healing old fears, 820–21
  shaman past and, 964–66
Feldenkrais Method, 777, 942
Felitti, Vincent, 33
Female energy system, 77–113, 389
  chakras and, 86–113
  earth's energy and, 84–86
  matter/energy continuum, 78–86
  menopause and, 692
  ovaries and, 243, 252, 267
  surgery and, 833–34
  uterine energy vs. ovarian, 257
Female genital mutilation (FGM), 7, 270,
    313, 316, 375–76, 601, 965
Female Patient, The (Nolan), 335
Female Pelvic Alchemy Jump Start
    Program, 374
Feminine intelligence, healing and, 29–55
Femme-Tasse, 129
FemSoft Insert, 385
Fenn, Mary Ellen, 589
Fertility, 464–532
  abortion, 466–75
  awareness, 483–90, 496
  BBT and, 484, *488*, 489–90, *489*
  drugs and ovarian cancer risk, 261
  emergency contraception, 476
  endometriosis and, 200, 202, 205
  fertile phase, 487
  freezing or donating eggs, 510–11
  infertility, 504–21
  letters to unborn potential beings, 210

  as metaphor, 531–32
  mucus checks, cervical, 484, 487
  See also Contraception
Fetal monitors, 572–75
Fiber, dietary, 144, 425, 429–30, 846,
    916
  estrogen metabolism and, 144,
    429–30, 846
  in program for healthy breasts, 429–30
  supplements for, 161
Fibrocystic breast disease, 400–401,
    437–38
Fibroid ablation, 223
Fibroid tumors, xxiii, 27, 215–36, *216*
  author's, 969–73
  common concerns, 219–23
  degeneration, 218
  energy blocks and, 80–81, 100–101
  heavy bleeding and, 181, 217–18
  hysterectomy alternatives, 223
  program for treating, 143–61
  relationships, security, creativity and,
    101, 737, 970
  risk factors, 216
  symptoms, 217–19
  treatment, 223–32
  types of, 217
  wisdom of, 223
  women's stories, 221–22, 232–36
Fibromyalgia, 361
Field, Tiffany, 546, 608, *656*
Fillod, Odile, 270
Finances and money, 195–96, 735–40,
    741–42
Fincher, Theresa, 391–94
Fire with Fire (Wolf), 635
Fisch, Harry, 515
Fish, 144, 149, 433, 650, 701
  oil capsules, 149, 433, 892, 893,
    894
Fisher, W. A., 508
*Five Minutes to Orgasm Every Time You
    Make Love* (Hutchins), 300
Flamm, Bruce, 574
Flaxseed and flaxseed oil, 149, 150, 430,
    433, 544, 678, 701, 892
Flibanserin (Addyi), 293
Flourish! (radio show), 719, 785, 845
F.lux app, 151
Foldès, Pierre, 271

Folic acid, 914
  for adrenal restoration, 657
  in anticarcinogenic protocol, 330
  for brain health, 705
  for cervical dysplasia, 352, 354
  for fertility, 517
  methylate form, 900
  for pregnancy, 542, 543, 900
  recommended dose, 915
Food. *See* Nutrition
Food (Hyman), 840
Forgive Assholes (video), 784
Forgive for Good (Luskin), 784
Forgiveness, healing and, 513, 783–90,
  965
Forks Over Knives (film), 839
Fo-ti, 679
Fourth Trimester, The (Johnson), 292
Fox, Matthew, 75
Frampton, Susan, 796
Frank, Barb, 526–28
Freakonomics (Levitt and Dubner), 467
Freud, Sigmund, 271, 465
Fritchie, Robert, 758, 830, 927
  At Oneness Healing System Advanced
    Protocol, 760
From Housewife to Heretic (Johnson),
  xxii
FSD (female sexual dysfunction), 293
FSH (follicle-stimulating hormone), 122,
  126, *138*, 434, *505*, *509*, *645*
  menopausal production, 643, 663–64
Fuller, Buckminster, 14
Functional medicine, 210, 445, 799, 800,
  858, 900
Fung, Jason, 247, 427–28, 839, 840,
  860–62
Future Health Now Encyclopedia
  (Dean), 339

Gabriel, Jon, 842–43, 876
Gadsby, Hannah, 958
Gall bladder, third chakra issues and,
  102
Game of Life and How to Play It, The
  (Shinn), 753
Gangwisch, James, 895
Gardasil and Gardasil 9, 331–39, 548
Gardnerella, 360
Garland, Cedric, 435

Garlic, 345
Gaskin, Ina Mae, 559, 561, 577, 598,
  616, 735
  Safe Motherhood Quilt Project,
    563–65
  Sphincter Law, 569
Gastrointestinal system, 58–59, 105,
  916
Gawande, Atul, 14
Gene therapy, 797
Genetic disorders, 112
  in utero gene editing and, 534
Genetic testing, 782–83, 838
Genital area
  affirmation for, 331, 346
  cancers of, 105
  changing perception, 346, 356–57,
    359
  cultural taboos and beliefs, 316–21,
    359
  naming, 734–35
  screening test for microbiome of, 346
  warts, 24, 49, 108, 318, 325–40
  wisdom of, 386
Genomic (genetic) profiles, 445
George, Demetra, 123
Gerow, Frank, 454
Gershon, Michael, 58–59
Gestational diabetes, 543
Getson, Philip, 413
Giamario, Daniel, 954
Gia Milagro program, 394
Gibney, Alex, 722
Gimbutas, Marija, 4
Ginseng (Siberian), 548, 679
Giving Birth Naturally, 565
Global Consciousness Project, 955
Global Fund for Women, 8
Glow 15 (Whittel), 862
Glutamates (including MSG), 867–68,
  908
Gluten intolerance, 857–59
GnRH (gonadotropin-releasing
  hormones), 207–8, 224–25, 227,
  972
Goals, lifetime, 794–95
Goddesses Never Age (Northrup), 647,
  672, 937
Gokhale, Esther, 212–13, 278, 298,
  941–42, 943

Gokhale Method, 278, 284, 941–42
Goldberg, Natalie, 761, 763, 812
Golden handcuff syndrome, 259, 446
Gonadotropins, 260–61
Gonzales, Nick, 839
Goodman, Ellen, 634
Good Mother, The (Bercov), 469
Gornick, Vivian, 966
Gottfried, Sara, 839
Gotzsche, Peter, 405
Grain Brain (Perlmutter), 704, 840, 859
Green, Glanda, 731
Green Mountain Doc blog, 337
Green tea, 330, 517
Grief, 20, 25, 32, 80, 106, 186, 210, 236, 359, 388, 390, 699, 730, 820, 959
  abortion and miscarriage, 466, 468–71, 522, 526–28
  breakdown to break through, 720
  midlife and loss, 640–42, 697
  stillbirth, 525–28
  surgery and, 494, 832–33, 834, 969
Groening, Bruno, 757, 758
  Circle of Friends, 757–58
Grossinger, Richard, 75
G-spot (sacred spot), 271, 274–76, 276
Guendelman, Sylvia, 540
Guerin, Maude, 49–50
Guided imagery (visualization), 53–54, 210, 252, 358
  for achieving goals, 794
  breast enlargement, 461–63
  CDs and MP3 files for, 545
  for fertility, 515
  health benefits, 545
  Inner Child Rescue exercise and, 81–82
  for labor, 546
  for meditation during pregnancy, 545–56
  restoring birth energy flow and bond, 594
  surgical outcome, 824
Guilt, 88, 91, 317, 319, 328, 359, 763
Gundry, Steven, 839
Gupta, Aditi, 188
Gynecologists, 323

Hacking of the American Mind, The (Lustig), 302, 848
Hair, thinning, 678, 695
Half the Sky (Kristof and WuDunn), 9, 974
Hamer, Ryke Geerd, 390
Hammer, Scott, 370
Happiest Baby on the Block, The (Karp), 617
Happiness, 794
Hardy, Benjamin, 794
Hargrove, Joel, 668
Harper, Diane, 332, 334
Harvey, Judie, 415
Haskell, Molly, 387
Hay, Louise, 40, 45, 331, 346, 358, 702, 779, 841
Hay, Sheila Kamara, 546–47
Hays, Bethany, 555, 560, 570, 590–92, 595–99, 610
Healing and creating health, xxiii, 22, 24–28, 713–95, 954–78
  acknowledging a higher power or inner wisdom, 753–61
  actively participate in life, 790–95
  Adverse Health Effects of Cluster B Individuals on Those in Relationships with Them, 721–23
  appreciating and accepting your body, xxiv, 749–50, 751–52, 842–43, 877
  balance in life, 732–33, 739
  beliefs, examining, 728–42
  body image and, 875–76, 877
  body work in, 777–78
  causes of health, creating health, 727–28
  commitment to, 508, 787, 974–78
  curing vs., 48–52, 266
  Divine Love and, 757–61, 813, 830, 927
  Einstein Time, 738–39
  emotional pain, 470
  emotional release and, 34, 59, 60–63, 525–26, 742–46
  energy transformation and, 236
  exercise: spiritual wisdom to keep you on track, 717–18
  exercise: three questions to create your future reality, 715–16
  family history, 718–21

Healing and creating health (*cont'd*):
  female anatomy, knowing, 734–35
  feminine intelligence and, 29–55
  food and, 836–927 (*see also* Nutrition)
  forgiveness and, 783–90, 965
  Four-Cycle Breathing, 759–60
  future, imagining, 714–16
  "healer quotient," 801
  Health Inventory, 724–26
  help or therapy, getting, 769–76
  information gathering for, 778–83
  inner guidance and, 715, 794, 812
  "letting go," 787
  listening to your body, 58–61, 135,
    136, 202, 243–44, 259, 748–51,
    972–73
  living in the present and, 112
  media avoidance, thirty day break,
    793
  medical records, 734, 808
  menstrual cycles and, 127–28
  mind/body connection, 733–34
  music and, 793
  obstacles to, 731–32
  personal/planetary, 968
  post-abortion trauma, 469–72
  prescription drugs and mental health,
    768
  priorities for time, 732–33, 739, 949
  by proxy, for a loved one, 760, 761
  a purposeful life and, 739–40
  reclaiming fullness of mind, 761–69
  respecting our body, 751–52
  self, 976–78
  self-care, 732–33
  self-pride, 740, 741
  self-sacrifice, 739, 743
  shamanic imprint removal, 746–48
  spontaneous remissions, 758
  statements for surgery, 827–28
  unblocking energy and, 80–81
  Violet Flame for, 747–48
  visualizing, 824
  See also specific disorders
Healing Back Pain (Sarno), 750
Healing the Family Tree (McAll), 783
Healing Hypertension (Mann), 553
Healing Into Life and Death (Levine), 63
Healing Love Through the Tao (Chia
  and Chia), 307

Healing Mind, Healthy Woman (Domar),
  515
Health care provider, choosing, 798–808
Health Inventory, 724–26
Health Outcomes, 942
Healthy for Life (Strand), 850
*Healthy Pregnancy and Successful
  Childbirth, The* (Naparstek), 545–46
Heart and Soul of Sex, The (Ogden), 269
Heart coherence, 792
Heart disease, 84, 361, 700–702, 926–27
  body fat and, 877
  exercise and, 701
  homocysteine levels, folic acid, and,
    900
  hormone therapy and, 666, 701–2
  hysterectomy and, 231
  increased risk of, 256, 650
  inflammation and, 105
  magnesium and, 907, 910
  nutrition and, 700–702, 836, 839, 846
  resentment and, 784
  reversal of, 784
  soy protein and, 890
HeartMath, 655, 702
Heart palpitations, arrhythmias, 72, 95,
  120, 163, 439, 554, 702, 726, 907,
  910, 941
Heed, Ellen, 292
Heller, Rachel S. F., 90
Hemp seed and oil, 701
Hendricks, Gay, 4, 110, 735, 738, 845
  Ultimate Success Mantra, 792
Hendricksen, Danielle, 5
Henes, Donna, 643
Hepatitis B vaccination, 600, 609
Hepatitis C, 797
Her Blood Is Gold (Owen), 142
Herbs (botanicals)
  for adrenal/thyroid/sex steroid
    restoration program, 659
  for bone health, 685
  for breast cancer, 700
  for fertility, 517
  for gynecological problems, 149–50
  for hair, thinning, 696
  for herpes, 345
  for menopausal symptoms, 679, 681,
    697, 701
  post surgery, 829

during pregnancy, what to avoid, 548
for UTIs, 380
vaginal thinning and, 681, 682
Heredity
breast cysts/cancer, 261, 263, 443–47
diseases that "run in the family," 719
endometriosis and, 204
environmental influence on, 719, 956
fibroid tumors and, 219–20
"genetic determinism," 719
ovarian cancer and, 257, 261, 263
stress urinary incontinence and, 384
transgenerational beliefs, DNA, and,
43, 465, 719, 961
Herpes, 18, 20, 49, 318, 322, 340–47
common concerns, 14, 342–44
danger to newborns, 343–44
diagnosis, 342
immune system and, 341
symptoms, 341
treatment, 344–47
woman's story, 346–47
Herrera, Isa, 277, 284, 374
HGSIL (high-grade squamous
intraepithelial lesion), 352
Hicks, Esther and Jerry, 85–86, 655,
742, 796
Hidden Messages of Water, The (Emoto),
31, 927
Highwater, Jamake, 4
Hikel, Katharine, 337
Hilakivi-Clarke, Leena, 432
Hill, Napoleon, 737
Hillman, James, 56
History
collective, 954–61
family legacy, 718–21
reclaiming, 961–64
See also Heredity
HIV/AIDS, 7, 8, 293, 315, 350, 368,
369–70, 548–49
Holick, Michael, 660, 688
Holistic Movement Program for Healthy
Pelvis and Pelvic Floor, 278–84,
279–83
Holland, Mary, 337
Holy Hunger (Bullitt-Jonas), 882
Homeopathy, 154
cream (Emuaid), 374–75
fibroid tumor treatment, 223

gynecological problems, 154
lichen sclerosus treatment, 374–75
menopause and, 648, 694
post surgery remedy, 829
Hormones
for adrenal/thyroid/sex steroid
restoration program, 659
breast cancer link, 425
breast-feeding and, 621
emotions and, 34, 42, 135, 136–40,
626
endometriosis treatment, 207–9
fibroid tumors, and, 224
menopause and, 649, 650, 663–64,
673–77
menstrual cramps and PGF2, 140
miscarriage and, 521
ovarian production of, 241–42,
257
primer, 673–77
production sites, 648–50, 649
program for hormonal balance,
143–61
stress hormones, 42, 317
testing levels, 670
UTIs and, 381
See also Estrogen; Progesterone;
Testosterone
Hormone therapies, 665–72, 812
alcohol and, 700
Alzheimer's and, 703–4
anti-aging and, 672
bioidentical, 667–72, 702
breast pain and, 440
cancer risk, 480, 700
for depression, 697–98
ELITE study, 671
for endometriosis, 207–9
evaluation of, 665–67
getting off, or changing from,
707
history of, 665–67
hysterectomy and, 230
individualized, 668–72
KEEPS study, 671
for loss of sexual desire, 230
menopause and, 649, 650, 659, 663,
665–72, 674–76, 699–700, 701–2,
707
for PCOS, 249

Hormone therapies (*cont'd*):
  Premarin, 385, 665–67, 668, 671, 700,
    703–4, 707, 780
  Prempro, 666, 702, 706, 780
  primer, 673–77
  progestin, 155, 174–75, 176, 180, 182,
    207, 482–83, 503, 666, 667
  See also specific hormones
Hot flashes, 24, 231, 650, 677–81
Houston, Jean, 38–39
Howes, Lewis, 75
*How to Live Happily Ever After "Down
  Under"* (Quick), 375
How to Prevent Heart Attacks (Sandler),
  846
HPV Vaccine on Trial, The (Holland,
  Rosenberg, Iorio), 337
Hsi Lai, 242, 268, 735
Hubbard, Barbara Marx, 957
Huddleston, Peggy, 822–23, 830
Human by Design (Braden), 956
Human papilloma virus (HPV), 325–40,
  373
  common concerns, 327–28
  diagnosis, 326–27
  Pap test and, 322, 350
  prevention, 339–40
  symptoms, 326
  treatment, 328–31
  vaccines, 331–39
Hurley, Janette, 461
Hutchins, Claire, 300–301
Hwang, Shelley, 423–24
Hydration Foundation, 716
Hyman, Mark, 810, 839, 840, 858
Hyperestrogenism, 400
Hyperprolactemia, 175
Hypertension, 84, 552–54, 781, 836,
  877, 880, 910
Hyperthyroidism, 681
Hypnobabies, 546
Hypnotherapy (hypnosis), 461–63, 546,
  614, 821, 925
Hypoglycemia (low blood sugar), 171
Hypothyroid disease, 110, 660–62
Hysterectomy, 193–94
  alternatives, fibroid tumors, 223
  artificial menopause and, 664–65
  chronic pelvic pain and, 199–200
  deciding on treatment, 199

for endometrial hyperplasia, 175
  endometriosis treatment, 209–10
  energy anatomy, second chakra issues,
    and, 194–96
  fibroid tumors treatment, 228–31
  for heavy periods, 182
  loss, grief and, 833–35
  oophorectomy during, 263
  ovarian cancer risk reduced by, 261
  sexual response after, 229–31
  surgery, 193–94, 833–35
Hysteroscopy, 225

Ibuprofen (Motrin, Advil), 547
Ilibagiza, Immaculée, 976–77
Illness
  abuse and, 7, 20, 24–25, 104, 105
  common symptoms associated with
    emotions, 72
  as cry for help, 554
  emotions as factor, xxiii, 20, 22,
    24–28, 35–37, 41–43, 72, 109,
    199–200, 249–50, 257–58, 316–21,
    355–56, 389–90, 403–4
  as energy leak, 78
  first-chakra issues and, 98–99
  health-damaging statements, 91
  inflammation and, 847–65, 892, 897
  messages from, 731
  mind/body connection, 40–45, 49–52
  purpose of, xxiii, 730–31
  response to, 52–55, 731
  as wisdom of the body, 27, 51, 71–76
I Love You Project, 393–94
Immune system, 207, 790
  archetypal forms of wounding and,
    38
  autoimmune disease and, 41
  cells, 35, 317
  drugs which suppress, 325
  emotions, stress, and suppression of,
    35, 36, 41, 42–43, 81, 325, 365–66
  endometriosis and, 206–7
  herpes and, 341
  HIV/AIDS and, 370
  HPV and, 325, 327, 328, 332
  infertility and, 505
  mucosal openings and, 315, 317, 361,
    369
  music and, 828

newborns, 627–33
nutritional support, 180, 352, 460, 632
relaxation and, 823–24
righteous indignation and, 84
social support and, 37
STDs and, 368
supplements for, 207, 369, 460
Immunizations, 14, 16, 627–33
Gardasil and Gardasil 9, 331–39
"well baby" checks and, 16
Improving Birth Coalition, 565
Ina May's Guide to Childbirth (Gaskin), 559, 598
Inconceivable (Indichova), 509
Indichova, Julia, 509
Infante-Rivard, Claire, 521
Infertility, 42, 63, 292, 504–21, *505*
adhesions and, *158*, 519–20
age and, *505*, 506, 512
ambivalence about, naming, 514
ART, *506*, 603
deep tissue massage, 519
ephistogram and, 513
factors, 504–5, *505*
fibroids and, 220–21
freezing or donating eggs, 510–11
healing oneself and, 508–9
integrative program to enhance, 511–14
male factor (sperm count), 504, 515
new modalities for, 518–20
psychological factors, 506–10
second-chakra energy and, 506
stress and, 92, 507, 514–15
TCM for, 518–19
technology and, 506
tubal problems, 518
women's stories, 520–21
Infertility Cure, The (Lewis), 518
Inflammation, 428, 847–65, 892, 897, 908
catecholamine levels and, 540
cytokines and, 777
estrogen and, 205
interleukin 6, emotional wounds, and, 37–38, 105
as root of autoimmune conditions, 41
See also Thermography
Inner Child Rescue exercise, 78, 81–82

Inner guidance, xxii–xxiii, 9, 10, 14, 17, 18, 19, 21, 25, 26, 27, 36, 40, 44, 51, 56–76, 452–53, 976
birth control pill and, 135, 136–40
body's message and, 748–51
Divine Love and, 757–61
dreams as, 64–65, 452–53, 733, 920
emotional cleansing and, 62–63
enteric nervous system, the gut, and, 58–59
God box and, 756
healing and medical decisions, 811, 812
how it works, 67–76
intuitive guidance, 66–67, 124, 699
listening to the body and its needs, xxiii, 58–61, 135, 136, 202, 243–44, 259, 748–51, 972–73
lunar information and, 124, 756
on mammography, 410
medical care, choosing, 804
negative information overload and impediment to, 793
personal needs vs. others, 739
sources of, 57–58
spiritual messages, 753–61
for your heart's desire, 715
Institute for Functional Medicine, 339, 445
Institute of HeartMath, 655, 792
Insulin, 141, 144, 165, 248, 427–28, 429, 653, 696, 701, 860–61, 882, 883, 894, 895, 901, 907, 909, 910, 926, 930, 931–32, 935
androgen increase and, 261
blood sugar and, 926
body fat and, 851
DUB and, 175
intermittent fasting and, 861
sensitivity, increasing, 144, 930, 931–32
Insulin resistance (Syndrome X or metabolic syndrome), 427, 695, 701, 702, 851–64, 894, 930, 931–32
Integrins, 30
Intention Experiment, The (McTaggart), 955
Interferon, 373
Interleukin 6 (IL-6), 37–38, 105
International Childbirth Education Association (ICEA), 572

Interstitial cystitis, 318, 371, 374, 377–79, 479

Intestinal dysbiosis, 363, 917

Intuition, 66–67, 88, 699
exercise and, 932–33
menstrual cycle and, 124, 135–40

Iodine, 149
for adrenal/thyroid/sex steroid restoration program, 658
benefits, 400, 428, 437–39, 543, 658, 696, 901
supplements recommended, 438, 901
tests for, 438–39

Iodine (Brownstein), 437

Iorio, Eileen, 337

Iron, 181, 542, 901, 915

Irritable bowel syndrome (IBS), 102, 105, 361, 916–17

Isoflavones, 430–32

I Support the Girls, 129

It Didn't Start with You (Wolynn), 43, 465, 719

It's My Pleasure (Rodale and Rodale), 304

It's Not Your Money (Silver), 736

James, William, 37

Jessel, David, 39

Jesus, 753, 954

Jetha, Cacilda, 289

Ji, Sayer, 837

Johnson, C. J., 513

Johnson, Dana, 69–70

Johnson, Emma, 477

Johnson, Jack, 744

Johnson, Karen, 836

Johnson, Kimberly, 292

Johnson, Magic, 292

Johnson, Sonia, xxii, 450, 967

Johnson, Trudy, 466, 468, 469

Johnston, Jack, 301–2

Jolie, Angelina, 263, 423

Journal-keeping, 71, 150–51, 154, 357, 761
appreciation, 791
dream diary, 442
moon journal (menstrual cycle), 190

Jung, Carl, 100, 296, 766, 955

Kabat-Zinn, Myla and Jon, 605

Karp, Harvey, 617

Karras, Nick, 376

Kassai, Kathryn, 383

KEEPS (Kronos Early Estrogen Prevention Study), 671

Kegel exercises, 213, 277, 278, 384

Keller, George, 40

Keller, Leah, 619

Keltner, Dacher, 956

Kennell, John, 12, 580, 607–8

Kent, Tami Lynn, 196, 197, 592, 593, 729–30, 779

Ketogenic diet, 144

Keys, Ancel, 860

Kickass Single Mom, The (Johnson), 477

Kidney stones, 689, 905, 908

Kinesiology, 918

King, Richard, 520

Kirshenbaum, Mira, 78

Kiyosaki, Robert, 737

Klaus, Marshall, 12, 580, 607–8

Klein, Luella, 464

Koch, Liz, 765

Komisaruk, Barry, 559

Kramer, Barnett S., 405

Kristof, Nicholas D., 9, 954, 974–75

Kübler-Ross, Elisabeth, 55, 526, 744

!Kung women, 677, 847

Kushi, Michio, 85, 838–39

Kussman, Leslie, 730

Labiaplasty, 375–76

Labor and birth, 565–604
accessing birth energy, 592–95
age and, 557
biofeedback and, 573
bonding with newborn, 576, 579, 605–11
Bradley Method, 584
breech presentation, 554–55, 556
Calm Birth Methods, 545, 584
cervix is a sphincter, 569
childbirth choices, 565
clamping the cord, 609–10
cultural inheritance, 562, 565–66, 567
ecstasy and, 269, 598
embracing the process, 584
epidurals, 578–79, 584
forceps delivery, 571, 573, 577, 579

Friedman curves, 583
home birth, 561–62, 597–99
hospital interventions/birth
    technologies, 13, 564, 566, 568–69,
    572–85
husbands, partners and, 568, 570–71,
    606
imprinting of, on baby, 561
induction, 550, 555, 573, 587
infant mortality, 566
labor experience and mother's life,
    connection between, 566–69
labor support, 12, 566, 580–81
magic of, 558–65
maternal death, 8, 563–65
midwife support, 590–92
mothering the mother, 566, 580–81
movement during, 932'
natural, safety of, 534, 561–62
newborn medical treatment and
    vaccines, 599–603, 609–10, 627–33
pain, working with, 589–99
preparing for, 545–47, 584
reclaiming birth power, 604
"rescue" from, 571
risk factors, 569–70
Safe Motherhood Quilt Project,
    563–65
sexuality and, 559–61, 596, 598
shaking and, 61
as spiritually transforming, 558–65,
    604, 617
stress urinary incontinence and, 383
supine position, 579–80
women's stories, 585–92, 595–99
See also Cesarean sections; Doulas;
    Episiotomies
Lakota Native Americans, 85
Lamott, Anne, 763
Lampe, Astrid, 100
Landers, Ann, 294
Lane, Nancy, 949
Langer, Ellen, 46, 647, 936
Langevin, Helene, 30, 942
Lanou, Ann, 686
LaPorte, Danielle, 69
Laser treatment, 329
Latthe, Pallavi, 100
Lauer, Matt, 5
Laurel's Kitchen (Laurel), 633

Law of attraction, 30–31, 74, 112, 223,
    397, 742–43, 791, 806–7
Layden, Mary Anne, 303
Lazare, Jane, 633
LCIS (lobular carcinoma in situ), 422
Lee, Sin Hang, 336–37
LEEP (loop electrode excision
    procedure), 330, 347, 350, 352, 353
Left to Tell (Ilibagiza), 976
Le Guin, Ursula, 778
Lemon, Henry, 674
Let's Eat Right to Keep Fit (Davis), 838
Levine, Amir, 90
Levine, Barbara, 750
Levine, Stephen, 63, 788, 961
    meditation on forgiveness, 788–90
Levitt, Steven, 467
Levonorgestrel, 476
Levy, Becca, 47
Lewis, Randine, 518–19
LGSIL (low-grade squamous
    intraepithelial lesion), 352
LH (luteinizing hormone), 122, 126, 138,
    434, 643, 645, 663–64
Lichen sclerosus, 374–75
Licorice root, 548, 659
Life-Changing Foods (William), 837
Life Magic (Bushnell), 297, 751–52
Life purpose
    chakras and, 111–12
    following, 735–40
    lifetime goals, 794–95
LifeSpa website, 438
Life Touches Life (Ash), 528
Light
    adrenal function and, 652
    for adrenal/thyroid/sex steroid
        restoration program, 660
    blue, from electronic screens, 151
    carbohydrate cravings and, 882
    "electronic sundown," 151
    elimination of, from bedroom, 151
    f.lux (app) for screens, 151
    full-spectrum lightbulbs, 152
    infertility and, 516
    natural, outdoor, 151, 152
    PMS and, 164
    for pregnancy, 546
    therapy for gynecological problems,
        152

Lignans, 430, 460
Lindsey, Timmie Jean, 454
Linton, David, 135
Lipton, Bruce, 17, 29, 719, 779, 781, 956
Liver, 102, 480, 652, 900, 916
LLETZ (large loop excision of transformation zone), 330
Longevity, 47, 931
Lorde, Audre, 268, 968
Louis C.K., 5
Love
    accepting nurturing and affection, 656–57
    addiction, 367
    Divine, 757–61, 813, 830, 927
    romantic love and the brain, 767–68
    for self, 359, 513, 954–61, 973–74
    wanted child and, 466
Love, Medicine, & Miracles (Siegel), 12
Love Happens (film), 390
Love Without End (Green), 731
Low GI Diet Cookbook, The (Brand-Miller), 853
Loye, David, 9
Ludwig, David, 247, 839, 840, 857
Lupron, 207
Lupus erythematosus, 41, 42, 479
Luskin, Fred, 784
Lustig, Robert H., 302, 848, 875
Lymphedema, 448

Maca, 230, 675, 680
Macadamia nuts/oil, 149, 433, 544, 701, 892
Macones, George, 573
Magnesium, 900–901, 906–12
    for adrenal function, 657–68
    for bone health, 689, 900–901
    for breast health, 428
    calcium and, 908
    for cardiac arrhythmias, 936
    chocolate cravings and deficiency, 165
    deficiency, effects of, 909–10
    deficiency, rise in, 908–9
    Epsom salts and, 658, 911
    food sources, 909
    for Gardasil side effects, 338
    for gynecological problems, 148–49, 165, 178

    for heart disease, 907
    Meyer's formula, 907
    need for, 907–8
    for pregnancy, 542
    recommended dose, 915
    ReMag and ReMyte supplement supplements, 338–39, 658–59, 910–11
    for surgical healing, 829
Magnesium Miracle, The (Dean), 657, 907, 909, 911
Maharishi Mahesh Yogi, 954
Maines, Rachel, 304
Male Biological Clock (Fisch), 515
Mama Gena's School of Womanly Arts, 296, 306, 765, 766
Mammography, 405–10, 416–18, 424, 444, 456–57, 667
    three-dimensional (DBT), 406
Mandrola, John, 801
Manganese, 542, 658, 689, 900, 901, 915
Mann, Samuel J., 553
Margulis, Jennifer, 632
Marijuana, 541, 621–22
Martial arts, 946–47
Martin, Doreen, 834
Martinez, Mario, 37, 84, 646–47, 705, 727, 783
Mask of Masculinity, The (Howes), 75
Massage, 12, 777–78, 942
    for adrenal/thyroid/sex steroid restoration program, 656–57
    for cramps/gynecological problems, 157–58
    hair restoration and, 696
    Maya traditional, 158, 520, 524
    monthly self-care breast ritual, 399
    during pregnancy, 546
    for tubal problems, infertility, 518, 519
    Wurn, 157, 200, 230, 518–19, 524
Master Program for Optimal Hormonal Balance and Pelvic health, 143–61
    affirmations, 154
    castor oil packs, 154–55
    detoxification, 159, 161
    diet, 144–48
    energy medicine, 152–53
    homeopathy, 154

manual therapies, 157–59
nutritional, herbal supplements,
    148–50
progesterone, natural, 155–57
reestablish cyclic emotional flow,
    150–51
reestablish cyclic ovulatory flow,
    151–52
stress reduction, 153–54
Maté, Gabor, 743
Mather, Kelly, 822
Mattes, Jane, 477
Matthews, Hope, 212, 941, 944
Mawson, Anthony, 629–30
McAll, Kenneth, 783
McCain, Marian Van Eyk, 698
McClellan, Myron, 744
McClelland, Sara, 294
McDonald, Evy, 731
McGarey, Gladys, 155, 472, 706
McGraw, Phil, 51
McKeown, Patrick, 941
McKinlay, Sonja, 696
McTaggart, Lynne, 955, 957
Mead, Margaret, 606
Mead, Michael, 39
Meade, Michael, 713
Meaning and Medicine (Dossey), 235
Medical care, xxii, 9, 15, 27–28,
    796–835
  becoming an adult, 805
  choosing provider, 798–808
  choosing treatment, 809–14
  complementary, integrative, 799,
    810–11
  conflicts of interest in, 15
  conventional, 13–15, 37, 809–10
  financial interests influencing, 37,
    780–82, 796–97
  functional medicine, 210, 445, 799,
    800, 810, 858, 900
  "healer quotient," 801–4
  health insurance, 798, 807
  holistic dentistry, 815–17
  hospitals, new generation of, 822
  iatrogenic illness, adverse drug
    reactions, and unnecessary surgeries,
    797–98
  inner guidance and, 811
  mainstream, xxii

medical records and, 734, 808
"the myth of diagnosis," 810
overdiagnosis, 14, 78
overprescribing meds for women, 811
placebo, power of, 802–3
power to choose and, 807–8
responsibility for, 796–98, 804–6
second opinions, 817–18
for sleep apnea, 813–14
surgery, 817–35
unnecessary CT and MRI scans, 14, 78
"well baby" checks, 16
women doctors, percentage of, 17
Medication Madness (Breggin), 782
Medicine Cards (Sams and Carson), 764
Meditation, 25, 266, 699, 761, 882, 920,
    954
  attuning your pelvic bowl, 198–99
  for breast cancer, 429
  breathing and, 940
  Calm Birth, 545, 584
  deciding to get pregnant and, 477
  Divine Love, 221
  for fibroids, 221
  on forgiveness, 788–90
  guided imagery for, 545–46
  for gynecological problems, 153, 232
  healing the world and, 954
  for IBS, 917
  illness as, 730
  for menopausal symptoms, 681
  for pregnancy, labor, and birth,
    545–46
  TM, 954
*Meditation to Promote Successful
    Surgery, A* (Naparstek), 823–24
Mehl-Medrona, Lewis, 550–52, 555, 569
Melanin, 865
Melatonin, 441
Melissa extract, 345
Memorial Sloan Kettering Cancer Center,
    nomograms and, 448–49
Menarche, 22
  celebrating, "period party," 187–88
  rituals for, 129–30, 133
Menastil, 150
Menofem, 679
Menopause, 16, 637–709
  adrenal glands function, 650–60
  Alzheimer's disease and, 702–4

Menopause (*cont'd*):
  artificial (surgical), 664–65, *745*
  breast cysts after, 401
  climacteric and, 637, 662
  creating health during, 648, 650
  as a crossroads for change, 638–43
  cultural inheritance, 644–47, 728
  as "deficiency disease," 242
  encoded wisdom in, 118
  fibroid tumors after, 231
  fuzzy thinking and, 663, 698–99
  GnRH agonists and, 224
  health concerns, long-term, 699–706
  hormone level testing, 670
  hormone primer, 673–77
  hormone replacement, 707
  hormones and, *649, 650*
  hot flashes, 650, 677–81
  hypothyroid disease, 660–62
  hysterectomy and, 231
  loss of sex drive, treatment, 680,
    692–95
  mood swings and depression, 696–97
  natural and perimenopause, 662–64
  as new beginning, 708–9
  osteoporosis and, 683–91
  ovaries and, 241
  premature, 42, 664
  products, environmentally friendly, 129
  progesterone for, *649, 650, 659,* 663,
    674–76, 699
  self-care during, 655–60, 708
  sexuality and, 691–93, 708
  symptoms, *650,* 663, 676–706
  treatment, deciding on, 707
  vaginal changes, 677, 678, 681–82
  wisdom of, 120, 640, 643, *645*
Menopret (Klimadynon), 679
Menorrhagia. *See* Menstruation
Menstrual cramps, xxiii, 140–61
  acupressure for, 159, *160*
  birth control pills for, 141
  diet and, 141, 144–48, 902
  energy medicine, 152–53
  herbs, 149–50
  Maya traditional massage, 158
  medication, 141
  nutritional treatment, 144–48
  program for treating, 143–61
  Pueraria mirifica for, 141, 149

  TENS for, 150
  women's stories, 141–43
Menstruation, xxiv, 22, 117–90, *123,*
  126
  cold, aversion to and, 131–32, 153
  cramps (dysmenorrhea), 140–61
  cultural inheritance of, 129–35, 728
  cyclical nature of, 121–28
  deodorized pads, tampons, 316, 362,
    363
  emotions and hormones, 125–26
  follicular, luteal phases, 122–27
  healing through, 127–28
  heavy periods (menorrhagia), 143–61,
    181–82, 217–18
  honoring, 132–33
  irregular periods, 121, 172–73, 178
  Lakota Native American women and,
    85
  light exposure and, 121
  lunar cycle and, 118, 121, *123,* 124,
    126, 129–30, 150–51
  menstrual cups, 129
  mind/body/soul connection, 172–73
  molimina, 173
  "ovarian sisters," 140
  "period poverty," 128–29
  premenstrual syndrome (PMS), 161–72
  preparing our daughters, 183–90
  program for menstrual health, 143–61
  regular periods, 173
  seed rotation for, 150
  spotting and breakthrough bleeding, 36
  taboos and, 130
  TCM and, 131–32, 152–53
  Victorian beliefs, 130, 132
  wisdom of, 118, 170, 172, 179
  women's stories, 177–80
Menstrupedia Comic, 188
Mentharil, 917
Mercier, Hugo, 783
Merck Pharmaceuticals, 331–39
Mercola, Joseph, 631
Messina, Mark, 431
Metabolism
  dieting and, 845, 849–50
  exercise and, 877–78
  factors influencing, 837
  fat vs. muscle and, 935
  insulin resistance, 851–64

intermittent fasting and, 861
rehabilitating, 877–96
reset program, 856–57
stress hormones and, 842
Metcalf, Linda Trichter, 38, 761, 762
#MeToo movement, 6, 109, 110, 288, 958
Microbiome
  foods recommended for, 346
  genital area, 318, 327, 342, 345–46
  gut, 248, 917
  vaginal seeding and, 585
  whole, natural foods and, 837
Microcosmic orbit, 285, 286
Mifepristone (RU486), 469–70
Migraine headaches, 59–60, 61, 155,
    163, 663, 771, 824, 858, 878, 900,
    908, 910, 916, 919, 969
Miklos & Moore Urogynecology, 214
Miller, Alice, 785
Miller, Edgar, III, 898–99
Mills, Dian Shepperson, 148
Mills, Dixie, 388
MindBody Code, The (Martinez), 37,
    646
MindBody Self, The (Martinez), 646
Mind/body/soul connection, 29, 30–37,
    56, 88, 730–31
  ALS and, 69–70
  amenorrhea and, 248–49
  books about, 779
  brain/pelvis interactions, 138
  breast health and, 389–94
  breast size and, 461–63
  cancer and, 390
  cellular level, 35, 831
  coauthoring each other's biology,
    37–38
  consciousness and (see Consciousness)
  curing vs. healing and, 48–52, 266
  emotions (see Emotions)
  endometriosis and, 206–7
  energy and, 31
  female body and mind, 734–35
  feminine intelligence and healing, 29–55
  fertility and, 504, 506–14
  fibroids and, 232, 234–35
  healing emotional pain and, 25–28
  hormones and, 34
  illness and, 40–45, 49–52, 730–31
  information about, 778–83

labor and birth preparation, 545–47
  menstruation and, 127, 172–73
  pelvic bowl and, 197
  PMS and, 164
  PNI and, 34
  pregnancy and, 550
  sexuality and, 693–94
  vaginitis, UTIs, and, 18, 105, 293,
    317, 365–68, 381–82
  vulvodynia and, 372, 373–74
Mind-body therapies
  for breast cancer, 429
  for childbirth, 545
  for fertility, 511–14
  for interstitial cystitis, 378
  for lichen sclerosus, 375
  for surgery, healing from, 822–25
  for vulvodynia, 371, 373–74
Mind-Body Unity (Dreher), 105
Mind of Your Own, A (Brogan), 614,
    697, 768, 811
Mind Over Back Pain (Sarno), 750
Minerals, 542–43, 900–901, 914, 915
Minger, Denise, 839
Miracle Moms, Better Sex, Less Pain
    (Wurn and Wurn), 157
Miracle Moms, Better Sex, Less Pain
    (Wurn, Wurn, and King), 520
Mirena IUD, 135
Miroestrol, 149
Mirren, Helen, 647
Miscarriage, 119, 172, 206, 210, 220,
    225, 494, 496, 513, 517, 521–23,
    532, 538, 556, 575, 724, 923
Misoprostol, 469
Mists of Avalon, The (Zimmer Bradley),
    300
Mittelschmerz, 246, 484
Moir, Anne, 39
Molecules of Emotion (Pert), 956
Molybdenum, 542, 658, 915
MonaLisa Touch laser, 215, 377
Money, A Love Story (K. Northrup), 736
Monolaurin, 345
Montagu, Ashley, 76, 623
Mood, 696–97, 881, 882
Moon
  inner guidance and, 124, 756
  menstruation and, 117, 121, 123, 124,
    126, 129–30

Moon (cont'd):
  "moon journal," 190
  ovulation, conception and, 121
  phases, tracking emotional flow,
    150–51
  planning work, rest time and, 118, 122
Moon Dance (Rose), 117
Moore, Jimmy, 861
Morais, Joan, 483
Moran, Marilyn, 611–12
Morris, Donette, 615–17
Morse, Melvin, 927
Moseley, Bruce, 802
Moss, Carrie-Anne, 640–62
Mother-Daughter Wisdom (Northrup),
    612, 627, 635
Motherhood, 605–36
  bonding with baby, 579, 605–11
  breast-feeding vs. formula, 619–27
  child's natural calming reflex and, 617
  dominator society and, 633–36
  early touching, 606–10
  postpartum period, 611–17
Mothering from Your Center (Kent),
    592
Mothering the Mother, 581
Mothers Naturally, 565
MRgFUS (MR-Guided Focused
    Ultrasound), 226–27
MRI (magnetic resonance imaging),
    411–12
Muir, Caroline and Charles, 273
Multiorgasmic Couple, The (Chia and
    Abrams), 307
Multiorgasmic Man, The (Chia and
    Abrams), 307
Multiple sclerosis, 41, 112, 332, 730,
    785, 893–94
Multivitamin-mineral supplements, 148
  for adrenal function, 657
  for birth control pill use, 517
  for cervical dysplasia, 354
  for gynecological health, 148
  for immune function, 369, 460
  postpartum, 614
  for UTIs, 382
  for vulvodynia, 372
Music, 793
  for surgery, 828
Myofasical release, 778

Myomectomy, 227–28
Myss, Caroline, 88, 96, 104, 109, 140,
    172, 216, 252, 254, 317, 318, 389,
    450, 473, 493, 494, 506, 540, 647,
    754, 776, 831, 969

Nabothian cysts, 322
Nadeau, Joe, 240
NAET (Nambudripad Allergy
    Elimination Therapy), 373, 378,
    521, 918
Nambudripad, Devi, 918
Nanette (Netflix special), 958
Naparstek, Belleruth, 515, 545, 823–24
  website, 546
"Narcissistic supply," 108
Nascent Iodine, 438
National Association for Continence,
    214
National Association for Incontinence,
    386
National Cancer Institute's Breast Cancer
    Risk Assessment Tool, 407
Natural Healing for Women, 426
Navajo people, 85, 130, 677
Nelson, Miriam, 687, 878, 935
Neural therapy, 831
Neuro-linguistic programming (NLP), 814
Neuropeptides, 35
#NeverAgain movement, 6
New Feminine Brain (Schulz), 698
New Glucose Revolution, The (Brand-
    Miller), 853
New Thought movement, 956
Ng, Stephanie V., 184
Nicholson, Barbara, 609
Nitric oxide, 30, 35, 269, 302, 305, 693
Noble, Vicki, 598
Nolan, Thomas, 335
Nonviolent Communication (Rosenberg),
    60
Norman Parathyroid Center, 684
Northrup, Kate, 736
NovaSure, 182
NSAIDs, 141, 163, 182, 706, 916
Nutrafem, 679
Nutrition, 836–927
  addictive eating, 848, 856, 866, 867,
    881–83
  adrenal restoration, 657–58

Alzheimer's and, 704
anti-inflammatory diet, 207, 372, 403, 517, 885
artificial sweeteners, 919–20
blood sugar/inflammation connection, 141, 847–65, 892
bone density and, 685–87
brain-boosting smoothie, 152
breakfast, lunch, and dinner, 862–63
breast cancer link, 427–28
for breast health, 428, 429–43
for cervical dysplasia, 354
chronic vulvar pain, 371–72
contradictory claims about, 839–40
cultural programming and, 870–72
dairy foods (see Dairy foods)
dieting, dieting mentality, 843–47, 850
"Diet Mentality" self-quiz, 844
endometriosis and, 204
exosomes and, 837
expectations, food preparation, 870–72
food/emotion connection, 865–69
"food fundamentalism," 837
food manufacturers and food supply, 204
food preparation, cultural roles, 870–72
gluten and, 704, 857–59
glycemic stress and insulin resistance, 851–64
for healthy teeth, 816
heart health and, 701
for herpes, 345
high-and low-glycemic foods, 850–53
history of human diet, 847–48
hormonal balance, pelvic health, 144–48
for hot flashes, 678
hydration, 878–81
infertility and, 516–17
intermittent fasting and, 860–62
for interstitial cystitis, 378
light energy from leafy greens, 864–65
low-acid diet for osteoporosis, 685–87
macrobiotic diet, 154, 168, 233, 745, 786, 838–39, 843, 854
Maine blueberries, 837
male sperm and, 516, 517

mealtimes, body's natural rhythms, 152
menopause and, 650
menstrual cramps and, 141, 144
metabolism and, 837, 877–96
Metabolism Reset program, 856–57
organic foods, 145, 380, 838, 884, 896, 902, 903, 906, 909, 927
ovarian cancer and, 259–60
Paleolithic diet, 847
PCOS and, 177, 247
phytoestrogens, 430–32
PMS and, 165
postpartum, 613–14
potatoes, 837
for pregnancy, 540–44
processed foods, glutamates, 848, 867–68
seed rotation program for menstrual regulation, 150
soy foods, 144, 430–31, 678–79, 885, 886–91
for stable blood sugar, 849, 962–63
for stress urinary incontinence, 384–85
thinning hair and, 696
trigger goods, 867
USDA dietary guidelines, 899
for UTIs, 380–81
vaginitis and, 363, 365
water-rich foods, 878–80
what and when to eat, 856, 862–63
whole, natural food as basic, 837
See also Carbohydrates; Fats, dietary; Protein; Sugar
Nutritional Magnesium Association, 912
Nutrition and Physical Degeneration (Price), 836
Nutritious Movement for a Healthy Pelvis (Bowman), 283–84

Obama, Barack, 9
Obesity, 33, 165, 177, 204, 384, 866, 868, 895
Obesity Code, The (Fung), 861–62
Obstetrics, 534
O'Connell, Helen, 269, 270
Ogden, Gina, 269, 287, 692
O'Hara, Kristen, 310–13
O'Keefe-Kanavos, Kathleen, 66, 442, 765

Oliver, Eloise, 834
Olsen, Ole, 405
O'Mara, Peggy, 624–25
On Death and Dying (Kübler-Ross), 526
One More Girl (film), 334
On Our Moon, 290
OPC (pycnogenol), 898
Opioids, 825–27
Oral sex, 293–94, 317, 341, 365
Orenstein, Peggy, 294
Orgasm. *See* Sexual response
Orgasmic Birth website, 561
Origin Collective, 118, 122
Orlando, Gina, 494
Orman, Suze, 737–38
Ornish, Dean, 839
Ortelee, Anne, 713
Ortner, Nick, 772
Osbourne, Sharon, 423
Oski, Frank, 902
Osteoporosis, 123, 231, 646, 653,
    683–91, 708, 720, 858
  calcium and dairy, 147, 685, 686,
      903–4
  depression and, 41, 906
  early, 948–49
  Fosamax, Actonel, Boniva warning,
      690–91
  fractures and, 650, 683, 688, 690,
      890, 905, 935, 947
  GnRH agonists and risk for, 224
  hormones and, 242, 673
  low-acid diet for prevention, 685–87
  magnesium deficiency and, 908, 910
  NTx test and Pyrilinks test, 684
  oophorectomy and, 257
  phosphate, soft drinks and, 688, 906
  Premarin and, 666
  program for bone health, 684–89, 804
  Pueraria mirifica to prevent, 680
  risk factors, 123, 212, 231, 257, 650,
      653, 673, 683, 684, 688, 883, 897,
      906, 920, 923
  soy for, 890
  testing, 683–84
  treatment, 242, 684–89, 947
  vitamin D for, 685, 688, 804, 904
Othering, 170–72
Otosclerosis, 674
Our Bodies, Ourselves, 779

Outrageous Openness (Silver), 717
Outwitting Multiple Sclerosis (Worth),
    785
Ovarian cancer, 105, 243–44, 256–66
  breast-feeding and reduced risk, 620
  dairy food link, 145, 259–60
  diagnosis, 261–63
  emotional trauma or loss and, 243
  familial, 219–20, 263
  golden handcuff syndrome, 259
  possible contributors to, 259–61
  prophylactic ovary removal, 263,
      264–65
  rapidity of growth, 259
  second chakra problems and, 243,
      257
  treatment, conventional, 265–66
  women's stories, 266
Ovarian cysts, 24, 49, 239, 245–47
  benign neoplastic, 246–47
  "chocolate," 202, 206
  egg production, new research, 239
  emotional influence on, 251–54,
      740
  follicular, 245–46
  luteal, 246
  solid, other, 247, 251–52
  stress and, 244
  wisdom of, 254, 740
Ovaries, 237–67
  anatomy, 239–44
  benign growths in, 243, 255–56
  caring for, things to do, 266–67
  creativity and, 237–39, 266, 740
  energy of, 239, 692
  heart disease risk and removal of, 231
  hormone production, 241–42, 257
  inner stroma, 241
  oophorectomy, 231, 256–57, 263
  PCOS, 177, 247–48
  prophylactic removal of, 263, 264–65
  recovering fertility, egg growth,
      239–40
  relationships and health of, 239
  risks of removal, 263
  second chakra and, 100
  sexual desire and, 231
  sexual energy and chi of, 242
  theca regression, 241
  tumors of, 255–56

uterine problems, relationship with, 239

wisdom of, 118, 242, 254, 256, 259, 481

Overeaters Anonymous, 774, 867

Ovulation, 121–24, 240–41
Daysy and app, 485
emotions and, 125–26, 172–73
fertility awareness, 483–90, *488, 489,* 496
freezing or donating eggs, 510–11
indicators, 484, 487
lunar phase and, 121–22
Natural Cycles app, 485
online community, 485
OvaGraph app, 485
Ovulation Method, 484–86
OvuSense app, 485
reestablishing cyclic flow, 151–52
salivary ovulation testing, 484

Owen, Amanda, 740

Owen, Lara, 142

Oxytocin (Pitocin), 308–9, 550, 555, 573, 587, 778, 956

Pain
as body's wisdom, 60–61, 67, 72
collective, 954–61
emotions and, 72, 750–51
innate ability to deal with, 61
labor and birth, 587, 589–92
massage for, 657
opioids and, 825–27
See also specific types

"Pain body," 127, 167, 613, 866

Papanicolaou, George, 348

Pap test, 322, 324, 330, 348–52
HPV vaccine and, 334, 350
recommended frequency, 322, 349
results, interpreting, 50, 348, 350–51

Parathyroid abnormalities, 684

Parker, Lysa, 609

Parkinson's disease, 257

Parton, Dolly, 752

Passion Prescription, The (Berman), 304

Patterson, Lisa Chase, 290

Paul, Pamela, 302–3

Pauling, Linus, 689

Payne, Niravi, 206, 509, 510, 513–14, 750

Peak 8 Workout (or Sprint 8), 937–38

Peay, Pythia, 753

Pelvic bowl, 196–99
attuning, 198–99
"the birthing field" and, 197–98
"trauma imprints," stress, and, 197

Pelvic examination, 323–24

Pelvic floor muscles (PFM), 196–99, 298, 464, 577–78
ApexM Pelvic Floor stimulator, 284
exercises, 212, 278–84, *279–83,* 373
Female Pelvic Alchemy Jump Start Program, 374
vaginal cones for strengthening, 384
yoni egg and, 284, 285–87, *286,* 298, 694

Pelvic mesh implants (slings), 214

Pelvic pain, xxiii, 26, 49
causes, 199–200, 470–71
chronic, 24, 64, 199–200
sexual abuse and, xxii, 100, 200
shame and, 105
wisdom of, 200, 254, 470–71

Pelvic pressure, 218–19

Pepogest, 917

Perelli, Kim, 383

Perimenopause, 637, 639, 643, 644, 648, 661, 662, 670, 674–75, 698, 699, 701

Period.org, 129

Perlmutter, David, 704, 839, 840, 859

Pert, Candace, 29, 956

Pessaries, 213

Petals (Karras) and video, 376

Peterson, Gayle, 568

Pheromones, 257, 308–9

Phytoestrogens, 149, 430–32, 678–79

Picasso, Pablo, 958

Pico-Silver Solution, 338–39

Pilates, 212, 687–88, 778, 798, 935, 941–42, 944

Pineal gland, 275, 276

Pittman, Frank, 369

Pituitary problems, 175, 179

Placebo, 15, 35, 802–3

Planetree, 800, 822

Planned Parenthood, 470, 478

Pliny the Elder, 130

Podofilox (Condylox), 329

Podophyllin, 329

Polycystic ovary syndrome (PCOS), 177, 247–48
mind/body connection, 246–47, 248–49
program for, 143–61, 177
treatment, 247, 249–50
women's stories, 250–56
Ponder, Catherine, 737
Pornified (Paul), 302–3
Pornography, 249, 302–3
Postel, Thierry, 559
Postpartum period, 607, 611–17
depression, 612–17, 662
diastasis recti and, 618–19
eliciting a child's calming reflex, 617
nutrition for, 613–14
Post-traumatic stress disorder (PTSD), 42, 614, 869
Posture, Primal posture, 212–13, 277–78, 942
Gokhale Method website, 278
Potassium, 543, 915
Potatoes Not Prozac (DesMaisons), 881
Power of Eight, The (McTaggart), 956
Power of Now, The (Eckhart), 127
Power of Receiving, The (Owen), 740
Prayer, 12, 477, 829–30
Predict, 448
Preeclampsia (toxemia), 164, 540, 543, 544, 546, 552–54, 893, 904
Pregnancy, 533–65
appropriate age for, 557
author's, 537–40
cellphones and, 549–50
childbirth preparation programs, 546–47
child's prenatal memories, 529, 534, 537
cultural inheritance, 533–34
death of mother, 524
ectopic, 523–24
emergency mindset of, 555–58
encoded wisdom in, 119
exercise and, 932
fibroid tumors and, 220–21
gestational diabetes, 543
herpes and, 343–44
HIV antiretrovirals and, 548–49
HPV and, 328
-induced hypertension, 552–54

loss of, miscarriage, 521–28
medications, vaccines, and, 547–48
preeclampsia (toxemia), 543, 552–54
premature birth, preventing, 550–52
prenatal bonding with infant, 533, 605
progesterone for, 534, 547
program for creating optimal, 540–55
psychological factors and poor outcomes, 550–51
reducing C-section risk, 540
stress and, 539–40
stress urinary incontinence and, 383
terminating without abortion, 476
testing, 523
transforming power of, 533–35
tribal memories and HCG, 533
in utero gene editing and, 534
weight gain, optimal, 540–41
why we have children, 535–36
wisdom of, 119
See also Labor and birth
Pregnenolone, 704
Premarin, 384, 665–67, 668, 671, 681, 700, 703–4, 707, 780
Premature birth, preventing, 543–44, 547, 550–52
Premenstrual syndrome (PMS), xxiii, 26, 161–72
alcoholism in family and, 170–72
charting symptoms, 162
diagnosis, 162–65
events associated with onset, 164
exercise for, 932
factors contributing to, 133, 164–65
menopause symptoms and, 662
mind/body connection, 71, 123, 128, 164, 167–70, 639, 745
nutrition and, 164–65
"othering" and, 170–72
"pain body" and, 127, 167, 613
Pueraria mirifica for, 141, 149
SAD and, 166–67, *168*
symptoms, 162–63, 171
treatment program, 143–61
tubal ligation and, 164, 491
women's stories, 167–70
Prempro, 666, 702, 707, 780
Prenatal and birth memories, 465, 529, 534

Prepare for Surgery, Heal Faster (Huddleston), 822–23
Prescott, James, 608–9
Price, Weston A., 836–38
Primal sounds, 744
Prior, Jerilynn, 644, 675, 699
Proanthocyanidins (pycnogenol, OPC), 331, 354, 372, 705–6, 898
Probiotics, 207, 346, 365, 380, 382, 434, 887, 888, 916, 917
Progesterone, 126, 155–57, 241, 650
  for bone health, 689
  breast cancer and, 439–40, 700
  breast health and, 439–40
  cream, 156, 209, 663, 675, 676
  DHEA restoration and, 659
  for DUB, 176
  for endometrial hyperplasia, 174–75
  for endometriosis, 208–9
  for estrogen dominance, 663, 674–75
  for fibroid-caused bleeding, 224
  for heart health, 701–2
  for heavy periods, 182
  hot flashes and, 682
  libido restoration and, 230
  for menopause, 649, 659, 663, 674–76, 699, 707
  for menstrual-related problems, 155–57, 165, 169, 176, 949
  pregnancy and, 534, 547
  Pueraria mirifica for balancing, 157
  synthetic progestin vs., 155–56
Progestin, synthetic
  for contraception, 135, 482–83, 503
  DUB therapy, 176
  for endometrial hyperplasia, 174–75, 180
  for endometriosis, 207
  heart disease risk and, 666, 702
  for heavy periods, 182
  hormone replacement, 666
  as "medical D&C," 175
  natural progesterone vs., 156
  PMS worsened by, 156
  See also Premarin; Prempro
Program to Promote Healthy Breast Tissue, 397
Prolactin, 175
Proprioceptive Writing Center, 761

Prostaglandin F2 alpha, 140, 141, 163, 165
Protein, 144, 147, 657, 883–91, 892
  arachidonic acid (AA) and, 147, 885
  calculating daily requirement, 883–84
  organic meats and, 884
  red meat, ovarian cancer and, 259–60
  soy, 886–91
Protein Power (Eades), 849
Provera, 155, 174, 176, 182, 666, 675, 702
Psoas Book, The (Koch), 765
Psychoneuroimmunology (PNI), 34
Psychotherapy, 379, 523, 769–76, 814
Pubococcygeous (PC) muscle, 277, 324
  exercises for, 308
Pueraria mirifica (Thai kudzu), 141, 149, 157, 175, 176, 178, 681
  for adrenal/thyroid/sex steroid restoration program, 659
  Amata Life company as source, 680
  for androgen level increase, 676
  bone health and, 680, 685
  for endometriosis, 208–9
  for fibroid-caused bleeding, 224
  for menopausal symptoms, 663, 675, 680
  miroestrol in, 149, 209, 659, 680, 685
  for mood swings, 697
  for PCOS, 249
  prostate health in men and, 680
  sexual response and, 230–31, 692, 694
  for thinning vaginal tissue, dryness, 213, 215, 309, 351–52, 381, 682
  for urinary control, 385
Pumpkin seeds, 150
Pushed (Block), 535
Pussy (Thomashauer), 306, 735
Pycnogenol, Proflavonal, 331, 354, 372, 705–6, 898

Quay, Thomas E., 408
Queen of My Self (Henes), 643
Queen's Code, The (Armstrong), 39
Quench (Bria and Cohen), 716
Quench (Cohen), 879
Quick, Tammie, 375

Radiation, preparing for, 822–33
Radical Remission (Turner), 391

Radical Remission Project, 391
Radical surrender, 390
Radner, Gilda, 263
Rafter, Annie, 775
Rape, 6, 8, 105, 106, 168, 200, 293
    archetype, 103–4, 258
Ratey, John, 932
Real Wealth of Nations (Berrett-
    Koehler), 8–9
Reclaiming the Menstrual Matrix
    (Slayton), 643
Red clover, 679
Redemption Circle, 475
Redmond, Layne, 561
*Reducing Infant Mortality and
    Improving the Health of Babies*
    (Takikawa), 562
Red Web Foundation, 186
Redwine, David, 201, 205, 206
Reflexology, 158–59, 298, 299, 696, 778
Reiki treatments, 232–33, 777
Reis, Patricia, 48, 189, 293–94, 755
Reiter, Robert, 100
Relationships
    addictive, 19
    Adverse Health Effects of Cluster B
        Individuals on Those in
        Relationships with Them, 721–23
    attachment style, 89, 90–91
    chakras and, 90–91, 99–101, 194–96
    dependency/codependency, 19
    "de-selfing," 171
    doctor/patient, 51
    energy vampires, 68, 74, 107, 258,
        306, 553, 722
    fibroids and, 232
    getting needs met and, 11, 20, 74,
        75, 90
    high heart, low heart and, 106
    infertility and, 507–8
    love addiction, 169, 233, 356, 367
    marriage rates, 196
    menopause and change, 640, 691–92
    narcissism and, 108, 258
    "othering," 170–72
    ovarian health and, 239, 243–44, 254
    positive, happy people and, 794
    rape archetype and, 103–4, 258
    resources, living with a narcissist or
        borderline personality, 769
    speaking your truth, 111
    stress from, cervical cancer and,
        320–21
    stuck emotions and, 81
    unsupported, 233–34
    woman's health and, 32, 64, 196,
        367–68
Relaxation, 514–15, 681, 823–24
Relman, Arnold, 781
Remifemin, 351, 679, 682
Renew Physical Therapy, 374
Renfrow, Chris, 941, 944
Resistance stretching, 778
Rest-Based Training (RBT), 938–39
Reticular activating system (RAS), 794
Revival products, 679, 681
Rheumatoid arthritis, 41, 105
Rich, Adrienne, xxiv, 761
Richardson, Cheryl, 732
Rich Dad, Poor Dad (Kiyosaki), 737
Riley, David, 797
Ritchie, Margaret, 432
Ritual, 54
    Blessing Way, 709
    coming of age, 129–30, 189
    reclaiming, 961–64
Rituals of Healing (Achterberg and
    Dossey), 817
Robèrt, Karl-Henrik, 812
Robin, Lori, 757
Robin, Vicki, 736
Rodale, Maria and Maya, 304
Rodale, Robert, 838
Rose, Charlie, 5
Rose, Sioux, 117, 121
Rosenberg, Kim Mack, 337
Rosenberg, Marshall, 11, 60, 975–76
Rosenthal, Marge, 189
Ross, Joseph S., 780
Roth, Geneen, 836
RU486. *See* Mifepristone
Rubenstein, Boris, 125
Ryan, Christopher, 289

Sacred Pleasure (Eisler), 305, 779
SAD (seasonal affective disorder),
    166–67, *168*, 881
Sagan, Leonard, 32
Saint John's wort, 548, 697, 702
Sales, Mary Jo, 183

Salt, salts, 880, 881
Salt Fix, The (DiNicolantonio), 880
Sams, Jamie, 764
Sandler, Benjamin, 846
Sarno, John, 750–51
Saunas, 159, 161
Savetsky, Carla, 426
Saying No to Vaccines (Tenpenny), 632
Schaef, Anne Wilson, 5, 10, 19, 357,
    763, 952, 959
Schauss, Alexander, 926
Schiff, Isaac, 699
Schulz, Mona Lisa, 698
Schwartz, Bob, 844
Schwartz, Gary, 758
Schweitzer, Albert, 835
Science of Orgasm, The (Komisaruk,
    Beyer-Flores, and Whipple), 559
Scott-Maxwell, Florida, 718
Sears, Barry, 849
Second Brain, The (Gershon), 58–59
Secret Pleasures of Menopause, The
    (Northrup), 296, 693
*Secret Pleasures of Menopause Playbook,
    The* (Northrup), 296
Secunda, Brant, 512
Seidelmann, Sarah Bamford, 305
Selenium, 165, 434, 543, 658, 705, 899,
    901, 915
Self-esteem/self-respect, 292, 811, 978
    accidents and, 32
    body image, 5, 288, 877
    exercise and, 931
    health, weight loss, and, 842–43
    menopause and, 647
    personal power and, 91, 101, 807–8
    third chakra and, 91, 102
    uterus and, 242
Self-harm, 10
Self-Nurture (Domar), 515
Sense and Sensibility (film), 75
Serotonin, 30, 59, 166, 167, 302, 371,
    614, 656, 661, 848, 881–82, 900,
    908
Sesame seeds, 150
"7 Steps of Rebirth" (Cohen), 82
Sex and Love Addicts Anonymous, 169,
    233, 356
Sex as Nature Intended It (O'Hara),
    310–11

Sex at Dawn (Ryan and Jetha), 289
Sex on the Brain (Amen), 287
Sex trafficking and sexual slavery, 7
Sexual addiction, 18, 169, 233, 289, 356
Sexuality, 268–314
    abuse of, 293–94
    adolescents, social media, texting and,
        183–84
    adrenal gland function and, 651
    affirmations, 297
    being in touch with your, 289
    "big bang" theory, 289
    birthing and, 269, 596, 598
    circumcision and, 310–13
    clitoral system, 269–72, 273
    conflicted feelings and illness, 317–18
    contraception and, 295
    cultural inheritance, 288–95
    double standards and stereotypes, 184
    education about female sexuality,
        184–85
    energy and health, 298–99
    finding women's true, 296–310
    fourth chakra and, 106
    "hookup" culture and, 106
    masturbation and, 189
    menopause and, 691–93
    men's attitudes towards, 295
    menstrual cycles and, 172
    mind/body connection, 693–94
    nature and, 297, 299–300
    nursing mothers and desire, 139
    rape archetype and, 103–4
    rethinking: concluding thoughts,
        313–14
    safe sex and, 369
    universal feminine and, 180
    UTIs and, 381
Sexual response, 268–69, 512
    abuse and flashbacks, 274
    affirmation for orgasm, 301
    after hysterectomy, 229–31
    amrita, 272
    botanicals for, 681, 692
    brain as sex organ, 287, 676
    childbirth and, 269, 559–61, 598
    clitoris and, 269–72, 273, 300, 301,
        307, 311
    community, creating, and, 306
    DHEA for, 676–77

Sexual response (*cont'd*):
 ecstasy, 305, 558, 559–61
 enhancing, 301–4
 erectile dysfunction (ED), 303
 erotic reclaiming program, 296–310
 Extended Sexual Orgasm (ESO), 304
 female sexual dysfunction, 293, 296
 G-spot (sacred spot), 271, 274–76, 276
 kissing and, 271
 loss of desire and treatment for, 139,
  309, 257, 483, 676, 681, 692–95
 lubricants for, 300, 309, 682
 male erectile dysfunction and, 693
 medication and libido, 298–99
 nipple sensation and, 271
 nitric oxide and, 269, 296, 302, 693
 orgasm, 229–31, 268, 270, 271, 287,
  289, 291, 300–306, 308, 507
 ovarian breathing and, 242
 painful intercourse, 203, 291–92,
  294–95
 partner, working with, 307–8
 pelvic floor exercises, 277–84, 278–83
 pheromones for, 257, 308–9
 pornography and, 302–3
 postpartum, 611
 primal sounds and, 744
 restoration program for, 654–60
 sense of smell and arousal, 300, 308–9
 sexuality-spirituality connection, 305
 tantra and, 512
 time to reach climax, 300–301
 vaginal dryness and, 309
 vibrator, 301, 304–5, 682
 videos, 307, 310
 without intercourse, 289
*Sexual Teachings of the White Tigress,
 The* (Hsi Lai), 242, 735
Sexy Years, The (Somers), 672
Shaking, 61
Shakti Woman (Noble), 598
Shaman, shamanic healing, 66–67, 79,
 964–66
Shame, 37, 92, 105–6, 133, 135, 328,
 359
Sharma, Geeta, 619
Shaw, Farida, 637
SHBG (sex hormone binding globulin),
 480
Shealy, Norman, 88

Sheets, Kayla, 603
Sheldrake, Rupert, 955, 965
Shifren, Jan, 293
Shinn, Frances Scovell, 753
Shoenfeld, Yehuda, 629
Shriver Report, The, 870, 872
Side Effects (film), 782
Siegel, Bernie, 12, 54, 358, 623, 754,
 828
Silver, Tosha, 717, 718, 736, 757
*Simple Truth About the Gender Pay
 Gap, The* (AAUW), 196
Simpson, Lani, 684, 905
Single motherhood, 477
Single Mothers By Choice (Mattes),
 477
Skin brushing, 161
Slattery-Moschkau, Kathleen, 782
Slayton, Tamara, 186, 643
Sleep, 656
 adrenal balance and, 656
 for breast health, 441
 Buteyko breathing and, 941
 insomnia and disorders, 79, 919
 obesity and, 895
 postpartum, 614
 reestablishing cyclic ovulatory flow,
  151
 tips for better sleep, 151–52
Sleep apnea, 813–14
SmartJane microbiome screening test,
 346
Smith-Rosenberg, Caroll, 467, 469
Smoking, 18, 898, 921–25
 Alzheimer's prevention and, 706
 asthma and, 923
 bone density and, 688
 cervical dysplasia, cancer, and, 350,
  353, 354, 355
 fertility and, 505, 517
 gum disease and, 816
 health risks for women, 922–24
 miscarriage and, 521, 923
 ovarian cancer and, 260
 pregnancy and, 541, 552, 923
 quitting, 828, 924–25
 sperm counts and, 504
 stress urinary incontinence and, 384
Social Costs of Pornography, The
 (Eberstadt and Layden), 303

Sociopath Next Door, The (Stout), 721–22

Somers, Suzanne, 672

Soul knowledge, 112

Soul on Fire (Calhoun), 746

Soy foods, 886–91
　allergies and, 886
　breast health, 430–31
　hormonal balance and pelvic health, 144
　for hot flashes, 678–79, 886
　as protein source, 885

Spacey, Kevin, 5

Spangler, David, 753, 755, 953

Spark (Ratey), 952

Spear, Deena, 78

Sperber, Dan, 783

Spiegel, David, 775

Spirit and spirituality
　affirmation for connection with, 79–80
　angels and, 753, 754, 756
　energy as, 31
　God box, 756
　higher power guidance, 753–61, 976–78
　motherhood and, 526–27
　physical vs., 88
　pregnancy and birth as transformational, 533–35, 545, 598–99, 617
　second Saturn return, 977
　sexuality and, 297, 313–14, 316
　surgery and "spiritual initiation," 820–21
　See also Divine Love; Mind/body/soul connection

Spiritual Alliance to Stop Intimate Violence, 9

Spiritual Fertility (Von), 506, 514

Spontaneous Evolution (Bhaerman and Lipton), 781

Spotlight (film), 294

Stanford, Joseph, 484, 486

Stapleton, Peta, 772

Starfield, Barbara, 797

St. Claire, Olivia, 307

STDs (sexually transmitted diseases), 7, 294, 368–70

Steinem, Gloria, 968

Steroid cream (Valisone), 374

Stevenson, Betsey, 535

Stevenson, Robert Louis, 56

Stevia, 380, 920

Stillbirth, 525–28, 532, 541, 575
　Jakob's Room, 525–26

Stout, Martha, 721–22

Stover, Sara Avant, 473–75

Strand, Ray, 850

STREAM (Scar Tissue Remediation Education and Management), 292

Streep, Meryl, 290, 778

Stress
　adrenal gland function and, 651–62
　amenorrhea and, 248–49
　androgen production and, 261
　autoimmune disease and, 42
　blood pressure and, 553–54
　blood sugar and, 926
　bone loss and, 688
　cancer and, 43–44
　of cancer diagnosis, 33
　changing perceptions and, 44–45
　conditions associated with, reversing, 784
　emotional, unresolved, 651–52
　environmental, fertility and, 504
　environmental and physical, 653
　exercise for, 932
　"flight-or-flight" response, 869
　food-emotion connection, 865–69
　genital area, susceptibility of, 317, 325
　heart focus exercise, 655–56
　herpes outbreaks and, 341
　hormones, 42, 317, 608
　illness and unresolved, 78, 124, 325
　immune suppression and, 366
　infertility and, 508, 514–15
　magnesium depletion and, 657
　master program for hormonal balance and pelvic health and, 153–54
　menopausal symptoms and, 681
　menstrual cramps and, 141, 153–54
　miscarriage and, 522
　ovarian problems and, 242, 244
　pregnancy and, 539–40, 552, 553–54
　psychosocial and BV, 317
　reduction, a purposeful life and, 739–40
　severe, breast cancer and, 389, 429
　side effects, 869

Stress (cont'd):
  suppressed emotions and, 743
  thinning hair and, 696
  uterine problems and, 242
  vaginitis and, 362, 366
  weight gain and, 842, 926
  in women, first three chakras and,
    91–92
Stress urinary incontinence (SUI), 383–86
Strong Women, Strong Bones (Nelson),
    687
Subtle Body, The (Dale), 86
Sucralose (Splenda), 919
Suffragette (film), 290
Sugar, 80, 141, 144, 145, 152, 171, 302,
    327, 346, 363, 365, 380, 382, 445,
    651, 657, 678, 696, 704, 815, 840,
    846, 847, 848, 851, 852, 856, 859,
    862, 878, 880, 881, 894, 903, 908,
    913, 921, 926
  addiction, cravings, 61, 171, 361, 843,
    850, 856, 867, 869, 881–83
  breast cancer link, 391, 427–28, 429
  self-test for sugar sensitivity, 882
Suicide, 7, 8, 84
Sunflower seeds, 150
Supplements, 896–915
  Alzheimer's prevention and, 705–6
  anticancer protocol, 330
  for birth control pill use, 480
  for bone health, 685, 688–89
  for breast health, 429–43
  for cervical dysplasia, 351–52, 354
  for fertility, 517
  for heart health, 701
  for herpes, 345
  for hormone balance, pelvic health,
    148–50
  for hot flashes, 678
  for HPV, 330, 331
  for menopause, 657–59, 688–89, 696
  for menstrual cramps, 148–50
  Meyer's formula, 907
  postpartum, 613–14
  post surgery, 828–29
  for pregnancy, 541–44
  during pregnancy, what to avoid, 548
  program for supplementation, 913–15
  recommended dosages (chart), 915
  for sexual health, 298

for sperm count increase, 516
for thinning hair, 696
for thyroid disease, 661–62
tips for choosing, 913–14
for UTI's and, 380–81
for vaginitis, 365
for vulvodynia, 372
Support and support groups
  accepting, 442–43
  for breast cancer, 428–29
  for breast health, 442–43, 452
  for cancer treatment, 448
  friendship, need for, 732, 742, 821
  groups or community, 774–76
  online, 448–49
  positive, happy people and, 794
  for pregnancy, 545
  for stopping smoking, 925
  for surgery, 821, 824–25
  women's groups, 775–76
Surgery, 817–35
  anesthesiologist, meeting, 825
  artificial menopause and, 664–65
  banking blood for, 818
  creating health through, 817–35
  fasting-before-surgery advice, 818–19
  grieving lost part, 494, 832–33, 834,
    969
  healing opportunity of, 817, 819–20,
    972
  hospitals, new generation of, 822
  Monroe Institute's Surgical Support
    series, 824
  Neural therapy for healing, 831
  opportunity to heal old fears, 820–21
  past surgeries, healing, 833–35
  prayer for, 829–30
  preparing for, 820–33
  second opinion, 817–18
  supplements for healing, 828–29
  support and, 821, 824–25
Surviving Chaos (Fritchie), 927
Sweeteners, 625, 848, 856, 862, 919–20
Swimme, Brian, 790, 929–30, 967
Swimming with Elephants (Seidelmann),
    305
Synarel, 207, 208, 224, 972

Tai chi, 393, 799, 946–47, 950
Takikawa, Debby, 562

Taking Charge of Your Fertility (Weschler), 485
Tamoxifen, 421, 423, 429, 430, 444, 780
Tampons, 135, 316, 362, 364–65, 380, 385
Tannen, Deborah, 39
Tantra (Muir and Muir), 273
Taoism, 298, 300, 493, 512, 694
Tapping Solution (Ortner), 772
Taubes, Gary, 851
TCM (Traditional Chinese Medicine), 12, 22, 30, 153, 474
    hormonal balance, pelvic health, 152–53
    for infertility, 518–19
    for menopausal symptoms, 681
    menstruation and, 130, 131–32
Tea, 862, 880
    Whittel's Autopha Tea recipe, 862
Technology of Orgasm, The (Maines), 304
Teeth and gums
    amalgam fillings, 816
    holistic dentistry, 815–17, 836
    natural toothpaste for, 816
    nutrition and supplements for, 816
    ways to keep your mouth healthy, 815–17
Telfer, Evelyn, 239–40
Telomeres, 428–29
Temoshok, Lydia, 105
Temple of Ara, 964
Tenpenny, Sherri, 632
Tension myosistis syndrome (TMS), 750
Testosterone, 122, 177, 230, 298, 299, 309, 480, 648, 676, 682, 694
Teta, Keoni and Jade, 938
Therapy for Black Girls website, 770
ThermIva radiofrequency treatment, 215, 377
Thermography, 412–15, 418–20, 424, 442
Thieriot, Angelica, 822
Think and Grow Rich (Hill), 737
Think Before You Pink, 426
Thinking
    ability, reclaiming, 761–69
    affecting cells, 779
    cottonhead or foggy, 72, 663, 698–99

male, 39–40
    multimodal and women's brain, 38–40
    negative, how to avoid, 791–92
    positive vs. negative, 743
    self-fulfilling prophecies and, 783
    "think with your heart," 655, 784
    Vital Mind Reset Program, 614, 769, 840, 856, 882
Thomas, Caroline, 84
Thomas, Lewis, 112
Thomas, Paul, 632–33
Thomashauer, Regena, 296, 306, 735, 741, 766
Thompson, Susan Peirce, 867
Thurman, Howard, 267, 977–78
Thyroid, 41, 651, 696
    cancer, 136
    Hashimoto's thyroiditis, 437
    hyperthyroidism, 681
    hypothyroidism, 110, 660–62
    iodine for, 658, 901
    medication (Synthroid), 662, 901
    replacement (natural), 662, 696, 901
    restoration program, 654–60
    soy and, 890–91
    testing, 901
    TG 100 Natural Glandulars, 661–62, 696, 901
Tilly, Jonathan, 512
Tims, Bill, 865
TMJ (temporomandibular joint disease), 94, 110
Tolle, Eckhart, 127, 166–67
Tonetti-Vladimirova, Elena, 561
Touching
    neonatal, 607–9
    primal need for, 608
    therapeutic, 12, 777–78, 824–25
Touch Research Institute, 546, 608, 656
Toxic masculinity, 75
Traffic Safety (Evans), 32
Traister, Rebecca, 196
Transcendental Meditation (TM), 954
Transformation Through Menopause (McCain), 698
Transverse myelitis, 42
"Trauma imprints," 197
Tribal mind, 37–38, 97, 102

Trichloroacetic acid, (TCA), 329
Trichomonas, 360–61
Truth About the Drug Companies, The (Angell), 630, 780
Tryptophan, 882
Tsao, Fern, 378
Tubal ligation, 478, 490–95, 503, 676
  artificial menopause and, 664–65
  ovarian cancer risk reduced by, 261
  PMS and, 164
  women's stories, 493–95
Tums, 689, 905–6
Tupper, C., 522
Turkeytail (*Coliolus versicolor*), 330
Turner, Kelly, 390–91
Tuttle, Carol, 752
Twelve step programs, 44–45, 169, 172, 356, 776, 831, 881
227 Ways to Unleash the Sex Goddess Within (St. Claire), 307
Two Moon Junction (film), 310
Type C Connection, The (Temoshok and Dreher), 105

UAE (uterine artery embolization), 226, 227
Ulcers, 102
Ulipristal acetate, 476
Ultrasound breast screening, 410–11
Umbilical cord clamping, 609–10
Union of Concerned Scientists, The, 531
Universe Is a Green Dragon, The (Swimme), 929–30
Urethra, 315, 321
Urinary control inserts, 385
Urinary frequency and stress incontinence, 212, 215, 218–19, 231, 318, 385
  vaginal thinning and, 681–82
Urinary tract infection (UTI), 318–19, 379–83
  anger, repressed, and, 317, 318, 382–83
  sex and, 379, 381
  treatment, 380–83
  vaginal thinning and, 381, 681–82
  wisdom of, 120, 317
  women's stories, 382–83
  See also Interstitial cystitis

Uterine cancer, 105, 249, 350
Uterine prolapse, 197, 211–15
Uterine transplant, 518
Uterus, 191–236, *192*
  caring for, things to do, 266–67
  cultural inheritance, 193–94
  cystic and adenomatous hyperplasia, 471
  endometriosis, 200–210
  energy anatomy, 194–96
  fibroid tumors, 215–36
  hysterectomy and, 193–94
  Mayer-Rokitansky-Küster-Hauser syndrome, 518
  second chakra and, 100, 194
  wisdom of, 118, 236, 481
Uva ursi, 380, 381

Vaccine-Friendly Plan, The (Thomas), 632–33
Vaccines, 548, 600, 609, 627–30
  helpful or harmful, 627–33
  for HPV, 331–39
Vagifem, 381
Vagina, 17, 315, 317, 364, 541
  cancer, 350
  cosmetic surgery for, 375–77
  douching, 316, 317, 362, 365, 541
  dryness, irritation, thinning of, 208, 213, 309, 351, 385, 677, 678, 681–82
  estrogen cream or *Pueraria mirifica* for, 213, 215, 309, 351–52, 381, 385, 682
  nonsurgical rejuvenation, 215, 377
  pelvic floor exercises, 277–84, *278–83*, 298
  pessaries and, 213
  pH and semen, 361–62
  plastic surgery for, 215
  reflexology and, 298, 299
  Remifemin for dryness, 351, 679, 682
  repeated intercourse, effect of, 361
  tampons and, 213, 316, 362, 364–65, 385
  wisdom of, 120
  yoni egg and, 284, 298, 385, 682
Vagina (Wolf), 272, 288, 289
Vaginal cones, 284, 384

Vaginal seeding, 585
Vaginismus, 374
Vaginitis, xxiii, 18, 24, 42, 49, 64, 319, 360–68
  diagnosis and treatment, 363–65
  dietary approach, 363, 365, 845, 902
  psychological, emotional aspects, 18, 64, 105, 293–94, 317–18, 365–68
  symptoms, causes, 361–63
  wisdom of, 64, 367–68
  women's stories, 365–68
Vaginosis, bacterial (BV), 317, 326, 541, 543, 904
Valacyclovir (Valtrex), 344
Vanadium, 543, 900, 915
Vanishing twin syndrome, 603
Vaxxed (DVD), 632
Vegetables, 144, 429, 460, 544, 650, 840
  phytoestrogens in, 430–32, 678
  program for healthy breasts, 429
  program for hormonal balance, pelvic health, 144–48
  top hydrating vegetables, 879
Vegetarianism, vegan diet, 144, 165, 430, 839, 850, 851, 884
Venereal warts, 18, 24, 49, 108, 318, 322, 325–40
Verny, Thomas, 537
Vestibulitis, 374
Villoldo, Alberto, 714, 964
Violet Flame, 747–48
Vital Choice Seafood, 701
Vital Mind Reset Program, 614, 769, 840, 856, 882
Vitamin A, 148, 330, 331, 434, 688–89
  pregnancy caution, 548
  recommended dose, 915
  for surgery, healing from, 828
Vitamin B5, 657, 915
Vitamin B6, 148, 165, 915
Vitamin B12, 165, 517, 915
Vitamin B complex, 148, 354, 480, 542, 657, 705, 900, 914
  recommended dose, 915
  for surgery, healing from, 829
Vitamin C, 148, 165, 338, 434, 516, 517, 542, 657, 689, 705
  "bowel tolerance," 338
  recommended dose, 899, 915

for surgery, healing from, 829
for UTIs, 380–83
Vitamin D, 207, 298, 340, 435–37, 543, 660, 904–5
  for bone health, 685, 688, 901, 904–5
  for breast health, 410, 425, 428, 434, 435–37
  for pregnancy, 542, 543–44
  recommended dose, 435, 915
  sunlight for, 434–35, 660, 904–5
  testing for, 436, 905
Vitamin E, 148, 165, 434, 542, 678, 705, 898–99, 914
  recommended dose, 899, 915
  safety of, 898–99
  for surgery, healing from, 829
Vitamin K, for pregnancy, 542
Vitex agnus-castus, 679
Voell, John, 390
Vogel, Marcel, 758
Von, Julie, 506, 514
Von Willebrand disease, 181–82
Vulva, 315, 316–21
  encoded wisdom in, 120
Vulva Gallery, The (website), 376
Vulvar cancer, 350
Vulvar dampness, chronic, 362
Vulvar dysplasia, 355–56
Vulvar pain, chronic (Vulvodynia), 318, 326, 370–74, 378

Walker, Alice, 6, 315
Walker, Barbara, 191
Walnut oil, 149, 433
Water, 878–79
  alcoholic drinks and, 921
  amount per day, 878, 881
  dehydrating foods, 880
  "eating your water," 878–79, 881
  electrolytes and, 879–80
  healthy teeth and, 816
  hydrating, hydrating salts, 878–81, 911
Water retention, 869, 877, 880
Watkins, Linda, 826
Watts, Kate Northrup, 118, 122
Way of the Happy Woman, The (Stover), 473
Webb, Sharon, 457
Weed, Susun, 708

Weeks, David, 269
Weight, body, 841–927
  acceptance and ideal weight, 842–43,
    872, 873, 875–76
  author's keys to losing weight, 841
  BMI and, 872, 874
  body fat, measuring, 876–77
  body frame size, 850
  body image and, 5, 873, 875–76, 877
  calories and, 895
  contradictory claims about, 839–41
  cortisol and, 869
  dieting, failure of, 841–47, 850
  "eat less, exercise more" fallacy, 875
  emotional component, 865–69
  excessive, endometriosis and, 204
  excessive, PMS, and estrogen, 165
  food restriction, results of, 843, 860,
    861
  Gabriel Method for weight loss, 842–43
  genetic link, 838
  glutamates, warning, 868
  glycemic stress and, 851–64
  height/weight ratios, 838
  hydration for weight loss, 878
  intermittent fasting and, 247
  Ludwig's approach to weight loss, 840
  massage for normalizing, 657
  PCOS and, 177
  PMS and, 165
  pregnancy and, optimal gain, 540–41
  sleep and, 895
  soy protein and losing, 678
  stress hormones and, 842, 865–69
  USDA suggested, 872
  what and when to eat, 846, 862–63
  writing down what you eat, 866
Weil, Andrew, 923–24
Weil, Robert J., 522
Weinstein, Harvey, xxi, 5, 109
Welch, H. Gilbert, 421
Wentz, Izabella, 437
Weschler, Toni, 485
Western culture, 4–9, 51
  awareness of acculturation, 18, 43
  baby's crying in, 62, 89
  body as inferior to mind, 12
  body image in, 751–52, 873, 875–76,
    877
  breasts in, 387–94
  characteristics of addictive system,
    22–23
  creativity in, 735–38
  dependency in, 19
  devaluing of females in, xxiv, 4–9, 102
  as dominator society, 9–10
  emotional control, suppression in, 62,
    75
  external vs. inner guidance in, 57–58
  female body as abnormal, 15–17,
    728–29
  fundamental beliefs of, 11–17, 89
  genital areas, taboos and beliefs,
    316–21
  "getting stuff done" valued in, 60
  healing and, 25–28
  illness in, 11–13, 731–32
  labor and birth in, 565–66, 567
  male approval in, 4, 243–44
  medical science and, 11, 13–15, 571
  menstruation, menopause, and xxiv,
    728
  naming and healing, 21, 24–25
  patriarchy and addiction, 10
  power of naming, 18–21
  pregnancy as illness in, 533–34, 555–58
  rape archetype rife in, 103–4
  reclaiming authority in, 17–28
  sexuality in, 288–95
  uterus and, 193–94
  victim model, 25
  violence against women in, 6–9
  women and sexual self-image, 183
  women and sports, 929–30
  women's careers, 536
  women's caring for others, 103,
    195–96, 639, 696
  women's place in, 51, 68–69, 107
  work ethic, 623, 735–40
Weston A. Price Foundation, 147
What the Bleep Do We Know? (film), 31
What the Health (film), 839
Wheat Belly (Davis), 839, 859
When the Body Says No (Maté), 743
When the Drummers Were Women
    (Redmond), 561
Whipple, Beverly, 559
Whittel, Naomi, 862
Whole 30, The, 856
Whole-Body Dentistry (Breiner), 817

Whole Person Fertility Program, The (Payne), 509
Wicca healers, 67
Wicca Made Easy (Curott), 964
Wiesner, Denise, 512
Wild Creative (Kent), 779
Wilde, Oscar, 891
Wild Feminine (Kent), 196
Wild Mind (Goldberg), 763
William, Anthony, 41, 837
Willpower Doesn't Work (Hardy), 794
Wira, Charles, 361
Wisdom
  anatomy of women's, 118–19
  of the body, 51, 67, 72–76, 554–55, 737, 748–51, 786 (*see also* Illness)
  of breast cancer, 393
  of breast pain, 404
  collective women's, 970
  of endometriosis, 202, 203, 211
  of fibroids, 223
  of genital and urinary regions, 386
  of menopause, 640, 643
  of menstrual cycles, 172, 179
  of the ovaries, 242, 254, 259, 481
  of pelvic pain, 200, 255
  of the uterus, 236, 481
  of vaginal problems or UTIs, 318–19, 367–68
  of the vulva, 120
  of vulvar pain, 374
Wisdom of Menopause, The (Northup), 640, 697, 973
Witches (the burning times), 964
Wolf, Andrew, 408
Wolf, Naomi, 184, 272, 288, 289, 461, 635
Wolynn, Mark, 43, 465, 719
Womack, Belinda, 109
Woman Heal Thyself (Blum), 159
Wombology (Johnson), 513
Women's Health Initiative (WHI), 428, 666, 668, 702, 780, 905
  Memory Study (WHIMS), 703
Women Who Love Psychopaths (Brown), 106, 258, 722
Wonder, Stevie, 55
Woodman, Marion, 25
World Service Institute, 339, 760, 761, 758, 813, 830

Worth, Bill, 785
Writing, 761–63
  dialogues with body, 763
  food consumption, 866
  letters to unborn potential beings, 210
  proprioceptive, 761–62
  recording past creations, 266
Writing Down the Bones (Goldberg), 763
Writing the Mind Alive (Metcalf and Simon), 761
Wszelaki, Magdalena, 150
WuDunn, Sheryl, 9, 954, 974–75
Wurn, Larry and Belinda, 157, 200, 230, 519, 520
Wurn technique, 157, 200, 230, 292, 298, 518, 519, 524
Wyeth Pharmaceuticals, 780

Yams, wild, 156, 676, 679
Yeast infection, 41, 316, 360–61, 363, 364, 365, 366
Yin and yang, 107–9, 127
Yoga, 88, 159, 374, 429, 515, 616, 688, 798, 799, 881, 935, 943, 951
  Iyengar yoga, 942
Yoga for Fertility Handbook (Dumais), 515
Yoni egg, 284, 298, 385, 682, 694
  Yoni Egg Practice, 285–87, 286
You Can Heal Your Life (Hay), 40, 45, 779
Young, Clayton, 333, 334
Your Body Believes Every Word (Levine), 750
Your Body's Many Cries for Water (Batmanghelidj), 878
Your Money or Your Life (Dominguez), 736
Yunnan baiyo, 829
Yurok people, 129

Zenji, Dogen, 795
Zinc supplements, 148, 516, 517, 543, 658, 901
  recommended dose, 915
  for surgery, healing from, 829
Zulresso (brexanolone), 613
Zuckerman, S., 172
Zurbriggen, Eileen, 183

ABOUT THE AUTHOR

CHRISTIANE NORTHRUP, M.D., an ob-gyn physician, is a leading authority in the field of women's health and wellness and the *New York Times* bestselling author of *Women's Bodies, Women's Wisdom: Creating Physical and Emotional Health and Healing, The Wisdom of Menopause: Creating Physical and Emotional Health During the Change,* and *Goddesses Never Age: The Secret Prescription for Radiance, Vitality, and Well-Being.* In *Making Life Easy: How the Divine Inside Can Heal Your Body and Your Life,* Dr. Northrup reveals her secrets to mind-body-spirit well-being. *Dodging Energy Vampires: An Empath's Guide to Evading Relationships That Drain You and Restoring Your Health and Power* offers radical "upstream" preventive medicine.

Internationally known for her empowering approach, Dr. Northrup embraces medicine that acknowledges the unity of mind, body, emotions, and spirit and teaches women to create health by tuning in to their inner wisdom. After spending decades transforming women's understanding of their sacred bodies and processes, Dr. Northrup now teaches women how to thrive at every stage of life.

drnorthrup.com
Facebook.com/DrChristianeNorthrup
Twitter: @DrChrisNorthrup

ABOUT THE AUTHOR

CHRISTIANE NORTHRUP, M.D., an ob-gyn physician, is a leading authority in the field of women's health and wellness and the *New York Times* bestselling author of *Women's Bodies, Women's Wisdom: Creating Physical and Emotional Health and Healing, The Wisdom of Menopause: Creating Physical and Emotional Health During the Change,* and *Goddesses Never Age: The Secret Prescription for Radiance, Vitality, and Well-Being.* In *Making Life Easy: How the Divine Inside Can Heal Your Body and Your Life,* Dr. Northrup reveals her secrets to mind-body-spirit well-being. *Dodging Energy Vampires: An Empath's Guide to Evading Relationships That Drain You and Restoring Your Health and Power* offers radical "upstream" preventive medicine.

Internationally known for her empowering approach, Dr. Northrup embraces medicine that acknowledges the unity of mind, body, emotions, and spirit and teaches women to create health by tuning in to their inner wisdom. After spending decades transforming women's understanding of their sacred bodies and processes, Dr. Northrup now teaches women how to thrive at every stage of life.

drnorthrup.com
Facebook.com/DrChristianeNorthrup
Twitter: @DrChrisNorthrup